L.J. Fredericks DVM

VETERINARY DRUG THERAPY

D1118410

THOMAS B. BARRAGRY

Department of Small Animal Clinical Studies
Faculty of Veterinary Medicine
University College, Dublin
Veterinary College
Ballsbridge, Dublin 4
Ireland

With the assistance of Thomas Powers, D.V.M., Ph.D.
Department of Veterinary Pharmacology and Physiology
Ohio State University
Columbus, Ohio

VETERINARY DRUG THERAPY

LEA & FEBIGER

PHILADELPHIA · BALTIMORE · HONG KONG
LONDON · MUNICH · SYDNEY · TOKYO

A WAVERLY COMPANY

1994

Lea & Febiger
Box 3024
200 Chester Field Parkway
Malvern, Pennsylvania 19355-9725
U.S.A.
(215) 251-2230

Executive Editor—Caroll Cann
Development Editor—Susan Hunsberger
Project/Manuscript Editor—R. Lukens
Production Manager—Samuel A. Rondinelli

Library of Congress Cataloging-in-Publication Data

Barragry, Thomas B.
    Veterinary drug therapy / Thomas B. Barragry : with the assistance of Thomas Powers.
        p.   cm.
    Includes index.
    ISBN 0-8121-1447-7
    1. Veterinary drugs. 2. Veterinary chemotherapy. I. Powers, Thomas E., 1925– .
II. Title.
SF917.B37   1994
636.089′558—dc20

93-28262
                                                                                    CIP

NOTE: Although the author(s) and the publisher have taken reasonable steps to ensure the accuracy of the drug information included in this text before publication, drug information may change without notice and readers are advised to consult the manufacturer's packaging inserts before prescribing medications. Because of the international focus of this book, the reader ought to be aware that not all drugs mentioned in the text and the tables have been approved for use within the U.S. market, and that this book does not endorse their use in any way. It is also important to note that manufacturers may use different corporate names outside the U.S. market.

Reprints of chapters may be purchased from Lea & Febiger in quantities of 100 or more. Contact Sally Grande in the Sales Department.

Copyright © 1994 by Lea & Febiger. Copyright under the International Copyright Union. All Rights Reserved. This book is protected by copyright. No part of it may be reproduced in any manner or by any means without written permission from the publisher.

PRINTED IN THE UNITED STATES OF AMERICA

Print number: 5   4   3   2   1

FOR MAEVE, RUTH, AND MIRIAM.

■|PREFACE

A sole authored text such as this can make no real attempt at comprehensiveness. It must rely heavily on the research undertaken by other specialists, and then try to provide a practical synthesis of existing knowledge, capturing relevant therapeutic information in a readable fashion. The author is painfully aware of inadequacies in style and content in this text, such that some vital areas seem to be either omitted, dismissed, or misrepresented. Beginning from the disease aspect, this book attempts to provide useful therapeutic guidelines for the veterinary undergraduate, clinician, veterinarians in state service, in research, industry and the regulatory sphere. It is intended neither as a basic pharmacology text, nor as a medicine text. It does try to bridge that gap. I have also assumed that the reader has a grasp of basic pharmacology. Each chapter is intended to be self standing so that it can be read on its own. This inevitably leads to elements of duplication of which I am aware.

In writing "Veterinary Drug Therapy" the intention was to provide a practical approach in drug therapy, beginning from the clinical symptoms, while at the same time, acknowledging the highly regulated world we live in, with regard to approved drugs and residue avoidance. Available scientific information doubles every six years. This inevitably leads to a vast array of new disciplines, sub-disciplines, and narrowly focused specializations. Necessary as this may be, it does carry the attendant hazard of a receding general knowledge. Because of this fragmentation, specialties can become disconnected instead of being a complementary part of the clinical overview. Because so much specialist knowledge is now available, the real challenge is to try to encapsulate this into clinically usable generalist material.

The aim in writing this book was to at least provide a coherent overall therapy guide, create a stimulus and direction for greater in-depth study on particular topics, and contribute a useful compilation of existing practical therapeutic knowledge for the clinician.

I am indebted to all of my many colleagues for their assistance with this work. I wish in particular to thank Professor Kevin Kealy for his enthusiasm in sparking the initiation of this project. I am indebted also to Professor Tom Powers for his painstaking proofreading, advice, evaluation, and valuable opinions on the manuscript, and also to many other veterinary colleagues overseas. Special appreciation is due to the efficient library service at University College Dublin, and also to Ms. Barbara Clarke and Ms. Eilis O'Connell for their excellent work in typing the manuscript.

Finally, a word of thanks to Lea and Febiger for their constant encouragement to this author to proceed in the face of a large task. It is, in a sense, appropriate that Lea and Febiger, sited for so long in Philadelphia, a city rooted in the publishing tradition of Ben Franklin, would be partial to a Dublin veterinary graduate. After all, Lea and Febiger was founded by another Dubliner, Matthew Carey, in 1785.

CONTENTS

Part I

GENERAL CLINICAL PHARMACOLOGY

1. Drug Development and Regulatory Clearance — 3
2. Controlled-Release Delivery Systems — 32
3. Biotechnology Drugs and Vaccines — 61
4. Clinical Pharmacology of Endoparasiticides — 80
5. Drug Therapy of Respiratory System Disorders — 119
6. General Therapy of Gastrointestinal Disease — 133
7. Practical Fluid Therapy — 166
8. Treatment of Poisoning — 194
9. Beta Lactam Antibiotics — 220
10. Aminoglycosides, Macrolides, and Lincosamides — 241
11. Tetracyclines, Chloramphenicol, and Quinolones — 263
12. Sulfonamides — 294
13. Public Health Concerns of Veterinary Drug Residues — 314
14. Current Residue Concerns and Tolerances — 355
15. Drug Distribution, Pharmacokinetics, and Residues — 382

Part II

THERAPEUTICS

Section A EQUINE

16. Drug Therapy of Equine Colic — 401
17. Therapy of Parasitism in Horses — 428
18. Therapy of Equine Joint Disorders — 446

19. Reproductive Therapy in the Horse: Bacterial Endometritis 470
20. Therapy of Miscellaneous Equine Conditions 486
21. Nonsteroidal and Steroidal Anti-inflammatory Drugs in Horses 514
22. Drug Clearance and the Doping Problem 546

Section B FOOD ANIMAL

23. Mass Medication and Diseases of Swine 565
24. Growth-Promoting Agents 597
25. Bovine Mastitis 655
26. Drugs and the Bovine Genital Tract 689
27. Disease of Sheep 717
28. Trace Element Deficiencies 734
29. Therapy of Endoparasites in Cattle and Sheep 759
30. Therapy of Bovine Respiratory Disease 780

Section C SMALL ANIMAL

31. Cardiac Disease 811
32. Parasitic Dermatoses and Otitis Externa 839
33. Pyodermas and Flea Infestation 855
34. Therapy of Endoparasites in Dogs and Cats 879
35. Heartworm Disease 898
36. Cancer Chemotherapy 919
37. Antimicrobial Chemotherapy in Small Animals 941
38. Medical Therapy of Uroliths in Dogs and Cats 970
39. Prescription Diets 982
40. Therapy of Epileptic Seizures 990
41. Drug Therapy of Behavior and Reproductive Disorders in Dogs and Cats 1002
Index 1025

PART I

GENERAL
CLINICAL
PHARMACOLOGY

CHAPTER

1

DRUG DEVELOPMENT AND REGULATORY CLEARANCE

1.1 Introduction
1.2 Drug Discovery and Screening
1.3 Drug Development
1.4 Toxicity Studies
1.5 Target Animal Studies
1.6 Regulatory Clearance—Federal Laws
1.7 Role of FDA in Drug Approval
1.8 Residue Monitoring

1.1 INTRODUCTION

The development of a new veterinary product is a costly, time-consuming, and complicated process involving the coordination of many scientific experts from varied disciplines, e.g., organic and analytical chemists, pharmacists, pharmaceutical specialists, microbiologists, pathologists, toxicologists, pharmacologists, veterinarians, and many others. Expansion of scientific and technologic possibilities for developing safer, more effective drugs has been accompanied by increases in the regulatory requirements that must be fulfilled before a new drug can be marketed in the field. Most product research and development (R&D) is conducted in the research laboratories of the major pharmaceutical industries committed to continuous R&D. Major costs are involved in developing a new drug. Considerable investment in time, revenue, and labor is expended both from investigative work in new molecules that are subsequently discarded and in the necessary evaluation and field testing of the final candidate molecule. At least 95% of drugs that are first shown to possess pharmacologic activity in laboratory animals are subsequently rejected before they reach target animal trials. Even those drugs that do survive to this stage may never be marketed.

Any R&D program is essentially a high-risk activity—there can be no guarantee of a successful outcome. In discovering a useful veterinary product, the overall costs of registration and compliance with regulatory authorities make the entire process capital intensive and high risk. Development of a new anthelmintic agent for cattle, for instance, can necessitate investing $100–150 million and take 7 to 8 years for completion. Toxicity testing to ensure drug safety may cost $25 million. For drugs used in food animals, the additional cost of extensive residue studies must be considered. R&D extends over many years, during which time financial investment in the product increases, while the patent protection period continues to decrease. Development of truly novel products is an expensive process, and in many instances anticipated market returns do not exceed the costs of development, safety testing, and regulatory clearance; thus unique products

in the animal health marketplace are becoming less frequent. Nonetheless, substantial economic gains can be achieved if a new drug proves especially successful, and this constantly stimulates ongoing research.

The objective of any product research is to isolate a new compound that is safe, effective, and economically successful. A basic concern not only of industrial research, but also of regulatory agencies and consumers is that a safe and adequate food supply be available. For a development program to succeed, market needs must be clearly identified. Selection criteria for a candidate compound must also take account of varying legislative requirements by government agencies and current advances in analytical detection methods.

1.2 DRUG DISCOVERY AND SCREENING

New drugs may be discovered quite by accident—penicillin being the classic example—or after many years of tireless pursuit. In the past, major reliance has been placed on plants as sources of potential new drugs (e.g., morphine, digitalis). Following extraction, isolation, and identification of active ingredients from plants, semisynthetic derivatives may be prepared whereby the organic chemist may use these substances as starting materials in the creation of a slightly different molecule. Such derivatives may have superior pharmacologic properties and fewer side effects. Only slight structural changes may be associated with disproportionately greater pharmacologic activity. Other natural sources include animal tissues (steroids) and microorganisms (antibiotics). Natural products were once the source of all drugs, but with technologic advances within the pharmaceutical industry, the organic chemist now plays a key role in developing new drugs. Not only can chemical modification of existing molecules be achieved, but also the synthesis of totally new agents. Exploitation of side effects of existing drugs is another approach. Molecular manipulation or "molecular roulette" can be effected by chemical modification of a known molecule or by screening of natural products for biological activity and subsequent semisynthetic production.

Structural modification improves selectivity of action by finding molecular changes to increase a desired biological action relative to its side effects. Altered patterns of absorption, distribution, or elimination may be achieved with resultant improvements in therapeutic efficacy and safety. Sometimes the molecule may be a member of a well-studied family of chemicals with predictable pharmacologic actions. The new compound may rival a successfully marketed drug. It also may eliminate or reduce the intensity of unwanted side effects. Some benzimidazole parasiticides are prepared using molecular manipulation with the ultimate candidate drug displaying slower clearance from the body and greater overall anthelmintic activity against migratory or hypobiotic larvae. Some benzimidazoles can be prepared as pro-drugs, releasing the active benzimidazole carbamate nucleus within the animal body.

Other types of drugs, the so-called designer drugs, are of known structure-activity relationship. Although the actions of most drugs have been discovered accidentally, the possibility of producing a drug to have specific effects has recently become real in the era of the receptors. Selective binding of drugs to receptors implies a highly complementary chemical structure. To bind a receptor site, the drug molecule must possess a configuration complementary to the structure of the receptor. Receptors themselves can have slight structural differences, and so drugs can be designed to interact with all receptor types within a system or with only certain receptors. Using "receptor mapping," the distribution of the major receptors and the functions they control are known. Drug molecules can therefore be designed with affinity for specific receptor types and subtypes so pharmacologic effects can be accurately predicted.

With the advent of computer technology, and micro electronics new methods are being applied to pharmaceutical research. Computers are now used to store large numbers of chemical structures from which new molecules can be designed. On screen they can be displayed three-dimensionally and turned and rotated as required. Pictures of similar drug substances can be superimposed and compared. In this way new molecules can be designed and visualized. Also, the computer's databank supplies a correlation between a given molecular structure and its likely effects.

The computer also allows the scouting out of those receptors in the body which match the drug molecule in a complementary fashion. In addition, once a particular receptor can be visualized on computer, it is no longer difficult to design a matching drug molecule. This selective designing of a drug on the electronic drawing board is called molecular modelling. In the future the computer will undoubtedly reduce the costs of the primary screening research for new molecules.

With genetic engineering, new products based on submicroscopic manipulation of the DNA double helix can be produced. This involves recombinant DNA and monoclonal antibody production. Each technique possesses the capability to elaborate specific proteins, which can represent an almost infinite source of new, more selective drugs. Vaccines, antibodies, and antibiotics will become more abundant, less expensive to produce, and more specific when prepared by such techniques.

When a compound has been isolated and found to possess potential veterinary application, many investigations must take place before a final decision can be made to enter the more detailed development phase (Table 1–1). The initial steps in the predevelopment phase to determine whether or not the drug molecule possesses useful biological properties are called screening. A pharmacologic screen is a series of procedures to which the test compound can be subjected. These preliminary tests must be relatively quick, simple, and inexpensive. Screening procedures must be carefully designed to retain and identify compounds of pharmacologic potential, while allowing compounds of little potential to be discarded. Blind screening evaluates compounds of unknown pharmacologic potential with unknown biologic activities. The objective is to uncover any pharmacologic activity in the molecule. Even if the molecule is from a family of well-studied chemicals with common structural properties, screening is necessary to demonstrate unsuspected side effects or to reveal undiscovered therapeutic activity.

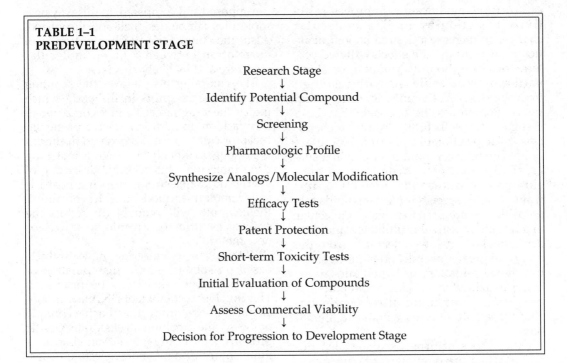

TABLE 1–1
PREDEVELOPMENT STAGE

Research Stage
↓
Identify Potential Compound
↓
Screening
↓
Pharmacologic Profile
↓
Synthesize Analogs/Molecular Modification
↓
Efficacy Tests
↓
Patent Protection
↓
Short-term Toxicity Tests
↓
Initial Evaluation of Compounds
↓
Assess Commercial Viability
↓
Decision for Progression to Development Stage

A pharmacologic profile can be drawn up based on the screening tests indicating the primary activity of the drug and the direction to follow in the later, more detailed investigations. Quantitative and qualitative bioassay forms the bulk of these screening procedures, i.e., the type of effect it elicits in the laboratory animals and the dose response. This bioassay is used to detect therapeutic and toxic properties. Based on these tests, molecular modification may be necessary to attain more desirable pharmacokinetic properties, selectivity of action, or diminution of side effects. This provides a "lead" compound, i.e., a leading candidate for further exploration as a successful veterinary drug. At this point, the necessary patent application will be made, to confer on the manufacturer exclusive "ownership" of the test compound for a fixed period (usually 15 to 20 years), ending in a monopoly after regulatory requirements are met. A patent permits the manufacturer to proceed, unhindered by rival competition, with R&D and marketing of the compound and serves as a form of compensation for costs incurred. If such patent protection did not exist, all R&D would be financially pointless.

1.3 DRUG DEVELOPMENT

Once laboratory screening tests have indicated useful pharmacologic activity and acceptable toxicity profile, the candidate drug enters the development stage (Tables 1–2, 1–3, 1–4). At this point, a decision is made to follow up the "lead" compound and reject others for various reasons. The decision to proceed to further investigation commits scarce and expensive resources. Even at this stage, initially promising compounds may have to be discarded, resulting in a considerable investment in time and money also being discarded. This development stage (Table 1–5) is a high-risk enterprise, and patent protection is vital. Before it can be decided to enter the development stage, the company or research institution addresses a number of key questions:

1. What is the ultimate therapeutic activity of the compound?
2. How good a product is it likely to be?
3. How expensive will the entire developmental procedure be?
4. Will it produce a good return on investment?
5. Will it be better than competitive products?

TABLE 1–2
STAGES OF RESEARCH AND DEVELOPMENT

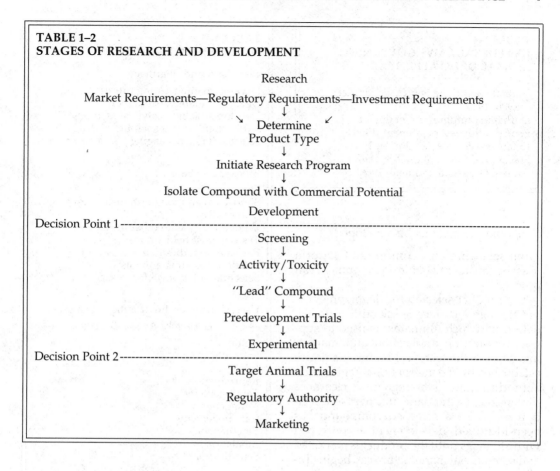

Research

Market Requirements—Regulatory Requirements—Investment Requirements
↓
Determine
Product Type
↓
Initiate Research Program
↓
Isolate Compound with Commercial Potential

Development

Decision Point 1 --

Screening
↓
Activity/Toxicity
↓
"Lead" Compound
↓
Predevelopment Trials
↓
Experimental

Decision Point 2 --

Target Animal Trials
↓
Regulatory Authority
↓
Marketing

TABLE 1–3
PHASES IN DRUG DEVELOPMENT

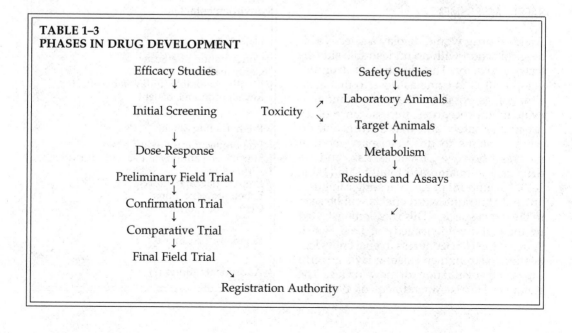

Efficacy Studies   Safety Studies
↓   ↓
Initial Screening   Toxicity   Laboratory Animals

Target Animals
↓
Dose-Response   Metabolism
↓   ↓
Preliminary Field Trial   Residues and Assays
↓
Confirmation Trial
↓
Comparative Trial
↓
Final Field Trial

Registration Authority

TABLE 1–4
US FEDERAL LAWS GOVERNING ANIMAL DRUG APPROVAL

Federal Food Drug and Cosmetic Act,
 1906/1938
Durham-Humphrey Amendment, 1951
Food Additives Amendment, 1958
Kefauver-Harris Amendment, 1962
Freedom of Information Act, 1967
Animal Drugs Amendment, 1968

TABLE 1–5
DEVELOPMENT STAGE

Chemistry and Pharmacy

Develop manufacturing process
Develop suitable formulation
Develop suitable analytical methods
Study stability and shelf life of drug
Select suitable packaging
↓

Efficacy and Safety

Dose-response studies
Short-term and longterm toxicity and
 tolerance
Compatibility with other drugs
Tests against field strains
Resistance studies (was necessary)
Safety in breeding animals
Selection of use level for dosage
↓

User, Consumer, Environmental Safety
 Laboratory Animal Toxicity

Acute
Subacute
Life span
Reproduction
Teratogenicity
Mutagenicity
Carcinogenicity
Percutaneous
Inhalation
Sensitization
 Pharmacokinetic Studies

Metabolism and residues
Analytical methods
Environmental fate
↓

Field Trials

Confirmation of efficacy
Confirmation of safety
Identify favorable/unfavorable effects
Reveal economic benefit
↓

Premarketing Stage

Prepare technical literature
Specify precautions in use, withdrawal
 times
Prepare package inserts
Labeling instructions
Claims for product
↓

Regulatory Authority
↓

Additional Studies (?)

6. Should the product be developed?

Thus scientific and commercial criteria must be considered before development can proceed.

The product selected for development is put through a battery of scientific tests, the data from which ultimately is used to support registration application and marketing. Most of the technical requirements are established by the international registration authorities, and so the regulatory clearance dimension is a fundamental part of development. Once a screened compound has been identified, development is concerned with all stages until the product is marketed and commercial manufacture can begin (Table 1–6).

SAFETY ASSESSMENT

An ideal drug would display a selective biological action with no undesirable side effects or toxicity. The objective of drug development is to come as close to this ideal situation as possible. The goals of modern evaluation procedures are assurance of efficacy and safety and that a drug will do what it claims to do. Veterinary medical progress, however, involves risk, and no drug can be guaranteed totally safe (Table 1–7). No amount of safety testing can guarantee that no untoward effects will be seen in the target species. This was demonstrated by the thalidomide tragedy of 1960, which spurred the U.S. Congress to enact new legislation to strengthen existing laws governing safety evaluation of new drugs. The Kefauver-Harris Amendment of 1962 was

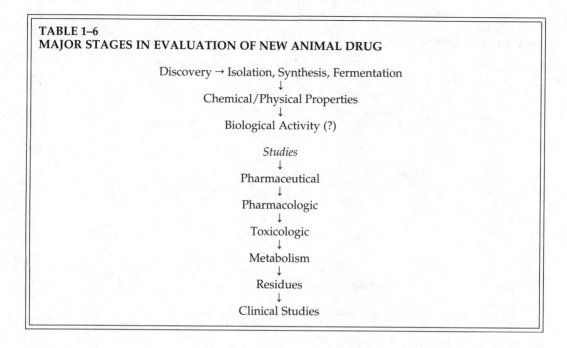

TABLE 1–6
MAJOR STAGES IN EVALUATION OF NEW ANIMAL DRUG

Discovery → Isolation, Synthesis, Fermentation
↓
Chemical/Physical Properties
↓
Biological Activity (?)

Studies
↓
Pharmaceutical
↓
Pharmacologic
↓
Toxicologic
↓
Metabolism
↓
Residues
↓
Clinical Studies

passed to ensure greater safety in all new drugs. For veterinary drugs, safety requirements fall into four major categories (Table 1–8):

1. To the animal receiving the drug
2. To the consumer of animal products
3. To handlers of the compound
4. To the environment

The toxicity study reveals the potential toxicity of the product, its metabolites, or residues, together with any side effects that may occur when the product is used as recommended in the target species. Initial safety/toxicity testing is performed in laboratory animals. This is based partially on the assumption that the drug will behave similarly in target animals and humans as it does in experimental animals. Although the ability to extrapolate data confidently from laboratory animals to target animals and humans has limitations, it does possess

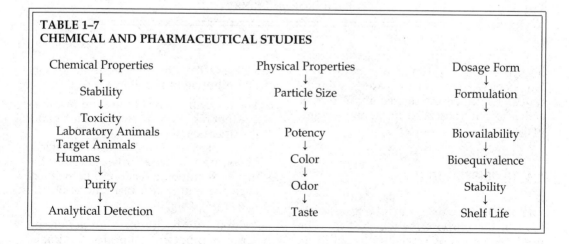

TABLE 1–7
CHEMICAL AND PHARMACEUTICAL STUDIES

Chemical Properties	Physical Properties	Dosage Form
↓	↓	↓
Stability	Particle Size	Formulation
↓	↓	↓
Toxicity		
Laboratory Animals	Potency	Biovailability
Target Animals	↓	↓
Humans	Color	Bioequivalence
↓	↓	↓
Purity	Odor	Stability
↓	↓	↓
Analytical Detection	Taste	Shelf Life

TABLE 1–8
SAFETY STUDIES

To Animal

Acute LD50	Rat and target species
Subacute study	90-day rat feeding
Longterm study	2 years rat
	Carcinogenicity
	Reproduction
	Teratogenicity
	Mutagenicity

$$\textit{Calculate} \quad \frac{\text{Toxic dose}}{\text{Final use dose}}$$

- -

To Consumer

Radiolabeled studies
Metabolism of compound
Identification of quantity and type of metabolites
Are metabolites more or less toxic: extractable or nonextractable
How long do residues remain
Establish tolerance and withdrawal times

- -

To Handlers of Product

Local irritation	Guinea pig skin
	Rabbits
Dermal studies	LD50
Inhalation toxicity	

- -

To Environment

Fecal excretion
Effect on animal/vegetable life
Stability
Buildup along food chain

---

high predictive value as a general rule. Nonetheless, many factors exert a significant influence on the degree and extent of active toxicity observed in laboratory animals.

1.4 TOXICITY STUDIES

The toxicity of a drug must be assessed in light of the purpose for which it is to be used, the period over which it is be given, and the effective dosage to be used. Toxicity can be subdivided as follows:

1. The toxic effects resulting from overdosage that represent an exaggeration of the therapeutic effect.
2. Toxic effects referred to as side effects. These are not necessarily related to the drug's therapeutic action, but their occurrence may place restrictions on the use of the drug.

Preliminary toxicity tests are performed in large numbers of laboratory animals,

---

TABLE 1–9
FACTORS INFLUENCING LD50 BIOASSAY

Species	Metabolic differences
Strain	Deficiencies in enzyme pathways
Sex	Hormonal levels/pregnancy
Age/weight	Liver/kidney function: microsomal enzyme activity
Environment	Housing/management factors/activity/disease status
Diet	Protein: fat ratio
Mode of Administration	Route/rate of delivery
Formulation	Vehicle, volume, pH, osmolarity

---

commonly the rat and sometimes nonrodent species. Particularly sensitive species may be needed to investigate special long-term toxicity effects, such as teratogenicity or carcinogenicity. Laboratory animals are easy to handle and house, possess short breeding intervals, produce large litters, and have short life spans. Large numbers facilitate detection of infrequently occurring side effects as well as statistical extrapolation of data. The evaluation assesses the likely hazards of the new drug when tested in accordance with a knowledge of its pharmacologic actions and the circumstances in which it will be used.

ACUTE TOXICITY, SINGLE-DOSE TOXICITY, LD50 TESTS

These preliminary tests reveal the type and extent of adverse effects a compound produces when administered as a single increased dose (Table 1–9). The quantitative dose-response curve provides the LD50, which can be used to establish the spectrum of pharmacologic activity. A more useful index is the ratio of lethal to effective dose (LD50:ED50), which is called the therapeutic index. In these quantitative bioassays, large numbers of laboratory animals, equal numbers of males and females, and different dosage rates and routes are used. Single-dose tests generate data on the no-effect dose, the maximum dose at which a toxic effect is never seen; the minimum lethal dose, the smallest dose required to kill any animal; and the median lethal dose, the dose that kills 50% of the animals.

Thus the derived data are used to provide:

1. The numerical dose-response reference values LD50
2. The therapeutic index and safety factors

Dose levels for the LD50 assay are determined by range finding, a series of exploratory doses between which the log interval is reduced progressively according to effect. The route for the test is selected according to the eventual field use; also, a route that ensures systemic absorption (IV, IM) is used to give some indication of absorption. For economic and practical reasons, rodents are the conventional test species. These doses are then used to calculate a starting dose for trials that will be performed in the target species.

Acute toxicity is tested to determine the degree of toxicity of a chemical substance (that is, the relationship between dose and adverse effects), to establish its toxicity relative to other chemical substances whose acute toxicity is known, and to determine specific toxic effects and provide information on the mode of toxic action. A suitably designed acute toxicity study also provides information from which a median lethal dose (LD50) can be calculated. By studying the effects after administration by different routes, the relative hazards of different pathways of exposure can be assessed. By using animals of both sexes, sex differences in toxic response can be detected.

Acute toxicity studies thus identify highly toxic chemicals and provide information on the possible hazards that could occur when humans are exposed. The slope of the dose-response curve and the type of toxic response in experimental animals are useful in human health hazard evaluation; exposure to single, acutely toxic doses of a chemical represents an abnormal or accidental situation for general human exposure.

Studies of single-dose toxicity evaluate functional and morphologic changes owing to a single administration of the test substance(s). These studies may give some indication of the likely effects of acute overdosage in the target animal(s) and may be useful for the design of repeated-dose toxicity studies on the relevant animal species.

The single-dose toxicity tests should be conducted so that signs of acute toxicity are revealed and the mode of death assessed as far as reasonably possible. In suitable species, a quantitative evaluation of the approximate lethal dose and information on the dose-effect relationship should be obtained, but a high level of precision is not required.

Single-dose toxicity tests are carried out in well-known strains of at least two mammalian species using equal numbers of both sexes. Rodents such as the mouse, rat, and hamster are suitable for the qualitative study of toxic signs and the quantitative determination of the approximate lethal dose. One mammalian species may be replaced, if appropriate, by an animal species for which the medicinal product is intended.

The dose levels should be chosen to demonstrate the range of toxicity. The maximum tolerated dose (MTD) and the minimum lethal dose (MLD) should be shown. LD50 tests need not be done when suitable adequate alternatives are available.

Although several accepted methods for determining the LD50 values have been developed, many important observations of toxicity are not represented either by these values or by slopes of dose-response curves for lethality. These observations are integral to an evaluation of acute toxicity and thus should be made during the course of an acute toxicity study.

Morbidity and pathogenesis may have more toxicologic significance than mortality.

The numerical value of the median lethal dose (LD50) is widely used in toxicity classification systems, but it should not be regarded as an absolute number that identifies the toxicity of a chemical substance. LD50 values for the same chemical may vary from study to study and between species or within a species because acute toxicity is influenced by both internal and external factors.

At least two different routes of administration are normally used. One route should be identical with or similar to that proposed for use in the target animal, and one should ensure systemic availability of the substance(s). If it is likely that the user of the finished product will be substantially exposed to the test substance(s) (e.g., by dermal or inhalation exposure), the potential routes of exposure should be included in the single-dose toxicity studies to ensure operator safety. Dose levels should ensure that the entire spectrum of toxicity is revealed.

1. Animals should be observed at regular intervals, usually for 14 days but not less than 7 days. Observation should continue, however, as long as signs of toxicity are apparent but without exposing animals to unnecessary prolonged suffering.
2. All animals dying during the period of observation and all animals surviving to the end of the study should be subjected to autopsy. Histopathologic examination should be considered on any organ showing macroscopic changes at autopsy. Generally all reasonable attempts should be made to obtain the maximum of scientific information from the animals used in the study.

Sub-acute and Repeat-dose Toxicity

These studies reveal any physiologic or pathologic changes induced by multiple dosing with the active substance and determine how these changes are related to dosage. This is especially important when a drug will be used repeatedly in the target animal or when residue formation is likely to occur. Subacute studies involve 90-day feeding programs in rats. Species differences between the rat and the final target species must be considered. These studies assess further the safety of the compound in use. Idiosyncratic reactions are difficult to identify in laboratory animal tests because the reaction may occur at a very low incidence frequency in a particular target species and be impossible to predict in advance.

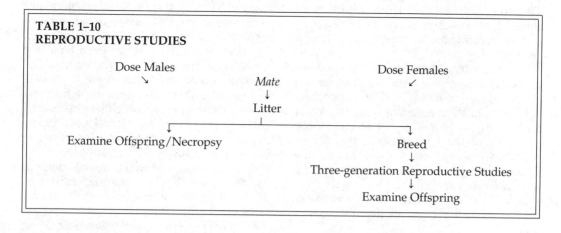

TABLE 1–10
REPRODUCTIVE STUDIES

Dose Males   *Mate*   Dose Females
         ↓
         Litter

Examine Offspring/Necropsy   Breed
         ↓
       Three-generation Reproductive Studies
         ↓
         Examine Offspring

Chronic or Longterm Toxicity Tests

These 2-year studies use the rat as well as a nonrodent species. Usually the experimental animals are blocked into four groups: one control and three treatment groups. Low, medium, and high doses are administered to the three treatment groups. The 2-year period is chosen because this accounts for the life span of the rat. During the trial period, high doses are administered frequently enough to ensure high plasma levels throughout the exposure period. Kinetic studies may be performed during this phase of testing, and routine hematologic/biochemical parameters are monitored. At the end of the drug exposure period, animals are sacrificed, and extensive pathologic examinations (macroscopic and microscopic) are conducted on body tissues and organs. Complete clinical observation, including terminal sacrifice and histopathology, is part of the study. In addition to the clinical biochemical and pathology tests, special tests are conducted to assess potential for teratogenic, mutagenic, or carcinogenic activity.

Teratogenicity

Since the discovery of teratogenic effects in children as a result of thalidomide medication in early pregnancy, it has become mandatory to test new drugs for possible adverse effects on the fetus. The rabbit is the experimental animal of choice because of the ease with which teratogenic effects can be induced in this species.

Different dosage levels of the candidate drug are given to test groups at various stages of pregnancy. Animals are sacrificed at various stages and the internal organs and litters examined. In the event of abortions, more intensive investigation may be necessary. Reproductive function and three-generation reproductive studies may also be performed (Table 1–10).

Mutagenicity

Bacterial mutagenicity tests are performed because extensive data exist on the correlation between results in such tests and carcinogenicity as determined by longterm whole animal studies. These data indicate that mutagenicity in bacteria is a generally reliable indication that a chemical is likely to be carcinogenic in vivo. It appears, however, that some chemical classes of carcinogens fail to be detected as mutagens in bacterial and other mutational assays.

A high positive correlation has been observed between the results of point mutational and DNA repair tests with in vivo bioassays for carcinogenicity. Unfortunately, negative test data in the mutagenicity assays do not correlate as well. Positive data from the less time-consuming and less expensive short-term tests, however, are considered useful for determining resources for longterm bioassays for carcinogenicity. The threshold assessment uses short-term test data.

The full mutagenic potential of a chemical is unlikely to be assessed in any single test for either technical or design reasons.

Therefore information from a battery of short-term tests is required to evaluate as fully as possible the mutagenic activity of a chemical.

The short-term tests generally used include (1) a bacterial gene mutation assay, the Ames *Salmonella* assay; (2) a mammalian cell gene mutation assay, of which the most widely employed are the thymidine kinase system and the Chinese hamster ovary (CHO) assay and, to a lesser extent, the Chinese hamster lung cell assay; and (3) a generalized assay for DNA repair (unscheduled DNA synthesis [UDS]) in mammalian cells, the UDS rat hepatocyte system.

Many of the short-term tests that may be considered as screens for carcinogenicity are, in fact, tests for mutagenicity. Although the hypothesis that the initiation of tumor growth results from mutations in somatic cells is a reasonable one, the validity of using mutagenic tests as screens for carcinogenicity does not depend on the validity of this hypothesis. The facts that most known carcinogens are mutagenic in at least some test systems and that most mutagens that have been adequately tested are carcinogenic provide the primary rationale for the inclusion of mutagenicity tests in the battery of screening tests for carcinogenicity. Evidence exists that some carcinogens do not yield a positive response in a particular short-term test. Therefore when a compound is of a structural class for which it is possible that a particular short-term test is inadequate as a screen for carcinogenicity, its use will not be accepted to reduce the concern for carcinogenicity.

All tests used in this battery should be conducted with a demonstrated metabolic activation system. Although the cell systems used in short-term tests do not possess the full metabolic capabilities of whole animals, incorporation of liver enzyme systems is considered the most reliable approach for overcoming this limitation in evaluating routinely chemicals of unknown carcinogenic activity. Some test systems (*Drosophila*, rat hepatocyte) have these enzyme systems; for others, an exogenous enzyme system must be added.

Because the metabolic capabilities of cell lines are limited, an exogenous system for metabolic activation must be added for the assay to be valid. Both of these problems are overcome in the UDS assay using primary rat hepatocytes. The freshly isolated nondividing liver cells that are used have the capacity to metabolize carcinogens. The sex-linked recessive lethal test in *Drosophila* is a suitable alternative gene mutation test when circumstances preclude the use of either of the above-mentioned gene mutation assays. An example of such a situation is when an antimicrobial or antifungal animal drug possesses such extreme toxicity in the Ames test that use of sufficiently high doses for significant negative results in bacterial tests is precluded.

In general, reproducible data indicating that a sponsored compound is positive in one or more of the tests in the battery result in a requirement for carcinogenicity testing in whole animals. Factors such as dosage, metabolism, test sensitivity, and reproducibility are considered in the Food and Drug Administration's (FDA) evaluation of data submitted.

Carcinogenicity

Carcinogenicity testing is conducted particularly when a drug has a close chemical similarity to known carcinogens or co-carcinogens; the number of tumors, their nature, and time of appearance are carefully noted over a 2-year period. Absence of tumor formation during this period cannot be taken as absolute evidence of lack of carcinogenic properties. Frequently carcinogenicity tests are required over a longer test period using either dogs or primates, especially with substances that give rise to suspect signs during the repeat-dose toxicity studies.

The studies evaluate carcinogenic potency of the drug and its metabolites. These studies should allow an extrapolation from experimental results to a true risk for the health of the consumer exposed to a possible contamination of food by such residues. Longterm studies on carcinogenicity in laboratory animals represent the most suited experimental approach to expose the carcinogenic potency of a substance.

The relationship between structure and activity, short-term mutagenicity tests, and toxicologic and biological information may be evaluated before making a decision.

Criteria on which a substance may be defined as carcinogenic in evaluating the results of the chronic bioassay are an increase in the incidence of tumors as compared with the untreated control animals, the development of tumors earlier than in control animals, and the occurrence of types of tumors usually not seen in untreated control animals.

Attempts to quantify a carcinogenic potency should take account of the number of sensitive animal species, the number of the types of tumors induced in the treated animals, the dose-effect relationship, the malignancy of the induced tumors, and the genotoxicity shown by an appropriate battery of tests.

Absorption, Distribution, Metabolism, and Elimination ("A,D,M,E") Studies

Data from "A,D,M,E" studies aid in the evaluation of test results from other toxicology studies and in extrapolation of data from animals to humans. "A,D,M,E" studies also provide data for selecting appropriate dose levels for chronic toxicity and carcinogenicity studies by providing information about dose-dependent kinetics.

The best time to do a "A,D,M,E" study varies with the need for data to evaluate the safety of the test chemical. In certain cases, initial experiments for determining absorption, distribution, and elimination of the test chemical may be done soon after acute toxicologic studies. Further experiments establishing the metabolic fate of the compound may be needed for chemicals that are likely to undergo chronic testing. If the results of toxicologic studies indicate that further information on the metabolism of the test chemical is needed, identification and characterization of major metabolites in blood and urine should be done. For some purposes, dose-related "A,D,M,E" studies may be carried out. In pregnant animals, a kinetic analysis assesses the amount of placental transfer of the parent compound and its metabolites at critical periods of organogenesis in relation to maternal exposure.

In addition to the preclinical toxicologic work, preliminary metabolism studies are conducted in at least two species to evaluate:

1. The rate of absorption of the drug from the site of administration (e.g., oral, parenteral)
2. Its distribution throughout the animal body
3. Its metabolic rate
4. Its rate of excretion
5. The extent of residue formation in the body

These studies are supplemented by radiotracer techniques and precede comprehensive metabolism studies in both laboratory and target species.

At this interim stage, a meeting with the FDA may take place at which a written protocol is discussed, perhaps modified, and, it is hoped, approved by the FDA. Most of the subsequent testing is carried out in accordance with rigidly fixed protocols. Field testing requirements, species, number of animals per group, dosages, and parameters to be studied are all standardized as much as possible to ensure that the results are acceptable to the regulatory authorities. In the United States, approval for field testing may be obtained as soon as basic toxicology and efficacy have been established from in-house studies. Product data submitted to the regulatory agency for field testing approval must be related to the stage the product has reached in development and indicate the number of animals to be included in the trial program. This minimizes delay and ensures that products can be developed under conditions in which they will be used in the field.

When the drug product is to be tested in food-producing animals, the FDA must be notified to the effect:

1. A commitment that edible products will not be used for food without authorization of the FDA
2. Approximate dates of start and end of trial
3. Maximum daily dosing, duration of administration, method of administration, and withdrawal time

1.5 TARGET ANIMAL STUDIES

Because the pharmacokinetic properties of a compound vary from one species to another, it is always necessary to study the behavior of the candidate drug in the target species. Such studies provide not only information on safety and distribution in the body, but also the likely occurrence and accumulation of residues. Using radiolabeling techniques and radiotracer studies, the distribution and sequestration of drug can be measured. Formulation and bioavailability studies can be investigated in conjunction with kinetic studies. Formulation studies should begin as soon as the route of administration and range of proposed dosages are known. Target animal studies also include large-scale efficacy trials and the compatibility of the candidate drug with other drugs that may be used with it. Animal trials begin when toxicity tests have established the apparent safety of the drug.

In designing an animal trial, certain guidelines must be clearly established:

1. Clear objectives must be stated.
2. There must be proper selection of suitable subjects.
3. Diagnostic criteria must be unambiguously defined.
4. Bias should be minimized or eliminated.
5. Test and control groups must be comparable.
6. Results and raw data must be properly generated, statistically analyzed, and scientifically interpreted.
7. High and uniform standards are needed for (a) supervision and administration of the trial and (b) quality of assessment and observation of effect.

EFFICACY AND SAFETY TRIALS

Studies on target animals are conducted at the proposed dose rate and at three to four times that level. Concurrently additional efficacy work is done. Field trials can be operated at three levels of investigation:

1. **Phase (I)**: Determines whether the target animal displays a significantly different response to the drug than the laboratory species used in preclinical testing (i.e., in the target species does the drug possess a pharmacologic action that may be useful in therapy?).
2. **Phase (II)**: Studies the drug in animals with the target disease to determine efficacy and safety (i.e., is the pharmacologic action useful in therapy of the diseased animal?).
3. **Phase (III)**: Comprises a large-scale, extensive full trial designed to ensure that the beneficial effect can be expected in animals at different locations under varying conditions of housing and management. It indicates the reliability of the drug as well as the frequency of unwanted side effects under field conditions of use.

The objectives of animal field trials are to ascertain the therapeutic effect of the product, to specify its indications and contraindications according to species and age, to identify side effects it may have, and to ensure its safety under general conditions of use.

Field trials are performed at various locations and may be repeated several times to provide data on the continuous use of the product over time as well as over area. This may identify any geographic, seasonal, or management factors affecting product performance. It also determines whether the magnitude of the drug-induced response is uniform and can be maintained with continual usage.

To eliminate both subjective and environmental bias, animals are selected at random. The frequent practice is to block animals into different groups based on breed, sex, weight, age, or origin and then select them randomly into a number of comparable groups. Trials in intensively managed livestock are in many ways easier to organize because animals are often already in groups that can be used to make comparisons. Field trials are performed using control animals whenever this is practicable, and the clinical or therapeutic effect obtained is compared with a placebo, absence of treatment, or a competitor product of established therapeutic value when appropriate. Only in the field using target species can proper assessments be made of variations in expense arising from breed management or nutritional factors. Unexpected but beneficial side actions may also be identified under field conditions, e.g., weight gain, increased appetite.

KINETIC STUDIES AND SAFETY TO HUMANS

These studies facilitate not only a comparison of the absorption of the drug and its tissue distribution, but also the number and kinds of metabolites formed in the animal body. Testing may have to be done on particular metabolites as well as the parent compound. Drug residue data and establishment of tolerances can be obtained only from these studies in the target species. From these data, withdrawal times are then laid down. This frames an important portion of the risk assessment for humans as consumers of animal-based products. Safety to humans is also examined in regard to actual contact with drugs during manufacture and handling.

A recent addition to the requirements imposed on the registration of a new animal drug is the determination of its effects on the environment; i.e., the drug must not adversely affect soil, water, or animal or vegetable life: It must not be adversely concentrated along food chains. The amount of compound in the feces of the animal to produce contamination of the pasture must be considered whether applied directly by the animal or by spreading onto the pasture when animals are housed. Analytical methodology is another major area now affecting product development. Methods must be developed and described by which the drug can be easily detected in the formulation, in feed, and in animal tissues.

On completion of these studies, precautions to protect animals, users, and consumers are defined. This includes establishment of withdrawal times. When the comprehensive trial program and all of the various experimental studies have been concluded, an application is filed with the regulatory clearance authority for product licensing and marketing authorization. All the technical data are then drawn up in accordance with a step-by-step protocol. Some additional studies may be requested even at this stage. If early communication and liaison with the FDA has been good throughout development and evaluation, however, additional requirements should be minimal.

1.6 REGULATORY CLEARANCE— FEDERAL LAWS

RELEVANT LEGISLATIVE CONTROL OF ANIMAL DRUGS IN THE UNITED STATES

The Federal Food Drug and Cosmetic (FD&C) Act of 1906 was the first national legislation exercising controls over drugs in the United States. Since its enactment, this law has been amended many times. The present legislative basis of regulatory control over new animal drugs and medicated feeds is embodied in the Federal FD&C Act of 1938, as amended. This act defined the authority and responsibility of the government to safeguard public health and to protect the interests of the consumer. Enforcement is the responsibility of the FDA. Some of the relevant legislation pertaining to animal drugs follows:

1. **The Federal Food Drug and Cosmetic Act (1938)**: Extended coverage of the 1906 Act to animal drugs and enabled the FDA to prohibit marketing of new animal drugs and medicated feeds unless their safety in the target species was clearly demonstrated.

2. **The Durham-Humphrey Amendment (1951)**: Governed the labeling of drugs and established two major categories: (a) prescription (Rx) drugs and (b) over-the-counter (OTC) drugs.

OTC drugs are bought and used by the public without veterinary supervision. Rx drugs require veterinary supervision for use. These products must bear this cautionary legend: "CAUTION. Federal Law restricts this drug to use by or on the order of a licensed veterinarian."

In 1989, a bill was passed by Congress to prevent questioning the FDA's authority to determine Rx drugs. Such Rx drugs must bear a label containing the following information: name and address of prescribing veterinarian, instructions for use, cautionary statement.

3. **The Food Additives Amendment (1958)**: The Delaney Clause of this amendment prohibits the use in food of any compound that is carcinogenic in humans or animals. Such carcinogenic compounds can be permitted in food animals only if no residues remain in the tissues of treated animals at the time of slaughter. "Zero tolerance" or "zero residue level" is applicable to such drugs. The 1958 Delaney Amendment (Food Additives Amendment) to the FD&C Act sets to zero the permissible residue level in foods for any substance shown to be carcinogenic in any species. The Delaney

Amendment applies to any compound that causes an increase in tumor response either in animals or in humans. This amendment is currently being invoked to determine whether sulfamethazine (Sulfamezathine) should continue to be used in food animals.

An exception to the Delaney clause, the so-called DES Proviso—"Sensitivity of the Method" rule (SOM)—has been invoked to account for increased sensitivity of residue detection methods. This exception permits the approval of the use of a carcinogenic compound in food-producing animals provided that there are no residues. Because in practice the FDA has been unable to conclude that no trace of any given substance will remain in edible products, the new procedure provides an operational definition of "no residues." It is designed to determine the concentration of residue of a carcinogenic compound that presents an insignificant risk of cancer to the consuming public. The concentration is defined in the regulations as a "maximum lifetime risk of cancer to the test animal in the order of 1 in 1 million." In addition to the operational definition of no residue, the regulations and guidelines identify the procedures and the criteria that "if followed will permit the approval of carcinogenic compounds intended for use in food-producing animals, provided that the level of any residue remaining in edible tissues is so minimal that it would not present any significant risk of cancer."

The new policy, which has been in the regulatory pipeline for many years (the original SOM procedures were first proposed in 1973), provides new assay standards for proposed animal drugs that are potential carcinogens. Drug manufacturers are required to submit with new animal drug applications a suitable method to test for residues. The test must be sufficiently sensitive to reveal a level of residue that would ensure that a maximum lifetime risk of 1 in 1 million is not exceeded, a risk that is essentially zero in the view of the FDA.

At present, some debate is taking place on the possibility of repealing the Delaney Clause, because it is now seen to be too inflexible. The term "negligible risk" has been proposed to replace the original wording of "zero risk". The problem lies in defining "negligible risk" for residues of potential carcinogens.

The Rose Bill (HR 3742) establishes a specific criterion of 1×10^6 maximum increase in risk from lifetime dietary exposure to a residue. The Kennedy/Waxman Bill (S1074/HR 2342) provides criteria as to how the risk should be calculated while the Bruce/Bliley Bill (HR 3216) leaves it to the discretion of the Regulatory Authority to decide on the level of acceptable risk.

4. **The Kefauver-Harris Drug Amendment (1962)**: Required for the first time that in addition to the establishment of drug safety, efficacy must also be demonstrated. This made it incumbent on drug manufacturers to prove to the FDA the effectiveness of products before marketing. Under this amendment, a sponsoring drug company must file a New Animal Drug Application (NADA) in accordance with a defined study protocol. The NADA must provide all relevant data validating safety, efficacy, and label claims. Other controls introduced under the Kefauver-Harris amendment governed the inspection and approval of manufacturing premises, registration of pharmaceutical firms, and establishment of manufacturing control standards. Reporting of adverse effects and removal of drugs from the market are also provided for under this amendment.

5. **The Animal Drugs Amendment (1968)**: Laid down particular requirements and restrictions on the sale of animal drugs per se and of animal feeds containing drugs. It also reinforced that animal drugs placed on the market at the time of or after the Kefauver-Harris Amendment of 1962 must be shown to be safe and effective for their intended usage—implied or stated.

1.7 ROLE OF THE FDA IN DRUG APPROVAL

The FD&C Act of 1938 is the primary legislation affecting the regulatory process. The FDA publishes various regulations in the Federal Register. Another layer of control is the policy and compliance guides is-

TABLE 1–11
FDA REGULATORY CLEARANCE PATHWAY

CVM Guidelines Issued
↓
Discussion with Sponsoring Company
↓
File NADA
↓
Drug Trials/Evaluation/Field Testing
↓
Protocol Submission
↓
NADA Processing
↓
Approval Notification
↓
Conditions of Use
↓
FOI Summary
↓
Residue Monitoring
↓
Field Monitoring

sued by the Center for Veterinary Medicine (CVM) through the FDA.

The FDA is responsible for the enforcement of federal law as it relates to the safeguarding of public health. The agency acts to protect the public on the basis that the public should not unknowingly or needlessly be exposed to injurious substances. This involves not only regulatory clearance and control of drugs used in human medicine, but also drugs used in animals. Within the FDA, the responsibility of ensuring the safety and efficacy of animal drugs lies with the CVM (Tables 1–11, 1–12).

The objective of animal drug registration is to ensure the safety, efficacy, and quality of veterinary medicines. Before any drug can be legally marketed in the United States, the sponsoring company must submit a NADA to the FDA.

Approved drugs are those for which data supporting safety and efficacy have been submitted to the CVM by the manufacturer or sponsor. The approved drug is then granted a NADA by the CVM. An unapproved drug is one that does not have a NADA.

The basic concept embodied in the CVM approval process is an assurance that in accordance with the Federal FD&C Act, marketing authorization will not be granted if a candidate drug is misbranded or adulterated. "Misbranded" refers to statements or label claims that are incorrect or misleading; "adulterated" refers to products that are manufactured under substandard conditions of quality, are unsafe, or are potentially defective.

Review and approval are the responsibility of the CVM, and submission of a NADA is required for drugs intended to be administered directly to animals or added to the feed. Evidence of the safety and efficacy of a product must be provided by the sponsoring company in the NADA. This is applicable to each species of target animal for which approval is being sought. Current

TABLE 1–12
GENERAL ROLE OF CVM AND FDA

PREMARKETING

Guidelines of safety/efficacy criteria for animal drug evaluation
Publish "federal register"
Inspection of manufacturers' premises
Manufacturing/quality control standards
Meet with sponsoring drug company re candidate compounds
Establish tolerance concept
Define "violative" residue
Evaluate assay methodology
NADA processing
Compliance with clearance criteria
Validation of label claims
New animal drug approval
FOI summary

POSTMARKETING
(With FSIS and EPA)

Inspection of animal food products, premises, and animal feed
Monitoring of samples
Coordinates nationwide residue monitoring
Violative residue investigation
Seizure/condemnation of animal feed/carcasses
Impoundment of future shipments
Mount surveillance program
Monitor adverse reactions/extralabel uses
Drug withdrawal (?)

legislation is detailed and explicit in its requirements for protocol submission, NADA processing, and approval. Unless all requirements are met, the FDA must withhold approval. For this reason, sponsors of NADA candidate drugs are encouraged to meet and discuss protocols and requirements with the CVM before beginning drug trials and studies to ensure that the FDA criteria will be met.

The NADA must contain all proposed labeling, including a full description of methods, facilities, and controls for manufacturing, processing, and packing of the drug or its metabolites; evidence to establish safety and effectiveness; environmental assessment; a statement that the studies were conducted in compliance with good laboratory practice regulations; and a summary basis of approval, commonly known as the freedom of information summary (FOI) (Table 1–13).

This usually voluminous application contains all details and results of the research protocols carried out by the pharmaceutical company and addresses major issues such as animal safety and efficacy, mutagenicity and carcinogenicity potential, consumer safety, operator safety manufacturing procedures, and environmental impact. The product sponsor indicates and the FDA decides the written contents of the label, bottle, carton, and package inserts.

A NADA must contain specific information on:

1. Safety and efficacy of drug for the animal
2. Safety for the environment
3. Safety of food for humans if it is used in food-producing animals

Regulatory clearance of a new animal drug takes place in accordance with a standardized protocol approach:

1. Filing of a NADA and subsequent preliminary field testing
2. Submission of documentation by the sponsoring drug company
3. Establishment of safety to treated animals and to humans when the drug is administered to food animals
4. Establishment of efficacy by means of controlled field trials that validate label claims

The FDA developed a series of guidelines to inform sponsors of the type of scientific data that the agency believes provides a reasonably acceptable basis for determining the safety and efficacy of the new animal drug. Reliance on these guidelines by sponsoring drug companies ensures that they describe procedures acceptable to the FDA. The guidelines describe the types of studies appropriate to the development of a study protocol for experimental work necessary for the preclearance evaluation of drugs and food additives used in animal production. The NADA contains all of the studies carried out to substantiate the safety, efficacy, and label claims of the new product. All cited data must be obtained from extensive, well-controlled, scientifically sound studies. The detailed and rigorous approach is necessary to generate scientific data establishing the definitive biological properties of the compound being tested.

For drugs intended for direct administration to food animals or in a feed premix, form FD 356 NADA is used. Animal feeds containing a new drug cannot be marketed without an approved animal feed application, form FD 1800. Feed additive drugs must state exact levels of feed inclusion, specific purposes of use, and assay levels for the drug in the final feed. A veterinarian is entitled to prescribe a drug for incorporation as a feed additive only if the feed mill has an approved NADA form 1800 on file. The feed level must comply with the level stated in the NADA form 1800.

Before approval of NADA, two basic criteria must be met:

1. A drug must be safe and effective for the intended target species when used as recommended.
2. If the drug is intended for use in food-producing animals, edible products must be safe for human consumers.

For food-producing animals, the NADA must include evidence of safety of residues of the drug and its metabolites. The Animal Drug Amendments of 1968 require the submission of acceptable methods of analysis for the recovery and measurement of residues from edible tissues to facilitate government regulatory agencies in residue monitoring programs.

TABLE 1–13
REGISTRATION DOSSIERS FOR REGULATORY AUTHORITY

Must possess full details regarding the following:

1. *Chemistry and Pharmacy*

Concerned with chemical and pharmaceutical aspects of the drug and formulation. Control tests on starting materials and the finished products. Manufacturing methods and controls, stability data, batch analysis, quality/purity of active/inactive ingredients, analytical assay techniques, shelf life, degradation products, specifications, containers

2. *Pharmacokinetics*

a. *Fate of drugs in animals*

Absorption, distribution, metabolism elimination, (radiolabeled studies). Laboratory animals and target animals. Metabolite isolation and characterization

b. *Residues*

Edible tissues assayed for residues. Target tissue identified as the tissue in which drug-related metabolite persists for longest time. Correlation between validity of chemical methods. Assay method must be specific for marker substance in target tissue and be sufficiently sensitive to measure lowest level of acceptable residue. Confirmatory assay procedure may also be required. Assays are necessary:

(1) To establish safe withdrawal times
(2) To provide a means of monitoring animal products entering human food supply

3. *Biological/Toxicologic Studies*

a. *Toxicity to target species*

Data necessary to ascertain safety of compound for pregnant animals, breeding animals. Safety claims must be validated. Label claims subject to dose scrutiny

b. *Safety to handler/operator*

c. *Safety to consumer*

Toxicity studies must be conducted not only on the parent compound, but also on metabolites that may be present in tissues

4. *Pharmacologic Studies*

To define the activity of the drug within the animal body, i.e., central nervous system, gastrointestinal tract, cardiovascular system, respiratory system, genitourinary system, autonomic nervous system. Side effects must be identified

5. *Toxicity Studies*

a. *Acute toxicity, subacute toxicity, chronic toxicity, specific toxicity studies*

Depending on the product, these may or may not be compulsory. The ultimate arbiter is the regulatory agency

b. *Tests*

Teratogenicity, reproductive studies, fertility studies, mutagenicity, carcinogenicity, local irritation, inhalation, relay toxicity

6. *Environmental Safety*

An Environmental Import Analysis Report (EIAR) must be included in the NADA submitted to the FDA

7. *Drug Resistance*

For antimicrobial compounds data on:

Spectrum of antibacterial activity
Resistance induction
Cross resistance
Transfer of resistance

8. *Assessment of Human Safety*

Establishment of withdrawal times
Approved tolerance levels, i.e., those exceeding what is considered negligible. Tolerances are usually based on chronic toxicity studies in rodents and nonrodents
Safety factors and acceptable daily intake calculations

9. *Labeling*

a. *Indications for use*
Disclaimers, dosages, forms, routes of administration
b. *Precautions in use*
Safety, side effects, contraindication

All label claims must be based on the scientific data used to support the NADA

Initially protocols designed to establish animal safety and drug effectiveness are reviewed by the CVM. Optimally the government receiver (evaluator) consults and participates in protocol review with the sponsoring company.

Statutorily the requirements for a NADA are as follows:

1. Safety to the animal: Toxicologic profile to establish the margin of safety relative to the therapeutic dose includes comprehensive clinical observations, hematology, blood chemistry, urinalysis, and fecal examination. (The CVM issues a guideline, "Target Animal Safety Guidelines for New Animal Drugs.")
2. Efficacy: Data from a minimum of two well-controlled studies conducted in accordance with section 21 CFR 514.111 of the regulations are necessary to prove that the drug is effective for the purpose indicated on the label. Dose titration studies are necessary to determine the optimal dosage.
3. Published articles from peer-reviewed publications can be used to support safety and efficacy, provided that the information is obtained in accordance with standards laid down in Section 512 of the Federal FD&C Act and Section 21 CFR 514.111 of the regulations.
4. Once safety and quality studies are conducted, methods of drug preparation, analysis, and control are used to ensure adequate identification of the test substance.
5. Environmental impact: All sponsoring drug companies are required to complete an environmental impact assessment of the proposed drug substance, in terms of excretory pathways, effect on environment, biodegradation, effect on ecology, and any other relevant actions.
6. Food safety: Safety of ingested meat, milk, and eggs from treated animals is of critical importance. The FDA addresses (among others) the following matters:
   a. What type of residues are found, and what are their potential effects on the consumer?
   b. How can the occurrence of these residues be minimized?
   c. Must the residues of these drugs in food be monitored? Is an acceptable method of analysis available that can be used for monitoring, surveillance, and enforcement?
7. With regard to identifying and evaluating the residues of veterinary drugs, the FDA requires the sponsoring drug company to do the following:
   a. Metabolism residues, especially those of toxicologic concern, must be identified.
   b. Test species (optimum) for toxicity studies must be identified.
   c. Target tissues, marker residues, and the lower limit of reliable measurement of other marker residues must be identified.
   d. A routine analytical regulatory assay must be identified.
   e. A regulatory assay to measure the marker residues must be available.

Section 512 (d) (2) of the Federal FD&C Act sets out the criteria to be considered in evaluating the safety of a new animal drug under its proposed conditions of use and directs that the FDA "shall consider among other relevant factors:

1. The probable consumption of such drug and of any substance formed in or on food because of the use of such drug.
2. The cumulative effective on man or animal of such drug taking into account any clinically or pharmacologically related substance.
3. Safety factors which in the opinion of experts, qualified by scientific training and experience to evaluate the safety of such drugs, are appropriate for the use of animal experimentation data.
4. Whether the conditions of use prescribed, recommended or suggested in the proposed labeling are reasonably certain to be followed in practice."

Another section of the Act requires that a tolerance or withdrawal period be established to ensure the safe use of the drug. Once FDA criteria are met and after approval of the new drug in accordance with a defined step-by-step protocol, section 512 (i) of the Federal FD&C Act requires that the Secretary of Health and Human Services publish a notice of approval in the Federal Register.

The Freedom of Information Act of 1967 required that all government agencies publish their policies, rules, procedures, and guidelines for public perusal. Following approval of a NADA, the FDA publically releases its FOI summary. This is a summary of the data regarding the safety and efficacy of an approved drug as produced by the sponsoring drug company and is accompanied by the approved labeling instruction. The FOI summary informs the public of the basis on which the agency approved the NADA, the clinical indications and specific conditions applicable to the use of the drug. Once the drug has been approved and marketed, the FDA becomes involved in postmarketing surveillance to monitor the safety and efficacy of animal drugs.

The agency has also adopted a "fast-track" review system whereby the time for review of a NADA can be shortened. CVM guidelines have been published to clarify the eligibility of a new animal drug for fast-track evaluation. Entitlement to this speedier review system depends on the sponsoring drug company demonstrating that the drug should obtain priority review status. Fast-track status does not mean that the evaluation procedure is any less rigorous than normal.

RESTRICTIONS

Prescription Drugs

Under Section 512 of the FD&C Act, the FDA may restrict approval of a new animal drug to the specific conditions for which it has been shown to be safe and effective. This may include appropriate restrictions on its use. Section 502 (F) (1) of the Act deems all drugs misbranded unless their labeling bears adequate direction for use. All drugs used in animals possess the capability of inducing undesirable or harmful effects, especially if misused. The FDA interprets this risk-benefit potential in its decision-making processes. The basis for distinguishing OTC animal drugs from Rx drugs is whether adequate written instruction for lay use can be prepared. Rx products must be used only by personnel adequately trained and skilled to use such products. For OTC use, products must have clear and adequate labeling instructions such that safe and effective use is assured.

Specific factors to be considered in deciding whether adequate directions for lay use can be written include:

1. Safety of the drug to the target animal
2. Safety of the drug to humans
3. Nature of the disease being treated (is it readily recognizable?)
4. Type of drug, its potential for misuse, and its route of administration

The Durham-Humphrey Amendment of 1951 established the criteria for distinguishing between OTC and Rx classes of drug. Rx drugs must be labeled: "For use by or on the order of a licensed veterinarian." Products without these words on the label may be sold to anyone. Some drugs are labeled: "For sale to veterinarians only." This does not reflect Rx drug status but simply company sales policy.

Extralabel Uses

A major problem for veterinarians is the extralabel use of animal drugs. Before 1983, the declared policy of the FDA was that in the course of normal day-to-day practice a veterinarian could use any drug that was legally obtained. Such professional discretion by veterinarians, however, was accompanied by the legal, ethical, and moral responsibility of:

1. Ensuring that no harmful residues occurred in treated food animals
2. That they accepted liability in the event of adverse reactions after the use of a drug for purposes not stated on the label

Subsequently the FDA stated that veterinarians in food-animal practice could use drugs only in the precise manner stated on the label. Following intervention by the American Veterinary Medicine Association (AVMA), a compromise was agreed on, permitting veterinarians to use FDA-approved drugs for extralabel purposes in food animals only when no appropriate FDA-approved product is available or when such approved products are shown to be clinically effective in individual situations. The major exception to this ruling is chloramphenicol, which was totally prohibited for use in food animals in 1984. Also, clenbuterol, DES, furazolidone, dimetridazole, and other nitromidazoles are banned in food animals.

Because of the limited array of FDA-approved drugs, dosages, and indications, veterinarians are often compelled to use medicines in a manner outside of the label recommendations.

Although this is a contentious issue, several highly specific conditions must be met before a veterinarian may legally use or prescribe drugs in an extralabel fashion.

''Extralabel usage'' refers to using an OTC or Rx drug in a form other than that specified on the manufacturer's label. This means that the user deviates from the specific instructions as written on the label.

Extralabel usage is a violation of the Federal FD&C Act. Nonetheless, the CVM in the FDA recognizes, as does the AVMA, that some degree of extralabel usage is unavoidable in the course of food-animal practice.

The CVM policy for extralabel drug usage is detailed in the Compliance Policy Guide 7125.06. This guide states interalia that, in the context of a valid veterinarian-client relationship, extralabel usage is permissible:

1. When there is no marketed drug specifically labeled to treat the condition diagnosed
2. When drug dosage at the labeled dosage recommended has been found clinically ineffective
3. When appropriate records of treated animals are kept.
4. When significantly extended withdrawal times are applied.

The decision to use a drug in an extralabel fashion (in accordance with certain stringent conditions) is the prerogative of the veterinarian. The FDA does not normally consider punitive regulatory action if certain exact criteria have been met in such cases.

Similarly nitroimidazoles such as dimetridazole and ipronidazole must not be used in food animals. Sulfamezathine cannot be used in dairy cattle more than 20 months of age.

If illegal residues occur and are attributable to extralabel usage, liability rests with the veterinarian. The Food Animal Residue Avoidance Database (FARAD) is of great importance to the veterinary practitioner when engaged in extralabel usage. This computes pharmacokinetics and withdrawal times for extralabel usage of a drug. Although a definitive answer may not be possible, the toxicologic and pharmacokinetic experts can normally provide sufficiently accurate information to indicate a responsible withdrawal time. The FARAD can translate the veterinary field requirements into kinetic data, thus suggesting a reasonable withdrawal time. When using drugs in an extralabel fashion, it should be remembered that doubling the drug dose adds at least one half-life to the withdrawal time. It takes eight half-lives to eliminate over 99% of an administered dosage.

1.8 RESIDUE MONITORING

The FDA has specific responsibilities to protect public health. Through the CVM, new animal drug approval attains high priority in this endeavor. The Agency is also responsible for inspection, monitoring, and surveillance. Its role includes monitoring animal feeds to ensure correct composition and the imposition of labeling, manufacturing, and quality control standards. Animal feed placed on the market and feed manufacturers' premises are liable for FDA inspection. The CVM is involved also in supervising, coordinating, and directing surveillance and compliance programs for the detection of illegal drug residues. Nationwide residue monitoring protects consumers from exposure to adulterated meat and poultry products. Part of the drug approval process requires manufacturers to submit a reliable assay method for detecting drug residues in slaughtered animals. These analytical methods are reviewed before drug approval. Residues that may persist after animal drug use are carefully evaluated toxicologically as well as legally. Tolerances for acceptable levels of residues are set by the FDA, and the discovery of residue levels in excess of the legal tolerance—the so-called violative residues—is an offense under federal law. Together with the United States Department of Agriculture (USDA), Food Safety and Inspection Service (FSIS), the FDA is responsible for ensuring the absence of violative residues in animal tissues. The FDA and FSIS monitor the correct use and application of animal drugs at the postmarketing phase. This involves inspection of animal food products and premises and laboratory examination of samples to ascertain whether edible animal tissues contain unacceptable levels of residue.

The FDA and Environmental Protection Agency (EPA) are responsible for establishing tolerances of drugs and chemicals in animal tissues. The USDA, through FSIS, enforces the tolerances established by the FDA. The FSIS also reports violative residues of drugs in meat and poultry to the FDA, which then investigates and prosecutes the responsible people.

Withdrawal time is the interval required for the residue of toxicologic concern to reach safe concentration as defined by the tolerance. Withdrawal times are established to ensure that illegal concentrations of drugs do not occur. A veterinarian using a drug in an extra label fashion must also comply with Section 503 (c) of the Federal Food, Drug and Cosmetic Act which states, "a drug would be considered misbranded if at the time of dispensing by a licensed veterinarian the drug does not bear a label containing the name and address of the practitioner, and directions for use and cautionary statements specified by the practitioner."

There are a number of exceptions to this extra label drug prescribing policy. Chloramphenicol and diethylstilboestrol may not be used in any food animals.

The maximal residue limit (MRL) (as defined by the Codex Alimentarius) is the maximum permissible level or concentration of a drug that can be present in food for human consumption.

In accordance with the FD&C Act, the FDA is responsible for establishing tolerance levels of drugs and chemicals in animal products. (The concept of Good Veterinary Practice has been introduced by the Codex Alimentarius Commission). Failure to observe appropriate withdrawal times has been cited as the most common failing leading to the occurrence of drug residues in food. Inadequate record keeping and inadequate cow identification are among the common causes of failure to observe withdrawal times.

In addition to the activities of the FDA in monitoring drugs currently on the market, the USDA, FSIS inspects and samples meat products to establish whether illegal drug residues are present. The USDA's program can be divided into monitoring and surveillance, to identify the incidence and trend of violative residues. This is then followed up by the FDA on a surveillance basis to determine the cause of the residues.

Another level of regulation is imposed by the State Department of Health or Department of Agriculture boards, which have the authority to regulate the safety and wholesomeness of food products being sold within the state. The Pasteurized Milk Ordinance (PMO) sets standards of quality for milk to be transferred freely interstate.

The FSIS assumes primary responsibility for the wholesomeness of the meat supply, and all animals slaughtered at federally inspected plants are subject to random sampling of carcasses for residue determination. Detection of violative residues is reported by the FSIS to the FDA and the CVM. The Agency then makes a followup investigation at the animal producer level to uncover the original source and cause of the contamination problem. Seizure of animal feed and seizure and condemnation of carcasses may result. In accordance with federal law, offenders may face prosecution if found guilty of contravening FDA tolerance levels. Producers of animals harboring violative residues may find future shipments impounded unless they can clearly demonstrate compliance with residue standards. If violative residues are demonstrated as a recurring problem on a particular premises, a surveillance program may be mounted. This intensive monitoring scheme is instigated when animals are known to belong to producers responsible for reaching illegal residue levels previously. Such surveillance programs involve a regular, routine sampling program that continues until the residue problem is deemed to be under control. Usually failure to follow label instructions and withdrawal times are the primary reasons for carcass contamination with illegal drug residues.

The FDA, USDA, and EPA each have a distinct role in residue monitoring. The EPA cooperates in programs in which pesticide residues are deemed to be involved and ensures that pesticides are used according to label instructions. Although the FSIS of the USDA assumes primary responsibility for the wholesomeness of the meat supply, the FDA has final authority for enforcement of the laws governing the use of animal drugs and the acceptability of medicated fields. The law is explicit in its requirements for veterinary drug approval, and the FDA must withhold approval until all scientific criteria are met. Once a drug is marketed, the FDA continues through post-marketing surveillance to oversee the safety and efficacy of drugs. In this role, however, FDA control over the usage is reduced considerably. For the most part, monitoring and surveillance programs are based on a ranking of drugs that offer priority potential to threaten human health if incorrectly used. It is now incumbent on manufacturers to submit for review by the FDA and FSIS a reliable assay method for detecting drug residue in slaughtered animals. The FDA then sets tolerances for acceptable levels of drug residue in animal tissues based on the no-effect level, i.e., the highest level at which the drug produces no measurable physiologic effects.

The Delaney Amendment of the Federal FD&C Act applies to drugs that are considered to be carcinogens and require zero tolerance. Advances in analytical chemistry have made the concept of zero tolerance less useful because increasingly smaller amounts of residue can be detected. Because of this constantly changing level of zero, the FDA proposed a new scientific rationale for establishing the sensitivity of an analytical method required for carcinogenic drug residues and their metabolites. This SOM approach implements the DES proviso, an exception to the Delaney anticancer clause that permits approval of use of carcinogenic compounds in food-producing animals, provided that the level of any residue remaining in edible tissues is so minimal that it would not present any significant risk of cancer for human consumption. According to the Federal Register, the SOM approval represents the FDA's perception of an acceptable method of demonstrating that a carcinogenic compound may be safely used in food.

RESIDUES AND TOLERANCES

Advances in pharmacokinetic studies have illustrated that a rapid initial decrease of drug concentration in the animal body is followed by an extremely slow phase of depletion. The latter phase often remained undetectable as long as sensitive analytical methods were generally unavailable. Only since the advent of improved analytical capabilities has this slow elimination phase become evident. Therefore the presence or absence of residues following the administration of any drug is really an academic question—residue detection depends on the sensitivity of the analytical method employed. Although the use of animal drugs must always be subject to stringent and judicious controls, nonetheless any attempt to produce food completely free of residues is a practical and biological impossibility. The concept of "zero tolerance" is no longer useful on account of the advances in analytic chemistry because increasingly smaller amounts of residue can be detected. Thus the scientifically zero tolerance concept has been replaced by a system of tolerances based on toxicologic evaluation of residues.

Because analytical methods have reached a high degree of sophistication, it is now possible to detect tissue levels in ever-decreasing amounts. It is not easy to assess the health significance of these minute levels that are becoming more routinely measurable. Thus the setting of tolerances and the establishment of withdrawal requirements that ensure that the intended drug will not pose a threat to human health are among the most important of the FDA's responsibilities in animal drug evaluation.

Drug-related residues must be identified and demonstrated to be nondetrimental to the consumer at the anticipated levels of dietary inclusion. Pharmacokinetic studies are necessary for identification of residues and play an extremely crucial role in safety assessment. To comply with additional FDA requirements, a reliable assay method for detection of residues in slaughtered animals must be submitted by drug manufacturers. This stated assay method must be sensitive to the established tolerance level. The term "violative residue" is used to describe a detected residue in excess of the legislatively permissible tolerance level.

"Tolerance" refers to approved finite residue levels, i.e., those exceeding what is considered negligible. A tolerance is established by finding the concentration that has no adverse effects in the most sensitive test species used in toxicity studies. The use of the term "tolerance" applies only to the legally permissible level of exposure; it does not imply the maximum residue that can be safely tolerated. In calculating a tolerance, all residues, including parent drug, metabolites, or other decomposition products, are taken to be of toxicologic significance. The FDA is charged with consumer health protection, and thus the safety of any residues that may persist from animal drug use must be carefully evaluated toxicologically as well as legally. Under the FD&C Act and its accompanying regulations, the agency must consider:

1. "[T]he probable consumption of such drug and of any substance found in or on food because of the use of such drug"
2. The cumulative effects on humans or animals of such drug, taking into account any chemically or pharmacologically related substance
3. Safety factors that, in the opinion of experts qualified by scientific training and experience to evaluate the safety of such drugs, are appropriate for use of animal experimental data
4. "Whether the conditions of use prescribed, recommended or suggested in the proposed labeling are reasonably certain to be followed in practice."

In the regulations, the types of tolerances and the conditions that govern their establishment are described.

Finite Tolerance

This is a measurable amount of residue that is permitted in food. Such a tolerance is permitted when residues persist beyond a reasonable withdrawal time, and analytical methodology does not support negligible tolerance. Two animal species—one a non-rodent—are used to set a finite tolerance. Lifetime studies in the rat and mouse, 6-month studies in dogs, and three-generation reproduction studies with a teratologic phase are incorporated as the study base. The no-effect level must provide for at least a 100-fold margin of safety.

Negligible Residue Tolerance

This is assigned when a toxicologically insignificant amount of residue resulting in a daily intake that is a small fraction of the maximum accepted daily intake is likely to occur. Following 90-day feeding trials in which the generated toxicologic data reveal a no-effect level, a 2000-fold safety margin is established, and the analytical methods proposed must be adequate to measure at the level that permits the margin of safety. The implication of negligible tolerance is toxicologic insignificance.

Zero Tolerance

The Delaney Amendment of the Federal FD&C Act applies to drugs that are considered to be carcinogens and thus require zero tolerance. No residue of any such drug is permissible in any edible tissue or in any food derived from the treated animal. Under the Delaney Clause, potential carcinogens may be used in animals if the drug does not adversely effect the animal and if no residue of the compound is detectable by an analytical method prescribed or approved by the Secretary of Health, Education, and Welfare. Under this amendment, the presence or absence of residues is obviously a function of the residue detection technique employed. This causes problems because each time more sensitive methods are developed, the term zero residue must be redefined. The concept of zero tolerance was originally developed to embrace three specific situations:

1. When no residue was allowable
2. When toxicologic data were insufficient to support a wider tolerance
3. When no residue could be detected using the most sensitive analytical method

A combination of events revolving around the Delaney Amendment, diethylstilbestrol, and improved sensitivities of detection methods led to a re-evaluation of zero tolerance.

On account of the constant redefining of "zero," the FDA proposed a new scientific approach to surmount the associated problems. This involved the establishment of the sensitivity of an analytical method used for detection of carcinogenic drugs or their metabolites. The SOM approach has now been adopted by the FDA.

SETTING OF TOLERANCES

The criteria for ultimate consumer safety include the no observable effect level (NOEL), the acceptable daily intake (ADI), and a safety factor. To calculate a tolerance level, information is needed to define:

1. The NOEL
2. The safety factor
3. The food factor
4. The ADI

No Observable Effect Level

Information on the no-effect concentration in the most sensitive species is required to calculate the tolerance level. Such studies may be performed in vivo on experimental animals or, currently to a limited but steadily increasing extent, on cultured mammalian cells or on microorganisms in vitro. Establishing a tolerance requires demonstration of proof of safety at an excessive tissue level. This is usually based on chronic toxicity studies in rodents as well as nonrodent species and a three-generation study.

These toxicologic data provide information of the hazards to the target species and to some extent for humans. Disadvantages are that species variation and individual susceptibility are not taken into account, and many variations can exist between different strains (e.g., half-lives) of laboratory animals. The aims of the study are:

1. To establish the nature of toxicity of the drug (qualitative dimension) and to relate this to humans
2. To measure its magnitude (quantitative dimensions) for the purpose of setting tolerance levels in food

From these data, the NOEL is derived. The NOEL is the highest dosage level leading to no observable morphologic or functional changes in the test animals. To define

this dosage, feeding studies at different dosage rates are performed on laboratory animals of both sexes. Usually this figure is derived from 90-day studies, but if other studies, such as mutagenicity, produce positive effects at lower concentrations, the NOEL is pitched to account for those findings.

Safety Factor

The safety factor reflects the quality of the toxicologic investigations and the degree of certainty with which results can be extrapolated to humans. The ADI is the amount of residues that can daily be ingested for a lifetime without fear of deleterious health effects. The safety factor that is applied to the no-effect concentration is a margin of safety that is determined by the tolerance requested and by the type of toxic effect observed in laboratory animal studies. In the case of a finite tolerance, a factor of 100 is applied for effects observed in the chronic toxicity study, but if teratogenicity is observed, the factor is normally increased to 1000. Safety factors are calculated by determining the quantity of residue ingested by humans and then relating it to the no-effects level established in subacute, chronic, or teratogenic studies. Generally a safety factor of 1000 to 2000 based on subchronic studies suffices. If this is not possible, chronic toxicity data are required, and a 100-times factor is minimal for approval. The latter are also necessary for establishing a tolerance.

Food Intake Factor

Any tolerance level for residues in food is obviously a function of the amount of food items ingested by the consumer. Human exposure is based on the residue in target tissues, and for this purpose a market basket approach is usually adopted.

This approach presumes that an average person weighing 60 kg consumes an average of 1.5 kg of food per day, which is further reduced by the fraction of the diet comprising meat products. Traditionally the FDA conservatively estimates meat as equivalent to one third of the diet. This is on the basis of an average intake per adult person of 300 g meat (muscle tissue), 100 g liver, 50 g kidney, and 50 g tissue fat (500 g).

Acceptable Daily Intake

Once the NOEL, safety factors, and food factors are determined, the ADI is calculated as follows:

$$ADI = \frac{NOEL \times 60}{SF} = mg/day$$

Where ADI = acceptable daily intake; NOEL = no observable effect level; 60 = average weight (kg) of human; and SF = safety factor.

Total Daily Consumer Intake =

$$\frac{Residue\ (ppm) \times Food\ Consumption}{Average\ Weight\ of\ Human}$$

Expressed as parts per million in food:

$$ADI = \frac{NOEL}{SF} \times$$

$$\frac{Weight\ of\ Human}{Food\ Consumption} = ppm$$

Having established the ADI, the withdrawal time can be calculated. This is the time (t) required for drug residues to decline below the ADI.

The withdrawal time is based on the time for the average human to ingest 1/100 or 1/2000 of the NOEL. The 100-times safety factor includes a 10-times factor for age differences and a 10-fold factor for extrapolation from laboratory animals to humans. The withdrawal period is the time required for the residue of toxicologic significance to reach a safe concentration as defined by the tolerance.

It is therefore possible to arrive at a maximal residue tolerance that is based on the ADI and the average consumption of meat, offal, and meat products:

$$\frac{safe\ concentration}{(Tolerance)} = \frac{ADI \times 60\ kg}{500\ g \times Food\ Factor}$$

Tolerances cannot be established for (genotoxic) carcinogenic substances or frequently for teratogenic substances.

GUIDELINE FOR ESTABLISHING A TOLERANCE

Food Factors

The FDA assumes that, muscle or eggs constitute 500 g of a 1500-g diet and that organ meats are consumed in lesser quantities. The FDA also assumes that milk may constitute the total diet of some individuals.

The FDA uses consumption factors in calculating the tolerance. These factors are summarized as follows:

EDIBLE PRODUCE	FOOD FACTOR
Cattle	
Milk	3
Muscle	1
Liver	1/2
Kidney	1/3
Fat	1/4
Swine	
Muscle	1
Liver	1/3
Kidney	1/4
Fat	1/4
Sheep	
Muscle	1
Liver	1/5
Kidney	1/5
Fat	1/5
Poultry	
Eggs	1
Muscle	1
Liver	1/3
Fat/skin	1/2

Establishing Tolerance (Maximal Residue Limit)

The tolerance establishes the concentration of marker residue permitted in the target tissue of a treated animal.

Safe Concentration =

$$\frac{ADI\ (\mu g/kg/day) \times 60\ kg}{FOOD\ FACTOR \times 500\ g/day}$$

MRLs must be proposed for the various edible tissues and produce in which residues of the substance concerned could occur. Proposals for MRLs should be based on the ADI of the substance established from safety studies. This evaluation of safety covers not only toxicologic properties, but also pharmacologic properties, possible allergenic potential, and, for antimicrobial substances, possible effect of residues on the human gut flora. The ADI is defined as the quantity of residue that can be ingested daily over a lifetime without appreciable health risk. It is derived from the NOEL for the most sensitive parameter in the most sensitive appropriate test species:

ADI (mg/day) =

$$\frac{\text{NOEL (mg/kg body weight)} \times \text{Standard Human Weight (kg)}}{\text{Safety Factor}}$$

The MRLs set for individual tissues should reflect the relative distribution of residue between the tissues observed in residue studies, so practical withdrawal times can be set for products containing the active substances concerned. This is an important point that distinguishes the approach used to set MRLs in the Europe from the approach used by the FDA to set residue tolerances. The FDA uses food consumption data and food factors in conjunction with the ADI to set safe concentrations of residues in edible tissues. This "safe concentration" of residue can be considered equivalent to a MRL.

1. Calculation of acceptable daily intake:
   NOEL: 0.25 mg/kg body weight
   Safety factor: 100
   ADI: 150 mg per person per day
2. FDA determination of safe concentration of total residue in cattle tissues:

	FOOD FACTOR	SAFE CONCENTRATION
Muscle	1.0	0.3 ppm
Liver	0.5	0.6 ppm
Kidney	0.33	0.9 ppm
Fat	0.25	1.2 ppm
Milk	3.0	0.1 ppm

For example, to calculate the muscle tolerance above.

Safe Concentration =

$$\frac{250 \text{ mcg/kg} \times 60 \text{ kg.}}{100 \text{ (S.F.)} \times 1 \text{ (F.F.)} \times 500 \text{ GM}}$$

$$= \frac{15000 \text{ mcg}}{50000 \text{ G}}$$

$$= \frac{1.5 \text{ mcg}}{5 \text{ G}}$$

$$= 0.3 \text{ mcg/G. (0.3 ppm)}$$

SELECTED REFERENCES

Anonymous: Veterinarian convicted on chloramphenicol charge. J. Am. Vet. Med. Assoc., *198*:1492, 1991.

Center for Veterinary Medicine: FSA and the Veterinarian. Washington, D.C., U.S. Government Printing Office, 1989.

Code of Federal Regulations: Title 21, Chapter 1, Part 556.20–556.70, 1982.

Code of Federal Regulations: Title 21, Parts 200–299 and Parts 500–599, 1982.

Council on Biologic and Therapeutic Agents: AVMA guidelines for supervising use and distribution of veterinary prescription drugs. J. Am. Vet. Med. Assoc., *193*: center pages, 1988.

Food and Drug Administration: Extra Label Use of New Animal Drugs in Food Producing Animals. Food and Drug Administration Compliance Policy Guide. 7125.05. Chapter 25. Rockville, MD, Center for Veterinary Medicine, 1984.

Goulding, R.C.: Know your drug restriction. California Vet., *44*:16, 1990.

Guest, G.B., and Paige, J.C.: The magnitude of the tissue residue problem, with regard to consumer needs. J. Am. Vet. Med. Assoc., *198*:805, 1991.

Hoffsis, G.F.: Regulatory issues: Drug residues avoidance in dairy cows. Compend. Contin. Educ. Pract. Vet., *12*:274, 1990.

Hoffsis, G.F.: Regulatory issues: The 1989 veterinary prescription drug amendment. Compend. Contin. Educ. Pract. Vet., *12*:1794, 1990.

Hoffsis, G.F., and Henry, S.C.: Extralabel use of veterinary drugs. Compend. Contin. Educ. Pract. Vet., *10*:1215, 1988.

Mercer, H.D.: Residue avoidance: Withdrawal times for drugs not labelled for food animals. *In* The Use of Drugs in Food Animal Medicine. Edited by J.D. Powers and T.E. Powers. Columbus, The Ohio State University Press, 1985.

Raef, T.A.: FDA re-evaluating labelling policy for dually classified drugs. J. Am. Vet. Med. Assoc., *196*:1743, 1990.

Sundlof, S.F.: Drug and chemical residues in livestock. Vet. Clin. North Am. [Food Anim. Pract.], *5*:411, 1989.

Sundlof, S.F.: Food Animal Residue Avoidance Databank (FARAD): Comprehensive Compendium of Food Animal Drugs. Gainesville, University of Florida, 1987.

Sundloff, S.F., Craigmill, A.C., and Riviere, J.E.: Food Animal Residue Avoidance Databank (FARAD): A pharmacokinetic-based information resource. J. Vet. Pharmacol. Ther., *9*:237, 1986.

Talbot, R.B., Haydee Fernandez, A., and Melendez, L.V.: 1987 list of FDA Approved Animal Drug Products. Blacksburg, Virginia Polytechnic Institute and State University, 1987. VA, Information Series 87–1.

The 1938 Food, Drug and Cosmetic Act as amended. Washington D.C., Superintendent of Documents, U.S. Government Printing Office, 1985.

Toxicological Principles for the Safety Assessment of Direct Food Additives and Color Additives Used in Food. U.S. Food and Drug Administration, Bureau of Foods, 1982.

Van Dressen, W.R., and Wilcke, J.R.: Drug residues in food animals. J. Am. Vet. Med. Assoc., *194*:1700, 1989.

Wilson, D.J.: Antibiotic and sulfonamide residues in bobveal calf tissues: Frequency of agents detected in Cast. positive calves. October 1987–September 1988. *In* An Epidemiological Study of Antimicrobial Residues in Tissues of Bob Veal Calves. Doctoral Dissertation, University of California, 1990 [submitted].

APPENDIX

Office of Information & Education (HFV-11), Center for Veterinary Medicine, Food and Drug Administration, 5600 Fishers Lane, Rockville, MD 20857

Some Centers for Veterinary Medicine Guidelines

Title
Anticoccidial Guidelines
Anthelmintics
General Principles for Evaluating the Safety of Compounds Used in Food-Producing Animals (SOM)
Guidelines for Efficacy Studies for Systemic Sustained Release
Sulfonamide Boluses for Cattle
Stability Guidelines
Guidelines for Submitting NADAs for Generic Drugs Reviewed by NAS/NRC
Antibiotic Residues in Milk, Dairy Products, and Animal Tissues: Methods, Reports, and Protocols
Guidelines for Toxicological Investigations
Preclearance Guidelines for Production Drugs (amendment) Section II (G) (1) (b) (4)
BVM Environmental Guidelines
BVM Policy and Procedure Guidelines: Export of New Animal Drugs for Investigational Use
Cattle Medicated Block Guidelines
Guideline and Format for Reporting the Details of Clinical Trials Using An Investigational New Animal Drug in FOOD Producing Animals
Guideline and Format for Reporting the Details of Clinical Trials Using An Investigational New Animal Drug in NON-FOOD Producing Animals
FOI Summary Guideline
Working Guidelines for Assigning Residue Tolerances
Antibacterial Drugs in Animal Feeds: Human Health Safety Criteria
Antibacterial Drugs in Animal Feeds: Animal Health Safety Criteria
Antibacterial Drugs in Animal Feeds: Antibacterial Effectiveness Criteria
BVM Position Statement—Status of Nutritional Ingredients in Animal Drugs and Feed
Guideline Labeling of Arecoline Base Drugs Intended for Animal Use
Guidelines for the Manufacture and Control of Medicated Blocks
Guidelines for Drug Combinations for Use in Animals
Guidelines for the Efficacy Evaluation of Equine Anthelmintics
Guidelines for the Preparation of Data to Satisfy the Requirements of Section 512 of the Act Regarding Animal Safety, Effectiveness, Human Food Safety and Environmental Considerations for Minor Use of New Animal Drugs
New Animal Drug Determinations
"FAST TRACK" Drug Classification Guideline
Guidelines for the Effectiveness Evaluation of Swine Anthelmintics
Guidelines for Anti-infective Bovine Mastitis Product Development
Guidelines for the Evaluation of Bovine Anthelmintics
Guideline for Threshold Assessment
Target Animal Safety Draft Guidelines for New Animal Drugs
BIOMASS Guideline—Guideline for New Animal Drugs and Food Additives Derived from a Fermentation; Human Food Safety Evaluation
BIOEQUIVALENCE Study Guideline (draft)
Guideline for Efficacy Evaluation of Canine/Feline Anthelmintics
Guidelines for Evaluation of Effectiveness of New Animal Drugs for Use in Poultry Feeds for Pigmentation
Guideline for Effectiveness Evaluation of Topical/Otic Animal Drugs

CHAPTER 2

CONTROLLED-RELEASE DELIVERY SYSTEMS

2.1 Introduction
2.2 Advantages of Controlled-Release Systems
2.3 Polymers
2.4 Polymer Design and Manufacture
2.5 Drug Release from Polymer Systems
2.6 Biodegradable Polymers
2.7 Nonbiodegradable Polymers
2.8 Matrix Devices
2.9 Reservoir Devices
2.10 Specialized Delivery Systems
2.11 Veterinary Applications
2.12 Oral Delivery Systems for Ruminants
2.13 Design Principles for Ruminant Boluses
2.14 Anthelmintic Devices
2.15 Growth-Promoting Boluses
2.16 Trace Element Supplementation
2.17 Controlled-Release Glasses
2.18 Pulsed-Release Systems
2.19 Antimicrobial Boluses
2.20 Parenteral Delivery Systems
2.21 External Application Systems
2.22 Miscellaneous Developments
2.23 Future Developments

2.1 INTRODUCTION

Major advances in the science of biotechnology have heralded a new era in veterinary pharmaceuticals and animal health product systems. Rapid changes have been especially evident in the development of controlled-release and novel delivery systems. Technologic progress in this sector has proliferated at such an unprecedented rate that it is likely to remain one of the most dominant and dynamic areas of development over the next decade.

The application of controlled-release delivery techniques to the specific problems encountered in animal health and production allows for unparalleled medication control. This is especially significant when the economic benefit of the treatment program can be established. Sustained-release techniques now comprise a significant component of modern veterinary medical methods. With expanding emphasis on the economic viability of livestock production, the benefits of delivery of therapeutically useful drugs in the most effective, efficient manner possible become self-evident. Improvements in prophylactic strategies of medication and optimization of livestock performance are beneficial consequences of the new technologies.

A current preoccupation of the international pharmaceutical research industry is to facilitate an easy care system of animal treatment. Such an approach envisages the widespread use of sustained-release delivery systems to minimize the inconvenience inherent in the repeated, frequent administration of conventional drug formulations. With labor costs soaring, time-efficient and manpower-sparing practices will inevitably attain a high priority in the animal health industry. Most likely future adoption of the technology will be unavoidable.

Marked changes have occurred not only at the level of delivery system design, but also with regard to the type of biologically active agent incorporated into the system. Such agents include hormonal substances and growth promoters (estradiol, testosterone, progesterone, zeranol, trenbolone), internal and external parasiticides, minerals, trace elements, and antimicrobial substances. Further developments can be anticipated for the sustained release of the tropic peptide hormones (including somatotropin-bovine growth hormone [bGH]), immunostimulators, and immunomodulators.

Erodible matrices, degradable polymers, and controlled-release glasses (CRG) have helped focus on the possibilities for programmed-release surges of drugs at preset time intervals. This so-called pulsed-release approach creates a new dimension in the manipulation of animal production and disease control, especially when potent bioactive agents, such as vaccines, antibodies, parasiticides, hormones, or antibacterial drugs, can be administered in an automated pulsed fashion.

Novel drug delivery systems involve not only the mechanical device employed to administer the drug dose, but also the control device that meters the rate of drug release to the host. The control device includes the physical system and the sustained-release pharmaceutical formation, which together govern the release of active drug molecules into the body for extended periods of time.

2.2 ADVANTAGES OF CONTROLLED-RELEASE SYSTEMS

Controlled-release drug delivery possesses a number of advantages over the conventional systems of single or multiple dosing. Ideally the administration of any drug substance provides effective therapeutic levels at the site of action (biophase) for a suitable period of time commensurate with the therapeutic objective. With traditional single-dose administration of conventional formulations, the concentration in the blood stream reaches a peak level quickly after parenteral delivery. As the free unbound fraction of drug in the blood stream diffuses to its site of activity in the tissues to initiate the pharmacologic response, it is simultaneously presented to the liver, where biotransformation usually, but not inevitably, inactivates the molecule, and also to the kidney, from where it is primarily excreted. Biliary excretion, fecal elimination, and mammary passage are other important portals of exit from the body. The rate of absorption of the drug from its original site of administration diminishes in accordance with the amount of drug remaining at this deposition site. Additionally, the formulation of the drug, type of salt or ester, particle size, vehicle type, solubility, and physiochemical properties modulate the absorptive pattern. Much of the drug is lost through rapid excretion, and duration of action is relatively short because of the rapid decline of high initial plasma levels and exhaustion of the drug reservoir at the injection site. Accordingly the shortcomings associated with traditional formulation systems are the direct result of the rapid disposition and elimination kinetics of the drug, leading to considerable wastage, perhaps unnecessarily high initial blood levels, and frequent redosing intervals.

Controlled-release delivery systems modify the release rate of a drug so the normal exponential plasma decay curve is not attained. These new delivery systems are characterized by rate-controlled drug release profiles capable of producing relatively constant concentrations in the blood stream or other sites in the body. This predetermined release rate can be rendered constant for hours, days, or months, exposing the recipient's tissues to constant drug levels for extended exposure periods. The peak and valley plasma fluctuations associated with conventional dosage forms in concentration-time profiles are thus avoided.

Controlled release of oral medications conventionally affects duration of action of drugs. The duration of action would superficially appear to be a function of rates of distribution, metabolism, and elimination. It may also, however, depend on rate of absorption. This can be visualized by considering a drug with a short elimination half-life. If a controlled-release preparation is designed so its rate of absorption is slower than its rate of metabolism or elimination, the rate of absorption is the deciding factor in the duration of action. The rate of disappearance of the drug from the blood appears to be slower, but the rate of elimination in this simple case is the sum of the absorption process and the metabolism and elimination process. Thus a drug with a short half-life can be given an apparently longer half-life by production of a sustained-release medication.

In general, oral controlled-release preparations deliver drugs to the gastrointestinal tract at a rate controlled by the formulation rather than by physiologic process. Extended-release preparations release drug over a period of time. Delayed-release preparations have a long period before beginning to release drug. Extended-release preparations contain an element of rapid release of drug to produce a rapid onset together with a prolonged release of drug.

Formulations with controlled-release delivery characteristics possess a number of advantages over conventional types of single or repeat dose treatment:

1. Extended duration of drug action is provided.
2. Frequent and repeated dosing is avoided.
3. Side effects associated with peak blood levels or fluctuating levels are minimized.
4. The total amount of drug required may be reduced.
5. More desirable and more effective kinetic profiles are obtained.
6. Premature inactivation and elimination of the drug dose are avoided.
7. Targeting of drugs to specific sites and selectivity of action are optimized.
8. Prophylactic and therapeutic programs are more effective.

Table 2–1 summarizes the advantages of these systems.

The essentials of any controlled-release system are the pharmacologically active macromolecule and the matrix—usually a polymer. Polymer systems enhance the activity of drugs with short half-lives, and by optimizing therapy, a new lease of therapeutic life can be conferred on pre-existing drug substances.

An ideal controlled-release system results in the drug substance being independent of the variable factors in the environment of the device.

2.3 POLYMERS

Fundamental to the concept of any controlled-release delivery system is the principle of diffusion or molecular transport of the active macromolecule from the polymer matrix. Many of the matrices currently employed in such systems are polymers (nat-

2.4 POLYMER DESIGN AND MANUFACTURE

The intrinsic physiochemical properties of the polymer must allow the desired release rate and diffusion of the active agents. Manufacture should be an inexpensive, efficient, reproducible process. The polymer must not induce local reactions in the host animal tissues. If the polymer is biodegradable, the end product must be nontoxic to the host animal. The manufacturing process should not disturb either the mechanical properties of the polymer matrix or the biological activity of the included substance. The polymer must be capable of accommodating large concentrations of the active macromolecule. There must be no detrimental chemical interaction between the matrix and the active agent. The polymeric device should retain its desired properties for a suitable period of time and must not decompose on storage (Table 2–4).

Many different manufacturing techniques exist. They may involve complex polymerization processes, molding, extrusion, dispersion, film casting, or injection

---

TABLE 2–1
ADVANTAGES OF CONTROLLED-RELEASE DRUG DELIVERY

Extends therapeutic efficacy of drugs of short half-life
Rapid biotransformation prevents toxic buildup in the body
Constant blood levels attained
Extended blood/tissue levels attained
Avoids peak and trough plasma fluctuations
Reduces host toxicity; less cumulation
Improves therapeutic efficacy
Promotes efficient prophylactic medication
Facilitates strategic dosing
Less frequent administration
Reduced trauma
Convenience
Targeting of drugs to specific organs/tissues
Greater tissue contact time
Potential for pulsed-release delivery
Reduction in total amount of drug required
Enhanced drug stability

---

ural or synthetic); because of the advances in polymer science, so many sophisticated precision release devices are now available.

Polymers are linear molecules built up from simple repeating units termed "monomers." Chemical polymers are created by polymerizing a mixture of monomers, producing a distribution of chain lengths and a random sequence, if more than one type of monomer is used. Branching three-dimensional structures can be created by a series of cross linkages (Tables 2–2 and 2–3).

The variety of polymers is almost infinite, and laboratory synthesis of such compounds can achieve desired characteristics of diffusion and degradation, prerequisites for a reproducible, efficient controlled-release system. Release patterns from these types of systems are based on migration to the surface by diffusion either through the matrix pores or through the polymer phase itself. For this purpose, matrix polymer materials must be biocompatible with tissues and possess proper permeability characteristics. Generally polymer systems can be divided into biodegradable and nonbiodegradable systems.

TABLE 2–2
TYPES OF POLYMERS

Natural
  Carboxymethylcellulose
  Ethylcellulose
  Starch
  Gelatin
  Waxes
  Proteins
  Shellac
  Polylactic acid
  Hydrogels
Synthetic
  Polyethylene
  Polypropylene
  Polyether
  Polyester
  Polyamide
  Polyvinylchloride
  Polyvinylacetate
  Ethylene vinylacetate (EVA) copolymer
  Silicone rubber
  Butyl rubber
  Hydrogels

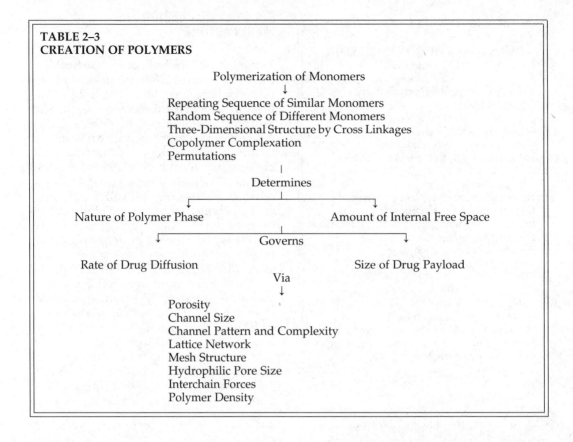

TABLE 2–3
CREATION OF POLYMERS

Polymerization of Monomers
↓
Repeating Sequence of Similar Monomers
Random Sequence of Different Monomers
Three-Dimensional Structure by Cross Linkages
Copolymer Complexation
Permutations
|
Determines

Nature of Polymer Phase   Amount of Internal Free Space
Governs

Rate of Drug Diffusion   Size of Drug Payload
Via
↓
Porosity
Channel Size
Channel Pattern and Complexity
Lattice Network
Mesh Structure
Hydrophilic Pore Size
Interchain Forces
Polymer Density

molding. Frequently the active agent is dissolved or dispersed within the monomeric substance before proceeding to the polymerization stage. In other systems, the entire payload of active drugs may be deposited within the final matrix by a process of soaking. The various stages of manufacturing procedure must be precisely controlled

TABLE 2–4
DESIRABLE PROPERTIES OF POLYMER MATRIX SYSTEMS

Ease of manufacture
Patentability
Compatibility with body tissues
Capacity for optimal drug payload
Suitable physiochemical properties
Attainment of desired release rate
Compatibility with entrapped active
    macromolecule
Stability during manufacturing process

to prevent degradation of the potentially labile macromolecules that are being incorporated into the system. Not only must the polymer complex ultimately deliver the desired release pattern, but also the biological reactivity of the released drug in the body must be assured. Thus the design of any polymer system must address such factors as stability, release rate, efficacy, bioavailability, sterility, ease of manufacture, patentability, and competitive cost. The drug and vehicle must be nonirritating and nontoxic to the animal. Tissue depletion studies and residues must be given a high priority, especially from the standpoint of regulatory clearance.

2.5 DRUG RELEASE FROM POLYMER SYSTEMS

Optimal drug therapy requires that a constant level of the pharmacologically active substance be maintained throughout the course of the treatment. A controlled-release system facilitates the use of many drugs, especially those that have a short half-life. Predetermined concentrations may thus be achieved for a specified period of time. Delivery from the device should be zero order (constant rate), with the release rate being constant and independent of time. Release rates can be affected by the process of diffusion, dissolution, or erosion from fabricated formulation or device. Successful attainment of zero order release rates is a function of the formulation and device interaction. With release by erosion, the release rate is constant as long as the surface area does not change during the erosion process.

Some polymer matrix systems, especially the monolithic and laminated type, achieve release patterns that are not zero order. This may not be a drawback, however, because in some cases, an initial release surge followed by a slower rate of release may be necessary.

The chemical composition of the polymer can be varied to optimize the release rate. With hydrophilic polymers, such as cross-linked polyacrylamide, polyvinylpyrrolidone, ethylene vinylacetate copolymer, and polyvinyl alcohol, release is governed by the design of the monolithic polymer and the molecular weight of the diffusing macromolecule. This relates in turn to the dissolution of drug particles within the polymer matrix and the diffusion pattern of the dissolved drug through the polymer phase. Micronization of drugs ensures rapid dissolution, whereas large particle size can retard the rate of release.

If release mechanisms depend on the process of leaching by a solvent, the porosity of the polymer is important. In such cases, the inward movement of water partitions the agent, which then migrates outward in accordance with the pore or channel structure of the polymer. Systems using leaching for release are usually characterized by shorter life spans when compared with polymer systems in which release is effected by diffusion or dissolution. Advances in polymer design have facilitated a high degree of control of the process of molecular transport and diffusion through polymeric materials. Usually the active agent is dissolved in the polymer or elastomer matrix until saturation is achieved, and the release pattern proceeds along a diffusional concentration gradient as drug is removed from the outer surface layer. The solute is removed by diffusion through the matrix phase or through the polymer pores.

Structural design of polymers creates a variable amount of free space or unoccupied volume within the matrix. Expansion or contraction of this volume by cross linkages or copolymer complexation governs not only the drug payload that can be accommodated, but also its delivery rate. Certain polymers possess weak interchain forces that confer properties of elasticity on them. These are known as "elastomers," and they stretch under tension. When an active molecule is soluble in the elastomer owing to the intermolecular forces, rate controlled release is of a diffusion-dissolution type. If the compound is insoluble in the elastomer, release is by the process of leaching, whereby inward movement of water or fluid solvent partitions the agent and draws it outward, following the pore structure. The porosity of the elastomer is one of the main rate-controlling factors together with the solubility of the macromolecule in water. If the slow rate of release characteristic of the diffusion-dissolution type is desired, a polymer in which the active molecule is soluble must be selected or designed.

FACTORS AFFECTING DRUG DELIVERY

To establish a uniform rate of release of active drug, (1) the agent must be incorporated in a matrix, and (2) it must migrate through the matrix at a controlled rate. A number of factors are critical for attaining a metered delivery rate (Table 2–5).

Concentration of Active Material

Carrying capacity of the system influences not only the release profile, but also the physical design of the device. Most pharmacologic agents incorporated into controlled-release devices are relatively potent agents and are unlikely to exceed payload of the system. This built-in payload determines the maximal concentration that can be released as well as the ultimate biological life span of the system. Many drugs dissolved in the polymer matrix are released

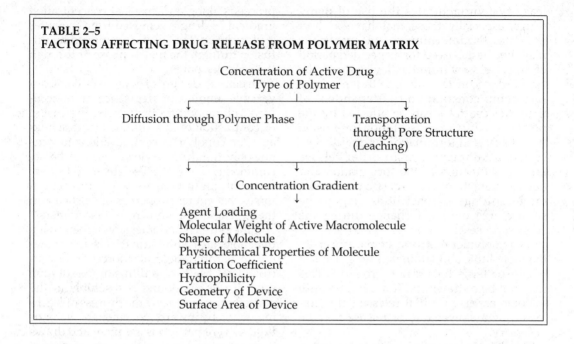

TABLE 2–5
FACTORS AFFECTING DRUG RELEASE FROM POLYMER MATRIX

Concentration of Active Drug
Type of Polymer

Diffusion through Polymer Phase   Transportation
                                              through Pore Structure
                                              (Leaching)

Concentration Gradient

Agent Loading
Molecular Weight of Active Macromolecule
Shape of Molecule
Physiochemical Properties of Molecule
Partition Coefficient
Hydrophilicity
Geometry of Device
Surface Area of Device

by outward diffusion through the polymer phase along a concentration gradient. In such cases, the initial matrix concentration is a key element governing release rate. Similarly, for systems dependent on molecular transport through the porosity of the polymer network, the release rate increases with the loading concentration. As the drug is removed from the surface of the formulation, more of the agent diffuses from the deeper layers along the decreasing concentration gradient.

Diffusion Coefficient

The rate of drug delivery is also a function of the diffusion coefficient of the macromolecule. Release of the macromolecule occurs by diffusion through the matrix phase or through the structural porosity. Successful passage through the interconnecting channels is determined by the shape of the diffusion molecule, its molecular weight, and the physiochemical properties of the polymer.

Partition Coefficient

Transfer from the polymer phase to the aqueous phase is vital for the delivery of the active molecule into the surrounding body fluids. This is an inherent property of the molecule conferred on it by its molecular structure and its physiochemical properties.

Solubility

Intermolecular forces and chemical bonding between the active drug matrix and the inflowing solvent affect release rates. Release rates can be predetermined from data studies of the thermodynamic relationships for drug-polymer systems.

The kinetics of drug release can be summarized as:

1. Drug blended into polymer matrix
2. Diffusion through polymer
3. Solubility in water
4. Absorption into tissue compartments

Geometric Configuration

The structure, design dimension, and shape of the device influence release of the included drug. Selection of a particular device depends on the active molecule, its lipophilicity, desired release rate, stability, desired duration of effectiveness, and route of administration. Most devices are cylindrical, spherical, or slab shaped. The geometry of the device is controlled by the dimensions of the mold or other manufacturing process. Usually the geometric configuration can be varied to suit the desired release rate. In many nonbiodegradable systems, the amount of drug delivered depends on the surface area, which can be modified depending on the dosage desired. If release is effected by surface erosion, the rate is constant (zero order) as long as the surface area does not change during the process of erosion. Cylindrical shaped erodible devices display a constant change in their geometry as the surface area decreases with time. Thus delivery decreases with time, and zero order kinetics are not maintained. Alteration of device size and shape therefore modifies the biological performance of the formulation.

Filler Materials

The physical properties of polymers can be affected by the incorporation of inert filler materials, such as silica, to improve structural integrity. Filler materials may retard drug transport by adsorbing the macromolecule or hindering its diffusion.

2.6 BIODEGRADABLE POLYMERS

Biodegradable polymers are based on release of active ingredients by erosion or a combination of erosion and diffusion. (In the nonbiodegradable system, the polymer acts as an inert matrix using a fixed pore structure to achieve the desired release rate.)

When natural biodegradable polymers are used, the intrinsic properties of the polymer itself are important. Factors such as molecular weight, degree of cross linking, polydispersity, and copolymer ratios influence the development and generation of large hydrophilic zones through which the active macromolecules diffuse. The ultimate degradation of the polymer in the body depends on such factors also. Covalent cross linkages confer a three-dimensional structure on a water-soluble polymer, a method by which a sparingly soluble hydrogel can be formed. Such a matrix facilitates the outward passage of small molecules but tends to hinder diffusion of

---

**TABLE 2–6
BIODEGRADABLE POLYMERS**

Lability
Solubility
Molecular Weight
Ratio of Copolymers
Degree of Cross Linkages
↓
Susceptibility to Body Degradation
   Erosion
   Hydrolysis
   Solubility
   Leaching
↓
End Products Nontoxic
↓
No Physical Residue

---

larger molecules, which can be released only as the hydrogel matrix is gradually degraded. Thus careful attention to the polymeric design and structure can accurately modulate the ultimate payout of the drug from the complex (Table 2–6).

For a biodegradable system, the above-mentioned properties of the polymer are important in determining the overall efficacy of the device. The quality of the manufacturing process controlling such variables determines the performance and reliability of the system in vivo. Some matrix systems combine the principles of both degradation and diffusion, whereby the diffusion rate increases as the matrix is eroded.

Many biodegradable systems use natural polymers, such as carboxymethylcellulose, gelatin, paraffins, waxes, starch, shellac, or polylactic acid. Polyorthoesters have the advantage that in the body, small monomers result from sequential cleavage, and these substances can be rapidly metabolized by the animal body. A new class of polymers, hydrogels, allows incorporation of many drugs and proteins (including bGH), which are then released by hydrolysis and erosion of the polymer rather than by diffusion of the macromolecule itself.

2.7 NONBIODEGRADABLE POLYMERS

Synthetic nonbiodegradable polymers act in general as inert matrix bases. In such systems, matrix pore structure is critical. A

TABLE 2–7
NONBIODEGRADABLE POLYMERS

Synthetic Polymers
Synthetic Elastomers
↓
Density
Tight Mesh Structure
Permutation of Cross Linkages
Complexity of Polymer Skeleton
Modified Pore Size, Channel Structure
Added Proteins
Monomer Ratio Manipulation
↓
Variation of Permeability, Stiffness, Flexibility
↓
Retardation of Diffusion of Active Molecules
↓
Physical Residue of Device

suitably designed system compound of EVA copolymer can achieve a metered release of active agents through its network of large hydrophilic pores or channels. By varying the particle size or by the loading of added proteins to the polymers, control can be exercised over the pore structure and thereby the rate of drug release. Additionally, permutations in the extent or type of cross linking within the polymer skeleton can be varied to obtain a tailor-made release pattern (Table 2–7). For instance, as the number of cross linkages increases, the smaller mesh structure created retards the egress of many entrapped active macromolecules. Substitution of labile polyesters into the structure can increase the release rate by rendering the resultant polymer more susceptible to hydrolysis in the body.

Although the final size and structure of the matrix pores can be manipulated by sophisticated advances in polymer technology, the determinants of desired polymer structure on the amount of active drug that is to be included, the physical form of this macromolecule, and the manufacturability of the desired complex.

Silastic silicone rubber is an elastomer that acts as a dense polymer to facilitate the longterm delivery of many steroidal substances. The mechanism of movement is retarded diffusion, with the dense polymer resisting the outward movement of the active molecules. Filling the silicone tubing with silica filler not only structurally reinforces the device, but also decreases transport. Silicone rubber displays relatively high permeability for many drugs of low water solubility, such as progesterone and other steroids.

Other polymers, such as the EVA copolymer system, offer a number of advantages of sustained-release devices. Small changes in the ratio of monomers result in controlled variation of permeability characteristics, stiffness, flexibility, and tensile strength. Such devices have been employed in human medicine as ocular delivery systems to obviate frequent local application of therapeutic agents to the eye.

Polymeric matrices composed of certain hydrophilic monomers are capable of imbibing water, resulting in the establishment of a stable three-dimensional network. These polymeric materials, known as "hydrogels," control the rate of movement of active material across them, in accordance with the water solubility of the agent. They are ideal for rate-controlled transport of water-soluble materials. Permeation rather than diffusion characterizes the system. Such rate-controlling membranes are employed most frequently in reservoir-type systems.

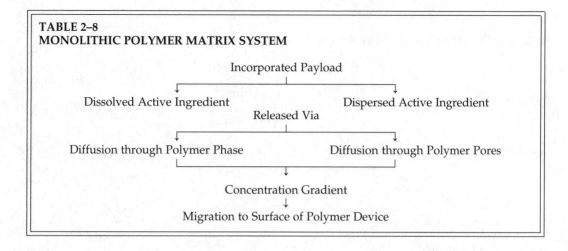

TABLE 2–8
MONOLITHIC POLYMER MATRIX SYSTEM

Incorporated Payload

Dissolved Active Ingredient   Dispersed Active Ingredient

Released Via

Diffusion through Polymer Phase   Diffusion through Polymer Pores

Concentration Gradient

Migration to Surface of Polymer Device

2.8 MATRIX DEVICES

This involves dispersal of the pharmacologically active agent in an inert polymer matrix. Such systems are commonly referred to as "monolithic" devices (Table 2–8). The solubility of the drug in the polymer and in water and the physical properties of the matrix determine the kinetics of drug release. Most monolithic systems depend on degradation or erosion. As the polymer degrades in the body, the active agent is released by a process of diffusion; if the matrix is fully biodegradable, no residue of the device remains. If surface erosion occurs by hydrolysis or some other mechanism, the active agent in the deeper layers of the device is gradually released. Although theoretically a zero order rate of release is aimed for, in practice the rate of release diminishes as the surface area contracts. The geometric configuration of the device is therefore important in determining the rate of release.

Other versions of these systems incorporate a microporous matrix within which the active agent is dispersed and from where it gradually diffuses to the surface. Such systems are not usually biodegradable, do not give a linear rate of release, and remain permanently in the tissues. Pore structure of nonbiodegradable polymers has a major influence on release rates in such systems, and this in turn is determined by the amount of active drug incorporated, the physical form

of the macromolecule, the method of preparation, and the desired release rate.

A development from the basic monolithic system is the laminated polymer matrix, which usually consists of three polymeric films laminated together. The central layer contains the active agent, and the outer layers function to control the release rate and to confer structural integrity on the polymeric sandwich.

2.9 RESERVOIR DEVICES

The reservoir type of controlled-release system is characterized by a storage depot that maintains the payload drug concentration in a stable form and a surrounding membrane (polymer) that modulates release by way of a rate control mechanism (Table 2–9). Transport of the active molecule from the reservoir occurs by permeation through the surrounding membrane (by absorption, solution, and diffusion along a concentration gradient). The molecular weight of the diffusate is important for this process to occur. To facilitate diffusion of many useful macromolecular drugs, the boundary membrane must be microporous. Hydrogels are frequently used as rate-controlling membranes when transport across the membrane depends on the water solubility of the active agent. An advantage of such systems is that zero order kinetics (control release rate) can be achieved because a fixed con-

TABLE 2–9
RESERVOIR MATRIX SYSTEM

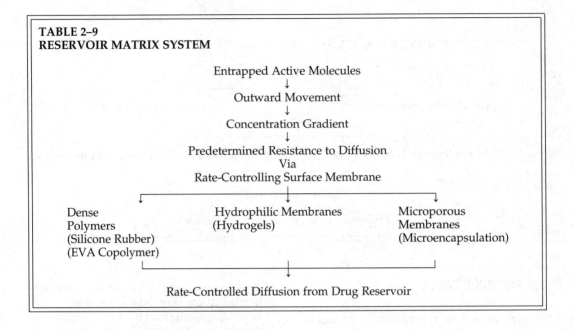

Entrapped Active Molecules
↓
Outward Movement
↓
Concentration Gradient
↓
Predetermined Resistance to Diffusion
Via
Rate-Controlling Surface Membrane

| Dense Polymers (Silicone Rubber) (EVA Copolymer) | Hydrophilic Membranes (Hydrogels) | Microporous Membranes (Microencapsulation) |

Rate-Controlled Diffusion from Drug Reservoir

centration of diffusible drug can be maintained in the reservoir at the interface of the boundary layer. The rate-controlling membrane is nondegradable because it permits a constant rate of release. Such nonbiodegradable systems, however, remain as a permanent residue in the tissues.

2.10 SPECIALIZED DELIVERY SYSTEMS

Certain medically important drugs present difficulty in formulation, i.e., in providing a dosage form that is stable, is well tolerated, and has adequate water solubility. Water solubility, in particular, is important because if a drug is not sufficiently soluble in water, little or no absorption occurs after oral dosing. If a poorly soluble compound is injected, it has lower and slower therapeutic activity.

A potential method of resolving these difficulties is molecular encapsulation technology, in which the drug is encircled with a well-tolerated, highly water-soluble substance. Solubility, stability, and palatability are all improved by encapsulation techniques.

Encapsulation techniques are receiving a lot of attention, particularly in the context of specific drug targeting. Basically drugs

are incorporated in microparticulate carrier systems, such as microemulsions, lipoproteins, liposomes (lipid vesicles), or microspheres. These may be of small diameter (from about 20 ng upward). They may be injected close to the intended site of action or remote from it, with the intention of them being trapped and preferentially released at the site of action. An example would be the physical entrapment of drug microparticles in the capillary bed of a tumor-bearing organ, with resulting sustained release of locally high concentrations of drug.

MICROENCAPSULATION

This is a type of reservoir system in which pharmacologic substances can be microencapsulated by polymeric materials, which then act as semipermeable membranes providing a rate-controlled release of active agent. These microcapsules are small, varying in diameter from 5 to 100 μm. Once introduced into the body, the active substance enclosed with the microcapsule is released at a controlled rate, in accordance with the concentration of active molecules within the microcapsule, the nature and thickness of the polymer coat, the size of the capsule, and the solubility of the entrapped substance. Many microcapsules are not biodegradable and may remain within the tissues. Microencapsulation is used most often to enhance drug stability and to control the rate of release and the site of absorption. Microencapsulation techniques are employed by pharmaceutical companies to exploit the enormous potential of modern technology and thus overcome problems of formulation and delivery. Many orally administered active materials are acid labile and on exposure to acidic conditions are denatured or chemically modified such that they lose activity. Entrapment or immobilization of active molecules within a core structure and coating of the solid core with a rate-retarding membrane result in the formation of microcapsules stable to gastric degradation and capable of sustained target delivery within the intestine or other body cavity. Microencapsulation not only enhances drug stability, but also masks a possible unpleasant taste.

Microencapsulation is a controlled-release technique that helps to accommodate a variety of lipophilic organic compounds. Parenterally microencapsulation:

1. Helps to assist solubilization and increases water solubility
2. Stabilizes compounds and hence improves shelf life
3. Reduces tissue irritation

Orally microencapsulation:

1. Increases bioavailability of drugs that have poor water solubility
2. Reduces stomach irritation
3. Masks bitter taste and unpalatability

Approximately one third of all available drugs have characteristics that make them poor candidates for parenteral product forms. These compounds are usually highly lipid soluble with no appreciable water solubility. As a result, these drugs are available only in oral dosage forms. Further, the first-pass effect by the liver on drugs given orally, can greatly diminish blood concentrations, plasma half-life, and overall usefulness.

Microdroplet technology is a delivery system composed of minuscule droplets of pharmaceutically accepted oil, encapsulated by a monomolecular layer of phospholipid. The drug can be in its oil phase or dissolved in the oil phase. The kinetics of drug release are controlled by the partition coefficient of the drug between the microdroplet and the interstitial water. Drugs with high lipid solubility and tissue affinity can be designed to provide a safe, long duration of effect. Microdroplet technology also provides a means of establishing high drug concentrations in specific target tissues.

The technology works well with highly lipid-soluble drugs that have the following characteristics:

- No appreciable water solubility
- Must be taken orally
- Large first-pass effect by the liver
- High degree of serum protein binding
- Long plasma half-life
- High degree of hepatic metabolism
- Systemic toxicity

Microdroplet technology enables the formulation chemist to incorporate large quantities of oil-soluble drugs into tissue-compatible dosage forms so the drug can be injected into target tissues intramuscularly and intravenously.

LIPOSOMES

Liposomal delivery systems are developments of the microencapsulation technique and offer exciting prospects for targeting and delivery of useful drug substances. Liposomes are microscopic spherical particles that consist in essence of phospholipid vesicles within which active molecules can be entrapped. Such lipid carrier systems assist the transportation of drugs into cells of the lymph nodes, liver, and spleen. By modifying the lipid composition of the vesicle, its lamellarity, or membrane potential, liposomes with different surface charges, pH sensitivities, and release kinetic patterns can be prepared.

The composition of the liposome facilitates intracellular drug delivery because reticuloendothelial cells phagocytose these particles, as they would any foreign matter, and thus ingest the enclosed drug substance. Liposomes may also fuse with cell membranes and introduce active substances by a process of injection. Insofar as the vesicle encapsulation comprises natural substances, such as phospholipid or cholesterol, the coating eventually is broken down by normal metabolic processes of the body. Reduced toxicity is therefore an important feature of liposomal delivery systems. A major application of liposome is the capacity to deliver and internalize antibiotics for the treatment of intracellular infections. In human brucellosis, for example, one of the major problems in treatment is the difficulty of introducing antibiotics into the reticuloendothelial system because the reticuloendothelial system membranes are impermeable to the therapeutically indicated antibiotics. Liposomal-associated streptomycin has been shown to overcome this problem experimentally in the treatment of splenic brucellosis in guinea pigs. Similarly, liposomal encapsulated cephalothin increases the intracellular antibiosis against *Salmonella typhi*. Liposomes appear to be tailor-made for transportation of drugs across cell membranes not normally permeable to the free form. The attainment of high intracellular concentrations of chemotherapeutic agents after the administration of the liposomal formulation creates vast potential not only for the treatment of intracellular infections, but also in the therapy of tumors of the reticuloendothelial system. Because liposomes are engulfed by the reticuloendothelial system, they provide a useful method of targeting therapeutic agents selectively to the body's natural defense system. Another aspect of this delivery technique is the suitability of liposomal microencapsulation for the intracellular targeting and transportation of peptide hormones (e.g., bGH).

Commercialization of this technology requires the production of liposomes with high trapping, efficacious regulated release kinetics, and acceptable shelf lives that are cost-effective and easily manufactured.

Possible applications of liposomes are geared toward taking advantage of the natural fate of these vesicles, which is internalization by phagocytic cells of the reticuloendothelial system. Hence the treatment of intracellular brucella infections could be attempted more successfully by encapsulating antibiotics within a liposome, which then targets the intracellular infection site. A similar approach could be used for antineoplastic therapy.

Liposomes have been used experimentally for delivery of albendazole. When administered parenterally, liposomes carry the encapsulated drug to the liver and are thus particularly suited for fluke treatment.

OSMOTIC PUMPS

The osmotic pump comprises an outer semipermeable membrane and internally a water-soluble drug substance and an osmotic core containing a water attractant, such as NaCl. When in contact with the aqueous tissue fluids, water is drawn inward by osmosis, and during this process of osmotic imbibition, the water-soluble active agent is expelled at a constant rate by way of a small delivery orifice. The delivery rate remains constant (zero order) as long as a saturated solution is maintained within the system. Swelling of the osmotic core compresses the drug reservoir, resulting in a controlled rate of drug release.

For relatively insoluble drugs, the device can be modified to incorporate a polymeric hydrophilic compression department that actively expands following ingress of water. The small physical size of these pumps, however, restricts the payload that can be incorporated. They are most useful for highly potent drugs, with which rate of delivery can be modified by increasing the thickness of the semipermeable membrane.

Many of the systems have been introduced into human medicine and designed on the premise of constant rate delivery to achieve optimal therapy. Infusion pumps, osmotic pumps for therapy with beta-blocking autonomic agents, intrauterine contraceptive devices, ocular inserts for eye medication, and microencapsulation have all received widespread application as a consequence of the new biotechnologic advances in pharmaceutical research. One of the particular advantages of the osmotic delivery system is the high shutdown rate, with 99.8% drug expulsion being achieved. The potential also exists for pulsed release of one or more drugs.

Osmotic pumps have been used in veterinary medicine to delivery metered amounts of ivermectin in nematode control programs. Such pumps function by absorbing water through an outer semipermeable membrane; increasing in internal pressure, and forcing the drug solution, held in a collapsible sac, through an orifice at one end at a regular rate. With this type of device, ivermectin can be delivered intraruminally to release active drug over an extended period.

2.11 VETERINARY APPLICATIONS

In veterinary medicine, controlled-release devices are usually restricted to diseases that lead to significant economic loss to the producer or to situations in which tangible cost-effectiveness to the producer is achieved. Prolonged-release characteristics can afford efficient control over many conditions that might otherwise be impractical to treat. In addition, it may be the only system for drug administration to large numbers of grazing animals in extensive areas. On a worldwide basis, parasitism is probably the most economically significant disease of animals, and slow release of anthelmintics is one important aspect of sustained delivery methodology. Other important applications of this new technology include delivery of hormones for growth promotion purposes, antibiotic substances for prophylaxis, and trace elements for specific deficiency situations. Not only does such an approach facilitate a more uniform pharmacologic response, but also labor costs, trauma to animals, and the necessity for repeat treatment are correspondingly reduced.

Many situations arise in which controlled-release drug delivery may be the only pragmatic method of administration of therapeutic agents to animals. For example, medication can be provided almost continually with the significant practical advantage that repeat treatments, especially to animals under extensive grazing conditions, become unnecessary. Such animals can be subject to prophylactic medication strategies under conditions in which they would otherwise be inaccessible. Specialized delivery systems are particularly useful in veterinary medicine because of the variety of animals kept under varying husbandry conditions, large numbers of which must be treated in relatively short periods of time.

Economics also play an important role in animal health care, and therefore the potential applications of the new systems lend themselves to those situations and diseases in which there is likely to be a potential economic gain for the animal producer. Cost-effectiveness is a major consideration in this context; devices and systems displaying retarded release rates of active agents are restricted to relatively potent compounds. This includes the delivery of hormonal substances to initiate accelerated growth rates or to achieve estrus synchronization, the longterm delivery of trace elements and nutrients (e.g., copper, cobalt, selenium, zinc, amino acids, vitamins), and the longterm administration of anthelmintic or antibacterial agents. Another, perhaps significant, aspect is that controlled-release delivery system is one method by which the continued usage and clinical application of an existing compound can be extended. Advances in formulation technology can often confer new clinical properties on a particular drug with a consequent dramatic effect on their pharmacologic properties and overall usefulness in animals. This is of particular significance today because of the high cost of time and research necessary to develop novel products and to satisfy the international regulatory agencies. Maintenance of marketability and turnover from existing products thereby increases in importance. Reformulation of such products is thus quite common.

Special considerations apply to the design of any controlled-release system for animal use (Table 2–10) because of the variety of animal species likely to be treated with such devices, their differing therapeutic or nutritional requirements, and dissimilar pharmacokinetic properties of drugs on an interspecies basis. Different release rates may be required from species to species to render the device effective for its intended purposes. Anatomic differences necessitate design types displaying contrasting sizes, shapes, and structures. Regulatory requirements necessitate that due cognizance be given to the possibility of residue formation after prolonged presence of the released drug in the food animal's tissues. Table 2–11 summarizes some examples of current controlled-release systems used in veterinary medicines.

TABLE 2–10
SPECIAL CONSIDERATIONS IN DESIGN OF SUSTAINED-RELEASE VETERINARY FORMULATIONS

Intended species application
Desired species release rate
Duration of effectiveness
Retrievable or nonretrievable
Biodegradable or nonbiodegradable
Cost-effectiveness
Continual or pulsatile release
Site of deposition in body
Safety to animal, user, environment
Regulatory requirements
Residue formation

2.12 DESIGN TYPES

Design of controlled-release systems for animals differ considerably from those intended for human use. Taking account of the wide variation of animal species, body systems, and requirements, considerably more flexibility exists with regard to the nature and physical structure of the veterinary device. Many such devices need to be biodegradable, for instance. Also, different release rates are indicated for different drugs or different species. Many systems are designed to be pulsatile, allowing for the release of surges of active drugs at predetermined intervals. In ruminants, active drugs may be released directly into the rumen for gastrointestinal or systemic effect. Alternatively, subcutaneous implants may be deposited in nonvascular sites for retarded release into the blood stream.

Current technology takes the form of rumen delivery systems, implant systems, or external application systems. For the ruminant species, the device must be released at a specific location so it can function as a drug reservoir.

In designing a controlled-release system for veterinary use, the nature of the compound to be delivered is of prime consideration, but in addition cognizance must be taken of the best route of delivery, the animal species, optimum release rate, desired duration of response, cost, manufacturability, and the potential hazards of violative

residue formation. Biodegradable polymers are receiving increasing attention for implant systems and for vaccine bullets. To overcome problems of physical and biological residues, many biodegradable polymers have been synthesized. An advantage with some of the more sophisticated devices is that they release active material not across a diffusional concentration gradient but at a constant rate.

The rate of release from polymer matrices is determined by the molecular weight distribution in the polymer, level of payload, nature of the drug-matrix interaction, geometry of the device, and mechanism of its degradation. For oral delivery systems, the range of devices includes soluble glasses, metallic cylinders, polymer matrix cores, and corroding alloys. Most of these deliver active drug content by diffusion.

2.12 ORAL DELIVERY SYSTEMS FOR RUMINANTS

Oral dosing in ruminants is frequently unsuccessful owing to the activities of the rumen flora. Degradation of the active compounds results in low bioavailability. Alternatively, the active ingredient may interfere with the function of the rumen microorganisms.

Considerable latitude exists with respect to the design of oral sustained-delivery systems for administration to ruminant species, in which the unique anatomic features of the alimentary tract facilitate the entrapment of controlled-release devices. The critical concern in the design of any suitable ruminant bolus system is to ensure retention of the drug reservoir within the reticulorumen and to prevent its elimination by regurgitation or intestinal expulsion. Ruminal retention is achieved either on the basis of density or the variable geometric configuration of the device. The minimum size is determined by the dimension of the esophageal and omasal orifices. Although sustained-release rumen devices for mineral or trace element supplementation have been used for years, only relatively recently has pharmaceutical technology developed methods of ensuring reliable delivery of organic drugs, such as anthelmintics, from

TABLE 2–11
SUSTAINED DELIVERY VETERINARY DEVICES

Drug Classification	Formulation or Device	Examples
Antibiotics	Boluses, microencapsulations, liposomes, osmotic pumps, ocular inserts	Penicillins, tetracyclines, cephalosporins, clindamycin, gentamicin.
Anthelmintics	Boluses:	Morantel tartrate, oxfendazole, dichlorvos, metallic cylinders, polymer matrices, corroding alloys, pulsed release, electronic delivery
	Resin pellets	
	Osmotic Pumps	Ivermectin
Hormonal growth promoters	Implants	Estradiol, progesterone, testosterone, zeranol, trenbolone acetate
Nonhormonal growth promoters	Boluses	Monensin
Insecticides	Impregnated collars, ear tags	Organophosphates, pyrethroid
Reproductive hormones	Vaginal sponges, silastic coils, subcutaneous implants estradiol, progesterone, testosterone, norgestomet	Medroxyprogesterone acetate
Sulfonamides	Boluses	Sulfamezathine, sulfadimethoxine
Trace elements	Bullets, corroding alloys, soluble glasses, gelatin-encapsulated needles	Cobalt, copper, selenium, iodine, iron, manganese

such systems. With conventional anthelmintic treatment, repeat dosing is necessary, which offers no preventive or residual effect, and so animals may be reinfested relatively soon after dosing. Controlled release of anthelmintics from sustained delivery rumen systems provides a useful alternative approach whereby continuous anthelmintic output protects animals from overwintered pasture infestation and prevents a subsequent pasture buildup of eggs and infective larvae. For effective prophylactic or therapeutic applications, a reliable, well-designed delivery system must contain a potent agent that is effective at relatively low dosage levels.

2.13 DESIGN PRINCIPLES FOR RUMINANT BOLUSES

Zero buoyancy is the most important factor affecting retention of boluses in the ruminoreticular sac. Weight, size, and, especially, density of the device are critical in this regard. Density of 2.5 g/ml is the critical limit for successful longterm retention to be obtained. Incomplete retention and loss by regurgitation are associated with bolus densities of less than 2.5 g/ml. The density of zero buoyancy principle was originally applied in the development of weighted cobaltic oxide boluses for the prevention and treatment of cobalt deficiency in ruminants.

If a ruminant drug entity formulation is of particularly low density, it may not be practical to include it in a zero buoyancy ruminal bolus. In such cases, variable geometry systems can be employed in which the expanded configuration hinders regurgitation. The device is administered in compact form, and ruminal residency is maintained by expansion of the bolus within the rumen. Hinged systems are used to ensure sievelike retention by exceeding the diameter of the esophageal and omasal orifices.

2.14 ANTHELMINTIC DEVICES

Anthelmintic ruminal devices are exemplified by the morantel tartrate sustained-release bolus. This consists of a large metal cylinder (Paratect Bolus) approximately 10 cm long and 3 cm in diameter that is administered by balling gun into the ruminoreticular sac. The reservoir payload is composed 13.5 g of morantel tartrate in polyethylene glycol. The ends of the cylinder are capped with two microporous sintered polyethylene discs impregnated with hydrogel, which confers a rate control capacity. The bolus is designed to deliver approximately 90 mg/day at constant rates over a 90-day period. The device is administered to young cattle at turnout and provides efficacious gut lumen levels of anthelmintic over the duration of the grazing season. A disadvantage of this nonbiodegradable bolus is that the metallic shell remains in the rumen for the lifetime of the animal.

A development of the morantel bolus led to the introduction in many countries of the paratect "Flex" bolus. This is a nonmetallic wormer bolus for cattle that uncoils in the rumen to ensure ruminal residency. The bolus is a rolled sheet of laminated EVA that unrolls in the rumen, preventing regurgitation. When anthelmintic has all been released, the bolus becomes more pliable and eventually breaks up. No physical residue is left from the biodegradable polymer (EVA).

A new variable geometry device containing albendazole (Captec, Proftril) ("captec") release active ingredient in the rumen

of sheep for 90 to 110 days. The principle of drug release depends on the entry of ruminal liquid into the capsule through the orifice leading to swelling of a sucrose ester. An internal spring pushes the gel thus formed containing albendazole through the capsule orifice and into the rumen interior. The rate of swelling and gel formation depends on the composition of the excipients of the tablets. The rate of penetration of the ruminal fluid and the rate of extrusion of the gel depend on the size of the orifice. Any change in the rate of release may therefore be attended by a change in the formulation, which affects the gel consistency, and by a change in the orifice diameter. (This is available in some countries only; the same design principle is being studied for monensin.)

Oxfendazole is another anthelmintic agent that possesses broad-spectrum activity in cattle and sheep. This is also available in ruminal bolus form. In this case, however, bioengineering advances have resulted in the development of a pulsed-release system. The cylindrical oxfendazole pulsed-release system consists of a steel weight from which extends a magnesium alloy core rod. Six plastic segments are arranged sequentially along this core, five of which hold an annular tablet containing 750 mg oxfendazole. Following deposition in the rumen by a balling gun, corrosion of the central core initiates the release of an encapsulated oxfendazole segment. The first dose is released approximately 3 weeks after administration, and the four remaining doses are released at regular predetermined intervals in accordance with the core corrosion rate. The anthelmintic life span of the system is up to 130 days. Pulsed release of five discrete doses of active ingredients removes the necessity for alternative repeat dosing programs (Table 2–12).

A novel development from this type of corrosion-based, pulsed-release system is the electronic bolus ("E. Bolus," Smithkline Beecham). Powered by two manganese batteries, the bolus is administered at turnout. Shortly after ruminal deposition, biosensors located on the bolus switch the device on, and a microprocessor chip commences countdown to drug release. At zero time, an electronic impulse is emitted to a CO_2-generating pressure expulsion mechanism,

TABLE 2–12
SUSTAINED-RELEASE INTERNAL PARASITICIDES

Product Name	Active Ingredient	Manufacturer	Duration
Paratect	Morantel tartrate, 22.7 g	Pfizer	90 days (continuous)
Autoworm/Redidose	Oxfendazole, 750 mg	Coopers (Pitman Moore)	130 days (pulsed every 21 days)
Synanthic Multidose 130	Oxfendazole, 750 mg	Syntex	130 days (pulsed every 21 days)
Ivomec SR.	Ivermectin	Merck Sharp & Dohme	135 days (osmotic pump)

which expels the anthelmintic into the rumen. After this expulsion, the chip automatically resets, and a 31-day countdown recommences. The system is potentially applicable to pulsed release of other drugs, such as growth promoters and mineral supplements. The drug release intervals can also be modified. The heavy bolus is constructed of polypropylene, which encases the active constituents and release mechanisms in a safe waterproof environment. With the marked increase in miniaturization of microprocessors, developments of bolus, implants, and pulsatile systems will undoubtedly involve more of this electronic-type technique.

Osmotic pumps administered by the oral route using a balling gun have been investigated with respect to longterm delivery of potent anthelmintic agents, such as ivermectin. Such devices, weighted to a specific gravity of 2.9 to ensure retention in the ruminoreticulum, have been loaded to release 2 mg ivermectin per day over a 30-day period in calves. Results from this approach have been encouraging to date. A 135 day slow release osmotic pump bolus of ivermectin is now commercially available. A disadvantage of most osmotic pump–type devices is that the container remains in the body and is not retrievable after oral administration. Complete elimination of drug from the osmotic reservoir, however, is usually attained.

Mini-osmotic pumps have been employed to investigate the pharmacokinetics of many drugs in both experimental animals and target animal species. Less sophisticated sustained-release formulations of parasiticides use impregnated resin pellets as the controlling device. Dichlorvos, a volatile organophosphate, in the form of resin pellets provides a stable, slow release of anthelmintic activity after oral administration. As the organophosphate pellets traverse the gut, the active principle dichlorvos is gradually released from the plasticized pellets. The release rate is designed to provide maximum anthelmintic activity, while assuring toxicologic safety by protecting the host animal from sudden, excessively high exposure levels.

2.15 GROWTH-PROMOTING BOLUSES

Monensin, a rumen active growth promoter, was one of the first nonhormonal feed additives used in cattle. As a feed additive substance, monensin is not easily supplied to grazing beef cattle. A ruminal delivery device (Rumensin RDD, Elanco) containing 16.5 g of monensin sodium, designed to deliver the active ingredient over a period of 150 days, is now available for beef cattle. The bolus comprises a cylindrical core containing a controlled-release formulation of monensin admixed with copolymer matrix. A polyethylene shell with rounded perforated ends envelopes the core. After ruminal deposition by a balling gun, the aqueous fluids dissolve the copolymer at the two exposed faces of the cylindrical core, and monensin is released at a uniform rate. The plastic-covered metal cylindrical bolus is of sufficient density to prevent regurgitation. The growth-promoting device remains effective for 5 months after administration.

2.16 TRACE ELEMENT SUPPLEMENTATION

Trace element deficiencies in ruminants require longterm supplementation to deliver both therapeutic and prophylactic levels of the required element. Many of the currently available trace element formulations do not provide sustained protection against mineral deficiencies. Some years ago, magnesium alloy bullets and boluses containing cobalt were introduced, which by virtue of their high density (>3 g/cm³) could become entrapped in the reticulorumen sac of cattle and sheep. After gradual dissolution in the rumen, these bullets provided adequate protection against cobalt and selenium deficiency in sheep for many months. The bullet was found to be effective as thrice-weekly drenching with 1 mg cobalt per day. Release from this high-density, slow-release bullet by abrasion and dissolution could, however, be quite variable. Similar boluses containing selenium have also been prepared, with beneficial results.

Large magnesium boluses with densities more than 4.5 g/cm³ have been evaluated as prophylactic measures against hypomagnesemia. Because of the higher daily requirements of magnesium (>3 g/day), such boluses have not been uniformly successful; the amount of magnesium released is inadequate to prevent grass tetany in cattle.

With many of the trace element boluses, the rate of release of the active agent declines substantially within a few weeks of administration. The dissolution rate from such boluses can also be adversely affected by formation of various salts on the bolus surface (e.g., calcium salts, iron salts). Problems of retention have been associated with many high-density, slow-release metallic bolus systems. In addition to variable release patterns, the formation of biologically inactive substances in the rumen has occurred (e.g., copper sulfide).

When copper deficiency has been recognized, attempts to remedy it by provision of extra oral copper have generally been found unsatisfactory because of the unpredictable intake, rapid excretion, and variable effect. With an element such as copper, which is a cumulative poison, the risk of chronic copper poisoning from a parenteral or oral copper treatment is positively correlated with its effectiveness in combating deficiency. Existing methods of treatment for copper deficiency have limitations. Mineral licks and supplements are unpredictable because of the individual refusal of some animals and overindulgence of others. Copper sulfate drenches are not only astringent, but also more than 90% of the copper is rapidly excreted onto the pasture. Boluses of copper that lodge in the rumen or reticulum can form unusable complexes with molybdenum sulfur and iron. Compounding copper salts with concentrate rations is effective as long as animals receive such rations regularly as part of their winter diet. Some injectable forms of copper are so acutely toxic that doses must be limited: Others are less toxic but only because the dose is partly encapsulated at the injection and thus prevented from achieving its objective. In both instances, repeated injections are needed to control deficiencies.

Gelatin capsules containing copper oxide needles have been administered to sheep and cattle and provide more longterm protection against copper deficiency than many of the conventional patented preparations. The sustained activity after oral dosing with copper oxide needles as a means of alleviating hypocupremia in ruminants has been widely reported. These gelatin capsules contain thousands of minute, blunt copper oxide rods. When given orally, the gelatin capsule dissolves in the rumen, releasing the copper oxide rods, which then lodge in the abomasum. There they release copper for the animal's immediate requirements and reserves. These rods dissolve completely over a period of time.

Copper oxide needles are brittle rods (5 to 10 mm long) made by oxidizing fine copper wire. They are nontoxic when given orally, and they can be given in doses sufficient to establish long-lasting reserves of copper in the liver. Their properties were discovered by Australian scientists, who found that a combination of small particle size and high specific gravity caused them to become trapped in the folds of the abomasum. Subsequent experiments showed that they are retained there for 30 to 60 days in sheep and cattle and slowly release copper in absorbable forms. The accumulated hepatic stores of the absorbed copper can protect the animal against copper deficiency for periods of months, usually a season's protection. The copper capsules for sustained-release delivery are administered by means of conventional balling guns.

2.17 CONTROLLED-RELEASE GLASSES

Many conventional release systems rely on diffusional processes through materials that are not inherently biodegradable. Also, they do not display zero order kinetic release patterns. For trace element supplementation, modern controlled-release glasses dissolve with a zero order release rate and leave no residues. Controlled-release glasses are phosphate glasses within which monovalent or divalent cations can be distributed. The cation loading may constitute up to 65 mole % of the glass. The glass consists of a polyanionic framework of phosphate that accommodates cations of any electropositive element within its interstices. It dissolves completely in aqueous solutions, and the rate of solution can be modified by varying the preparations of monovalent and divalent cations associated with the phosphate base. During the dissolution process, breakdown of phosphate cross linkages occurs, releasing the polyphosphate anions and their admixed cations into solution. Dissolution rate is also affected by the pH of the aqueous surrounding fluid and the surface area of the glass. Thus phosphate-based glasses can be fabricated with tailor-made solubility rates to ensure a metered release of specific trace elements to suit individual animal requirements. Cations can therefore be released at near constant predetermined rates for long periods.

The solubility of controlled-release glass depends on the relative concentrations of the major constituents, calcium, sodium, and phosphate ions. The glasses vary from being deliquescent to totally insoluble. The proportions of trace elements included also affect the solubility of the glass. Glass solubility is determined by the glass composition: An increase in the ratio of monovalent to divalent cations tends to increase solubility. As the controlled-release glass dissolves, the component elements are released into the surrounding media in proportion to their concentration in the original glass.

Trace elements can be incorporated into controlled-release glasses, which then provide almost steady-state delivery rates for periods of up to a year for protection against trace element deficiencies. To date, glass boluses containing copper, cobalt, and selenium with density greater than 2.5 g/cm^3 have been available for use in cattle and sheep. Although glass normally contains 60 to 70% silica, the trace element glass boluses consist of constituents that occur naturally in the ruminant diet—sodium, phosphorus, calcium, and manganese oxides as well as copper, selenium, and cobalt. Hence they leave no residue.

2.18 PULSED-RELEASE SYSTEMS

Controlled-release glasses as delivery systems are not restricted to trace element delivery; they have many other novel, potentially useful applications in veterinary medicine. Organic macromolecules with various therapeutic properties, such as anthelmintics or growth-promoting agents, can be enclosed within a sintered block of phosphate glass, giving a constant rate release profile as the controlled-release glass dissolves in the ruminal fluids. The physical properties of these glasses also facilitates the development of useful pulsed-release systems. Variations in the dissolution rates of synthetic phosphate glasses can be used to govern the release of active constituents within an assembly of glass tubules. The interval between release pulses can be controlled to modify the geometric configuration of the tubular assembly and the solution rate of the various glass tubules. Alternatively, a sequential arrangement of cells of active ingredients immersed in relatively insoluble glass may be separated by cores of controlled-release glass of high solubility. Pulse intervals are a function of the

---

TABLE 2–13
PRINCIPLES OF PULSED-RELEASE SYSTEM

Weighted High-Density Bolus
↓
Sequential Series of Cells Containing Active Drugs
↓
Cells Separated by Degradable Spacer Cores
↓
Surface Erosion of Spacer Cores
↓
Release of Drug Cell Compartment
↓
Pulse Intervals: Size/Dissolution Rate of Spacer Cores

---

size of the spacer cores and its dissolution rate (Table 2–13).

Such pulsed-release systems show great promise for the programmed delivery of chemotherapeutic agents and immunomodulators. Using a surface erosion controlled system, pulsed release can be achieved by alternating the layers or spacers.

2.19 ANTIMICROBIAL BOLUSES

Many sulfonamide slow-release boluses are available for use in ruminants (Table 2–14). The preparations that provide extended blood level–time profiles are frequently employed for treatment of shipping fever, pneumonias, metritis, foot rot, enteritis, and septicemia. The magnitude and duration of plasma sulfonamide concentrations are critical for therapeutic effectiveness. Because the plasma half-life of many sulfonamides is short, conventional sulfonamide preparations must be administered daily to be therapeutically effective. Sustained-release sulfonamides have several advantages over repeated administration of nonsustained-release preparations; including less peak and valley fluctuation in the plasma, less risk of overdosing, and less handling of the animals.

In 1967, a sulfamethazine bolus was introduced for cattle. The bolus was later modified into a bilayered preparation (Spanbolet II, Norden), which allowed both immediate and prolonged release of the sulfonamide. At a dose of 180 mg sulfameth-azine/lb body weight, the bolus produced continuous plasma concentrations of 5 mg/dl for up to 5 days. Because of its size, however, the bolus was unsuitable for use in smaller calves. Consequently, a smaller bilayered bolette (CalfSpan, Norden) was developed for use in calves.

Some of these formulations contain a rapid-release component for quickly establishing high blood concentrations and a slow-release component for prolonged maintenance of blood concentrations in excess of the minimum therapeutic levels (5 mg/100 ml). Frequently a long-acting sulfonamide, such as sulfadimethoxine, is incorporated into a bolus with a slow dissolution rate, ensuring high plasma levels for 76 hours. Alternatively, a sulfonamide in a fast and a slow granulation is twinned within a bolus admixed with carriers such as bismuth subcarbonate or subnitrate and cellulose. Such a preparation provides both high and prolonged blood levels.

Other sulfa boluses are formulated with sulfamezathine, which gradually releases the active drug on digestion within the ruminant gut. Bilayered bolettes of sulfamezathine consist of two layers of drug programmed for different release rates. One layer contains sulfamezathine compounded for rapid disintegration; the other layer contains a higher inclusion rate for more gradual release. Such boluses can provide sulfamezathine exceeding minimum therapeutic levels within 4 hours and up to 72 hours after administration. Such sustained-release forms eliminate the inconvenience

TABLE 2-14
SULFONAMIDE PROLONGED-RELEASE BOLUSES

Product Name	Active Ingredient	Manufacturer	Dose	Duration of Action
CalfSpan	Sulfamethazine, 8 g	Norden/SKB	1 bolus/45 lb	Bilayered bolus combining rapid and sustained release 4 days activity
Spanbolet II Tablets	Sulfamethazine, 27 g	Norden/SKB	1 bolus/150 lb	Bilayered bolus combining rapid and sustained release 5 days activity
Sustain III	Sulfamethazine, 32.1 g	Osborn	1 bolus/200 lb	3 days activity
Albon—S-R	Sulfadimethoxine, 12.5 g	Roche	1 bolus/200 lb	4 days activity (rumen dissolution)
Hava-Span	Sulfamethazine, 22.5 g	Haver	1 bolus/100 lb	5 days activity (bolus digested)
Sustain III Calf Bolus	Sulfamethazine, 8.02 g	Osborn	2 boluses/100 lb	3 days activity

and inconsistencies of more frequent administration of conventional sulfonamide preparations. Because of the prolonged action of the drugs, special care must be exercised to observe the recommended withdrawal times to avoid violative residue deposition in food animals.

Slow-release tetracycline boluses have been developed for treatment of sheep infected with *Corynebacterium pyogenes* and *Streptococcus pyogenes*.

IMPLANTS

As a reliable method of sustained drug delivery, the implant is restricted to active molecules of relatively high potency, and the devices of most current interest incorporate hormonal substances for growth promotion. Oral doses of estrogens necessitate rather large amounts (milligrams) per day to promote anabolism effectively. Higher bioavailability is attained by subcutaneous deposition, and efficacious delivery of only micrograms per day from this rate is necessary for growth promotion.

Implant pellets can therefore be small to accommodate an hormonal payload for a 90-day period. Implant designs commonly involve dispersal of the drug into a polymer matrix with or without coating or laminates to affect rate control delivery.

A typical implant consists of a sterile tablet manufactured by processes of compression or thermal molding. In its simplest form, the powdered active constituent without excipient is compressed under aseptic conditions. It may also be mixed with an inert carrier, such as lactose, and then pelleted as a subcutaneous implant. Adjuvants or other excipients may be included to modify the absorption rate. Following deposition of such implants on the dorsal surface of the ear, release of the active agent is by diffusion. Ideally the release rate would be zero order (constant rate). For many reasons, this state is not usually attained. Frequently the implant becomes encapsulated in connective tissue, and the consequent back diffusion pressure of drugs in the tissues adjacent to the implant creates an intermittent and episodic rate of release. In addition, as the implant tends to be absorbed, a contracting surface area is presented for absorption. Because release is by diffusion alone and the rate is not controlled by other processes within the device, the overall rate of release declines with time. The most rapid release of hormone is therefore initially with an ever-decreasing rate as the pellet erodes, dissolves, or becomes encapsulated within the body. Safety margin is therefore an important factor to take into account to permit the initial peak release of active ingredients from the pellet. Assuming a first-order rate of dissolution of the compressed tablet, relatively high levels of hormone must be released early on from the pellet payload to ensure adequate levels at the end of the release period.

A number of formulations are available in which estradiol-17β is combined with testosterone or progesterone. The improved efficacy of such products is due to the relatively slower release of estradiol from the implant in the presence of the second steroid. This is possibly a physical effect attributable to the intimate mixing of the estradiol with larger concentrations of the other steroids. It has also been established that the half-lives of many steroids can be extended by the presence of other steroids that are competitive at the hepatic microsomal site of enzymatic biotransformation.

Attempts to achieve new zero order release rates from pelleted implants have resulted in the development of impregnated Silastic polymers. Lilly research has developed a cylinder of silicone rubber in implant form that incorporates micronized crystals of estradiol-17β. In this system, the drug is enclosed or distributed throughout a polymer in which the active component is soluble and permeable. Silicone rubber has been extensively studied as a matrix base and its useful properties of permeability and tissue compatibility render it an excellent drug delivery system. The cylindrical implant is composed of an inert silicone rubber core surrounded by an outer silicone rubber matrix impregnated with 45 mg (or 24 mg) of micronized crystals of estradiol-17β. The rate of drug transport through or across the medicated silicone layer is contingent on the concentration in the polymer matrix, the lipophilicity of the drug, the permeability and porosity of the polymer, the surface area, and the thickness of the encapsulating polymer. The implant can deliver up to 60 μg of estradiol per day to steers for approximately 400 days. The amount of drug delivered depends on the surface area, and both the length and the diameter of the device can be varied to suit requirements, depending on the dosage required and the desired payout period. Such polymer systems are not usually biodegradable, and the silicone rubber implant retains its structural integrity indefinitely. The duration of release is controlled by the thickness of the medicated encapsulating layer, and implant length governs the payload capacity. The objective of zero order release is not completely achieved by this improved delivery system because of an initial surge of active material released from the superficial tissue boundary interface of the polymer. After this initial burst, extended release depends on diffusion from within the impregnated matrix to achieve a controlled, extended period of payout of efficacious levels of hormones. Finaplix (trenbolone acetate) and Ralgro (zeronal) are also widely used and FDA approved asynthetic hormonal ear implants for growth problems.

Implant systems for veterinary use are not restricted to hormonal growth promoters. Norgestomet, a suspension of steroid particles in a hydrogel/water polymer, has been employed in implant form for the synchronization of estrus. This implant is withdrawn from the ear after a 9-day period. Table 2–15 lists some commonly used hormonal implant systems.

Sustained-release reproductive hormones deposited intravaginally have been widely used as labor-saving devices for breeding control programs in cattle and sheep. Sponges or Silastic coil polymers impregnated with progesterone deliver a metered payout of steroidal hormones, facilitating the synchronization of estrus and the optimization of reproductive performance. Polymers of various structural design and dimension have been administered intravaginally as sponges or coils for delivery of many synthetic gestagenic agents. As a nondegradable reservoir in an accessible body cavity, they can be removed when the drug is no longer required.

2.20 EXTERNAL APPLICATION SYSTEMS

Slow-release pesticides for external application can take many forms, including tags, strips, and collars (Table 2–16). In farm animal species, polyvinyl chloride (PVC) tags are impregnated, usually with potent pyrethroids, such as cypermethrin, permethrin, or fenvalerate. Outward diffusion of the impregnated insecticide provides longterm protection against many economically important ectoparasites, a significant improvement over the more conventional dipping or spraying techniques. Resin collars for flea and tick control in dogs and cats contain various volatile organophosphate agents (e.g., dichlorvos), which by vaporous activity are lethal to the ectoparasite but relatively harmless to the host animal. Extended protection periods are commonly claimed by manufacturers for these preparations. Other collar insecticides act by way of a direct contact mechanism wherein insecticidal effect is generated by surface diffusion from the resin and movement through the coat of the animal, especially in the neck area.

2.21 MISCELLANEOUS DEVELOPMENTS

Biodegradable polymers, glasses, liposomes, and microcapsules have many uses and advantages, including development of pulsatile release, intracellular delivery, and potential for minimal residue formation. Such systems are being increasingly investigated and tested for the delivery of growth hormone, immunomodulators, vaccines, antibodies, anthelmintics, and antibiotics as well as regarding sustained ocular and sustained intramammary drug targeting. Encapsulation technology is growing prodigiously, and advances in membrane research are now on the verge of changing the face of the pharmaceutical industry. Veterinary liposome-encapsulated drugs under development include products for brucellosis, mastitis, and infectious keratoconjunctivitis. Topical liposomal ocular devices can provide continued deposition of entrapped drug at high concentrations in

TABLE 2–15
SUSTAINED-RELEASE HORMONAL FORMULATIONS

Product Name	Active Ingredients	Administration	Indication
Steer-oid	Progesterone USP, 200 mg Estradiol benzoate USP, 20 mg	Subcutaneous ear implant	Growth promotion in steers
Synovex C	Progesterone USP, 100 mg Estradiol benzoate, 10 mg	Subcutaneous ear implant	Growth promotion in calves
Synovex H	Testosterone propionate, 200 mg Estradiol, benzoate, 20 mg	Subcutaneous ear implant	Growth promotion in heifers
Synovex S	Progesterone, 200 mg Estradiol, 20 mg	Subcutaneous ear implant	Growth promotion in steers
Ralgro	Zeranol, 36 mg	Subcutaneous ear implant	Growth promotion in beef cattle
Finaplix	Trenbolone acetate, 300 mg	Subcutaneous ear implant	Growth promotion in heifers/steers
Syncro-Mate B	Norgestomet, 3 mg	Hydrophilic polymer ear implant (Removable at 9 days)	Synchronization of breeding in cycling heifers
Compudose 200	Estradiol, 24 mg	Silicone rubber ear implant	Growth promotion in steers
Compudose 365	Estradiol, 45 mg	Silicone rubber ear implant	Growth promotion in steers

TABLE 2-16
EXAMPLES OF SUSTAINED-RELEASE EXTERNAL PARASITICIDES

Product Name	Active Ingredient	Manufacturer	Duration of Activity
	Large Animals		
Expar Insecticide Ear Tag	Permethrin 10%, w/v	Coopers/Pitman Moore	5 months
Ear Force Tags	Permethrin 10%, w/v	Bioceutic	Season protection
Tirade Fly Tags	Fenvalerate 8.5%, w/w	Hoechst	Season protection
Stockguard Insecticidal Ear Tag	Flucythrinate 7.5%, w/w	M.S.D.	5 months
	Small Animals		
Dermaton Dog Collar	2-Chlor-1-(2-4-dichlorphenyl) vinyl diethyl phosphate, 15%	Coopers	$4-6\frac{1}{2}$ months
Sprecto Cat Insecticide Collar	0, Isopropoxyphenyl methyl carbonate, 9.4%	Pitman Moore	5 months
Marmaduke Flea and Tick Collar for Dogs and Cats	Propoxur, 9.4%	Norden/SKB	5 months
Flea Collar for Cats	2,2-Dichlorovinyl dimethyl phosphate, 4.8%	Solvay	3 months
Flea Collar for Dogs	2,2-Dichlorovinyl dimethyl phosphate, 9.6%	Solvay	3 months

the eye for long periods. Other ocular polymeric matrices acting as rate-controlled systems have the advantage over eye drops insofar as prolongation of drug contact time with the eye is assured. Ocular inserts, aqua polymers, colloidal dispersal systems, and medicated contact lenses have been investigated in many species and are particularly useful in that they can be easily removed from their site of application. Microencapsulation of veterinary drugs is promising for increasing the efficacy of intramammary infusion of antibiotics.

In dry cow therapy, the retention time of more rapidly absorbed antibiotics is sometimes increased by using insoluble salts, e.g., benzathine or procaine salts, or by formulating them in slow-release bases, such as peanut or mineral oil gelled with aluminum monostearate. Chloramphenicol, cephacetrile, and clindamycin have been shown to be rapidly absorbed from the bovine udder.

Studies have demonstrated that when these antibiotics were infused at drying off, suspended in conventional intramammary formulations, antibiotic activity in the udder did not persist beyond 3 to 5 days. Encapsulated preparations of these antibiotics, however, maintained total drug concentrations within the udder equal to or higher than the respective minimal inhibitory concentration for udder pathogens for at least 21 days.

Microencapsulated intramammary antibiotic formulations can be prepared by entrapping the drug as a dispersion in a spherical matrix or by encapsulating spherical particles as a central depot surrounded by a polymeric membrane barrier. Microencapsulation techniques also possess appreciable potential for oral delivery of labile substances, antibiotics, enzymes, and growth promoters. The use of encapsulation techniques is well suited to the field of peptide delivery, and microencapsulated boluses of growth hormones have given encouraging results in many reports.

Topical delivery through the skin provides another role for polymeric systems, in which a drug reservoir laminate, a rate control membrane, and an adhesive interface for skin attachment modulate a transcutaneous absorption pattern at a controlled speed. Innumerable classes of drugs are applicable to such a technique. Slow-release topical skin preparations (especially for cardiovascular conditions) are common in human medicine.

Pulsed-release systems will undoubtedly be of considerable benefit regarding immunologic compounds, especially when booster doses are required. Perhaps bovine somatotropin possesses the greatest future potential of all the hormones, and the arrival of a protected delivery system for this compound will have unparalleled impact on animal production systems.

2.23 FUTURE DEVELOPMENTS

This is an active research area, and there will certainly be further developments. Oral formulations are likely to retain their position as the more widely used.

New peptides and their analogs are likely to provide much material for research and development. Nonoral routes will receive increasing attention, and novel injectable products, including biodegradable implants, will be used for prolonged actions. Also important is the possibility of specific targeting of drugs perhaps to cancer-bearing tissue or to the sites of other pathologic processes.

Systems for transdermal delivery and by way of other topical sites, which are important in human medicine, will probably see some development for animal use, albeit on a limited scale.

Many patented drug delivery systems are now used to put new life into old or well-established drugs. Rather than reinventing the wheel, the wheel is simply being rethreaded. Microdroplet technology allows oil-soluble drug compounds to be made into ingestables.

Among the types of product under investigation are long-acting local anesthetics that can be administered along the incision of suture line to provide anesthesia for 6 or 7 days. Slow-release oxytetracycline formulations have also been prepared to deliver 3 days of sustained-release oxytetracycline from a single dose without significant irritation or pain at the injection site.

The need to deliver animal drugs in the most economic and productive manner is leading to a new phase of drug delivery systems. The new technology sectors in which most current investment is being made fall into a number of categories:

1. Growth enhancers
2. Management aid products
3. Delivery system technology
4. Electronic technology
5. Immunologic developments

Optimization of rate of growth and efficacy of feed conversion continue to be primary objectives. Growth promoters, hormones, and immunologic agents are the critical areas in which agriculture is likely to see the greatest impact of biotechnology in the near future. The number and diversity of compounds that can now be linked to controlled-release technology systems are almost limitless, and such delivery systems may become the preferred means of dosing in the future.

Inherent in the development of any modern technologic system capable of ensuring extended drug release, however, is the necessity to address the issues of efficacy and safety. Safety issues apply not only to the recipient target animal, but also to the consumer of food animal products. For this reason, tissue depletion studies are important to minimize the occurrence of violative drug residue formation.

SELECTED REFERENCES

Anderson, N., Laby, R.H., Prichard, R.K., and Hennessy, D.: Controlled release of anthelmintic drugs: A new concept for prevention of helminthosis in sheep. Res. Vet. Sci., 29:333, 1980.

Bakan, J.A., and Powell, T.C.: Stability of controlled release pharmaceutical microcapsules. In Controlled Release Delivery Systems. Edited by T.J. Roseman and S.Z. Mansdorf. New York, Marcel Dekker, 1983.

Bowen, J.M.: Recent advances in methods of drug administration for animals. J. Am. Vet. Med. Assoc., 185:1102, 1984.

Breimer, D.D.: Potential of new drug delivery systems in veterinary medicines. Proceedings of Third Congress of European Association of Veterinary Pharmacologists and Toxicologists, Ghent, 1985.

Breimer, D.D., De Leede, L.G.J., and De Boer, A.G.: New drug delivery systems as tools in clinical pharmacology. In Proceedings of the Second World Conference on Clinical Pharmacology and Therapeutics. Edited by L. Lemberger and M.M. Reidenberg. Washington, D.C., American Society for Pharmacology & Experimental Therapeutics, 1984.

Byford, R.L., River, J.L., and Hair, J.A.: A sustained release oxytetracycline bolus for ruminants. Bovine Pract., 15:91, 1981.

Cadarelli, N.F.: Compound methods for controlled release elastomers. In Proceedings of Controlled Release Pesticide Symposium. Akron, University of Ohio, 1976.

Cardinal, J.: Controlled drug delivery: Veterinary applications. J. Contr. Rel., 2:393, 1985.

Donald, A.D.: New methods of drug application for control of helminths. Vet. Parasitol., 18:121, 1985.

Drug Delivery Systems. Pharm. Tech. Springfield, Aster Publications Corp., 1983.

Esker, M., and Boersma, J.H.: Delay in timing of the oxfendazole pulse release bolus in calves in the Netherlands Vet. Quarterly. 11:210, 1989.

Flynn, G.L.: Considerations in controlled release drug delivery systems. Pharm. Tech., 6:33, 1982.

Flynn, G.L.: Influence of physiochemical properties of drug and system on release of drugs from inert matrices. In Controlled Release of Biologically Active Agents. Edited by C.A. Tanquay and R. Lacey. New York, Plenum Press, 1974.

Goldman, P.: Rate controlled drug delivery. N. Engl. J. Med., 307:286, 1982.

Herman, E.H., Rahman, A., Ferrans, V.J., et al.: Prevention of chronic doxorubicin cardiotoxicity in Beagles by liposomal encapsulation. Cancer Res., 43:5427, 1983.

Hopfenberg, H.B.: Controlled release for erodible slabs, cylinders and spheres. In Controlled Release Polymeric Formulations. ACS Symposium Series 33. Edited by D.R. Paul and F.W. Harris. Washington, D.C., American Chemical Society, 1976.

Hutchinson, F.G., and Furr, B.J.A.: Biodegradable polymers for the sustained release of peptides.

Jacobs, D.E., Gowling, G., Foster, J., et al.: Chemoprophylaxis of bovine parasite bronchitis using an oxfendazole pulse release intraruminal device: A preliminary study. J. Vet. Pharmacol. Ther., 9:337, 1986.

Jubaro, R.L.: Drug delivery systems: A brief review. Can. J. Physiol. Pharmacol., 56:683, 1978.

Kydonieus, A.F.: Controlled Release Technologies: Methods, Theory and Applications. Vol. I, Boca Raton, FL, CRC Press, 1980.

Laby, R.H.: Australian Patent Application, No. 35908/78, 1978.

Linder, C., and Ziv, G.: Encapsulated forms of slow release dry cow products of rapidly absorbed antibiotics. J. Vet. Pharmacol. Ther., 6:33, 1983.

Manston, R., Sansom, B.F., Allen, W.M., et al.: Reaction cements as material for the sustained release of trace elements into the digestive tracts of cattle and sheep. I. Copper release. J. Vet. Pharmacol. Ther., 8:368, 1985.

Miller, G.E., et al.: Blood concentration of a sustained release form of sulfamethazine in cattle. J. Am. Vet. Med. Assoc., *154*:773, 1969.

Morgan, D.W.T., and Rowlands, D.T.: A pulsed release device for the administration of oxfendazole to cattle. Proceedings of 14th Congress on Diseases of Cattle, Dublin, 1986.

Murphy, J., Wong, M., and Ray, W.H.: The advantages of a timed release sulfamethazine bolette for calves. Vet. Med. Sept. 1986, pp. 882, 1986.

Pope, D.G.: Specialized dose dispensing equivalent. *In* Formulation of Veterinary Dosage Forms. Edited by J. Blodinger. New York, Marcel Dekker, 1983.

Pope, D.G.: Animal health specialized delivery systems. *In* Animal Health Products. Edited by D.C. Monkhouse. Washington, D.C., American Pharmaceutical Association, 1978.

Schwartz, J.B., and Ando, H.Y.: New drug delivery system: Controlled release. Am. Druggist, *188*:43, 1983.

Urquhart, J.: Controlled Release Pharmaceuticals. Washington, D.C., Ed. Amer. Pharm. Assoc., 1980.

CHAPTER

3

BIOTECHNOLOGY DRUGS AND VACCINES

3.1 Genetic Engineering
3.2 Recombinant Technology
3.3 Hybridoma Technology
3.4 Production of Pharmaceutical Agents by Biotechnology
3.5 General Applications
3.6 Modern Pig Vaccines
3.7 Future Trends in Biotechnology

3.1 GENETIC ENGINEERING

Genetic engineering technology is the major scientific revolution of the 20th century. Rapid developments are occurring, especially in veterinary medicine. Genetically engineered vaccines and monoclonal antibodies are already on the market for veterinary use. Many other animal health care products are being tested.

Biotechnology is an interdisciplinary field of activity. Chemists and biochemists, biologists and microbiologists, and genetic engineers and process engineers cooperate closely in research. Defined briefly, biotechnology in its original concept uses the biochemical metabolism of living cells—microorganisms, plant cells, and animal cells—for yielding or transforming substances that can be produced on an industrial scale. Although a new scientific field, biotechnology has its roots in the dawn of history. Two of the best-known products of biotechnology are wine and beer. In the fermentation process, microorganisms convert grape and malt sugars into alcohol. This classic fermentation process is imitated in present-day industrial-scale fermentation. Other products that are manufactured by fermentation include valuable antibiotics such as penicillins, synthetic vitamins C and B_{12}, yeasts, and citric acid.

Through the use of genetic engineering techniques, the desired characters can be introduced into a microbe by appropriately changing its genetic information, or genotype. In agriculture, genetic engineering is focusing on manipulation of organisms to produce animal vaccines, hormones, amino acids, chemicals, enzyme assays, and drugs. These technologies will have the greatest impact on improved livestock production by:

1. Reducing animal losses through prevention of infectious diseases, using effective genetically engineered vaccines and antitoxins
2. Increasing production of meat and milk through use of growth promotants
3. Improving the nutritional values of animal feed

TECHNOLOGY

Two major developments in genetic engineering, recombinant DNA and monoclonal antibody technology, have been used to address problems in animal health care and production. The DNA molecule is an extremely long chain (polymer) made up of four chemical subunits, called "nucleotides," joined end to end. In addition, the long DNA molecule consists of two polynucleotide chains intertwined as a double helix. Biotechnology involves manipulation of genes and cells, using five basic techniques or innovations learned in the past few years.

1. **Isolating genes**. Knowing the genetic code and the common structural features of DNA has made possible the delineation of general principles to identify and purify DNA fragments containing genes of interest.
2. **Recombinant DNA**. Molecular biologists can take a gene from one DNA molecule and chemically splice it to another. This feat is often called recombinant DNA technology because new combinations of genes are made. Genetic engineers can isolate a gene from one organism and put it into the DNA of another, e.g., combine the DNA of a simple bacterium with the gene encoding a surface antigen of a virus. This simple bacterium then can become a factory, churning out the specific viral surface antigen encoded by the spliced-in gene. This new source for a viral antigen (in the absence of the original virus) makes possible vaccines that are novel, safe, and inexpensive.
3. **Gene transfer**
4. **Cell culture**
5. **Cell fusion**. Certain classes of white blood cells produce antibodies. Such antibody-producing cells usually die quickly in the test tube. Certain cancer (myeloma) cells are immortal and divide continuously in the test tube as long as they are fed regularly. So by fusing a single antibody-producing cell with a single cancer cell, immortal hybrids can be made. Such cells are called "hybridomas," and because they were derived from one antibody-producing cell, they produce a monoclonal antibody.

Recombinant DNA technology, the essence of genetic engineering, is not a single discipline; it represents a fusion of ideas and techniques from biochemistry, molecular biology, genetics, organic chemistry, immunology, and medicines. This scientific breakthrough involves restructuring and editing genetic information and constructing microorganisms with new genetic information. The technology allows us to isolation of genes from any source (viruses, bacteria, fungi, plants, or animals) and amplifying of these genes to unlimited quantities.

3.2 RECOMBINANT TECHNOLOGY

"Recombinant technology" is the joining of DNA sequences from different sources, usually genes from two different organisms (recombinant DNA). Ideally desired genetic traits from one organism—a bacterium, for example—can be transferred to another, thereby endowing a cell with new characteristics that enable it to produce a sought-after compound, including vital proteins and enzymes. To alter a cell, biologists first use enzymes to "cut away" critical fragments of DNA isolated from any one type of cell. The DNA fragments are then attached to a plasmid, a small circular DNA molecule that carries the new genetic material into another, or target, cell.

Once new DNA is inserted into a suitable host—often a harmless bacterial cell—that cell produces millions of copies of itself, and with them comes the ability to make the desired protein or enzyme by following the cell's new genetic instructions. Scientists are now using recombinant DNA technology to produce human insulin, growth hormone, interferon, and hepatitis B vaccine. New medical, chemical, and agricultural products are also forthcoming.

With the aid of genetic engineering, it is possible to carry out selective modification of the genes of simple organisms or in isolated body cells and to "reconstruct" them at will. The information stored in the DNA determines the way in which proteins are built from their components, the amino acids. This structure in turn determines the function of the protein within the organism.

The genetic alphabet consists of only four letters, the DNA building blocks. Three of these building blocks make up a triplet or codon—a "word." To put it another way, three nucleotides constitute a unit of information that is "translated" into an amino

acid. Several hundred "words" are necessary to make a "sentence," i.e., a protein molecule. This genetic code is universal.

The stored information has to be "translated" into a genetic product, a process known as expression. Generally genetic information is transmitted to the progeny of a cell—"inherited"—during cell division by doubling the DNA strands. This process is known as identical reduplication. The double DNA strand is opened like a zipper, and each strand acquires a complementary second strand—a "negative" copy of the first. Each individual strand is capable of creating its "other half" from the plentiful supply of nucleotides in the cell. The result is that once cell division is complete, there are two completely identical double strands. This means that every new cell contains all the genetic information required. DNA is the only substance known to be capable of producing identical copies of itself.

Another type of nucleic acid called "ribonucleic acid" (RNA) is responsible for transferring the message. RNA is closely related to DNA and is in fact copied from it using the two RNA strands as templates. It functions as a mold for the protein molecule that is to be constructed and transmits the chemical message contained in the DNA to the ribosomes, where the protein is synthesized. This task gives it the name "messenger RNA" (mRNA). Molecular biologists use the term "translation" to describe the step by which the arrangement of mRNA building blocks is transferred to the corresponding arrangement of amino acids according to the genetic code.

In the next step, another substance related to RNA, called "transfer RNA" (tRNA) fishes the necessary amino acids out of the cell plasma, where they are floating freely, and carries them to the mRNA matrice and thus to the site of synthesis. There the amino acids are built up into the proteins, which, according to the DNA information, are designated for this location in the genetic program of the organism.

Recombinant DNA technology transfers DNA from the genetic stock of a foreign (e.g., animal) cell and "smuggles" it into a bacterial cell, with the aid of a suitable vector. The infiltrated cell is "reprogrammed" by the foreign DNA in such a way that it forms not only its own genetic products, but also the foreign genetic products.

One method that genetic engineers use to incorporate pieces of DNA into plasmids involves restriction (cutting at certain points) and ligation (fusing) of DNA. They use special enzymes, mostly of bacterial origin, as chemical "scissors" to cut the DNA strands at particular points. Now scientists know of more than 200 different enzymes (called restriction endonucleases) that can be used in this way. With these indispensable aids, the genetic engineer can cut into the genes at will. He combines the fragments obtained in this way with other fragments and fuses them using another type of enzyme known as DNA ligases.

If a single breakthrough in gene splicing were to be identified, it would be the identification and isolation restriction endonucleases, which enable the isolation of specific genes or gene fragments. Because these restriction endonucleases make staggered breaks in DNA at sites exhibiting twofold rotational symmetry, the result is a piece of DNA with complementary cohesive ends that can then, by virtue of these "sticky" ends, be inserted or recombined with another piece of DNA that has been cut by the same enzyme.

The essential ingredients in this technology include:

1. A DNA vector that generally represents the chromosome of either a plasmid, which is an autonomously replicating DNA molecule found in bacteria and yeast, or a virus, which can infect bacteria or higher organisms. Vectors must be able to replicate in living cells after foreign DNA is inserted into them.
2. A DNA fragment to be inserted into the vector.
3. A method of introducing the joined molecules (recombinants) into a host that can replicate them.
4. A method of detection of those cells that carry the desired recombinant DNA molecule.

Once the vector carrying the inserted foreign DNA molecule is placed into an organism, such as bacteria or yeast, it replicates to make many copies of itself, the foreign gene inserted thereby providing an unlimited supply of the gene of interest.

The results of recombinant DNA research provide the means by which the strands of the DNA of one organism can be inserted into the DNA of another unrelated organism, thus endowing the recipient with a biological property that it did not hitherto possess. These revelations led to an unprecedented explosion of scientific knowledge, the most recent of which includes the biotechnologic developments of recombinant DNA technology or gene splicing (altering heredity by transplanting genes from one organism to another). Further advances in immunology have been responsible for the development of hybridoma technology, in which highly specific antibody molecules termed "monoclonal antibodies" have been responsible for an additional component of the new biotechnology.

Genetic engineering is the culmination of three main lines of research, all begun several years ago:

1. Recognition and isolation of extrachromosomal DNA.
2. Manipulation of DNA with enzymes so it can be cut into fragments and the fragments then rejoined in novel patterns.
3. Ability to reinsert manipulated DNA into living cells so it becomes part of the hereditary information carried by that cell.

ISOLATION OF EXTRACHROMOSOMAL DNA FROM BACTERIA

The greater part of a bacterium's DNA exists as a single chromosome—a piece of DNA that contains about 10,000 genes. This piece of DNA is a single circular molecule with a molecular weight of about 2×10^9. In addition to the chromosome, most bacteria also carry extrachromosomal DNA. This often consists of virus particles, yet more important from the point of view of in vitro recombination studies are plasmids—circular pieces of DNA, rarely more than 5% the size of the chromosome, which replicate in the cell independently of the chromosome.

It is now easy to prepare plasmid DNA uncontaminated with chromosomal material. This allows one to manipulate plasmid DNA as though it were a chemical in a test tube, but one can be sure that it will retain its informational function on transfer to a different living cell.

Plasmid DNA is isolated by centrifuging the crude DNA (which contains both plasmid and chromosomal DNA and is obtained by breaking open bacterial cells with detergents) in a density gradient of cesium chloride to which the drug ethidium bromide has been added. The centrifugation ensures that the plasmid DNA forms a band in the centrifuge tube at a position clearly separate from that of the chromosomal DNA. Once separated in this way, the plasmid DNA can be collected uncontaminated by other DNA.

There are three methods available. First, all the DNA in a cell can be cut into fragments using "scissors" and then incorporated directly into plasmids. Second, the mRNA can be isolated and used to produce a copy of the DNA (cDNA) by reverse transcription with the aid of an enzyme. It is now also possible to produce fully synthetic genes, provided that the amino acid sequence of the required protein is known and the gene is not too large.

Third, DNA can be cloned. Cutting DNA into pieces naturally produces a mixture of DNA fragments coding thousands of different proteins. These fragments are incorporated into a certain type of plasmid, and in this way genetic engineers obtain another mixture of recombinant (newly combined) plasmids. This is then introduced into a specially pretreated culture of *Escherichia coli* bacteria, the individual cells of which each take up different plasmids. As the *E. coli* culture grows, the plasmids naturally multiply. The result is a mixed population of cells, i.e., one in which the plasmid content of the various cells is different. These cells can be individualized by appropriate dilution techniques. Each individual cell then grows into a colony or cell clone, in other words, a population of completely identical daughter cells derived from a single mother cell. At this point, the painstaking part of the genetic engineering process begins: gene screening. The gene with the desired properties must be sought from among 10,000 or more clones.

Once the right clone has been located, it is possible to reproduce in cultures, isolate the plasmids, cut out the gene with restriction enzymes, and incorporate it into an expression vector. This vector is also based on a plasmid, or on a suitable virus if expression is to take place in an animal cell. This "Trojan horse" is then smuggled into a host cell as an *E. coli* bacterium, which then takes on a kind of "midwife" function.

This transforms the host cell in such a way that, provided that the necessary conditions have been created, it can reproduce the foreign gene product perfectly and effortlessly. Because of its tendency to divide, it is surrounded by masses of identical copies of itself within a short time. These cells also transform the "inherited" foreign genetic information into the corresponding product, for example, a valuable human protein, such as insulin or interferon.

ENZYMIC MANIPULATION OF DNA

Two classes of enzymes active on DNA are used in in vitro recombination experiments: restriction endonucleases, enzymes that cut the DNA backbone at certain specified points along its length, and ligases, enzymes that rejoin lengths of DNA cut by restriction endonucleases. In practice, most restriction endonucleases cut DNA in a specific way that facilitates subsequent rejoining. Moreover, they allow junctions to be formed between DNA molecules that previously were not in contact.

It follows that each restriction enzyme opens DNA only at those points where the appropriate base sequence is to be found. Each time the DNA is cut, however, the sticky ends formed are characteristic of the enzyme; where restriction enzymes cut circular DNA molecules, they produce linear products.

DNA ligases work in the opposite direction and with much less specificity. They join any two molecules with the same sticky ends; that is, they can splice together any two DNA fragments generated by restriction enzymes with the same specificity. Cutting DNA from different sources with the same enzyme generates the same cohesive termini and allows the joining of DNA fragments from diverse organisms.

The power of the technique lies in the fact that DNA can be inserted by this means into vectors capable of autonomous replication in host cells. Most of the original experiments were done in *E. coli* because the molecular genetics of this organism were well understood. There are two main types of vector of *E. coli*: those based on plasmids (these are modified forms of naturally occurring antibiotic resistance plasmids) and those based on bacteriophages.

The procedure is called "cloning" because each bacterial colony resulting from the transformation, growing on the agar plate, contains millions of bacteria each containing the same piece of inserted DNA. Provided that a way is available for selecting a particular DNA fragment, it is possible to isolate (clone) complete genes in this way. By transferring specific genetic information in this way, genetic engineering is opening up new perspectives in biotechnology.

SUMMARY OF RECOMBINANT TECHNIQUE

Isolation of Gene

The gene can be synthesized by chemically stringing the required nucleotides together. Alternatively, the required section of DNA may be isolated from the organism by using restriction enzymes, which act as "biological scissors," allowing DNA to be cut into predetermined fragments.

Incorporation of Gene into a Vector

Plasmids, consisting of a circular duplex of DNA, are most commonly used as the vector for transfer of the gene into a host. Restriction enzymes are used to cut the plasmid and insert the foreign gene. The two DNA fragments are then bonded using ligase, resulting in the formation of a recombined plasmid containing a foreign gene.

Transfer of Vector into a Recipient

The K12 strain of the *E. coli* bacterium is most often used as a host organism for vectors in the rDNA process. Transfer of a plasmid into a recipient organism may be achieved by mixing the two in the presence of free calcium, rendering the bacterial membrane permeable, and allowing the plasmid to enter the cell.

Selection and Cloning of Host Cells Carrying the Gene

Not all of the bacterial cells take up the plasmid when they are mixed, so it is necessary to identify only those bacteria containing the gene-carrying plasmid. This may be achieved by tagging the vector with a specific antibiotic resistance gene. Placed in a solution containing the antibiotic, only those cells containing the plasmid grow.

Expression of the Gene

For the protein to be produced by the bacteria, the gene must be expressed. In some cases, the bacteria secrete the protein out of the cell, but more often the cells must be broken open to obtain the product. The foreign protein must then be separated from the other bacterial proteins present.

Scaling-Up Production

The bacteria containing the required genes are produced using large-scale fermentation processes.

3.3 HYBRIDOMA TECHNOLOGY

The other major biotechnologic development that will have an impact on animal health and production is hybridoma technology. This technique, which results in the generation of monoclonal antibodies by cell fusion procedures, will be useful for the diagnosis of specific diseases as well as the prevention and cure of diseases affecting the morbidity and mortality of farm animals. Moreover, because of their tremendous specificity, these monoclonal antibodies will be useful for the purification of various genetically engineered products after fermentation in bacteria or yeast.

The body's immune system is a complex network of cell types and secreted chemicals that defends against anything the body recognizes as foreign. An invading bacterium and one of the body's own cells each has a variety of surface structures (for their own use) recognizable as antigens of differing uniqueness and reactivity. The immune system must keep track of these millions of different antigens, distinguish between its own cells and invaders, and destroy only the invaders.

These antibodies are Y-shaped proteins with the two short ends constructed to mate and bind with only one specific antigen. Antibodies are secreted by B cells. In the 1960s and 1970s, mixes of antibodies were prepared by injecting an animal with a known antigen preparation and then harvesting blood plasma containing the antibodies. These were used in laboratory tests to identify the original microbe or injected into another animal to give brief, passive immunity. The usefulness of these polyclonal antibodies was limited. Because each injected animal produced a different mix of antibodies, the product was neither standardized nor as specific as current monoclonal products.

A scientific breakthrough, allowing today's progress in immunology, was made in 1975 by fusing a rapidly dividing mouse tumor cell with a mouse B cell that produced only one type of antibody. The resulting cell, a hybridoma, establishes an "immortal" cell line that can be grown as a factory producing one specific (monoclonal) antibody.

The starting point of the preparation of monoclonal antibodies was the knowledge that any one antibody-producing cell and its progeny would produce identical antibody molecules. The cell and its progeny constitute a clone of functionally identical cells that, if isolated, would give a homogeneous antibody population. The desire to produce such functional clones was inspired both by an interest in dissecting out the genetics and mechanisms of the immune system and by the practical advantages that their products, "monoclonal antibodies" (MAb) might offer.

Spleen cells from an immunized mouse are mixed together with special myeloma cells in the presence of a fusing agent, such as polyethylene glycol. Fusion produces "hybridoma" cells, which contain the genetic material of both of the spleen cells, which carry the information required for the production and export of specific antibody, and of the myeloma cells, which have the characteristic ability to grow and proliferate in vitro.

The procedure involves fusing spleen cells from mice immunized with an antigen to which a MAb is desired to mouse myeloma cells in culture and screening fused cells for production of the specific MAb with the labeled (radioactive or dye) antigen. The myeloma cells serve to immortalize the spleen cells so they may be maintained indefinitely in cell culture. Special procedures are employed, such as the use of myeloma cells requiring certain growth factors provided by the spleen cells fused over unfused myeloma cells. The MAbs can then be obtained by harvesting the liquid medium from the cell cultures or by inoculating the fused cells into the peritoneum of mice and collecting the fluid present after ascites tumors have developed. MAbs have also been generated for protection of newborn calves and swine against enteric *E. coli* bacillosis responsible for neonatal diarrhea or scours.

Antibodies have been essential reagents in many diagnostic and analytical tests for decades. The introduction of the single, highly specific, pure antibody by cell hybridization techniques can greatly increase the precision and sensitivity of such procedures. Their use includes assays of biological activity, blood grouping, tissue typing, and identification of pathogens and their antigenic variation as well as for therapeutic purposes. The unique specificity that can be produced in a MAb provides new possibilities for their use.

3.4 PRODUCTION OF PHARMACEUTICAL AGENTS BY BIOTECHNOLOGY

Biotechnology in the pharmaceutical industry is already well established in the production of antibiotics and steroids by fermentation. Increasing the yields of microbial strains and creating new ones by gene transfer and hybridization have been early goals of genetic engineering. The search is also on for the "new avermectin": Screening of new microbial isolates and use of unusual precursors in culture broths to generate novel analogs of existing chemical are now commonplace.

E. coli and *Bacillus* species are used to produce materials of interest, but there is a move away from these prokaryotes, stimulated by their inability to secrete proteins in a form that is biologically active in animals and their all-too-efficient degradation of foreign materials before these can pass through the bacterial cell wall. Yeasts and vertebrate cells are now increasingly used to manufacture and release desired products in an active form.

Similar to more traditional pharmaceuticals, the proportion that will be developed specifically for veterinary use is likely to be small, and consequently most products will be "borrowed" from human use. Nevertheless, there is a great deal of research in the extension of use of these materials into animal health.

Significant advances have been made in the areas of agriculture, pharmaceuticals, industrial chemicals, food science, and insect management. Products already available include:

- **Human insulin**. This was the first recombinant DNA–derived product to become commercially available. It was first marketed in 1982.
- **Human growth hormone**. Protropin became the second recombinant drug to reach the market. Primarily indicated for children afflicted with pituitary dwarfism, human growth hormone was formerly available only in small quantities from human pituitary glands. Humatrope became commercially available in 1987.
- **Hepatitis B vaccine**. Recombivax-HB, released in January, 1987, was the first human vaccine to be made available through biotechnology. It is indicated for the prevention of hepatitis B infection in individuals at high risk for the disease.
- **Human interferon**. Interferon-alpha is a protein that may prove useful in treating some cancers and viral infections.

The harnessing of a cell's genetic machinery to produce a protein such as insulin does not simply involve inserting the insulin gene into a bacterial cell because the gene would not be replicated or transcribed. The gene must be incorporated into a vector (e.g., a plasmid), which, when transferred into a bacterial cell, replicates at each division of the bacterium. Thus, producing a specific protein by recombinant DNA techniques requires the following:

1. A gene (for the protein required)
2. A vector

3. A suitable recipient organism

The major biotechnology products are:

- **Human insulin**
- **Human growth hormone**
- **Interferons**
- **Interleukin-2**

Of all the cytokines, interleukin-2 has shown the most promise as an anticancer agent.

Other products of biotechnology that will make their mark over the next few years include tissue plasminogen activator (tPA), tumor necrosis factor (TNF), MAbs for diagnostic and therapeutic use, factor 8, acquired immunodeficiency syndrome (AIDS) vaccines, hepatitis vaccines, and other anticancer agents, such as müllerian inhibitory factor. Using recombinant DNA, researchers are developing microorganisms for production of less expensive and more nutritious feed ingredients.

Some antibiotics are produced naturally in environments so hostile that the antibiotic is rapidly destroyed. It is possible to use recombinant DNA technology to produce these antibiotics from transformed organisms in more conducive environments. Amplification of productive capability through recombinant technology could be used to increase concentrations.

VACCINES

When administered to a patient, antigens in a vaccine stimulate the production of antibodies, conferring resistance to subsequent infection. One problem with this method is that these vaccines are not always 100% safe. Sometimes vaccines revert to an infectious form and can cause the disease they are intended to prevent. Preparations made from disease organisms often contain an uncharacterized mix of antigens, some of which confer no protection and actually reduce the effectiveness of the vaccine. An immediate and valuable prospect from recombinant DNA research is the production of new, inexpensive, safe vaccines for viral diseases of humans and animals.

For the production of subunit vaccines, specific steps are required: (1) Identify protective proteins or epitopes on the proteins.

Once this is done, an individual can produce a subunit vaccine either by recombinant DNA technology or by synthetic peptide technology. (2) Identify gene coding for the protein. (3) Clone the gene coding for the specific protein and express it is a suitable expression system. (4) Purify the protective protein to homogeneity.

An advantage of using the subunit vaccine approach, especially for viruses such as herpesviruses, which can induce latency, is the possibility of developing tests to differentiate animals that are latent carriers of the virus from those that are immunized with a subunit vaccine and are protected from subsequent challenge but are not latent carriers of the virus. Recombinant DNA technology has simplified the large-scale production of antigen for the preparation of vaccines and enables the production of "subunit" vaccines containing part of an organism that is itself noninfectious but that nevertheless stimulates the production of neutralizing antibodies in the recipient animal.

Recombinant Vaccine Production

Production of the specific proteins required for a subunit vaccine involves the following steps:

1. Identification of the antigenic protein required to stimulate the immune response and its isolation (or synthesis) of the gene coding for it
2. Incorporation of the gene into a vector
3. Transfer of the vector (carrying the gene) into the recipient (host)
4. Selection and cloning of the host cells carrying the gene
5. Expression of the gene
6. Extraction of the protein
7. Scale-up of the laboratory technique into a full-scale production process

Rather than introducing the specific protein into various expression systems, it is possible to identify the specific epitopes involved in inducing protective immunity and synthesize the peptide. For example, the identification and characterization of the major neutralizing antigen of bovine rotavirus can be alluded to. Using MAbs against different proteins of bovine rotavirus, scientists have identified an immuno-dominant neutralizing epitope on the outer coat glycoprotein of bovine rotavirus. This epitope was identified by the ability of MAb directed against it to neutralize virus in vitro as well as prevent diarrhea in animals in vivo.

Another example is *E. coli*. Enterotoxicogenic *E. coli* (ETEC) strains differ from other *E. coli* strains in that they express immunogenic surface appendages, known as adhesion fimbriae or antigens, which are responsible for attaching the organisms to the gut wall. ETEC also secrete one or more enterotoxins that induce the diarrheal symptoms. A small but increasing number of immunologically distinct adhesion antigens have been identified on ETEC isolated from different animals: e.g., the K88 and 987P antigens of porcine isolates and the K99 and F41 antigens of bovine isolates. These antigens can be readily extracted from the surface of *E. coli* by heating, and they have proved to be effective vaccine components. The first commercially available ETEC vaccines were based on the K88 antigen, and these have been improved to include other adhesion antigens. Gene cloning has been used to characterize these antigens, and this has led to the development of *E. coli* strains that express improved yields of antigen and that can express more than one antigen simultaneously. On completion of the preparation of the vaccine by producing solely the immunogenic protein in *E. coli*, the costly tests of innocuity of the vaccine are unnecessary, and the ever-present suspicion is removed that sporadic outbreaks of the disease in circumstances of low prevalence might have been due to traces of surviving infective virus.

In the veterinary field, there are still many viral diseases with no adequate means of protection because of inherent problems, and there are others in which the current methods could be greatly improved. The technology of genetic manipulation may provide the means of solving some of these problems and for developing new markets of great potential.

Apart from the live "deleted" vaccines, new vaccines appear containing only the immunogenic part of the virus, or what is mainly understood as such today, the envelope glycoprotein fraction. These vaccines are called subunit vaccines.

An alternative way to produce components for subunit vaccines has been developed from the finding that short synthetic peptides can be used to raise an immune response against the polypeptide from which the sequence was derived. In the case of Aujeszky's disease, for the gI-negative (glycoprotein-deleted) vaccine, control of the genome confirms the absence of the gI gene as well as the gp63 gene. The glycoprotein technique also helps in the development of diagnostic methods. The competitive gI-(ELISA) is one of the most recent developments.

GENE DELETION VACCINES

In a gene deletion vaccine, the virus used has a part of its genome deleted, which has two major advantages:

• Decreased virulence, produced by deletion of specific genes, giving better control than conventional attenuation methods
• Differentiation of vaccinated and naturally infected animals by use of appropriate diagnostic reagents, making monitoring of eradication campaigns easier

gI-NEGATIVE VACCINES

Many gI-negative vaccines exist based on naturally occurring viral strains. Diagnostic tests, which detect antibodies to the gI protein, can be used together with such vaccines.

The basic protocol for developing genetically engineered vaccines includes:

1. Identification of the major surface antigen of the pathogenic organisms of interest that induce antibody capable of neutralizing or inactivating the infectious organisms
2. Identification of the surface antigen gene or its specific antigenic determinants
3. Isolation and transfer of this gene into a plasmid vector capable of expressing large amounts of its product in fermentable organisms, such as bacteria or yeast

Such methods have been employed to generate large amounts of vaccine proteins against bovine papillomavirus, porcine par-

vovirus, canine parvovirus, foot-and-mouth disease virus, and K99 *E. coli*.

GI deleted Aujeszky's vaccine is now popular in field use. The primary requirement for the production of novel vaccines, whether replicating or not, is to identify the immunogenic protein(s) of the microorganisms and the gene(s) that code for such protein(s). The gene for the immunogenic protein or polypeptide is cloned into a suitable expression vector, which can then be transfected into a prokaryotic or eukaryotic cell. Preparation of a viral vaccine involves identifying the nucleic acid sequences responsible for the production of the specific antigenic function of the virion and isolating and inserting these into a bacterium, within which there is expression of the protein, isolation of that protein, and its formulation into a potent vaccine.

Previously available vaccines have several drawbacks, such as virulence, which cause occasional outbreaks and problems with herd testing because all vaccinated animals are seropositive. Vaccines are protein surface antigens, encoded by a synthetic gene that is cloned and expressed at high levels in *E. coli*. So far these new vaccines have been reported as safe and effective.

Several different recombinant DNA approaches have been used in developing safer, more effective vaccines. The most straightforward is the "harmless antigen" approach, in which a gene coding for a surface protein is cloned and expressed. The merit of this approach is eliminating the danger of virulent vaccines. The second approach is "directed attenuation," achieved by removing specific regions of the pathogen's genome. This can weaken the reproductive ability of the pathogen to a point at which it is safe as a vaccine. Additionally, using ELISA tests, antibodies from deleted vaccines can be discriminated from antibodies arising from field infections.

3.5 GENERAL APPLICATIONS OF BIOTECHNOLOGY

(1) VACCINES

Conventional vaccines are normally based on either inactivated preparations of whole, dead organisms or live preparations that have been extensively cultivated outside of their natural host so as to render them non-pathogenic, a process known as "attenuation." The principles of these approaches have been established for many years. Molecular biology has opened new avenues to the development of novel vaccines. The reasons for this are multifold. Considerable information is now available about the molecular structure of many bacterial, viral, and parasitic pathogens, especially in regard to their vital surface components. Such surface and extracellular components often play vital roles in the establishment of infection of the pathogens and in the subsequent development of disease symptoms in the infected host animal. These surface components are also often antigens that can be recognized by host's immunologic defense systems. Only some of these antigens, however, known as "protective antigens," are usually required to induce protective immunity. Once the protective antigens of a pathogen have been identified, methods can be developed to modify their immunologic or biological properties, to purify them from other cellular components, or simply to monitor their production under different growth conditions. Such procedures can be used in the development and eventual production of more effective vaccines. Subunit vaccines are likely to be less reactogenic than whole-cell vaccines. Defined genetic lesions can also be introduced into the genome of virulent pathogenic organisms to construct attenuated strains.

Many existing vaccines are less than ideal because they show poor efficacy in the field, they are reactogenic, or both. Efficacy can be improved by monitoring the levels of protective antigen in vaccine batches rather than total antigen. Reactogenicity could be reduced by constructing mutant strains that are missing toxic components.

OTHER SUBUNIT VACCINES

Molecular approaches are being used to study a wide range of veterinary bacterial and parasitic pathogens, and a consequence of this work may be the development of subunit vaccines. The genetic determinant for the pili genes of *Bacteroides nodosus*, one of the causes of ovine foot-rot, has been cloned and expressed in *E. coli*. A number of feline vaccines are now of the subunit type.

(2) DIAGNOSTIC PROBES

Synthetic DNA probes can also be used to identify, quickly and accurately, a variety of pathogens, including bacteria, fungi, and viruses. The cells to be diagnosed are first disrupted, and intact DNA is isolated. The DNA is then denatured into single strands, which are bound to a filter matrix. Labeled DNA probes are added and allowed to hybridize to the bound DNA. After washing off unhybridized probes, the hybridized probe is identified and quantitated. The probe can be labeled with an enzyme catalyzing a sensitive and easy-to-assay reaction or with a radioactive compound. Such diagnostic tests can be completed in about 3 hours, as opposed to the days required for other techniques.

(3) GROWTH PROMOTANTS

The development of natural growth hormones for livestock and poultry represents a major means of improving animal production, and genetic engineering techniques have made this development a reality both for logistical and for economic reasons. Several groups have now cloned bovine growth hormone (bGH) to expression in bacteria and yeast. The recombinant DNA procedures employed were similar to those used for cloning virus genes pertinent for subunit vaccination production. A mRNA species from pituitary gland enriched for bovine growth hormone nucleotide sequences is first reverse transcribed into DNA, and this DNA copy is inserted into plasmids for expression in bacteria and yeast. Because this bGH gene lacks the required regulatory features necessary for these microorganisms to express this gene, some additional restructuring of the gene is required. One of these maneuvers results in the addition of an amino acid (methionine) at the beginning of the bGH gene, so it differs slightly from naturally occurring bGH.

(4) MONOCLONAL ANTIBODIES

E. coli bacteria causing intestinal problems in calves have two common features:

1. They have and use the pilus (hairlike structure) attachment mechanism to adhere to the animal's gut wall.
2. A common pilus structure (that to the calf is the actual antigen) exists called K99.

The first 12 hours postpartum are by far the most critical in terms of preventing pathogenic *E. coli* bacteria with the K99 antigen from adhering to the intestinal gut wall surface. A specific K99 *E. coli* antibody that can be administered directly to calves to prevent K99 pilus attachment is now available. (Genecol/Molecular Genetics)

MAbs against K99 antigen of *E. coli* have been commercially available in the last few years. Usually such antibodies are given within 12 hours of birth to preempt antigen attachment to the intestinal mucosal surface. A small fraction of antibody is absorbed to provide a level of systemic protection. After 24 hours, however, no further absorption occurs, and protection is restricted to the intestinal lumen only. Such MAbs are intended as prevention rather than treatment agents, and timing of administration is critical.

Oral use of genetically engineered monoclonal *E. coli* K99 antibody (Generol 99, Molecular Genetics) within the first 12 hours of life can reduce losses from scours caused by *E. coli*.

(5) IMMUNOASSAYS

The impact of new immunoassay technology in veterinary diagnostic medicine has been dramatic. Immunoassays for proteins and haptens are now well established in clinical chemistry, microbiology, oncology, therapeutics and toxicology, and hematology and blood transfusion, and home-use assays are beginning to be used in pregnancy testing.

Once it was thought that an antibody was specific for the whole of the antigen cell, but now it is known that the unit recognized by the antibody, the "epitope," may consist of as few as six to eight amino acids. So, for example, when a mouse's lymphocytes produce antibodies to an invading *E. coli* cell, a range of MAbs is involved, each specific for only a part of the *E. coli* cell. If the hybridoma cell is injected intraperitoneally into a mouse, one single animal can produce enough antibody for more than a million diagnostic kits.

At the heart of these systems is an antibody. This should be selected based on its affinity for the antigen in question together with its specificity for that antigen. Whether to use monoclonal or polyclonal antibodies, or a combination of the two, as might be the case with the sandwich ELISA, depends to a large extent on the nature of the antigen to be detected. The immune response to a particular antigen is heterogeneous. Even in response to a simple hapten, a large number of different clones of antibody-producing cells are stimulated. The description of a general method for the production of MAbs by cell fusion overcame the problem of proteins of undefined specificity and has already been of enormous benefit.

Polyclonal antibodies were the first to be exploited in terms of immunoassay. Such antibodies are raised by injecting a purified form of the antigen into a host animal, e.g., a sheep. MAbs by comparison are raised by taking the spleen cells of an animal previously immunized with the antigen in question and fusing these in culture with myeloma cells. The resulting hybridoma has the advantage of immortality because it is drawn from the myeloma cell line. Of equal importance is the fact that the antibody secreted by the hybridoma is of single specificity.

The polyclonal and monoclonal antibodies thus produced form the basis of immunodiagnostics. They can be used in their native state or purified to "capture antigens," i.e., function to pull antigen out of solution and immobilize it on a so-called solid phase, e.g., plastic tube or microwell, or, conversely, they can be used as "detectors," whereby the antibody is labeled (conjugated) with a signal generator, e.g., isotope, or enzyme.

The breakthrough was to couple antibodies to the surface of plastic wells, hence the "immunosorbent" title. Either antibody or antigen can be fixed, so antigen or antibody can be sampled. The high specificity of the test is due to the development of "monoclonal antibodies."

ENZYME IMMUNOASSAYS

These are the sandwich ELISAs, which are commonly used to measure multivalent antigens, e.g., proteins, viruses; the indirect ELISA, which is used to measure circulating antibodies, e.g., antibodies to rhinotracheitis virus; and the competitive enzyme immunoassay, which is used to measure small-molecular-weight compounds (haptens), e.g., aflatoxin, drug residues, progesterone.

In antibody detection tests, known antigen is used to capture antibody from the sample in Step 1. Step 2 detects the presence of antibody by adding a second, labeled antibody directed against the immunoglobulin captured in step 1. If antigen is adsorbed to the wall of the test well, it binds with antibody in the sample. Enzyme-conjugated, anti-immunoglobulin antibodies are then incubated in the well. These latch on to the bound antibody. Small molecules, such as drugs that have a limited number of antigenic sites, are best detected using competitive assays.

In noncompetitive assays, labeled antibody reacts with antigen so the minimum response is at zero binding, and amount of signal (color development) increases in direct proportion to the concentration of material in the sample. In competitive assays, unlabeled antigen in the sample and labeled antigen compete for a limited number of binding sites on the capture antibody. The maximal response is at zero binding, and color development decreases in proportion to the concentration of material in the sample.

The choice of enzyme to generate signal has largely been between three candidates: horseradish peroxidase (HRP), alkaline phosphatase, and beta-galactosidase.

When substrate is added, the enzyme acts on it to give a color change. The material for assay is sandwiched between the antigen bound to the well wall and the antibody enzyme-linked molecule. The unbound enzyme remains in solution and is washed away before substrate is added so the color intensity is directly proportional to the amount of antibody that is being assayed.

These "sandwich assays" can be used to detect antigen or antibody, the converse molecule being bound to the well wall, but they are not sufficiently sensitive for milk progesterone assay because the concentration of progesterone being sought is tiny.

To increase the sensitivity of the test, the competitive enzyme immunoassay has been developed. In this test, antiprogesterone is bound to the well wall. The sample is incubated along with a measured amount of progesterone-enzyme conjugate.

The unknown quantity of progesterone in the sample competes with the measured amount of progesterone-enzyme complex for the binding sites on the well wall. The more progesterone in the sample, the fewer sites are left for the progesterone-enzyme complex to bind to, so more of it is washed away, and less color finally develops. Thus high progesterone samples give pale end points.

Swine and cattle health managers have also begun to take advantage of new biotechnology-based diagnostic products. For example, most testing in the United States for Aujeszky's disease, caused by herpesvirus in swine, is now done with immunoassays developed only 2 to 3 years ago. Tests are available to distinguish between vaccinated and infected animals. This resolves a long-standing issue that has hampered eradication efforts for a disease that causes the swine industry high economic losses each year.

New biotechnology-based tests are also being used to detect aflatoxin, salmonella, and other contaminants in both animal feed and animal-derived food, such as beef, poultry, pork, and milk. Novel kits for Johne's disease, respiratory diseases, mastitis, leukemia, and other infectious agents are expected to see increasing use by bovine practitioners and veterinary laboratory diagnosticians. Reproduction-oriented tests also have begun to emerge as an important application of MAbs and other biotechnology products. Examples are laboratory and cow-side tests for progesterone and DNA probes for determining the sex of bovine embryos.

There are two areas, however, in which the investment in appropriate MAb production and selection is now beginning to offer marked improvements in assay performance. The first is the microdetermination of proteins for which MAbs are now making practicable. The second is the immunoassay of specific antigens present in pathogenic microorganisms, in which the ability to limit the antigenic site to a single determinant offers diagnostic specificity that has not been possible with conventional antibodies.

After injecting a mouse with an antigen (e.g., feline leukemia virus [FeLV]), a collection of mouse B cells producing differing antibodies in response to the numerous FeLV antigens are gathered and fused with tumor cells. Each hybridoma produces just one type of antibody. The challenge is testing the thousands of hybridomas to find the antibody that binds most strongly to the FeLV and only FeLV. Once that cell line is finally identified and tested, kit chemistry is developed, and the new test is compared with standard laboratory tests for accuracy.

Extremely accurate, rapid, and easy-to-use tests for canine heartworm, parvovirus, FeLV, and other applications have become common in veterinary clinics. Veterinarians can expect further advances in immunoassay technology to lead to even easier, more convenient, and more accurate testing capabilities for an expanded range of health care applications. Nucleic acid probes can be used to identify the presence of microorganisms in tissue by hybridization. Although sensitivity is greater than the use of MAbs, the cost and time required at present are greater.

Biotechnologic approaches are used to develop diagnostic and detection methods. Manipulation of viral and cellular genomes together with analysis of the mechanisms involved in pathogenicity and immunity will lead to the preparation and production of cheaper, more effective vaccines against infectious pathogens.

To be commercially viable, biotechnology must produce a large range of new products; it must result in reduced production costs; it has to be socially and politically acceptable; environmental acceptability has to be achieved; and finally, it has to have a pervasive effect throughout the economic system. Biotechnology's impact on the agricultural sector was seen as being as far-reaching as that in the public health sector but taking place at a slower pace.

3.6 MODERN PIG VACCINES

Traditionally live vaccines against Aujeszky's disease have been produced by taking a field isolate and attenuating it by serial passage. This procedure produces major changes in the viral genome, with a total loss of some individual proteins (epitopes) and modification of others. Such modifications not only reduce virulence, but also affect the immunogenicity of the attenuated virus. The dominance of the thymidine kinase gene in determining virulence in pigs, however, and the availability of technology to inactivate this gene have raised the possibility of deleting it from a fully virulent virus, to produce a virus that is nonpathogenic for pigs yet retaining its full immunologic potential. Further, the deletion of a gene that does not contribute to immunogenicity, but that is highly conserved and induces a strong antibody response in natural infections, raises the possibility of being able to discriminate between vaccinated and infected pigs.

Using recombinant DNA technology, it has been possible to construct deletion mutants against many animal herpesviruses, including pseudorabies and bovine herpesvirus-1, whose virulence and ability to induce latency are dramatically reduced after deletion of some genes. Although a number of genes have been associated with virulence, the thymidine kinase gene has received the most attention. Deletion of these genes not only reduces neurovirulence dramatically, but also it reduces the virus' ability to induce latency. Based on these observations, a number of pseudorabies virus vaccines are either licensed already or are in the process of being licensed. The next logical step is to insert genes from other viruses into the region of the deleted TK genes or other nonessential herpes glycoprotein genes.

Some envelope glycoproteins of the pseudorabies virus proved to be nonessential for the induction of a protective immune response. The production of vaccines that do not contain some envelope glycoproteins (so-called deleted vaccines) distinguishes infected animals from both noninfected and vaccinated ones without losing efficiency. ELISA kits were developed to perform this distinction.

In recent years, several deletion mutant vaccine viruses of Aujeszky's disease virus have been constructed by means of recombinant DNA technology. Another group of investigators has developed a vaccine strain, starting from an iododeoxyuridine-resistant mutant of the Aujeszky strain of Aujeszky's disease virus, with deletions in the thymidine kinase gene and in the gene coding for the nonstructural glycoprotein gX.

AUJESZKY'S DISEASE AND DELETED SUBUNIT VACCINES

A subunit biological is one that contains only those immunogenic components necessary to elicit an immune response. A requirement for subunit products is knowing which particular immunogen is responsible for the production of immunity by the host.

Methods of Production

Three methods are available for large-scale production:

1. Large-scale production of the biological agent followed by extraction and purification of the subunit immunogen. This method has been used successfully with influenza types A and B. Its major disadvantage is high cost.
2. Synthesis of the specific immunogen by chemical means. This requires high technology that does not yet have a practical application. In this technique, the determinant sites, which involve only a few amino acids, can be coupled to a carrier protein, such as bovine serum albumin. This coupled hapten is then used as the subunit vaccine.
3. Identification of vaccinates. Serologic test procedures can be developed to differentiate vaccinates from infected animals.

The ideal vaccinal strain should be inactivated or, if live, genetically stable. If living, the vaccinal strain should undergo only limited replication and then should be completely eliminated by the recipient's defense mechanisms with no opportunity for spread to other animals. Its use should not interfere with the host's ability to respond to other antigens in the vaccine or to other infectious agents regardless of the dosage used. It should be free from local and systemic adverse reactions.

Vaccines of two type are available at present. Both have major shortcomings. Live vaccines, produced by passing virus through tissue culture, usually prevent the symptoms and resultant economic loss. They run a risk of turning virulent or of contamination with wild virus. Killed vaccines are safer but not as effective against the disease. Both types do not prevent the entry of disease into the herd and subsequent spread.

The modern live vaccines have been developed using recombinant DNA technology. Scientists took the Aujeszky wild virus strain and genetically altered it so it would not only protect against disease, but also would be unable to revert to virulent or wild-type virus strain. In addition, because it is different from the disease organisms, vaccinated pigs can be distinguished from pigs infected with the disease. The modified virus has the gene holding the DNA code for virulence removed. Removing this gene, called the thymidine kinase (tK) gene, makes it virtually impossible for the virus to revert to wild status.

To distinguish the vaccine from the disease organisms, the viral glycoprotein (gX) gene also has been removed. The precise function of this gene is unknown, but it allows infected pigs to be separated from vaccinated pigs. Vaccinated pigs do not produce antibodies to gX. Using an ELISA, infected and vaccinated pigs may be identified.

Many companies are in the process of introducing these new gI deleted vaccines for Aujeszky's disease. Their major advantage is not only safety, but also allowing vaccinated animals to be identified with animals infested by the wild strain under field conditions.

Research has demonstrated that the immunogenic proteins of the virus that favor the installation of protection are composed of envelope glycoproteins, whereas those proteins responsible for hypersensitivity reactions are made up of capsid proteins. The pseudorabies virus glycoproteins used for Aujeszky's vaccine production are devoid of glycoproteins 1 and 63 (= Gp V). This offers the possibility of differential diagnosis between commercially vaccinated and infected animals.

Because deleted vaccines use only determinants that deal with immunogenicity, those viral subunit vaccines, represent an original contribution to the medical prophylaxis for Aujeszky's disease. Conventional vaccines can lead to economic losses owing to reproduction disorders or local reactions at the site of injection. Many of the modern deleted vaccines are inactivated, oil-adjuvanted, purified, and concentrated vaccines containing only the immunogenic subunits of the Aujeszky's disease virus.

3.7 FUTURE TRENDS IN BIOTECHNOLOGY

The impact of these technologies has been far-reaching, with the most rapid developments in human pharmaceuticals and agriculture. Developments have allowed the isolation of genes and parts of genes and their recombination within and between species. The consequences are manifold: the analysis of gene structure and function, the production of polypeptides and proteins in large quantities, the manipulation of microorganisms, and the production of transgenic animals.

Interferon is also being studied as a potential treatment for AIDS and as a nasal aerosol to prevent the common cold. Examples of other potential new medications are recombinant sources of interleukin-2, a protein that gives a boost to the immune system; tPA, a substance that dissolves blood clots with the advantage that it acts mainly at the site of the clot; calcitonin, which regulates the calcium content of bones; and future generations of an inhibitor of the kidney enzyme renin that may provide more effective treatment of high blood pressure.

Also in development are new, more effective recombinant vaccines against both human and animal diseases; DNA probes that can hunt for (and therefore help diagnose) abnormal genes of viral infections;

and MAbs, pure antibodies of a single type, rather than the mixtures usually found in nature. Antibodies are immune system proteins—natural defenders of the body—that can be put to a variety of uses, including detecting the presence in the body of small quantities of foreign substances, such as meningitis and venereal disease micro-organisms.

Biotechnology is hastening change in agriculture. For example, bovine somatotropin can now be produced using recombinant DNA techniques and used to increase the efficiency of milk production in lactating dairy cows. The substance could eventually reduce the herd size, land requirements, and feed needed to produce a given amount of milk. Pseudorabies, a herpesvirus, is a contagious disease of swine and has a major economic effect on the pork industry. Vaccines are being developed that contain the swine pseudorabies virus lacking a gene necessary to produce disease.

Researchers also are studying ways to confer resistance to disease on plants, to develop better herbicides (weed killers), and to reduce insect and frost damage. Production of improved hybrid seeds is another important scientific and commercial goal.

Genetic engineering in agriculture will continue to be directed toward manipulation of microorganisms to produce animal vaccines, hormones, amino acids, and other chemicals or drugs with the ultimate aim of improving the quality, health, and production of farm animals. Genetically engineered products, such as vaccines, antitoxins, growth promotants, and interferon, will be introduced on the veterinary market in the near future. Many of these products are now being tested in animals, for example:

1. **Vaccines**, particularly those that were impractical or impossible to produce by traditional means; e.g., control of hematotropic disease in cattle, control of coccidiosis in poultry, protection against endoparasites and ectoparasites.

2. **Therapeutic and productivity improvers**. Natural hormones and synthesized compounds with similar actions now play an important part in veterinary medicine to correct deficiency or control estrus; e.g., insulin, sex hormones (hormones that have not been available for

commercial use are now becoming possible through recombinant DNA). Thus we would hope to see naturally occurring hormones used to an increasing extent to enhance fecundity, food conversion, growth, and meat quality.

3. **Antibiotics**. The need will continue for novel antimicrobial compounds to keep ahead of resistance problems and provide the veterinarian with product characteristics that particularly meet his requirements.

4. **Interferon**. The marketplace clearly needs products with antiviral activity. Whether interferon can fill this need remains to be seen, but, as more becomes known about it and production techniques improve, it should stand a good chance of achieving some use in veterinary medicine.

5. **Monoclonal antibodies**. The potential for products of real value from this area and look forward to further progress in improved yields from cell cultures, renders this a major area of development.

The first generation of MAbs has been used outside the body to test blood or other samples for the presence of disease antigens. Further applications being developed include the injection of antibodies into the body to supplement, assist, or manipulate the immune system. The first of the foreign (e.g., mouse produced) antibodies combined with chemicals to tag or treat cancers and infections should reach the market over the next 2 years.

Rational drug design is one of the most exciting and fastest growing areas of pharmaceutical research. The current cost of discovering a successful new drug and gaining regulatory approval is some $120 million and 10 years' time. Much of this is spent in the traditional cycles of synthesizing thousands of candidate molecules and testing their activity. Drug receptor interaction can be studied using anti-idiotypic antibodies.

In some cases, antibodies themselves are treated as antigens by other antibodies ("anti-antibodies"). The anti-antibodies are called anti-idiotypic antibodies. For example, a rabbit immunized with a human antibody will form antibodies against it.

Anti-idiotypic antibodies can be made to mimic a variety of molecular interactions, which form the basis of nearly all immunologic, pharmacologic, endocrine, and other biological processes.

Anti-idiotypes may permit the accurate mimicking of drug receptor interactions. Receptors are proteins on cell surfaces that bind messenger molecules, such as hormones. Drugs often mimic these messenger molecules by binding to specific cell receptors.

Researchers in the pharmaceutical industry are using receptor molecules in the laboratory to screen new drugs and predict the optimum structure of new drug molecules. Naturally occurring receptors, however, are not obtainable. Anti-idiotypes, by mimicking the structure of the receptors, may supply a highly effective alternative.

Anti-idiotypic antibodies may also prove useful in treating autoimmune diseases, such as lupus erythematosus, and rheumatoid arthritis. These debilitating conditions are caused when the body erroneously manufactures antibodies to its own cells, leading to attack by the immune system and widespread tissue damage.

Genetic engineering can provide better, more efficacious vaccines and antitoxins against many more diseases. Developments as a result of genetic engineering include:

- Interferons
- Additional animal hormones
- Cheaper feed supplements, antibiotics
- Fertility control, sexing
- Improvements in animal feed
- Antitoxins
- Growth promotants
- Bovine interferons
- bGH, porcine growth hormone

Vaccines include those acting against canine parvovirus, foot-and-mouth disease, Aujeszky's disease, K-99 (scours), bovine papillomavirus, porcine parvovirus, K-99, K-88, and K-987.

Regarding antibiotics, through recombinant technology, organisms that now produce in such low concentrations that it is not practical to recover the antibiotic can be altered to produce much larger quantities for the marketplace.

SELECTED REFERENCES

Allen, C.E.: New horizons in animal agriculture: Future challenges for animal scientists. J. Anim. Sci., 57 (suppl. 2): 16, 1983.

Beale, A.J.: Biotechnology: Impact of immunization. Vet. Rec., *113*: 77, 1983.

Beck, E., and Stohjmaier, K.: Subtyping of European foot-and-mouth disease virus strains by nucleotide sequence determination. J. Virol., *61*: 1621, 1987.

Ben Porat, T., De Marchi, J.M., Lomniczi, B., et al.: Role of glycoproteins of pseudorabies virus in eliciting neutralizing antibodies. Virology, *54*: 325, 1986.

Bittle, J.L., Houghten, R.A., Alexander, H., et al.: Protection against FMDV by immunization with a chemically synthesized peptide predicted from the viral nucleotide sequence. Nature, *298*: 30, 1982.

Bittle, J.J., and Murphy, F.A.: Vaccine biotechnology. Adv. Vet. Sci. Comp. Med., *33*: 1, 1989.

Brown, F., and Underwood, B.O.: Identification of FMD virus isolated by ribonuclease T1 fingerprinting of their RNA. Foot-and-Mouth Disease Committee Proceedings of the 16th Conference of the Office International des Epizooties, Paris, 14–17 Sept. 1982.

Brun, A., and Vannier, Ph.: Essais de vaccination par la voie dermique chez le porc. J. Rech. Porcine en France, *20*: 147, 1988.

Chappuis, G., Fargeaud, D., and Brun, A.: Industrial production and control of a subunit vaccine against Aujeszky's disease. *In* Vaccination and Control of Aujeszky's Disease. Edited by J.T. van Oirschot. Dordrecht, Holland, Kluwer Academic Press, 1989.

Cheung, A.K., and Kupper, H.: Biotechnological approach to a new foot and mouth disease virus vaccine. *In* Biotechnology and Genetic Engineering Reviews. Vol. 1. Edited by G.E. Russell. Newcastle upon Tyne, Intercept, 1984.

Clifford, M.N.: The history of immunoassays in food analysis. *In* Immunoassays in Food Analysis. Edited by B.A. Morris and M.N. Clifford. New York, Elsevier Applied Science Publishers, 1985.

Cohen, S.N.: The manipulation of genes. Sci. Am., *233*: 24, 1975.

Crevat, D., Fornes, A., Lacoste, F., et al.: Evaluation of a competition ELISA for the differentiation between pigs infected by Pseudo-rabies virus or vaccinated with gI-negative vaccines. 11th International Pig Veterinary Society Congress, Lausanne, 1990.

Cuello, A.C.: Monoclonal antibodies to neurotransmitters. *In* Monoclonal Antibodies in Clinical Medicine. Edited by A. McMichael and J. Fabre. London, Academic Press, 1982.

Cuello, A.C., Milstein, C., and Priestly, J.V.: Use of monoclonal antibodies in immunocytochemistry with special reference to the central nervous system. Brain Res. Bull., *55*: 575, 1980.

Eliot, M., Fargeaud, D., Vannier, P., et al.: Development of an ELISA to differentiate between animals either vaccinated with gI negative vaccines or infected by Aujeszky's disease virus. Vet. Rec., *124*: 91, 1989.

Emery, A.E.H.: Recombinant DNA technology. Lancet, 2: 1409, 1981.

Enquist, L.W.: Genetic engineering. 1. An emerging technology. Veterinary Medicine/Small Animal Clinician, *79*: 689, 1984.

Feldkamp, S.C., and Smith S.W.: Practical guide to immunoassay method evaluation. *In* Immunoassay: A Practical Guide. Edited by D.W. Chan and M.T. Perlstein. New York, Academic Press, 1987.

Ganong, W.F.: Review of Medical Physiology. Los Altos, CA, Lange Medical Publications, 1971.

Gerlis, L.S., and Daniels, V.G.: Biotechnology—From Microbe to Market. Cambridge, Cambridge Medical Books, 1986.

Glass, R.E.: Gene Function: E. coli and Its Heritable Elements. London, Croom Helm Ltd., 1982.

Glover, D.M.: Genetic Engineering: Cloning DNA. London, Chapman & Hall, 1980.

Goeddel, D.V., Heyneker, H.L., Hoxumi, T., et al.: Expression in Escherichia coli of a DNA sequence coding for human growth hormone. Nature [Lond.], *281*: 544, 1979.

Goeddel, D.V., Kleid, D.G., Bolivar, F., et al.: Expression in E. coli of chemically synthesized genes for human insulin. Proc. Nat. Acad. Sci., U.S.A., *76*: 106, 1979.

Goeddel, D.V., Yelverton, E., Ullrich, A., et al.: Human leucocyte interferon produced by E. coli is biologically active. Nature [Lond.], *287*: 411, 1980.

Greene, C.E.: Immunoprophylaxis and immunotherapy. *In* Infectious Diseases of the Dog and Cat. Edited by C.E. Greene. Philadelphia, W.B. Saunders, 1990.

Grimont, P.A.D., Grimont, F., Desplaces, N., and Tchen, P.: DNA probe for Legionella pneumophila. J. Clin. Microbiol., *21*: 431, 1985.

Hampl, H., Ben Porat, T., Ehrlicher, L., et al.: Characterization of the envelope proteins of pseudorabies virus. J. Virol., *52*: 583, 1984.

Hardy, K.: Bacterial Plasmids. Walton-on-Thames, Surrey, Thomas Nelson & Sons, 1981.

Henderson, L., Levings, R., Davis, A., and Sturtz, D.: Recombination of pseudorabies virus vaccine strains in swine. Am. J. Vet. Res., *52*: 820, 1991.

Itakura, K., Hirose, T., Crea, R., et al.: Expression in E. coli of a chemically synthesized gene for the hormone somatostatin. Science, *198*: 1056, 1977.

Katz, J.B., Henderson, L.M., and Erickson, G.A.: Recombination in vivo of pseudorabies vaccine strains to produce new virus strains. Vaccine, *8*: 286, 199.

Kehoe, M., Sellwood, R., Shipley, P., and Dougan, G.: Genetic analysis of K88 mediated adhesion of enterotoxigenic Escherichia coli. Nature, *291*: 122, 1981.

Kleid, D.G., Yansura, D., Small, B., et al.: Cloned viral protein vaccine for foot and mouth disease: Responses in cattle and swine. Science, *214*: 1125, 1981.

Kohler, G., and Milstein, C.: Continuous cultures of fused cells secreting antibody of predefined specificity. Nature, *256*: 495, 1975.

Krakowka, S., et al. Canine parvovirus infection potentiates canine distemper encephalitis attributable to modified live virus vaccine. J. Am. Vet. Med. Assoc., *180*: 137, 1982.

Lacoste, F., Languet, B., Brun, A., et al.: Safety and activity of a live glycoprotein gI deleted vaccine against pseudorabies. 11th I.P.V.S. Congress, Lausanne, 1990.

Lehninger, A.L.: Biochemistry. New York, Worth, 1970.

Lerner, R.A.: Tapping the immunological repertoire to produce antibodies of predetermined specificity. Nature, *299*: 592, 1982.

Maniatis, T., Fritsch, E.F., and Sambrook, J.: Molecular Cloning—a Laboratory Manual. Cold Spring Harbor, NY, Cold Spring Harbor Laboratory, 1982.

Marchioli, C.C., Yancey, R.J., Wardley, R.C., et al.: A vaccine strain of pseudorabies virus with deletions in the thymidine kinase and glycoprotein X genes. Am. J. Vet. Res., *48*: 1577, 1987.

Mercola, K.E., and Cline, M.J.: The potentials in inserting new genetic information. N. Engl. J. Med., *303*: 1279, 1980.

Miller, W.L., and Baxter, J.D.: Recombinant DNA—a new source of insulin. Diabetologia, *18*: 431, 1980.

Milstein, C., Clark, M.R., Galfre, G., and Cuello, A.C.: Monoclonal antibodies from hybrid myelomas. Prog. Immunol., *4*: 17, 1980.

Moore, D.M.: Introduction of a vaccine for foot and mouth disease through gene cloning. Beltsville Symposia in Agricultural Research, Genetic Engineering in Agriculture, Remonbinant Technology, Allanheld Osmun, Montclair, 1982.

Morris, B.A.: Principles of immunoassay. In Immunoassays in Food Analysis. Edited by B.A. Morris and M.N. Clifford. New York, Elsevier Applied Science Publishers, 1985.

Muscoplat, C.C.: Genetic engineering. 2. Applications for animal health care. VM/SAC, *79*: 832, 1984.

Muscoplat, C.C.: What's in store in immunology: Immunomodulators, genetic engineering, new vaccines. Bov. Proc., No. 15, 8, 1983.

Old, R.W., and Primrose, S.B.: Principles of Gene Manipulation. 2nd ed. Oxford, Blackwell Scientific Publications, 1983.

Old, R.W., and Primrose, S.B.: Principles of Gene Manipulation: An Introduction to Genetic Engineering. Oxford, Blackwell Scientific Publications, 1982.

Paul, J.K.: Genetic Engineering Applications for Industry. New Jersey, Noyes Data Corporation, 1981.

Pouwels, P.H., Enger-Valk, B.E., and Brammar, W.J. (eds.): Cloning Vectors. Amsterdam, Elsevier, 1986.

Rees, A.R., and Sternberg, M.J.S.: From Cells to Atoms: An Illustrated Introduction to Molecular Biology. Oxford, Blackwell Scientific Publications, 1984.

Scharff, M.D., and Roberts, S.: Present status and future prospects for the hybridoma technology. In Vitro, *17*: 1072, 1981.

Schirvel, C., Brun, A., Lacoste, F., et al.: Vaccination of sows, maternal antibodies and interference with active immunity. First International Symposium on the Eradication of Pseudorabies (Aujeszky's Disease) Virus, St. Paul, 1991.

Scott, A.L., et al.: Monoclonal antibodies against somatic antigens of Dirofilaria immitis. Fed. Proc., *42*: 1089, 1983.

Secher, D.S., and Burke, D.C.: A monoclonal antibody for large scale purification of human leukocyte interferon. Nature, *285*: 446, 1980.

Sherman, D.M.: Protection of calves against fatal enteric colibacillosis by orally administered Escherichia coli K99. Specific monoclonal antibody. Infect. Immun., *42*: 653, 1983.

Shine, J., Fettes, I., Lan, N.C.Y., et al.: Expression of cloned beta-endorphin gene sequences by Escherichia coli. Nature [Lond.], *285*: 456, 1980.

Spinks, A.: Targets in biotechnology (the Phillips Lecture, 1981). Proc. R. Soc. Lond., *B214*: 289, 1982.

Stokes, C.R., Newby, T.J., Huntley, J.H., et al.: The immune response of mice to bacterial antigens given by mouth. Immunology, *38*: 497, 1979.

The Commercial Exploitation of Biotechnical Processes in Western Europe over the Next Twenty Years. London, Information Research Limited, 1981.

Tijssen, P.: Quantitative enzyme immunoassay techniques. In Practice and Theory of Enzyme Immunoassays. Edited by P. Tijssen. New York, Elsevier Applied Science Publishers, 1988.

Tizard, I.: Risks Associated with use of live vaccines. J. Am. Vet. Med. Assoc., *196*: 1851, 1990.

Tizard, I.: General principles of vaccination and vaccines. In Veterinary Immunology: An Introduction. 3rd Ed. Philadelphia, WB Saunders, 1987.

Valenzuela, P., Median, A., Rutter, W.J., et al.: Synthesis and assembly of hepatitis B virus surface antigen particles in yeast. Nature, *298*: 347, 1982.

Vandeputte, J., Chappuis, G., Fargeaud, D., et al.: Vaccination against pseudorabies with glycoprotein gI + or glycoprotein gI-vaccine. Am. J. Vet. Res., *51*: 1100, 1990.

van Oirschot, J.T., Houwers, D.J., Rziha, H.J., et al.: Development of an ELISA for detection of antibodies to glycoprotein I of Aujeszky's disease virus: A method for serological differentiation between infected and vaccinated pigs. J. Virol. Methods, *22*: 191, 1988.

van Oirschot, J., Moormann, R., Berns, A., and Gielkens, A.: Efficacy of a pseudorabies virus vaccine based on deletion mutant strain 783 that does not express TK and gI. Am. J. Vet. Res., *52*: 1056, 1991.

Williamson, R. (ed.): Genetic Engineering. Vols. 1–4. Academic Press, 1982–84.

Zweig, M.H., and Robertson, E.A.: Clinical validation of immunoassays: A well-designed approach to a clinical study. In Immunoassay: A Practical Guide. Edited by D.W. Chan and M.T. Perlstein. New York, Academic Press, 1987.

CHAPTER **4**

CLINICAL PHARMACOLOGY OF ENDOPARASITICIDES

4.1 General Principles
4.2 Benzimidazoles
4.3 Imidazothiazoles—Levamisole
4.4 Organophosphates
4.5 Tetrahydropyrimidines—Pyrantel, Morantel
4.6 Avermectins
4.7 Salicylanilides and Substituted Phenols—Flukicides
4.8 Miscellaneous Parasiticides
4.9 Resistance

4.1 GENERAL PRINCIPLES

INTRODUCTION

Modern research has provided a considerable array of highly effective, highly selective drugs with which to attack helminth parasites. These agents must be used correctly and judiciously if a favorable clinical response to treatment is to be obtained.

Most of the older anthelmintic compounds had narrow margins of safety; the more modern drugs possess considerably improved activity against the immature or larval stages of the parasite, have a higher margin of safety, and have a broader spectrum of activity. Many factors limit the usefulness of anthelmintics in practice, including features relating to the inherent efficacy of the drug itself, its mechanism of action, its pharmacokinetic properties; features relating to the host animal, such as the operation of the esophageal groove reflex; or features relating to the parasite, such as its location in the body, its degree of hypobiosis, or whether it has acquired anthelmintic resistance. Before discussing general principles of anthelmintic activity and the individual compounds, the major characteristics that should be looked for in a new anthelmintic agent are listed:

1. It should have a broad spectrum of activity against mature, immature, and, if possible, arrested larvae.
2. It must be easy to administer to a large number of animals.
3. It must have a wide margin of safety and be compatible with other compounds.
4. It should not present a residue problem requiring long withdrawal periods.
5. The compound should be economical for the livestock producer to use.

Anthelmintics must be selectively toxic to the parasite. This is usually achieved either by the inherent pharmacokinetic properties of the compound itself causing the parasite to be exposed to higher concentrations of the anthelmintic than the host cells or by inhibition of metabolic processes vital to the parasite.

MECHANISM OF ACTION OF ANTHELMINTICS

Although the primary physiologic mode of action of all drugs used against parasites is not fully understood, it remains possible to indicate general sites of action and biochemical mechanisms. Life support mechanisms of parasites are based on maintaining an advantageous feeding site and using the acquired foodstuff to generate chemical energy. Parasitic helminths must maintain an appropriate feeding site, and nematodes and trematodes must actively ingest and move food through their digestive tracts to maintain an appropriate energy state. These functions require proper neuromuscular coordination. The common pharmacologic basis of the treatment of helminths generally involves interference with one or more of these functions vital to the parasite, i.e., disruption of (1) energy process and subsequent starvation of the parasite or (2) neuromuscular coordination, with paralysis of the parasite and subsequent expulsion by peristalsis (Table 4–1).

Energy Processes

Several chemical classes of compounds and many different types of metabolic inhibitors are found within the group of commonly used anthelmintics in veterinary practice.

Inhibitors of mitochondrial reactions (fumarate reductase) or glucose transport include benzimidazoles—albendazole cambendazole, parbendazole, mebendazole, fenbendazole, oxibendazole, oxfendazole, thiabendazole, and flubendazole. The probenzimidazoles thiophanate and febantel are metabolized in vivo to active benzimidazoles and thus act in the same manner.

Uncouplers of oxidative phosphorylation include salicylanilides—oxyclozanide, rafoxanide, niclosamide, clioxanide, closantel, and brotianide—and substituted phenols—nitroxynil, bithionol, niclofolan, and hexachlorophene.

The benzimidazoles inhibit the enzyme fumarate reductase and thus inhibit energy generation. These compounds are broad spectrum in activity and are often effective against adult larvae and eggs. Being chemically quite similar and affecting the same metabolic pathway in the parasite, cross resistance frequently exists among the benzimidazoles. Mebendazole and flubendazole interact with tubulin in the intestinal cells of nematodes, resulting in the disappearance of microtubules from the cells and

TABLE 4–1
CHEMICAL GROUPS AND MECHANISMS OF ACTION OF COMMONLY USED ANTHELMINTIC AGENTS

Group	Chemical Name	Mode of Action in Parasite	Effect
Benzimidazoles	Thiabendazole Parbendazole Cambendazole Mebendazole Oxibendazole Fenbendazole Albendazole Oxfendazole	Interfere with energy production Inhibit fumarate reductase Block tubulin synthesis Inhibit glucose transport	Starvation of parasite (slow process) Ovicidal
Probenzimidazole	Thiophanate Febantel Netobimin	Metabolized in vivo to benzimidazole carbamates	As above
Imidazothiazoles	Tetramisole Levamisole	Ganglionic stimulants	Spastic paralysis
Pyrimidines	Pyrantel Morantel	Cholinergic agonists (ganglionic)	Spastic paralysis
Salicylanilides	Rafoxanide Oxyclozanide Niclosamide	Uncouple oxidative phosphorylation	Energy depletion
Substituted Phenols	Nitroxynil Niclofolan Bithionol Hexachlorophene	Uncouple oxidative phosphorylation	Energy depletion
Organophosphate	Trichlorphon Dichlorvos, Coumaphos, haloxan Fenthion	Cholinesterase inhibition	Spastic paralysis
Piperazine	Piperazine Diethylcarbamazine	Neuromuscular hyperpolarizers	Flaccid paralysis
Avermectin	Ivermectin Doramectin Moxidectin	GABA potentiation	Flaccid paralysis
Sulfonamide	Clorsulon	Inhibits glycolysis	Energy Depletion

decreased absorption and digestion of nutrients such as glucose.

For these benzimidazoles, it has been shown that one important factor in ensuring their efficacy is the prolongation of contact time between the drug and the parasite. The requirement that this contact be prolonged for as long as possible is a consequence of the mode of action of this group. Because they act on the energy systems within the nematode cell, death occurs after the stored energy sources are exhausted. This is a slow process compared with the much quicker actions of other anthelmintics, which act on the neuromuscular coordination system of the parasite.

Uncoupling of oxidative phosphorylation processes has been demonstrated for a number of compounds, especially the fasciolicides. Many of these compounds are ineffective in vivo against nematode species of parasites, apparently owing to a permeability barrier because isolated nematode mitochondria are equally susceptible to them. Because these compounds are general uncouplers of oxidative phosphorylation, their safety indices are not as high as the benzimidazoles although adequate if used as directed. Looseness of feces and slight loss of appetite may be seen in some animals after treatment at the recommended dosage rates. High doses may cause blindness, hyperthermia, convulsions, and death—classic symptoms of uncoupled phosphorylation.

Neuromuscular Coordination

Interference with this process in the parasite may occur by inhibiting the breakdown of excitatory neurotransmitters or by mimicking the action of the excitatory transmitter, resulting in spastic paralysis of the parasite. Other mechanisms are mimicking the action of the inhibitory transmitter or causing hyperpolarization, with an ensuing flaccid paralysis of the parasite. Either spastic or flaccid paralysis of an intestinal helminth allows the normal peristaltic action of the host to expel the parasite.

The following agents affect neuromuscular coordination: Cholinesterase inhibitors include organophosphates—haloxon, trichlorfon, dichlorvos, and coumaphos (spastic paralysis). Cholinergic agonists include imidazothiazoles—tetramisole and levamisole—and pyrimidines—morantel and pyrantel. Muscle hyperpolarization is caused by piperazine. Potentiation of inhibitory transmitters is caused by avermectins.

Thus anthelmintic mode of action is closely related to the unique life-support parasite requirements. Drug efficacy is generally based on interference with energy generation or neuromuscular coordination. Differential toxicity between host and parasite is based on the presence of a unique parasite system or on an effective concentration of drug that inhibits the parasite system without interfering with the comparable host system (selective toxicity).

ADMINISTRATION OF ANTHELMINTICS

Anthelmintics can be administered in many ways. Generally, drench, paste, and injectable preparations allow greater control over the amount of anthelmintic that is administered to an animal than in feed or medicated block preparations. Whichever method of administration is selected, it is important to read the manufacturer's instructions with particular regard to:

1. The types of worm against which the anthelmintic is active

2. The class of stock for which the product is recommended and any limitations to its use that may be advised
3. The dosage rate to be used and any increase in dosage rate that may be recommended to deal with different developmental stages or different species or types of worm
4. The withholding period

The solubility of an individual anthelmintic compound governs the choice of route of administration. Insoluble anthelmintics usually have to be given orally as suspensions, pastes, or granules. The more soluble compounds may be given orally as a solution, topically in the pour-on form (organophosphates, levamisole) or subcutaneously as an injectable solution (nitroxynil, rafoxanide, levamisole). Particle size is an important consideration in determining the behavior and subsequent efficacy or toxicity of an orally administered agent. Small particle size determines the rate and extent of absorption from the gastrointestinal tract and may increase the efficacy of compounds that must undergo metabolism in the liver before exerting their anthelmintic effect. Conversely, large particle size coupled with insolubility minimizes gut absorption, may reduce systemic toxicity, and ensures increased efficacy of the parent drug against lumen-dwelling parasites further down the alimentary tract.

The route of administration of these drugs also determines their persistence in the body and their antiparasitic efficacy. In ruminants, administration directly in the abomasum by way of the esophageal groove bypass may increase the rate of absorption and excretion of an anthelmintic. This resultant lack of persistence may reduce the efficacy of the compound by reducing the period of contact between the drug and the parasite. Lowered efficacy may occasionally occur owing to an unexplained direct passage of the drug into the abomasum and a more rapid flow of drug through the alimentary tract. Operation of the rumen bypass acts to reduce the efficacy of certain benzimidazole anthelmintics, such as oxfendazole. It has been deduced experimentally that immediate arrival of the compound in the abomasum after dosing reduced its efficacy from 91 to 45%

against a thiabendazole-resistant strain of *Haemonchus contortus*. Absorption of levamisole is not affected by the route of administration because this drug is highly soluble, unaffected by the operation of the ruminal bypass, and thus superior to benzimidazoles in this particular respect.

Most of the benzimidazoles are most effective if injected or deposited directly into the rumen; efficiency is lower if injected into the abomasum. Deposition in the rumen tends to prolong the passage of the insoluble compound through the alimentary tract, slows the rate of absorption, and so maintains the level of circulating anthelmintic. The rumen acts as a type of drug reservoir from which plasma concentrations can be sustained for long periods and slows the passage of unabsorbed drugs through the alimentary tract.

Drench and Paste Preparations

Many anthelmintics, particularly the benzimidazoles and certain flukicides, are available as suspensions. Therefore the containers must be well shaken both before and during use to ensure that adequate dispersion of the chemical throughout the liquid is continuously maintained.

Injectable Preparations

Certain soluble anthelmintics, notably levamisole, ivermectin, and diethylcarbamazine for the treatment of stomach worms, intestinal worms, and lungworms and rafoxanide and nitroxynil for the treatment of liver fluke, are available as injectable preparations. They are as effective as drench or paste preparations against different worm types and they ensure that the full recommended dose is administered. In some situations, notably with cattle and pigs, they have an added advantage of ease of administration. Local reactions at the injection site may occasionally be noticed. These are regarded as of little consequence if the site for injection is not an area from which prime cuts of meat are taken. This is particularly true of levamisole.

Pour-on Preparations (Topical)

The pour-on preparations currently available contain levamisole ivermectin/organophosphates and are licensed for use only in cattle. In these preparations, the drug is contained within a liquid or vehicle that is rapidly absorbed through the skin after application. As with injectable preparations, high blood levels of the anthelmintic are achieved rapidly, and they offer the advantage of ease of administration.

In-feed Preparations

Many of the benzimidazoles are available for mass medication as in-feed preparations. In-feed preparations allow little control over the amount of anthelmintic that individual animals consume, unless they are fed separately or in small supervised groups. Therefore a risk exists that some animals will receive less than the recommended dose for their weight and that others will receive more. On account of the high safety margin of the benzimidazoles, however, this should not be a problem.

Dosing Paste Syringes

Many anthelmintics for equine use are presented in paraffin-based oral dosing syringes. The precalibrated amount of paste is deposited carefully on the animal's tongue. This is now a popular method in horses because it is less troublesome than stomach tubing and is more convenient and labor saving.

Sustained-release Formulations—Boluses

Slow-release devices represent a new approach to the way in which anthelmintics may be administered and the manner in which they can be used to control parasitic disease. With all parasiticide boluses, retention in the rumen is critical for efficacy. To minimize the risk of boluses being coughed up and lost, a critical density is incorporated into the bolus design to ensure that the weighted delivery device remains continually in the gut. The morantel sustained-release bolus is a cylindrical metal bolus comprising an inner drug reservoir and a microporous barrier permeable to drug passage by diffusion. The pores of the material in contact with the drug reservoir contain a hydrogel and provide controlled, predictable release rates of drug for an extended period. The bolus is loaded with 13.5 g of morantel tartrate in polyethylene glycol, the active principle escaping across the cellulose acetate end-discs at a constant rate of approximately 90 mg/day for the duration of the grazing season. The bolus is given prophylactically at turnout, and the continuous low-level release of morantel suppresses worm egg output by treated animals, reduces larval infection on pasture, and prevents appearance of clinical parasitism. Through the strategic use of the bolus, the normal epidemiologic pattern of bovine gastrointestinal nematodiasis is effectively disrupted.

Oxfendazole is available in the form of a pulsed-release bolus for use in cattle between 100 and 200 kg body weight. The bolus is designed to release oxfendazole not continuously but intermittently as full therapeutic dose (750 mg) five times at approximately 21-day intervals. The bolus device is made up of a polyvinyl chloride segment, five individual cells, a corroding central alloy core, and a steel end weight to prevent regurgitation from the rumen. Each individual cell comprises a circular tablet containing 750 mg oxfendazole and a silicone rubber sealing washer. In the rumen, corrosion of the central steel-magnesium alloy spring leaves the polyvinyl chloride caps between the oxfendazole tablets unsupported. As the divider drops off, the oxfendazole tablet is left exposed. This process is repeated at approximately 23-day intervals, giving a life span of 130 days to the bolus. Pulsed-release systems are claimed to possess fewer problems than the continued-release-type bolus, in which constant subtherapeutic levels of anthelmintic are leached out.

The electronic bolus containing albendazole is encased in a weighted polypropylene shell. This device delivers three full therapeutic doses of albendazole at 31-day intervals. Similar to other boluses, it is administered by balling gun at turnout. In the rumen, rubber biosensors within the bolus powered by two manganese batteries switch the device on, and a silicon chip microprocessor triggers an impulse to three carbon-dioxide-generating drug expulsion mechanisms, which drive the drug out of the device into the rumen. The microprocessor then automatically resets and begins a countdown to the next 31-day interval release time.

The levamisole bolus is a compact polymeric bolus containing 22 g of levamisole. Encased in an outer impermeable shell, the polymeric matrix becomes slowly impregnated with water, increasing the internal surface area and ultimately expelling the levamisole through the single outer pore. A sustained-release formulation of ivermectin is currently being developed for use in ruminant animals. To date, osmotic pump delivery systems containing ivermectin have been investigated with a view to ensuring rate-controlled release of ivermectin over prolonged periods of time. This slow-release preparation which releases ivermectin for 135 days is now available in some countries.

ABSORPTION AND DISTRIBUTION OF ANTHELMINTIC COMPOUNDS

After administration, anthelmintics are absorbed from the stomach and intestines (oral preparations), from the subcutaneous tissues (injectable preparations), or through the skin (pour-on preparations) and enter the blood stream. In the blood, they are transported to different parts of the body, particularly the liver, where they are broken down (metabolized) and eventually passed out (excreted) in the feces and urine. With some anthelmintics, e.g., probenzimidazoles, antiparasitic activity lies not with the chemical that was originally given, but with the compound that results from its breakdown in the body. The speed with which an anthelmintic is metabolized and excreted from the body tissues and fluids determines the length of the withholding period, which is required by law before an animal can be slaughtered or milk sold for human consumption after treatment. The rate at which chemicals are metabolized and excreted can vary among animal species; it may also be affected by the route of administration and the dose rate.

Absorption

Although many parasites reside in the gut lumen or close to the gastrointestinal mucosa, other major parasites dwell at tissue sites more remote from the gut, i.e., liver and lungs. Thus absorption from the gut is usually required for anthelmintic action against these latter parasites. Intestinal parasites come in contact with the anthelmintic not only from the unabsorbed drug passing through the digestive tract, but also from the absorbed fraction of the dose that is carried to the intestinal mucosa by way of the circulation. This has been shown to be of major importance with many of the benzimidazole compounds.

Absorbed oxfendazole is at least as important in achieving efficacy against nematodes in the abomasum and small intestine as the unabsorbed drug passing down the gastrointestinal tract. Once in the blood stream, oxfendazole recycles across the gut wall between the vascular system and the gastrointestinal tract. Worms in the mucosa of the abomasum and small intestine may be exposed to this recycling anthelmintic to a greater extent than to drug contained in the passing digesta in the lumen of the gastrointestinal tract. It is now clear also that much of the anthelmintic activity of albendazole and fenbendazole is associated with their sulfoxide metabolites formed after metabolism in the liver.

Oxfendazole is a sulfoxide and is identical to the sulfoxide of fenbendazole. Most tests of anthelmintic activity have shown oxfendazole to be more potent than fenbendazole. After oral administration of fenbendazole, appreciable levels of its active metabolite oxfendazole are present in the abomasal fluid, indicating gut recycling and passive diffusion from the blood stream into the abomasum. Thus absorbed benzimidazoles are extensively secreted into the gastrointestinal tract by way of the circulation. Oxfendazole is the active metabolite of albendazole, fenbendazole, and febantel after their absorption from the gut, biotransformation in the liver, and resecretion into the alimentary tract. The persistence of high blood concentrations of such active benzimidazoles has been shown to be of importance for activity against both tissue-dwelling parasites, such as arrested *Ostertagia ostertagi* larvae, and parasites on the gut mucosa, such as *Haemonchus* and *Trichostrongylus*.

The efficacy of benzimidazole anthelmintics is related to the duration of exposure of the parasite to the drug, with prolongation of contact time being required to ensure effective action. A rapidly absorbed, rapidly metabolized, and rapidly excreted drug such as thiabendazole is anthelmintically less potent than the more slowly metabolized, slowly excreted benzimidazole such as fenbendazole. Because this group of anthelmintics acts on microtubules within the nematode cell, thereby interfering with the cellular energy systems, cell death within the parasite occurs after all energy sources are exhausted. This process is slow and requires prolongation of contact time between the drug and the parasite. It is a lengthy process compared with the much quicker actions of anthelmintics such as levamisole, which acts on the nematode's nervous system, inducing paralysis. Many of the more recent, more effective benzimidazoles (fenbendazole, albendazole, oxfendazole) have been synthesized by modifying the side chains of the basic benzimidazole nucleus, characterized by the prototype drug thiabendazole. The pro-drugs or benzimidazole precursors, such as thiophanate and febantel, have been shown to be metabolized into true benzimidazoles within the target animal. The increased efficacy of these compounds arising from this chemical modification renders them less soluble and more difficult to absorb, so they take longer to achieve peak blood levels and take longer to be eliminated. Operation of the esophageal groove reflex after oral administration may contribute to variation in field efficacy of many benzimidazoles against various parasites, especially those in the arrested state. If benzimidazole anthelmintics for the treatment of abomasal infestations were administered routinely by the intraruminal route, it would be expected that efficacy against inhibited ostertagia larvae would be improved.

Metabolism and Excretion

Metabolism of anthelmintics is important in determining whether the end product (metabolite) is pharmacologically active or inactive. Metabolism may occur in the alimentary tract, as in the case of albendazole and fenbendazole, which are reduced from sulfide to the active sulfoxide in the rumen. In flukicides such as diamphenethide, this metabolism within the gastrointestinal tract may be important for full efficacy. (Nitroxynil is metabolized by rumen bacteria that destroy its activity and so restrict administration to injection.) The more usual site of metabolism is the liver, where oxidation and cleavage reactions commonly take place. Thiabendazole is rapidly metabolized in the liver, with the sulfate and glucuronide metabolites being increasingly soluble in water and rapidly excreted by the kidney.

Frequently resecretion of active metabolites back into the alimentary tract may occur. Many of the more modern benzimidazoles re-enter the gastrointestinal tract by passive diffusion in the active metabolite form—the sulfoxide. The biliary route may also be important in recycling benzimidazoles such as albendazole to the gastrointestinal tract. Resecretion by way of the liver and bile is especially important, however, for drugs active against adult *Fasciola hepatica*.

Many flukicides, such as the salicylanilides and the substituted phenols, appear to bind strongly to plasma proteins. The fasciolicidal effects of salicylanilides, such as rafoxanide in sheep, were found to depend on the persistence of the drug in the plasma. This association with plasma protein is important for their transport throughout the body as well as in reducing the rate of elimination from the host animal. Associated with the persistence of such compounds, however, is the necessity for long withholding periods. Oxyclozanide also is bound to plasma protein and is then metabolized in the liver to the anthelmintically active glucuronide and excreted in high concentration in the bile duct, where it encounters masses of the mature flukes. Immature flukes in the liver parenchyma ingest mainly liver cells containing little anthelmintic; the high protein binding of the drug limits its entry into the tissue cell. As the flukes grow and migrate through the liver, they cause extensive hemorrhaging and come into contact with plasma-protein-bound anthelmintic. When the parasites reach the bile ducts, they are in the main excretory channels for the flukicides present in the active metabolite form and thus are exposed to high concentrations. This may explain why the mature fluke is more vulnerable to the effects of these flukicides than the immature fluke. Because higher concentrations of flukicides and their metabolites are found in feces than in urine, it is reasonable to assume that the bile ducts are the main excretory pathways for these anthelmintics.

Diamphenethide is metabolized in the gut as well as to a greater extent in the liver to an active metabolite, which can enter the tissue cells of the liver and exert its antiparasitic effect against young stages of the parasite. The low plasma protein binding of this compound coupled with the rapid excretion of its active metabolite necessitates only a short withholding time for this particular preparation. A recent benzimidazole anthelmintic, triclabendazole, has been discovered to be efficient against mature and early immature *F. hepatica* infections in cattle and sheep. At a recommended dose of 10–12 mg/kg orally, triclabendazole possesses potent antiparasitic action against the early parasite in the liver parenchyma and maintains this high level of activity against the parasites as they reach maturity in the bile ducts. The maximum tolerated dose in the target species is 200 mg/kg; thus the compound has a working safety margin of 20. This is a useful feature in any flukicide.

Of the other benzimidazoles, such as fenbendazole, mebendazole, and albendazole, which are used for nematode control, some possess marginal efficacy at elevated dosage rates against liver flukes. Only albendazole, however, is recommended for use against *F. hepatica*, and its activity is directed against flukes at least 12 weeks of age. Because of the lack of efficacy against the immature stages, benzimidazoles generally are not useful for treatment of acute fascioliasis or for strategic control of the disease. Triclabendazole, however, is unique among the presently available benzimidazoles in possessing high activity against the immature and mature stages.

Withholding Times

Modern benzimidazoles are retained in the body much longer than earlier members of the group; they therefore have longer withholding periods. Thiabendazole is absorbed from the gut and excreted from the body so quickly that only a short withholding period is required after its use in cattle and sheep. In contrast, fenbendazole, oxfendazole, and albendazole are absorbed from the rumen more slowly and excreted over a longer period, necessitating long withholding periods for meat and milk. The longer persistence in the body of fenbendazole, oxfendazole, and albendazole is thought to be one of the reasons why they possess greater activity against immature worms, particularly those arrested in their development, than other members of the group. A similar relationship between the rate of metabolism of an anthelmintic and its activity against immature parasites exists with certain flukicides. After administration, rafoxanide, nitroxynil, brotianide, and oxyclozanide are all absorbed into the blood stream, where they become bound to proteins in the blood. In this bound state, they are transported to the liver, where they are metabolized and excreted in the bile, i.e., the environment inhabited by adult liver flukes. Rafoxanide, nitroxynil, and brotianide bind more strongly to blood proteins than oxyclozanide and therefore remain for longer periods in the blood. This longer persistence in the blood stream is associated with greater activity against immature liver flukes.

Safety in Use

In general, modern anthelmintics have high safety margins; the maximum dose that can be given to an animal before adverse effects are noticed is much higher than the dose recommended for use. For benzimidazoles, the safety index is invariably high. This safety margin is not so high for levamisole (safety index = 6) or for the chemicals active against liver fluke (safety indices = 3 to 6). It should also be noted that if for any reason the dosage rate of an anthelmintic is increased, the safety margin is correspondingly decreased; if the dosage rate is doubled, the safety index is halved.

Many situations occur also in which animals may, inadvertently, receive less than the full dose of anthelmintic recommended by the manufacturer. As a result, the efficiency of the anthelmintic may be lowered.

4.2 BENZIMIDAZOLES

Many related compounds, all based on the prototype parent compound thiabendazole, are now available on the market, each one claiming distinct advantages and applications for antiparasitic use. The ever-increasing number of benzimidazoles appearing regularly is a good example of so-called molecular manipulation or "molecular roulette," whereby individual pharmaceutical companies endeavor to compete with a rival company's successful product without breaching the patent rights of a particular compound. The benzimidazole parasiticides constitute the largest chemical family of veterinary drugs used for treatment of endoparasitic diseases in domestic animals. They are characterized by broad-spectrum activity against a range of parasites and high safety indices in target species. Their high degree of clinical efficacy under field conditions of use is related both to pharmacodynamic and to pharmacokinetic characteristics. The benzimidazoles of immediate interest are thiabendazole, cambendazole, parbendazole, mebendazole, fenbendazole, triclabendazole, oxfendazole, oxibendazole, albendazole, flubendazole, luxabendazole, thiophanate, febantel, and netobimin. Of the wide number of these drugs used in veterinary medicine, only thiabendazole and mebendazole have been used as anthelmintics in humans. In veterinary medicine, both albendazole and triclabendazole possess activity against liver flukes. Table 4–2 depicts the spectrum of activity of commonly used benzimidazoles.

CHEMISTRY

The benzimidazole group is derived from the simple benzimidazole nucleus and includes the thiabendazole analogs and the benzimidazole carbamates. Substitution of various side chains and radicals on the parent nucleus gives rise to the individual members of this group. Modification of the kinetics of a particular benzimidazole indirectly affects clinical potency because such factors as relative insolubility, slow elimination, and persistent circulation of parent drug or active metabolites increase the drug-parasite contact time. On account of

TABLE 4–2
BENZIMIDAZOLES AND THEIR GENERAL ANTIPARASITIC SPECTRUM

Group	Chemical Name	Gastrointestinal Tract Nematodes	Inhibited Larvae	Lungworm	Fluke	Mode of Action in Parasite	Effect
Benzimidazoles	Thiabendazole	+	−	−	−	Interfere with energy production	Starvation parasite (slow process)
	Parbendazole	+	+	−	−	Inhibit fumarate reductase	
	Fenbendazole	+	+	+	−	Block tubulin synthesis	
	Oxfendazole	+	+	+	−	Inhibit glucose transport	Ovicidal
	Albendazole	+	+	+	+		
	Triclabendazole	−	−	−	+		
Probenzimidazoles	Febantel	+	+	+	−	Metabolized in vivo to benzimidazole carbamates	As above
	Thiophanate	+	±	−	−		
	Netobimin	+	+	+	+		

the pharmacodynamic mechanism of action of these drugs, such prolongation of contact time increases both antiparasitic efficacy and spectrum.

Thiabendazole was the first commercially available benzimidazole introduced for use in domestic animals in 1961. Metabolism of this prototype compound occurs by way of hydroxylation to the 5-hydroxy compound, which is then rapidly eliminated in the urine as the glucuronide. Efforts to prolong the presence of this substance in the body (to amplify potency) led to the introduction of a substituent to prevent rapid hydroxylation. From this development, the related compound cambendazole was produced. Further studies on the chemical classes of substituents paved the way for newer benzimidazole molecules characterized by longer half-lives in the animal body, distinct biotransformation pathways, and greater potency (see Table 4–2). Inherent in this tendency toward slower body clearance was the necessity to observe longer tissue and milk withholding times. Subsequently many new benzimidazoles with increased potency have been developed, facilitating lower dosage rates (mg/kg) and an increased spectrum of activity to include both lungworms and tapeworms. Fenbendazole was the first anthelmintic with high efficacy against arrested *O. ostertagi* larvae.

Most of the modern benzimidazoles possess a carbamate substituent. Variations in efficacy between these carbamates is principally a function of their different kinetics. A number of benzimidazoles exist as pro-drugs. Their anthelmintic activity is due to the fact that they are metabolized in the animal body to the biologically active benzimidazole carbamate nucleus. Febantel, thiophanate, and netobimin are examples of such pro-drugs. Synthesis of benzimidazole carbamates depends on a cyclization process. Metabolic or chemical activation generates an active benzimidazole in vivo from an inactive pro-drug precursor. Cyclization occurs in the case of thiophanate. Febantel is hydrolyzed to the active metabolite fenbendazole. Netobimin undergoes a process both of reduction and of cyclization to yield the active compound albendazole. Netobimin is a nitrophenylguanidine that is cyclized to albendazole after reduction of the nitro group to an amino group, and febantel

is a phenylguanidine that is hydrolyzed by removal of a methoxyacetyl group and then cyclized to fenbendazole.

Newer benzimidazole carbamates are characterized by novel substituents on the benzimidazole nucleus and the replacement of the thiazole ring by methylcarbamate. Such molecular modifications have spawned a new benzimidazole generation, with much slower rates of elimination, higher potencies, broader spectra, and complex metabolic pathways. Inherent in these developments is the attendant risk of greater biological reactivity of their metabolites and the possibility of their heightened toxicologic significance.

Early benzimidazoles, such as thiabendazole, were quite soluble and quickly eliminated from the body. The most effective compounds of the group are the less soluble compounds, such as oxfendazole, fenbendazole, and albendazole, which remain as solid precipitates within the gut for a longer time. As the solid form slowly dissolves, effective concentrations are maintained for an extended period both in plasma and in the gut, increasing the efficacy of these compounds against immature and arrested larvae and adult nematodes. The following points regarding benzimidazole usage should be noted.

1. Benzimidazoles are more effective in ruminants and horses, in which their kinetics are slowed by the presence of a rumen or caecum.
2. Abomasal parasites are less susceptible to abomasally administered drug than to the same drug given orally.
3. Divided doses are more effective than a single dose because the nature of their antiparasitic action depends on prolongation of contact time.
4. The most effective benzimidazoles are less soluble than earlier compounds; i.e., their kinetics are slowed. Efficacy against lungworm has also been noted for these insoluble benzimidazoles (Table 4–3).
5. Benzimidazoles are much less effective parenterally and are given only orally.

Extending the period of exposure by administering the more soluble drugs such as thiabendazole over a prolonged period of time improves their efficacy.

TABLE 4–3
GENERAL SPECTRUM OF ACTIVITY OF SOME COMMONLY USED ANTHELMINTICS IN RUMINANTS

Group	Chemical Name	Gastrointestinal Tract Nematodes	Inhibited Larvae	Lungworm	Fluke
Benzimidazoles	Thiabendazole	+	–	–	–
	Parbendazole	+	±	–	–
	Fenbendazole	+	+	+	–
	Oxfendazole	+	+	+	–
	Albendazole	+	+	+	+
	Triclabendazole	–	–	–	+
Probenzimidazoles	Febantel	+	+	–	–
	Thiophanate	+	±	+	–
Imidazothiazoles	Levamisole	+	–	+	–
Pyrimidines	Morantel (bolus)	+	Prevents establishment	Prevents establishment	–
Avermectins /Milbemycins	Ivermectin	+	+	+	–
	/doramectin	+	+	+	–
	/moxidectin	+	–	–	–
Organophosphates	Haloxan/Coumaphos	+	–	+	+
Piperazine	Diethylcarbamazine	–	–	–	–
Salicylanilides	Rafoxanide	–	–	–	–
	Oxyclozanide	–	–	–	–
Substituted phenols	Nitroxynil	–	–	–	+
	Niclofolan	–	–	–	+
	Bithionol sulfoxide	–	–	–	+
	Hexachlorophene	–	–	–	+
Aromatic amide	Diamfenetide	–	–	–	+
Sulfonamides	Clorsulon	–	–	–	+

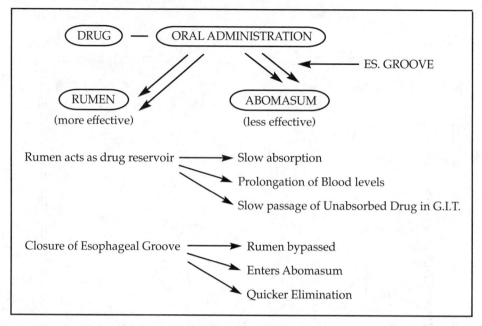

FIG. 4–1. The significance of the esophageal groove reflex.

For many of the potent benzimidazoles, anthelmintic activity is related to the sulfoxide metabolite. Oxfendazole is the sulfoxide metabolite of fenbendazole, and fenbendazole owes much of its activity to the oxfendazole formed from it. Albendazole requires metabolism to the sulfoxide in the liver to be active, whereas febantel requires metabolism to fenbendazole and the oxfendazole to be active.

Potency also increases with the arrival of newer members of the benzimidazole group. This is reflected by a decrease in dosage rate, i.e., from 50 mg/kg for thiabendazole to 20 mg/kg for parbendazole, 15 mg/kg for mebendazole, and 5–7.5 mg/kg for fenbendazole. Because of the relatively slow excretion rate, the newer insoluble benzimidazoles have fairly long withholding times for milk and meat in contrast to the less effective, more rapidly excreted thiabendazole. Strict observance of these withholding times is always necessary because of the potentially toxic and teratogenic effects of some of these parent compounds and their metabolites.

In ruminant animals, oral dosing with the benzimidazoles removes all the major adult gastrointestinal tract parasites and many of the larval stages. Albendazole, fenbenda-

zole, oxfendazole, and febantel possess activity against inhibited *Ostertagia* fourth-stage larvae. The degree of efficacy of these compounds in the prophylaxis of ostertagiasis type II may be related to the degree of hypobiosis of the larvae; i.e., those with a low metabolic rate have a low energy requirement and thus are not amenable to disruption by the benzimidazoles, and also to the operation of the esophageal groove bypass effect (Figs. 4–1 and 4–2).

PHARMACOKINETICS

Being sparingly soluble in water, most benzimidazoles are given orally in suspensions, pastes, or powders. Differences in the rate and extent of absorption from the alimentary tract depend on such factors as species, dosage, formulation, bioavailability, and operation of the esophageal groove reflex. The differences in kinetics of the benzimidazoles, especially the sulfoxide metabolites that are thought to be the most anthelmintically active forms, between sheep and cattle and goats account for the different efficacy of the drugs in each species and thus the higher dosages recommended for cattle and goats for single

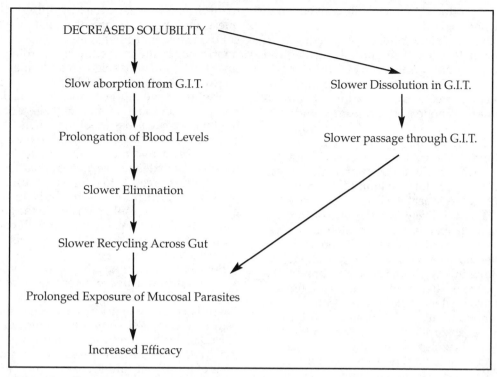

FIG. 4–2. The effect of benzimidazole solubility on potency.

administration. Benzimidazoles display large kinetic differences between ruminant and monogastric species.

Anatomic features, such as the rumen and caecum of ruminant and equine species, which slow the passage and digesta in these species, may enhance the activity of the benzimidazoles by extending their transit time. This has been confirmed in sheep after oral and intra-abomasal administration of fenbendazole, whereby the drug maintains high plasma concentrations for a prolonged period when given orally. The kinetics of the benzimidazoles differ between species of ruminant. Thiabendazole achieves higher plasma concentrations in sheep than in cattle and goats. This may reflect a reduced capacity for oxidative metabolism in the sheep because a higher proportion of parent thiabendazole than its major metabolite 5-hydroxythiabendazole is excreted in the urine of sheep than cattle.

For most members of the benzimidazole group, extensive biotransformation occurs primarily in the liver, although extrahepatic sites may be involved in metabolic conver-

sion. Metabolism takes the form of oxidative or hydrolytic cleavage processes, resulting in free water-soluble metabolites. These metabolites concentrate in the plasma, tissues, bile, and urine. Biliary secretion of metabolites and conjugates may occur, and the more polar metabolites are readily excreted in the urine. Elimination through the milk and feces is observed also; some enterohepatic circulation takes place. Biological activity can be associated with the parent drug alone, its metabolites, or in some cases both. For thiabendazole and cambendazole, anthelmintic activity resides with the parent drug nucleus alone.

For more recent benzimidazole carbamates, the processes of biotransformation and metabolic interconversion are more complex. Metabolites are associated with anthelmintic activity and biological reactivity. This is especially true of many of the sulfoxide and sulfone derivatives. For prodrugs, such as febantel, thiophanate, and netobimin, biological activity resides in the resultant benzimidazole carbamate metabolites produced by metabolic conversion in the body.

Oxfendazole and fenbendazole are both known to be anthelmintically active and metabolically interconvertible. After administration of oxfendazole to the horse, however, greater concentrations of both oxfendazole and fenbendazole (area under the curve [AUC] 3.17 and 2.32 µg/ml) were achieved in the plasma than after the administration of the same dose (10 mg/kg) of fenbendazole alone, after which oxfendazole was below the limit of detection and fenbendazole achieved an AUC of only 1.77 µg/ml. It is likely that the rate of metabolism of fenbendazole into oxfendazole was exceeded by the subsequent conversion of oxfendazole into oxfendazole sulfone, resulting in low plasma concentrations of oxfendazole after administration of fenbendazole. Oxfendazole is more soluble than fenbendazole, and this may explain its greater absorption in the horse. In the dog, benzimidazoles are absorbed and excreted rapidly, reducing the length of time parasites are exposed to the drugs, and divided dosage regimens (usually once daily for 5 days) are recommended.

The sulfoxide of albendazole (albendazole oxide) is also marketed as an anthelmintic. Although albendazole, netobimin, and albendazole oxide have activity against *F. hepatica*, they are useful only against older stages of the parasite. Only triclabendazole has good efficacy against all stages of the liver fluke, but unfortunately it is ineffective against parasitic nematodes. A new benzimidazole, luxabendazole, with activity against nematodes, cestodes, and trematodes, has been marketed.

The pharmacokinetics of fenbendazole in serum or plasma have been examined in a variety of mammalian species after oral or intragastric administration. Several of these studies have also identified or quantified the four known metabolites of fenbendazole. The major metabolite is fenbendazole sulfoxide (oxfendazole), which also possesses anthelmintic activity. Considerable information is available on the disposition and elimination of fenbendazole and its metabolites. Little of the parent drug or any of its metabolites are excreted in the urine of any species. Likewise, the sulfoxide and sulfone metabolites are present in feces and urine in small quantities, bringing into question the importance of fenbendazole sulfoxide (oxfendazole) as an active anthelmintic metabolite in the lower gastrointestinal tract. Fenbendazole is readily metabolized to its sulfoxide, oxfendazole, which is also an active anthelmintic. This oxidation occurs in the liver and may also occur in other organs or tissues of mammals. The sulfoxide can be further oxidized to the sulfone, a less active metabolite. The fenbendazole and oxfendazole metabolites have been found to recycle to the gastrointestinal tract after absorption, particularly to the abomasum. As a result, parasites in the gastrointestinal tract are exposed to high concentrations of fenbendazole and its metabolite oxfendazole.

Both oxfendazole and fenbendazole are anthelmintically active, whereas the sulfone metabolite has no anthelmintic activity. There is some evidence from the metabolism of the related sulfide benzimidazole, albendazole, that the sulfoxide has good activity per se because the plasma concentrations of the parent sulfide are extremely low compared with the sulfoxide metabolite, whereas systemic anthelmintic activity of this compound is high.

Albendazole and triclabendazole are both metabolized to their sulfoxide metabolites, and because negligible amounts of the parent drug are found after oral administration, they are assumed to undergo first-pass oxidative metabolism in the liver. Low concentrations of albendazole have been detected in the plasma of sheep after the intraruminal administration of netobimin. It is subsequently oxidized to albendazole sulfoxide and sulfone as noted earlier for fenbendazole.

In clinical trials, oxfendazole is generally found to have similar efficacy at a lower dosage rate, and this results in the recommended therapeutic dosage rate for cattle being higher for fenbendazole than for oxfendazole. Most of the anthelmintic activity of fenbendazole is due to the oxfendazole metabolites. Oxfendazole, in a test of anthelmintic efficacy in mice, was more active than were fenbendazole and the sulfone. As with albendazole, the sulfoxide, oxfendazole, is the result of hepatic metabolism, and its presence in the abomasum is due to passive diffusion from the systemic compartment.

PHARMACODYNAMICS AND TOXICOLOGY

Active benzimidazoles are considered to have a similar mode of action and to be relatively equipotent. Differences in their efficacy in vivo have been attributed to different pharmacokinetics in the host and in vitro to their solubility and consequent absorption by the parasite from the culture medium. Benzimidazoles act by inhibiting the uptake of low-molecular-weight nutrients by the parasite, which then starves. This is brought about by a binding process between the active benzimidazole and tubulin, a structural protein. Blockage of polymerization of tubulin into microtubules damages the integrity and function of the absorptive cells within the parasite. Enzymes of energy metabolism, such as fumarate reductase, are also inhibited by benzimidazoles, and so the parasite can neither absorb nor use its foodstuffs. The antiparasitic effect is accordingly a lethal but relatively tardy process.

All benzimidazoles are thought to have a similar mode of action, and differences in efficacy of the drugs reflect differences in bioavailability. Studies to investigate the mode of action of the benzimidazoles have concentrated on the antimitotic properties of some members of the group. The antimitotic activity was suggested to be due to disruption in the formation of the mitotic spindle. Rat brain tubulin studies suggested that the antimitotic activity of the benzimidazoles was due to binding to tubulin. The attachment of benzimidazoles to tubulin molecules caused inhibition of the formation of microtubules, resulting in disruption of cell division. A similar mechanism of tubulin binding and disruption of the microtubular framework within cells was suggested as a possible reason for the anthelmintic activity exhibited by the benzimidazoles.

The anthelmintic action of benzimidazoles is due to differences in the sensitivity of host and parasite cells to the tubulin binding effects of the benzimidazoles. Microtubules are considered essential for enzyme secretion by parasites. Binding of benzimidazoles to tubulin is a reversible and saturable effect. An association has been established between antitubulin activity and teratogenicity for a number of compounds, including griseofulvin colchicine and vincristine. Mutagenic activity can also be associated with antitubulin activity. Antimitotic and genotoxic effects have been documented for many benzimidazoles. In the light of experimental work revealing genotoxic effects, such as chromosome nondisjunction, the question of potential carcinogenicity must be addressed.

The antimicrotubular effect of the benzimidazole compounds may cause disruption of the mitotic spindle. This could lead to nondisjunction of chromosomes during cell replication, and the benzimidazoles are suspected of having a mutagenic effect. In mammals, however, changes in the number of chromosomes usually lead to cell death. This may be why there is no correlation between the antimitotic activity and the mutagenic effect of the benzimidazole compounds.

The high safety margin of benzimidazoles for target animals is due to the greater selective affinity for parasitic tubulin than for mammalian tissues. Nonetheless, some toxic effects based on antimitotic activity (teratogenicity/genotoxicity) do occur in target species. Hence the selective toxicity of benzimidazoles is not absolute. Therefore differences in binding of these benzimidazoles to tubulin from parasites and mammalian tissues may account for the differential toxicity of the benzimidazoles between host and parasitic cells. The benzimidazole anthelmintics have very high margins of safety, e.g., for fenbendazole and oxfendazole; lethal doses cannot be established during evaluation. The low solubility of the more potent benzimidazole compounds could account for this low toxicity because insufficient drug is absorbed to have a toxic effect. The main toxic effect of the benzimidazole compounds, however, involves their teratogenic effect. This effect varies with structure of the benzimidazole, and there is species variation in susceptibility.

Teratogenicity

The possible teratogenic effect of the benzimidazoles was identified first with parbendazole in sheep. The main congenital defects identified in the lambs were skeletal malformations, occurring mainly in the long bones, pelvis, joints, and digits; there were no central nervous system lesions identified.

Cambendazole, oxfendazole, albendazole, and febantel are also teratogenic in this species, whereas fenbendazole, mebendazole, and oxibendazole are not. Teratogenic effects occur at relatively low dosage rates, much lower than those associated with acute toxicity states in target species. Species differences occur in domestic animals and in laboratory animals, as regards susceptibility to teratogenic effects. Dosage rate, specific benzimidazole, and stage of embryonic development are major influencing factors. Cattle seem to be unaffected by most benzimidazoles that are teratogenic in sheep. A similar relationship exists between rats and rabbits. These species differences in the sensitivity to the teratogenic activity of the benzimidazoles may be due to the kinetics and metabolism of the drug in the various species.

Fenbendazole is not teratogenic, probably because of poor intestinal absorption (5% in the rat) and metabolic considerations. Oxfendazole has poor antitubulin activity in vitro but is teratogenic in the rat and sheep. The bioavailability of oxfendazole is greater than that of fenbendazole, and it is metabolically interchangeable with fenbendazole intracellularly. Many benzimidazoles teratogenic in sheep are also teratogenic in rats.

Although benzimidazoles all possess similar pharmacodynamic effects (antitubulin), species differences in terms of sensitivity to embryotoxic effects are attributable to metabolic and pharmacokinetic disposition factors. Benzimidazoles can be classified as:

- Those that are not teratogenic per se and have no teratogenic metabolite (oxibendazole)
- Those that are not teratogenic and give rise to a teratogenic metabolite (fenbendazole)
- Those that seem to be teratogenic per se and have no teratogenic metabolite (oxfendazole)
- Those that are possibly teratogenic per se and have additionally a metabolite that seems to be more toxic than the one of the parent compound (mebendazole)

TISSUE CLEARANCE

Thiabendazole is rapidly absorbed and metabolized by the liver. In cattle and sheep, peak plasma levels are attained in approximately 4 hours, with metabolites accounting for up to 30% of the total concentration. The major primary metabolite is the 5-hydroxy component, which further conjugates with sulfate and glucuronide to increase water solubility and the rate of renal clearance. The duration of pharmacologic activity of thiabendazole is short. Nonetheless, using 35S-thiabendazole, levels are still detectable in the brain, heart, liver, kidney, and pancreas of sheep 5 days after dosing. At 16 days post-dosing, radioactivity is detectable in the liver and muscle. Similar findings have been reported for calves and pigs. Using 35S-thiabendazole in calves, radioactivity-associated levels have been detected in the liver 59 days after administration. This hepatic incorporation is indicative of metabolic incorporation into the endogenous pool, rather than drug storage, binding, and residue burden deposition.

The metabolism and excretion of thiabendazole is more extensive in cattle than in sheep. The bovine species seems to possess greater capacity for oxidative metabolism for benzimidazole parasiticides. Systemic anthelmintic activity is greater in sheep than in cattle for thiabendazole. Clinically this is exemplified by the fact that although thiabendazole is ineffective against lungworm infestation in cattle, it does possess useful activity against the ovine lung parasite. The brief duration of action of thiabendazole in animals is attributable to its solubility and rapid metabolism to pharmacologically inactive metabolites.

Residues of albendazole, oxfendazole, fenbendazole, febantel, and thiabendazole concentrate primarily in liver tissue in cattle and sheep and persist longest in this tissue. At therapeutic dosage rates, residue levels in liver exceed those of muscle and kidney. Residues are more persistent for fenbendazole, oxfendazole, and febantel than for albendazole or thiabendazole. Although residues are detectable in milk for these drugs, their presence is relatively short-lived.

The use of oxfendazole in cattle is associated with low levels of residues in milk. Using high performance liquid chromatography (HPLC) after oral administration at 5 mg/kg, oxfendazole is not detectable beyond 72 hours. In sheep, oxfendazole reaches peak plasma concentration at 30 hours, whereas albendazole sulfoxide peaks at 20 hours.

Nine metabolites of albendazole were identified in the urine of cattle and sheep that were given the labeled drug orally. Metabolic conversions included oxidation at sulfur, alkyl, and aromatic hydroxylation; methylation at both nitrogen and sulfur; and carbamate hydrolysis. All detectable urinary metabolites were sulfoxides or sulfones; unchanged albendazole was present in only minor amounts.

After dosing of cattle with 2.5% suspension of febantel at a dosage rate of 7.5 mg/g, febantel sulfone, fenbendazole, and oxfendazole were detectable in milk. At 12 hours, levels were 0.16 ppm for the parent compound, 0.035 ppm for fenbendazole, and 0.105 ppm for oxfendazole. At 60 hours post-dosing, levels were approximately 0.01 ppm.

In various tests, triclabendazole showed no mutagenic effects, and no embryotoxicity or teratogenicity was observed in rats, sheep, and cattle. After oral administration, triclabendazole is satisfactorily reabsorbed and biotransformed, the two main metabolites formed being the sulfoxide and sulfone derivatives. More that 95% of the quantity administered orally is eliminated in the feces, about 2% in the urine, and less than 1% in the milk. After oral doses of 10 mg/kg in sheep and 12 mg/kg in cattle, residues of triclabendazole and its metabolites are detectable in edible tissue (muscle, liver, kidneys) over a prolonged period. The residue concentrations in edible tissue drop to below 0.4 mg/kg within 28 days in sheep and 14 days in cattle.

Parbendazole C14 administered orally to sheep at 45 mg/kg resulted in peak plasma levels of C14 activity at 6 hours. Plasma levels dropped continuously until 48 hours, at which time concentrations less than 1 μg/ml were detected. Seven urinary metabolites were identified. Liver residues remained elevated at 1.41 ppm after 16 days. Poor absorption and low tissue concentrations were recorded in lambs given C14 mebendazole. Liver concentration was highest and radioactivity in this organ was still de-

tectable at day 15 post-dosing. In the case of C14 cambendazole in calves, liver radioactivity was detectable 30 days after administration, and a fraction of this was in the bound form.

Residual Fractions

Three types of residues rapidly appear after drug administration:

1. Total residues, determined by overall quantitative assessment of residual radioactivity after administration of the labeled compound. This value is often used but has the major disadvantage of expressing a nonspecific radioactivity. In this way, residues, the nature of which is unknown or different from that of the initial molecule, are sometimes given an acceptable daily intake (ADI), which is relative to the initial compound. This practice is often disadvantageous.

2. Extractable residues, a fraction that, as the name implies, can be extracted from biological tissues or fluids using various solvents (water at varying pH, organic solvents) before and after denaturation of macromolecules. This fraction includes all compounds, i.e., the parent compound and the metabolites, in free form or loosely bound to tissues.

3. Nonextractable or bound residues, the fraction of radioactivity that persists in tissue extracts after the above-mentioned treatments. The nature of these residues can be determined only after almost complete breakage, particularly of proteins (enzymatic or acid hydrolysis, for instance); it may or may not be related to that of the initial molecule.

Bound Residues and Bioavailability

The bioavailability and toxicity of this bound-residue fraction often differs from that of the parent compound. Bound residues may contain degradation products of the parent compound in intermediary metabolism or new compounds resulting from covalent binding of the parent drug or metabolites to endogenous macromolecules. Recently an increasing number of drugs have been reported for which metabolism includes some covalent binding of metabolites to macromolecules. Several veterinary drugs belong to this list and give rise to nonextractable bound residues in tissues. This tissue-bound residue is of considerable interest because of the possible participation of this binding process in target species toxicity as well as its potential toxicologic significance in terms of food safety for humans.

The binding of reactive metabolites to biological macromolecules has been implicated in several toxic manifestations, including carcinogenicity, allergenic effects, hepatotoxicity, nephrotoxicity, neurotoxicity, lung toxicity, bone marrow toxicity, and teratogenicity. The mechanism of covalent binding of metabolites to macromolecules generally involves a preliminary metabolic oxidative reaction. It is not possible, however, to draw conclusions about the toxicologic significance of bound residues from absolute values of residue levels.

As is true of many xenobiotics, electrophilic reactants arise from biotransformation processes. This is also true of benzimidazoles, and resultant electrophilic metabolites undergo nonextractable binding. although the basic benzimidazole ring structure is relatively stable, for thiabendazole and cambendazole thiazole ring metabolism leads to incorporation into endogenous metabolism and hepatic tissue protein. Binding at the hepatic site has also been noted with albendazole.

Bound residues are believed to result from tissue reaction with a chemically reactive metabolite. The subsequent bioavailability of bound residues is known to be poor. Mebendazole and cambendazole are specific examples of benzimidazoles that form bound residues. With cambendazole, it is difficult to assess the precise nature of the bound form. The principal binding site is through interaction of the thiazole moiety with endogenous compounds. The toxicologic assessment of this nonextractable fraction is difficult. Residual radioactivity also depends on the type and position of radiolabeling. Bound residues of parbendazole found in the liver of sheep after 15 days have been attributed to incorporation of radioactivity into amino acids. In thiabendazole, liver radioactivity is also found in proteins, lipids, nucleic acids, and glycogen.

Early studies on the mode of action of benzimidazole anthelmintics indicated that they disrupt normal glucose metabolism by inhibition of key enzymes, such as fumarate reductase. More recent studies, however, have demonstrated that many benzimidazoles have an ability to bind to tubulin and thus interfere with normal microtubule function. Many benzimidazoles also prevent normal embryonation and hatching of nematode and trematode eggs, a process dependent in part on normal microtubule function. Fenbendazole, through its metabolite oxfendazole, possesses embryotoxic potential. Unchanged oxfendazole is responsible for the observed teratogenic effects through a mechanism that probably does not involve covalent binding of metabolites to tissues. The toxicity of these anthelmintics appears to be related to pharmacokinetics of their free metabolites. Bound residues for these compounds do not appear to have toxicologic significance for the target animal with respect to teratogenic effect.

Toxicologic assessment of bound residues can be attempted by bioavailability studies and relay toxicity methods. With cambendazole and albendazole, bound residue bioavailability is low. Experiments in rats demonstrated that after administration of calf liver treated with cambendazole, only 15% of total radioactivity was absorbed. Relay embryotoxicity studies for these two benzimidazoles in rats after feeding of liver residue tissue revealed no toxicity. Bioavailability of albendazole bound residues is 4 to 5% from beef liver.

Mebendazole has a poor oral bioavailability, owing to the extremely poor solubility in aqueous systems and the slow dissolution rate in the gastrointestinal tract. This is reflected by low plasma levels and the high fecal excretion of unchanged parent drug during the first 2 days after treatment. Maximal radioactivity remains in the gastrointestinal tract. The small amount of systemically absorbed mebendazole is distributed throughout the body.

Bound residues, although toxicologically potentially significant, could also theoretically be considered relatively nontoxic for many reasons. Once bound, it is possible that the fixed residue may no longer possess biological reactivity and become "unbound." When the risk involves allergenicity, bound residues may possess the potential to trigger off hypersensitivity reactions. Distinguishing between drug-related residues bound to macromolecules and fractions that have entered the normal metabolic pool is difficult.

Present evidence suggests that because of the low residue levels in target animal tissues and the observed low bioavailability, covalently bound residues should not present a major hazard. In the light of current scientific knowledge, their toxicologic significance is speculative.

Extractable Residues

Extractable residues of benzimidazoles undoubtedly constitute a relatively higher toxicologic risk. Concern regarding extractable residues is related to the established toxicologic properties of this group. The basis for the anthelmintic action of benzimidazoles is the inhibition of microtubular assembly by specific binding to tubulin. Because microtubules are involved in a variety of cellular activities, any disruption of this process affects important cellular activities (e.g., secretion, absorption, digestion). In contrast, degenerative changes are not observed in the host cells. This selectivity is based on the fact that parasite tubulin is much more susceptible for binding than mammalian tubulin. The anthelmintic activity of benzimidazoles is probably not based exclusively on this mechanism because numerous compounds with antitubulin activity, such as colchicine, vincristine, podophyllotoxin, and griseofulvin, are all teratogenic but have not been described as anthelmintics. Some benzimidazoles also inhibit enzymes of energy metabolism, such as fumarate reductase. The mechanism of the teratogenic effect of these compounds may be related to their reversible inhibitory activity against cell microtubulins, as for colchicine, vinblastine, and griseofulvin, which are teratogenic but not anthelmintic.

The antimicrotubular effect of benzimidazole compounds may cause disruption of the mitotic spindle. This could lead to nondisjunction of chromosomes during cell replication, and benzimidazoles are suspected of having a mutagenic effect. The selective toxicity of benzimidazoles for the parasites is not absolute because the toxic effects observed in mammals are, for the most part, antimitotic (teratogenicity, genotoxicity, alopecia, leukopenia, testicular lesions).

Residues of benzimidazole compounds in animal products and tissues may be important in the consideration of public health. The unbound drug or metabolites are likely to exert toxic effects in mammals, and the tightly protein-bound residues that persist in the tissues for longer periods of time are thought to be of lower significance toxicologically.

The free metabolites account not only for the primary and desirable anthelmintic activity, but also for the observed undesirable secondary toxic effects (embryotoxicity or teratogenicity) in specific compounds. A biological relationship exists between many metabolites and teratogenicity. Albendazole is embryotoxic in rats when the dosage exceeds 6 mg/kg. The urinary sulfoxide metabolites display embryotoxic properties, and these have bioavailability of 73%. The bioavailability of bound residues in edible tissue is 3 to 4.4%. Although extractable residues (parent drug, or free metabolites, or both) can be correlated with definitive toxicologic potential, safety margins can be defined. Some benzimidazoles, other than thiabendazole and fenbendazole, have been found to have high affinity for mammalian tubulin; this may result in a higher level of host toxicity, and some have been used successfully as anticancer drugs.

The consumer may be exposed to many active and inactive drug metabolites. Some of the inactive metabolites could conceivably be converted to active metabolites within the body. To determine the ADI in food, therefore, is an extremely complex exercise for benzimidazole residues. Although the ADI is computed based on the lowest no effect level (NOEL), in the most sensitive species studies, toxicologists and regulatory agencies differ in their interpretation of the most suitable safety margins applicable. Some countries adopt a safety margin of 1000 to 2000 for drugs that are known or possible teratogens.

For benzimidazoles, NOELs are low. Teratogenic metabolites, however, have been identified and measured in edible animal products. Although ADIs can be determined, agreement is necessary internationally to standardize safety margins and to harmonize toxicologic criteria. Withdrawal periods for benzimidazoles are calculated based on metabolic and toxicologic data, taking into account the bioavailability of the residues. The extractable residues (parent drug, or free metabolites, or both) are chemical species with defined toxic potential for which safety margins may be defined.

4.3 IMIDAZOTHIAZOLES—LEVAMISOLE

Levamisole is the laevo isomer of DL-tetramisole, which is a racemic mixture. The parent compound tetramisole was first marketed as an anthelmintic in 1965, but it was soon noted that its anthelmintic activity resided almost entirely in the Laevo-isomer, levamisole. Thus it was determined that the dosage could be reduced by one half using the L-isomer alone. Reducing the dosage in this way also appreciably increased the margin of safety, while leaving the anthelmintic potency unchanged. Levamisole is widely used as an anthelmintic agent, and although it is less toxic than tetramisole, some preparations of tetramisole are still available. Levamisole possess a broad spectrum of activity against a wide range of gastrointestinal helminths and lungworms. It is commonly used in cattle, sheep, pigs, goats, and poultry and occasionally in the horse, dog, and cat.

Levamisole is normally administered orally or by subcutaneous injection in the soluble hydrochloride form, and generally the two routes are considered equivalent in efficacy. Topical preparations for cattle have been introduced. Levamisole slow-release boluses are available in some countries. Levamisole is a ganglion stimulant of nematode nerves, leading to neuromuscular paralysis of the parasites. (Hexamethonium, a ganglionic blocker, inhibits the action of levamisole.) As such, it would be expected that the maximum concentration achieved, rather than duration of concentrations, would be more relevant to anthelmintic activity. According to this hypothesis, the effect obtained after administration through drinking water would seem less reliable than that obtained after drenching or intramuscular injection of the drug.

Because it acts on the roundworm nervous system, levamisole is not ovicidal. Its broad spectrum of activity against nematodes, ease of use being water soluble, reasonable safety margin, and lack of teratogenic effects have allowed it to be used successfully in a wide range of hosts. Owing to its mechanism of action, the peak concentration of levamisole achieved in the blood rather than the duration of concentrations is more relevant to its antiparasitic activity. Thus comparing the routes of administration, it would be expected that subcutaneous administration rather than oral administration would provide better efficacy against lungworms by virtue of the higher plasma (and therefore lung) concentrations achieved. In addition, because of its different mechanism of action, levamisole possesses activity against benzimidazole-resistant parasites.

Levamisole is rapidly absorbed from the gastrointestinal tract after oral administration to mammals. When given intramuscularly to animals, peak blood levels are approximately twice those achieved after oral administration of the same dose. Peak blood levels of levamisole occur within 30 minutes of subcutaneous administration. These concentrations decline over a period of 6 to 8 hours, with 90% of the total dosage being excreted in 24 hours, largely in the urine. After oral dosing in cattle, levamisole residues are present in muscle, fat, liver, and kidney at 2 hours postmedication but are below the limits of assay detectability (0.1 ppm) at 48 hours after treatment. Blood and urine levels of levamisole peak at 2 to 6 hours postmedication but are below the 0.1 ppm level of detectability at 36 and 72 hours after treatment. Muscle fat, liver, kidney, blood, and urine contain levamisole at 2 hours postmedication following injectable levamisole. No residues are detectable 7 to 8 days after injection, in the tissues, blood, or urine. Highest residue levels appear in the liver.

Levamisole hydrochloride residues in milk averaged 0.50, 0.55, 0.58, and 0.32 ppm 12 hours after the administration of levamisole drench (8 mg/kg), pellets, bolus, and injectable formulation. Residues were below 0.01 ppm in milk at 48 hours after drench treatment and at 60 hours after treatment with the other three formulations. In sheep, levamisole at a dose rate of 7.5 mg/kg produced mean plasma concentrations of 3.1, 0.7, and 0.8 μg/ml after administration by the subcutaneous, oral, and intraruminal routes.

Levamisole residues in edible tissues from sows given 8 mg/kg orally were less than 0.1 mg/kg of muscle and fat in sows killed on post-treatment day 3 and less than 0.1 mg/kg of kidney in sows killed on post-treatment day 5. Liver residues averaged 0.78 mg/kg in sows killed on day 3 and were reduced to 0.31 mg/kg in sows killed on day 5. In contrast to the benzimidazoles, excretion is rapid, and the consequent withholding times are shorter than the insoluble benzimidazoles. Mammalian toxicity with levamisole, or especially with tetramisole, is usually greater than for the benzimidazoles, although toxic signs are not usually seen unless the normal therapeutic dosage is exceeded. Levamisole toxicity in the host animal is largely an extension of its antiparasitic effect, i.e., cholinergic-type symptoms of salivation, muscle tremors, ataxia, urination, defecation, and collapse. In fatal levamisole poisoning, the immediate cause of death is asphyxia from respiratory failure. Atropine sulfate can alleviate such symptoms in the host animal.

It is recommended that cattle are not treated concurrently with a systemic organophosphorus warble dressing and levamisole. It is possible that the simultaneous use of levamisole and an organophosphorus compound may have an increased toxic effect on the nervous system. Levamisole may cause some inflammation at the site of subcutaneous injection, but this is usually of a transient nature. The compound is widely used in cattle, sheep, pigs, and poultry for all the major parasites. It possesses good activity against adult and immature parasites of the gastrointestinal tract and lungs. It has no activity against fluke and tapeworms. Its toxicity is sufficiently high in the horse, cat, and dog to preclude general use in these species, although it is used against heartworm as a microfilaricide. Levamisole has been found experimentally to possess immunostimulant effects, and it has been used clinically in humans and to a limited extent in animals in a variety of disease conditions. The use of levamisole in the treatment of brucellosis in humans has been described, and experimental work has shown that levamisole exerts its immunostimulant effects

by restoring the number of T lymphocytes to normal when these are depleted. Several clinically measurable parameters of immune status are restored to normal by the drug. The significance of the immunologic potential of levamisole residues has yet to be assessed.

The immune-potentiating activity of levamisole has been demonstrated in many laboratory systems, however, some of which are biphasic and subject to variations under different experimental conditions. The possible application of levamisole as an immune regulant in cancer therapy and rheumatoid arthritis has received a lot of attention because of an antirheumatic effect in humans, but its clinical use is limited by its low incidence of severe hematologic toxicities, such as leukopenia and agranulocytosis. (Another widely used anthelmintic agent, thiabendazole, has mild anti-inflammatory and weak immune adjuvant activity.)

STUDIES ON IMMUNOLOGIC EFFECTS

There are several reports regarding the effects of levamisole on established tumors or tumor cells in experimental animals. Levamisole failed to activiate macrophages against syngeneic tumor cells in Balb/c mice after intraperitoneal injection. The beneficial effects, where noted, have been ascribed to the potentiation of cellular immunity by levamisole.

OBSERVATIONS IN HUMANS

Various nonspecific effects have been noted after humans have been given therapeutic doses of levamisole, including nausea, vomiting, abdominal pain, taste disturbances, fatigue, headache, confusion, dizziness, fever, insomnia, arthralgia, muscle pain, hypotension, vasculitis, and skin rashes. Administration of levamisole has resulted in both neutropenia and thrombocytopenia. One of the most common and probably the most severe side effect of levamisole in humans is agranulocytosis.

Levamisole-induced agranulocytosis appears to be an idiosyncratic reaction, which in some instances may be associated with

HLA-B27, seropositive rheumatoid arthritis, or otherwise abnormal immune function. It is reversible, although corticosteroids may be required to initiate the recovery process. The highest incidence was noted in patients with rheumatoid arthritis. There are no data on which to base a dose response or NOEL for levamisole-induced agranulocytosis in humans. (It has recently been employed in the therapy of colon cancer in humans.)

4.4 ORGANOPHOSPHATES

A number of organophosphates have been used as anthelmintics in recent years. Although originally they were extensively employed as insecticides, now agents such as dichlorvos, trichlorfon, haloxon and coumaphos are used as anthelmintics in sheep, cattle, horses, and dogs. Organophosphates inhibit many enzymes, especially acetylcholinesterase by phosphorylating its esterification site. This has the effect of blocking cholinergic nerve transmission in the parasite, resulting in spastic paralysis. The cholinesterases of humans, host, and parasite and those of different species of parasite vary in their susceptibility to organophosphorus drugs. Because of such variations in susceptibility, attempts have been made to produce organophosphate products with maximum effects against the parasite and minimum toxicity to the host and handler. In the host animal, the susceptibility of its cholinesterase enzymes to the organophosphate, the rate at which the inhibition can be reversed, and the rate of inactivation of the various organophosphate compounds largely determine their relative toxicity to the different species.

The organophosphates tend to be labile to varying extents in alkaline medium and may be partially hydrolyzed and inactivated in the alkaline region of the small intestine. Thus, for example, the oral dosage rate for trichlorfon (metrifonate) in cattle is 4.5 times that when given subcutaneously. In ruminants, organophosphates generally have satisfactory efficacy for nematodal parasites of the abomasum (especially *Haemonchus*) and small intestine but lack satisfactory efficacy for parasites of the large bowel. Organophosphates are usually rapidly oxidized and inactivated in the liver. Their margin of safety is generally less than that of other broad-spectrum anthelmintics (benzimidazoles), and thus strict attention to dosage is necessary.

Haloxon is probably the safest organophosphorous anthelmintic for use in ruminants. Its primary action is against parasites of the abomasum and small intestine. Similar to other compounds of this group, haloxon interferes with the neuromuscular system of the parasite, resulting in paralysis, detachment from the wall of the digestive tract, and expulsion by the peristaltic movement of the host. The concentration of haloxon required to inhibit cholinesterase activity of the parasite is extremely low, hence its wide margin of safety, in addition to which mammals possess cholinesterase that forms unstable complexes with haloxon. Haloxon is administered orally in the form of a paste, bolus, or drench and displays exceptional efficacy against adult forms of *Haemonchus, Trichostrongylus, Cooperia,* and *Strongyloides*. Its activity is somewhat less but still good against *Osteragia, Bunostomum,* and *Nematodirus*. Haloxon is rapidly absorbed from the gut, metabolized fairly rapidly, and excreted in the urine.

Dichlorvos is a particularly versatile organophosphate because of its high volatility. It can be incorporated as a plasticizer in vinyl resin pellets. The volatile dichlorvos is released slowly from the undigestible pellets as they pass through the digestive tract. This allows for a therapeutic concentration against parasites all along the digestive tract. This controlled release governs the concentration of dichlorvos available to the host and parasite and increases the safety margin by enabling the host animal to detoxify small quantities of the drug rather than being exposed to a sudden concentrated dose when not formulated in a resin. When passed out in the feces, the pellets still contain approximately 45 to 50% of the original drug. Dichlorvos is rapidly absorbed and metabolized in the animal body.

Dichlorvos and trichlorfon are particularly effective against bots and ascarids, with broad-spectrum effects against other intestinal helminths also. Their principal problem is organophosphate-induced adverse reactions owing to cholinesterase inhibition. Contraindications in general are any respiratory diseases; parturition within 30 days; evidence of diarrhea or other gastrointestinal tract problems; and the use or contemplated use of insecticides, muscle relaxants, phenothiazine-derived tranquilizers, or central nervous system depressants.

Organophosphate compounds, which may be nerve agents or insecticides, combine with acetylcholinesterase (AChE), inactivate the enzyme, and permit the buildup of excess acetylcholine (ACh) at synapses. Thus the signs of organophosphate poisoning include a variety of effects of excess ACh in certain regions of the central and peripheral nervous system. Mildly exposed animals may have lethargy, anorexia, and diarrhea for several days or more. Most assays designed to measure AChE activity are based on the observation that the initial velocity of an enzyme-catalyzed reaction is proportional to the amount of active enzyme in a given sample. Blood or brain AChE activity determination is currently in widespread use as an aid in the diagnosis of organophosphate and carbamate insecticide poisoning in domestic species. Atropine is used as an antidote to organophosphate toxicity.

Bound residues (indicated by prolonged radioactivity) are found in the tissues of some animal species after administration of dichlorvos. This persistent radioactivity, however, is believed to be associated with the incorporation of the radiolabel into endogenous metabolism. When 14C-vinyl-dichlorvos is orally administered to rats, the compound is rapidly metabolized. At day 4, 40% is eliminated in expired air (carbon dioxide) and 12% in urine (hippuric acid and urea). At day 5, 75% of liver radioactivity is nonextractable material; 14C is incorporated in endogenous compounds, such as glycocol, serine, and cysteine (derived from carbon dioxide), and thus in proteins.

Organophosphates can provide hazards to humans. Being lipid soluble, they are well absorbed through unbroken skin. Cholinesterase inhibition can occur in humans after accidental organophosphate exposure. These drugs also have the propensity toward interaction with many other drugs. Although relatively rapidly degraded in the animal body, tissue residues are unlikely to pose a serious consumer hazard if specified withholding times are enforced. Perhaps the major risk arises from contamination of the environment, from fecal excretion or accidental drug spillage. Fish are particularly susceptible to organophosphate poisoning, and many instances of serious water pollution and fish kills have been attributed to careless disposal of organophosphate pesticides. Sprays, collars, and washes of organophosphates used in small animals can present significant hazards to infants following ingestion, inhalation, or transcutaneous absorption of the active principle.

Fenthion induces lethal inhibition of cholinesterase activity in the flea. Owing to its spatial configuration, the active ingredient molecule binds ideally to the insect cholinesterase. Because of the molecular shape and weaker membrane penetration, fenthion has less inhibitory effect on mammalian cholinesterase. For this reason, enzyme inhibition is considerably less pronounced in warm-blooded organisms. This selective action results in a combination of highly effective parasite destruction and low mammalian toxicity. The cholinesterase inhibitions occuring at higher concentration levels are fully reversible.

Fenthion is a yellowish brown substance of oily consistency. It is readily soluble in most organic solvents but sparingly soluble in water. It is characterized by a weak garliclike odor. In contrast to other insecticides, the fenthion parasiticide does not take effect immediately but after a few hours when the active ingredient has been almost completely absorbed. The systemic effect can be observed, with affected fleas falling off the animal. A significant reduction in the level of flea infestation can be observed after only 4 hours; it may take up to 2 days for complete eradication of all the fleas on a dog.

During extensive clinical research, no side effects occurred in either laboratory or field tests. No side effects are to be expected following applications of the recommended doses. In some cats, the typical smell of the active ingredient may cause salivation, and restlessness, and overdoses correspond to the symptoms of parasympathetic irritation. Spontaneous vomiting and diarrhea may occur. Neurologic symptoms with fibrillary muscular twitching in the head and neck regions are reversible.

In normal circumstances, incompatibility reactions disappear without antidote therapy. 0.2 to 0.5 mg/kg of atropine should be applied intravenously or intramuscularly to treat acute toxicologic reactions in dogs and cats. If there is no effect after 15 to 20 minutes after intramuscular application, the treatment should be repeated. Oximes should not be used to reactivate cholinesterases, if this is necessary, until potentially fatal symptoms (bronchial spasms, laryngospasms) have been overcome (obidoxime, 5 mg/kg intravenously or intramuscularly; pralidoxime, 10 mg/kg intravenously or intramuscularly).

4.5 TETRAHYDROPYRIMIDINES— PYRANTEL, MORANTEL

Pyrantel was first introduced as a broad-spectrum anthelmintic in 1966 for use against gastrointestinal parasites of sheep. It subsequently has been used for cattle, horses, dogs, and pigs. It is prepared for use as a tartrate embonate or pamoate salt. Aqueous solutions are subject to photoisomerization on exposure to light with a resultant loss in potency. Suspension should therefore be kept out of direct sunlight. Pyrantel is not recommended for use in severely debilitated animals because of its levamisole-type pharmacologic action.

Pyrantel tartrate is well absorbed in the pig and dog. There is less absorption of the drug by ruminants. Metabolism is rapid, with the metabolites being excreted in the urine (40% of the dose in the dog) and some unchanged drug being excreted in the feces (principally in the ruminant). Peak blood levels are usually attained 4 to 6 hours after oral administration. The pamoate salt of pyrantel is poorly soluble in water, which offers the advantage of reduced absorption of this particular salt from the gut, allowing the drug to reach and be effective against parasites in the lower end of the large intestine, hence its application for human, equine, and canine use. Pyrantel is usually delivered for oral use in the form of a suspension, paste, or drench. Similar to levamisole, excretion is rapid. Pyrantel is effective against large and small ascarids, strongyli, and pinworms.

Morantel is the methyl ester analog of pyrantel, and in ruminant animals, morantel tends to be somewhat safer and anthelmintically more effective than pyrantel. The drug is absorbed rapidly from the abomasum and upper small intestine of sheep. The drug is rapidly metabolized in the liver, and about 17% of the initial dose is excreted in the urine as metabolites within 96 hours after dosing.

Oral dosing of sheep with morantel tartrate (10 mg/kg) resulted in peak liver residues (1.92 ppm) 48 hours after administration. Lowest liver residues (0.27 ppm) occurred at 216 hours, after which time they were no longer detectable. No residues were detectable in muscle tissue of cattle 14 days after dosing with morantel drench (sensitivity of method, 0.01 ppm).

Both pyrantel and morantel have higher efficiency against adult gut worms and larval stages that dwell in the lumen or on the mucosal surface; activity is much less against the stages found in the mucosa and is low against arrested osteragia larvae. A sustained-release ruminal bolus of morantel has been introduced for use in cattle that acts as a controlled drug delivery system, releasing morantel over a 90-day period. This appears to be quite successful in preventing buildup of infective larvae on pasture and thus the development of parasitic gastroenteritis and lungworm infestation. The sustained-release morantel bolus effects a sustained delivery of active agent into the gut lumen. Relatively little morantel is absorbed into the systemic tissue from the bowel.

4.6 AVERMECTINS

CHEMISTRY

The avermectins, which are isolated from the mycelia of *Streptomyces avermitilis*, are a family of antiparasitic compounds that are potent broad-spectrum agents at low dosage levels. Since the original finding that 0.002% of the avermectin complex in the diet completely cured mice infested with specific gastrointestinal nematodes, activity has been demonstrated against a wide range of nematode and arthropod parasites.

Avermectins have neither antibacterial nor antifungal activities. Ivermectin was introduced as an antiparasitic drug in 1981, and abamectin was introduced as an agricultural pesticide (and as an antiparasitic drug) in 1985. Abamectin is in commercial use as an agricultural pesticide, and its applications continue to expand.

Avermectins are active when given orally or parentally, at dosages of a fraction of a milligram per kilogram, against many immature and mature nematode and arthropod parasites of sheep, cattle, dogs, horses, and swine. Avermectins appear to paralyze nematodes and arthropods in a unique manner. Although there are a number of naturally occurring avermectins arising as fermentation products of the actinomycete, the derivative of most interest is avermectin B 1, a chemically modified derivative known as ivermectin. This particular compound is active against arrested and developing larvae and adults of the important cattle and sheep nematodes. Avermectins are naturally occurring fermentation products elaborated by the morphologically distinct soil organism *Streptomyces avermitilis*. Early studies on the broth culture from this mold indicated the presence of a substance of unparalleled anthelmintic potency. Further, this new substance displayed high potency and high safety in the crude form as it occurred in nature and without chemical modification. Early chromatographic studies yielded four separate entities, and on thin-layer chromatography these were seen to represent compounds with varying degrees of anthelmintic efficacy. The complex was seen to contain four components designated A1, A2, B1, and B2 in varying proportions. These major components existed as two variants designated *a* and *b*. The *b* series was the lower homologue of the corresponding major *a* component (i.e., A1a more potent than A1b). Component B1a was outstanding, being active against nematodes in sheep at a dosage rate of 0.025 mg/kg. The basic chemical structure of the avermectins is that of a macrocyclic lactone with two sugars attached. (The milbemycins are structurally related but are missing the disaccharide substituent.)

Removal of the sugar fraction from the molecule results in marked diminution in potency and in the anthelmintic activity. Analogs have been developed chemically, and such derivatives can be compared with the parent compound in relation to activity and safety. The derivative of most interest

in this context is 22, 23 dihydroavermectin B1, or ivermectin. This compound displayed good characteristics of efficacy and safety in early laboratory and in vivo studies and was therefore selected for further study and development. Ivermectin comprises at least 80% 22.23 dihydroavermectin B1a and not more than 20% of the B1b homologue. Its efficacy in human onchocerciasis has made it a promising candidate for the control of one of the most insidious and intractable of tropical diseases. The product that is being developed for agricultural use is designated abamectin. It refers to a mixture of not less than 80% avermectin B1a and not more than 20% avermectin B1b.

MECHANISM OF ACTION

Gamma-aminobutyric acid (GABA) is the neurotransmitter substance mediating transmission of inhibitory signals from the interneurons to the motor neurons in the ventral nerve cord of the parasites. It is now established that ivermectin acts as a GABA agonist. The function of the GABA transmitter is to open the chloride channels on the postsyaptic function, allowing inflow of chloride ions and the induction of the resting potential. Ivermectin potentiates this effect by stimulating the presynaptic release of GABA and by increasing its binding to the postsynaptic receptors. In the presence of ivermectin, the chloride channels are open when they should be closed, the net effect being that signals and impulses are not received by the recipient cell. Although the motor neuron and muscle cells are both capable of individual excitation, passage of electrical impulse across the synapse is blocked.

The overall GABA-mediated chloride ion conductance effect may be due to (1) ivermectin acting as a GABA agonist either at the GABA binding site or elsewhere on the protein, (2) stimulation of presynaptic GABA release, or (3) potentiation of GABA binding to its receptors. In experimental work, it was further observed that washing neurons with picrotoxin (an antagonist of GABA) abolished this ivermectin-induced paralysis.

Paralysis is the most evident effect of ivermectin in parasites, but suppression of reproductive function has also been observed in ticks. Ivermectin displays no activity against cestodes or trematodes because these parasites do not use GABA as a neuroransmitter. This is consistent with the hypothesis regarding mode of action.

Arthropods used GABA as a neurotransmitter but tend to use it not between two sets of nerve cells, as in nematodes, but between nerve and muscle cells. Prolonged stimulation and GABA release render the effects of ivermectin sustained and irreversible. For most parasites, this results in neuromuscular blockade, paralysis, and death.

Paralysis is the most evident effect of ivermectin in parasites, but suppression of reproductive function has also been observed in ticks. Ivermectin displays no activity against cestodes or trematodes because these parasites do not use GABA as a neurotransmitter. This is consistent with the hypothesis regarding mode of action.

Cattle

Ivermectin is effective against all of the gastrointestinal nematodes that are of pathogenic or economic importance in cattle. It is available as a 1% parenteral injection, topical pour-on form (0.5%), and oral controlled-release bolus (135-day release osmotic pump). At dosage of 0.2 mg/kg, ivermectin has been shown to be highly effective against at least seven species of gastrointestinal nematodes, including the adult and larval stages of *Ostertagia, Trichostrongylus, Oesophagostomum*, and *Haemonchus* as well as the lungworm *Dictyocaulus viviparus*.

Immature larvae, hypobiotic fourth-stage larvae, and strains with established resistance to other anthelmintics are also susceptible. The drug is equally effective against nematodes when administered orally or parenterally. A dosage rate of 0.2 mg/kg by subcutaneous injection is used commercially for field conditions. A feature of many anthelmintics is poor or variable activity against early hypobiotic fourth-stage *Ostertagia* larvae. At the recommended dosage rate, ivermectin is effective against these parasites by either the oral or the parenteral route. A useful feature of parenteral treatment in cattle is the persistent efficacy against the immature stages of certain ne-

matodes. This period of protection depends on the susceptibility of the nematode species to ivermectin, but it can be up to 21 days. Such longevity of efficacy is consistent with the plasma and tissue kinetics of the drug. Trials have indicated that the protection period against *Dictyocaulus viviparus* is of longer duration than for gastrointestinal nematodes. Ivermectin also displays activity against many economically important arthropod parasites of cattle. Lice, mange mites, ticks, and warble grubs are susceptible to ivermectin. As a systemic ascaricide, ivermectin is fairly slow in attaining maximum efficacy, and attempts have been made to simulate controlled-release systems to optimize therapy.

Sucking lice tend to be more consistently susceptible than biting lice, presumably reflecting the more superficial or intermittent feeding habits of the latter. *Sarcoptes* is usually affected within 7 days, and *Psoroptes*, a more superficial parasite, is eliminated after 14 days. Death of ticks normally occurs 2 to 3 days after treatment. Numerous studies have demonstrated exceptional activity against parasitic larvae (grubs) of warble flies. A single dose of ivermectin (0.2 mg/kg subcutaneously) is 100% effective against first-, second-, and third-stage larvae of *Hypoderma bovis*.

The new sustained-release ivermectin bolus provides season-long control of lungworm, roundworms, and external parasites. Indicated for cattle between 100 kg and 300 kg, each bolus contains 1.72 g. of ivermectin. The bolus remains in the rumen/reticulum, and 12 mg of active ingredient per day is released continuously over approximately 135 days through osmotic action. In countries where it is authorized, animals may not be slaughtered for human consumption until 180 days after the last administration, and it is not permitted for use in dairy cattle.

Sheep

As an oral drench in sheep, ivermectin displays 93 to 100% efficacy against immature and adult stages of commonly occurring endoparasites, including *Haemonchus contortus, Ostertagia, Trichostrongylus, Cooperia, Nematodirus, Chabertia ovina, Trichuris*, and *Strongyloides papillosus*. Efficacy is maintained against benzimidazole-resistant strains of *Haemonchus* and *Trichostongylus*. Some metabolism to less potent products occurs in the rumen, and this may explain the relatively lower efficacy of oral ivermectin when compared with subcutaneous injection against body lice in sheep. High potency against larvae of *Lucilia* has been reported, but activity against *Melophagus ovinus*, the sheep ked, is variable. All three larvae of the nasal bot fly *Oestrus ovis* are completely removed at the standard dosage rate.

Infestations caused by mange mites, *Sarcoptes scabiei*, and itch mites, *Psorergates ovis*, also are controlled by ivermectin given subcutaneously. In contrast to the oral formulation, which does not control *Psoroptes ovis*, sheep given the injectable formulation experience marked reductions is *Psoroptes* numbers and clinical signs. A second injection 7 days later may be required to eliminate all living mites.

Swine

For routine use in swine, ivermectin is presented as 1% injection for subcutaneous administration at a dosage of 0.3 mg/kg. In this species, the spectrum of action includes the adult and larval stages of *Ascaris suum*, *Hyostrongylus rubidus*, *Oesophagostomum*, *Trichuris*, and the lungworm *Metastrongylus apri*. The treatment of pregnant sows can block the transcolostral transmission of *Strongyloides ransomi* to the piglets. Ivermectin is highly efficacious against the porcine mange mite *S. scabiei* as well as the sucking louse *Haematopinus suis*.

Horses

As an oral paste in horses, ivermectin displays an efficacy greater than 98% against *Gastrophilus*, *Trichostrongylus axei*, *Parascaris equorum*, *Oxyuris equi*, *Strongylus vulgaris*, *Strongylus edentatus*, *Habronema muscae*, *Draschia megastoma*, *Strongyloides westeri*, *Dictyocaulus arnfieldi*, and *Onchocerca*. In *Habronema*, *Draschia*, and *Onchocerca*, ivermectin exerts a larvicidal action.

Initially studies indicated that ivermectin was active at dosages as low as 0.02 mg/kg, but as in the case of many other host species, a dosage of 0.2 mg/kg was shown to provide broad-spectrum efficacy and was selected for commercial use. Although an intramuscular formulation was originally employed for the equine species, the oral paste formulation containing 1.87% of the active ingredient is now the only preparation approved for use in the horse. The oral route is claimed to be marginally more effective than the parenteral route regarding efficacy against *O. equi*. Other reports indicate that the parenteral route extends for approximately 2 weeks the efficacy of ivermectin in reducing strongylus egg production and in reducing subsequent pasture contamination.

Arterial larval stages of *Strongylus* tend to be refractory to most equine anthelmintic agents. Intensive therapy with certain members of the benzimidazole class has been reported useful against these migratory pathogenic strongylus stages. Many studies have indicated 100% efficacy against arterial larvae using a single dose of ivermectin at the recommended dosage rate. Such treatment has prevented vascular damage following experimental infection, reduced the size of cranial mesenteric aneurysms, and increased circulation to arteries distal to the aneurysm. Resolution of arteritis has been reported following such treatments. The ubiquitous but less pathogenic "small strongyli" are equally susceptible to ivermectin therapy. All stages of bot fly larvae are removed also. Ivermectin efficacy against adult *P. equorum* has been confirmed, and although the drug is ineffective against migratory *Parascaris* larvae, ascarids that return to the bowel are susceptible to treatment.

Administration to mares at foaling protects offspring against *Strongyloides westeri* infection received through the mare's milk. Good clinical response has been documented in the treatment of *Onchocerca* infection. Cutaneous habronemiasis responds well to orally administered ivermectin. Ivermectin displays high clinical potency against a wide range of benzimidazole-resistant parasites. This would be anticipated considering its unique structure and mode of action.

Dogs

Hookworms are particularly susceptible to ivermectin, with efficacy of 96 to 100% being demonstrated against adults and larval stages of *Ancylostoma caninium* and *Uncinaria stenocephala* at dosages of 0.002 mg/kg orally. Doses of 0.2 mg/kg are necessary for control of adult *Ascaris, Strongyloides,* and *Trichuris* infections. Ivermectin is not active against the adult form of *Dirofilaria immitis,* but efficacy has been demonstrated against microfilariae and precardiac stages of the heartworm at dosages of 0.005 mg/kg orally or 0.2 mg/kg subcutaneously. Reports have indicated that more than 99% of *Trichuris vulpis* infections are expelled at dosages of 0.1 mg/kg or greater, and 0.2 mg/kg removes 90% of all adult stages and 97% of the intestinal larval stages of *Toxocara canis.* High doses (1 to 2 mg/kg) are required to produce an effect against tissue-dwelling stages of *T. canis* in dogs. Against canine ectoparasites, a single dose of ivermectin at 0.2 mg/kg gave complete cure of natural infection of *Otodectes cynotis* and *S. scabiei.* In severe cases of sarcoptic mange, two treatments at 14-day intervals have been advocated.

TARGET ANIMAL SAFETY

Cattle

The breeding performance, including semen quality of bulls, was evaluated before dosing with ivermectin at 0.4 mg/kg (twice the normal dosage level) and for 70 days thereafter. No adverse effects were observed. No ill effects during early, mid, or late pregnancy were noted in cows treated at a similar dosage. Oral doses of 2 mg/kg caused no adverse effects but 8 mg/kg administered subcutaneously resulted in listlessness, ataxia, and death in some cases. One calf died as a result of bloat during an efficacy trial with ivermectin. Eosinophilic esophagitis apparently had developed in response to death of *Hypoderma* larvae. Posterior paresis was recorded in other infected cattle as a result of spinal cord hemorrhages following treatment.

Sheep

Sheep given 4.0 mg/kg ivermectin in propylene glycol displayed ataxia and depression, with hemoglobinuria evident in a number of cases. The control animals given the vehicle alone, however, displayed similar effects. Propylene glycol can give rise to hemoglobinuria in calves.

Swine

Clinical signs of toxicosis, including lethargy, ataxia, mydriasis, tremors, and lateral recumbency, were observed in swine receiving 30 mg/kg ivermectin. No adverse effects of breeding performance were noted.

Horses

Adverse reactions in horses have been associated exclusively with intramuscular administration of ivermectin. Such reactions are unrelated to GABA potentiation. The most frequently reported problems have included the development of local abscessation, transient midventral edema associated with death of *Onchocerca* microfilariae, and swelling at the injection site. Clostridial infection at the injection site and anaphylactoid reactions to the vehicle polysorbate 80 have been observed in some cases. Impaired vision, ataxia, and depression have been recorded after oral administration of 2 mg/kg ivermectin to horses. Rarely post-treatment drowsiness has been observed.

Dogs

The safety of ivermectin in dogs after extralabel usage must not be assumed. Both overdosage and breed susceptibility are involved in canine toxicity states. Collies are adversely affected by ivermectin, and this breed idiosyncrasy is manifested by depression, muscle weakness, blindness, coma, and death. Many cases of ataxia progress to paralysis and decreased consciousness. Relatively higher brain concentrations of ivermectin are found in Collies than in Beagles, mice, cattle, sheep, and pig. Thus, greater penetration across the blood-brain barrier occurs in the Collie. Reports have indicated that picrotoxin infusion might be a useful antidote in such cases. Anaphylactic reactions attributable to polysorbate 80 in the injectable formulation have been described in the dog.

TISSUE DISPOSITION

Ivermectin is well absorbed when administered orally or parenterally. The route of administration and the formulation employed affect its disposition profile. High levels of ivermectin are reached in the lungs and skin regardless of the route of administration. Efficacies greater than 95% have been achieved against parasites of the skin, respiratory system, and blood after oral treatment. Concentrations of ivermectin are maintained in body fluids for prolonged periods of time.

The results of the experiments of subcutaneously administered ivermectin reveal a short distributive phase in cattle; a biological half-life of 2.8 days; a large volume of distribution, 1.9 liter/kg (consistent with the lipophilicity of this compound).

After intravenous delivery of 0.2 mg/kg ivermectin in sheep, a terminal half-life of 178 hours was detected. This relatively long half-life is related to the high potency of the compound, as studies with other anthelmintics have indicated that efficacy is profoundly effected by the kinetic profile. In sheep, low bioavailability was reported when ivermectin was administered into the rumen. Some degradation in the rumen may account for this reduction in bioavailability. The monosaccharide and aglycon derivatives (two possible metabolites of rumenal degradation) are less potent than the parent drug. The lower efficacy and shorter duration of action of orally administered ivermectin (compared with parenteral dosing) may explain the less potent effect against certain ticks (*Boophilus*) in cattle and body lice in sheep. There is ample evidence of the prolonged half-life of ivermectin, based on antiparasitic trials. Cattle did not become infected when exposed to infective stages of gastrointestinal parasites, lungworms, and mange mites 14 to 21 days after subcutaneous treatment. Blood-sucking lice and flies died after feeding on cattle treated 10 to 14 days earlier.

Most of the administered dose of ivermectin is excreted in the feces and the remainder in the urine. Minimal residues are present in the muscle and kidneys, highest concentrations being detected in the liver and fat tissues. Residues in all tissues are extractable in nature with little or no macromolecularly bound drug or metabolites present. The major single component in the edible tissues of cattle, sheep, and pigs is the unaltered parent drug. Ivermectin is also excreted through the milk of lactating cattle.

Although mammals use GABA as a central neurotransmitter, they are generally not adversely affected by ivermectin. This is because being a macrolide of large molecular weight, ivermectin does not readily cross the blood-brain barrier of the mammal to affect GABA within the central nervous system.

In tests of brain concentration of the drug in cattle, radioactive residue assays revealed only minute traces of ivermectin. This was the lowest concentration of all tissues analyzed. Many cases of central nervous system depression in purebred and crossbred long-haired Collies have been cited. The reason for this breed susceptibility is not known. It has been postulated that the blood-brain barrier in the Collie may be more permeable to ivermectin than in other species, allowing ivermectin to enter the central nervous system.

TOXICITY ASPECTS

Ivermectin is teratogenic in rats, rabbits, and mice but only at or near maternal toxic dose levels. Mice are the most sensitive species, at a dosage of 0.2 to 0.4 mg/kg/day. Reproduction and multigeneration studies have demonstrated that neonatal rats are more susceptible to the toxic effects of ivermectin than adult rats. An acceptable daily intake (ADI) of 1 μcg/kg has been established by JELFA.

Based on the relationship of the ADI to residue levels in edible tissues from pharmacokinetic studies, the current withdrawal times for sheep and cattle have been established. On account of its high potency and elimination through milk, however, ivermectin preparations are contraindicated for use in lactating cattle producing milk for human consumption. Year-round parasite control programs can involve three to four treatments per year in young stock. The impact on the environment from the use of ivermectin in farm animals is the excretion of the drug by treated animals through feces and urine. Ivermectin in feces/soil degrades at a slow but significant rate. In a winter environment, decomposition is slow, necessitating a period of 13 weeks for ivermectin levels to deplete by 50%. When exposed to an outdoor summer environment, ivermectin in soil decomposes with a half-life of 0.8 weeks.

Ivermectin possesses little adverse effect on fresh water algae, but only limited information is available on the application of the drug to plant foliage or roots. Studies with the dung beetle have shown that although ivermectin residues in feces from treated animals do not adversely affect the adult beetles, larvae in the treated dung do not complete their development. Larval development of the buffalo fly in fresh feces of treated cattle is prevented for up to 14 days after treatment.

The concentration of ivermectin and metabolites in the accumulated waste of cattle and sheep is approximately 18 to 19 ppb. Assuming that normal spreading practices are observed on pasture, concentration of dung and metabolites in soil is estimated to be less than 0.1 ppb. From laboratory experiments, exposure levels of 300 mg/kg of soil (ppm) are necessary for toxicity to earthworms. Thus a margin of 3 million exists between anticipated pasture/soil levels and toxic levels for earthworms.

Ivermectin and abamectin have an effect on some important dung fauna, such as the larval stages of *Diptera* and of some dung beetles. The use of ivermectin ruminal boluses in calves has been shown to affect dung degradation in implanted animals.

The results of trials reported appear to indicate that there is a difference with regard to ivermectin formulations and degradation of cattle fecal pats (i.e., pour-on or oral bolus versus parenteral dosing). Dung samples collected from calves fitted with ruminal boluses delivering ivermectin at 40 μg/kg/day contained a total of only 17 adult dung beetles, 35 dipterous larvae, and 44 earthworms after 100 days compared with controls, which yielded 780 dung beetles, 267 dipterous larvae, and 46 earthworms over the same period. Although these dung-induced effects may vary with the manner in which the drug is administered as well as with the geographic location and climate, the routine use of ivermectin in cattle may pose an ecologic threat

to those insects (particularly *Diptera*) that have evolved to exist uniquely in conjunction with cattle dung. Failure of dung degradation may be attributable to the absence of insects that are eliminated by the insecticidal effects of ivermectin. Widespread use of ivermectin may have important environmental consequences for pastureland in certain geographic locations. Strong soil binding and lack of mobility could result in the accumulation of ivermectin in soil.

4.7 SALICYLANILIDES AND SUBSTITUTED PHENOLS—FLUKICIDES

The salicylanilides and substituted phenols include:

- *Salicylanilides*—oxyclozanide, rafoxanide, clioxanide, closantel, and brotianide
- *Substituted phenols*—hexachlorophene, bithionol, niclofolan, nitroxynil, and disophenol
- *Aromatic amide*—Diamphenethide

All the members of these chemical groupings possess clinical efficacy against liver fluke. The activity of oxyclozanide was reported in 1966, rafoxanide in 1969, substituted phenols (disophenol) in 1961, and nitroxynil in 1966. Diamphenethide is unique in that it possesses exceptionally high activity against the youngest immature stages of the liver fluke in sheep, with a diminution of its activity as the flukes mature. (Triclabendazole, one of the benzimidazole family, displays high potency against all stages of liver fluke. This undoubtedly is due to its unique mechanism of action.)

The salicylanilides and substituted phenols act to uncouple or disconnect the mitochondrial reactions involved in electron-transport-associated events from adenosine triphosphate (ATP) generation. In vivo mainly the adult flukes are affected with variable activity against the immature flukes in the liver parenchyma. The lowered efficacy of a number of the salicylanilides and substituted phenols against the immature flukes may be due to the high protein binding of these drugs in the blood, which bathes the immature stages in the liver tissue. A number of these compounds, however, do possess activity against 6-week-old flukes in cattle and sheep. Metabolism may affect the pharmacologic activity of various fasciolicides, and some of this metabolism may occur in the gastrointestinal tract. In diamphenethide, which is given orally, this metabolism may be important for full efficacy.

Nitroxynil is used parenterally because its nitro group is reduced to an inactive metabolite by rumen microorganisms if given orally. Nitroxynil is metabolized by rumen bacteria, which destroy its activity and restrict administration to injection. Diamphenethide following absorption is further metabolized in the liver to an amine metabolite, which is active against fluke. It is not active against liver flukes in vitro unless incubated in the presence of enzymatically functional liver cell.

Parent diamphenethide is inactive in vitro; however, the high concentrations of the metabolite formed in the liver parenchyma are extremely effective against immature fluke at this site. The active amine metabolite may undergo further metabolism within the parenchyma to an inactive compound, which is neither toxic to the host nor the parasite, and this may explain its high therapeutic index and poorer efficacy against bile-duct-dwelling stages of *F. hepatica*. It is almost 100% effective against 1-, 3-, and 5-week-old *F. hepatica*. The efficacy of diamphenethide decreases as the parasites mature, and it is more than 80% effective against 7-week-old parasites and more than 60% effective against 10-week-old stages, although these efficacies can be improved if the dosage rate is increased.

Oxyclozanide is metabolized in the liver to the anthelmintically active glucuronide and is excreted in the bile in high concentrations in the vicinity of the adult fluke. Biliary excretion is an important pathway for fasciolicides active against the adult parasite in the bile ducts. Most of the available fasciolicides are administered in the form of oral suspensions or occasionally as solutions by subcutaneous injection. Increasing the dosage of these compounds above the therapeutic rate frequently results in increased activity against the later parenchymal stages, but where such elevated dosages are employed, cognizance must be taken of the inherent safety margin of the particular drug in use.

Nitroxynil is well tolerated at the recommended therapeutic dosage rate of 10 mg/kg. At higher dosages of more than 40 mg/kg, however, toxicity can occur, and the signs of hyperpnea and hyperthermia that have been reported suggest that the mechanism of toxicity may uncouple oxidative phosphorylation in the mammalian cells. The biochemical mode of action is probably by the uncoupling of oxidative phosphorylation because nitroxynil increases ATPase activity of rat liver mitochondria and stimulates the rate of oxygen uptake by intact flukes at concentrations that correlate well with the lethal concentrations for fluke.

The bile ducts are important in the excretion of many of these compounds, as is evidenced by the high proportion of these and their metabolites excreted in the feces rather than the urine. The increased susceptibility of the developing flukes is largely related to the pharmacokinetic behavior of the individual compounds. Because they are bound to plasma proteins, many of the individual compounds are slowly excreted and possess long plasma half-lives, and so lengthy withholding times must be observed in many cases. The fasciolicidal activity of salicylanilides depends on the extent to which they persist in the plasma. For example, rafoxanide is fully absorbed, and plasma levels of approximately 29 μg/ml are found 24 hours after sheep receive the recommended dose. The plasma half-life is about 4 days, and it binds to plasma proteins with a high affinity. Plasma dissolves up to 2 mg/ml, whereas it is virtually insoluble in water. Relatively high levels of residues are found in plasma even 42 days after dosing, but residues in other tissues are negligible. The plasma half-life of disophenol is even longer, 7 to 14 days in dogs and more than 30 days in sheep. The penalty for high efficacy associated with long plasma half-life is the need for long withholding periods.

The high efficacy of many salicylanilides and substituted phenols against blood-ingesting parasites, such as *Haemonchus contortus* and hookworms, may be related to their attachment of plasma proteins. Presumably they are released to poison the parasite after ingestion of blood. Binding to plasma proteins reduces incorporation into host cells and toxicity. Young flukes probably ingest mainly liver cells containing little anthelmintic. As they grow and migrate through the liver, they cause extensive hemorrhage and come into contact with plasma-bound anthelmintic. Finally, when they reach the bile ducts, they are in the main excretory channel for the salicylanilides and exposed to even greater toxic concentrations. The salicylanilides are known to be uncouplers of oxidative phosphorylation in mammals and in liver fluke. It might be expected that as flukes mature and move from more anaerobic conditions in liver parenchyma to more aerobic conditions in bile ducts, the increased efficacy of uncouplers of oxidative phosphorylation against mature flukes would be explained. Pharmacokinetic data for many modern fasciolicides is sparse.

Peak plasma levels, which may be an indicator of efficacy, are reached in 12 to 24 hours for salicylanilides and 3 to 4 days for bithionol sulfoxide. The absorption of fasciolicides given parenterally (nitroxynil) is rapid and complete, peak plasma levels being achieved 30 to 60 minutes after dosing. The relatively high residue of nitroxynil found in milk is due to the relatively high dosage rate, parenteral administration, and tendency to form complexes with serum and body proteins.

Nitroxynil is retained in the liver and plasma of sheep at detectable levels for 66 days after a single dose of 10 mg/kg. Although binding to serum albumin occurs, longterm exposure to the drug is critical for antiparasitic activity. Plasma levels associated with activity against the mature fluke are greater than 55 ppm. Nitroxynil has been shown to cause stunting of flukes that survive treatment, and these parasites had reduced oogenesis and spermatogenesis. Plasma and tissue pharmacokinetic studies indicate that nitroxynil has a long plasma elimination half-life of approximately 8 days and that plasma concentrations remain considerably higher than tissue concentrations for at least 9 weeks after a single subcutaneous administration of 10 mg/kg.

Closantel, rafoxanide, and oxyclozanide have long terminal half-lives in sheep (14.5, 16.6, and 6.4 days). These long half-lives are related to the high plasma protein binding of these three drugs (>99%), and residues in liver are detectable for extended periods (weeks) after administration. It has been suggested that the long terminal elimination half-life of some of the salicylanilides may reflect turnover of plasma albumin, to which they are bound because the plasma albumin turnover rate is about 16.6 days.

The antiparasitic activities of closantel and rafoxanide are related to protein-bound drug, and their activity against other hematophagous parasites, such as *H. contortus*. There may be opportunities to give these drugs as extended release preparations minimizing any toxicity hazards to the host animal, or to incorporate such drugs in continuous-release rumen bolus formulations. It has also been suggested that the poor activity of oxyclozanide against immature *F. hepatica* may be due to its high protein binding in blood, which bathes the immature flukes in the liver parenchyma at a stage at which they are thought to feed on liver cells rather than blood.

The benzimidazole triclabendazole possesses flukicidal activity and is also highly bound to plasma protein in the form of its sulfone and sulfoxide. (This is in contrast to other nematocidal benzimidazoles, such as albendazole, in which binding is less than 50%.)

Salicylanilides and substituted phenols are potent uncouplers of oxidative phosphorylation. Their selective toxicity for the parasite is determined by their rates of absorption and metabolism, the pathways of excretion, their affinity for plasma protein, and their persistance in the blood stream. Because they are general uncouplers of oxidative phosphorylation, their safety indices are usually not as high as many other anthelmintic agents but nonetheless are more than adequate if used as directed. Commonly a slight loss of appetite and looseness of feces may be seen after treatment at the recommended dosage rates. High dosage rates may cause blindness and classic symptoms of uncoupled phosphorylation: hyperventilation, hyperthermia, convulsions, tachycardia, and ultimately death. Adverse effects are most commonly seen in severely stressed animals, animals in poor condition nutritionally or metabolically, or animals with severe parasitic infestations. Niclofolan is known to induce teratogenic effects, including spina bifida in hamsters, when used at elevated dosages.

On account of their narrow safety margins, pharmacodynamic effects, long half-lives, high binding to plasma protein, deposition in the liver, and excretion in detectable quantities in milk, consumer concerns arise. Because these fasciolicides are used no more than two or three times per year, however, residues are unlikely to occur in milk with any great frequency. Nonetheless, the ADI could possibly be exceeded in the case of infants or small children, consuming 1 liter of milk per day and with a body weight of 10 kg or less, even at the end of the withholding period.

4.8 MISCELLANEOUS PARASITICIDES

Clorsulon is a sulfonamide that inhibits certain glycolytic pathways of trematodes. Given orally at the rate of 4 mg/kg, clorsulon is 91 to 96% effective in the treatment of 56-day-old *F. hepatica* infections. In addition to effective fluke removal, clorsulon displays a stunting effect on flukes that remain post-treatment. Clorsulon also is effective as an injectable formulation for liver fluke infection in cattle. Immature flukes (8 weeks old) require a higher dose (7 mg/kg) than adult flukes (3.6 mg/kg). In plasma, clorsulon is bound to protein, which when ingested by liver flukes inhibits enzymes of the glycolytic pathway. It acts on the parasite energy metabolism as a competitive inhibitor of 3-phosphoglycerate kinase and inhibits glucose oxidation to acetate and propionate, thereby blocking glycolysis and inhibiting ATP formation. It is thought that the parasites also ingest clorsulon bound to host erythrocytes. Clorsulon has a wide therapeutic index in domestic animals. It is a sulfonamide derivative with the chemical formula 4-amino-6-trichloroethenyl-1,3-benzendisulfonamide. It is usually given orally at a dosage of 7 mg/kg.

Piperazine is a compound that when given orally is rapidly absorbed from the gastrointestinal tract. Piperazine base can be detected in the urine as early as 30 minutes after the drug is administered: The excretion rate is maximal at 1 to 8 hours, and urinary excretion is practically complete within 24 hours. Piperazine acts to block neuromuscular transmission in the parasite by hyperpolarizing the nerve membrane, leading to a state of flaccid paralysis. It also blocks succinate production by the worm.

The parasites, thus paralyzed and depleted of energy, are expelled by peristalsis. The spectrum of activity of piperazine is largely directed against ascarid parasites in all species and also esophagostomum species. There is variable activity against hookworms and strongyli but no effect against whipworms or tapeworms. Although a safe compound, toxicity has occasionally been reported in pups.

Diethylcarbamazine citrate also acts to paralyze nematodes by interfering with nerve function. It is employed largely in the treatment of prepatent hoose in cattle and given for 3 consecutive days by intramuscular injection. The drug is relatively ineffective against the mature form of *D. viviparus* in established cases of lungworm infestation. It is also a long-established drug for heartworm infection.

Praziquantel displays high efficacy against cestode parasites at a relatively low dosage rate but possesses no effect on nematodes. In dogs, praziquantel is rapidly absorbed, maximum blood levels being reached as early as 30 to 60 minutes after administration. After absorption into the blood stream, it is believed to be re-excreted back into the intestinal lumen by the mucous membrane. This may explain the extremely high efficacy even against 3-day-old *Echinococcus granulosus*. Cestode parasites buried in the crypts of Lieberkühn surrounded by mucous and inflammatory exudate are usually rather inaccessible to anthelmintic agents working from the lumen of the gut. Delivery to the sites of infestation from the blood stream makes for more effective action as in the case of praziquantel. The resecretion into the gut is a rapid process. Studies have identified the active drug present in the ileum within 8 minutes of administration when the bulk of the administered dose still remained far higher up the alimentary tract. Praziquantel exerts its antiparasitic effects in many ways, impairing both motility and the proper functioning of the suckers of the cestode. In vivo studies have indicated that praziquantel induces spastic paralysis of the parasite. Thus praziquantel joins the number of anthelmintics that act primarily on the target of neuromuscular coordination. The compound also influences the tegument of the worm making it permeable to excessive glucose loss. Epsiprantel is available in tablet form for the treatment of Dipylidium Caninum and Taenia species in dogs.

Bunamidine is another anticestodal compound used in small animals. It is most effective if given on an empty stomach. Bunamidine is absorbed and metabolized in the liver and brings about digestion of the tapeworms in the gut of the host. Vomiting and mild diarrhea may be seen in a proportion of treated animals.

Niclosamide is poorly absorbed from the digestive tract. The bulk of the dose remains in the lumen of the gut, where it brings about its taeniacidal effect by inhibiting glucose uptake by the parasite.

Nitroscanate is one of the broad-spectrum anthelmintics introduced for use in small animals against *Toxocara, Taenia, Dipylidium, Ancylostoma, Uncinaria,* and *Echinococcus*. Vomiting occasionally occurs after dosage.

4.9 RESISTANCE

The development of resistance to chemical groups of anthelmintics by nematodes of domestic animals is now considered as a potentially major problem. Until recently, resistance to anthelmintics in nematodes has been slow to develop under field conditions (in comparison to antibiotic resistance in bacteria). Resistance, however, is likely to become more widespread because relatively few chemically dissimilar groups of anthelmintics have been introduced over the past decade. Most of the commonly used anthelmintics belong to two or three chemical classifications, within which all individual compounds act in a similar fashion. Thus resistance to one compound spreads to all other members of the group because of the similar mechanisms of action within the parasite. Although resistance to *Haemonchus* is becoming a global problem, resistance to *Trichostrongylus* and *Ostertagia* is also increasing. After application of anthelmintics, resistant strains of nematodes are derived from the initial population by the selective mortality of the more susceptible genotypes. The continued application of highly efficient anthelmintics selectively removes the majority of susceptible genotypes, with the resultant progeny of succeeding generations being composed of resistant strains.

Examination of management practices has shown that resistance is not an important problem on farms where different chemical classes of anthelmintics are used in a rotation program. Resistance may be expected to be minimized by using an appropriate anthelmintic at a dosage rate not less than that recommended by the manufacturer. Also, no one chemical group of anthelmintics should be used for prolonged periods.

Resistance in sheep and goat nematodes to the effects of benzimidazoles and other anthelmintics is of economic importance in Australia, New Zealand, South Africa, and countries in South America. Resistance to anthelmintic is expressed by increased egg laying by the parasite, higher establishment rates of adults in the host, and greater larval availability on the pasture. Development of significant resistance seems to require 9 or 10 generations of helminths, and the general consensus is that anthelmintics of different chemical grouping or of differing modes of action should be alternated between generations of "seasons" to prolong their worthwhile therapeutic existence.

If resistance to one drug in the benzimidazole group occurs in a nematode population, there is usually resistance to all benzimidazoles. This is designated "side-resistance." Resistance to these broad-spectrum anthelmintics developed and was reported initially from the United States in a strain of *H. contortus*. Further reports of resistance to benzimidazoles in *H. contortus* in Australia followed. Benzimidazole-resistant cyathostomes appear to be widespread in horses, and they are likely present in all animals in which benzimidazoles have been used extensively. Anthelmintic-resistant nematodes in a flock or herd of animals come from two sources: They are either introduced with purchase of animals, or they are selected, as anthelmintics are used, from small numbers of naturally tolerant worms on the farm. Among the nematodes of sheep, resistance to benzimidazoles has been found, and it has been demonstrated that this resistance is caused by a reduction in the binding of benzimidazoles to the tubulin of these nematodes. Changes in carbohydrate metabolism in benzimidazole-resistant parasites have been noted compared with metabolism in susceptible parasites. All benzimidazoles are side-resistant. One exception to this appears to have been the control of benzimidazole-resistant small strongyli in horses by oxibendazole.

Three mechanisms of avoiding parasiticide action are common in parasites: reduced drug uptake, increased drug metabolism, and alteration of the drug receptor site. Cross resistance is frequently seen between members of the benzimidazole group because of their similar mechanism of action. Control of benzimidazole-resistant parasites by, for example, levamisole can be expected because of the different modes of action of the two types of drug. Although there is no cross resistance between levamisole and benzimidazoles, this does not mean that worms resistant to both kinds of drugs will not evolve. In addition, cross resistance between levamisole and morantel can occur as a result of the similarities of their mechanisms of action. Levamisole and pyrantel/morantel are cross resistant, and morantel does not control levamisole-resistant nematodes, although levamisole controls morantel-resistant nematodes.

Evolution of anthelmintic resistance may be delayed by using chemicals with different modes of action. The current recommendation is for a slow rotation of the different chemical groups. This alternation must occur between the generation interval because the latter usage may hasten the development of resistance to more than one chemical. This means that no individual worm should be repeatedly subjected to a multiple selection of anthelmintics from more than one chemical group. Because there are usually only one or two generations of parasite per annum in practice, rotation of anthelmintics from different groups should be carried out annually between dosing seasons. In the control of parasites, there is no doubt that permanent economic benefit is obtained only by planned treatment of a whole flock or herd, taking into account the biology of the parasite present. Good results should be obtained, provided that the correct control measures are directed against the parasitic phase in the body of the host at the appropriate time, coupled with attention to the free living nonparasitic stages in the environment.

Three approaches underpin any program geared to avoid resistance: reduced use of anthelmintics, use of a full dose, and alternation of types of anthelmintics. Field studies with thiabendazole and levamisole in Australia have shown that increased frequency of dosing increases the rate at which resistance appears. Changing within chemical types (e.g., the benzimidazoles) or between drugs with a similar mechanism action (e.g., levamisole and morantel) is of no benefit. Present information dictates continued use of an anthelmintic for at least a whole season, provided that it is effective. Changing within a season is not recommended. Management systems that require the intensive use of anthelmintics promote resistance.

SELECTED REFERENCES

Anderson, N., and Waller, P.J. (eds.): Resistance in Nematodes to Anthelmintic Drugs. Glebe, NSW, CSIRO Division of Animal Health, 1985.

Anthelmintics for Cattle, Sheep, Pigs and Horses. Northumberland MAFF Publications, 1983.

Averkin, E.A., Beard, C.C., Dvorak, C.A., et al.: Methyl 5(6)-phenylsulfin 1-2-benzimidazole carbamate, a new potent anthelmintic. J. Med. Chem., *11*:1165, 1975.

Baker, N.F., Miller, J.E., Madingan, J.E., et al.: Anthelmintic action of ivermectin, oxibendazole and pyrantel paomate against thiabendazole-resistant small strongyles of horses. Equine Pract., *6*:8, 1984.

Bardana Jr., E.J.: Recent developments in immunomodulatory therapy. J. Allergy Clin. Immunol., *74*:423, 1985.

Barragry, T.B.: A review of the pharmacology and clinical uses of ivermectin. Can. Vet. J., *28*:512, 1987.

Barragry, T.B.: Anthelmintics: A review. N.Z. Vet. J., *32*:161, 1984.

Barragry, T.B.: Anthelmintics: Review part II. N.Z. Vet. J., *32*:191, 1984.

Barton, N.J.: Development of anthelmintic resistance in nematodes from sheep in Australia subjected to different treatment frequencies. Int. J. Parasitol., *13*:125, 1983.

Behm, C.A., and Bryant, C.: The modes of action of some modern anthelmintics. *In* Resistance in Nematodes to Anthelmintic Drugs. Edited by N. Anderson and P.J. Waller. Glebe, NSW, CSIRO Division of Animal Health, 1985.

Bennett, D.G.: Clinical pharmacology of ivermectin. J. Am. Vet. Med. Assoc., *1*:100, 1986.

Bernier-Valentin, F., Aunis, D., and Roussett, B.: Evidence for tubulin-binding sites on cellular membranes: Plasma membranes, mitochondrial membranes and secretory granule membranes. J. Cell Biol., 97:209, 1983.

Blakley, B.R., and Rousseaux, Cl.G.: Effect of ivermectin on the immune response in mice. Am. J. Vet. Res., 52:593, 1991.

Bogan, J.A., Armour, J., Bairden, K., and Galbraith, E.A.: Time of release of oxfendazole from an oxfendazole pulse-release bolus. Vet. Rec., 121:280, 1987.

Bogan, J.A., Benoit, E., and Delatour, P.: Pharmacokinetics of oxfendazole in goats: A comparison with sheep. J. Vet. Pharmacol. Ther., 10:305, 1987.

Borgers, M., De Nollin, S., De Brabander, M., and Thienpont, D.: Influence of the anthelmintic mebendazole on microtubules and intracellular organelle movement in nematode intestinal cells. Am. J. Vet. Res., 36:1153, 1975.

Boyd, M.R., and Burka, L.T.: In vivo studies on the relationship between target organ alkylation and the pulmonary toxicity of a chemically reactive metabolite of 4-ipomeanol. J. Pharmacol. Exp. Ther., 207:687, 1978.

Britt, D.P.: Benzimidazole-resistant nematodes in Britain. Vet. Rec., 110:343, 1982.

Brown, H.D., Matzak, A.R., Ilves, I.R., et al.: Antiparasitic drugs. IV. 2-(4'-thiazolyl)-benzimidazole; a new anthelmintic. J. Am. Chem. Soc., 83:1764, 1961.

Burgat, V., Delatour, P., Benard, P., et al.: Metabolism and residues toxicity of benzimidazole drugs. Presented at 22nd World Veterinary Congress, Perth, Australia, 1983.

Burke, T.M., and Robertson, E.L.: Critical studies of fenbendazole suspension (10%) against naturally occurring helminth infections in dogs. Am. J. Vet. Res., 39:1799, 1978.

Campbell, W.C.: Ivermectin: An update. Parasitol. Today, 1:10, 1985.

Campbell, W.C.: An introduction to the avermectins. N.Z. Vet. J., 29:174, 1981.

Campbell, W.C., and Benz, G.W.: Ivermectin: A review of efficacy and safety. J. Vet. Pharmacol. Ther., 7:1, 1984.

Campbell, W.C., and Blair, L.S.: Efficacy of avermectin against Dirofilaria immitis in dogs. J. Helminthol., 52:308, 1978.

Campbell, W.C., Fisher, M.H., Stapley, E.O., et al.: Ivermectin: A potent new antiparasitic agent. Science, 221:823, 1983.

Carnes, S.A., and Watson, A.P.: Disposing of the US chemical weapons stockpile: An approaching reality. J.A.M.A., 262:653, 1989.

Clara, R., and Germanes, J.: Levamisole and agranulocytosis. Lancet, 1:47, 1977.

Coles, G.C.: Anthelmintic resistance in sheep. Vet. Clin. North Am. [Food Anim. Pract.], 2:423, 1986.

Coles, G.C.: Benzimidazole resistant nematodes in sheep. J. Am. Vet. Med. Assoc., 183:166, 1983.

Coles, G.C., and Briscoe, N.G.: Benzimidazoles and fluke eggs. Vet. Rec., 103:301, 1978.

Confer, A.W., and Aldinger, W.K.: The in vivo effect of levamisole on PHA stimulation in normal and Marek's disease virus inoculated chickens. Res. Vet. Sci., 30:243, 1981.

Craig, T.M., and Huey, R.L.: Efficacy of triclabendazole against Fasciola hepatica and Fascioloides magna in naturally infected calves. Am. J. Vet. Res., 45:1644, 1984.

Dawson, P.J., Gutteridge, W.E., and Gull, K.: A comparison of the interaction of anthelmintic benzimidazoles with tubulin isolated from mammalian tissue and the parasitic nematode Ascaridia galli. Biochem. Pharmacol., 33:1069, 1984.

De Caprio, A.P., Olajos, E., and Weber, P.: Covalent binding of a neurotoxic n-hexane metabolite: Conversion of primary anines to substituted pyrrole adducts by 2, 5-hexandione. Toxicol. Appl. Pharmacol., 65:440, 1982.

Delatour, P.: Pharmacokinetics and metabolism of anthelmintics in ruminants. Presented at 12th Conference of the World Association for the Advancement of Veterinary Parasitology, Montreal, 1987.

Delatour, P., Caudon, M., Garnier, F., and Benoit, E.: Relationship of metabolism and embryotoxicity of febantel in the rat and sheep. Ann. Rech. Vet., 13:163, 1982.

Delatour, P., Garnier, F., and Benoit, E.: Kinetics of four metabolites of febantel in cows milk. Vet. Res. Commun., 6:37, 1983.

Delatour, P., Garnier, F., Benoit, E., and Longin, C.H.: A correlation of toxicity of albendazole and oxfendazole with their free metabolites and bound residues. J. Vet. Pharmacol. Ther., 7:187, 1984.

Delatour, P., and Parish, R.: Benzimidazole anthelmintics and related compounds: Toxicity and evaluation of residues In Drug Residues in Animals. Edited by A.G. Rico. New York, Academic Press, 1986.

Delatour, P., Parish, R.C., and Gyurik, R.J.: Albendazole: A comparison of relay embryotoxicity with embryotoxicity of individual metabolites. Ann. Recherches Vet., 12:159, 1981.

Drudge, J.H., Lyons, E.T., and Tolliver, S.C.: Benzimidazole resistance of equine strongyles—critical tests of six compounds against population. Am. J. Vet. Res., 40:590, 1979.

Duncan, W.A.M., Lemon, P.G., and Palmer, A.K.: The effects of methyl-5(6)-butyl-2-benzimidazole carbamate (parbendazole) on reproduction in sheep and other animals. IX. Effect of administration to the pregnant rabbit. Cornell Vet., 64(suppl. 4):104, 1974.

Duwel, D.: Fenbendazole II. Biological properties and activity. Pest. Sci., 8:550, 1977.

Epstein, W.V., Michalski, J.P., and Talal, N.: Corticosteroids in levamisole-induced agranulocytosis. Lancet, 2:245, 1977.

Food and Drug Administration: Freedom of Information Summary. NADA No. 127–443. Rahway, NJ, Eqvalan, MSD-Agvet, 1983.

Friedman, P.A., and Platzer, E.G.: Interaction of anthelmintic benzimidazoles and benzimidazole derivatives with bovine brain tubulin. Biochem. Biophys. Acta, 544:605, 1978.

Gordon, G.B., Spielberg, S.P., Blake, D.A., and Balasubramanian, V.: Thalidomide teratogenesis: Evidence for a toxic arene oxide metabolite. Proc. Nat. Acad. Sci. U.S.A., *78*:2545, 1981.

Hayes, R.H.: Toxicity investigations of fenbendazole and anthelmintic of swine. Am. J. Vet. Res., *44*:1108, 1983.

Hoebeke, J., Van Nijen, G., and De Brabander, M.: Interaction of oncodazole (R17934), a new anti-tumoral drug, with rat brain tubulin. Biochem. Biophys. Res. Comm., *69*:319, 1976.

Ireland, C.M., Clayton, L., Gutteridge, W.E., et al.: Identification and drug binding capacities of tubulin in nematode Ascaridia gulli. Mol. Biochem. Parasitol., *6*:45, 1982.

Irons, R.D., Dent, J.G., Baker, T.S., and Rickert, D.E.: Benzene is metabolized and covalently bound in bone marrow in situ. Chem. Biol. Interact., *30*:241, 1980.

Jallow, D.J., Mitchell, J.R., Potter, W.Z., et al.: Acetaminophen-induced hepatic necrosis. II. Role of covalent binding in vivo. J. Pharmacol. Exp. Ther., *187*:195, 1973.

Kelly, J.D., and Hall, C.A.: Resistance of animal helminths to anthelmintics. Adv. Pharmacol. Chemother., *16*:89, 1979.

Kinabo, L.D.B., and Bogan, J.A.: Pharmacokinetics and efficacy of triclabendazole in goats with induced fascioliasis. J. Vet. Pharmacol. Ther., *11*:254, 1988.

Kohler, P., and Bachmann, R.: Intestinal tubulin as possible target for chemotherapeutic action of mebendazole in parasitic nematodes. Mol. Biochem. Parasitol., *4*:325, 1981.

LeJambre, L.: Egg hatch as an in-vitro assay of thiabendazole resistance in nematodes. Vet. Parasitol., 2:385, 1976.

Lovell, R.A.: Ivermectin and piperazine toxicoses in dogs and cats. Vet. Clin. North Am. [Small Anim. Pract.], 20:453, 1990.

Lyons, E.T., Drudge, J.M., and Tolliver, S.C.: Antiparasitic activity of ivermectin in critical tests in equids. Am. J. Vet. Res., *41*:1069, 1980.

Malone, J.B., Ramsey, R.T., and Loyacano, A.F.: Efficacy of clorsulon against 8-week-old experimentally induced and mature naturally acquired Fasciola hepatica in cattle. Am. J. Vet. Res., *45*:851, 1984.

Malone, J.B., Smith, P.H., Loyacano, A., et al.: Efficacy of albendazole for treatment of naturally acquired Fasciola hepatica in calves. Am. J. Vet. Res., *43*:879, 1982.

Marriner, S.E., and Bogan, J.A.: Pharmacokinetics of fenbendazole in sheep. Am. J. Vet. Res., *42*:1146, 1981.

Marriner, S.E., and Bogan, J.A.: Pharmacokinetics of oxfendazole in sheep. Am. J. Vet. Res., *42*:1143, 1981.

Marriner, S.E., and Bogan, J.A.: Pharmacokinetics of albendazole in sheep. Am. J. Vet. Res., *41*:1126, 1980.

Martin, P.J., and Le Jambre, L.F.: Larval paralysis as an in-vitro assay of levamisole and morantel tartrate resistance in Ostertagia. Vet. Sci. Commun., 3:159, 1979.

Martz, F., Failinger III, C., and Blake, D.A.: Phenytoin teratogenesis: Correlation between embryopathic effect and covalent binding of putative arene oxide metabolity in gestational tissue. J. Pharmacol. Exp. Ther., *203*:231, 1977.

Meerdink, G.L.: Organophosphorus and carbamate insecticide poisoning in large animals. Vet. Clin. North Am. [Food Anim. Pract.] 5:375, 1989.

Meuldermans, W., Michiels, M., Woestenborghs, R., et al.: The metabolic fate of closantel after intramuscular and oral administration in sheep. *In* Comparative Veterinary Pharmacology, Toxicology and Therapy. Proceedings of the 3rd EAVLT Congress, Ghent (Part I). Edited by A.M. van Miert, M.J. Bogaert, and M. Debackere. Utrecht, EAVPT, 1985.

McKellar, Q.A., Scott, E.W.: The benzimidazole agents—a review. J. Vet. Pharmacol. Therap., *13*:223, 1990.

McKellar, Q.A., Kinabo, L.D.B.: The pharmacology of flukicidal drugs. Br. Vet. J., *147*:306, 1991.

Miller, J.A., Drummond, R.O., and Oehler, D.D.: A sustained-release implant for delivery of ivermectin for control of livestock pests. *In* Proceedings 8th International Symposium Controlled Release Bioactive Materials, Ft. Lauderdale, 1981.

Miller, J.A., and Miller, E.C.: The metabolic activation of chemical carcinogens. Recent results with aromatic amines, safrole and aflatoxin B1. IARC Scientific Publications, *12*:153, 1976.

Mitchell, J.P., Potter, A.Z., and Jollow, D.J.: Furosemide-induced hepatic and renal tubular necrosis. I. Effects of treatments with alter drug metabolizing enzymes. Fed. Proc., *32*:305, 1973.

Mohammed-Ali, M.A.K., and Bogan, J.A.: The pharmacodynamics of flukicidal salicylanilides, rafoxanide, closantel and oxyclosanide. J. Vet. Pharmacol. Ther., *10*:127, 1987.

Morris, D.L., Dykes, P.W., Dickson, B., et al.: Albendazole in hydatid disease. B.M.J., *286*:103, 1983.

Nerenberg, C., Runken, R.A., and Martin, S.B.: Radioimmunoassay of oxfendazole in bovine, equine or canine plasma or serum. J. Pharm. Sci., *67*:1553, 1978.

Ngomuo, A.J., Marriner, S.E., and Bogan, J.A.: The pharmacokinetics of fenbendazole and oxfendazole in cattle. Vet. Res. Commun., *8*:187, 1984.

Parker, S.W.: Allergic reactions in man. Pharmacol. Rev., *34*:85, 1982.

Paul, A.J., Tranquilli, W.J., Todd, K.L., et al.: Evaluating the safety of administering high doses of a chewable ivermectin tablet to collies. Vet. Med., 623, 1991.

Prichard, R.K.: Anthelmintic resistance in nematodes: Extent, recent understanding and future directions for control and research. Int. J. Parasitol., *20*:515, 1990.

Prichard, R.K.: Anthelmintics for cattle. Vet. Clin. North Am. [Food Anim. Pract.], 2:489, 1986.

Prichard, R.K.: The fumarate reductase reaction of Haemonchus contortus and the mode of action of some anthelmintics. Int. J. Parasitol., 3:409, 1973.

Prichard, R.K., Hennessy, D.R., and Steel, J.W.: Prolonged administration a new concept for increasing the spectrum and effectiveness of anthelmintics. Vet. Parasitol., 4:309, 1978.

Prichard, R.K., Hennessy, D.R., Steel, J.W., and Lacey, E.: Metabolite concentrations in plasma following treatment of cattle with five anthelmintics. Res. Vet. Sci., 39:173, 1985.

Prichard, R.K., Steel, J.W., and Hennessy, D.R.: Fenbendazole and thiabendazole in cattle: partition of gastrointestinal absorption and pharmacokinetic behaviour. J. Vet. Pharmacol. Ther., 4:295, 1981.

Pulliam, J.D., Seward, R.L., Henry, R.T., and Seinberg, S.A.: Investigating ivermectin toxicity in Collies. Vet. Med., 80:33, 1985.

Rew, R.S.: Mode of action of common anthelmintics. J. Vet. Pharmacol. Ther., 1:183, 1978.

Sampson, D., Peters, D.G., Lewis, J.D., et al.: Dose dependence of immunopotentiation and tumour regression induced by levamisole. Cancer Res., 37:3526, 1977.

Sanz, F., Tarazona, J.M., Jurado, R., et al.: An efficacy study with the new compound Netobimin (Totabin-Sch) against Dicrocoelium dendriticum in sheep. In Abstracts, World Association for the Advancement of Veterinary Parasitology, 1985.

Seiler, J.P.: Toxicology and genetic effects of benzimidazole compounds. Mut. Res., 32:151, 1975.

Seward, R.L.: Reaction in dogs given ivermectin [letter to editor]. J. Am. Vet. Med. Assoc., 183:493, 1983.

Short, C.R., Barker, S.A., Hsieh, L.C., et al.: The disposition of fenbendazole in the goat. Am. J. Vet. Res., 48:811, 1987.

Short, C.R., Flory, W., Hsieh, L.C., and Barker, S.A.: The oxidative metabolism of fenbendazole: A comparative study. J. Vet. Pharm. Ther., 11:50, 1988.

Song, M.D.: Using ivermectin to treat feline dermatosis caused by external parasites. Vet. Med., 86:498, 1991.

Steel, J.W., Hennessy, D.R., and Lacey, E.: Netobimin (Totabin-Sch.): Metabolism and pharmacokinetics in sheep. Communication to the Congress of the World Association for Advancement of Veterinary Parasitology, Rio de Janeiro, 1985.

Swenson, D.H., Miller, E.C., and Miller, J.A.: Aflatoxin B1-2-3-oxide; evidence for its formation in rat liver in vivo and by human liver microsomes in vitro. Biochem. Biophys. Res. Commun., 60:1036, 1974.

Thornes, R.D.: Febrile side-effects. Lancet, 2:90, 1977.

Tripodi, D., Parks, L.C., and Brugenans, J.: Drug-induced restoration of delayed hypersensitivity in anergic patients with cancer. N. Engl. J. Med., 289:354, 1973.

Wall, R., and Strong, L.: Environmental consequences of treating cattle with the antiparasitic drug ivermectin. Nature, 327:418, 1987.

Watts, S.A.M.: Colchicine binding in the rat tapeworm. Hymenolepis diminuta. Biochem. Biophys. Acta, 667:59, 1981.

Williams, I.A.: Levamisole and agranulocytosis. Lancet, 1:1980, 1980.

CHAPTER

5

DRUG THERAPY OF RESPIRATORY SYSTEM DISORDERS

5.1 Bronchodilators
5.2 Removal of Secretions
5.3 Cough Suppressants
5.4 Anti-Inflammatories
5.5 Antihistamines
5.6 Miscellaneous Measures
5.7 Small Animals—Respiratory Infections
5.8 Nasal Aspergillosis
5.9 Feline Respiratory Disease

The therapy of respiratory disease warrants a wide spectrum usage of therapeutic agents.

> Constriction of the airways, which may be mediated by various inflammagens such as histamine, kinins, prostaglandins, and leukotrienes, or by cholinergic stimulation, is important in many respiratory diseases. Because tidal volume varies with airway diameter, bronchoconstriction, together with a buildup of mucus or exudate in the bronchi, can readily lead to hypoxemia, hypercapnia, and respiratory acidosis.

> Alveolar ventilation may be maintained by the control of secretions, relief of airway constriction/compression, and when indicated, short-term oxygen therapy and/or ventilatory support. In theory, mucosal edema and bronchospasm may be relieved by decongestants and bronchodilators.

Central to any successful therapeutic strategy is identification of the underlying cause, be it infectious, parasitic, allergic or multifactorial. Regardless of the underlying cause, certain basic principles underpin any successful therapy program. Many of these principles embrace the concept of treating resultant symptoms to increase oxygenation of the alveolar tissues in the affected animal. Thus, once the cause has been identified and treatment initiated, it is imperative to use pharmacologic agents to relieve respiratory distress and improve the process of gaseous exchange. In this way, one can attempt to restore the tidal volume to normal. Drugs used for symptomatic relief include bronchodilators, expectorants, mucolytics, decongestants, anti-inflammatories, antihistamines and antitussives.

In the dog, heparin has been advocated for use in pulmonary thromboembolism and for DIC. If severe interstitial edema is present the animal may benefit from a diuretic such as furosemide. Oxygen therapy may be warranted in some cases.

PHARMACOLOGICAL AGENTS

5.1 BRONCHODILATORS

There are three classes of action for bronchodilators: (1) anticholinergics such as atropine, glycopyrrolate, and other belladonna alkaloids; (2) Beta-adrenergic agonists such as clenbuterol and ephedrine; and (3) methylxanthines, such as theophylline, which are phosphodiesterase inhibitors, though that may not be their mode of bronchodilation.

The adrenergic agents most widely used in the treatment of asthma include epinephrine, ephedrine, isoproterenol, and a number of $Beta_2$-selective agents. Because epinephrine and isoproterenol cause greater cardiac stimulation (mediated by $Beta_1$ receptors), they should probably be reserved for special situations.

A new generation of adrenergic drugs, effective after oral administration, with a long duration of action and a significant degree of $Beta_2$ selectivity, has recently become available.

$BETA_2$-ADRENERGIC DRUGS

Numerous $beta_2$-adrenergic receptor stimulants have been developed for use in human asthmatic patients, such as terbutaline, salbutamol or albuterol, fenoterol, clenbuterol.

Several adrenergic agents have been used to elicit bronchodilation through $Beta_2$-receptor action and the cAMP mechanism. Selective $beta_2$ activity produces bronchodilation without significant cardiostimulatory effects.

Stimulation of the local $Beta_2$ receptors in the bronchi will increase the production of cyclic AMP which counteracts any spasm in the area and so causes bronchodilation. Being selective agents for the $beta_2$ receptors in the bronchi, they are freer of side effects than many other mixed-action sympathomimetics such as adrenaline or ephedrine. Sympathomimetic amines act on adrenergic receptors that may be divided into alpha- and beta-receptors. Beta receptors can be further divided into $beta_1$ or cardiac receptors, and $beta_2$ or smooth muscle receptors. Specific $beta_2$ stimulants will therefore produce bronchodilation with considerably fewer side effects than less specific mixed-receptor action drugs. Salbutamol (Ventolin) is one of the better known $beta_2$ bronchodilators used in man.

In general, stimulation of $beta_2$ receptors relaxes airway smooth muscle, inhibits mediator release, and causes skeletal muscle tremor as a toxic effect. Beta-adrenergic drugs stimulate cilia and can also alter the viscosity of mucus.

Clenbuterol (Ventipulmin) is used in the horse, especially in cases of C.O.P.D., where it brings about a marked improvement in the clinical condition lasting 4 to 8 hours. There are usually no side effects at the therapeutic dose in the horse.

> **Dose:** Clenbuterol (Ventipulmin) is given orally or parenterally i.v. to the horse at a dosage of 0.8 μg/Kg b.i.d. for 10 days.
> **Intravenously:** 1.25 ml/50 Kg.
> **Orally:** 10 Kg measure/200 Kg. (Clenbuterol also increases the clearance of bronchial secretions by ciliary action).

Clenbuterol currently is widely used in Europe and Canada for chronic obstructive pulmonary disease in horses, but is not currently available in the U.S.

The nonselective sympathetic stimulant ephedrine was first introduced into human medicine in 1924. The first selective beta-adrenoceptor agonist was isoprenaline, which although a very effective bronchodilator, had the disadvantage of cardiac stimulation. Following the sub-division of beta receptors into beta$_1$ and beta$_2$ subtypes, selective beta$_2$ agonists were introduced. These latter drugs were essentially devoid of cardiac stimulatory properties.

Many beta$_2$ receptors are distributed through the bronchial tree. Following stimulation of these receptors, adenyl cyclase is activated by a nucleotide regulatory protein within the bronchial smooth muscle cells. This leads to increased production of cyclic AMP locally which then induces bronchodilation. Increased mucociliary clearance of the bronchial tree, reduction of bronchial edema and reduction of elevated pulmonary artery pressure as a result of beta$_2$ receptor-mediated vasodilation of the pulmonary arteries are secondary effects. The primary indication for treatment with a beta$_2$ agonist is reversible airflow obstruction.

These effects may result from stimulation of adenylate cyclase, which catalyzes the formation of cAMP, although the exact role of increased intracellular concentrations of cAMP is still uncertain.

The beta$_2$-adrenergic agonists include such drugs as albuterol, hexoprenaline (Salbutamol), clenbuterol, fenoterol, and terbutaline. None is approved for use in horses at present in the United States, although clenbuterol has been approved for horses in other countries. These drugs dilate airways by stimulating the airway beta$_2$ receptors, which results in an increase in cyclic AMP concentrations in the smooth muscle cells and relaxation. They also may enhance mucociliary activity. Side effects can include excitement, trembling, sweating, tachycardia, and ileus and increase with higher dosages.

Because beta receptors are not only found in the bronchial tree but also in other tissues such as vascular smooth muscle, some minor side effects may accompany the use of beta$_2$ agonists, such as tremors, blood pressure changes and altered biochemical function. Although most veterinary preparations are in the form of injections or granules for oral treatment, they should ideally be delivered to the airways by inhalation.

XANTHINES

Xanthines possess several pharmacologic actions including central nervous system stimulation, myocardial stimulation and bronchodilation. Two of these compounds, aminophylline and etamiphylline, possess very potent actions on the bronchioles, making them very effective bronchodilators. They act to inhibit the enzyme phosphodiesterase that normally catalyzes the breakdown of cyclic AMP. Because phosphodiesterase hydrolyzes cyclic nucleotides, this inhibition results in higher concentrations of intracellular cAMP.

The theophylline preparation most commonly used for therapeutic purposes is the theophylline-ethylenediamine complex (aminophylline). This is a phosphodiesterase inhibitor and this prevents degradation of cyclic AMP. It may be given intravenously or per os and apparently helps some horses with chronic obstructive pulmonary disease.

Aminophylline, or its active form, theophylline has long been used in man for treating bronchospasm. In man, horses, and dogs, it decreases the work of breathing and increases diaphragmatic contractility.

Etamiphylline camsylate is a popular xanthine available for clinical use, and is presented as an injection, powder or tablets. The half-lives of these xanthines are relatively short (about an hour in the dog), and it is possible that the central nervous system stimulant action contributes to the improved respiratory function as does the improved circulatory and renal function.

Methylxanthines can increase mucociliary clearance by stimulating the ciliary beat frequency, increasing water flux toward the airway lumen, and increasing secretion of mucus in the lower airways.

Etamiphylline camsylate (Millophylline) Dose: Injectable prep. 700 mg/5 ml Horse/Cattle: 10 ml i.m. S/C—repeated at 8 hour intervals. Dog/Cat: 1–2 i.m. S/C repeated at 8 hour intervals. *Oral*: Horse/Cattle: 3 × 300 mg. sachets in feed or as a drench. Dog/Cat: 1–2 tablets (100 mg. each) every 8 hours.

Bronchodilator drugs, e.g. aminophylline (5–10 mg/kg p.o. bid), terbutaline (0.02–0.06 mg/kg p.o. bid) or clenbuterol (0.8 µg/kg p.o. or i.v. bid) are sometimes administered parenterally or orally to severely pneumonic foals on a empiric basis and can prove beneficial.

Since beta$_2$ agonists promote the synthesis of cAMP through adenylate cyclase, and the methylxanthines prevent the inactivation of cAMP by phosphodiesterase, it is rational to use bronchodilators from both classes when dealing with a refractory case.

PARASYMPATHOLYTICS

Anticholinergic drugs include atropine, glycopyrrolate, ipratropium, and oxytropium. These are parasympatholytic and bronchodilatory. Atropine is useful as an immediate bronchodilator in horses in certain situations, but it has a short duration and is not appropriate for continuous or frequent use because of its side effects. It can cause ileus, mydriasis, tachycardia, and excitement, particularly in ponies. Anticholinergic drugs decrease submucosal gland and goblet cell production of mucus, but atropine can also thicken the secretions.

When given intravenously, atropine, the prototype muscarinic antagonist, causes bronchodilatation at a lower dose than that needed to increase heart rate. Systemic side effects limit the quantity of atropine sulfate that can be given.

In the respiratory tract, parasympatholytic agents (e.g., atropine) reduce the volume of secretions and relax the bronchial and bronchiolar smooth muscle. The rationale for their use as bronchodilators is that they antagonize muscarinic bronchoconstriction. Although atropine can be given orally or parenterally, its attendant side effects (notably tachycardia, increased viscosity of secretions and reduced bowel motility) have tended to preclude its use as a general bronchodilator other than for temporary relief of dyspnea in a severely affected case.

Atropine has long been used as a bronchodilator. It decreases airway resistance, increases dead space and blocks reflex bronchoconstriction.

Atropine Sulphate. Dose: S/C 30–100 µg./Kg.

Atropine's quaternary ammonium congeners, atropine methonitrate, glycopyrrolate, ipratropium bromide, and oxytropium bromide, have been reported to be very effective bronchodilators in man. Ipratropium is commercially available as an inhalant for human use and is especially helpful for asthma and in preventing exercise-induced bronchospasm.

Glycopyrrolate is a quaternary ammonium compound that inhibits acetylcholine's action at receptors on postganglionic cholinergic neurons and smooth muscle. As a charged molecule, it displays a low volume of distribution, fewer side effects in other organs and tissues, and high potency.

SYMPATHOMIMETICS

Ephedrine is a mixed action amine (alpha and beta receptors) producing its effect by direct receptor activation and release of noradrenaline. Pedriatic preparations containing ephedrine are used in small animal cases to induce bronchodilation. Compared to epinephrine, ephedrine has a longer duration, more oral activity, more pronounced central effects, and a much lower potency. Because of the development of more efficacious and beta$_2$-selective agonists, ephedrine is now infrequently used.

Ephedrine syrup 5 mg./ml., is an effective bronchodilator given orally in small animals. It is usually administered 2 or 3 times a day, 25 mg. per dose.

Adrenaline may be valuable as a drug of emergency for intramuscular or intravenous administration in severe anaphylaxis.

Adrenaline acid tartate (1 mg./ml.)
Dose: Horse/Cattle 0.2–0.4 ml./50 Kg. i.m. S/C; i.v. 0.1–0.2 ml./50 Kg/ Dogs: S/C.m./i.v. 0.05–0.15 ml./10 Kg.

5.2 REMOVAL OF SECRETIONS

Expectorants: These are designed to increase the removal of secretions from the respiratory tree by increasing the volume and reducing the viscosity of respiratory secretions. The inhalant types are occasionally used. Water vapor is an effective expectorant—small animals may be exposed to steam for short periods and the increase in humidity provided by the vaporization will present a less-viscous accumulated secretion for removal. Vaporization also has a soothing effect on the irritated respiratory surfaces.

Benzoin is the aromatic resin incorporated in Friars' Balsam, and eucalyptus oil has also been used. Both are placed in boiling water and inhalation takes place in a confined space, or a face mask may be used.

Steam has often been used to add water to mucus, and thus decrease its mucosal viscosity.

Bland aerosol therapy (e.g., sterile 0.9% NaCl) has been suggested as means of loosening secretions and thereby facilitating their clearance.

Fluid therapy with balanced electrolyte solutions is indicated in some cases to maintain hydration and promote mucociliary clearance and expectoration by reducing the viscosity of tenacious bronchial secretions. "Hyper-hydration" is practiced by some clinicians to further assist in mobilizing secretions but such therapy should be closely monitored by central venous pressure measurement because animals with pneumonia are susceptible to the development of pulmonary edema.

Large doses of intravenous fluids have been used to loosen secretions in the airways and treat horses with COPD. Intravenous administration of isotonic saline (20 to 40 L per day at a rate of 10 L per hour for 3 to 5 days) was reported to be of benefit in the treatment of equine COPD. However, there can be significant adverse side effects, such as excitement, dyspnea, tachycardia, discomfort and ataxia.

Fluid therapy for dehydration is extremely important. Not only will rehydration improve clearance mechanisms, but volume expansion remains the foremost therapy for the toxemia and endotoxic shock associated with pasteurellosis.

Expectorants may be beneficial in alleviating the thick mucous plugs in the airways. Included in this group are: ammonium chloride, acetates, acetic acid, creosote, guaiphenesin, ipecacuanha, potassium iodides, sodium citrate and squill. Although iodides have long been used for their apparent secretolytic action to aid expectoration, iodide can increase proteolytic digestion of mucus by enzymes present in purulent sputum.

Expectorants such as the iodides, guaiacol, and volatile oils are often beneficial by helping mobilize respiratory secretions. Mucolytics such as Bromhexine hydrochloride or a newer derivative, Sputolosin can also be beneficial in cases with large amounts of mucopus in the airways.

Orally administered hypertonic electrolyte solutions, such as ammonium carbonate and ammonium chloride, are claimed to be effective expectorants as they depolarize complex proteins in sputum and attract water from cells and blood vessels of the mucosa into the mucus in the airways.

Locally acting systemically administered expectorants are typified by saline type, such as ammonium chloride and sodium iodide. These are administered orally and are then excreted locally through the bronchial mucosa where they loosen the secretions. Ammonium chloride is incorporated in many proprietary cough preparations.

Mucolytic Agents: These substances act to break down long-chain glycoproteins found in the more viscous secretions of the respiratory tract. Mucus is a normal defense mechanism and is produced in a variety of cells within the wall of the respiratory tract. It is propelled by ciliary activity to the pharynx where it is usually swallowed. Mucus humidifies inspired air, traps and transports inhaled foreign particles and protects the mucoid surface from dehydration and injury by physical, chemical and infectious agents. In respiratory disease, mucus undergoes a physical change in its constituents and becomes extremely viscous. Cilia become overloaded, are unable to function adequately and effective mucus clearance ceases. Many microorganisms (viruses, mycoplasma, etc.) can destroy whole areas of cilia resulting in further impairment of the mucus clearance. The thick tenacious material not only restricts the passage of air into and out of the lungs but also inhibits treatment and recovery in respiratory disease. The ability of antibiotics and the host's defense mechanisms to penetrate adequately to the site of infection is impaired. This results in delayed recovery and bacterial recolonization.

Mucous 'viscosity' is related to the structure and content of the mucopolysaccharides (MPS) present. The long continuous strands of MPS fibers present in abnormal mucus produce a tenacious feltwork that is difficult to expectorate. Bisolvon acts by increasing the body's production of lysosomes that fragment the MPS fibers into small, noncontinuous units. The volume of bronchial secretions is also increased by Bisolvon. This mucolytic effect thus helps to re-establish normal mucociliary clearance and speed recovery when used in the treatment of respiratory disease.

Mucolytic drugs include acetylcysteine, bromhexine, dembrexine, proteolytic enzymes, and expectorants such as iodide salts. Depolymerization of glycoprotein molecules or hydrolysis of protein or nucleoprotein strands are the usual mechanisms involved.

N-acetylcysteine and S-carboxymethylcysteine are effective in depolymerizing mucus and also act on DNA. These substances act through free sulfhydryl groups that effectively open the disulfide bonds of mucous glycoproteins. Acetylcysteine breaks disulfide bonds and decreases viscosity of mucus. Two features of concern are its tendency to cause bronchospasm, ciliary inhibition, and severe coughing, and its propensity to inactivate antibiotics, particularly the penicillins.

The properties of mucus depend on the glycoproteins, around which water is organized and bound. With purulence there is increased crosslinkage of glycoproteins by disulfide bonds, and these bonds differ in cleavage properties. Mucoid sputum becomes less viscous with addition of water, and as it dries, viscosity increases. All are irritating to mucous membranes and can cause bronchospasm and bronchial edema.

The mucous layer itself contains substances that aid in airway protection. These include: lactoferrin, an iron-binding protein that inhibits bacterial iron metabolism; lysozyme, a bacteriocidal enzyme that may function with immunoglobulin (lg) A and complement in the process of bacteriolysis; lg, primarily lgA (which can neutralize bacterial toxins and viral and bacterial enzymes, and aid in agglutination, immobilization, and adherence of bacteria) and lgG (which is capable of agglutination, neutralization of toxins), and with complement, opsonization, and bacteriolysis.

In respiratory disease, the mucous coat is generally dehydrated, diminishing the ability of cilia to move. Fibrin adds significantly to the viscosity and elasticity of mucus. Treatments aimed at optimizing the mucous escalator have been directed toward alteration of mucus production and character and enhancing the activity of ciliary action. Mucolytic therapy is aimed at decreasing the viscosity of mucous to enhance the effectiveness of the mucous escalator.

The viscosity and elasticity of tracheobronchial mucus is due primarily to polymerization, an aggregation of glycoproteins. Polymerization takes place through the formation of disulfide bonds involving cysteine. The ability to polymerize and aggregate depends on glycoprotein concentration, which increases in dehydration.

Thick, tenacious mucus not only restricts passage of air into and out of the lungs, but also inhibits treatment and recovery in respiratory disease. The ability of antibiotics and the body's own defenses to penetrate adequately to the site of infection is impaired.

Dehydration is common in animals with lung disease because of diminished water intake and excessive insensible water loss associated with pyrexia and hyperpnea. Water and saline solutions are the practical mucokinetic diluents used to liquify hyperviscous mucus; oral rehydration, administration of parenteral fluids, and inhalation of water vapor (vaporization or "steaming") or saline aerosols (nebulization) are the approaches used. With iodide salts, direct stimulation occurs because iodides concentrate in the glands.

Bromhexine is another mucolytic expectorant that increases bronchial secretions and decreases their viscosity. It also results in an increase in immunoglobulin levels in airway secretions.

Bromhexine hydrochloride (*Bisolvon*) is a mucolytic compound used in conditions where excessive or tenacious sputum is a problem. Normally mucus is secreted in the respiratory tract in small amounts and it transports bacteria, irritants, dust, and cell debris from the lungs. The secretions consist of mucopolysaccharide fibers, but in the presence of infection, a highly viscous secretion is produced which often overcomes the system of expectoration, ciliary transportation and cough, thus obstructing the airways and impairing gas exchange. Bromhexine renders the secretions less viscous and more easily cleared, and following its administration at therapeutic dose levels, the activity of the secretory cells of the respiratory epithelium is increased, and a less viscous secretion is produced, improving expectoration. At high doses, Bisolvon has an antitussive action. In addition it alters the permeability of respiratory mucous membranes and of the local capillary supply so that there is an increase in the concentration in the bronchial mucus of certain antibiotics, especially oxytetracycline, sulphonamides and erythromycin. Bisolvomycin for injection contains bromhexine hydrochloride, oxytetracycline and lignocaine, a combination that provides the mucolytic and antibiotic concentrating properties of Bisolvon, together with the broad spectrum activity of oxytetracycline for respiratory disease.

Dose (a) *Bisolvomycin* (Bromhexine hcl. 3 mg: Oxytet. hcl. 50 mg.: (mucolytic & antibiotic) Lignocaine 20 mg./ml.)

Cattle: i.m./5 ml./50 Kg. B.W. 3–5 days.
(b) *Bisolvon* (Bromhexine hcl. 3 mg./ml.) i.m./
(mucolytic alone)
Horse: 25–30 ml. (L. 1–0.25 mg./Kg.)
Cattle: 25–30 ml. (0.2–0.5 mg./Kg.)
Dog: 1–2 ml. (1 mg./Kg.).
(Bisolvon powder for oral administration is also available.)

Humidifiers, nebulizers, mucolytic drugs and surface acting wetting agents have been used to attempt to decrease viscosity of secretions. Steam and most vaporizers probably affect only the extreme upper airways, but their benefit there can be considerable.

Nebulization is helpful in foals with tenacious secretions and/or a nonproductive cough but is probably contraindicated in foals with voluminous moist secretions. The major functions of nebulization are to liquify secretions, relieve bronchospasm, decrease mucosal oedema and kill bacteria. Ultrasonic nebulizers which disperse droplets less than 5μ in diameter should be used since larger droplets are filtered out in the upper respiratory tract and do not reach the terminal airways. Nebulized agents include bland carrier solutions, bronchodilators, mucolytics and antibiotics.

Particle size of the inhalant is the most important factor in deposition and nebulizers which produce particles less than 3 μm diameter will deliver moisture deeper into the tract. The most commonly used drugs nebulized in small droplet size are bronchodilators, especially the xanthines, which include theophylline and aminophylline, mucolytic, and the sympathomimetics such as epinephrine, isoproteronol, and salbutamol. Xanthines inhibit hydrolytic degradation of 3,5 cyclic AMP, and sympathomimetics stimulate conversion of ATP to 3,5 AMP.

Decongestants: These will help to reduce the production and accumulation of inflammatory edema in the local area. Vasoconstrictor drugs are used—especially pseudoephedrine—which is similar to ephedrine in its functions: however it has less bronchodilatory action and greater vasoconstrictor action than ephedrine.

Alpha agonists such as phenylephrine and phenylpropanolamine are useful as decongestants due to their vasoconstrictive properties. They should not be used systemically because they are bronchoconstrictors, but as effective nasal sprays.

5.3 COUGH SUPPRESSANTS

If a cough is productive, it should not be abolished. It is a protective reflex and if productive will allow removal of secretions. If the cough is not productive and particularly if it is chronic and continuous, the cough in itself may initiate chronic respiratory parenchymal changes such as emphysema and fibrosis.

A productive cough produces phlegm or sputum, and is essentially a protective device to clear the lungs which might otherwise become congested with plugs of mucus providing sites for infection and disturbance of effective gaseous exchange. Such cough may be encouraged by expectorants.

A dry, irritating or ticklish cough, producing little or no sputum (which if present should be white in color and nonpurulent) is common in tracheitis, in post-viral conditions such as the common cold and sometimes in chronic bronchitis. It can be distressing and exhausting, preventing sleep at night and irritating other people by day. Such a cough may be treated with cough suppressants.

Cough suppressants may act at any one of the sites in the cough reflex. Examples of centrally acting agents are codeine, dextromethorphan, pholcodine and noscapine. Antihistamines, as central nervous system depressants, will also exert a sedative effect on the cough center. Note that diphenhydramine has a potent antitussive effect.

Antitussive drugs can help fulfill only one of the basic needs in treatment for respiratory disease. For cough suppression two types of agents may be used: (a) local antitussives or (b) central antitussives.

Local Agents: These are the demulcent compounds—sweet syrupy vehicles in which other active principles are dissolved. Demulcents such as honey, glycerin, menthol or syrup act to coat, protect and soothe the raw eroded inflamed mucosa for a short period. Many cough mixtures, elixirs or electuaries include cough depressants, such as Benadryl, in a demulcent base of honey or glycerine. These demulcents act by coating the mucosa and, especially when it is dry and inflamed, will protect the upper respiratory tract above the level of the trachea from noxious physical irritants.

Central Antitussives: Opiates and several of their derivatives are potent inhibitors of the medullary cough center at subanalgesic doses and are used specifically as antitussives. Examples of narcotic antitussives include the following: codeine, hydromorphone, hydrocodone and butorphanol. Non-narcotic antitussives include pholcodine, benzonatate and noscapine.

Narcotic-like drugs such as codeine and dehydrocodeinone have a definite place in the treatment of dry, irritating, nonproductive coughs. Such coughing wastes energy and is self-perpetuating because of its continual irritation of tracheobronchial mucosa. The rationale for antitussive therapy in early stages of acute tracheobronchitis is that suppression of coughing breaks the irritation cycle, thereby allowing natural healing to occur. Codeine is the major central antitussive that depresses the cough center in the brain. It is well absorbed orally and has a slow rate of metabolism in the body. Codeine is effective at an oral dose of 1 to 2 mg./Kg. Dihydrocodeine is essentially similar to codeine, and pholcodeine is about twice as potent.

A number of human pediatric preparations are now frequently used in small animal practice. The continuing search for compounds with potent antitussive properties to relieve the dry hacking cough of canine tracheobronchitis has resulted in the widespread use of newer, more potent, drugs to replace codeine for the relief of cough.

Butorphanol was developed to minimize side effects associated with earlier opiates such as morphine or codeine. The drug is classified as a narcotic agonist-antagonist because it can either activate or block opiate receptors. In relative potency terms, butorphanol possesses 5 to 7 times the analgesic activity of morphine and 20 times that of pentazocine. It is approximately 20 times more potent than codeine as an antitussive agent, with minimal side effects, and relief lasts for twice as long as codeine. Butorphanol is a potent selective antitussive agent with little potential for abuse. Unlike other narcotics, butorphanol does not produce profound respiratory depression or cardiovascular changes. The specific site of action of butorphanol is unknown. Butorphanol probably exerts analgesic and antitussive effects through the central nervous system (subcortical, possibly in the hypothalamus). Clinically it displays potential as an analgesic for equine colic, as an analgesic component in balanced anesthesia, and also as a cough suppressant in horses. (Cats *appear* to tolerate the drug well.) Butorphanol has potent antiemetic and antitussive activity. Given subcutaneously to dogs, its antitussive potency is reported to be 100 times that of codeine, 10 times pentazocine, and four times morphine. It is indicated in dogs for relief of acute or chronic, nonproductive cough associated with tracheobronchitis, tracheitis, tonsillitis, laryngitis and pharyngitis originating from inflammatory conditions of the upper respiratory tract.

The usual antitussive dosage in dogs is 0.025–0.05 mg./lb. subcutaneously of the tartrate salt b.i.d. Therapy can be followed up by butorphanol tartrate tablets 0.25 to 0.5 mg./lb. In many cases a 3 to 4 day course of treatment is necessary. Sometimes, cough suppression is accompanied by mild sedation although this can be dose-related. Like other centrally acting opiodal antitussives, butorphanol should not be used in conditions of the lower respiratory tract associated with copious mucus production. When using central cough suppressants the very important protective reflex of coughing will be abolished—the animal may have respiratory secretions that must be removed. However, central suppression may be necessary with severe paroxysmal coughing to avoid severe fatigue and active propagation of the disease complex. (Cough suppression may also be attained by reducing the local need to cough. This can be achieved by reducing secretions or their viscosity, removing them, increasing the diameter of the airways and reducing the inflammation in that area, i.e., by reducing the local cause of the cough, so the need for coughing will be reduced.)

5.4 ANTI INFLAMMATORIES

(a) Corticosteroids

Arachidonic acid is released from reactive cells in tissue inflammation, and is converted to a number of derivatives. Inflammatory mediators of bronchoconstriction include histamine, serotonin and arachidonic acid derivatives. Prostaglandins, PGE1 and PGE2, leukotrienes, vasoactive intestinal peptide and histamine, all of which are increased in respiratory disease, have been demonstrated to increase mucus, water and electrolyte secretion by respiratory epithelium.

The most effective therapy of interacting with prostaglandin, thromboxane, and the leukotriene system in inflammation, is the use of glucocorticoids. Glucocorticoids exert their anti-inflammatory action through induction of synthesis of lipocortins: peptides generated by cells containing glucocorticoid receptors. Lipocortins, through inhibition of phospholipase A2, prevent mobilization of arachidonic acid from membrane lipids, and thus block the synthesis of its derivatives.

Because of the ability of corticosteroids to inhibit phospholipase enzymes in cell membranes, they prevent formation of prostaglandins and leukotrienes—powerful endogenous bronchoconstrictive substances. It should be recognized, however, that glucocorticoids significantly blunt natural defense mechanisms against bacterial and viral infections. Their widespread actions include interference with antigen processing, inhibition of T-lymphocyte responses to antigens, and suppression of tissue response to IgE-mediated release of histamine from mast cells.

Inhibition of pulmonary macrophage function (adhesion, phagocytosis, intracellular killing, degradation), for example by viral infection and corticosteroid use, has a major role in the development of secondary bacterial infections. Glucorticoids should not be used in situations in which bacterial infections are not adequately treated with antimicrobials, nor in infections known to be viral.

In viral respiratory disease, the main emphasis should be on adequate antibiotic treatment to counter secondary bacterial infection, with fluid therapy in more severe cases if dehydration may become a problem. Corticosteroids are contraindicated because they may potentiate the virus infection.

Some undesirable side effects of steroids are adrenal suppression and an apparent predisposition to laminitis and infections. Low doses minimize some of the potential ill effects but do not preclude development of laminitis in horses.

Corticosteroids administered parenterally are sometimes used in the treatment of certain respiratory conditions. In cases of acute pneumonia or aspiration pneumonia, they may be occasionally used to relieve respiratory distress, reduce pulmonary effusion and improve the general well-being of the animal. These effects are mediated mainly by their anti-inflammatory effects and mild euphoric action. However, corticosteroids should be used with extreme caution as their effects are simply palliative; by their immunosuppressive properties, they may propagate the cause of the disease (as in calf pneumonia), lead to premature termination of antibiotic therapy on account of the apparent improvement, or lead to subsequent relapse and disease recurrence. Systemic corticosteroid administration leads to suppression of the immune system and therefore it is important to provide adequate antibiotic cover during corticoid therapy and for at least 3 to 4 days thereafter. The selected antibiotic should have bactericidal rather than bacteriostatic properties, to minimize the recurrence of infection after cessation of antibiotic therapy. In general, the use of corticosteroids is contraindicated in all but very severe cases of respiratory infections. Side effects are related to duration of action; so short-acting corticoids such as Dexamethasone, sodium phosphate, or betamethasone are safer than the longer-acting depot type preparations such as Methyl Prednisolone acetate and Dexamethasone Trimethyl acetate (Depo-Medrol type).

Preparations (Soluble formulations)

1. Dexamethasone sodium phosphate 2 mg./ml. DEXADRESSON—(Intervet) Dose, Cattle/Horses: 10 to 30 mg. (5 to 15 ml.) i.v., i.m. S/C.

2. Betamethasone sodium phosphate Betsolan soluble (Glaxo) 2 mg./ml. i.m., i.v. Cattle/Horses: 5 to 20 ml.

(b) Nonsteroidal Anti-inflammatory Drugs (NSAIDs)

The synthesis of prostaglandins and thromboxanes are inhibited by nonsteroidal anti-inflammatory drugs (NSAIDs) such as aspirin, phenylbutazone, oxphenbutazone, dipyrone, isopyrin, piroxicam, ibuprofen, naproxen, meclofenamic acid, acetaminophen, and flunixin. The NSAIDs are also potent inhibitors of the biologic effects of endotoxin, but without the immunosuppressive properties. In addition, they are also potent analgesics and antipyretics.

This group of compounds has been overlooked in bovine practice but combine the advantages of anti-inflammatory action, antipyresis and analgesia without the unwanted immunosuppressant effects of the corticosteroids. Their antiprostaglandin effects reduce local inflammation and exudation. Acetylsalicylic acid (aspirin), Flunixin (Banatune) and phenylbutazone-isopyrin are of value in giving relief from the stress of acute edema and inflammation.

Kinetic studies in the cow indicate that a loading dose of 2.2 mg/Kg followed by maintenance doses of 1.1 mg/Kg every 8 hours should provide levels similar to those required for analgesia and prostaglandin inhibition in the horse. Aspirin is available for use in cattle; the recommended dosage is 100 mg/Kg orally twice daily. Phenylbutazone can be given at 6 mg/Kg for loading, followed by 3 mg/Kg daily for maintenance, i.v. or p.o.

Finadyne: Flunixin Meglumine (50 mg./ml.)
Cattle: 2 ml./45 Kg. i.v. at 24 hour intervals for up to 5 days.
Tomanol: (Intervet/Bayer) (Isopyrin 240 mg.: PBZ 120 mg./ml.) Cow 20 to 30 ml. i.m. or slowly i.v. Horse: 20 to 40 ml. slowly i.v.

(c) Dimethyl Sulfoxide (DMSO)

DMSO is another compound with possible anti-inflammatory properties. One of its main beneficial effects is thought to be its ability to scavenge oxygen radicals. It is therefore of use as a possible means to prevent neutrophil-mediated tissue damage in pasteurellosis. DMSO may also have analgesic effects, may reduce platelet aggregation and coagulation, and improve tissue perfusion.

Methylsulfonylmethane, a metabolite of DMSO with anti-inflammatory activity, has been effective in stopping cough in horses with suspected allergic airway inflammation when administered at a dosage of 18 to 22 mg/Kg (8 to 10 mg/lb) orally twice a day. It appears that superoxide dismutase, and other agents, by scavenging O_2 in extracellular fluid, prevent activation of the superoxide dependant chemoattractant, which represents the basis for the anti-inflammatory activity of these agents.

5.5 ANTIHISTAMINES

Histamine release in inflammatory or hypersensitive states can cause contraction of the bronchial smooth muscle and extravasation of fluid. Histamine exerts its effects on respiratory smooth muscle through two distinct H1 and H2 receptor types. H1 receptors mediate bronchiolar constriction and H2 receptors mediate bronchodilation. H1 receptors dominate in respiratory smooth muscle, so that the effect of histamine is bronchoconstriction. H1 blocking agents, such as promethazine, pyralamine and diphenhydramine are effective antihistaminics, resulting in bronchodilation in histamine induced bronchoconstriction.

Many respiratory diseases have definite histamine involvement and antihistamines may be employed to counteract the local bronchoconstriction. The antihistamines also possess parasympatholytic, local anesthetic and CNS depressant effects all of which may be beneficial in cough control, especially in small animals. Diphenhydramine hydrochloride (Benadryl) is commonly incorporated in cough remedies for dogs and cats where its antihistamine effects reduce local bronchoconstriction and production of secretions. Its atropine-like activity also widens the airways; its local anesthetic effect reduces respiratory irritation, and it possesses also a strong sedative effect. Antihistamines have long been used

to suppress coughing and to treat COPD. Large doses can inhibit the secretory activities of the bronchial glands because of their anticholinergic-like effect and this, in theory, could result in drying of secretions and adversely affect mucociliary clearance. Antihistamines are only partially beneficial when mediators other than histamine are released and have no effect on established bronchoconstriction.

Benylin Expectorant (Parke Davis) contains diphenhydramine Hcl, together with ammonium chloride, sodium citrate and menthol. Dose: 7.5 ml. orally per 10 lbs. in the dog.

Trepelennamine Hcl. is a useful antihistamine for use in cattle where it possesses a useful central stimulant action. However, antihistamines have a tendency to dry up bronchial secretions, and make them more viscous and more difficult to expel. Trepelennamine given intravenously at commencement of therapy may be of use in acute pulmonary edema or aspiration pneumonia.

Trepellenamine (20 mg./ml.) i.m. or slowly i.v.
Horse/Cattle 1 ml./45 Kg. Calf 3 to 5 ml.

5.6 MISCELLANEOUS MEASURES

Asthmatic bronchospasm might be reversed or prevented, for example, by drugs that prevent mast cell degranulation (cromolyn, calcium channel antagonists), block the conduction along sensory or motor nerves to the airways (topical anesthetics), inhibit the effect of acetylcholine released from vagal motor nerves (muscarinic antagonists), or directly relax airway smooth muscle (adrenergic agents, theophylline).

Disodium cromoglycate differs from most antiasthmatic medications in that it is only of value when taken prophylactically. Its main use is in the prevention of C.O.P.D.

Cromolyn prevents antigen-induced release of histamine and other mediators of anaphylaxis from sensitized mast cells and lung fragments, by preventing the transmembrane influx of calcium provoked by IgE antibody-antigen interaction on the mast cell surface.

5.7 RESPIRATORY INFECTIONS—SMALL ANIMALS

A common presentation is one of a chronically coughing patient suffering from some form of respiratory disease. The primary etiology may sometimes be difficult to establish: it may be infective, environmental or multifactorial. A chronic nonproductive continual cough may develop in the animal, and if left untreated, may progress to a condition of chronic respiratory disease with development of emphysema and generalized fibrosis. A chronic cough will create fatigue in the animal and also interfere with normal breathing and feeding. It may induce bronchiectasis, atalectasis, emphysema and severe secondary tracheobronchitis.

Tracheobronchitis is an inflammatory process where a decrease in the number of active cilia, hypertrophy of the mucus-secreting glands, an increase in the production of mucus and an increase in the viscosity of the mucus occurs. There is a decrease in the water content of the airway surfaces and secretions, and if mucopurulent secretions are present, the inflammatory cells will also increase the viscosity. In short, there will be increased production of drier, more tenacious secretions into a respiratory tree with depleted ciliary capacity. This in turn will lead to obstruction of the airways, with a consequent reduced filling capacity of the lungs.

Additional changes will also be attributable to the inflammatory process—local swelling, edema, irritation and bronchial spasm. The presence of bronchospasm, edema and increased tenacious secretion accumulation will reduce the diameter of the bronchi and its ability to carry adequate air. The reduced ciliary activity and exaggerated cough reflex will give rise to continual chronic coughing and fatigue. Bronchiolar spasm and the viscous mucus accumulation significantly reduces airflow to the lungs. The chronic coughing is purposeless, insofar as the viscous secretions are difficult to move, and the reduced ciliary activity renders this movement almost impossible. In small animals, a number of classic clinical conditions are commonly encountered which can give rise to respiratory symptoms.

The dry hacking cough associated with canine tracheobronchitis is both a nuisance and a medical concern for which the owner expects the veterinarian to provide prompt effect relief. Butorphanol tartrate (Torbutrol—Bristol) represents a synthetic analgesic compound with both potent and fast-acting antitussive properties. Butorphanol was developed in an attempt to minimize the side effects associated with such classic narcotic analgesics as morphine and codeine.

5.8 NASAL ASPERGILLOSIS

Nasal aspergillosis is a common upper respiratory tract infection in dogs. Aspergillus species acts as an opportunist pathogen causing sneezing and a nasal discharge. Signs of CNS involvement can be seen in advanced cases if severe infestation of the sinuses are involved. Amphotericin B has been widely recommended in treatment of aspergillosis but the drug has several disadvantages. Treatment must be given intravenously, three times weekly for 2 to 4 months and the drug itself is high nephrotoxic.

Ketoconazole, a synthetic imidazole-dioxolane derivative, is a potent oral antifungal agent. It has been used in human medicine, and also for many superficial and deep mycoses where *Candida spp.* is involved. Ketoconazole possesses in vitro activity against several strains of Aspergillus, yeasts, dermatophytes, Nocardia, Blastomyces, Coccidioides and Histoplasma. Treatment for nasal aspergillosis consists of ketoconazole 30 mg./Kg. orally for 8 to 11 weeks. Thiabendazole 20 mg./Kg. b.i.d. for 7 days can also be effective. While Miconazole, an imidazole related to ketoconazole looks promising, it is not as potent as Ketoconazole for aspergillosis. Additionally, miconazole is not as readily distributed throughout the body by the gastrointestinal tract. An alternative is intranasal infusion of 0.1% natamycin.

5.9 FELINE RESPIRATORY DISEASE

Feline viral rhinotracheitis (FVR virus) and feline calici virus (FCV) are two of the prime causes of respiratory disease in cats. Feline

Calicivirus is involved, either alone or with FVR, in 40 to 45% of cat flu cases.

Feline Chlamydia psittaci can be a significant pathogen where predominant clinical signs are those of persistent conjunctivitis. Bacteria and mycoplasmas are implicated commonly as secondary invaders. Immunosuppression arising from intercurrent illness from feline leukemia virus or feline immunodeficiency virus can exacerbate the pathogenicity of the various primary or secondary pathogens.

Feline respiratory vaccines are commonly used but protection is not always complete. Breakdown can occur from an overwhelming challenge of virulent viruses, or the presence of interfering material passively acquired antibodies. Occasionally, apparent vaccine breakdowns may be caused by Chlamydia psittaci infection.

In cases of outbreaks of feline respiratory viral disease, adequate antimicrobial therapy is necessary against the secondary bacterial infection. In *C. psittaci* infection, oxytetracycline, minocycline or doxycycline are the antimicrobials of choice. Therapy should be intensive, both parenteral and oral, and may have to be continued for 3 to 4 weeks to adequately eliminate the infection. Eradication can be difficult and underlying stress related causes (dietary or parasitic management) should be addressed. Fluid therapy may be warranted in debilitated cases where dehydration from anorexia may be a problem. Corticosteroids are contraindicated as they may potentiate spread of the virus infection. NSAID tablets can be considered as alternatives. Although no suitable antiviral agents for veterinary use are commercially available for the cat, IUDR has occasionally been used for ulcerative keratitis accompanying the feline viral rhinotracheitis syndrome. Idoxuridine has been used also in horses for its antiherpetic effects in ocular problems.

SELECTED REFERENCES

Anthony, V.B., Sahn, S.A. and Repine, J.E. Effect of dimethyl sulfoxide on chemotaxis of phagocytic cells. Ann NY Acad. Sci. 411, 321, 1983.

Aubier, M. and Roussos, C. Effect of theophylline on respiratory muscle function. Chosl. 85, 915, 1985.

Ayres, J.W., Pearson, E.G., and Riebold, T.W. Theophylline and dyphylline pharmacokinetics in the horse. Am. J. Vet. Res. 46(12), 2500, 1985.

Ayres, J.W., Pearson, E.G., Riebold, T.W., et al. Theopylline and dyphylline pharmacokinetics in the horse. Am J Vet Res. 48, 423, 1987.

Bauck, L.B. Treatment of canine nasal aspergillosis with Ketoconazole. Vet. Med/SAC. XX, 1713, 1983.

Beech, J. Respiratory problems in foals, Comp Cont Educ Pract Vet. 8S, 284, 1986.

Borelli, D. Ketoconazole, an oral antifungal: Laboratory and clinical assessment of imidazole drugs. Post Grad J Med. 55, 657, 1979.

Boyd, E.M. and Sheppard, P. On the expectorant activity of Bisolvon. Arch Int Pharmacodyn Ther. 163, 284, 1966.

Burgi, H. Sputum mucopolysaccharides. Ther. Umsch. 22, 331, 1965.

Cavanaugh, R.L. Antitussive properties of butorphanol. Arch Int Pharmacodyn Ther. 220, 258, 1976.

Christie, G.J. Butorphanol tartrate: A new antitussive agent for use in dogs. Vet Med/SAC, 75, 1559, 1980.

Deegan, E. Massive intravenous infusion: A novel secretolytic therapy for horses with chronic obstructive pulmonary disease. (COPD) Proc AAEP. XX, 27, 1981.

Eldridge, F.L., Millhorn, D.E. and Waldrop, T.G. Mechanisms and respiratory effects of methylxanthine. Respir Physiol. 53, 239, 1983.

Gaskell, R. and Knowles, J. Feline respiratory disease. In Pract. 23, 1989.

Gaskell, R.M. Feline respiratory disease complex. *In* Manual of Small Animal Infectious Diseases. Ed. by J.E. Barlough, New York, Churchill-Livingstone, 1988., pp. 135.

Gaskell, R.M. Feline viral respiratory disease—present attitudes towards and problems with vaccination. Bull Fel Adv Bur. 18, 4, 1980.

Gingerich, D.A., Rourke, J.E. and Strom, P.W. Clinical efficacy of Butorphanol injectable and tablets. Vet. Med/SAC 78, 179, 1983.

Gross, N.J., and Scoradin, M.S. Anticholinergic antimuscarinic bronchodilators. Am Rev Respir Dis. 129, 856, 1984.

Jenkins, W.L. Concurrent use of corticosteroids and antimicrobial drugs, in the treatment of infectious diseases in large animals. JAVMA. 185, 1145, 1984.

Knifton, A. Drug therapy for respiratory disease in calves. Vet Ann. 23, 56, 1983.

Lambert, H.P. Clinical significance of tissue penetration of antibiotics in respiratory tract. Scand J Infect Dis Suppl. 14, 262, 1978.

Leff, A. and Munoz, N.M. Interrelationship between alpha dn beta adrenergic agonists and histamine in canine airways. J Allergy Clin Immunol. 68, 300, 1981.

Leid, R.W., and Potter, K.A. Inflammation and mediators of lung injury. *In* Veterinary linics in North America. Food Animal Practice, Symposium in bovine Respiratory Disease. Ed. by R. Breeze. Philadelphia, W.B. Saunders, 1985. P. 377.

Lieberman, J. and Kurnick, N.B. The induction of proteolysis in purulent sputum by iodides. J Clin Invert. 43, 1892, 1964.

Littenberg, B. and Gluck, E.H. A controlled trial of methylprednisolone in the emergency treatment of asthma. N Engl J Med. 314, 150, 1986.

Lundgren, J.D., Hirata, F., Marom, Z. et al. Dexamethasone inhibits respiratory glycoconjugate secretion from feline airways in vitro by the induction of lipocortin (lipomodulin) synthesis. Am Rev Respir Dis. 137, 353, 1988.

Marom, Z., Shelhamer, J.H., Alling, D. et al. The effects of corticosteroids on mucous glycoprotein secretion from human airways in vitro. Am Rev Respir Dis. 129, 62, 1984.

Matthews, A.G., Hackett, I.J. and Lawton, W.A. The mucolytic effect of Sputolysin in horses with respiratory disease. Vet Rec. 122, 106, 1988.

McKiernan, B.C., Koritz, G.D., Scott, J.S. et al. Plasma throphylline concentration and lung function in ponies with recurrent obstructive lung disease. Eq Vet J. 22, 194, 1990.

Nadel, J.A. and Davis, B. Parasympathetic and sympathetic regulation of secretion from submucosal glands in airways. Federation Proc. 39, 3075, 1980.

Orsini, J.A. Butorphanol tartrate: Pharmacology and clinical indications. Comp Cont Educ Pract Vet. 10, 849, 1988.

Potthof, A. and Carithers, R. Pain and analgesia in dogs and cats. Comp Cont Educ Pract Vet. 11, 887, 1989.

Roth, J.A. and Frank, D.E. Recombinant bovine interferon famma, as an immunomodulator in dexamethasone-treated and non-treated cattle. J Interferon Res. 9, 143, 1989.

Sasse, W., and Deegan, E. Efficacy of Sputolysin (ambroxol) inb chronic bronchitis of horses. Tierartzl Umsch. 39, 941, 1984.

Schurig, J.E. Effects of butorphanol and morphine in pulmonary mechanics, arterial blood pressure, and venous plasma histamine in the anaesthetised dog. Arch Int Pharmacodyn Ther. 223, 296, 1978.

Soma, L.R., Beech, J. and Gerber, N.H. Effects of cromolyn in horses with chronic obstructive pulmonary disease. Vet Res Commun. 11, 339, 1987.

The Use of Drugs in Food Animal Medicine. Proceedings of the 10th Annual Food Animal Medicine Conference. Ed. by Powers, J.D. and Powers, T.E. Columbus, OH, Ohio State Univ Press, 1984. P. 62.

Wanner, A. Effects of methylxanthine on airway mucociliary function. Am J Med. 79, 16, 1985.

Wanner, A. Effects of methylxanthine on airway mucociliary function. Am J Med. 79, 16, 1985.

Webb, A.I., Coons, T.J., Koterba, A.M. et al. Developments in management of the newborn foal in respiratory disease. 2. Treatment. Eq Vet J. 16, 319, 1984.

Wong, G.A., Pierce, T.H., Goldstein, E. et al. Penetration of antimicrobial agents into bronchial secretions. Am J Med. 59, 219, 1975.

CHAPTER 6

GENERAL THERAPY OF GASTROINTESTINAL DISEASE

6.1 Emetics
6.2 Antiemetics
6.3 Antiulcer Drugs
6.4 Protectives and Absorbents
6.5 Central Antiemetics
6.6 Narcotic Analgesics
6.7 Anticholinergics
6.8 Spasmolytic Drugs
6.9 Locally Active Drugs
6.10 Antisecretory Drugs
6.11 Laxatives, Cathartics, Purgatives
6.12 Diarrhea
6.13 Neonatal Diarrhea in Calves
6.14 Coliform Calf Scour
6.15 Antimicrobial Therapy
6.16 Protectives and Adsorbents
6.17 Antisecretory Drugs
6.18 *Lactobacillus* and Other Bacterial Inocula (Probiotics)
6.19 Motility-Inhibiting Drugs
6.20 Fluid Replacement
6.21 Role of Colostrum
6.22 Immunologic Approaches

Disturbances of the gastrointestinal tract in any of the domestic species may present a variety of clinical signs, including vomiting, diarrhea, dehydration, malabsorption, loss of weight, impaction, spasm, and visceral pain. These symptoms can be treated by a range of drugs that alter motility or simply modify certain functions of the gastrointestinal tract. Pharmacologic aids may influence motility and absorptive and digestive processes and treat pain. Objectives of therapy are to treat the clinical signs and to restore normal function as soon as possible. Attention must also be paid, however, to treating and controlling the predisposing factors as well as correcting and maintaining the fluid/electrolyte and acid-base balance, also taking into account dietary and management factors.

Drugs influence motility, absorption, digestion, pain, and infection. General aims of therapy (e.g., for diarrhea) are as follows:

- Treat cause
- Control motility
- Protect inflamed or eroded mucosa
- Relieve pain
- Fluid/electrolyte replacement

Types of drugs active on the gastrointestinal tract are:

- Emetics and antiemetics
- Drugs affecting motility (parasympatholytics, antispasmodics)
- Locally acting drugs (protectives/opiates)
- Laxatives
- Analgesics
- Antisecretory agents

6.1 EMETICS

Emesis is a complex reflex action that is usually confined to carnivores and humans. Vomiting can be induced by irritation of the gastrointestinal tract (particularly the pharynx), middle ear disturbances, motion sickness, or drugs or toxins that act centrally to activate motor nerves to the abdominal muscles and diaphragm. Emetic agents may act centrally by affecting the chemoreceptor trigger zone or vomiting center; locally acting emetics act by inducing local irritation of the pharynx or gastric mucosa.

CENTRAL EMETICS

Apomorphine Hydrochloride

This agent may be used in dogs but is contraindicated in cats. Vomiting usually occurs in about 4 to 5 minutes and lasts for 20 to 25 minutes. After vomiting, the animal becomes depressed and narcotized, and for this reason great care must be exercised in treating a case of poisoning caused by a central nervous system depressant because summation of depression may occur. Overdosage is characterized by rapid respiration, running in circles, and tetanic convulsions (dopaminergic activity). This may be treated by a phenothiazine derivative, such as chlorpromazine.

Dosages in dogs are as follows:

Subcutaneously, 0.08 mg/kg (effect, 3 to 5 minutes)
Intravenously, 0.04 mg/kg (effect, 1 to 4 minutes)
Ocular or oral administration, 0.25 mg/kg (effect, 5 to 12 minutes)

Ipecac

This is another centrally active emetic that contains an alkaloid emetine and has a dual action producing chemoreceptor trigger zone stimulation and peripheral gastric irritation. It is given orally usually as a glycerine-based syrup at a dose of 2.2 to 6.6 ml/kg of 7% solution. Vomiting is usually seen in 10 to 15 minutes. The use of syrup of ipecac in cats is controversial, but the drug is probably safe if used cautiously.

LOCAL EMETICS

These irritate the gastric mucosa or pharynx, e.g., household detergents, soap, mustard, common salt, and 50 ml 1% copper sulfate, or zinc sulfate, (effective in 10 minutes in dogs).

XYLAZINE (HYDROCHLORIDE)

This is a predictable and safe emetic agent following intramuscular administration of 1 mg/kg. Emesis is followed by sedation for 30 to 90 minutes. Xylazine is also useful in cats for emesis. Xylazine consistently induces emesis in cats 3 to 5 minutes after the administration of a low dose and is not associated with central nervous system depression. The mechanism of vomiting appears to involve alpha$_2$-adrenoreceptor stimulation.

6.2 ANTIEMETICS

Although it is often desirable to induce vomiting after ingestion of a poison, it is often desirable to suppress vomiting, as, for instance, in severe gastritis, in which prolonged vomiting may lead to intense dehydration, loss of chloride, and metabolic alkalosis. Simple preparations with protective or absorbent functions may be of value in controlling gastritis (or enteritis) by protecting the ulcerated and eroded mucosae.

6.3 ANTIULCER DRUGS

ANTACIDS

These are widely used in human and veterinary medicine for the neutralization of the hydrochloric acid of the stomach. Antacids are weak bases that neutralize or remove acid from the gastric contents. They are categorized as systemic or nonsystemic (which neutralize gastric contents without causing systemic alkalosis). These compounds include calcium carbonate and many aluminum and magnesium salts. The purpose of therapy with these drugs is to maintain the gastric pH above 4 to 5 and to decrease diffusion of acid back through the gastric wall or prevent it from reaching the duodenum. Slow-acting antacids are the less soluble compounds, such as magnesium hydroxide (milk of magnesia), aluminum hydroxide, aluminum trisilicate, and calcium carbonate. The antacid effects of some of these are only temporary, however, because the carbon dioxide released by the chemical neutralization reaction causes distention of the stomach and thereby may cause reflex secretion of acid and digestive enzymes (acid rebound). Rapid-acting agents are those soluble in water, such as sodium bicarbonate. Proprietary preparations often also contain absorbents and protectives.

Antacids are useful in treating severe gastritis, reflex esophagitis, and gastric or duodenal ulcers. Side effects include acid rebound and the laxative (magnesium) or constipatory effects (calcium, aluminum) of many antacids. The duration of action depends on the gastric emptying time and on the volume of acid secretion.

Aluminum hydroxide and magnesium hydroxide can be used as antacids or phosphorous binders (aluminum hydroxide) in cats. Cimetidine (Tagamet) and ranitidine (Zantac) are histamine (H$_2$)-receptor blockers that can be used in cats to control gastric acid secretions. Although both drugs are probably equally effective in controlling gastric acid secretion, ranitidine is associated with fewer adverse affects in humans.

The chain of events leading to acid secretion is complex, but gastrin is believed to be the major stimulus and to function through release of histamine. The parietal cells possess receptors for histamine, gastrin, and acetylcholine. Histamine receptors on these parietal cells (H$_2$ receptors) differ from histamine receptors elsewhere in the body (H$_1$ receptors). Cimetidine and ranitidine are competitive H$_2$ receptor antagonists that decrease gastric acid output by 70 to 90%. These drugs are effective in gastric or duodenal ulcers, controlling upper gastrointestinal ulcers. Both drugs have proved to be equally effective in human ulcer therapy, and both have been used successfully in treating foals with ulcers. Research in foals has shown that ranitidine is more effective than cimetidine in suppressing gastric acid production. Recent research suggests that previously used doses may have been inadequate.

Histamine blockers cimetidine or ranitidine block the H$_2$ receptors on gastric parietal cells, resulting in a marked decreased in gastric acid secretion. In dogs, 10 mg/kg i.v. cimetidine, 5 mg/kg orally, is given every 6 to 8 hours, or 0.5 mg/kg intravenously. Ranitidine is given orally at 0.5 mg/kg twice daily. In foals oral doses are: cimetidine 8.8 mg/kg every 8 hours; ranitidine 4.4 mg/kg every 8 hours. Clinical signs of ulceration may resolve within a few days, but complete healing of the ulcers usually takes 10 to 14 days, and therefore treatment should be continued for 2 weeks.

OMEPRAZOLE

Omeprazole is a potent inhibitor of gastric acid secretion and has a long duration of action. Therapeutic effect is obtained with a single daily dose. Traditional antisecretory drugs, such as the histamine H_2-receptor blockers cimetidine and ranitidine and the muscarinic receptor blocker pirenzepine, require multiple daily doses.

Omeprazole blocks the proton pump and inhibits gastric secretion. Omeprazole inhibits the final step in hydrogen ion production, thereby preventing the secretion of gastric acid that is stimulated by various secretagogues (e.g., histamine, gastrin, and acetylcholine). This mechanism of action differs from that of the histamine H_2-receptor blockers, which have no inhibitory effect on secretagogues other than histamine. Omeprazole appears to be safe in dogs and is 10 times more potent than cimetidine, with a longer duration of action. Omeprazole is given orally or by way of a gastrostomy or jejunostomy tube at a dosage of 0.7 mg/kg once daily for 10 to 14 days. Omeprazole is a substituted benzimidazole and is superior to ranitidine.

MUCOSAL AND ORAL PROTECTIVES

The other commonly used drugs are called mucosal protectives. Sucralfate, a mucosal protective, forms a viscous paste in the acid environment of the stomach. This paste adheres to the base of an ulcer, protecting it from the normal acid secretions. Also, sucralfate is thought to enhance other mucosal defense mechanisms. The dosages used in foals are based on those used in humans (1 to 2 g/70 kg body weight, given by mouth four times per day). It is common for ranitidine and sucralfate to be used in combination for treatment of foal ulcers. Because sucralfate requires an acid environment for activation, it should be administered an hour before ranitidine. Sucralfate effectively treats duodenal or gastric ulceration in humans by forming a protective barrier against gastric acid at the ulcer site. The drug has yet to be fully evaluated in small animals, and no dose is available for the dog.

Oral protectives, e.g., kaolin, kaopectate, or bismuth preparations, are rarely indicated for gastric ulceration. (Both aluminum hydroxide and magnesium hydroxide may inhibit the absorption of orally administered cimetidine.)

6.4 PROTECTIVES AND ABSORBENTS

Protectives and absorbents are insoluble compounds that coat the inflamed gastrointestinal mucosa and absorb or bind toxic agents. Kaolin, a widely used antidiarrheal, is a hydrated aluminum silicate that can absorb large quantities of bacteria and toxins. Kaopectate (Upjohn) contains 25% kaolin and 1% pectin. Kaolin-containing compounds decrease the frequency of defecation. The most widely used compounds contain combinations of kaolin and pectin.

Protectives, such as sucralfate, and absorbents, such as kaolin and pectin, can generally be used safely in cats. Bismuth subsalicylate preparations contain salicylic acid, which potentially can be absorbed to toxic concentrations in cats after repeated administrations. The antiprostaglandin effects of subsalicylate and the gastroprotective effects of bismuth, however, warrant its use for the treatment of acute gastroenteritis accompanied by vomiting or diarrhea.

Bismuth subnitrate and magnesium trisilicate act to protect and coat the inflamed, eroded mucosa. Demulcents, such as dextrose, glycerine, and egg albumin, also possess this property and soothe the gastric mucosa.

ABSORBENTS

These are substances that bind with toxic agents and carry them out of the digestive tract. Aluminum silicate (kaolin), aluminum hydroxide, activated charcoal, and pectin are absorbents that also act as inert mechanical coating agents. Many of these are incorporated into commercial antidiarrheal mixtures, e.g., kaolin-pectin mixture—30 to 60 ml given to a dog or cat after each bowel movement. Activated charcoal is a valuable agent for the emergency treatment of poisoning—20 to 120 mg/kg mixed in water as a drench.

ASTRINGENTS

These cause precipitation of proteins but have little penetrating ability: Tannic acid and catechu precipitate alkaloids into insoluble complexes in the stomach in cases of poisoning. In chronic gastritis, absorbents, e.g., kaopectate every 4 to 6 hours; parasympatholytics (atropine/scopolamine type); and local sedatives, such as amethocaine, have been used in conjunction with fluid and electrolyte therapy.

6.5 CENTRAL ANTIEMETICS

TREATMENT OF THE VOMITING DOG

Emesis of vestibular origin can be treated with antihistaminergic drugs, such as diphenhydramine or its chlorotheophylline salts, dimenhydrinate, meclizine, or cyclizine. Peripherally active antiemetics include metoclopramide; domperidone; centrally active anticholinergics atropine and aminopentamide; and peripherally active anticholinergics glycopyrrolate, hyoscine, isopropamide, and propantheline. The aims of treatment are to correct or remove the primary cause of the vomiting; control the vomiting episodes; and correct any fluid, electrolyte, or acid-base abnormalities.

Peripherally acting agents (anticholinergics and metoclopramide) are useful in treating vomiting induced by inflammation and other diseases of the gastrointestinal tract or other abdominal organs. Centrally acting antiemetics effective at the chemoreceptor trigger zone (antidopaminergic drugs, such as phenothiazines and metoclopramide) are effective treatments for vomiting. Many centrally acting sedatives suppress the vomiting center in the medulla along with other centers and brain areas. The phenothiazine tranquilizers are also useful here; in addition to a central inhibiting action of the chemoreceptor trigger zone (vomiting center), some of them possess a peripheral antagonistic action to gastrointestinal irritation (antidopaminergic effects).

Phenothiazines tend to be potent, centrally acting antiemetics. They are principally antidopaminergic but are also antihistaminergic and at higher doses probably anticholinergic. Chlorpromazine is an effective antiemetic that has minimal tranquilizing action. Phenothiazines are contraindicated in dehydrated or hypovolemic animals because of their alpha-adrenergic action, which causes arteriolar vasodilation and hence hypotension.

Acepromazine tablets (0.5 mg/lb) are useful as is chlorpromazine. Phenothiazine tranquilizers are effective in prophylaxis and control of mild nausea and vomiting associated with a wide spectrum of disease. At low dosages, these compounds inhibit the chemoreceptor trigger zone, whereas at higher dosages, they depress the emetic center. They do not, however, block peripheral visceral afferent impulses to the emetic center. Hence control of vomiting associated with severe gastrointestinal disease may require a combination of a phenothiazine derivative and an anticholinergic. These compounds should not be used in hypotensive patients because they are alpha blockers and predispose to vasodilation. Examples are prochlorperazine, promazine, and chlorpromazine. Prochlorperazine, used in combination with the anticholinergic isopropamide, is an effective combination antiemetic. Chlorpromazine and prochlorperazine have significant activity at dopaminergic, muscarinic, cholinergic, and histaminic (H_1) receptors.

The phenothiazine and butyrophenone tranquilizers have similar chemical structures to gamma-aminobutyric acid (GABA). Phenothiazines block the chemoreceptor trigger zone at low doses and depress the emetic center at higher doses. Phenothiazine derivatives are able to produce other effects in the body including, alpha-adrenoceptor block, anticholinergic actions, and stimulation of the extrapyramidal system. Chlorpromazine may be used orally to prevent motion sickness at a dosage rate of 0.5 to 1.0 mg/kg, but such doses induce sedation as well. Animals showing signs of gastrointestinal disease may be medicated with chlorpromazine at a low dose to prevent emesis, but acepromazine should be used only if it is certain that there is no decrease in circulating blood volume.

Fluphenazine, droperidol, and haloperidol are all potent dopamine antagonists, but fluphenazine also has significant antihistaminic and anticholinergic activities. Opiates can be effective antiemetics but must be chosen carefully because they have emetic properties as well. Morphine and apomorphine consistently cause vomiting in the dog. Apomorphine's emetic action can be blocked by dopamine antagonists, but morphine's is blocked only by naloxone. Morphine, however, possesses antiemetic activity when it binds to opiate receptors in the medullary vomiting center. Fentanyl penetrates more rapidly than morphine and is an antiemetic that can even prevent vomiting caused by other narcotics.

Anticholinergics are another class of antiemetic. Although they have been considered as an illogical choice for antiemesis, they nevertheless appear to stop vomiting in some dogs. Considered ineffective because of their proposed peripheral action, there is now reason to believe that they may also have a central action.

Anticholinergic drugs inhibit gastric motility but do not inhibit apomorphine-induced emesis. Atropine and *dl*-hyoscine have two main actions in the body:

1. On the smooth muscle and secretory glands innervated by postganglionic cholinergic nerves
2. On the central nervous system

Their antiemetic activity is largely due to their central activity.

Parasympatholytic drugs, such as atropine, isopropamide, methscopolamine, and propantheline, inhibit cholinergically mediated impulses along visceral afferent nerves. These compounds are believed to modify emesis associated with irritation or spasm of gastrointestinal smooth muscle.

By far the most common anticholinergic drug used is hyoscine hydrobromide. It has a short duration of action, and evidence suggests that it is thus of most value during short journeys. Similar to other anticholinergics it has numerous side effects, including drowsiness, blurred vision, dry mouth, constipation, and urinary retention. These side effects, however, are not generally marked at the doses used in the prevention of travel sickness.

Anticholinergics, which reduce motility by inhibiting peristalsis, may increase the time available for gut bacteria to multiply and invade other tissues. These disadvan-

tages, together with the lack of selectivity of these agents, limit their use in veterinary practice as antiemetics.

METOCLOPRAMIDE

Metoclopramide is similar chemically to procainamide and is an antidopaminergic agent with both peripheral and central actions. This acts on dopamine receptors in the central nervous system and raises the threshold of the chemoreceptor trigger zone (vomiting center). It also possesses a local spasmolytic action on the stomach and pyloric sphincter. The actions of metoclopramide are mediated by its antidopaminergic effects on the chemoreceptor trigger zone. Metoclopramide increases the tone and amplitude of esophageal and gastric contractions; relaxes the pyloric sphincter, thereby promoting gastric emptying; and increases duodenal peristalsis. It has no effect on gastric or intestinal secretions.

Clinical Pharmacology

Metoclopramide stimulates motility of the upper gastrointestinal tract without stimulating gastric, biliary, or pancreatic secretion, apparently through sensitizing smooth muscle to the action of acetylcholine. In the central nervous system, metoclopramide, similar to phenothiazines and related drugs (also dopamine antagonists), produces sedation, inhibits the effects of prolactin, and causes a transient release of aldosterone.

Gastrointestinal Effects

The effect of the drug on gastrointestinal smooth muscle is achieved primarily through its cholinergic properties. Inadequate cholinergic stimulation has been incriminated in a number of gastrointestinal motility disorders in humans, explaining why metoclopramide finds its most important clinical applications in diseases in which normal motility is diminished or impaired. The unique action of the drug lies in its ability both to stimulate and to coordinate gastric, pyloric, and duodenal motor activity.

Central Nervous System Effects

Metoclopramide has a variety of actions on the central nervous system, most important of which is its antiemetic actions. The drug, for example, is about 20 times more potent than phenothiazine derivatives in controlling vomiting induced by apomorphine and is much more effective than phenothiazine derivatives in controlling nausea and vomiting induced by cisplatin chemotherapy in human patients. The antiemetic effect of metoclopramide is thought to be exerted by way of blockade of receptors in the chemoreceptor trigger zone located near the fourth ventricle. The drug, however, also raises the threshold of activity in the vomiting center and decreases input from visceral nerves. In clinical situations associated with nausea and vomiting, the central antiemetic effect of metoclopramide generally is viewed as both supplementary and complementary to its direct effect on gastrointestinal smooth muscle. It most likely is due to its effect on motility, which overrides the stasis and retroperistalsis that precede vomiting.

The oral dosage is 0.1 to 0.3 mg/kg three times a day; the drug can also be given subcutaneously at the same dosage or intravenously. Intravenous boluses (2 to 10 mg as needed) are probably absorbed too quickly, but the drug may also be infused slowly intravenously in severe emesis (e.g., in parvovirus infection). The exact intravenous infusion dosage is undetermined, but 0.01 to 0.02 mg/kg/hour is usually effective. Metoclopramide would appear to be the antiemetic of choice for most clinical situations, unless sedation is required as well.

The short half-life of metoclopramide requires constant oral, subcutaneous, or intravenous administration to maintain effective therapeutic concentrations for a reasonable treatment period.

The usual effective oral dosage of metoclopramide in the dog and cat is 0.2 to 0.4 mg/kg administered every 6 to 8 hours.

Domperidone (Motilium, Janssen) is a similar antiemetic compound possessing antidopaminergic activity. It does not cross the blood-brain barrier. (0.1–0.5 mg/kg i.m., 0.5–1.0 mg/kg orally.)

Treatment of Motion Sickness

A number of drugs can be considered, including tranquilizers (acepromazine, promazine, chlorpromazine), antihistamines (promethazine, diphenhydramine [Benadryl]), diazepam (Valium), and hyoscine. As a general rule, the drug should be given about 30 minutes before traveling. Hyoscine is an excellent antimotion sickness agent and acts mainly as a parasympatholytic. It is used in doses of 0.3 to 0.6 mg in dogs by mouth. Some side effects, however, such as ocular disturbances and dryness of the mouth, may accompany long-term usage.

Antihistamines block the chemoreceptor trigger zone and depress input from the vestibular apparatus. Their main indication is for the control of vomiting associated with motion sickness or vestibular disease. They are generally less effective than phenothiazines. Antihistamines inhibit the chemoreceptor trigger zone and depress both labyrinth excitability and conduction in the vestibular-cerebellar pathways. Nausea and vomiting associated with motion sickness respond to these compounds, the best known example of which is Dramamine (Searle).

The use of diazepam to prevent motion sickness is increasing in popularity. This is an hypnotic agent, possessing muscle relaxant, anticonvulsant, and antianxiety properties. It is not established, however, whether it possesses specific antiemetic properties or whether the traveling sickness is abolished owing to antianxiety properties.

MOOD-ALTERING DRUGS

Mood-altering drugs may be useful antiemetics, especially when vomiting is a conditioned reflex. Diazepam and derivatives of tetrahydrocannabinal have been useful in selected human patients. Cannabinoids appear to be useful in preventing chemotherapy-associated vomiting in the cat. They act through stimulation of opiate receptors because naloxone blocks the antiemetic action. Cannabinoids, however, are not effective in preventing apomorphine-induced vomiting in the dog and may even prolong it. Further, neurotoxicity has been reported after prolonged exposure to high doses.

BEHAVIORAL MODIFICATION

Success of behavioral modification has been reported in cases devoid of organic causes of vomiting. Although most cases of vomiting are readily attributable to disease, behavioral vomiting is reported in the dog (epimeletic and limbic epilepsy) and probably must be considered in other circumstances as well. In one instance, a male dog with a history of vomiting for 5 years was successfully treated with a behavior-modifying drug (megesterol).

OTHER AGENTS

Some antiemetics have a predominantly peripheral action. These include bismuth subsalicylate and domperidone. The mechanism of action of the first is unknown. Domperidone is a dopamine antagonist that does not cross the blood-brain barrier.

Some antihistamines possess antiemetic activity. Promethazine has marked antihistaminic and anticholinergic properties and has been found to be capable of inhibiting apomorphine-induced emesis in dogs. Promethazine, at a dosage rate of 2 mg/kg twice daily, is used in small animal practice for prevention of motion sickness. It has also been found to be effective in increasing tolerance to radiation-induced emesis in dogs.

Butyrophenones are more potent antiemetic drugs than phenothiazines, but they are not widely used in veterinary practice because they may induce bizarre behavioral changes.

When vomiting is particularly severe or associated with a gastric outflow obstruction, a hypokalemic, hypochloremic metabolic alkalosis is suspected, and saline normal (0.9% NaCl) is the fluid of choice because replenishing the chloride deficit allows for the renal excretion of bicarbonate with conservation of potassium.

DRUGS AFFECTING MOTILITY

Motility modifiers fall into two broad groups: narcotics and anticholinergics.

6.6 NARCOTIC ANALGESICS

Narcotic analgesics, such as diphenoxylate (Lomotil, Searle), are widely used as antidiarrheals. In addition to their effect on intestinal secretions, they are believed to increase the frequency of rhythmic segmentation and decrease the speed of transit of luminal contents.

Opiate-type drugs act locally on the gastrointestinal tract and bring it to a standstill by a multiplicity of actions at different sites. They decrease gastric motility and delay emptying time. They are potent suppressants of all intestinal movements, particularly propulsive peristalsis. They increase the tone of the sphincters, and these effects are long lasting. The use of morphine itself has declined in recent years for a variety of reasons (both pharmacologic and legislative), but opiate-type drugs are still frequently used in low concentrations in many antidiarrheal preparations. Mixtures of morphine and chloroform (Chlorodyne) are still available.

Opioids, in contrast to anticholinergic agents, are useful in symptomatic treatment of diarrhea. Opioids stimulate increased segmentation and thus delay transit by causing increased resistance to flow of feces. In addition, these drugs provide analgesia and promote re-establishment of normal colonic secretion and absorption. Opioids may enhance the effects of other drugs used in colitis therapy by increasing their contact time in the colon. Paregoric, loperamide, and diphenoxylate are useful for short-term treatment of diarrhea. Opioids are contraindicated in cases of invasive or toxogenic bacterial infections of the gastrointestinal tract.

Powdered opium and paregoric (camphorated tincture of opium) are included in several proprietary mixtures that may also include anticholinergics, kaolin, and pectin. Diphenoxylate, a meperidine derivative, is available in combination with atropine (Lomotil) to lower the chances of its potential abuse by humans.

Diphenoxylate is a synthetic compound similar to opiates in structure and function. Diphenoxylate is a derivative of the analgesic pethidine, and its principal action is to inhibit gastrointestinal motility and thus control diarrhea. The gut active antibiotic neomycin is sometimes included in the mixture to control the infection. Diphenoxylate is given in dogs in doses up to 0.25 mg/kg.

In Lomotil, the combination of diphenoxylate with atropine increases efficacy because diphenoxylate acts directly on opiate receptors in smooth muscle and the mesenteric plexus, whereas atropine, originally included as an ingredient to prevent overdosing in humans, acts primarily on muscarinic receptors in the mesenteric plexus and mucosa. The oral dosage in dogs and cats is 0.2 mg/kg three to four times a day. Codeine, another effective antidiarrheal drug, is given orally at 0.25 to 0.5 mg/kg three to four times daily.

Loperamide (Imodium, Janssen) is one of the most potent available antidiarrheals. The development of loperamide resulted from the synthesis of a new chemical series of piperidine derivatives that lacks the pethidine moiety. Loperamide, a morphine derivative, has been shown to have an effect on secretion; it also inhibits motility of the intestine.

Loperamide hydrochloride, a piperadine derivative, is a potent, long-acting, oral antidiarrheal drug. Loperamide has been used for years for symptomatic control of acute and chronic diarrhea in humans. As a synthetic opioid with antidiarrheal properties, loperamide is similar to other opioids, such as morphine, codeine, and diphenoxylate hydrochloride.

Loperamide has been proved to increase segmental muscular contractions in the canine small intestine and colon while decreasing propulsive (longitudinal) contractions. The net effect is prolonged intestinal transit. Experimental studies in rats suggest that loperamide (1) inhibits prostaglandin-induced and cholera-toxin-induced intestinal secretion and (2) stimulates absorption of fluid, electrolytes, and glucose. The effects of loperamide are blocked by naloxone hydrochloride; this fact suggests that the mechanism is mediated by opiate receptors.

Loperamide is structurally similar to diphenoxylate but has distinctly different pharmacologic activity. Because it does not readily cross the blood-brain barrier, oral loperamide has minimal addictive or abuse potential. Loperamide might help to control chronic small or large bowel diarrhea in dogs. The agent should be considered, however, only after the underlying cause has been thoroughly investigated. The initial dose of 4 mg of loperamide is followed by 2 mg after each subsequent unformed stool; dosing should not exceed 16 mg/day. Usually any improvement of acute diarrhea should be observed within 48 hours.

Loperamide and morphinelike drugs have a direct local action on intestinal opiate receptors, which appears to be essential for their antidiarrheal activity. In binding studies, however, loperamide also shows high affinity binding of large capacity to other receptors. One of these has been identified as the calmodulin binding site, which is considered important in calcium-dependent hypersecretion in the intestine and to which loperamide, in contrast to morphinelike drugs, binds at low concentration.

6.7 ANTICHOLINERGICS

Atropine, tincture of belladonna, and many other anticholinergics are often used in treatment of diarrhea by decreasing fluid secretion and increasing absorption rather than by decreasing motility.

Initially it was considered that diarrhea was associated with hypermotility; atropine and methscopolamine were used to inhibit motility. It was subsequently shown, however, that diarrhea is associated with hypersecretion and hypomotility. Atropine (0.08 mg/kg) and methscopolamine (0 to 1 mg/kg) as well as other anticholinergics, such as benzetemide, may be effective clinically by inhibiting enterotoxin-induced hypersecretion.

Synthetic cholinolytics that may be used include aminopentamide, dicyclomine, glycopyrrolate, mepenzolate bromide, oxyphenonium bromide, pipenzolate, camylofine, propantheline, clidinium, isopropamide iodide, diphemanil methylsulfate, and tridihexethyl chloride. As well as playing a role in symptomatic treatment of diarrhea, these drugs are useful in controlling gastrointestinal problems that may have an underlying psychological basis. Such disorders probably exert their effect on the gut through excessive parasympathetic activity, and such effects are blocked by anticholinergics.

Atropine (dl-hyoscyamine) and scopolamine (hyoscine) inhibit the muscarinic actions of acetylcholine, resulting in relaxation of the gastrointestinal tract smooth muscle, reduction in tone, inhibition of ruminal motility, and blockage of secretions. The major indications for these types of drugs are:

1. Episodes of spasmodic colic in which intense smooth muscle contraction gives rise to considerable visceral pain.
2. Cases of mild or functional diarrhea. Many commercial antidiarrheal mixtures contain atropine-type parasympatholytics in combination with one or a number of the following types of drugs: protectives, absorbents, antibiotics, opiates, and astringents.

The main naturally occurring antispasmodic drugs are atropine and hyoscine, but owing to their widespread activity throughout the body, inhibition of peristaltic activity is accompanied by many other undesirable effects. Secretions in the mouth and respiratory and gastrointestinal tracts are blocked. Tachycardia due to vagal blockade and disturbances of ocular accommodation with mydriasis are found. The presence of these unwanted side effects has led to the introduction of less potent synthetic anticholinergics, such as isopropamide and methscopolamine. Methscopolamine is a slightly less potent semisynthetic alkaloid than hyoscine and is used in Neobiotic-P (Upjohn). Its major distinguishing feature is that, owing to a quaternary nitrogen, it does not cross the blood-brain barrier and produce the central excitement seen in cattle following hyoscine. (Atropine sulfate, 15 to 30 mg, can be administered subcutaneously to the horse, but side effects, especially on the eye, heart, and gastrointestinal tract secretions, are prominent.)

In canine colitis, short-term use of anticholinergics may be indicated when colonic spasm or severe straining is present. Propantheline bromide, dicyclomine hydrochloride, and clidinium bromide combined with chlordiazepoxide chloride are useful anticholinergics with relative specificity for gastrointestinal and urinary tract smooth muscle and minimal effects on the heart, glands, and central nervous system. These drugs are contraindicated in invasive or toxogenic bacterial enteritis or colitis, gastric atony or outlet obstruction, and paralytic ileus.

Antispasmodic/central nervous system depressant combination products used to treat psychomotor diarrhea in humans have benefited some cases of canine colitis. Isopropamide and prochlorperazine or clidinium and chlordiazepoxide may be useful if psychogenic or stress-associated colitis is suspected.

6.8 SPASMOLYTIC DRUGS

These are used in a variety of conditions ranging from spasmodic colic to diarrhea, esophageal obstruction, and dystokia—in fact, many conditions in which excessive acetylcholine activity results in hyperactivity of smooth muscle and spasm associated with pain. Effective antispasmodics are the belladonna alkaloids (e.g., atropine), anticholinergics (e.g., propantheline and isopropamide), and direct-acting smooth muscle relaxants (e.g., dicyclomine [Bentyl, Merrell Dow]). Antihistamines also fall into this category. Newer synthetic spasmolytic preparations are available, and these frequently combine analgesic agents with the spasmolytic ingredient to give more prompt relief of pain.

BUSCOPAN (BOEHRINGER)

Buscopan contains hyoscine (spasmolytic) and dipyrone (metamizole), a nonsteroidal anti-inflammatory drug (NSAID) related to phenylbutazone. The combination of the two active ingredients allows for the relief of pain and inflammation resulting from the diminution of muscle spasm.

Doses, intramuscular or intravenous, are as follows:

Horses, 20 to 30 ml
Cattle, 20 to 25 ml
Dogs, 1 to 2.5 ml

Local reactions occasionally follow its intramuscular usage in the horse.

ISAVERIN (BAYER)

Isaverin contains dipyrone (metamizole), an analgesic (NSAID), and methindizate, a spasmolytic. This is also given by intravenous or intramuscular injection, as follows:

Horses and cattle, 10 to 20 ml
Dogs, 1 to 4 ml

ACEPROMAZINE

This agent is frequently employed, particularly in the horse, for treatment of spasmodic colic, in which it possesses not only central sedative effects, but also appreciable spasmolytic activity at a dose of 0.05 mg/kg intravenously.

The use of spasmolytic agents remains highly speculative in view of the perception as to whether diarrhea involves an increase or decrease in gut motility. Drugs that simply reduce gut motility, whether centrally or peripherally, may not necessarily be indicated. If spasmolysis is combined with antisecretory activity, however, some benefit may occur.

Gastrointestinal tract sedatives, such as opium, loperamide, and diphenoxylate, have their place undoubtedly, as also do atropine and methscopolamine. Their role and effects, however, must not be oversimplified. Antisecretory activity typified by the anticholinergic agents (e.g., benzetimide) certainly can hasten recovery of calves from diarrhea with a consequent reduction in fluid and bicarbonate loss.

6.9 LOCALLY ACTIVE DRUGS

ABSORBENTS AND PROTECTIVES

Absorbents are nonabsorbable materials that can bind other substances onto their surfaces and thus prevent these substances from entering into chemical reactions or from being absorbed into the body. Many naturally occurring drugs contain colloidal aluminum silicate, which when hydrated forms into a gel. Fuller's earth, bentonite, and kaolin are examples. Activated attapulgite is a purified magnesium aluminum silicate with potent absorbent properties.

Pectin, a complex polysaccharide, is another absorbent frequently combined with kaolin (e.g., Kaopectate). Activated charcoal is probably one of the most potent absorbents of all with a rapid action and a high capacity for adsorption. It is a useful agent for the emergency treatment of poisoning (to absorb the toxin). It is frequently combined with kaolin to treat bacterial enteritis. Insoluble salts of bismuth are commonly used for their protective or demulcent properties.

Pectin is a polyuronic polymer consisting of purified carbohydrate extracted from citrus fruit. Up to 90% of the drug is degraded in the gastrointestinal tract, but it nonetheless does decrease absorption of several substances.

Kaolin and pectin are often used as protectives in diarrheic states. These act to coat the intestine and protect it from further irritation. By protecting the inflamed mucosa, they allow time for healing.

Activated attapulgite, magnesium trisilicate, aluminum hydroxide, and various bismuth salts are also employed to the same effect. Bismuth subsalicylate possesses antiprostaglandin activity that reduces the hypersecretion caused by *Escherichia coli* enterotoxin. Kaolin, attapulgite, and bentonite clays are also absorbent in nature, but perhaps one of the most potent is activated charcoal. Absorbents (or adsorbents) function by prevention of toxin binding to sites on the mucosal cells. Cholestyramine, a quaternary ion exchange resin, is a particularly potent enterotoxin absorbent.

6.10 ANTISECRETORY DRUGS

Antisecretory drugs are useful in therapy of hypersecretory diarrhea in animals especially diarrhea associated with *E. coli* enterotoxin. Enterotoxins are known to stimulate intestinal secretions. The mechanism of secretory activity is related to local calcium ion activity in the enterocytes and mucosal production of cyclic adenosine monophosphate (cAMP) or guanosine monophosphate (GMP). Enterotoxin raises cytoplasmic Ca^{2+}, thereby activating calcium-dependent regulators, which cause hypersecretion. Calcium channel blockers diminish net efflux of ion and water by modulating the concentration of intracellular calcium; however, because heat stable enterotoxin type a induced secretion may not be mediated by Ca^{2+}, there may be a second mechanism.

Calmodulin, a calcium-dependent regulator, is inhibited by the action of chlorpromazine, and this calcium entry blockade leads to more quiescent bowel function. Its use is accompanied by marked sedative activity.

A number of NSAIDs, especially salicylates (aspirin), reduce cAMP levels through inhibition of prostaglandin synthesis. Although this was first demonstrated against cholera toxin, aspirin and related compounds also possess this effect against *E. coli* toxins and can reduce the incidence of scouring. Flunixin meglumine, acting by the same mechanisms, can reduce severity of scouring in calves.

A curious, miscellaneous group of antisecretory agents is the alpha$_2$ agonists (clonidine, oxymethazoline, naphazoline, xylazine), which have been found to reduce intestinal secretion caused by *E. coli* toxins. Before becoming acceptable as calf scour therapies, however, such classes of drugs must become more receptor selective to minimize undesirable side effects attributable to receptor activity at sites other than the gastrointestinal tract.

Opioidal derivatives, such as loperamide and diphenoxylate, although traditionally regarded as antimotility agents, possess some antisecretory activity.

6.11 LAXATIVES, CATHARTICS, PURGATIVES

A cathartic produces more fluid evacuation; a laxative produces a soft-formed stool.

IRRITANT TYPE

Castor Oil

This is a bland triglyceride hydrolyzed by the small intestinal lipases to ricinoleic acid, which is then irritant. Castor oil acts mainly on the small intestine. Dosing is as follows:

Dogs, 4 to 25 ml
Cats, 2 to 15 ml

Pigs, 50 to 150 ml
Calves and foals, 50 to 100 ml

In small animals, effects begin 1 to 2 hours after dosing and last up to 7 to 8 hours.

Anthraquinones

Cascara and senna are examples. These glycosides are hydrolyzed in the large intestine, and the active principle, emodin, is released. There is a lag phase of 6 to 12 hours until effects are seen. These compounds are regarded as severe purgatives and should not be used in cases of obstruction, enteritis, or colitis. They are also excreted through the milk and could have a laxative effect on the young. Dosing is as follows:

Horses, 10 to 30 g
Cattle, 20 to 45 g
Calves and foals, 3 to 5 g

SALINE TYPE

These are nonirritant, inexpensive, and effective compounds in simple-stomached animals. They act as poorly absorbed soluble salts that retain water by osmotic action and thus distend the bowel.

Magnesium (Epsom Salts)

Isotonic solution contains 34.4 g salts per liter. Dosing is as follows:

Horses and cattle, 250 to 100 g
Foals and calves, 25 to 50 g
Sheep and pigs, 25 to 50 g
Cats, 2 to 5 g

BULK-FORMING LAXATIVES

These stimulate motility by distending the bowel. Most of these polysaccharide and cellulose derivatives dissolve or swell in water (hydrophilic), producing an increase in the indigestible mass within the intestine. Effects are usually apparent within 12 hours or so and persist for 2 days or more. Bran or linseed mashes are the safest and the most physiologic types used. Other indigestible hydrophilic colloids, such as sterculia granules and ispaghula husks, are available commercially. Sterculia granules can be used in diarrheic states to normalize gut function.

LUBRICANT OR EMOLLIENT TYPES

Generally these are the most commonly used and are pharmacologically inert agents.

Mineral Oil (Liquid Paraffin)

This is an indigestible hydrocarbon that acts to lubricate the gut. It may interfere, however, with absorption of fat-soluble vitamins and can disturb normal defecatory reflexes. Dosing is as follows:

Horses and cattle, 3 to 10 liters
Pigs, 25 to 300 ml
Dogs, 5 to 30 ml
Cats, 2 to 6 ml

Vegetable Oils (Linseed Oil)

Vegetable oils, such as linseed oil, are more expensive and are absorbed to a greater extent. Raw linseed oil has been used in the horse at a dose of 500 to 750 ml. Boiled linseed oil must never be used, it contains lead oxide.

6.12 DIARRHEA

Diarrhea is characterized by increased smooth muscle activity of the alimentary tract, passage of voluminous watery feces, inflammation and erosion of the intestinal mucosa, increased irritability of the bowel, and dehydration with acid-base imbalance. Treatment is geared toward relieving the clinical signs and restoring gut function to normal. Vigorous attention must also be paid, however, to the control of the underlying initiating causes, whether infectious or noninfectious. A general approach to therapy of diarrhea includes the following classes of drugs.

DRUGS AFFECTING MOTILITY

Atropine, hyoscyamine, scopolamine, methscopolamine, and methindizate are examples. Analgesics in some of these preparations may alleviate the visceral pain. These agents should be used with care, however, because diarrhea is not automatically associated with excessive smooth muscle movement.

Opiates include chloridyne (morphine/chloroform), codeine, diphenoxylate (Lomotil), and loperamide. These possess constipatory activity. It must always be remembered, however, that diarrhea can be beneficial in ridding the body of unwanted toxins. Hence inhibition of peristalsis is not always automatically desirable.

Antisecretory agents include NSAIDs and parasympatholytics.

PROTECTIVES AND ABSORBENTS

This group includes kaolin, pectin, bismuth subnitrate, attapulgite, and activated charcoal.

FLUID THERAPY

Most cases of diarrhea and dehydration give rise to metabolic acidosis through excessive loss of bicarbonate ions. Accordingly fluid replacement therapy should use alkalinizing fluids, such as Hartmann's solution (compound sodium lactate), Darrow's solution, or lactated Ringer's solution.

SPECIFIC CHEMOTHERAPEUTIC AGENTS

Generally, when it is appropriate to use chemotherapy for enteric disease, poorly absorbed aminoglycosides, such as gentamicin, neomycin, or streptomycin, occur in a variety of proprietary antidiarrheal preparations. Also, those sulfonamides that are poorly absorbed from the gastrointestinal tract are useful for treatment of infections in the tract, provided that the pathogens are susceptible to the action of sulfonamides. Among those in proprietary preparations are:

- Phthalylsulfacetamide
- Sulfamethazine, Sulfadiazine, Sulfadimethoxine
- Sulfathiazole, Sulfapyridine
- Sulfaguanidine

The potentiated sulfonamides given orally or parenterally have widespread applications, as also do the semisynthetic penicillins, ampicillin or clavulate-potentiated amoxicillin. The cephalosporins and especially fluoroquinolones (enrofloxacin) are now finding increased application and field success in treating salmonellosis. Yogurt may be helpful in certain forms of diarrhea in the dog.

ENZYME SUPPLEMENTS

Pancreatic exocrine insufficiency is a relatively common cause of chronic diarrhea and weight loss in young large-breed dogs. The disease is caused by degenerative atrophy of the pancreas and occurs mainly but not exclusively in German Shepards. Treatment is predicated on supplementation of endogenous enzymes with commercial enzyme preparations.

A severe form of maldigestion due to failure of production of digestive enzymes by the exocrine pancreas causes a failure of digestion and absorption of starch, triglycerides, and proteins. It produces a syndrome of ravenous appetite, weight loss, coprophagia, and steatorrhea. Tests include:

1. Sequential fecal smears to check for the presence of muscle fibers, starch granules, and fat globules.
2. Trypsin digest test. In this condition, trypsin secretion is diminished or absent. Sequential samples must be consistently negative before a diagnosis of pancreatic insufficiency can be made. If trypsin is being secreted, some should be present in the feces and be able to digest the gelatin of an undeveloped x-ray film. A suspension of 1 g. feces and mLs 1% sodium carbonate is diluted serially to give dilutions of 1:10, 1:20 etc. A drop of each solution plus controls are placed on undeveloped x-ray film and incubated at 37° C for 30 minutes. After it is washed, the last zone of complete clearing is the titer of pancreatic trypsin in the sample.
3. Para-aminobenzoic acid (PABA) absorption, accurate in diagnosis of pancreatic insufficiency.
4. Serum trypsinlike immunoreactivity—usually low in cases of exocrine pancreatic insufficiency and probably one of the most reliable tests for its diagnosis.

Therapy is expensive and in severe cases does not curb the weight loss or ravenous appetite, although it improves the diarrhea. Diet should be high protein, low carbohydrate, and low fat. (Prescription Diet) Large quantities of pancreatic extract must be added to the feed. A high percentage of this is thought to be denatured on passing through the stomach, so sodium bicarbonate or cimetidine can be given before feeding to enable a greater concentration of enzymes to reach the small intestine.

COLITIS IN DOGS

Symptomatic relief may be obtained with diphenoxylate, loperamide or anticholinergic drugs such as propantheline or clidinium. Of the antimicrobial drugs. Sulfasalazine is a combination of sulfapyridine and 5-acetylsalicylic acid (ASA), which is cleaved by colonic bacteria, resulting in the sulfa component being absorbed and ASA excreted in feces. ASA is probably the active ingredient owing to antiprostaglandin activity. The exact mechanism, however, is unknown. The drug is indicated primarily for ulcerative and granulomatous colitis. The major adverse effect, although uncommon, is keratoconjunctivitis sicca. Other occasional adverse effects include vomiting, allergic dermatitis, and jaundice. The drug has been used in cats at half the dose rate, but there is risk of toxicity owing to the ASA; therefore the drug should be used cautiously in this species.

Metronidazole is frequently used to treat colitis. The mechanism of action is not known but probably includes antiprotozoal action against *Giardia*, alteration of immune-mediated reactions in the bowel, and antibacterial action against anaerobes. (See also Chapter 37).

APPETITE STIMULANTS

Small animals react favorably to benzodiazepines, such as diazepam and oxazepam, as appetite stimulants. Both drugs can be administered orally; a more rapid effect can be achieved by intravenous administration of diazepam. Some veterinarians, however, may prefer to use oxazepam, a metabolite of diazepam, because it is associated with less central nervous system depression (manifested as sedation and ataxia) than diazepam, and it requires less hepatic metabolism.

6.13 NEONATAL DIARRHEA IN CALVES

Epidemiologic studies conducted in many countries have determined that most cases of gastroenteritis are caused by three groups of pathogenic infectious agents: enterotoxigenic colibacilli rotavirus and coronavirus. Some enzootics are caused by other microorganisms, some of which can affect not only newborn calves, but also older cattle: septicemic colibacilli, *Salmonella typhimurium* and *S. dublin*, cryptosporidiosis, and the virus of bovine viral diarrhea.

Diarrhea in calves has many causes. The differentiation of these is important in deciding which therapeutic agents and supportive treatment to use. Calves with a fermentative diarrhea caused by overfeeding have a different response to treatment than calves with a hypersecretory diarrhea caused by *E. coli* enterotoxin or calves with a destructive enteritis caused by coronavirus. Many enteric disease outbreaks are not clinically separable because of the involvement of mixed infectious agents and various environmental, nutritional, and hygienic factors. Dehydration, acidosis, impaired growth, and death are the major consequences. The cause of diarrhea is generally mixed and varies from herd to herd. Common viral diseases in calves are rotavirus, coronavirus, and bovine viral diarrhea (BVD) infections. Infection by parvoviruses, astroviruses, viruslike fringed particles, and the Breda virus has also been associated with calf diarrhea. Microbial agents routinely involved are *E. coli*, *Clostridium perfringens* type C, and *Salmonella*. *Campylobacter fetus* subspecies *jejuni* may also be involved in enteric disease. Protozoa, such as cryptosporidia and coccidia, can be primarily or secondarily involved. Coccidiosis is occasionally observed in calves under a month of age.

COLIBACILLI

Enterotoxigenic Colibacilli

Colibacillosis caused by enterotoxigenic *E. coli* (ETEC), one of the three principal causes of calf scours, occurs most often during the first week of life. After this time, calves generally become resistant to ETEC but continue to be susceptible to coronavirus and rotavirus, the two other main causes of calf scours.

In calves of 1 to 4 days of age, intense diarrhea characterized as very liquid and straw yellow with signs of dehydration is evidence of an attack of enterotoxigenic colibacilli. Enterotoxigenic colibacilli have two characteristics:

1. They have pili, which are thin filaments on the surface of the bacterial body. With them, the colibacilli can fix onto the brush border of epithelial cells of the small intestine. For this reason, these pili are called the adhesion factor. Of proteinic substance, these pili are antigenic. They induce the synthesis of specific antibodies and allow the identification of strains in the laboratory.

   These pili (fimbria) are composed of specific protein antigen, which has been identified and labeled as K99. K99 *E. coli* also produce exotoxins, which increase intestinal secretions and cause damage to the cells to which they are attached. Once attached, they multiply rapidly and secrete enterotoxins. The enterotoxins affect the secretory cells of the intestinal crypts, causing them to increase their secretion of fluid and electrolytes. In pathogenic colibacilli in calves, the most important adhesion factors are antigens K99, Y (Att 25), and F41.

2. As regards the intestinal mucuous membrane, they excrete a thermostable enterotoxin, which by direct action on enterocytes induces water and electrolyte flux in the gut. The consequences are diarrhea and dehydration.

Septicemic Colibacilli

Septicemia during the first days as well as respiratory localizations may be caused by septicemia colibacilli. These colibacilli have structures such as 31A factor or VIR factor enabling them to spread throughout the animal. The septicemic colibacilli invasion induces acute respiratory problems and diarrhea, rapidly leading to death.

Septicemic colibacillosis is an acute infection of the blood stream by *E. coli* that strikes suddenly and is most commonly fatal. The bacteria invade the blood stream, usually within the first 4 days of life, by way of the nasopharynx (mouth), the intestine, or the umbilical vessels. The *E. coli* rapidly multiply and are phagocytozed (engulfed) by white blood cells. Fragments of bacterial cell wall (endotoxins) are released into the blood stream, causing effects such as fever, intravascular coagulation, and endotoxic shock.

E. coli strains are classified by serologic typing to identify these structural antigens: O (somatic or cell wall) antigens, K (capsular) antigens, and H (flagellar) antigens. O and K antigens are most commonly used to identify ETEC serotypes in calves.

Pilus antigens were originally given K designations because of serologic similarities to capsular K (polysaccharide) antigens but are now known to be distinct from capsular (K) antigens. In the future, pilus antigens may be designated by the letter F to avoid this confusion (e.g., K99 is now F5). The most common *E. coli* serogroups involved in calf scours are 08:K25, 08:K85, 09:K30, 09:K35, and 0101:K28. The pilus antigen of major importance in calf scours is K99 (F5). The ileum is the first segment to be colonized by *E. coli* in diarrheic calves.

The factors that allow adhesion of organisms to the mucosa have been defined: in the pig, K88 antigen and 987P antigen; in the calf and lamb, K99 (Y, 31A, 47A). These can be seen under the electron microscope as surface structures on the bacterial surface. The K88 and K99 (pig and calf) are the most important, although the 987P adhesion factor may be more important in North American pigs.

E. coli are capable of producing various classes of enterotoxins: heat-labile enterotoxin (LT) and heat-stable exterotoxin (ST). The toxin binds to receptors on the epithelial lining; villous absorptive cells have about twice as many receptors as crypt cells. Once ST is bound to the intestinal epithelial cell, it induces hypersecretion, which results in loss of electrolytes, bicarbonate, and fluid. Death results from dehydration, metabolic acidosis, or both.

Considerable research has been done on the enterotoxins of *E. coli*, and it is now clear that there are at least three types of enterotoxin, each of which is distinct from the well-known gram-negative endotoxin that causes fever and shock. Endotoxin may play a role in systemic *E. coli* infections and in bowel edema.

E. coli enterotoxins are characterized as follows:

- LT—heat labile (65° C), large molecular weight, immunogenic
- STa—heat stable, methanol soluble
- STb—heat stable, not methanol soluble, not immunogenic

LT and cholera toxin (choleragen) are known to act through activation of adenyl cyclase, which raises the mediator cAMP. The mechanism by which ST produces the secretion of fluid appears to involve an increase in calcium ions within the cell, which stimulates calmodulin (also known as calcium-dependent regulator), and this causes the excretion of water and electrolytes.

The STa induces net secretion of Na^+ and Cl^- by activating guanylate cyclase. The role of intracellular Ca^{2+} and calmodulin is still controversial. Release of arachidonic acid and formation of prostaglandin also may occur. The Na^+-Cl-cotransport system in the enterocyte's membrane is disabled by STa.

E. coli toxins can have effects on cAMP and GMP, which may indirectly affect calmodulin. Enterotoxins produced by ETEC do not directly affect the digestion of disaccharides, the absorption of glucose and amino acids by the small intestinal mucosa, or the coupling of sodium absorption to these mechanisms. The total amount of glucose absorbed, however, may be affected by the decreased brush border function owing and the decreased intake of milk by the weakened calf or pig.

Vaccination or exposure of the dam to expected pathogens increases the amount of antibodies, which are then secreted in the colostrum. (Some species transfer antibodies transplacentally, but this is not true of swine or cattle.)

SALMONELLOSIS

The causative agent is usually *S. typhimurium*, but in some herds with frequent abortions it may be due to *S. dublin*. The latter is isolated in calves with diarrhea. *C. jejuni* has been isolated from calves with diarrhea, and infection of experimental calves results in mild diarrhea. *C. jejuni* and *Campylobacter coli* are now recognized as major causes of diarrhea in humans. The significance of these and other species of *Campylobacter* in the pathogenesis of diarrhea in calves is less certain because they can be commonly isolated from healthy calves.

ROTAVIRUSES AND CORONAVIRUSES

Among the causes of diarrhea in calves, the important interaction of colibacilli has been well established in the first days of life. It has been proved that viruses, rotaviruses and coronaviruses being among them, are also responsible for severe enteritis during the first days of life.

Rotaviruses are classified in the Reoviridae family. They are RNA viruses with no envelope. They are stable in the exterior environment and resistant to numerous chemical and enzymatic agents.

Coronaviruses are classified in the Coronaviridae family. They are RNA viruses with envelope characterized by the morphology of the spicules that surround the viral envelope forming a corona. Coronaviruses show a lower resistance in the external environment. Although thermolabile, they are resistant to some chemical agents. Almost all cows from infected herds have antirotavirus and anticoronavirus antibodies. Their level is not enough, however, to protect the newborn calf from infection.

In 20-day-old calves, rotavirus is associated with 50 to 80% of diarrhea cases and coronavirus with 40% diarrhea cases. During the first 4 days, the incidence is much lower because of maternal antibodies.

Numerous calves excrete some of the virus without clinical signs. This may contaminate the external environment. The contamination of animals is made through the orofecal route.

Rotaviruses colonize cells at the top of intestinal villi, where they multiply by destroying the enterocytes. Rotavirus infects epithelial cells covering the villi of the small intestine; the large intestine is spared. Loss of villous epithelial cells results in shortened villi covered by undifferentiated replacement cells from the crypts. These immature cells are deficient in brush border enzymes and absorptive function. Undigested, unabsorbed nutrients, subject to bacterial fermentation, create increased osmotic pressures that draw fluid into the intestinal lumen.

This fluid loss, in addition to the normal influx of fluids into the lumen through crypt cell secretion and other digestive secretions (salivary, gastric, biliary, pancreatic), is not countered by regular absorptive processes because the immature villous epithelial cells are not fully functional. Thus rotaviral diarrhea is primarily the result of maldigestion and malabsorption. Rotavirus infection, however, may occur in the absence of diarrhea, although there are lesions in the small intestine.

Calves that receive insufficient colostrum and that are housed in highly contaminated environments may scour within 24 hours. Consequently rotaviral diarrhea is often seen during the first few days of life under these conditions. Clinically apparent infection in calves older than 1 month is rare.

Antiviral compounds are not available for practical use in calves. Therapy is directed toward replacing fluid and electrolytes and supplying energy. Vaccinating cows with inactivated, adjuvanted rotavirus may increase antibody levels in colostrum and milk, and this is more likely to be of value in protecting calves.

Similar to enteric colibacillosis and rotavirus infection, coronavirus infection is also usually seen in calves 1 to 2 weeks old. As with rotavirus, small intestinal villous epithelial cells are infected; however, epithelial cells on the surface and lining the crypts of the colonic mucosa are infected as well. Coronaviruses are excreted in great quantity in the intestinal lumen and in the external environment, where they live for a long time owing to their great capacity for resistance.

The important pathogenic power of coronaviruses can be explained by the fact that similar to rotaviruses they colonize differentiated cells of the small intestine, colon, and rectum. Clinically their presence can induce mucoid elements and blood in the feces. Usually an irreversible malabsorption syndrome induces cachexia and leads to the death of the animal.

In viral diarrheas (rotavirus, coronavirus), there are probably at least two mechanisms involved. One is the flattening of the mucosal villi; the other is a direct stimulation of secretory activity through a mechanism so far poorly understood.

The flattening of the mucosa reduces the surface area for digestion and absorption, but in particular it can cause malabsorption by removing the disaccharidase enzyme activity, which is situated toward the tips of the villi. This interferes with normal digestion of lactose, which may then be broken down by organisms within the large intestine to produce fermentative diarrhea.

Several other infrequently encountered viruses have been associated with diarrhea in calves. Bredavirus and adenovirus in particular can be serious pathogens when first introduced into a herd.

BVD virus occasionally is detected in young calves with diarrhea, but its role in producing such disease is unclear. Some calves in which BVD virus has been detected also have been infected with other enteric and respiratory pathogens, and many have concurrent bacterial pneumonia. BVD virus infection has been observed and reported to increase susceptibility to, or to increase the relative severity of, concurrent *Pasteurella haemolytica* infection of the calf. This may or may not be a true example of immunosuppression.

Villous atrophy, fusing of villi, and inflammatory cell infiltrate are typical lesions caused by viruses and cryptosporidia. When brush-border enzymes (particularly lactase) are lost, lactose is not degraded in the small intestine.

Although rotavirus and coronavirus are the most familiar viral pathogens, astrovirus, Bredavirus, calici-like virus, and parvovirus have been isolated from diarrheic calves and have caused diarrhea in experimental calves.

CRYPTOSPORIDIOSIS

These protozoan parasites infect almost all mammals, birds, fishes, and reptiles. They have a cycle similar to that of *Coccidia* without a necessary passage by way of the external environment. Clinically the infection induces yellow diarrhea, usually nausea, with low or no general problems. Dehydration is moderate, and appetite is often normal. These parasites are frequently associated with other pathogenic agents.

The pathogenic power of cryptosporidia is caused by their fixation on the brush border on epithelial cells of the small intestine. Thus they induce a shortening of the villi and a modification in the enzymatic potency of parasitized cells.

Cryptosporidiosis chemotherapy continues to be a therapeutic challenge. Only lasalocid (8 mg/kg) is effective, but toxic, from a variety of antiprotozoal drugs used to treat experimental cryptosporidial infections in calves. Spiramycin or a combination of quinine and clindamycin may be effective in humans. Other drugs used experimentally include amprolium hydrochloride (Dohme), sulfadimidine, sulfadiazine-trimethoprim, dimetridazole, metronidazole, ipronidazole hydrochloride, quinacrine dihydrochloride, monensin sodium, and lasalocid.

6.14 COLIFORM CALF SCOUR

Factors to consider when treating calves with ETEC diarrhea include removing the *E. coli* from the intestine, and correcting dehydration and acidosis. A rapid, accurate, and economical enzyme-linked immunosorbent assay (ELISA) kit (Coli-Tect 99, Molecular Genetics) can be used in practitioner laboratories to detect *E. coli* K99, a major cause of neonatal diarrhea. Test interpretation is based on a color change directly proportional to the amount of pilus antigen in the fecal sample.

Because the cause of death in most cases of diarrhea is associated with dehydration, rehydration of the calf either by the intravenous or oral route is important. Other therapeutic agents that have been used in the treatment of calf diarrhea with varying success include antibiotics, modulators of intestinal motility, gastrointestinal protectives and absorbents, astringents, agents affecting secretion, *Lactobacillus* and other bacterial organisms, steroids, and recently the NSAIDs, such as flunixin.

TABLE 6-1
ROLE OF PROSTAGLANDINS IN SCOUR

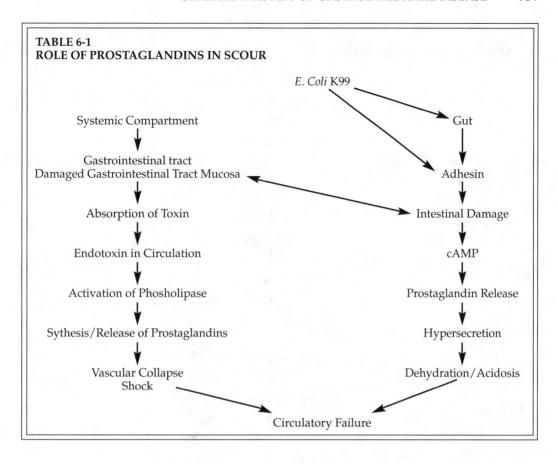

Activated charcoal also has been suggested for treating colibacillosis.

The most widely used, and probably the most overused, drugs for treatment of diarrhea of calves are the antimicrobial agents. Antimicrobial therapy can be empirical, using customary drugs and dosage regimens and based entirely on a presumptive diagnosis and a knowledge of the likely bacterial species involved and their usual antimicrobial susceptibility.

Antibiotics may be administered intravenously, intramuscularly, or orally. Boluses, liquids, and pastes have been used extensively.

Besides the problem of resistance, some antimicrobial agents have been shown to cause damage to the intestinal mucosa and may actually exacerbate the disease they are supposed to control.

E. coli enterotoxin causes hypersecretion in the mucosal cells of the small intestine by activating adenylate cyclase, thus elevating cyclic nucleotide levels within the secretory cells (Tables 6–1 and 6–2).

Salicylates (aspirin), bismuth subcalicylate, and flunixin reduce cAMP levels through blockade of prostaglandin synthesis. This alleviates the severity of scouring and the extent of hypersecretion. Other drugs, such as phenylbutazone, indomethacin, and ethacrynic acid, also cause reduction in secretion. Use of NSAIDs and other drugs, such as lidamidine, for this effect offers considerable promise. The antiprostaglandin effect of the NSAIDs is additionally useful in controlling any shocklike syndrome that might develop in severely affected calves.

Corticosteroids have often been recommended as antisecretory agents in diarrhea. It must be remembered, however, that steroids can depress the capacity of the intestine to absorb immunoglobulins and that they can markedly depress the cell-mediated immune response. Scouring calves,

TABLE 6-2
CHAIN REACTION IN DIARRHEA

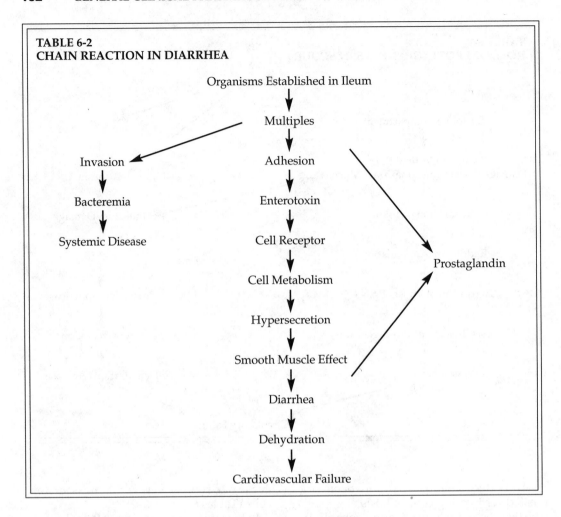

TABLE 6–3
DRUG THERAPY

Agent	Indication
Antibiotics	Bacteria
Antisecretory	Enterotoxins
Antiprostaglandin	Hypersecretion
Adsorbents	Diarrhea
Motility modifiers	
Loperamide	
Fluids	Dehydration

in fact, display already elevated blood glucocorticoid levels. The disadvantages of indiscriminate use of corticosteroids is that they are ulcerogenic to both normal and diseased gastrointestinal epithelium by impairing the normally protective effect of prostaglandins and inhibiting normal replication of mucosal cells.

Treating dehydration, acidosis, and hypothermia is critical in advanced cases of neonatal diarrhea. To estimate the liters of fluid needed to rehydrate a diarrheic calf, multiply the calf's weight in kilograms by the estimated percentage of dehydration and add maintenance needs (50 to 100 ml/kg/24 hours). The total 24-hour requirement is divided into equal doses given every 4 hours. Calves that have lost 8% or more of their body weight owing to dehydration usually require intravenous fluid therapy to prevent hypovolemic shock and to treat metabolic acidosis.

Vaccination programs are also valuable in controlling colibacillosis. Vaccinating cows before calving with a bacterin containing K99 pilus antigen enhances colostral antibodies and provides the calf with passive protection against K99 *E. coli* infection.

Bacteria must extract iron from their environment to survive and proliferate. Although it is not a widely used treatment, reducing the availability of usable iron to bacteria has been shown to inhibit proliferation of *E. coli*. Deferoxamine is an iron-chelating compound that absorbs iron from intestinal contents, making it unavailable for bacterial use.

An immunodeficient calf with an inadequate level of immunoglobulins usually becomes septicemic, and diarrhea may be one of the clinical signs. Such calves must receive aggressive antimicrobial therapy together with fluid and electrolyte replacement. Septicemic shock may warrant specific treatment, and the pharmacokinetics of antimicrobial agents, especially aminocyclitols, can be markedly affected in such cases, resulting in renal toxicity (Tables 6–3 and 6–4).

6.15 ANTIMICROBIAL THERAPY

Calves may have an *E. coli* bacteremia and should be treated with systemic broad-spectrum antibiotics, such as gentamicin, amikacin, ampicillin, amoxicillin, trimethoprim-sulfonamide combination, or other antimicrobial agents to which the clinician believes the organism is susceptible. Some antimicrobial agents, such as: eptomycin, neomycin, and gentamicin are poorly absorbed from the gastrointestinal tract and therefore of minimal value for calves with colisepticemia if given orally.

Parenteral antibiotic therapy is often an effective means of controlling susceptible ETEC. Parenteral antibiotics, however, may

---

TABLE 6–4
CALF SCOUR THERAPY PACKAGE

PREVENTION
 Adequate colostrum intake
 Maternal vaccination
 Monoclonal antibiotics
 Probiotics
TREATMENT
 Dehydration/shock
 Fluid/electrolytes
 Energy
 Plasma expanders
 NSAIDs
 Intestinal activity
 Adsorbents
 Protectives
 Antisecretories
 NSAIDs
 Motility modifiers
 Infection
 Antimicrobials

---

be indicated in patients with hemorrhagic diarrhea in which there is loss of the intestinal mucosal barrier and therefore the potential for bacterial invasion and septicemia. This is particularly so if leukopenia is also present, as in viral infection, or if the presence of leukocytosis and pyrexia may suggest systemic bacterial invasion.

Most practitioners believe that antibiotics are effective, provided that the outbreak in question is caused by a sensitive strain of *E. coli*. There must be some doubts, however, concerning efficacy of antibiotics in diarrhea, especially if viruses are implicated, although secondary bacterial involvement may still respond. The bovine practitioner is often called to attend many cases of diarrhea of nonspecific origins, particularly in the neonate, and the decision has to be made whether or not to employ antibiotic therapy in these cases. First is the choice of whether or not, and second is the route of administration, whether oral or parenteral. Neither choice can be made independent of the other. The choice of antibiotic depends on a number of considerations: degree of absorption of the antibiotic, whether nonabsorbed antibiotic or not, incidence of resistance against the antibiotic.

The major indication for parenteral bacterial therapy is if a bacterial septicemia exists or is suspected to exist. If this is the case, a broad-spectrum antibacterial, such as tetracycline, enrofloxacin, sulfonamide, or clavulanate/amoxicillin, is indicated. The use of oral antibiotics either in neonatal diarrhea or even in severe adult diarrheas, such as salmonellosis, has been debated over the years. In cases of salmonellosis, for example, it has been found that administration of antibiotics does nothing to hasten the recovery and in fact enhances the carrier state of a resistant organism or on occasion may provoke a carrier state into a systemic infection. In cases of neonatal diarrhea, the pathophysiology of the disease usually involves an interaction between viruses, bacteria, and an immune deficiency.

Because ETEC are noninvasive, the oral route for administration of antimicrobial drugs is preferred. Antibiotics may not be of value for viruses or problems of immune deficiency but have been efficacious for enterotoxic colibacillosis. This suggests that if oral antibiotics are going to be beneficial, results should be obtained within the first 36 hours, and prolonged use of these drugs should therefore be avoided. In a number of instances, however, oral antibacterials have proved to be of little use, and the decision whether or not to administer them must be based on cost relative to the value of the patient, coupled with history on the property of their effectiveness. If the decision is made to use them, a 2- to 3-day course should be adequate. Several limitations of antibiotic therapy are cited, including multiple causes of calf diarrhea, pharmacologic variation, development of resistant bacterial strains, residue problems, and increased cost to the producer. Indiscriminate use of antibiotics in many calf diarrheas is likely to be of no benefit and may actually compound the problem. In a rational approach, clinical efficacy of the therapy must first be established. Antibiotic therapy may best be reserved for those patients at risk of developing systemic gram-negative bacterial infections. A host of antimicrobials are available, including neomycin, apramycin, tetracycline, streptomycin, penicillin, streptomycin and neomycin combination, ampicillin, kanamycin, polymyxin-B, methicillin, nalidixic acid, gentamicin, amoxicillin, trimethoprim-sulfadiazine, sulfachlorpyridazine, spectino-

mycin, and erythromycin. Various studies have demonstrated the efficacy of these antimicrobial agents for calfhood diarrheas in the clinical setting. Calf diarrhea results from a variety of causes, including bacterial, viral, protozoan, nutritional, and mechanical. Often a combination may be secondary to these causes. Successful antibiotic treatment in calves, however, has been reported for apramycin, enrofloxacin, amoxicillin, clavulanate, and gentamicin. Trimethoprim-sulfadiazine was also found effective but only to a similar degree as milk reduction. This is rather similar to the finding that, in experimental infection in calves, amoxicillin treatment, although significantly superior to a placebo, was by itself similar in efficacy to an oral glucose glycine electrolyte formulation.

6.16 GASTROINTESTINAL PROTECTIVES AND ADSORBENTS

Even if all the pathogenic bacteria were instantly killed, this would not bring about an immediate remission of clinical signs because of the presence of bacterial toxins in the lumen of the bowel. In an attempt to remove these toxins, adsorbents have been used. Chief of these available to the bovine practitioner have been kaolin and attapulgite (available with electrolytes). These are valued by veterinarians and stock owners, although there is little evidence of efficacy.

Kaolin, pectin, and attapulgite have been used for many years as "toxin adsorbents." Adsorbents such as kaolin were popular until a decade ago for the treatment of diarrhea, but there is little evidence that they are useful, and hence their use has declined. Theoretically they absorb water and add bulk to the stool. In adults, they are normally combined with other agents (e.g., kaolin and morphine mixture), and it is difficult to differentiate their effects from those of the other agents. Other examples are pectin, attapulgite, and charcoal.

Adsorbents work by adsorbing toxin molecules, rendering them unavailable to attach to the intestinal wall, and possibly preventing toxin binding to receptor sites on the mucosal cells. Gastrointestinal protectives produce a coating or lining on the intestinal mucosa that protects from injury by harmful substances. Adsorbents bind chemical and bacterial compounds and prevent their absorption but may also interfere with the absorption of various pharmaceutical agents. Kaolin (natural hydrated aluminum silicate) and pectin (natural polygalacturonic acids) are used as protectives in calf diarrhea to protect the inflamed intestinal mucosa and allow time for healing. They reduce the volume of feces passed, but the total amount of water excreted in the feces is not significantly reduced. Commonly used agents are magnesium trisilicate, hydrated magnesium aluminum trisilicate (activated attapulgite), aluminum hydroxide, and phosphate and calcium carbonate. The insoluble bismuth salts, bismuth subcarbonate, bismuth subnitrate, bismuth subgallate, and bismuth subsalicylate, are also used. The subsalicylate portion has an antiprostaglandin synthetase action that reduces the hypersecretion caused by the *E. coli* enterotoxin. Activated charcoal has primarily absorbent properties. Kaolin, attapulgite, and bentonite clays are other adsorbents. Many antidiarrheal preparations contain kaolin, attapulgite, or other adsorbent agents. There are, however, few reports of experimental verification of their efficacy. The rationale for their use is adsorption of toxins within the lumen of the intestine, and evidence has been presented to show that *E. coli* enterotoxins can be adsorbed by attapulgite and charcoal.

Attapulgite, pectin, and kaolin function as luminal lining adsorptive agents, and kaolin in particular is especially effective in its capacity to adsorb *E. coli* toxins. Bentonite and cholestyramine are found in a number of commercial antidiarrheal preparations. Cholestyramine is a quaternary ammonium ion exchange resin of high molecular weight that is superior to kaolin, attapulgite, and bentonite clays as an enterotoxin binder.

6.17 ANTISECRETORY DRUGS

Most changes in small intestinal activity probably result from increased secretion causing dilation and reflex contraction. *E. coli* enterotoxin has been shown to cause hypersecretion by the mucosal cells of the small intestine. This is thought to be due to an effect on mucosal adenyl cyclase. There is evidence that prostaglandins play an important role.

A number of drugs have shown antisecretory activity in vitro. NSAIDS, alpha-adrenergic agonists, calcium channel blockers, opiates, phenothiazines, and other compounds reduce net loss of intestinal fluid in vitro. An interesting group of compounds has been found that reduce intestinal secretion caused by *E. coli* toxins. These are the drugs that stimulate adrenaline alpha$_2$ receptors (alpha$_2$ agonists). Examples include oxymetazoline, lidamidine, clonidine, and naphazoline, and these or related compounds may have a role in treatment of diarrheal secretion if side effects can be reduced to an acceptable level. (Alpha-adrenergic agonists reduce secretion by decreasing intracellular cAMP.)

For enterotoxins to exert their intestinal effects, a secondary cytoplasmic transmission system within the mucosal enterocytes is required. Cholera toxin (the classic model) is known to raise calcium-dependent regulators. Chlorpromazine inhibits this relay system and experimentally relieves diarrhea in human cholera.

Chlorpromazine, a phenothiazine derivative, may exert its antidiarrheal activity through its effect on calmodulin, cAMP, or membrane stabilization. This has been corroborated in work on pig diarrhea. A number of other chemically unrelated compounds, such as melperone (a butyrophenone), show this pharmacologic effect but lack the undesirable effects of chlorpromazine.

The heat stable enterotoxins of *E. coli* produce secretion of fluid by causing an increase in calcium ions within the cell, which in turn stimulates calmodulin, also known as "calcium-dependent regulator," and this causes the secretion of water and electrolytes. (*E. coli* toxins have effects on cAMP and GMP, which may indirectly affect calmodulin. Drugs that affect intracellular calmodulin or cyclic nucleotides may thus be used to reduce intestinal secretion.)

Chlorpromazine affects calcium-dependent regulators and thus reduces bicarbonate and water loss. Its sedative effects, however, are undesirable. Loperamide, an opiate derivative, possesses antisecretory activity, as also do many alpha$_2$-adrenoceptor agonists, such as clonidine, oxymethalozine, and xylazine.

Acidic anti-inflammatory agents are the most recent group of drugs to be used to treat diarrhea. These compounds act by inhibiting prostaglandins. Prostaglandins are known to play a role in the absorptive and secretory mechanisms of the gastrointestinal tract as well as a number of other cellular mechanisms throughout the body. Aspirin, indomethacin, and 5-ASA are a few of the acidic anti-inflammatory agents under study.

Experiments have described inhibition of colibacillosis in calves using flunixin meglumine, which, similar to aspirin and indomethacin, is a NSAID inhibiting prostaglandin formation. Current pharmaceutical research is directed at a better understanding of the inflammatory process and what can be pharmacologically controlled. It has been postulated that the cholera toxin involves a prostaglandin in raising intracellular cAMP as part of the inflammatory processes. Certain anti-inflammatory drugs, including aspirin and phenylbutazone and derivatives such as suxibuzone and indomethacin, are believed to inhibit prostaglandin, and they have been shown to reduce diarrhea. In humans, these drugs are considered to have a high proportion of undesirable side effects (20% or more for phenylbutazone and 13 to 15% for indomethacin). Newer drugs are being developed that are more specifically antiprostaglandin and that have relatively few side effects. These could well have a future in the treatment of diarrhea. One such drug is flunixin meglumine, an antiprostaglandin compound marketed for treating inflammatory conditions. Flunixin meglumine (1.1 mg/kg intravenously) reduces diarrhea in experimental calves challenged with live ETEC, and 2.2 mg/kg intramuscularly reduces total fecal output of calves receiving partially purified STa.

Numerous studies have demonstrated the benefits of bismuth subsalicylate as a preventive and treatment of diarrhea in humans. Proposed mechanisms of action include (1) binding of the enterotoxin, (2) prevention of attachment, (3) antimicrobial activity of bismuth, (4) antisecretory activity of salicylate, and (5) binding of bile acids.

Salicylates, such as aspirin and bismuth subsalicylate, are thought to reduce cAMP levels through the blockade of prostaglandin synthesis, and the use of such drugs has reduced the incidence of scouring in pigs. The potent nonsteroidal, anti-inflammatory flunixin meglumine, has been reported to reduce the severity of scouring in calves. Phenylbutazone and indomethacin have also been shown to be successful in the reduction of hypersecretion.

NSAIDs not only can drastically reduce the severity of mortality from severe intestinal disturbances, but also they may reduce the systemic shock-type syndrome accompanying many such states. Salicylates, flunixin, and phenylbutazone have long been used empirically to control enteric colibacillosis and to reduce the severity of peripheral circulatory collapse. This successful therapy is now known to be scientifically well based by virtue of inhibition of prostaglandin synthesis.

6.18 *LACTOBACILLUS* AND OTHER BACTERIAL INOCULA (PROBIOTICS)

Probiotics have been advocated for prevention of diarrhea when fed before disease is present and as an aid in enhancing recuperation if fed during convalescence. Theories proposed to explain the potential benefit of probiotics include alteration of pH in the intestinal lumen; production of enzymes, B vitamins, and antibiotics; alteration of intestinal flora through competition.

Changes in the gut environment cause changes in the types of organisms living there, which, in turn, are likely to make the animal more susceptible to infections causing diarrhea and other ill effects that reduce the animal's performance. *Lactobacillus acidophilus* cultures have been used to alter gut flora, but their efficacy is questioned. They function by increasing the number of beneficial intestinal bacteria and interfering with attachment of enteric pathogens to the intestinal mucosa. They also cause a reduction in intestinal pH by the production of lactic acid and may lower the intestinal oxidation reduction potential, thereby inhibiting aerobic intestinal pathogens. This may also reduce the production of undesirable by-products. The manufacturers of one product also claim that the inoculum may increase the rate of weight gain and feed efficiency under certain conditions and may decrease morbidity and mortality. Other organisms, such as *Streptococcus faecium* and *Lactobacillus bulgaricus*, have more specific antienterotoxic effect.

Increased weight gain, greater onset of recovery, and good prophylaxis are all claimed benefits of oral probiotic administration. Levels of *E. coli* challenge, however, and whether the enteric disturbance is attributable to toxin producing *E. coli* are critical determinants of the degree of clinical success that may be expected with such agents. Colostrum intake is important to maximize response of neonatal animals to probiotics.

The breakdown of milk sugar (lactose) to lactic acid is also facilitated by lactobacilli, which elaborate bacterial enzymes that assist digestion. Multiplication of lactobacilli tends to crowd out other pathogens, which have to compete for sites on the cell wall. In a sense, probiotics are the opposite to antibiotics insofar as they promote the multiplication of (beneficial) bacteria. It is not strictly a new concept—the benefits claimed for both humans and animals from eating fermented products (live yogurt) containing lactobacilli are well known.

6.19 MOTILITY-INHIBITING DRUGS

The use of drugs inhibiting motility (e.g., atropine, methscopolamine) is based on the assumption that diarrhea is caused by excessive smooth muscle movement. Present understanding suggests that, at least in the colon, the opposite is true, and diarrhea is associated with decreased motility. Initially it was considered that diarrhea is associated with decreased hypermotility: Atropine and methscopolamine were used to inhibit motility. It was later shown, however, that diarrhea is associated with a hypersecretion and hypomotility. Atropine (0.08 mg/kg) and methscopolamine (0.5 to 1 mg/kg) as well as other anticholinergics, such as benzetemide, may be effective clinically by inhibiting enterotoxin-induced hypersecretion. Other anticholinergics include hyoscyamine, homatropine, glycopyrrolate, isopropamide, and aminopentamide. Although these can be useful antisecretory agents, their clinical applications are somewhat debatable. Drugs that have a specific constipating effect are available, e.g., loperamide and diphenoxylate. These may have morphinelike actions—increasing smooth muscle tone and decreasing propulsion in the intestine. The opiates function by producing an increase in segmentation, while reducing propulsive movements in the intestine.

The antidiarrheal effects of opiates (e.g., morphine, codeine, and diphenoxylate) are attributed to the promotion of intestinal fluid and electrolyte absorption and to increased segmental (circular) contractions of the intestinal smooth muscle. This results in a resistance to passage of intestinal contents and therefore more complete absorption of water and nutrients.

Powdered opium and paregoric (camphorated tincture of opium) are included in several proprietary mixtures that may also include anticholinergics, kaolin, and pectin. Diphenoxylate, a meperidine derivative, is available in combination with atropine. It has an effective constipating action, as does loperamide, another congener of meperidine. Loperamide has also been shown to have potent antisecretory actions. This type of symptomatic approach is not without risks because diarrhea may be beneficial in removing toxins, and inhibition of movement may thus be counterproductive.

Opiates function by producing an increase in segmentation while reducing propulsive movements in the intestine. Such activity by way of local opioidal receptors, however, may be contraindicated because such bowel stasis can facilitate further absorption of enterotoxin and proliferation of bacteria, which may result in further hypersecretion.

Although many drugs have been used to suppress hyperactivity in diarrhea, this has been based on the mistaken assumption that hypermotility invariably accompanies such enteric disturbances. This is not necessarily so because hypomotility is often present. For this reason, anticholinergic drugs are most probably contraindicated in this regard. Opioidal derivatives that possess antisecretory and antimotility properties (e.g., loperamide) are probably better choices. (*E. coli* diarrhea is now considered to be associated with hypersecretion and hypomotility.) Opiates, however, are effective antidiarrheal drugs. Previously described as an antisecretory drug, loperamide is thought by some to exert its antidiarrheal effect primarily through its motility-modifying properties. Loperamide induces changes in motility of the gastrointestinal tract of calves. When compared with diphenoxylate plus atropine (Lomotil), attapulgite, or bismuth subsalicylate, loperamide was superior.

6.20 FLUID REPLACEMENT

In the normal calf intestine, there is a net absorption of fluid, but in diarrhea, there is a net secretion; the fluid loss contains electrolytes, notably bicarbonate, sodium, and potassium ions. Fluid replacement must be initiated as early as possible—the route of administration depends on the severity of dehydration. It is important that one appreciates the quantities of fluid required. A 50-kg calf should receive at least 4 liters of fluid per day.

The one inevitable effect of scour, regardless of its cause, is dehydration, i.e., the loss of excessive amounts of fluid from the calf's body. In severe cases of scour, dehydration and electrolyte loss lead to a number of other damaging effects, which may, if untreated, result in the calf's death. First, dehydration causes a reduction in blood volume, and the blood becomes thicker; this means that there is a reduced blood flow to the calf's brain, vital organs, and body tissues. Second, the calf's blood pH becomes acidic for two reasons:

1. Bicarbonate ions, which the body uses to prevent acid buildup, are lost through diarrhea.
2. Lactic acid is produced by those muscles not receiving an adequate blood supply.

The buildup of acid in blood is known as acidosis; unless reversed, the effects of acidosis and reduced blood flow damage heart and brain function and cause the calf's death.

The four major abnormalities or disturbances that can usually be identified in diarrheic calves are dehydration, acidemia, electrolyte abnormalities, and negative energy balance or hypoglycemia. Dehydration results from fecal fluid loss and is compounded by decreased fluid intake owing to anorexia or withdrawal of milk by the owner. Acidemia is caused by bicarbonate ion loss in the feces, lactic acid accumulation in poorly perfused tissues, reduced acid excretion by poorly perfused kidneys, and organic acid production in the colon as a result of fermentation of unabsorbed nutrients. Hypoglycemia is a frequent complication of diarrhea and dehydration.

Many dehydrated, acidemic calves are hyperkalemic, yet they often have a total body potassium deficit. This paradoxical situation arises because hydrogen ions in academic plasma diffuse along their concentration gradient into the intracellular fluid space. To maintain electroneutrality, potassium ions diffuse into the extracellular fluid space.

Maintenance fluid requirements for the neonatal calf are 50 to 100 ml/kg/day, whereas ongoing fluid loss can range from minimal amounts to as much as 4 liters in 24 hours.

In severe cases, especially the very young, there is no doubt that intravenous fluids are essential. After an initial intravenous infusion, the calf may recover sufficiently for oral therapy to be used to continue the treatment. The practical problems associated with prolonged intravenous therapy in calves, however, mean that only a small proportion of animals can justify such measures. Despite this, it seems probable that intravenous rehydration remains a necessary part of therapy in severely affected collapsed animals. Oral rehydration was first found effective in treatment of human cholera. The underlying principle was the continued active absorption of glucose, glycine, or both in the small intestine. This active absorption was accompanied by water and sodium, so there was a net increase in absorption, with associated reversal of rehydration. A similar situation exists in diarrheic calves and pigs, in which *E. coli* infection has been shown to have no effect on glucose or amino acid absorption. Thus oral rehydration should be an effective means of reversing dehydration, and this has been confirmed in diarrheic calves and in pigs. The basis for the choice of oral electrolyte replacement is much the same as for intravenous. Many different types and recipes are available. A number of authors do not recommend the inclusion of bicarbonate because the alkalinized abomasum slows the digestion of milk and favors bacterial growth. Also, it is much less palatable. This then rules out bicarbonate as an alkalinizing agent; hence citrate and lactate are usually recommended. Glucose is usually included in these preparations, but sucrose must be omitted because the calf is unable to digest this sugar, and its inclusion would induce an osmotic diarrhea.

It should be noted that neither sucrose nor maltose is suitable as a glucose replacer because neonatal calves do not have sucrase nor significant amounts of maltase in the brush border. Sucrose can even induce diarrhea.

Also, lactose is hardly usable because lactase in the brush border is a fragile enzyme, tending to be diminished in activity in many diarrheal diseases. Therefore glucose appears to be the carbohydrate of choice for inclusion in electrolyte mixtures.

Because dehydration and electrolyte loss are major factors in pathogenesis of diarrhea, fluid replacement has been recognized as important in therapy. Fluid therapy for diarrheic neonatal calves is increasingly recognized as the most appropriate and practical solution for providing life support. The major emphasis on fluid and electrolyte maintenance for diarrheic calves has become focused on the use of oral fluids. This is based on the outstanding success of oral glucose-electrolyte therapies for treatment of *Vibrio cholera* and infant diarrhea in humans. Associated with this beneficial effect is the recognition that the mechanism by which *E. coli* enterotoxin induces diarrhea is analogous to the pathogenesis of *V. cholera* diarrhea as well as diarrhea induced by other enterotoxigenic bacteria. Increased secretory activity is the initiating cause, yet absorption may continue and even be increased. In determining the fluid of choice, it must be remembered that, depending on the severity and duration of the diarrhea, there may be significant losses of sodium, potassium, chloride, calcium, magnesium, and bicarbonate. As the dehydration progresses and sodium and bicarbonate losses progress, water and ions are lost from the cells, and the chief intracellular cation is potassium. Thus the degree of hyperkalemia bears no relationship to the total potassium status of the animal but rather the degree of cellular loss in response to the increasing dehydration and metabolic acidosis. This loss of ions in both extracellular and intracellular fluids results in a loss of resting cell membrane potential. This causes, particularly in muscle cells, a state of reduced polarity and weakness and in the case of cardiac muscle leads to hypoirritability and fibrillation, as anoxia develops secondary to inadequate coronary circulation. Finally heart action ceases. The other important feature of diarrhea is the metabolic acidosis that accompanies it. Bicarbonate ions are lost from the extracellular fluid to the feces, the feces becomes alkaline, and the animal becomes severely acidotic. Intravenous fluids should therefore contain either bicarbonate ions or ions that will be metabolized to yield bicarbonate, e.g., lactate, citrate, or acetate.

The most practical way of rehydration is by the oral route. This is based on the combined uptake of glucose and glycine with sodium and water to cause a net rehydrating effect. Solutions for this purpose should be approximately isotonic (300 mOsm/kg) because before they can be absorbed, hypertonic solutions must first become isotonic by means of equilibration in the stomach and upper intestine. This is likely to aggravate the dehydration initially before rehydration can occur.

In oral rehydration solutions, glucose enhances sodium absorption in the small intestine by way of a transmembrane cotransport system. Once absorbed or injected, glucose also stimulates the release of insulin, which in turn enhances the movement of potassium from the extracellular fluid to the intracellular fluid. Lastly, glucose provides readily available energy.

Glucose helps reverse dehydration by stimulating absorption of water and sodium from the gut into the blood and body tissues. It also provides the calf with a valuable source of energy. The extra glucose in Lectade Resorb Plus means:

- Faster fluid absorption from the gut, to help calves get better sooner
- 41% extra energy, to help reduce setback

Glucose and amino acids (e.g., glycine) are absorbed from the lumen into the mucosal cells lining the small intestine by separate energy-dependent mechanisms. Both mechanisms are sodium dependent.

Sodium ions are actively extruded into the intercellular space, while glucose and amino acids diffuse out of the cell, resulting in increased osmolality within the interstitial fluid. The raised osmolality in the interstitial fluid causes water to move from the lumen through the intercellular ("tight") junction. Water from the intercellular space, together with glucose, amino acids, sodium, and other electrolytes, enters the circulation.

Citrate ions have a dual function. First, they stimulate water and sodium absorption through linked uptake mechanisms at the cell surface. Second, after absorption, citrate is metabolized to produce adenosine triphosphate (ATP) (so contributing to sodium transport) and to add bicarbonate to counter acidosis. In this way, the potentially lethal effects of acidosis on heart and brain function are minimized.

Trials using a commercially available glucose-glycine-electrolyte solution (GGES) showed that its use gave clinical results at least equivalent to those obtained using an antibiotic (amoxicillin). The inclusion of glycine in oral rehydrating solutions has also been shown under field conditions to be clinically beneficial.

There are many other oral proprietary and homemade scour remedies with a variety of constituents. Many contain adsorbents, such as kaolin and pectin; some contain antacids, charcoal, antispasmodics, or minerals. Finally, it should be remembered that nursing is vitally important, particularly ensuring that the calf is given extra heat.

6.21 ROLE OF COLOSTRUM

In contrast to humans, the transplacental transfer of antibodies does not normally occur in the majority of commercially important livestock. Cattle and other ruminants (including sheep and goats) are characterized by the possession of a thick syndesmochorial placentation that prevents the in utero transfer of large-molecular-weight immunoglobulins. Colostral immunoglobulins are derived largely from plasma proteins by selective transport from blood to milk without alteration and, to a lesser degree, from local production by mammary gland lymphocytes.

Because there is no transplacental transfer of immunoglobulins from the maternal to the fetal circulation in ruminants, the newborn calf is born agammaglobulinemic. All of the systemic and local humoral immunity of the newborn therefore depends on the passive transfer of maternal antibodies through the colostrum. The cells lining the mucosa of the small intestine of the newborn are capable of nonselective absorption of colostral immunoglobulin for the first 24 hours after birth (pinocytosis). The greatest absorption occurs in the first few hours after birth and declines thereafter.

There are three main types of immunoglobulins: IgG, IgM, and IgA. The IgG class is heterogeneous and can be further subdivided into IgG1 and IgG2. IgG is the major immunoglobulin in the sera of adult cattle. Colostrum is the primary source of passive natural protective antibody for the neonatal ruminant. Early ingestion of this immunoglobulin-rich milk is critical for neonatal calf survival; colostrum deprivation results in neonatal failure of passive transfer of antibody. Maternal serum IgG1 and IgG2 are concentrated in the udder as colostrum during the month before calving; IgG1 is the major antibody constituent of colostrum.

IgG1 is concentrated in colostrum by an active, selective, receptor-mediated transfer of IgG from the blood of the dam across the mammary gland secretory epithelium. As a result of this active transport, IgG1 is the predominant colostral immunoglobulin, whereas IgM, IgA, and IgG2 are present in considerably lower concentrations.

Although the young are capable of producing antibodies at birth, protective levels of these are not manufactured until the animal is several weeks or months old. Passive immunity acquired through colostrum is thus critical for the young until the antibodies they manufacture themselves reach protective concentrations.

Antibodies are proteins, and in normal circumstances they are too large to be absorbed whole from the gut. The special mechanism (pinocytosis) by which the calf can take in antibody exists only for a short time after birth, and for maximum absorption, colostrum must be received within the first 6 hours of life. This time scale correlates with the quality of colostrum produced by the cow. The concentration of antibody is highest immediately after calving and then declines after 6 to 12 hours.

Maternal immunoglobulin is transferred from the intestinal lumen to the circulation by the apical tubular system in intestinal absorptive cells for a limited time after birth. Maximum transfer is achieved by feeding at least 2 liters of colostrum within 4 hours of birth, or 6 pints in 6 hours.

The small intestine of the calf has the capability of absorbing and transferring colostral immunoglobulins into the intestinal lymph and subsequently to the circulation. This capacity exists for the first 24 to 36 hours after birth, following which ingested immunoglobulins are not absorbed and are lost as far as the circulatory immune system is concerned, although they may still have considerable importance in intestinal luminal activity. In normal calves, the closure times for immunoglobulin absorption are 27 hours for IgG, 16 hours for IgM, and 22 hours for IgA.

The number of pinocytotic cells is most efficient when the calf suckles naturally because closure of the esophageal groove results in more rapid delivery to the absorptive sites. In calves, absorption of antibodies is highest within the first 6 to 8 hours of life, and gut "closure" occurs at 25 hours.

Although little benefit, in terms of circulating immunoglobulin, is derived from feeding colostrum beyond 24 hours of age, there is clear evidence that colostral immunoglobulin can provide local immunity, within the gastrointestinal tract, against enteropathogens. Maternal vaccination schemes for the prevention of neonatal diarrhea depend on the presence of agent-specific antibody in the gut lumen during the time of exposure to the agent.

Colostral immunoglobulins provide both circulating antibody and antibody active at local surfaces, such as the gut. The transfer of colostral immunoglobulins to the calf is influenced by factors such as age at first feeding, method of feeding, the volume of colostrum ingested and its immunoglobulin concentration, the feeding of single versus pooled colostrum, a possible effect from the presence of the dam, seasonal influences, and individual calf variation in efficiency of absorption.

The immunoglobulin mass is the product of immunoglobulin concentration and the volume of colostrum and is the most important determinant of the calf's immunoglobulin concentration. The immunoglobulin mass decreases to two thirds and one third of the original mass by 6 and 24 hours after the first milking.

Mixing colostrum from different dams is commonly done to minimize the effect of poor-quality colostrum and to pool antibodies reflecting the antigenic experience of the herd. Considerable evidence has shown that colostral pools have lower immunoglobulin concentrations than fresh colostrum and that calves fed on the former have lower postfeeding serum immunoglobulin levels. Handling and processing of colostrum also affects the final product. Colostrum is relatively labile and cannot be kept for more than a few days at refrigerator temperatures. It is stable when frozen and can maintain its quality for more than 1 year at $-20°$ C ($-4°$ F). Colostrum may be stored by freezing, refrigeration, or the addition of chemical preservatives.

Colisepticemia occurs only in calves that are agammaglobulinemic or markedly hypogammaglobulinemic, and this disease can be completely prevented by instituting management changes that prevent the occurrence of failure of passive transfer. The severity of diarrhea in enteric disease of neonatal calves is influenced by serum immune globulin concentrations, and balance studies in groups of calves with diarrhea have demonstrated a significant negative relationship between fecal output and serum immune globulin concentrations. If either the quality of colostrum is poor or the amount ingested is small, the neonate may be hypogammaglobulinemic because there is a direct relationship between the concentration of antibodies in colostrum and the amount of antibodies absorbed during the period of maximum absorption.

Factors often listed as responsible for failure of passive transfer of colostral immunoglobulins into calves include (1) failure of calves to suckle, (2) delayed time of first suckling, (3) insufficient quantity of colostrum available from the dam, (4) temporary inability or inferior quality colostrum, (5) a short dry period, and (6) foremilking.

The spectrum of antibodies in colostrum is determined by the pathogens and vaccinations to which the dam has been exposed. If the dam has had limited exposure, the antibody spectrum she provides to her offspring is narrow. In cattle, colostrum quality is also influenced by the length of the dry period. Premature induction of parturition may reduce colostral quality. Prostaglandin administration reduces colostral IgG concentrations, and corticosteroids decrease colostral volumes, and absorption.

With regard to udder pathology, mastitis attributable to environmental pathogens is common in the periparturient dam. This can affect colostral intake because of reduced palatability or reluctance of the dam to allow suckling. Other factors that interfere with the intake of colostrum by calves include rejection of the calf by the dam (heifers particularly), trauma experienced by the calf from a prolonged or assisted delivery, and birth of the calf into unfavorable environmental conditions that may restrict its ability to nurse.

6.22 IMMUNOLOGIC APPROACHES

Acquisition and absorption of adequate amounts of colostral immunoglobulins are essential to the survival of the newborn calf. Protection against infection by ingested organisms may depend entirely on local gastrointestinal immunity or may be mediated by combinations of local and systemic immune mechanisms. Absorbed immunoglobulins protect against systemic invasion by microorganisms, but unabsorbed immunoglobulins also play an important role in protection against intestinal disease.

Vaccination of cows during gestation provides passive immunity to the calf during the first 2 to 3 weeks of life before it can produce its own antibodies. Vaccines to consider for dams are rotavirus-coronavirus-*E. coli* (Scourguard 3, Smithkline Beecham), *E. coli* K99 bacterin (Coligen, Fort Dodge), and types C and D *Clostridium perfringens* toxoid. Cows should be initially vaccinated about 6 weeks before calving, with the second given 2 to 3 weeks before the expected calving date. The second ro-

tavirus-coronavirus and *E. coli* vaccination should be given as close to calving as possible to ensure a high colostral antibody level at calving. Many of these vaccines become more effective the more often the cow is vaccinated.

Aluminum salts have been used extensively as adjuvants in veterinary biologics because of their ability to potentiate immune responses and because of their apparent safety. Although aluminum hydroxide is the most common adjuvant used in veterinary biologics there is a clear consensus that the most powerful experimental agent is Freund's complete adjuvant. The increased protection and duration of immunity produced by oil adjuvants have stimulated new interest in the use of oil emulsions when prolonged immunity from vaccination is desired.

Vaccination of cows during gestation periods passive immunity to the calf during the first 2 to 3 weeks of life, before it can produce its own antibodies. Of critical importance is the acquisition of the antibody-rich colostrum by the calf as early as possible post partem.

MATERNAL VACCINATION WITH *E. COLI* BACTERINS

Maternal vaccination with formalin-killed bacterins of enteropathogenic *E. coli* has been shown to give significant protection to calves challenged with the same strain. A surface antigen of *E. coli* termed K99 is strongly associated with enteropathogenicity. Considerable evidence indicates that K99 is a virulence factor allowing adhesion of the enteropathogenic *E. coli* strains to the intestinal wall.

In considering the practical aspects of vaccination, it is evident that a single dose is preferable to multiple doses. Also, a long period of immunity between vaccination and exposure is desirable. These considerations are especially important in the prevention of colibacillosis, wherein *E. coli* bacterins containing aqueous adjuvants require duplicate vaccination and undue stress to pregnant cows, often during times of adverse weather, shortly before calving.

Commercial bacterins containing K99 antigen are available. A number are combined with rotavirus and coronavirus. It has been demonstrated that the colostral rotavirus antibody titer can be substantially increased by maternal vaccination with a killed product containing adjuvant and that this gives significant protection to calves against rotavirus-associated diarrhea.

MONOCLONAL ANTIBODIES

The first 12 hours postpartum are by far the most critical in terms of preventing pathogenic *E. coli* bacteria with the K99 antigen from adhering to the intestinal gut wall surface.

An immunologically based preventive is monoclonal antibody against the ETEC K99 adhesin. This product is orally administered to the calf within the first 12 hours of life and appears to block colonization of the intestine by K99-positive *E. coli* strains.

Monoclonal antibodies against K99 antigen of *E. coli* have been commercially available for a number of years. Usually such antibodies are given within 12 hours of births to preempt antigen attachment to the intestinal mucosal surface. A small fraction of antibody is absorbed to provide a level of systemic protection. After 24 hours, however, no further absorption occurs, and protection is restricted to the intestinal lumen only. Such monoclonal antibodies are intended as preventives rather than treatment agents, and timing of administration is of critical importance.

Oral use of genetically engineered monoclonal *E. coli* K99 antibody (Genecol 99, Molecular Genetics) within the first 12 hours of life can reduce losses from scours caused by *E. coli*. Monoclonal antibodies directed against enteropathogenic *E. coli* (K99 strains) adhesive factors that permit attachment to the intestinal mucosa are more likely to be effective in the treatment of colibacillosis than are many antimicrobial drugs. Polyclonal antibodies are new additions to this range of immunologicals.

SELECTED REFERENCES

Adler, H.F., and Ivy, A.C.: Morphine atropine antagonism on colon motiligy in the dog. J. Pharmacol. Exp. Ther., *70*:454, 1940.

Aldridge, B., Garry, F., Adams, R.: Role of colostral transfer in neonatal calf management: failure if acquisition of passive immunity. Comp. Cont. Educ., *14*:265, 1992.

Amend, J.F., and Klavano, P.A.: Xylazine: A new sedative analgesic with predictable emetic properties in the cat. VMSAC, *68*:741, 1973.

Awouters, F., Niemegeers, C.J.E., Kuyps, J., et al.: Loperamide antagonism of castor-oil induced diarrhea in rats: A quantitative study. Arch. Int. Pharmacodyn. Ther., *217*:29, 1975.

Baker, J.C.: Bovine viral diarrhea virus: A review. J. Am. Vet. Med. Assoc., *190*:1449, 1987.

Barrett, K.E., and Dharmsathaphorn, K.: Pharmacologic aspects of therapy in inflammatory bowel diseases. Antidiarrheal agents. J. Clin. Gastroenterol., *10*:57, 1988.

Beeman, K.: The effect of Lactobacillus spp. on convalescing calves. Agri. Pract., *6*:8, 1985.

Berg, J.N.: Clinical indications for enrofloxacin in domestic animals and poultry. *In* Quinolones: A New Class of Antimicrobial Agents for Use in Veterinary Medicine. Lawrenceville, NJ, Veterinary Learning Systems, 1988.

Booth, A.J., and Naylor, J.M.: Correction of metabolic acidosis in diarrheal calves by oral administration of electrolyte solutions with or without bicarbonate. J. Am. Vet. Med. Assoc., *191*:62, 1986.

Boothe, D.M.: Drug therapy in cats: a systems approach. J. Amer. Vet. Med. Assoc., *196*:1502, 1990.

Bradshaw, M.J., and Harvey, R.F.: Antidiarrheal agents. Clinical pharmacology and therapeutic use. Drugs, *24*:440, 1982.

Brobst, D.: Pathophysiology of alterations in potassium homeostasis. J. Am. Vet. Med. Assoc., *188*:1019, 1986.

Buck, W.B., and Bratich, P.M.: Activated charcoal preventing unnecessary death by poisoning. Vet. Med., *81*:73, 1986.

Bueno, L., Fioramonti, J., Ruckebusch, M., et al.: Evaluation of colonic myoelectrical activity and functional disorders. Gut, *21*:480, 1980.

Burrows, C.F.: Treatment of gastrointestinal disease in small animals. Mod. Vet. Pract., *66*:181, 1985.

Burrows, G.E., Barto, P.B., Martin, B., et al.: Comparative pharmacokinetics of antibiotics in new born calves: Chloramphenicol, lincomycin and tylosin. Am. J. Vet. Res., *44*:1053, 1983.

Bywater, R.J.: Pathophysiology and treatment of calf diarrhea. Prac. World Cattle Congress, Durban, 1982.

Bywater, R.J.: Rehydration therapy. *In* Recent Advances in Neonatal Diarrhea in Farm Animals. 1980.

Bywater, R.J.: Evaluation of an oral glucose-glycine-electrolyte formulation and amoxicillin for treatment of diarrhea in calves. Am. J. Vet. Res., *38*:1983, 1977.

Collins, J.K., et al.: Shedding of enteric coronavirus in adult cattle. Am. J. Vet. Res., *48*:361, 1987.

Current, W.L.: Cryptosporidiosis. J. Am. Vet. Med. Assoc., *187*:1334, 1985.

deLeeuw, P.W., et al.: Rotavirus infections in calves. Efficacy of oral vaccination in endemically infected herds. Res. Vet. Sci., 29:142, 1980.

Donovan, G.A., Braun, R.K., and Littell, R.C.: Comparison of colostrial and serum antibody titres in cows vaccinated with E. coli K99 antigens. Bov. Proc., 18:196, 1984.

Duhamel, G.E., and Osburn, B.I.: Neonatal immunity in cattle. Bov. Proc., 71, 1984.

Du Pont, H., Ericsson, C., Du Pont, M. et al.: A randomized open-label comparison of nonprescription loperamide and attapulgite in the symptomatic treatment of acute diarrhea. Am. J. Med., 88(Suppl 6A):20S, 1990.

Fettman, M.J.: Hypertonic crystalloid solutions for treating haemorrhagic shock. Comp. Cont. Educ. Pract. Vet., 7:915, 1985.

Fettman, M.J., and Rollin, R.E.: Antimicrobial alternatives for calf diarrhea: Iron chelators or competitors. J. Am. Vet. Med. Assoc., 187:746, 1985.

Fioramonti, J., Fargeas, M., and Bueno, L.: Stimulation of gastrointestinal motility by loperamide in dogs. Dig. Dis. Sci., 32:641, 1987.

Fioramonti, J., Garcia-Villar, R., Bueno, L., et al.: Colonic myoelectrical activity and propulsion in dog. Dig. Dis. Sci., 25:641, 1980.

Glock, R.D.: Enteric pathology. Bov. Proc., 20:121, 1988.

Goto, Y., et al.: Sequential isolation of rotavirus from individual calves. Vet. Microbiol., 11:177, 1986.

Gross, M.E., and Tranquilli, W.J.: Use of alpha-2-adrenergic receptor antagonists. J. Am. Vet. Med. Assoc., 195:378, 1989.

Gryboski, J., and Kocoshis, S.: Effect of bismuth subsalicylate on chronic diarrhea in childhood: A preliminary report. Rev. Infect. Dis., 12(Suppl 1):S36, 1990.

Guard, C.L., and Tennant, B.C.: Rehydration of neonatal calves with experimental coli bacillosis: Oral v intravenous fluids. 1986.

Gupta, S.K., and Mitra, K.: Corticosteroids in asthma pharmacology and therapeutics. J. Assoc. Phys. Ind., 36:221, 1988.

Haggard, D.L.: Bovine enteric colibacillosis. Vet. Clin. North Am. [Food Anim. Pract.], 1:495, 1985.

Haskins, S.C.: Fluid and electrolyte therapy. Comp. Cont. Educ. Pract. Vet., 6:244, 1984.

Hunt, E.: Calculation of fluid and bicarbonate deficits for parenteral fluid replacement therapy. Vet. Clin. North Am. [Food Anim. Pract.], 1:657, 1985.

Ingram, D.M., and Catchpole, B.N.: Effects of opiates on gastroduodenal motility following surgical operation. Dig. Dis. Sci., 26:989, 1981.

Janke, B.H., et al.: Attaching and effacing Escherichia coli infections in calves, pigs, lambs and dogs. J. Vet. Diag. Invest., 1:6, 1989.

Jenkins, C.C., DeNovo, R.C.: "Omeprazole": a potent antiulcer drug. Comp. Cont. Educ. 1578, 1992.

Johnson, S.E.: Clinical pharmacology of antiemetics and antidiarrheals. Proceedings, 8th Kal Kan Symposium 1984.

Johnson, S.E.: Loperamide: a novel antidiarrheal drug. Comp. Cont. Educ. 1373, 1991.

Jones, R., et al.: Hypersomotic oral replacement fluid for diarrheic calves. J. Am. Vet. Med. Assoc., 185:1501, 1984.

Kasari, T.R., and Naylor, J.M.: Clinical evaluation of sodium bicarbonate, sodium L-lactate and sodium acetate for the treatment of acidosis in diarrheic calves. J. Am. Vet. Med. Assoc., 187:392, 1986.

Leib, M.S., Monroe, W.E., Codner, E.C.: Management of chronic large bowel diarrhea in dogs. Vet. Med., 86:992, 1991.

Levine, M.M.: Escherichia coli that cause diarrhea: Enterotoxigenic, enteropathogenic, enteroinvasive, enterohemorrhagic and enteroadherent. J. Infect. Dis., 155:377, 1987.

Macy, D.W., Gasper, P.W.: Diazepam-induced eating in anorexic acts. J. Am. Anim. Hosp. Assoc., 21:17, 1984.

McNulty, M.S., et al.: Effect of vaccination of the dam on rotavirus infection in young calves. Vet. Rec., 120:250, 1987.

Mebus, C.A., Stair, E.L., Inderdahl, N.R., et al.: Calf diarrhea of viral etiology. Ann. Rech. Vet., 4:71, 1973.

Mero, K.N., Rollin, R.E., and Phillips, R.W.: Malabsorption due to selected oral antibiotics. Vet. Clin. North Am. [Food Anim. Pract.], 1:581, 1985.

Michell, A.R.: Oral and parenteral rehydration therapy. In Practice, May:96, 1989.

Michell, A.R.: Drips, drinks, drenches: What matters in fluid therapy. Irish Vet. J., 42:17, 1988.

Michell, A.R., Bywater, R.J., Clarke, K.W., et al.: Veterinary Fluid Therapy. Oxford, Blackwell, 1989.

Moon, H.W., Woode, G.N., and Ahrens, F.A.: Attempted chemoprophylaxis of cryptosporidiosis in calves. Vet. Rec., 110:181, 1982.

Morgan, J.: Epidemiology, diagnosis, and control of undifferentiated calf diarrhea. In Practice, Jan.:17, 1990.

Muir, W.W.: Equine shock. Equine Vet. J., 19:1, 1987.

Mullowney, P.C., et al.: Therapeutic agents used in the treatment of calf diarrhea. Vet. Clin. North Am. [Food Anim. Pract.], 1:563, 1985.

Murdoch, P.: An Investigation of Solute Fluxes in Enterocytes and the Relevance of These fluxes to Diarrheic Disease. Doctoral Thesis, University of Bath, 1988.

Naylor, J.M.: Therapeutic approach to the diarrheic calf. Proc. 21 Ann. Conf. AABP, 1988.

Naylor, J.M.: Severity and nature of acidosis in diarrheic calves over and under one week of age. Can. Vet. J., 28:168, 1987.

Naylor, J.M.: Alkalizing abilities of calf oral electrolyte solutions. Proceedings of the Fourteenth World Congress on Diseases of Cattle, 1:362, 1986.

Naylor, J.M., and Forsyth, G.W.: The alkalizing effects of metabolizable bases in the healthy calf. Can. Vet. J., 50:509, 1986.

Palmer, G.H., Bywater, R.J., and Francis, M.E.: Amoxicillin: Distribution and clinical efficacy in calves. Vet. Rec., *100*:487, 1977.

Papich, M.G., Cavis, C.A., and Davis, L.E.: Absorption of salicylate from an antidiarrheal preparation in dogs and cats. J. Am. Anim. Hosp. Assoc., *23*:221, 1987.

Pearson, G.R., et al.: Pathological changes in the small intestine of neonatal calves with enteric colibacillosis. Vet. Pathol., *15*:92, 1978.

Phillips, R.W.: Fluid therapy for diarrheic calves. Vet. Clin. North Am. [Food Anim. Pract.], *1*:541, 1985.

Phillips, R.W.: Oral fluid therapy: Some concepts of osmolality, electrolytes and energy. *In* Veterinary Pharmacology and Toxicology. Edited by Y. Ruckebusch, P.L. Toutain, and G.D. Korits. Lancaster, MTP Press, 1983.

Phillips, R.W., and Lewis, L.D.: Intravenous high potassium therapy for diarrheic calves. Bov. Pract., *16*:79, 1981.

Reynolds, D.J., Morgan, J.H., Charter, W., et al.: Microbiology of calf diarrhea in Southern Britain. Vet. Rec., *119*:34, 1986.

Richter, K.P.: Therapy for vomiting patients with gastrointestinal ulcers. Vet. Med., *87*:819, 1992.

Richter, K.P.: Treating acute vomiting in dogs and cats. J. Vet. Med., *87*:814, 1992.

Roussel, A.J., and Brumbaugh, G.W.: Treatment of diarrhea of neonatal calves. Vet. Clin. North. Am. [Food Anim. Pract.], *7*:713, 1991.

Roussel, A.J., Sriranganathan, N., Brown, S., et al.: Effect of flunixin meglumine of Escherichia coli heat stable enterotoxin induced diarrhea in calves. Am. J. Vet. Res., *49*:1431, 1988.

Sanders, D.E.: Field management of neonatal diarrhea. Vet. Clin. North Am. [Food Anim. Pract.], *1*:621, 1985.

Sandhu, B.K., Tripp, J.H., Candy, D.C.A., et al.: Loperamide: Studies on its mechanism of action. Gut, *22*:658, 1981.

Snodgrass, D.R., Anmgus, K.W., Gray, E.W., and Keie, W.A.: Cryptosporidia associated with rotavirus and E. coli in an outbreak of calf scour. Vet. Rec., *106*:458, 1980.

Snodgrass, D.R., Terzolo, H.R., Sherwood, D., et al.: Aetiology of diarrhea in young calves. Vet. Rec., *199*:31, 1986.

Torres, A.: The pathogenesis and clinical management of neonatal diarrhea. Proceedings of Symposium on Bovine Neonatal Diarrhea. Western Veterinary Conference, Las Vegas, 1988.

Torres-Medina, A.: Effect of combined rotavirus and Escherichia coli in neonatal gnotobiotic calves. Am. J. Vet. Res., *45*:643, 1984.

van Wyk, M., Dormehol, I.C., Sommers, D.K., et al.: The influence of loperamide, codeine and naloxone on the gastric emptying of beagle dogs. Med. Sci. Res., *16*:575, 1988.

White, D.G.: Colostral supplementation in ruminants. Comp. Cont. Educ., *15*:335, 1993.

White, G.G.: Colostrum supplementation in ruminants. Comp. Contin. Educ. Pract. Vet., *15*:335, 1993.

Whitlock, R.H.: Therapeutic strategies involving antimicrobial treatment of the gastrointestinal tract in large animals. J. Am. Vet. Med. Assoc., *185*:1210, 1984.

WHO/UNICEF: The Management of Diarrhea and Use of Oral Rehydration Therapy. 2nd Ed. Geneva, 1985.

Wilcke, J.R., and Turner, J.C.: The use of adsorbents to treat gastrointestinal problems in small animals. Semin. Vet. Med. Surg. [Small Anim.], *2*:226, 1987.

Wren, W.B.: Probiotics: Fact or fiction. Anim. Health Nutr. 42:28, 1987.

Yeoman, G.H.: Recent advances in the chemotherapy of neonatal diseases in farm animals. *In* Recent Advances in Neonatal Diarrhea in Farm Animals. 1980.

Zeman, D.H., Thompson, J.U., Francis, D.M.: Diagnosis, treatment and management of enteric colibacillosis. Vet. Med., *84*:794, 1989.

Ziv, G.: Comparative clinical pharmacology of amikacin and kanamycin in dairy calves. Am. J. Vet. Res., *38*:337, 1977.

7 PRACTICAL FLUID THERAPY

7.1 Introduction
7.2 Body Compartments
7.3 Osmolarity and Tonicity
7.4 Acid-Base Balance
7.5 Evaluation of Dehydration
7.6 Therapy
7.7 Choice of Replacement Solution
7.8 Route of Administration
7.9 Guidelines for Fluid Therapy
7.10 Fluid-Responsive Conditions
7.11 Shock
7.12 Endotoxic Shock
7.13 Nonsteroidal Anti-Inflammatory Drugs
7.14 Miscellaneous Approaches for Shock Therapy

7.1 INTRODUCTION

Many diseases of large and small animals are characterized by severe acid-base and serum electrolyte disturbances as well as dehydration. When the disturbance is severe, parenteral or oral fluid and electrolyte replacement therapy must be initiated. Each of the water compartments of the body contains electrolytes, and the distribution and concentration of electrolytes in each compartment differs from that of the others. All fluid compartments are separated by semipermeable membranes that allow free passage of water in either direction but restrict particles and ions. The number of individual particles in the water is important, and it is independent of electrical charge, valency, or chemical formula of the substances. The electrolyte concentrations found in body fluids are expressed in milliequivalents rather than weight, and this gives a figure that is directly related to the number of ions. These particles in solution exert an osmotic pressure, and the unit of osmotic pressure is termed the milliosmol.

Dehydration denotes loss of water and electrolytes. Most cases of dehydration result from a loss of extracellular fluid, of which sodium constitutes the chief cation. An extensive loss of fluid not only changes the volume, but also the composition of the extracellular fluid. Because of this, distortions of the electrolyte pattern must also be considered in replacement therapy. When the animal body loses water at a rate exceeding intake, circulatory fluid tends to be depleted, resulting in decreased hydrostatic pressure and increased colloid osmotic pressure (plasma proteins). This depletion is rapidly compensated for by movement of fluid from the extracellular fluid into the plasma. Because of differences related to body fluid reserves and surface area, the young animal is far more susceptible than the adult animal to the effects of dehydration.

7.2 BODY COMPARTMENTS

Water is the largest single constituent of the body, representing about 70% of total body weight. Fifty percent of this water is intracellular, and 20% is extracellular. Of this extracellular fluid (ECF), 15% is present in the interstitial fluid and 5% in the plasma. The interstitial fluid acts as a cushion between the largest and the smallest compartments. Water is not retained rigidly in the compartments but is in a state of dynamic equilibrium with the opposing forces of hydrostatic and osmotic pressure. The electrolyte content of the intracellular fluid (ICF) and ECF is quite different:

	CATIONS	ANIONS
ECF	Na^+	CL^- HCO_3^-
ICF	K^+	PO_4^- protein

Sodium (Na^+) is the principal cation ($+$) in the ECF, whereas potassium (K^+) is the principal cation in the ICF. The predominant anions ($-$) of the ECF are chloride and bicarbonate and of the ICF phosphate and protein. The difference in cations results from active extrusion of sodium by living cells. This is the "sodium pump," and it requires considerable metabolic energy. A similar process enables sodium to pass from the intestine to the plasma against other prevailing forces. The ECF and plasma differ from each other principally in the higher concentration of proteins in the latter. The concentration of water, however, relative to osmotically active ingredients is the same in all compartments, and any net imbalance in osmolarity between two compartments either from a loss of fluid or loss of electrolytes results in a net shifting of water.

SHIFTS OF WATER WITHIN BODY COMPARTMENTS

For selective fluid distribution, a selectively permeable membrane is necessary. Between the plasma and the ECF, this membrane is the capillary wall, which is permeable to water, electrolytes, and small molecules but impermeable to plasma proteins. These proteins exert an osmotic pressure that results in the passage of fluid from the interstitial spaces into the circulation. The hydrostatic pressure of the circulating fluid within the capillary opposes this force, and fluid leaves the capillary as long as the hydrostatic pressure is greater than the osmotic pressure.

Therefore loss of plasma protein or increased hydrostatic pressure leads to an increased passage of fluid and electrolytes out of the capillaries and into the ECF. Similarly, venous obstruction or shock leads to passage of fluids and electrolytes in the same direction. In such cases, parenteral electrolyte infusions are of no value in expanding the blood volume because, as a result of the decreased osmotic pressure of the plasma proteins, they simply pass out into the ECF.

7.3 OSMOLARITY AND TONICITY

Osmolarity is usually expressed as the number of milliosmols per kilogram (or liter) of fluid. Isotonic means that the solution contains approximately 300 mOsm per liter of body fluid. Hypertonic solutions are more than 300 mOsm, and hypotonic solutions are less than 300 mOsm. The osmolarity is made up from all the particles in solution, each molecule (or ion if the substance is dissociated) contributing 1 mOsm. The number of individual particles in solution is important, and if it amounts to 300 per liter, the solution is isotonic: This is why 0.9% sodium chloride, 5% dextrose, or 1.3% sodium bicarbonate are all isotonic. Similarly, 100 mmol/liter each of sodium, chloride, and glucose (300 mmol in all) provide an isotonic solution. Thus dextrose/saline (4.3% dextrose, 0.18 (N/5) saline) is also an isotonic solution but one particularly low in sodium.

Tonicity, usually expressed in milliosmols, provides a measure of concentration of dissolved particles (e.g., ions, nutrients), in the body fluid. Ideally any rehydration treatment should be as near as possible isotonic with calf serum (approximately 300 mOsm/kg). If the solution is hypertonic (e.g., 407 mOsm/kg), it tends to produce an initial net secretion of fluid into rather than absorption from the small intestine.

A plasma substitute (dextran) is also isotonic and contains large molecules to help hold fluids in the blood stream. Hypertonic solutions include 50% dextrose, 3% saline (table salt or sodium chloride), and 10% calcium gluconate or 5% amino acid solution. Lactated Ringer's solution with 2% glucose, Peridial 1.5%, or Inpersol 1.5% are hypertonic solutions used for peritoneal dialysis.

7.4 ACID-BASE BALANCE

The acid-base balance of body fluids is important because the chemical and metabolic reactions of the body being controlled by enzymes are greatly influenced by small changes in pH. Despite the large amounts of acid production by normal endogenous cellular metabolism, blood pH is maintained within narrow limits in the range 7.35 to 7.45, with the mean figure of 7.4. Death results if the pH falls below 6.8 or rises above 7.8. The acid-base balance depends largely on the ratio between bicarbonate and carbonic acid in the blood. The carbonic acid level is controlled by respiration, and the bicarbonate concentration is controlled by renal and other nonrespiratory processes.

Acidosis may be caused by several factors:

1. Loss of bicarbonate ions into the feces by intestinal secretion
2. Buildup of lactic acid produced in underperfused tissues
3. Production of organic acids by an abnormal gut flora
4. Depressed renal excretion of hydrogen ions and reduced regeneration of bicarbonate in the kidney

During digestion in the normal animal, large volumes of secretions are produced mainly in the upper part of the gastrointestinal tract. These secretions contain the digestive enzymes and large amounts of water, sodium, potassium, chloride, and bicarbonate. Normally they are almost completely reabsorbed, so little remains in the feces. In cases of diarrhea, however, reabsorption is impaired, and the secretions are lost in the feces. Digestive secretions of the small intestine are alkaline, and hence when they are lost from the body acid-base equilibrium is disturbed, and acidosis results. This is a frequent complication of diarrhea in calves. Further, during periods of illness and dehydration, the animal's food intake is drastically reduced or totally absent. In many cases, the animal begins to break down reserves of fat, resulting in the accumulation of ketone bodies. This tends to worsen the already existing acidosis resulting from the original ionic loss and imbalance.

Other factors may also contribute to the development of acidosis. Decreased tissue perfusion and oxygenation accompany hypovolemic shock and result in increased anaerobic glycolysis and increased production of organic acids, such as lactic acid. Hypovolemia also causes reduced renal blood flow, which in turn decreases hydrogen ion excretion by the kidneys. Calves in deep hypovolemic shock may also have depressed respiration, resulting in additional hydrogen ion production and decreased hydrogen ion excretion by the kidney. All are implicated in the development of metabolic acidosis in the scouring animal. In contrast to this, the constituents of the gastric juice are acidic and are normally secreted into the stomach or abomasum. Normal fluid, electrolyte, and acid-base balance depend on reabsorption of this secretion, and whenever this process is impeded, gastric juice tends to be sequestered in the abomasum or vomited from the stomach.

This results in a loss of water and hydrochloric acid from the body, and a syndrome characterized by dehydration and metabolic alkalosis ensues with a low serum chloride and a high serum bicarbonate values. This alkalosis is more commonly seen in the vomiting animal, but it also occurs in animals with displacement or torsion of the abomasum. It may occur in other disorders in which there is atony or impaction of the abomasum. It is thus apparent that the disorders of the anterior portion of the alimentary tract are quite different from those of the posterior portion. Accordingly the fluid therapy chosen must be different also to correct the hypochloremia and alkalosis (seen in vomiting) or the hyperkalemia and acidosis (seen in diarrhea).

The effects of scours on potassium metabolism are complex. The starving animal responds to dehydration by release of intracellular potassium into the ECF in an attempt to maintain the volume of the latter. Normally excess potassium in the ECF is excreted in the urine, but when urine flow is reduced, as in dehydration, the ECF level of potassium may become quite elevated. Hyperkalemia is a common finding in calves with diarrhea, although the intracellular levels may be less than normal. An overall potassium deficit exists owing to potassium loss, but the contrasting levels in body fluids may interfere with cardiac function. Depletion of potassium from tissue cells, especially those of skeletal muscle, is manifested by skeletal muscle weakness. Administration of potassium to a hyperkalemic patient seems paradoxical, but the objective is to replace the total body potassium deficit that exists despite hyperkalemia.

Metabolic acid-base imbalance can be separated into two types, metabolic acidosis and metabolic alkalosis. In the former, HCO_3^- (carbon dioxide tension) concentration is low, and in the latter, it is high.

Two pathogenic mechanisms cause metabolic acidosis:

1. Loss of HCO_3-rich secretions
2. Endogenous production of excess organic acids, such as ketoacids, lactic acid, or uremic acids

Bovine diseases causing metabolic acidosis by loss of HCO_3-rich secretions are diarrheal diseases and diseases characterized by excessive salivation, rabies, actinobacillosis, upper digestive system foreign body, or organophosphate toxicity. Duodenal, pancreatic, and salivary secretions rich in HCO_3^- are produced with a net bodily gain in H^+ and net loss in HCO_3^-. Normally HCO_3^- in these secretions is reabsorbed so acid-base balance is maintained. Bovine diseases causing metabolic acidosis by endogenous production of excess organic acids are ketosis (ketoacidosis), shock, grain overload and septic metritis/mastitis (lactic acidosis), and uremic acidosis or renal failure.

There are four primary acid-base disorders: (1) Respiratory acidosis, (2) respiratory alkalosis, (3) metabolic acidosis, and (4) metabolic alkalosis. Respiratory disturbances affect the carbon dioxide tension in the blood whereas metabolic disturbances are reflected in the bicarbonate concentration. Thus excessive losses of bicarbonate or accumulation of hydrogen ions produces a metabolic acidosis, whereas excessive losses of hydrogen ions or excessive administration of bicarbonate causes a metabolic alkalosis.

METABOLIC ACIDOSIS

This condition arises owing to increased production and retention of acid metabolites or to abnormal losses of alkaline ions. Some examples are:

1. Diarrhea results in considerable losses of HCO_3^-, Na^+, and K^+ ions
2. Intestinal obstruction leads to sequestration of these same ions in the lumen of the gut
3. In inadequate tissue perfusion, as in shock, hypoxia leads to the production of acid metabolites
4. In renal disease or inadequate renal perfusion, as in severe shock, there is retention of H^- ions
5. In myositis, starvation, or severe infection, there is increased production of acid metabolites

RESPIRATORY ACIDOSIS

This condition arises when inadequate alveolar exchange results in retention of carbon dioxide:

1. In anesthesia, inadequate ventilation, increased dead space, or obstructed airway may be the cause
2. Lung pathology, such as congestion, pneumonia, or emphysema, also results in inadequate respiratory exchange

In the shocked surgical patient requiring prolonged anesthesia, the combined effects of metabolic and respiratory acidosis may depress pH to critical levels, and it is suggested that in such cases (e.g., the colic case in which surgery is performed) this factor contributes considerably to irreversible shock.

Many other features are common to cases of dehydration, chief among which is that in subnormal hydration in an animal, the body attempts to conserve sodium and water by reducing the output of urine. This reduced output of urine leads to a buildup of metabolic wastes that would normally be excreted. Blood urea and creatinine can build up to dangerously high levels.

Breakdown of body fat leads to accumulation of ketone bodies and metabolic acidosis. Normally the bicarbonate in the blood would tend to neutralize any acidosis that might develop, but in cases of diarrhea, bicarbonate is lost into the lumen of the bowel and so is not available to counteract this tendency adequately.

Overall metabolic acidosis is a commonly encountered disturbance and can arise in three distinct ways:

1. Excessive acid production (as in overeating of grain in cattle, ketosis in cattle and sheep, and diabetes mellitus in dogs)
2. Restricted acid excretion (renal acidosis or adrenal insufficiency)
3. Loss of bicarbonate from diarrhea

Acidemia can be corrected by administering bicarbonate ions or so-called bicarbonate precursors, salts of weak organic acids that generate bicarbonate ions when metabolized in the calf. The bicarbonate precursors include lactate, acetate, gluconate, and citrate.

Sodium bicarbonate is the most economical and readily available alkalinizing agent. Lactate is probably the most widely used alkalinizing agent in veterinary medicine. Lactate and acetate are poorly metabolized in calves that are more than 8% dehydrated, and they are less effective alkalinizing agents in these circumstances. Calves that are more than 8% dehydrated and that have moderate or severe acidosis (pH <7.2) are best treated with sodium bicarbonate because this gives a consistent alkalinizing effect.

If depressed dehydrated scouring calves are treated with oral fluids that do not contain an alkalinizing agent, acidosis persists, and improvement in attitude and strength is only partial. A more complete recovery is obtained if bicarbonate-containing oral electrolyte solutions are used. Sometimes, however, bicarbonate solutions are considered to be inappropriate because of their adverse effect of raising the pH of the stomach contents and destroying this natural barrier against further infection.

A convenient and effective oral treatment of acidosis is based on the conversion of citrate to bicarbonate in the liver, each citrate ion yielding three bicarbonate ions. Citrate ions have a dual function. First, they stimulate water and sodium absorption through linked uptake mechanisms at the cell surface. Second, after absorption, citrate is metabolized to produce adenosine triphosphate (ATP) (so contributing to sodium transport) and to add bicarbonate to counter acidosis.

A general feature of diarrhea and dehydration is that in all cases a contraction of the ECF occurs. Urinary output is reduced also, and as the condition progresses, sodium conservation is increased by the action of aldosterone. The diminishing volume of the ECF leads to the classic signs of dehydration in the affected animal, and hypovolemic shock (water withdrawn from the blood stream) and death from circulatory failure may occur in extreme cases. A scouring calf can produce up to 40 times the normal amount of feces. This increased quantity is almost entirely composed of fluid and electrolytes and has a dry matter content around 5% instead of the normal 23 to 35%. As the animal dehydrates, the volume of the circulating blood decreases (hypovolemia) until eventually all the fluid compartments of the body share in the water deficit. This is because loss of water and sodium from the plasma is followed by transfer of water and electrolytes from the intestinal fluid in replacement. As the loss continues water, is drawn from the tissue cells themselves. An animal may lose all of its glycogen and fat and a considerable amount of its protein without dying, but the loss of 10% of its water content results in serious metabolic disturbance.

7.5 EVALUATION OF DEHYDRATION

Continued loss of water and electrolytes in diarrhea leads to dehydration, and this occurs regardless of the cause of the diarrhea. The animal is losing fluid that approximates to plasma—it contains in particular sodium, potassium, and bicarbonate, and these are the constituents in which the animal is deficit. Symptoms of dehydration are seen when about 6% of body water has been lost, with collapse occurring when more than 8 to 9% is lost.

The loss of blood volume causes reflex release of aldosterone from the adrenal cortex. This causes the kidney to conserve sodium (and water) at the expense of potassium. Interestingly aldosterone also stimulates water absorption in the colon, which acts as a compensatory system (again with corresponding loss of potassium). There is a movement of water and ions from ICF to ECF, and as loss of bicarbonate produces acidosis, so potassium from cells enters plasma and often causes a rise in plasma potassium despite the overall net deficit.

Eventually hemoconcentration so impairs the perfusion of vital tissues, such as the brain, that there is inadequate oxygenation, which leads to death. Dehydration then is a vital part of the disease pathophysiology.

The degree of dehydration can be assessed by:

1. Consideration of the body weight
2. Clinical signs exhibited by the animal
3. Use of certain laboratory aids

BODY WEIGHT

Because 70% of the body weight is water, any change in the fluid status of the animal is reflected by a change in body weight. A useful method is to assess the level of dehydration as a percentage of the total body weight because this then gives an approximate guideline for the volume of replacement fluid required, e.g., a 400-kg horse that is 7% dehydrated requires a total fluid replacement volume of 28 liters (over 5 gallons).

i.e., 400 kg × 7% Weight Loss (Fluid)
= 28 kg = 28 Liters Required

CLINICAL SIGNS

The following signs may be helpful in determining the percentage of dehydration and electrolyte imbalance of affected animals. A calf with about 5% dehydration may appear thirsty and drink readily. The eyes should be bright and skin and extremities warm. Dehydration of 10% renders the animal more lifeless and unwilling to stand. The body may be warm but the extremities cold, and the skin begins to lose elasticity. Rectal temperature ranges from 90° to 94° F. If a finger is placed in the mouth, the calf does not suck.

As the condition becomes critical (i.e., dehydration exceeds 10% body weight), circulation deteriorates, and the extremities and mucous membranes become cold. Eyes are sunken, the corneas often appearing dry and dull. The calf is usually comatose, and a wet area is apparent around the mouth.

The extent of dehydration may be roughly assessed on the basis of losses of

5%, 7%, 10%, and 12% body weight loss. These figures are accompanied by definite clinical signs.

0 to 5% Fluid Loss: Little clinical change

7% Fluid Loss: Loss of skin elasticity (contraction of the lubricating ECF), dry mouth, injected conjunctivae, eyes dry and sunken, urine reduced in volume

10% Fluid Loss: Hidebound, apparent loss of weight, cold, weak, unable to stand, pale mucous membranes, temperature decrease, sluggish capillary refill time (hypovolemia), weak pulse, minimal urine formation, concentrated urine

12% Fluid Loss: Recumbent, weak pulse, rapid shallow respiration, unable to sit up unassisted, body weight loss, muscle tremors, subnormal temperature, hypovolemia, shock, circulatory failure

A rough estimate of the degree of dehydration may be made by examining the texture and elasticity of the skin and the appearance of the mucous membranes. Dryness of the oral mucous membranes may indicate primary water depletion, but panting also causes dryness without necessarily concomitant dehydration. Capillary refill is indicative of the adequacy of tissue perfusion. The normal pink color of the gum should return within 2 seconds of compression. A time of more than 3 seconds accompanied by tachycardia and cool extremities indicates hypovolemic shock, which, if caused by dehydration, indicates a large deficit (12 to 15%).

LABORATORY AIDS

The most direct indicator of the state of hydration that can be measured easily is the hematocrit. Using a microhematocrit centrifuge and heparinized tubes, it is possible to determine the hematocrit value (packed cell volume [PCV]) of an animal in only a few minutes, and this information is valuable in assessing the fluid balance of that animal. To assess the state of hydration accurately, it is necessary to measure the hematocrit value of the individual concerned and if

possible, that of another animal of similar breed and age in the same herd. The degree of abnormality can then be approximated. The pathogenesis of dehydration is such that following fluid loss, water is drawn from the tissues into the blood stream to restore the circulating blood volume toward normal. Further fluid loss then causes a reduction in the fluid content of the blood, resulting in reduction in the circulatory blood volume (hypovolemia) and a relative increase in the number of circulating erythrocytes (hemoconcentration). This hemoconcentration causes an increase in the viscosity of the blood and also causes the PCV to rise. Thus in cases of dehydration, the PCV tends to increase. The normal range of hematocrit values in cattle is 24 to 46%. Generally the greatest usefulness of the hematocrit lies with daily monitoring of critical cases in which day-to-day changes parallel the changing state of hydration. It should be apparent, however, that concurrent anemia in a dehydrated animal tends to mask this increase in the PCV, and a normal or near normal reading is obtained in such an animal. In these cases, the plasma protein concentration of the animal should be examined. Elevated levels of plasma proteins determined on the refractometer indicate dehydration. Normal plasma protein levels in cattle are as follows: under 1 year, 6 g/%; young adults, 7 g/%, adults (lactating), 8 to 9 g/%. Recorded values above normal are most frequently caused by dehydration. As with the hematocrit, day-to-day changes in plasma protein parallel changing states of fluid balance.

Urine specific gravity is another index that is useful in the evaluation of dehydration. When water is lost from the body, the osmolarity of the ECF increases. This increase in osmolarity tends to stimulate certain specialized ganglion cells of the anterior hypothalamus known as the osmoreceptors. Impulses from these osmoreceptors are transmitted from the hypothalamus through the pituitary stalk to the neurohypophysis, where they promote the release of antidiuretic hormone (ADH). This hormone on release into the blood stream then promotes increased water reabsorption from the distal tubules and the collecting ducts of the kidney. Hence normal values in cattle range from 1.025 to 1.045, with an approximate mean value of 1.035. Disease states accompanied by total body water deficit will result in stimulation of physiology mechanisms for conservation of water. Accordingly, renal conservation of water occurs: urine with altered specific gravity is produced. Because urine formation is reduced to minimal levels to conserve body fluids, there is a marked increase in metabolic end products in the plasma. In a scouring calf, the blood urea level increases from a normal 10 to 20 mg/100 ml to 30 to 45 mg/100 ml. This is another parameter that can be measured in the laboratory.

Plasma electrolyte concentrations may also be estimated by laboratory methods. Blood gas analysis and the anion gap are especially useful indicators. Sodium concentrations are elevated in predominant water loss, whereas in salt loss they are initially normal and fall only in advanced cases. Not all cases of hyponatremia, however, represent actual salt depletion: The cause may be dilution of the plasma, as in "overhydration." Plasma potassium levels may also be estimated, but the concentration of this electrolyte in the blood does not always reflect the body status with respect to this element. Generally hyperkalemia is a characteristic finding in scouring animals. Laboratory estimations of the various above-mentioned parameters serve to strengthen a clinical opinion based both on the history—principally the amount and source of fluid lost—and on the clinical condition of the patient.

7.6 THERAPY

Treatment of dehydration may be viewed as comprising four phases:

1. Correcting life-threatening hypovolemia
2. Restoring accumulated deficits of fluids and correcting electrolyte and acid-base disturbances
3. Providing sufficient fluids and electrolytes to meet continuing losses each day
4. Meeting normal daily requirements

The first step in fluid therapy is assessment of the needs of the animal. The needs include not only the fluid that has already been lost, and current dehydration, but also continuing fluid losses through diarrhea, maintenance requirements, and electrolyte imbalances. Dehydration is best estimated based on clinical signs, such as skin tension, sunken eyes, and dry mucous membranes. The next decision is the route of administration. Subcutaneous fluid therapy is fast and simple but ineffective in a severely dehydrated animal. Perfusion of the peripheral parts of the body is generally poor, resulting in poor absorption of the fluids. The volume of fluids that may be given by this method is limited and may be inadequate. The next possibility is intraperitoneally. This choice presents the risk of causing peritonitis, and the amount of uptake by this route is questionable. The best route in the severely dehydrated animal, greater than 6%, is intravenous. Although this route requires considerable care in administration with regard to cleanliness and technique, it offers the best advantage is getting the proper volume of fluid and electrolytes to the area where they are needed most. Intravenous therapy, although medically the best choice, may be economically prohibitive. This is especially true when dealing with a major herd problem or with pigs. Oral fluid therapy seems to be the method of choice when dealing with a large number of individuals that require treatment when the value of an animal does not warrant the expense involved in intravenous therapy. This is the most economical and effective method of treatment early in the disease. The need for sterility is eliminated, and the treatment can be administered by the owner rather than the veterinarian. There are contraindications for oral therapy, however. One is the moribund animal, in which oral therapy is simply too slow to save the animal. The other is malabsorptive diarrhea.

Fluid therapy for diarrhea should represent a combination of replacement and maintenance of ions and fluids. The replacement product selected should fulfill the need to reverse the dehydration and ion losses as well as provide necessary energy to correct the hypoglycemia and facilitate the movement of potassium from ECF to ICF.

The problems that must be corrected in the diarrheic and dehydrated neonatal calf are:

1. Hemoconcentration and decreased blood volume owing to extensive losses from the extracellular body fluids
2. Total body potassium deficit despite an above-normal level of potassium in the blood (hyperkalemia)
3. Total body deficits of sodium and chloride
4. Acidosis due to bicarbonate losses and anaerobic metabolism
5. Hypoglycemia and whole body energy deficit

ADJUNCTS TO FLUIDS

The use of fluids alone is satisfactory, but antibiotics; vitamins; extra electrolytes, such as sodium bicarbonate and potassium chloride; diuretics; steroids and NSAIDs; and analgesics are all useful. If indicated, patients should receive a broad-spectrum antibiotic for at least 5 days at the recommended dosage. Vitamin supplements can be given intravenously in the infusion to animals that have been anorexic for prolonged periods.

Sodium bicarbonate is used at a rate of 2 to 6 mmol/kg to overcome acidosis, especially in shock, although Ringer's lactate solution generally provides sufficient bicarbonate for body needs. Lactate or bicarbonate metabolizes in the liver in 2 to 6 hours, but sodium bicarbonate provides an immediate effect. This immediate effect is often of benefit in cases of diabetic ketosis to overcome the deficit of serum bicarbonate. Extra potassium can be added as potassium chloride, if the patient is passing urine satisfactorily, to replace potassium losses. For example, in profuse diarrhea or massive wound discharge. Excess plasma protein is normally excreted by the kidneys and if large quantities of this electrolyte were administered to an animal with impaired renal function, cardiac embarrassment might result, owing to its toxic effect on the myocardium. The normal daily requirement for potassium is 1.2 mmol/kg, so it is safe to administer 2 mmol/kg intravenously over 24 hours in the presence of diuresis, to a scouring animal.

ORAL FLUIDS

The following should be considered in determining appropriate formulation for oral use:

1. Absorbability of the fluid
2. Re-establishment of normal body fluid volume
3. Replacement of lost ions—anions (Cl^-, HCO_3^-); Cations (Na^+, K^+)
4. Acid-base correction—HCO_3^- or bicarbonate equivalent
5. Energy maintenance—glucose
6. Tonicity

Owing to the loss of body fluids, provision of large quantities of water is necessary. The ionic composition of oral fluid replacement therapy should be designed to approximate the ECF with added potassium. This approach is needed so crystalloids remain after energy substrates are used; otherwise, hypo-osmolarity may develop, or there may not be sufficient water retention. To be an ECF replacement, the fluid should contain sodium at 120 to 140 mEq/liter; chloride at 30 to 40 mEq less than sodium; and either bicarbonate or a bicarbonate equivalent, as represented by a readily metabolized organic anion.

The optimal quantity of bicarbonate (or equivalent) required should be the amount necessary to correct the acidosis. This is not easily determined, nor can it be readily accomplished in a single therapy. Provision of a crystalloid solution containing 120 to 140 mEq/liter of sodium, with 10 to 30 mEq/liter of potassium and approximately equal quantities of chloride and bicarbonate, or equivalent, helps to restore fluid volume and correct the acidosis.

Energy substrates are also a necessary component. Diarrheic calves almost always have some degree of hypoglycemia. Glucose corrects the hypoglycemia and serves as an energy source. Glucose also enhances potassium movement from plasma to the ICF. This alone would make glucose an important component because hyperkalemia is one of the more serious effects of diarrhea.

Complex carbohydrates may be of less value. Neonatal calves cannot digest sucrose or maltose because of a lack of brush-border enzymes. Lactose is of poten-

TABLE 7–1
COMPOSITION OF FLUIDS

	Na$^+$	K$^+$	Cl$^-$	HCO3$_3^-$	Glucose %	Ca/Mg	Other	Classification
Plasma	145	5	100	24	+	+	+	300 mmol/isotonic
Hartmann's	131	5	112	28	–	+	–	ECF alkalinizer isotonic (278)
Ringer's Lactated	147	4	155	–	–	+	–	ECF acidifer
Ringer's	131	5	111	29	–	+	–	ECF alkalinizer isotonic
Darrow's	120	36	104	52	–	–	–	Isotonic high K+
Saline	154	–	154	–	–	–	–	ECF acidifer isotonic
Dextrose 5%	–	–	–	–	5	–	–	ECF diluent isotonic
Ionalyte	145	11	105	57	0	+	–	ECF alkalinizer
Electrosol	138	8	83	68	2.5	+	–	ECF alkalinizer
Ionaid	75	26	75	0	2.1	+	Glycine	Promotes Na$^+$ uptake
Lectade/ Resorb	74	15	74	2	2.2		Citrate, Glycine (amino acetic)	Promotes Na$^+$ uptake (isotonic) (320 mOsm)
Duphalyte	18	3	3	18	5		Amino A vitamins	Maintenance only
N/5 Saline + 4.3% Dextrose	31	–	31	–	4.3	–	–	Maintenance isotonic
Dextrose/ Saline Full Strength	154	–	154	1	5	–	–	Hypertonic intravenous

tial benefit, but lactase in the brush border is a fragile enzyme and may be decreased in activity during diarrhea.

Hypoglycemia and a negative energy balance commonly occur. This is often associated with acidosis and ultimately results in the development of shock, leading to death.

7.7 CHOICE OF REPLACEMENT SOLUTION

Sodium acts as the osmotic skeleton of ECF, enabling it to resist the osmotic pull of the solutes in the much larger volume of the ICF. The end result of sodium retention is volume expansion, i.e., an increased ECF volume. Similarly, sodium loss results in volume depletion. In deciding on the intended use of the majority of commercial fluids, one must remember the following:

1. The general composition of plasma (sodium, 145; potassium, 5; chloride, 100; bicarbonate, 24 mmol/liter)
2. That isotonicity approximates 300 mmol/liter (Tables 7–1 through 7–4)

FLUID SOLUTIONS

Normal Saline (Isotonic Saline—0.9% Sodium Chloride)

This contains sodium and chloride ions in water at the same osmolarity as body ECF and so is useful for most cases of replacement therapy. It is bicarbonate-free and therefore acts as an ECF acidifier and is useful in correcting metabolic acidosis, especially after vomiting.

Isotonic Dextrose-Saline (0.18% Sodium Chloride (N/5 Saline) + 4.3% Dextrose)

This is also isotonic, but its low sodium and energy content make it suitable only for maintenance therapy (40 ml/kg/24 hours).

5% Dextrose

This is an isotonic fluid containing water and some energy in the form of glucose. It acts principally as a source of water only,

---

TABLE 7–2
CLASSIFICATION OF FLUIDS

ECF replacers	Hartmann's
	Ringer's lactate
ECF acidifiers	Normal saline (bicarbonate-free)
	Dextrose-saline (hypertonic)
	Ringer's solution
ECF alkalinizers	Lactated Ringer's, Hartmann's, Darrow's, 1.3% Sodium bicarbonate
ECF diluent	5% Dextrose
Maintenance solutions	N/5 Saline (0.18%) + 4.3% dextrose (isotonic)
Composite/nutrient fluids	Glucose, amino acids, (proprietary preparations)

---

as in a case of hypertonic dehydration resulting from water deprivation or heat stroke. Although it is poor as a source of calories, it may be used in an emergency to provide a transient alleviation of hypoglycemia.

Compound Sodium Lactate (Hartmann's Solution, Ringer's Lactate)

This is the universal replacement solution, and it approximates plasma without protein. It is isotonic and contains approximately 131 mmol/liter of sodium, 5 mmol/liter of potassium, 112 mmol/liter of chloride, and 25 mmol/liter of bicarbonate (precursor) together with a varying amount of calcium, magnesium, and so forth. Thus it is similar to plasma. The lactate is metabolized to bicarbonate by the liver and therefore is useful in treating metabolic acidosis (as in diarrhea). This solution can be given

to most patients initially for the replacement of losses owing to gastrointestinal dysfunction (vomiting, diarrhea,) hemorrhage, or burns.

Darrow's Solution

This consists of 0.4% sodium chloride, 0.27% potassium chloride, and 0.58% sodium lactate. It is similar in composition to lactated Ringer's but contains more potassium. The sodium lactate is metabolized to

---

TABLE 7–4
COMPOSITION OF FLUIDS: EXTRACELLULAR FLUID ALKALINIZERS

Hartmann's
Ringer's acetate
Rose's solution
    NaCl—4.5 g/liter
    KCl—1.4 g/liter
    Na HCO$_3$—4.5 g/liter
Hypertonic bicarbonate (>1.3%)
    5% bicarbonate can be used initially for severe acidosis (grain overload)
    Alkalinizing capacity of fluids such as Hartmann's can be increased by addition of 15–20 ml of 8.4% bicarbonate without affecting osmolarity significantly
Concentrate solutions should never be administered directly to an animal
Emergency solution (2 liters)
    1/2 tablespoon NaCl
    1 tablespoon Na HCO$_3$

TABLE 7–3
COMPOSITION OF FLUIDS: EXTRACELLULAR FLUID ACIDIFIERS

Saline
    NaCl—9.0 g/liter
Ringer's solution
    NaCl—8.6 g/liter
    KCl—0.3 g/liter
    CaCl$_2$—0.33 g/liter

Note: These solutions allow bicarbonate-free expansion of plasma, restoring circulating volume and correcting metabolic alkalosis.

sodium bicarbonate and so has an alkalinizing effect. It is used for treating metabolic acidosis associated with diarrhea dehydration and potassium loss.

Dextrose Saline (0.9% Sodium Chloride + 5% Dextrose)

This is a hypertonic solution for intravenous use indicated for emergency treatment of dehydration and the immediate treatment of hypoglycemia.

Sodium Bicarbonate (1.3%)

This is used for the treatment of severe acidosis when immediate results are required (i.e., not waiting for lactate to be metabolized to bicarbonate).

Whole Blood

This is a suitable replacement for blood loss in treating anemia. Blood transfusions are relatively successful, especially the first time, but in about 10% of second transfusions, reactions may occur owing to mismatching, which leads to destruction of the donor cells by the recipient.

PLASMA EXPANDERS

Dextran

This is a plasma substitute and expander derived from a glucose polysaccharide. It is relatively expensive but effective in the restoration of blood volume in cases of hemorrhage or shock. It is manufactured in different molecular weights—40, 70, 110, and 150.

Dextran 40 and 70 can be used in veterinary practice. Dextran 40 is infused at a rate of 10 to 20 ml/kg in 24 hours together with a suitable fluid replacement, such as Ringer's lactate. It is important to note that internal hemorrhage or shock, with an ensuing loss in the osmotic property of the blood, use of replacement fluids alone is worthless because they simply run out of the circulation and the hypovolemia (owing to reduced osmotic pressure) remains. Dextran's duration of action is approximately 24 hours.

Gelatin Colloidal Solution

This is a plasma substitute that is isotonic, manufactured from degraded gelatin, and contains sodium, potassium, calcium, sulfate, phosphate ions, and water. It is less expensive than Dextran and is suitable for use alone because it is isotonic and contains sufficient electrolytes. It should be infused at a rate determined by the condition of the patient, and it is recommended that the rate not exceed 20 ml/kg every 12 hours. It is useful in cases of hypovolemic shock, and its duration of action is 2 to 3 hours. This colloid is indicated for shock, burns, blood loss, and diarrhea.

MAINTENANCE FLUID SOLUTIONS

In these fluids, the concentrations of sodium and other electrolytes (potassium, chloride) are usually about one fifth of their concentration in plasma. These concentrations reflect only the daily requirements of water and electrolytes as opposed to the need to replace losses. A number of these commercial preparations sometimes contain small amounts of glucose, e.g., N/5 saline + 4.3% dextrose.

7.8 ROUTE OF ADMINISTRATION

ORAL THERAPY AND NEONATAL SCOUR

Oral rehydration solutions have become popular and effective for treating diarrheic calves. Most of these products contain electrolytes, glucose, and bicarbonate or a bicarbonate precursor.

Oral therapy is often successful in early cases of dehydration and diarrhea, and provided that the degree of dehydration is 7% or less, the animal is likely to respond favorably to oral fluid administration. Diarrhea is essentially a failure of intestinal fluid and electrolyte transport mechanisms. Solutions containing a specific range of concentrations of glucose and saline promote the intestinal uptake of sodium, which opposes the underlying pathologic change in electrolyte transport. Components such as glycine and acetate reinforce the uptake of sodium, and a number of formulations specifically designed to promote sodium absorption have become available for calf scour (e.g., Lectade/RE-SORB).

Most calves that succumb to diarrheal disease are not killed by the bacterial, viral, chemical, or nutritional agents that initiate the disease but are victims of dehydration, acidosis, electrolyte imbalances, and energy deficit. A proper formulation used in fluid therapy for correcting the imbalances that occur in neonatal diarrheic calves should provide fluid to reverse the dehydration, ion replacement, acid-base correction, and energy maintenance. When these needs are met, the clinical signs of acidosis, hyperkalemia, hemoconcentration, and hypoglycemia are eliminated, and the dehydrated calf can recover and begin to function normally.

The cause of diarrhea in young pigs and calves includes a number of bacterial and viral agents, with *Escherichia coli*, and rotavirus being the most important. It is now clear that enteropathogenic strains of *E. coli* produce diarrhea through secretion of enterotoxins that act on the small intestinal mucosa to cause fluid and electrolyte secretion.

Currently the emphasis on fluid and electrolyte therapy for diarrheic calves is focused on use of oral fluids. A principal basis for this approach is the outstanding success of oral glucose electrolyte therapies for the treatment of *Vibrio cholera* diarrhea in humans. Associated with this beneficial effect is the recognition that the mechanisms by which *E. coli* enterotoxin induces diarrhea is analogous to the mechanisms of *V. cholera* as well as other enterotoxigenic bacteria.

In severely diarrheic calves, hypoglycemia and lactic acidosis are an almost constant finding. Hypoglycemia and lactic acidosis are also pathognomonic signs of endotoxemia. Damage to the intestinal epithelial barrier allows both bacteria and endotoxin to enter the blood stream in increased quantities and thus endotoxemia is a common sequela to diarrhea. The hypoglycemia, hyperlactacidemia, and hyperkalemia seen in diarrheic neonates may represent a combination of altered epithelial transport and developing endotoxic shock. The relative role of each dysfunction, however, is not known.

During diarrhea, dehydration occurs with the greatest losses for the extracellular pool. Acidosis is seen as a result of bicarbonate loss and increased lactate levels; hypoglycemia is common; and major losses of sodium, chloride, and potassium occur. Intracellular-extracellular potassium imbalance may become severe, resulting in reduced resting membrane potential and altered cardiac and general muscular function.

The benefits of oral rehydration have been demonstrated in human medicine. Whether the cause of the diarrhea is infectious, nutritional, or environmental, oral rehydration has been shown to be effective in both the calf and the pig. Oral rehydration with glucose and glycine is an active process, with accompanied absorption of sodium and water. This linked absorption increases the net fluid and electrolyte uptake and offsets fluid losses of diarrhea, thus reversing dehydration. Further, this active transport of glucose and glycine may not be affected by *E. coli* enterotoxins. In one study, glucose and glycine uptake was unaffected by *E. coli* enterotoxin in loops of piglet intestine.

Normal calves have a limited capacity to absorb glucose. This amount is probably significantly less in calves with damaged villi. Special considerations should be given to possible harmful effects of giving large amounts of glucose to calves with a damaged bowel. A high concentration of glucose may cause an osmotic diarrhea on its own or may contribute to fermentative diarrhea by serving as a growth medium for bacteria in the large bowel.

Glycine also promotes intestinal absorption of water and sodium. Glycine is thought to be especially beneficial in stimulating water absorption in the distal small intestine, the area of maximum water loss associated with colibacillosis in calves. Glycine may also have a protein-sparing effect by increasing available nitrogen levels.

GLUCOSE AND GLYCINE CONTENT

Active absorption of glucose and the amino acid glycine is linked with water and sodium. As stated earlier, this linked absorption increases net fluid and electrolyte uptake and offsets fluid losses caused by diarrhea, reversing dehydration. Although some water enters the body by passive diffusion from the gut, more effective and rapid uptake of fluid can be achieved by means of active transport mechanisms.

Glucose and amino acids (e.g., glycine) are absorbed from the lumen into the mucosal cells lining the small intestine by separate energy dependent mechanisms (both mechanisms are sodium dependent). Sodium ions (Na^+) are actively extruded into the intercellular space, while glucose and amino acids diffuse out of the cell, resulting in increased osmolality within the interstitial fluid.

The raised osmolality in the interstitial fluid causes water to move from the lumen through the intercellular ("tight") junction. Water from the intercellular space, together with glucose, amino acids, sodium, and other electrolytes, enter the circulation. Amino acids, such as glycine, have been shown to stimulate intestinal absorption of sodium and water; however, they are less beneficial than glucose.

The increased water uptake in the presence of glucose and glycine over that from isotonic saline solution is especially marked in the cranial part of the small intestine, where glucose absorption occurs. Thus the combination of glucose and glycine is rational for therapy. The inclusion of citrate contributes significantly to water absorption, possibly by forming an energy source for the intestinal mucosal cells. Citrate not only helps to maximize absorption of water from the gut, but also reverses acidosis. When citrate is absorbed from the intestine, it is converted by the liver into bicarbonate.

Researchers disagree as to the optimal amount of glucose in oral rehydration solutions. One view is that oral rehydration solutions should contain high levels of glucose to provide energy. The additional glucose in such solutions renders them hypertonic. The opposing viewpoint is that oral solutions should contain the maximum amount of glucose, while still maintaining isotonicity of the solution. It is probably true to say that most oral fluids are deficient in glucose. It is better to err on the side of too much glucose to ensure adequate energy to the hypoglycetic calf.

Trials using a commercially available glucose-glycine-electrolyte solution (GGES) showed that it gave clinical results at least

equivalent to those obtained using antibiotic. The inclusion of glycine in oral rehydrating solutions has also been shown under field conditions to be clinically beneficial. Oral rehydration has benefits in that it can reduce the amount of antibiotic used in treatment of diarrhea, it gives no problems of resistance, and it is relatively easy to use under field conditions.

In rotavirus diarrhea, there is damage to the mucosa, but despite this it has been shown that virus-infected animals still respond to oral rehydration. This is important in view of the difficulty in clinically differentiating between the different causative agents and the fact that in many outbreaks, more than one pathogen may be involved.

Based on the absorption rates of glucose after either oral glucose or lactose administration and calculated rates of glucose transport, the small intestine in the normal calf can absorb larger quantities of glucose and presumably amino acids than are presented by most oral therapies. Further, to achieve a necessary provision of energy substrates to the young calf, the most appropriate approach physiologically is to have a slow constant provision of nutrients from the stomach. The fatal loss of large volumes of fluid in the scouring calf results in dehydration (which may progress to shock), metabolic acidosis, and depletion of Na^+, K^+, and Cl. When the acidosis is severe, a potentially dangerous hyperkalemia may also develop owing to a tissue-buffering effect, which forces intracellular K^+ out of the cell.

Even though these calves have a total K^+ deficiency, K^+ given to a hyperkalemic patient is potentially cardiotoxic. Although some have therefore recommended potassium-free solutions, it is generally thought that these calves should receive K^+ at 15 to 20 mEq/liter in at least a portion of the fluids being given. This level can be achieved by adding concentrated potassium chloride to commercial balanced multiple electrolyte solutions.

Because they increase the rate of movement of potassium back into the cell, glucose and insulin may be valuable in management of the K^+ abnormality. Potassium should be present to restore whole-body potassium deficits as hyperkalemia is corrected. An available energy supply in the form of glucose is important for several reasons. Diarrheic calves are hypoglycemic; glucose is readily absorbed in most cases; and following absorption, glucose facilitates movement of potassium into cells, correcting the hyperkalemia. Other carbohydrate sources may be of less value. Neonatal calves do not have sucrase nor significant quantities of maltase in the brush border, so sucrose and maltose are not digested and absorbed. Their inclusion is of negligible value. Therefore glucose appears to be the carbohydrate of choice for inclusion in therapies.

Glycine has also been shown to stimulate overall intestinal absorption of sodium and water and in addition may provide a protein-sparing effect by increasing available amino nitrogen. Lipids could be considered of possible benefit because of their high energy content. Lipids are less stable, however, and little information is available on their absorbability during diarrhea.

Balanced multiple electrolyte solutions should be used to repair the multiple deficits and correct the acidosis. Although Ringer's lactate solution has been commonly used in this type of patient, questions have been raised as to whether or not the lactate can be metabolized to bicarbonate in the severely dehydrated patient with poor liver perfusion or altered liver function. It has further been suggested that the administration of lactate may exacerbate the lactic acidosis that exists in most states of shock. In one study of calves with induced diarrhea, it was concluded that lactate in solutions used for treating diarrheic calves in shock is contraindicated. Some alternatives to Ringer's lactate solution in the patient would be Ringer's solution with a concentrated sodium bicarbonate source added or commercially available multiple electrolyte solutions containing bicarbonate precursors in the form of acetate alone or with gluconate.

Generally a diarrheic calf (5 to 6% dehydrated) should receive 2 liters of oral fluid three times a day. The nutrients these oral fluids contain, however, are not included as a source of energy—they are designed solely to increase the intestinal absorption of water and other solutes (they provide less than 15% of the energy requirement of the growing calf daily). Thus additional energy sources should be provided if the calf is still diarrheic after 2 days. Although oral administration of fluids is useful in moderately dehydrated animals, it is contraindicated in dehydration due to bowel obstruction. Lectade/RESORB (Beecham) is a popular oral rehydrating fluid available for use in calves, pigs, dogs, and cats. It comprises two sachets, A and B, which must be mixed together in warm water:

Sachet A—sodium chloride, potassium dihydrogen phosphate, potassium citrate, citric acid, aminoacetic acid
Sachet B—dextrose

Lectade/RESORB is a palatable solution and is approximately isotonic.

INTRAVENOUS ROUTE

The intravenous route is used in severe cases of dehydration. It gives rapid and sure addition of fluid to the circulation and is essential in treating shock. It also "rests" in the digestive tract. The rate of infusion is important when the intravenous route is used, and great care must be exercised when using potassium-containing solutions to avoid cardiac toxicity.

Intravenous fluids must supply daily maintenance requirements (40 to 60 ml/kg/day), correct any existing fluid deficit, and replace continued losses as they occur; 75% of the estimated fluid deficit may be replaced over 24 hours and the remainder over the following 12 hours. This route should be used when the fluid loss exceeds 8% or for weak, collapsed calves and those unable to suck. A number of solutions are available; those most commonly used are:

• Isotonic saline
• Glucose saline
• Darrow's solution

Hypertonic fluids for intravenous delivery have been developed, and despite their apparent physiologic contradiction, they appear to be highly effective in shocked animals.

SUBCUTANEOUS ROUTE

The subcutaneous route can be used if the volume is not too great, but hypertonic solutions must never be given by this route because fluid is likely to accumulate at the injection site as a result of osmotic factors. The rate of uptake is inadequate to treat shock, but the route may be useful in providing a sustained absorption depot (reservoir effect) after the acute deficit has been treated by the intravenous route.

INTRAPERITONEAL ROUTE

Large volumes may be given rapidly by this route, but in hypovolemia absorption is delayed. There is always a risk of peritonitis or damage to the viscera. The route is not commonly used except for piglets and kittens.

7.9 GUIDELINES FOR FLUID THERAPY

Guidelines are as follows:

1. Calculate fluid volume required.
   a. Deficit repair:

   Body Weight ×
       Percentage Dehydration =
           Liters Required

   b. Maintenance/continuing loss requirement:

       Body Weight × 40 ml/kg

   c. Total required:

       a + b

2. Decide route of administration:
   Mild dehydration—oral
   Moderate dehydration—subcutaneous
   Severe dehydration—intravenous
3. Determine rate of infusion:
   15 ml/kg/hour
4. Choose solutions (Table 7–5).
   a. Vomiting: metabolic alkalosis + dehydration + loss of Cl⁻

   Use Saline, dextrose saline, Ringer's solution.
   b. Diarrhea: metabolic acidosis + dehydration + loss of Na^+, K^+, HCO_3^-

   Use Darrow's, Hartmann's, lactated Ringer's solution.
   c. Shock: hypovolemia, dehydration, circulatory failure, loss of osmotic pressure of blood

---

> **TABLE 7–5**
> **FLUID THERAPY**
>
> *Vomiting*
> Normal saline or Ringer's solution
> *Diarrhea*
> Lactated Ringer's/Hartmann's (Darrow's in chronic cases in which K^+ decreases)
> *Bowel obstruction*
> Lactated Ringer's (+ colloid for shock)
> *Hemorrhage*
> Whole blood; lactated Ringer's and colloid
> *Peritonitis*
> Colloid and lactated Ringer's
> *Bladder/urethra*
> N/5 saline and dextrose
>
>   Rate of Infusion
> Severe dehydration—5 ml/kg/minute for 30 minutes until condition improves; otherwise 15 ml/kg/hour (1 ml ≈ 16 drops)

Use (1) Dextran + Hartmann's, Ringer's lactate, (2) gelatin colloid or (3) intravenous hypertonic solution (saline).

CALCULATION OF FLUID REPLACEMENT VOLUME

There are two aspects of this: deficit repair and provision for maintenance and continuing losses.

Deficit Repair

The 8% rule is often used to make an initial estimate of water volume replacement needs. This is based on the premise that any animal deemed by the clinician to be sufficiently dehydrated to need parenteral fluid therapy probably has a water deficit equivalent of at least 8% of its body weight. At this level, the patient shows significant clinical signs of dehydration. This 8% rule applies to any size animal.

Body weight × 8% provides an estimate of the amount of fluid required to replace the deficit. Thus the replacement volume

---

TABLE 7–6
ESTIMATION OF FLUID REQUIREMENT

Degree of Dehydration
    Slight: loss of 2.5%–5% body weight
    Moderate: 5–10% fluid loss
    Severe: >10% fluid loss
Evaluation of Requirement
    Based on:
        Weight of animal
        Percentage dehydration
        Continual maintenance requirements
For Example
    50-kg Calf − 5% Dehydration = 50 × 0.05 = 2.5-kg Weight Loss = 2.5-liter fluid loss
    Therefore *deficit* repair = 2.5 liters
Maintenance requirement = 40 ml/kg = 2 liters (50 kg × 40 ml)
Total fluid = 4.5 liters

---

calculation for an 80-lb calf or foal judged to be a candidate for fluid therapy is:

$$80 \text{ lb} = 40 \text{ kg (approximately)} \times 0.08$$
$$= 3.2 \text{ kg} = 3.2 \text{ liters water}$$

The deficit should be corrected during 12 to 24 hours with about 25% of the 3.2 liter estimate being given in the first hour or so, or even faster in a critically ill patient. Also, depending on the animal's condition or clinical response, a portion of the initial estimate could be given orally.

Provision for Maintenance and Continuing Losses

Some patients do not take food or water orally during the 12 to 24 hours of therapy. Maintenance requirements are about 40 ml/kg/day for most patients. For a 40-kg patient, the calculation is:

$$40 \text{ kg} \times 40 = 1600 \text{ ml} \ (1.6 \text{ liters}) \text{ water}$$

This 1.6 liter estimate for maintenance plus the original 3.2 liters for replacement brings the subtotal to 4.8 liters (Table 7–6).

CONTINUING ABNORMAL LOSSES

An estimate for continuing loss should be added to the previous subtotal. This is particularly important in a young patient with acute diarrhea.

ROUTE OF ADMINISTRATION

1. 0 to 5% dehydration (showing no clinical signs)—oral therapy
2. 6 to 10% dehydration (able to stand and walk but showing clinical signs of dehydration)—initial subcutaneous administration (or intravenous) with follow-up oral administration
3. 10% dehydration (recumbent and unable to rise)—intravenous therapy may be started at once; alternatively subcutaneous infusion may be given initially and after a few hours intravenous infusion may be started

RATE OF INFUSION

Regardless of the route or type of fluid given, it is essential to warm it to body temperature. Cold fluids may cause local vasoconstriction and thus retard the rate of absorption. Cold fluids given intravenously may produce cardiac arrhythmias or even cardiac arrest. Fluids should be administered rapidly at first and then at decreasing rates until the condition has stabilized. If given too fast, however, any solution can cause circulatory overload. There is much argument about safe rates of intravenous infusion—mainly reflecting a lack of data for providing sound guidelines. A general guideline for the intravenous route is to administer fluids at the rate of 15 ml/kg/hour.

The actual rate may be expressed as milliliters per minute or drops per minute. One milliliter represents 16 drops. Thus 15 ml/kg/hour becomes 240 drops/kg/hour. Thus a 20-kg dog should receive:

$$20 \times 15 \text{ ml/hour} = 300 \text{ ml/hour}$$

$$= \frac{300}{60} = 5 \text{ ml/minute}$$

$$= 5 \times 16 \text{ drops/minute}$$

$$(1 \text{ ml} = 16 \text{ drops})$$

$$= 80 \text{ drops/minute}$$

Most proprietary fluid preparations, which although used in veterinary practice are primarily intended for human use, indicate drop flow rates of 120 to 160 drops/minute. The corresponding rate for calves is somewhat higher—about 15 ml/minute (15 ml/kg/hour)—and this can be raised to 25 ml/minute in critical cases.

For example:

70/kg calf with 10% dehydration requires

7 liters (deficit) + 2.8 liters maintenance

$$(40 \text{ ml/kg}) = 9.8 \text{ liters total}$$

Rate of infusion:

15 ml/kg/hour = 70 × 15

$$= 1 \text{ liter (approximately)}$$

1 hour = 16 ml/minute/approximately

$$= 250 \text{ drops/minute}$$

$$= 180 \text{ to } 200 \text{ (in practice)}$$

The aim in replacement therapy is to provide half the requirements in 6 hours, three quarters in 24 hours, and all within 48 hours. Thus a 70-kg calf requiring 9.8 liters receives fluid at the rate of 1 liter/hour and should be reasonably well rehydrated within a few hours.

7.10 FLUID-RESPONSIVE CONDITIONS

Different diseases cause different ion imbalances, so the fluid type for therapy depends on the animal's condition. For ex-ample, vomiting causes loss of hydrochloric acid from the stomach. The Cl^- in hydrochloric acid is normally recycled by the body during digestion, so Cl^- that is lost by vomiting should be replaced by administering a fluid rich in Cl^-. If a solution low in Cl^- is given, the patient's condition would worsen rather than improve as a result of the therapy.

ALKALOTIC STATES

The following conditions render the bovine patient alkalotic:

1. Abomasal disorders
2. Intestinal obstructions
3. Generalized gastrointestinal stasis

All of these conditions inhibit or prevent the chloride ion being reabsorbed in the small intestine after being excreted in the abomasum. This causes a buildup of serum bicarbonate ion as well as hypochloremia. Therefore to correct the alkalotic state, a solution rich in chloride is needed. Saline, dextrose saline, and Ringer's solution are used to replace the entire volume deficit in alkalotic patients. Five to 10 gallons is usually sufficient if the underlying causes can be corrected (Tables 7–7 and 7–8).

ACIDOTIC STATES

The following conditions render the bovine patient acidotic:

1. Toxic mastitis
2. Toxic metritis
3. Grain overload
4. Diarrhea
5. Pharyngitis

TREATMENT OF THE ACIDOTIC PATIENT

Hartmann's solution is suitable for treating animals suffering from metabolic acidosis owing to shock, endotoxemia, or diarrhea. The sodium lactate is converted by the liver to sodium bicarbonate, thus helping to correct the metabolic acidosis. Fortunately, in animals suffering from these conditions, the degree of acidosis is linked in a reasonably

---

TABLE 7–7
CONDITIONS IN ANIMALS REQUIRING FLUIDS

    A. *Vomiting*
       Loss of H_2O, H^+, CL^-, K^1—metabolic alkalosis
    B. *Diarrhea*
       Loss of H_2O, NA^+, CL^-, HCO_3^-, K^1—metabolic acidosis
    C. *Bowel obstruction*
       Loss of H_2O, Na^+, HCO_3^-—metabolic acidosis
    D. *Ruptured bladder*
       Buildup of H^+—metabolic acidosis (K^+)
    E. *Urethral obstruction*
       K^+—metabolic acidosis (K^+)
    F. *Burns/Hemorrhage/peritonitis*
       Hypovolemic

---

predictable way to the degree of dehydration.

For example, a 500-kg cow that is 9% dehydrated would require 45 liters of Hartmann's solution and 2.5 liters of 4.2% sodium bicarbonate solution.

It takes 120 to 125 g of sodium bicarbonate to correct the acidosis of a 1000-lb cow. The sodium bicarbonate is added to the first gallon of Ringer's solution that is given. Once the acidosis is corrected, straight Ringer's solution is used if additional fluids are needed. It usually takes approximately 1 hour to administer 5 gallons. If administration approaches 2 to 3 hours, there is a chance the sodium bicarbonate may form a calcium carbonate precipitate.

An alternative solution that does not precipitate can be made by adding 50 g of sodium bicarbonate per gallon of water. This gives an approximately isotonic solution and would be used to correct the initial acidosis, followed again by Ringer's if more fluids are needed. Three to 4 gallons of isotonic sodium bicarbonate solution corrects the acidosis in most cows.

The majority of calves requiring fluid therapy are suffering from diarrhea and as a result are acidotic. It takes 26 g or 2 tablespoons of sodium bicarbonate to correct acidosis in a calf. This is usually given as an isotonic bicarbonate solution by mixing it with one half-gallon of water (i.e., 26 g in 2400 ml = 13 g in 1200 ml. 1.3% isotonicity). Balanced (isotonic) multiple electrolyte solutions should be used in such cases to repair the NA^+ and K^+ deficits and correct the acidosis (e.g., Hartmann's, Darrow's compound, sodium lactate, Ringer's lactate).

Although Ringer's lactate solution has been commonly used in this type of patient, it is often debated whether or not the lactate will be metabolized to bicarbonate in the severely dehydrated patient with poor liver function. It has further been suggested that the administration of lactate may exacerbate the lactic acidosis that may exist in shock. Ringer's solution with sodium bicarbonate added (6.5 g/liter) may be more appropriate initially. Another area of controversy involves management of potassium

TABLE 7–8
CHOICE OF FLUIDS

  ECF Repair
    Hartmann's (lactated Ringer's)
    Ringer's acetate
    Darrow's
  ECF Acidifier
    Saline 0.9%
    Ringer's
  ECF Alkalinizer
    Hartmann's
    Ringer's acetate
    Rose's solution
    Hypertonic bicarbonate solution
    Emergency solution
  Maintenance
    Isotonic glucose saline

abnormality. Even though these animals have a total potassium deficit, hyperkalemia may exist, and some potassium should be administered. Darrow's solution contains higher potassium levels (36 mmol/liter) than most other available fluids (average 4 to 5 mmol/liter) and hence is indicated for diarrhea. It must be given slowly, however, and with care. After correction of the initial deficit, maintenance solutions in the form of amino acid vitamin and electrolyte solutions, e.g., Duphalyte, Ionalyte, or dextrose saline, may be used.

Ketosis in Dairy Cows

An occasional ketotic cow develops metabolic acidosis owing to accumulation of acetoacetic acid and beta-hydroxybutric acid. In this event, approximately 5% sodium bicarbonate is helpful in addition to the standard ketosis therapy.

Acute Mastitis or Metritis in Dairy Cows

The generalized toxemia that may result from acute or peracute coliform mastitis or from severe uterine infection may cause septic shock accompanied by lactic acidosis. These patients need balanced isotonic, alkalinizing, multiple electrolyte solutions in large volumes.

TREATMENT OF THE ALKALOTIC PATIENT

Upper Gastrointestinal Obstruction in Cows

Hypokalemic hypochloremic alkalosis frequently occurs with upper gastrointestinal tract obstructions in cattle. This disturbance is often associated with abomasal displacement, impaction torsion, and stasis as well as intussusception and cecal displacement or volvulus. These animals become alkalotic and hypochloremic because they are unable to resorb the hydrogen and chloride ions secreted into the abomasum. They also become dehydrated because water cannot enter the intestine for absorption.

Instead of an alkalinizing solution, this patient should be given a solution high in potassium and chloride. Use of acidifying agents, such as ammonium chloride or dilute hydrochloric acid, has been suggested to counteract the alkalosis, but there is not strong evidence that this is necessary. A portion of the estimated requirement of electrolyte solution can be given orally to patients after the obstruction has been corrected.

FLUID THERAPY IN HORSES

Diarrhea

Diarrhea in the foal and the adult results in disturbances similar to those in the calf except that hyperkalemia is less likely to occur. A fluid and electrolyte regimen, similar to that for the calf, should be used.

Acute Intestinal Obstruction

Because large volumes of fluid are sequestered proximal to an obstruction, these horses often develop severe dehydration (which may progress to shock) fairly quickly. Concurrent metabolic acidosis and multiple electrolyte deficits must be corrected with a balanced multiple electrolyte solution containing bicarbonate or a usable bicarbonate precursor.

Lactated Ringer's solution, Darrow's solution, or Hartmann's solution can be used. As a general rule, Hartmann's solution is the solution of choice. The volume of fluid required in a shocked horse may be as great as 60 liters. It is vitally important also to restore the circulatory plasma volume rapidly, and dextran 40 or colloidal expanders can be valuable.

7.11 SHOCK

It is not always realized that in acute hemorrhage, the reduction in blood volume is more dangerous to life than the reduction in red cells. Shock may be defined as a pathogenic state involving a sustained inadequacy or ineffectiveness of tissue perfusion. This state can lead to irreversible tissue changes and ultimately to death if corrective measures are not taken.

TYPES OF SHOCK

Different types of shock are encountered clinically, but each has the same basic pathophysiologic defect. Types of shock include the following:

1. Cardiogenic shock
2. Hypovolemic shock, e.g., hemorrhage or fluid loss as in dehydration
3. Thermal shock
4. Traumatic shock
5. Surgical shock
6. Toxicologic shock, e.g., acute arsenic poisoning
7. Neurogenic shock, e.g., deep anesthesia
8. Septic or endotoxic shock
9. Anaphylactic shock
10. Addisonian shock

"Shock" is a term used to describe a situation of cardiovascular collapse. It can arise from several causes and is usually divided into several categories. These categories are broadly connected by the underlying ultimate failure of the cardiovascular system.

Traumatic injury and blood loss, endotoxic impairment of the myocardium, and loss of ECF volume all lead to decreased perfusion of vital organs. These organs then begin to fail from lack of nutrition or accumulation of waste products. The failure of critical organ systems further compromises cardiovascular function, and thus a vicious cycle is established.

Shock is a disease state characterized by inadequate blood flow or delivery of nutrient substances required to maintain normal cellular metabolism. As a result of prolonged reduction in tissue perfusion or inadequate nutrient delivery, various abnormalities in tissue metabolism, function, and structure occur at subcellular, cellular, and eventually systemic levels. Shock is therefore attributable to mechanisms that disturb and eventually destroy cellular function.

This phenomenon is fairly well understood, and the currently accepted treatments for shock are directed toward maintaining or re-establishing organ perfusion. In the initial phase of shock, peripheral blood vessels are the first affected by catecholamines: Arterioles and venules constrict, resulting in an increase in peripheral resistance and a decrease in cardiac output. Tissue perfusion decreases, and cell hypoxia begins. The first organs affected are the kidneys, bowel, liver, lung, and skin. Usually the blood supply is diverted to the vital cerebral and cardiac areas and to the muscle mass. This selective ischemia becomes

detrimental if shock continues. As shock progresses, there is continued venous constriction, greater increase in peripheral resistance, decreased venous return, and continued reduction in cardiac output. This causes a further decrease in perfusion, resulting in tissue anoxia, acidosis, edema, and pooling of blood—the last-mentioned further reducing circulating blood volume. Abdominal viscera, lung, and skin become poorly oxygenated, and with time even organs such as the heart and brain become somewhat hypoxic along with the muscle mass. When timely pharmacologic doses of corticoids (such as Solu-Medrone V, 30 mg/kg) are employed along with other conventional therapy, there is an improvement in microcirculation. This helps reduce peripheral resistance, improves venous return, and increases cardiac output. There naturally is an improvement in blood pressure and an increase in tissue perfusion. Vital organs respond to increased perfusion when microcirculation improves and an increase in cardiac output maintains adequate blood pressure. The function of the kidneys, skin, bowel, liver, and skeletal muscle improves. Shock is not simple ECF depletion, although this may occur, e.g., in hemorrhagic shock. It is the volume of circulating ECF that is reduced and is associated with failing tissue perfusion. In the treatment of shock, the restoration of plasma volume is of prime importance.

In many cases of severe dehydration (10 to 15% fluid loss), shock is well marked. Loss of plasma proteins, collapse of the circulation, and lowered blood volume may have occurred. In such a case, the administration of fluids is of no avail in expanding the circulation because they simply pass out into the ECF owing to the decreased osmotic pressure of the plasma proteins, leaving the circulating blood volume unchanged. In this case, colloidal solutions of plasma volume expanders must be given. These solutions contain proteins of large molecular weight, such as dextran, which, owing to their size, do not pass out from the circulation, increase its osmotic pressure, and accordingly readjust the blood volume to normal. These dextran solutions can be used in conditions of severe shock, hemorrhage, and acute fluid loss. An excessive rate of transfusion, however, or overinfusion, causes dyspnea and distention of the lingual and jugular veins. A practical alternative to dextran is whole blood or serum, which can be used to the same effect.

Early treatment of shock with a suitable plasma volume expander of high molecular weight is vital because the depletion of plasma colloids underlies the reduced plasma volume. Moreover, this treatment itself facilitates the correction of any other fluid and electrolyte derangements.

A variety of drugs are currently advocated for treatment of signs associated with shock. Corticosteroids (dexamethasone, methylprednisolone), antiprostaglandins (flunixin meglumine, phenylbutazone), antibiotics, and selective vasodilator agents (prazosin, phenoxybenzamine, phenothiazines, dopamine, verapamil) have been used experimentally and clinically with the hope of reversing the effects of shock and improving survival.

Fluid therapy, however, remains the foundation of the treatment of shock. In some instances, e.g., when using adrenergic blockers to relieve vasoconstriction and improve capillary flow, adequate volume replacement is an even more essential prerequisite, to avoid hypotension.

Dopamine and dobutamine (Dobutrex, Eli Lilly) are catecholamines that may produce beneficial effects by improving peripheral blood flow and helping to maintain systemic blood pressure. Their clinical use is generally reserved for causes of shock that result from cardiac failure. Both dopamine and dobutamine have been used clinically to treat hypotension in horses. There is now renewed interest in the possibility of using hypertonic solutions of either glucose or saline in the treatment of shock, although the mode of action of hypertonic saline appears to be unusual, possibly through interaction with baroreceptors and stimulation of cardiac output.

Hypertonic sodium chloride solutions have been demonstrated to produce beneficial hemodynamic effects in hypovolemic shock. Hypertonic (2400 mOsm) sodium chloride infused into hypovolemic sheep increases arterial blood pressure and cardiac output and improves peripheral blood flow. Although hypertonic saline solution may improve hemodynamics during hypovolemic shock in horses, also the poten-

tial longterm benefits and therapeutic guidelines for their use have not yet been fully determined. They have the advantage of small volumes being required.

Dextran

Because the fundamental problem is to restore plasma volume, colloids seem especially appropriate in treating shock. They mimic the normal function of albumin, which provides an osmotic gradient to return ECF from the interstitial spaces to the plasma, thus opposing the outward flow driven by the hydrostatic pressure.

Intravascular retention of fluids is improved by provision of artificial colloids to mimic the effect of albumin. Albumin itself is expensive and may have adverse effects on clotting, immune globulins, and respiratory function in shock.

The most extensively used artificial colloids have been dextran, gelatin, and hydroxyethyl starch. Dextran 70 (molecular weight 70,000) is usually given as a 6% solution in isotonic saline and pulls some additional fluid from the interstitial space. Dextran 40 (10% in isotonic saline) pulls in much more fluid from the interstitial fluid from the interstitial space but is half excreted in 6 hours and totally gone in 24 hours. Both of the dextrans can decrease blood viscosity and decrease platelet aggregation. The lower molecular weight dextran has a shorter half-life, only 3.5 hours compared with 72 hours for dextran 70. The dextrans cause a shift of body fluid from the intracellular compartment to the extracellular compartment as part of their mechanisms of blood volume expansion.

Dextran 40 is infused at a rate of 10 to 20 ml/kg in 24 hours along with another fluid, such as Ringer's lactate, at a similar rate. This avoids any tissue dehydration effect resulting from the hypertonicity of dextran. Its useful properties include reducing blood viscosity and preventing coagulation and venous thrombosis.

The main problems with dextran 40 are a tendency to impede clotting and blood matching and occasionally to cause allergy. The interference with clotting occurs at doses exceeding 20% of blood volume (20 ml/kg) and also arises with dextran 70 and hydroxyethyl starch. Bleeding may resume within 30 to 90 minutes of excessive infusion of these colloids. The other alternative is hydroxylethyl starch. This substance is composed of polymerized starch molecules. It has been used in human medicine as volume replacement for cases of hypovolemic shock. It compares favorably with albumin and is much less expensive.

Gelatin Polypeptide Colloidal Infusion (Haemaccel, Hoechst)

This is a plasma substitute that is isotonic, manufactured from degraded gelatin and containing sodium, potassium, calcium, sulfate and phosphate ions, and water. It is less expensive than dextran and is suitable for use alone because it is isotonic and contains sufficient electrolyte. It should be infused at a rate determined by the condition of the patient, and it is recommended that the rate not exceed 20 ml/kg every 12 hours.

7.12 ENDOTOXIC SHOCK (SEE ALSO SECTION ON EQUINE COLIC IN CHAPTER 16.)

Because the effects of endotoxins, or endotoxemia, are devastating, treatment methods are extensive and primarily aimed at the blood vascular system: large volumes of fluids to maintain adequate blood flow, glucocorticoids for cellular integrity and to raise blood glucose, and antiprostaglandins (e.g., Flunikin) to reduce the many effects of the prostaglandin cascade. Broad-spectrum antibiotics or antibiotic combinations are used to control the primary infection. Treatment must be administered early before a definitive diagnosis. No one drug is sufficient to control all the effects of endotoxins. Proper combinations of therapy, however, have greatly reduced the mortality rate following gram-negative septicemia. Antibiotics are essential for treating all forms of shock and are used to prevent or minimize the effects of invading organisms from a deteriorating or compromised intestinal barrier. Endotoxins are large molecular weight lipopolysaccharides (LPS) derived from gram negative bacteria.

To be toxic, endotoxins must gain access to the circulation. They are essentially nontoxic when given orally to an animal with a normal gastrointestinal mucosa, although large oral doses may cause diarrhea. Bile appears to help prevent the absorption of endotoxin from the normal gastrointestinal tract. Endotoxins can be absorbed by aerosol or through the gastrointestinal tract if the organisms are invasive (such as *E. coli*) or if the mucosa is compromised (such as with intestinal infarction).

The effects of endotoxin are varied and often profound. The severity of these changes are dose and rate dependent. Surprisingly endotoxins appear to have relatively little direct toxic effect; most of the severe changes are indirect, associated with cascades of biological processes initiated by endotoxin. (Horses are particularly susceptible to the effects of endotoxin.)

Endotoxins alter membranes in a variety of cell types and can trigger the alternate complement pathway. These effects may trigger intravascular coagulation. Microcirculatory disturbances include constriction of arterioles, dilation of venules, loss of erythrocyte plasticity, sticking and aggregation of granulocytes and thrombocytes to endothelium and each other, release of thromboxane A_2 from platelets, and increased permeability (loss of integrity) of capillary and venule walls.

The presence of endotoxin in the circulation initiates a series of circulatory, hormonal, hematologic, and metabolic changes that signal the need for therapy. Endotoxemia results in damage to the vascular endothelium and causes endothelial cells to separate from each and to slough from the underlying basal lamina. When the cell membranes are damaged, the fatty acid components of the phospholipids are cleaved by specific phospholipase enzymes. One of the fatty acids, arachidonic acid, serves as the substrate for at least two enzyme systems: cyclooxygenase and lipoxygenase. Cyclooxygenase converts arachidonic acid to the unstable endoperoxide intermediates, which may be modified further to form the classic prostaglandins, with effects on the local circulation, pain receptors, and thermoregulatory center (prostacyclin, thromboxane).

Although these specific arachidonic acid metabolites have different effects on different vascular beds in different species, generally prostaglandin E_2 is associated with vasodilation, fever, and a lowered pain threshold; prostaglandin I_2 causes vasodilation and inhibits platelet aggregation; prostaglandin F_2 alpha causes vasoconstriction; and thromboxane A_2 mediates intense vasoconstriction. Thromboxane B_2 concentrations increase early in the course of shock, in association with the initial drop in blood pressure, whereas 6-keto-prostaglandin F_1 alpha concentrations increase later, in association with terminal hypotension. Treatment using indomethacin or aspirin blocks the elevation in prostaglandin E and prostaglandin F_2 alpha. Treatment with flunixin meglumine blocks the increase in thromboxane B_2 and 6-keto-prostaglandin F_1 alpha.

The early cyclooxygenase-dependent effects of endotoxin (dyspnea, tachypnea, pulmonary hypertension) are related to the abrupt generation of the vasoconstrictive metabolite, thromboxane. Other characteristic responses to endotoxin (abdominal pain, systemic hypotension, increased capillary refill time) correlate with increases in plasma concentrations of prostacyclin metabolites. The involvement of arachidonic acid metabolism in clinical cases of intestinal ischemia in horses has been demonstrated with reported increases in plasma phospholipase activity in clinical cases of colic and substantially higher activity in horses that failed to survive.

PROSTAGLANDINS

Prostaglandins are endogenously secreted products of the arachidonic cascade. They have a variety of actions in the body, depending on the location. They are vasodilatory in some vascular beds and cause vasoconstriction in other areas. Therefore it is not surprising that both administration of specific prostaglandins and administration of prostaglandin synthesis blockers have been found to be beneficial in shock treatment.

Two of the prostaglandins, E_1 and I_2, have some of the same beneficial effects as corticosteroids, including improved cardiac output and increased membrane stability. In addition, prostaglandin E_1, may reduce platelet aggregation and preserve cell energy stores. One study has shown that prostaglandin E_1-treated dogs survived experimental hemorrhagic shock much longer than those treated with corticosteroids. Treatment with aspirin or indomethacin has also improved survival in several shock models. Both of these nonsteroidal anti-inflammatory drugs (NSAIDs) block prostaglandin and thromboxane synthesis or release. They also have other properties, including inhibiting the release of 5-hydroxytryptamine from platelets.

Considerable interest and research activity have been focused on the importance of the various metabolites of arachidonic acid as important mediators of shock. Studies using experimentally produced endotoxic shock in horses and ponies have demonstrated that the cyclooxygenase inhibitors phenylbutazone and flunixin meglumine produce anti-inflammatory and analgesic actions while preventing the rise of prostaglandin I_1, thromboxane A_2, and thromboxane B_2.

The administration of low-dose flunixin meglumine to ponies normalizes cardiopulmonary response, minimizes the hematologic and blood biochemical changes, and prolongs survival after endotoxin administration.

The arachidonic acid cascade results in the production of prostaglandins, thromboxanes, and other potential mediators of inflammation. Inflammatory stimuli activate phospholipases, which result in the eventual release of arachidonic acid from phospholipids in cell membranes. In the cascade, arachidonic acid can be considered to have three major fates:

1. The lipoxygenase pathway may produce leukotrienes and monohydroxy metabolites of arachidonic acid
2. Chemotactic lipids may be produced by way of the action of activated oxygen species or ultraviolet light
3. The prostaglandins and thromboxanes may be produced

Steroids may reduce the yield of all products of arachidonic acid. In contradistinction, the nonsteroidal agents act at the level of cyclooxygenase and reduce production of the thromboxanes and prostaglandins. After therapy with nonsteroidal agents, lipoxygenase products and chemotactic lipids may be unaffected or increased.

7.13 NONSTEROIDAL ANTI-INFLAMMATORY DRUGS

NSAIDs are a diverse group of pharmacologic agents that share certain actions. All of these agents reduce fever, reduce inflammation, and act as analgesics. All are known to cause inhibition of cyclooxygenase, resulting in decreased prostaglandin production. The drugs share common toxicities secondary to prostaglandin blockade: gastric and intestinal ulceration, disturbance of platelet function, prolongation of gestation, and renal damage. The major differences between these drugs are the severity of their toxic side effects and their relative abilities to act as antipyretics, anti-inflammatory agents, and analgesics. The reasons for the differences are poorly understood but probably result from differing actions on other pathways and on cellular sites of action.

In treatment of endotoxic shock, it has been demonstrated experimentally that animals given low-dose flunixin meglumine 24 hours after being given endotoxins intravenously had longer mean survival time and less severe blood changes than untreated animals or those given dexamethasone or prednisolone at therapeutic dosage. Flunixin by virtue of this antiprostaglandin effect assists in the maintenance of cellular integrity and blood flow to vital organs. Neither high-dose corticosteroids nor flunixin alone is suitable for treating endotoxic shock, but both are useful in combination with supportive therapy. Flunixin minimizes hemoconcentration, reduces plasma loss, and maintains normal blood volume in animals given endotoxin.

The overall benefits of cyclooxygenase inhibitors in shock, however, remain questionable, particularly because, similar to corticosteroids, they must be administered before or during the early stages of shock. Their ability to shunt arachidonic metabolism toward lipoxygenase metabolites (leukotrienes) and evidence supporting the role of leukotrienes as the major mediators of shock are of major concern at present.

Macrophages and other phagocytic cells produce a polypeptide called interleukin-1 in response to endotoxins. Interleukin-1, a polypeptide produced mainly by phagocytic cells, was discovered to be a mediator of the host's response to infection and inflammation. It is responsible for inducing prostaglandin synthesis, stimulating B and T lymphocytes, stimulating fibroblast proliferation for wound healing, causing neutrophilia, and inducing the production of acute-phase proteins. The stimulation of prostaglandin synthesis, in turn, causes clinical signs, such as fever and muscle and joint soreness. Prostaglandin inhibitors therefore prevent these signs but not the signs that involve interleukin-1 directly, such as sleepiness, neutrophilia, lymphocyte activation, and fibroblast proliferation.

Conflicting results have been obtained concerning the effects of NSAIDs on the acute decrease in blood pressure and increase in portal pressure that occur during canine endotoxemia. Some studies indicated that these events were blocked or ameliorated, whereas in other studies, no such effects were noted. The conflicting evidence indicates that other mediators as well as prostaglandins are probably responsible for the acute cardiovascular changes. Numerous studies have confirmed that NSAIDs block the secondary decrease in blood pressure that occurs from endotoxemia. Because prostacyclin is a vasodilatory prostaglandin, this effect is presumed to be caused by blockage of prostacyclin production. Other effects of treatment noted in some studies were decreased hemoconcentration, prevention of metabolic acidosis, and increased cardiac output.

STEROIDS

Steroids produce little effect on normal vascular tone, but in shock, in which vascular resistance is increased by abnormal vasoconstriction, they actively play a part. Inhibition of vasoconstriction along with volume replacement helps perfusion and provides for cellular protection. Steroids provide direct protection to cellular membranes, preventing cellular edema, mitochondrial damage, and lysosomal membrane rupture. Incorporation of steroids into the therapeutic regimen is important not only to survival, but also to preservation of organs such as the kidney, intestinal lining, and myocardium, which are easily damaged during shock.

...K THERAPY	Dose (mg/kg)	Duration of Action (hours)
...methasone in	5–10	10–15
	15–30	12–24
	15–30	12–24
	15–30	12–24
Hya... ...te	150	6–8

Corticosteroids have been used clinically to treat shock in all animals for more than 30 years, despite a lack of clear evidence of their effectiveness. Studies in humans, dogs, and ponies have demonstrated that corticosteroids antagonize the hemodynamic, hematologic, and blood biochemical changes induced by *E. coli* endotoxin. These beneficial effects are attributed to stabilization of lysosomal membranes; inhibition of phospholipase A_2, thereby inhibiting the formation of arachidonic acid metabolites; inhibition of complement-induced granulocyte aggregation; improved myocardial performance; a right shift in the oxygen-hemoglobin dissociation curve; and improved cellular metabolism.

The most important finding from experimental studies and clinical experience, however, has been that if a beneficial effect is desired, corticosteroids must be used in pharmacologic doses (15 to 30 mg/kg body weight methylprednisolone or prednisolone sodium succinate; 5 to 10 mg/kg body weight dexamethasone) and be administered before, or as early as possible after, the onset of shock. Corticosteroids provide short-term improvement and appear to prolong survival. These potential benefits must be considered carefully against studies in mature horses and ponies demonstrating suppression of adrenal function, delayed healing, and increased tendency to bacterial infections and a potentiation of biogenetic amines in the horse's limbs predisposing to laminitis.

The dose of steroid required to treat shock must be pharmacologically active and not just aimed at "replacement therapy" for a failing adrenal gland. Massive pharmacologic doses have proved to be optimal in treating shock.

The route of administration is also an important consideration. For therapy to be effective, large doses must be given for a relatively short period of time, eliminating the intramuscular, intraperitoneal, and subcutaneous routes from consideration. The ester to which the steroid analog is attached plays an important role. A water-soluble ester should be used for this purpose and the phosphate and succinate esters. Of the two, the succinate ester has proved superior because of its rapid uptake into the cellular compartment (Table 7–9).

INTENSIVE SHORT-TERM SHOCK THERAPY

The effects of glucocorticoids in all forms of shock are still controversial; however, some evidence suggests that early treatment (probably less than 4 hours postinduction in dogs) may lead to increased survival, particularly in hemorrhagic and septic shock. The nature of the formulation (particularly the ester) may affect the speed of cellular entry of glucocorticoids during shock.

Glucocorticoids improve hemodynamics and enhance survival in canine models of endotoxic and hemorrhagic shock. Therapy for shock, however, should also include aggressive fluid therapy. Suspected endotoxic shock should be treated with bactericidal broad-spectrum antibiotics, with or without glucocorticoids.

Corticosteroids have been incorporated into the successful treatment of shock for more than a decade. Several well-designed studies have shown increased survival rates with steroid use. The mechanism of action in shock therapy has often been elusive.

Corticosteroids, if administered before or immediately after exposure to endotoxin, act on macrophages to block production of interleukin-1. NSAIDs (antiprostaglandin) have no effect on interleukin-1 production. Corticosteroids have many of the same effects as antiprostaglandins, and they minimize lymphocyte activation, fibroblast proliferation, and degree of neutrophilia. In so doing, corticosteroids may help prevent endotoxic shock. They also, however, hinder clearance of bacteria, antibody production, and healing, which may be undesirable effects. Because NSAIDs do not hinder bacterial clearance, they may be indicated instead of corticosteroids in all but the most life-threatening situations.

7.14 MISCELLANEOUS APPROACHES FOR SHOCK THERAPY

These agents are currently only of experimental interest in treatment of shock in animals. These include calcium entry blockers, ACE inhibitors, hypertonic saline, ionophores, DMSO, and naloxone.

CALCIUM CHANNEL BLOCKERS

Calcium channel blockers include verapamil, nifedipine, and diltiazem. They are used for anginal disease in man where they induce vasodilation. These drugs act to inhibit the influx of calcium into the cell through the "slow channels." They are most recognized for their beneficial effect on the cardiovascular system. They act to depress cardiac contractility and heart rate and protect the myocardium from ischemic damage.

ACE INHIBITORS

CAPTOPRIL

Captopril is an inhibitor of angiotensin II formation. Because angiotensin II is a potent vasoconstrictor, it has been postulated that administration of captopril may be beneficial in shock.

HYPERTONIC SALINE

This produces hemodynamic effects in hypovolemic shock. Hypertonic, 2400 mOsm, increases arterial blood pressure, cardiac output and peripheral blood flow. It improves hemodynamics during hypovolemia. Usually it possesses a tonicity of 8 to 9 times that of plasma. (7.5% solution is commonly used.) This is given over 8 to 10 minutes. It can be given rapidly and improves tissue perfusion and urine production. Hypertonic saline has been reported to be of great benefit in stock. It is vaguely mediated.

IONOPHORES

Ionophores include monensin, narasin, lasalocid, maduramycin, and salinomycin. These compounds act by increasing intracellular calcium content and have been shown to increase coronary blood flow, myocardial contractility, cardiac output, and blood pressure. These possess vasodilatory activity. Monensin-treated dogs subjected to endotoxic shock showed dose-dependent increases in these parameters.

Monensin appears to have a selective coronary vasodilatory action. Some of the pharmacologic effects of monensin may be due to other mechanisms, such as release of endogenous catecholamines.

DMSO (DIMETHYL SULFOXIDE)

This possesses a variety of vasodilatory actions. DMSO is one of a class of compounds called the free-radical scavengers. Free radicals are possible mediators of cellular damage following ischemia. One source of these free radicals is the enzyme xanthine oxidase.

NALOXONE (OPIOID ANTAGONIST)

As a specific opiate antagonist, it acts by blocking the activity of endogenous endorphins. These endorphins are thought to cause some of the hypotension associated with shock. Administration of naloxone has been shown experimentally to reverse hypovolemic shock in dogs. It also improves survival in endotoxic shock models. There has been some controversy concerning the exact mechanism of naloxone used in such situations, and several authors have suggested that naloxone effects may be the result of a mechanism unrelated to its opiate antagonism. It has been shown that administration of both naloxone and cyproheptadine, an antiserotonin drug, is beneficial in traumatic shock. Both treatments resulted in decreased pulmonary platelet trapping and decreased platelet agreggability following traumatic shock. Only naloxone, however, prevents the hypotension associated with traumatic shock. Numerous experiments testify to this mechanism of action.

ADRENOCEPTOR AGENTS

These are also of use in the collapse of the circulation. Vasodilator drugs, such as prazosin (cefentolamine), may be helpful in increasing blood flow to vital organs. (Hypertonic saline and milrinone will also improve cardio-function.)

APPENDIX 7–1

GRAM CONCENTRATION	
NaCl	17 mEq/g
NaHCO$_3$	12 mEq/g
KCl/NaCl	15.5 mEq/g
KCl	14 mEq/g

ISOTONIC CONCENTRATION OF COMMON SALTS	
NaCl	9 g/liter
NaHCO$_3$	13 g/liter
KCl/NaCl	10 g/liter
Dextrose	50 g/liter

8

TREATMENT OF POISONING

8.1 Introduction
8.2 Preventing Further Absorption
8.3 Hastening Elimination
8.4 Supportive Therapy
8.5 Large Animal Intoxications
8.6 Small Animal Intoxications
8.7 General Therapy of Common Toxicoses

8.1 INTRODUCTION

Poisoning is a frequently encountered problem for the veterinarian and often one of the most difficult to manage. The veterinarian is frequently contacted by telephone concerning a suspected case of poisoning. The instructions given at this time are important to subsequent therapeutic success. The owner should be instructed to protect the animal, keep it warm, and avoid any other stress. It may be necessary to muzzle the animal. If exposure is believed to be topical, the animal's skin or eyes should be washed with large volumes of water. It may occasionally be useful for the client to induce vomiting in the animal. Vomiting must not be encouraged, however, if the suspected poison causes central nervous system depression or is a corrosive agent. Emetic techniques and preparations available to the layman include hydrogen peroxide, salt and water, and mustard and water. Nothing should be administered by mouth if the animal is severely depressed, unconscious, or convulsing. The owner should be instructed to bring the animal without delay to the hospital and to bring along any materials that may assist in the identification of the alleged intoxicant, e.g., vomitus, suspected materials, or their containers.

On initial presentation, adequate physiologic functioning must be ensured immediately. Antidotal measures are useless if the animal has lost one or all of the vital functions. A brief examination should be performed emphasizing those areas most likely to give clues to the toxicologic diagnosis. These include vital signs, eyes and mouth, skin, abdomen, and nervous system. Careful evaluation of vital signs (blood pressure, pulse, respirations, and temperature) is essential in all toxicologic emergencies.

First, the airway should be cleared of vomitus or any other obstruction and an oral airway or endotracheal tube inserted if needed. Adequacy of breathing can be assessed by observation and by measuring arterial blood gases. Circulation should be assessed by measurement of pulse rate, blood pressure, urinary output, and evaluation of peripheral perfusion. Every patient with altered mental status should receive fluids with concentrated dextrose. Patients comatose from hypoglycemia are rapidly and irreversibly losing brain cells.

Stabilization of the vital signs is the first priority: establishment of a patent airway, artificial respiration, cardiotherapy, and control of external hemorrhage, if necessary. Once stabilization has occurred, therapeutic measures can be instigated. If the poison is known, an antidote may be available. If unknown, general symptomatic therapy may be instituted. To estimate the severity of poisoning, it is important to estimate the time since ingestion.

BASIC CONCEPTS OF TREATMENT

The initial management of a patient with coma, seizures, or otherwise altered mental status should follow a standard approach regardless of the poison involved. Attempting to make a specific toxicologic diagnosis delays the application of supportive measures that form the basis of poisoning treatment. Because few specific "antidotes" exist, the treatment of toxicosis must be based first on the following principles:

1. Remove the source of poison and prevent further exposure
2. Delay further absorption
3. Hasten elimination of absorbed poison
4. Supportive therapy
5. Application of specific antidotes

When initiating therapy, the clinician should first treat the signs shown by the animal. It is important to stress that as little time as possible should be lost before beginning treatment (Table 8–1). First, as mentioned, the animal must be stabilized physiologically. The stabilized animal may then be treated in the following steps:

1. Preventing the animal from absorbing additional poison is a priority. Removal of the animal from the affected environment is the first step to prevent further absorption. This may also entail washing the skin to remove the toxicant. Protective clothing such as rubber gloves or aprons may be necessary for the handler to prevent contamination. Wash gently but thoroughly with toilet soap or detergent. Rinse with a large quantity of lukewarm water. Dry thoroughly and keep

TABLE 8–1
EARLY MANAGEMENT

Emetic
↓
Wash or Inactivator (Antidote)
↓
Saline Laxative
↓
Monitor Closely
↓
Prevent Further Access

warm. Decontamination involves removing toxins from the skin or gastrointestinal tract.

2. Judicious use of absorbents and cathartics aids the prevention of further absorption of toxic material from the gastrointestinal tract. Absorption may also be retarded by precipitation, inactivation, neutralization, oxidation, and chelation. Several of these effects may be accomplished by a carefully chosen, locally acting chemical antidote.

3. In ruminants, a rumenotomy may be considered because the rumen holds a large reservoir from which toxicants may be absorbed.

4. Use antidotes if available for specific or supportive therapy.

8.2 PREVENTING FURTHER ABSORPTION

EMETICS

To eliminate remaining poison or to prevent further absorption, emesis may be induced. Emesis must be instituted only when the animal is neither comatose nor convulsing. It is also contraindicated when ingestion of corrosive acids and alkalis is suspected because in such cases emesis would cause additional damage to the esophagus and oral cavity (Table 8–2).

Central or locally acting emetics can be used. If the airway is protected by a gag reflex, there is no ulceration of mucous membranes, and the patient is not having seizures, emesis can be induced.

Apomorphine is a useful central emetic agent. A dose of 0.04 mg/kg intravenously or 0.08 mg/kg subcutaneously is given. It can cause respiratory depression, however, and is contraindicated in animals in which additional central nervous system depression must be avoided.

Xylazine (0.4–1.0 mg/kg intramuscularly) is an effective, safe emetic for cats. Syrup of ipecac is another general emetic agent. It combines mainly a gastric irritant effect with some central stimulation. The dose for small animals is 1 to 2 ml/kg, repeated after 15 minutes if necessary. It is contraindicated in the presence of activated charcoal.

Local agents, such as copper sulfate, table salt, mustard, or hydrogen peroxide, may be used with varying effect.

Emetics are administered as follows:

1. Local emetics
   Saturated salt solution, 10 to 100 ml
   1% Copper sulfate solution, 10 to 60 ml (dog), 3 to 20 ml (cat)
   Washing soda crystals, 1 to 2 g

TABLE 8–2
ADVANCED MANAGEMENT

EMERGENCY ACTION
Anticonvulsant
↓
Respiratory Stimulant/Oxygen
↓
Establish Airway Patency
↓
Combat Shock
IDENTIFY POISON
Give Antidote
↓
Wash
PREVENT ABSORPTION
Gastric Lavage
↓
Inactivator
↓
Saline Laxative
↓
Diuretic
SUPPORTIVE THERAPY
Fluids
↓
Corticosteroids
↓
Guard Body Temperature
PREVENT FURTHER ACCESS

TABLE 8–3
GASTRIC LAVAGE

Use instead of emesis especially if
    depressed, convulsive, or unconscious
Pass endotracheal tube and inflate cuff
Lubricate stomach tube, pass it, and
    confirm
Raise tube end, run in lavage fluid
Tilt patient, so mouth below stomach
Aspirate fluid/lower tube so stomach
    contents flow out
Repeat until contents clear (5 to 15 flushes)
On final occasion, leave an inactivator/
    saline laxative in stomach

---

2. Central emetics
    Apomorphine hydrochloride, 0.08
    mg/kg, s.c. (not in cats)
    Xylazine, 0.4–1.0 mg/kg, intravenously,
    intramuscularly, or subcutaneously
    Syrup of ipecac, 1 to 2 ml/kg (not to ex-
    ceed 15 ml)

GASTRIC LAVAGE

This is a method of emptying the stomach
in patients who are anesthetized or sedated
(Table 8–3). It is a reliable technique when
undertaken within about 2 hours of ingestion of a poison. The animal should be unconscious or under light anesthesia. An endotracheal tube should be passed and the
cuff inflated. The patient is best placed on a
tilted table with the mouth below stomach
level. A stomach tube is passed, and 5 to 10
ml of water/kg body weight is then flushed
in and withdrawn using an aspirator bulb
or 50-ml syringe. The flushing process is repeated 10 to 15 times until the aspirate is
clear. Activated charcoal in the solution enhances the effectiveness of the washing-out
technique. Low pressure should be used at
all times to avoid forcing the stomach contents through the pylorus and into the duodenum.

PRECIPITANTS AND ASTRINGENTS

Table 8–4 summarizes some commonly
used precipitants. Tannic acid is a useful
general antidote. It can be given in the form
of strong tea, and it precipitates many alkaloids, including strychnine (and lead).
Milk and egg whites neutralize many poisons, such as heavy metals, and are useful
general antidotes owing to their demulcent
properties. Also, mixtures of sugar and
milk, eggs, and oatmeal gruel are useful.
For corrosive acids, lime water, milk of
magnesia, chalk, and baking powder are
useful. For caustic alkalis, vinegar (5%
acetic acid), lemon juice, citric acid (5 to
10%), or tartaric acid (5 to 10%) might be
considered. Potassium permanganate is a
useful local oxidizing agent in the gut for
lavage or for oral administration in alkaloid
poisoning.

LOCALLY ACTING GUT ANTIDOTES

Activated Charcoal

Activated charcoal is one of the best adsorbing agents available. It can be used with
emetic or gastric lavage techniques, and although it does not detoxify agents, it adsorbs them and makes them unavailable for
absorption. It is an excellent adsorbent for
strychnine, other alkaloids, and ethylene
glycol. It is administered as a slurry through
a stomach tube using either a funnel or a
large syringe. A cathartic of sodium sulfate
should be given simultaneously or as a follow-up after about 30 minutes. The importance of including a saline cathartic cannot
be overemphasized. Activated charcoal
given alone becomes stationary in the gas-

TABLE 8–4
INACTIVATORS AND ANTIDOTES

Adsorbents
    Activated charcoal; make slurry (1 g/5
        ml water), give 5 g/kg body weight
Precipitant
    Tannic acid; make strong tea, give
        15 ml/kg
Oxidizing agent
    Potassium permanganate
Precipitant/demulcent
    Mix milk and egg white
Acids or alkalis to neutralize ingested
    poisons

---

trointestinal tract, releasing its adsorbed toxin, which may subsequently be absorbed by the mucosa again to produce toxicosis. The saline cathartic promotes passage of the activated charcoal and adsorbed toxin by way of the feces.

Activated charcoal in combination with a saline purge is a useful treatment for a variety of poisonings, ranging from pesticide poisonings to rumen overload or to pharmaceutical toxicity. Activated charcoal absorbs a chemical or toxin and facilitates its excretion by way of the feces. It can be used when:

1. An animal ingests organic poisons or chemicals
2. Bacterial toxins are present or released in the gastrointestinal tract
3. Enterohepatic circulation of metabolized toxicants has occurred

It adsorbs pesticides, environmental hydrocarbons, pharmaceutical agents, mycotoxins, phytotoxins, bacterial toxins, feed additives, and antibacterials.

When treating grain overload (rumen acidosis), sodium bicarbonate 2 g/kg, mixed in a slurry with the activated charcoal is most effective.

Classes of poisons for which activated charcoal can be useful include anthelmintics, antifreeze (ethylene glycol), antimicrobials, feed additives, fungicides, herbicides, household chemicals, insecticides, molluscacides, parasiticides, rodenticides, bacterial toxins, plant alkaloids, rumen overload, hydrocarbons (PCB, PBB), pharmaceuticals, mycotoxins, and endotoxins. Activated charcoal is ineffective against caustic materials, fertilizers, heavy metal salts, iodides, nitrate, nitrite, sodium chloride, chlorate, ethanol and methanol.

Guidelines for Use

The recommended dose of activated charcoal for all species of animals is 1 to 3 g/kg body weight. In most instances, a saline cathartic, such as sodium or magnesium sulfate, should be added at a dose of 1 g/kg. The mixture should be made into a slurry with water and given by drench or stomach tube. Tablets, boluses, and capsules of activated charcoal are either less effective than slurries or not effective at all. Other types of charcoal, such as cooking briquettes, are ineffective and may contain impurities.

Sorbitol is an equally effective cathartic for use with activated charcoal in monogastric animals; however, it may not be advisable to use it in ruminants. Because it is a sugar, it could cause microfloral changes in ruminants that result in the release of bacterial toxins. For this reason, use either sodium or magnesium sulfate with activated charcoal when treating ruminants. An important exception is treatment of grain overload (ruminal acidosis). In these cases, sodium bicarbonate at about 2 g/kg mixed in a slurry with the activated charcoal is most effective. Because animals suffering from rumen overload usually already have a diarrhea, a saline cathartic is probably not necessary.

Activated charcoal is regaining favor as a treatment for poisonings and has been termed the most active single agent for the emergency treatment of oral drug poisoning in human medicine. The microporous structure of activated charcoal provides a large adsorptive surface onto which a variety of compounds are readily and rapidly adsorbed. Exceptions include caustic alkalis or mineral acids and alcohols. Although adsorption kinetics are reversible, adsorption occurs only when inadequate amounts of charcoal are present, i.e., when the charcoal-to-toxic compound ratio is slow.

Charcoal is best administered as soon as possible after ingestion of a poison but has been effective even 24 hours after poison ingestion. As a result of charcoal's adsorption of a compound in the gastrointestinal tract, some of the already absorbed compound passively diffuses back into the tract because of the lowered concentration of free compound present in the tract. This effect represents a form of gastrointestinal dialysis and has proved useful for treating toxicity of a number of absorbed toxic compounds.

Digoxin clearance in normal human subjects has been increased by 47% during charcoal treatment and by 200% in patients with renal failure. Because cardiac glycosides undergo enterohepatic recirculation, the presence of charcoal in the intestinal tract reduces reabsorption significantly.

Multiple oral doses are especially effective in accelerating rate of elimination. Charcoal may have value in terminating effects of oral sustained-release drugs.

Adverse effects of charcoal therapy are rare and are primarily related to aspiration of the charcoal. Charcoal adsorbs antidote compounds, rendering them ineffective, just as it adsorbs toxic substances.

A new petroleum-based activated charcoal is being marketed for human and veterinary use. This activated charcoal, as a result of a special manufacturing process, has 2 to 3.6 times greater adsorptive capacity than the conventional wood-based activated charcoal. The new charcoal preparations form a suspension in water more readily than the conventional charcoals.

Because it is desirable to make the initial dose of activated charcoal as large as possible, ideally at least 10 times the estimated amount of ingested poison, the new charcoal has a dose size advantage. Expense of the new charcoal is about twice that of conventional charcoal products. It is important to note that adsorptive capacity at least equivalent to the USP Pharmacopeia form should be used. Good quality charcoals adsorb 100 to 1000 mg of a drug per gram of charcoal.

In addition to effectiveness in adsorption of chemical poisons, activated charcoal can adsorb bacterial toxins. It has proved effective in combination with sodium bicarbonate for treatment of endotoxic shock associated with rumen autointoxication in cattle.

Activated charcoal can be incorporated into a "universal antidote" and can be prepared as follows:

10 g activated charcoal
5 g magnesium oxide
5 g kaolin
5 g tannic acid
(Make into slurry with water.)

8.3 HASTENING ELIMINATION

CATHARTICS AND LAXATIVES

Administration of a cathartic agent should hasten removal of toxins from the gastrointestinal tract and reduce absorption. Sodium sulfate is the preferred cathartic agent if heart failure is not present. Sodium sulfate can be used for evacuation of the bowel and is more effective and less toxic than magnesium sulfate, which could cause central nervous system depression. The dose of sodium sulfate is 1 g/kg. Mineral oil (liquid petrolatum) is inert and unlikely to be absorbed. Oil should be followed by a saline cathartic in 30 to 40 minutes. Enemas of warm water and soap can be useful to hasten elimination of toxicants from the gastrointestinal tract.

A saline laxative can be given if several hours have elapsed since a poison has been ingested. Make up 3.2% solution of sodium sulfate in water. Give 30 to 120 ml to dogs and 15 to 45 ml to cats (to be given after emesis or gastric lavage). Do not use an oily laxative or purgative. Alternatively, make up 4% solution of magnesium sulfate (isotonic) in water. Administer by drench or preferably by stomach tube, 100 to 200 ml to dogs and 25 to 100 ml to cats.

Absorbed toxicant can be eliminated in two main ways: by way of the kidneys or by way of the liver. Generally renal elimination is the most common. Renal excretion can be manipulated in many instances by alteration of the pH or the use of diuretics. The use of diuretics to enhance urinary excretion of substances requires adequate renal function and hydration of the animal. It is necessary to monitor urinary output, and it may be necessary to rehydrate the animal during the course of the treatment. The diuretics of choice are mannitol or furosemide at dosage rates of 1 g/kg/hour and 2 mg/kg.

Alteration of urinary pH to increase the excretion of toxicants relies on the fact that ionized compounds do not easily pass cell membranes and are not reabsorbed from the renal tubules. Acidic compounds, such as aspirin or barbiturates, remain ionized in an acidic urine. Ammonium chloride can be used to acidify urine.

Peritoneal dialysis is indicated in small animals but is obviously difficult in large animals. The procedure is time-consuming but effective. It requires the use of two separate solutions to be exchanged every 30 to 60 minutes. Examples of the solutions to be used are:

1. 5% dextrose in 0.45% sodium chloride with 15 mmol/liter of potassium as potassium chloride
2. 5% dextrose in water with 44.6 mmol/liter of bicarbonate and 15 mmol/liter of potassium added

The method is to infuse 10 to 70 ml/kg of solution no. 1 into the peritoneal cavity, wait 30 to 60 minutes, withdraw the first solution, and infuse the same quantities of solution no. 2 and wait the same period of time.

The cycle is maintained until normal renal function is restored or 12 to 24 hours. This method is indicated in cases of anuria or impaired renal function. The pH of the solution may be altered to keep the toxicant in an ionized state. The objective is to set up an osmotic gradient into the dialyzing solution. Potassium sodium and chloride ions are added to prevent their loss by the patient during the dialysis procedure.

8.4 SUPPORTIVE THERAPY

Management of poisoning requires thorough knowledge of how to treat hypoventilation, coma, shock, and seizures. Sophisticated toxicokinetic considerations are of little value if vital functions are not maintained. These measures are the most important. Many animals die as a result of shock or hypothermia. Measures include control of body temperature, maintenance of respiratory and cardiovascular function, control of central nervous system signs, and pain control.

BODY TEMPERATURE

Hyperthermia is controlled through use of ice bags, cold water baths, and cold water enemas. Whatever control system is used, however, it is vital to monitor the temperature so overcorrection does not occur. In cases of hypothermia, blankets, infrared lamps, heating pads, and hot water jars, may all be considered. Hypothermia is a common sequela to ingestion of a toxicant coupled with shock. Infrared lamps should be used with caution and under constant observation. It is easy to burn areas with excessive or prolonged heat.

RESPIRATORY SUPPORT

A patent airway must always be obtained. Usually a cuffed endotracheal tube assists the patient with respiratory embarrassment. An anesthetic machine can be used with manual compression of the bag to provide positive pressure ventilation. A mixture of 50% oxygen and 50% room air is usually suitable. In severe respiratory depression or apnea, analeptic drugs and respiratory stimulants should be used. Analeptics, such as bemegride (10 to 20 mg/kg) or pentylenetetrazol (6 to 10 mg/kg), are effective, but large doses can cause convulsions. It is better to use a pure respiratory stimulant with little or no side effects, such as doxapram (5 to 10 mg/kg intravenously).

CARDIOVASCULAR SUPPORT

This requires the presence of an adequate circulatory volume, adequate tissue perfusion, correct acid-base balance, and adequate cardiac output. If hypovolemia owing to fluid loss alone is present, lactated Ringer's solution or plasma expanders should be considered. In hypovolemia owing to loss of both cells and volume, whole blood is the necessary agent. Tissue perfusion must be monitored periodically, and in such cases it may be necessary to administer massive doses of corticosteroids intravenously to restore adequate tissue perfusion, e.g., 2 to 10 mg/kg dexamethasone. Cardiac activity can be modified by a number of pharmacologic agents. Intravenous calcium gluconate is a good nonspecific inotropic agent.

In hypovolemia, it is important not to overload the heart with too much fluid too rapidly, although animals seem to be able to withstand more than humans can. Tissue perfusion should be monitored by watching the capillary refill time. The normal pink color of the gum should return within 2 seconds of compression. A capillary refill time of more than 3 seconds with tachycardia and cool extremities indicate hypovolemic shock (12 to 15%). In severe hypovolemic shock, fluid should be replaced as quickly as possible, e.g., 50 ml/kg/hour for the first 20 to 30 minutes. After that, a rate of about 10 to 15 ml/mg/hour should be used.

TABLE 8–5
RESPIRATORY STIMULANTS

Convulsant in Large Doses
  Pentylene tetrazol, 6–10 mg/kg
  Bemegride (Megimide), 20 mg/kg
    intravenously
  Nikethamide (Coramine), 250–500 mg
    intravenously or intramuscularly
Latent Period for Effect
  Picrotoxin, 2–6 mg intravenously or
    intramuscularly
Safest
  Doxapram (Dopram), 5–10 mg/kg
    intravenously

Cardiac Activity

In the event of inadequate activity, chest massage should be undertaken initially, but cardiac stimulants may need to be used in many instances. Calcium gluconate can be infused slowly intravenously or intraperitoneally (20% solution 5 ml/kg) until heart rate returns to normal. Digoxin (0.2 to 0.6 mg/kg intravenously) may also be used. Care must be taken not to overdose because these agents are highly toxic to the myocardium. Dopamine ($2-10 \mu g/kg/min$) or dobutamine ($5-30 \mu g/kg$) provide for a more reliable cardiac inotropism.

CENTRAL NERVOUS SYSTEM

The type of treatment obviously depends on the presence of depression or hyperactivity. Either disorder can be turned into the opposite problem by overzealous therapeutic measures.

Central Nervous System Depression

This can be considered also as respiratory depression. Analeptics, such as bemegride, 10 to 20 mg/kg, or pentylenetetrazol, 6 to 10 mg/kg, are effective stimulants of the medulla. Overdosage, however, could induce convulsions. Better still is to use doxapram, 5 to 10 mg/kg, which is a specific and selective respiratory stimulant, with short-lived activity and no tendency toward convulsive action (Table 8–5).

Central Nervous System Hyperactivity

Convulsive activity may be controlled by the administration of central nervous system depressants and tranquilizers. Pentobarbital sodium is generally the agent of choice for convulsions and hyperactivity. A tranquilizing effect coupled with skeletal muscle relaxant activity is particularly useful, and intravenous diazepam (Valium), 0.5 to 1.5 mg/kg, is successful in many convulsive states associated with spasm of skeletal muscle. Methocarbamol (Robaxin) is a useful agent for relaxing skeletal muscle spasms, and it possesses a potent blocking effect at the level of the interneurons in the spinal cord. It is useful in strychnine poisoning. Regardless of the regimen of therapy, animals should always be kept in a darkened quiet room away from auditory or visual stimuli (Table 8–6).

ACID-BASE IMBALANCE, SHOCK, AND PAIN

Measures to take account of acid-base imbalance, pain, and shock are critical to patient survival. In correcting acidosis, lactated Ringer's solution, Hartmanns' solution, or sodium bicarbonate are the solutions of choice.

The most common acid-base disturbance seen in animals is acidosis, mainly of metabolic origin. Alkalosis may also occur. In

---

TABLE 8–6
ANTICONVULSANTS[*]

Valium (Diazepam), 0.5–1.5 mg/kg
  intravenously slowly or
  intramuscularly
Pentobarbital, 20–35 mg/kg slowing to
  effect for anesthesia
Pentobarbitone, 10–20 mg/kg
  intravenously slowly or
  intramuscularly for sedation
Acetylpromazine, 0.025 mg/kg
  intravenously
Methocarbamol (Robaxin), 40 mg/kg
  intravenously

---

[*]Place the animal in a warm, quiet room following sedation. Some poisons (e.g., chlorinated hydrocarbons) enhance barbiturates.

TABLE 8–7
FLUIDS, PAIN, AND SHOCK

Acidosis
   Lactated Ringer's, 20 mg/kg
   Sodium bicarbonate 1%, 50 ml/kg
      intravenously slowly
Alkalosis
   5% glucose saline
   Ammonium chloride, 100 g/kg orally
   Normal saline
Anemia
   20 ml whole blood/kg, intravenously
Pain
   Pethidine, 5 mg/kg intravenously or
      intramuscularly
   Pentazocine, 2 mg/kg
   Butorphanol, 0.2–0.4 mg/kg
   Flunixin, 1.1 mg/kg intravenously
Shock
   Dextran, 20 ml/kg intravenously
   5% glucose saline, 20 ml/kg
   Dexamethasone, 2–10 mg/kg

---

correcting acidosis not of respiratory origin, sodium bicarbonate administered intravenously (33 to 66 ml/kg of a 1% solution) every 15 minutes or lactated Ringer's solution (120 ml/kg) should be considered.

Alkalosis does not generally occur as frequently. If present, however, 0.9% sodium chloride (physiologic saline), 10 ml/kg intravenously, is usually sufficient for initial therapy. This can be followed with oral ammonium chloride (200 g/kg/day) in divided doses. Caution must be exercised when altering acid-base balance not to overcompensate.

If shock develops, corticosteroids, nonsteroidal anti-inflammatory drugs, balanced polyionic fluids, and plasma volume expanders need to be administered. Shock associated with internal hemorrhage must be treated with whole blood infusion, and many such cases also require analgesics of the opiate family. Pain itself can exacerbate shock in the traumatized animal.

Another supportive measure in patients with intoxication is the control of pain when this is a problem. The following agents may be considered: pethidine, 5 mg/kg intravenously, intramuscularly, or subcutane-

ously; pentazocine, 2 mg/kg; butorphanol, 0.2–0.4 mg/kg; phenylbutazone, 4.4 mg/kg intravenously or 20 mg/kg orally; and flunixin, 1 mg/kg intravenously (Table 8–7).

SYSTEMIC AND SPECIFIC ANTIDOTES

When a poison has been absorbed, if a systemic antidote is available, it should be used. Those available are shown in Table 8–8. A popular misconception is that there is an antidote for every poison. The opposite is true: Relatively selective antidotes are available for only eight classes of toxins.

TABLE 8–8
ANTIDOTES FOR COMMON TOXICANTS

Arsenic
   Dimercaprol
   Sodium thiosulfate
   Penicillamine
Barbiturates
   Doxapram
   Bemegride
   Amphetamine
Bracken
   DL-batyl alcohol
   Thiamine
Cholinesterase inhibitors
   Atropine sulfate
   Pralidoximes
Copper
   D-Penicillamine
   Molybdenum
Coumarin derivatives (anticoagulants)
   Vitamin K_1
Digitalis glycosides
   Propranolol
      (beta blockers)
Lead
   Calcium disodium edetate (EDTA)
Antifreeze
   Ethanol
Methemoglobinemia-producing agents
   (nitrates, chlorates)
   Methylene blue
Strychnine
   Pentobarbital
   Diazepam
   Methocarbamol

Chelating agents are the most versatile and effective antidotes for metal intoxication. These compounds are usually flexible molecules with two or more electronegative groups that form stable coordinate-covalent bonds with the cationic metal atom. The complexes thus formed are then excreted by the body. The action of these drugs provides an excellent application of the principle of chemical antagonism.

Specific Agents

Dimercaprol (2,3-dimercaptopropanol) is a useful antidote in arsenic, mercury, lead, and cadmium poisoning. Penicillamine is used chiefly for poisoning with copper or to prevent copper accumulation. It is also used as adjunctive therapy in the treatment of lead and arsenic poisoning. Ethylenediaminetetra-acetic acid (EDTA) (Versenate) is an efficient chelator of many divalent and trivalent metals in vitro. Metals such as lead and a few other heavy metals capable of binding EDTA and displacing Ca^{2+} are effectively chelated. Deferoxamine mesylate is isolated from *Streptomyces pilosus*. It binds iron avidly but essential trace metals poorly.

8.5 LARGE ANIMAL INTOXICATIONS

GRAIN ENGORGEMENT AND RUMEN ACIDOSIS

Sudden ingestion of large quantities of highly fermentable grain leads to lactic acidosis, acute dehydration, and depression. Change in the rumen microflora results in an overgrowth of gram-positive streptococci, lactobacilli, and clostridia. Increased lactic acid production contributes to metabolic acidosis coupled with endotoxin absorption from the rumen, and hypertonicity of the rumen contributes to hemoconcentration. The syndrome is really an endotoxic shock associated with dehydration and acidosis. Clinical signs include extreme weakness, depression, lowered blood pressure, anorexia, dehydration, diarrhea, and rumen stasis. Treatment includes:

1. Fluids to correct the dehydration (lactated Ringer's solution)
2. Oral bicarbonate in water to correct the rumen acidosis
3. Oral administration of activated charcoal (1 g/lb) to absorb endotoxins

Fluids should be alkaline in nature (sodium bicarbonate, lactated Ringer's, Hartmann's) to correct the acidotic state. Saline is acidic and is not indicated. Rumenotomy and general supportive therapy are also indicated. Barley poisoning has been successfully treated by intravenous injection of B vitamins.

UREA POISONING (AMMONIA TOXICOSIS)

Urea toxicosis in cattle may result from improper mixing of rations using a high-fiber, low-carbohydrate diet and feeding high levels of urea to animals whose digestive tracts are not adapted to the compound. Poisoning occurs when the hydrolysis of urea releases more ammonia than the rumen microorganisms are capable of dealing with. Animals most at risk are those abruptly given a diet with high levels of nonprotein nitrogen of urea as the major portion of dietary protein.

Urea poisoning results from the release of excess ammonia in the rumen. Hyperammonemia occurs with the rapid absorption of ammonia from the rumen, especially under conditions of alkaline pH. Only un-ionized free ammonia diffuses into the portal circulation. The liver is unable to convert the excessive amount of ammonia in the portal blood system back to urea. Systemic acidosis results from inhibition of the tricarboxylic acid (Krebs) cycle owing to hyperammonemia. Acidosis subsequently leads to cardiac shock and death owing to hyperkalemia.

Clinical signs may occur within 30 to 60 minutes after ingestion. Untreated animals can die within 4 hours of ingestion. Clinical signs include salivation, grinding of the teeth, abdominal pain, bloat, muscle tremors, ataxia, spasms, and convulsions. Clinical analysis is the key to definitive diagnosis. Ammonia concentrations greater than 2 mg/dl in the blood or greater than 80 mg/dl in the rumen contents are diagnostically significant. A ruminal content pH of 7.5 or greater is indicative of urea poisoning. Urea in ruminant feed is generally recommended at a level of 3% of the grain ration—not to exceed 1% of the total ration. Acetic acid has proved to be an effective antidote: 4 to 12 liters 5% (vinegar) given orally with 20 to 40 liters cold water.

ORGANOPHOSPHATE POISONING

Organophosphates are inhibitors of cholinesterase that are fat soluble and that can pass through the intact skin easily. The onset of clinical signs in cases of acute organophosphate poisoning may be as short as a few minutes after exposure, but alternatively signs may not be apparent for 3 to 4 days after exposure in some cases. Organophosphate compounds, which may be nerve agents or insecticides, combine with acetylcholinesterase (AChE), inactivate the enzyme, and permit the buildup of excess acetylcholine (ACh) at synapses. Thus the signs of poisoning include a variety of effects of excess ACh in certain regions of the central and peripheral nervous systems.

Mildly exposed animals may have lethargy, anorexia, and diarrhea for as many as several days or more. Ruminants often have fewer central nervous system effects from acute exposures than do other animal species. The interval between exposure and the onset of clinical signs is strongly influenced by the route of exposure, with possible delays of as much as a week or more for dermal application.

In most domestic animals, 80% or more of the total blood cholinesterase activity is associated with the erythrocytes; thus blood cholinesterase is a good indicator of blood AChE activity. Clinical signs are due to inactivation of AChE and consequent accumulation of ACh. The animals first tend to stay away from the herd and are slightly depressed and off feed. Clinical signs appear, such as lethargy, droopy ears, ruminal atony, bloat, diarrhea, excessive salivation, miosis, lacrimation, muscle tremors, and collapse with bronchoconstriction. Death occurs from hypoxia owing to bronchoconstriction and excessive respiratory secretions. Organophosphates, being fat soluble, can pass into the brain, where local accumulation of ACh can result in central nervous system stimulation. Some reports indicate that certain bulls can be unduly susceptible to pour-on organophosphates,

and this may be related to high circulatory levels of testosterone, which in some way render the animal more sensitive to the adverse affects of these insecticides.

Organophosphate and carbamate poisoning must be regarded as an emergency, with therapy instituted immediately:

1. Activated charcoal, given orally to prevent further absorption of any insecticide remaining in the gastrointestinal tract. Approximately 2 to 4 lbs for cattle is recommended in an oral slurry.
2. Atropine, 0.25 to 0.5 mg/kg. Give 25% intravenously and the rest subcutaneously. Repeat at 3 to 6 hourly intervals. Adequate atropinization is indicated by pupillary dilatation and lack of salivation.
3. Oximes, cholinesterase enzyme reactivating agents that cause dissociation of the enzyme-organophosphate bond. Obidoxime 5 mg/kg i.m., i.v.; pralidoxime 10 mg/kg, i.v., i.m.

In the event of dermal exposure, animals should be washed as quickly as possible (preferably with soap and water) to minimize further transcutaneous absorption. Anticonvulsant drugs, such as acetylpromazine, xylazine, and especially diazepam, can be used in addition to atropine or atropine-oxime combinations. Diazepam can prevent some of the central effects of accumulated Ach and the bradycardia produced by anticholinergics. Some antihistamines (e.g., diphenhydramine) have been shown to neutralize the effects of nicotine receptor overstimulation in dogs.

DELAYED NEUROTOXICITY

Delayed neurotoxicity is a distal axonopathy developing from 1 to several weeks after exposure. In delayed neurotoxicity, it is thought that the phosphorylated esterase is neurotoxic.

In the 1930s, this syndrome was seen in many people in the U.S. who ingested "Ginger Jake"—a drink that used an organophosphate in the extraction procedure. The axon is primarily effected—myelin sheaths are secondary.

NITRATE POISONING

Nitrate/nitrite toxicity occurs after ingestion of stored forage. The ruminal flora converts nitrate into nitrite. Intoxication is marked by methemoglobin formation. Nitrite also possesses vasodilatory action. Tissue hypoxia, low blood pressure, brown mucous membranes, dyspnea, rapid weak heartbeats, and muscular weakness are typical signs of nitrite toxicity. Treatment consists of slow intravenous injection of 1 to 2% methylene blue, 5 to 20 mg/kg in isotonic saline. This can be repeated after half an hour or so.

Methylene blue converts methemoglobin to hemoglobin. A recommended regimen of therapy is the administration of a vasoconstrictor, such as epinephrine or etamiphylline camyslate, intravenously, followed by 1 to 2 mg/kg body weight methylene blue administered intravenously as a 1% solution. Oral administration of formalin or antibiotics to destroy the rumen flora that convert nitrate to nitrite may also be indicated. Vitamin C, intravenously at 5 g/adult animal, is also useful ancillary therapy.

LEAD POISONING

Lead is one of the most common poisons to affect farm animals. Lead poisoning is commonly seen in calves, the source of lead usually being from paints, used oils, grease, batteries, machinery, industrial contaminants, and garbage. The most commonly observed symptoms of lead poisoning are blindness, twitching, head pressing, ataxia, circling, wall climbing, teeth grinding, and tenesmus.

The standard treatment is use of a loaded chelating agent, 1 to 2% calcium disodium edetate (in 0.9% saline or 5% dextrose) at 110 mg/kg (slowly intravenously) twice a day for 2 days. This is followed by no chelator treatment for 2 days and then 2 more days of treatment. The chelating agent acts to form a stable ring complex with lead, mobilizing it from the tissues and thus assisting in its urinary excretion. Thiamine (vitamin B_1) given subcutaneously at 3 to 5 mg/kg twice a day in conjunction with the chelating agent is also beneficial. Vitamin D and calcium borogluconate (subcutaneously) are important ancillary aids, and a sedative provides additional support. Thiamine alone, at doses of 20 mg/kg, has been shown to be an effective antidote given subcutaneously for up to 14 days. Oral magnesium sulfate may be beneficial given at a dose of 0.5 kg/500 kg body weight.

ARSENIC POISONING

Arsenic toxicity may be derived from herbicides, pesticides, insecticides (ant poisons), wood preservatives, paints, or detergents. The symptoms of toxicity are mainly those of a gastrointestinal problem with profuse watery diarrhea (tinged with blood), severe colic, dehydration, weakness, depression, subnormal temperature, edema, and blistering of the skin. Treatment consists of sodium thiosulfate intravenously and later orally (after charcoal administration), 20 to 30 g in 300 ml water or 8 to 10 g as a 10% solution intravenously. Dimercaprol (if available), at an intramuscular dose of 4 to 5 mg/kg, should also be considered. Supportive therapy includes oral activated charcoal (2 g/kg) with a saline cathartic, demulcent, restoration of blood volume, and correction of the usually significant dehydration. Dimercaptosuccinate (DMSA) and Dimercaptopropane sulfonate (DMPS), at 20 mg/kg parenterally, can be effective antidotes. Pethidine, (meperidine) 3 to 5 mg/kg, and dextrose saline should also be considered.

HERBICIDE POISONING

Dinitro herbicides give rise to severe hyperthermia, yellow skin discoloration, and central nervous system stimulation. The affected animal should immediately be placed in a cool shady place. Barbiturates can be used to sedate the animal and control hypothermia. Parenteral carbohydrates and vitamin A are usually considered useful adjuncts. Phenothiazine tranquilizers, especially chlorpromazine, must not be used as sedating agents. Atropine is contraindicated.

Paraquat and diquat (dipyridyls) herbicides are notorious for causing fatal accidents in humans. In animals, symptoms range from inappetence and depression to vomiting, incoordination, and sometimes sudden death. Pathologically lesions are present in the mouth, esophagus, and lungs. Dyspnea is a major feature of paraquat poisoning beginning 3 to 4 days after ingestion. Absorption and development of symptoms can be relatively slow.

Treatment is often too little and too late. Fluid therapy, intensive steroidal treatment, and diuretics to enhance excretion are indicated. These highly potent, commonly encountered herbicides can give rise to a variety of lesions and symptoms. Free radical release and tissue irritation typify their action. Pulmonary damage, severe gastrointestinal irritation, renal damage, or hepatic damage can be present. Occasionally toxicity is enhanced by selenium and vitamin E deficiency. Treatment includes intensive oral administration of adsorbents and cathartics. Furosemide (Lasix) or mannitol can be used to enhance diuresis and hasten excretion. Vitamin E and selenium can be given. Owing to slow absorption of these dipyridyl compounds, adsorbents and cathartics can be useful.

Sodium chlorate is a commonly used weed-killer that induces the formation of methemoglobinemia, and so tissue anoxia becomes a major problem in toxicity states. Specific therapy is with methylene blue 1% (10 mg/kg slowly intravenously). Blood transfusions are also indicated, and intravenous isotonic saline can help to accelerate elimination of the chlorate ion. Ataxia, dyspnea, and diarrhea also accompany sodium chlorate toxicity.

FURAZOLIDONE POISONING

The margin between the therapeutic and toxic dose of furazolidone for calves is not wide. It is generally accepted that furazolidone poisoning in calves appears in two forms: acute poisoning after administration of high doses for short periods of time, which causes central nervous system disturbances, and chronic toxicity, which causes hemorrhagic diathesis. Signs of acute poisoning include opisthotonos, muscle twitching, spasms, seizures, apparent blindness, walking on knees, and salivation. Disseminated petechial hemorrhages are seen on postmortem examination. The rational treatment of furazolidone poisoning is based on its chemistry, metabolism, and mechanisms of action. Oral sodium bicarbonate (14 g/liter in a 10% solution of glucose) is used to enhance the excretion of the acidic furazolidone. Vitamin B_1 (thiamine) is also used as a therapeutic agent owing to its effect on the conversion of pyruvate into acetyl CoA, to improve energy supply in the cells. Acepromazine and calcium solutions have also been used to good effect. Clearly labeled furazolidone concentrations and care in mixing or inclusion rates are essential to avoid toxicity in calves.

MONENSIN IN HORSES

Concentrations of monensin used for routine cattle feeding are not usually toxic to horses. Equine intoxications lasting several days are caused by exposure to concentrates or contaminated feed. Clinical signs include a stiff gait, nonspecific colic, and uneasiness, progressing to sternal and then lateral recumbency. Assays of serum glutamic-oxaloacetic transaminase (SGOT) and creatine phosphokinase (CPK) may help to diagnose the disorder because muscle (cardiac or skeletal) is the target site of toxic action. Serum levels of these enzymes double or treble within 24 hours of exposure. Vitamin E, 17 IU/kg; selenium, 0.25 mg/kg; and intensive fluid and electrolyte therapy may be of some benefit. (For more on ionophore toxicity, see Chapter 24.)

COPPER POISONING

Sheep are most susceptible to this toxicity. A number of factors that affect copper metabolism can influence chronic copper poisoning by enhancing its absorption or retention. Poisoning in cattle and sheep is characterized by an acute hemolytic syndrome resulting from the release of excessive copper stored in the liver. Molybdenum interaction, especially when the dietary ratio of copper to molybdenum increases above 10:1, usually triggers problems. Acute poisoning produces anemia, severe gastroenteritis, depression, weakness, anorexia, and hemoglobinuria.

Therapy for copper toxicity involves use of gastrointestinal tract sedatives and symptomatic treatment for shock. Ammonium tetra thiomolybdate can be successful (experimentally intravenously) by tying up copper and limiting its absorption. Administration of ammonium molybdate (50 to 100 mg) and sodium sulfate (0.5 to 1 g) can minimize losses in lambs. Penicillamine or EDTA can be useful if given early. Fluid, plasma volume expanders, hematinics, and whole blood transfusion may be necessary.

8.6 SMALL ANIMAL INTOXICATIONS

Cats are thought to be exposed less frequently than dogs to poisoning because of their selective eating habits. Anticoagulants, carbamates, and organophosphates are among the most frequently reported toxicants in dogs. Active ingredients involved in most of the anticoagulant exposures are warfarin, diphacinone, and pival. (These are used as rat or mouse baits.) Exposures to carbamates involve carbaryl, propoxur, and methiocarb, used to kill garden slugs, snails, and insects. Commonly encountered organophosphates include diazinon, fenthion, DDVP, disulfoton, and malathion. Other pesticides include metaldehyde and arsenicals (ant poisonings).

The U.S. Environmental Protection Agency has in recent years (in common with the situation in other countries) required that the formulation of metaldehyde baits be less attractive to dogs, and hence the incidence of poisoning with these has declined, although isolated cases still occur. Also, many of the organochlorines have been phased out internationally.

ALPHA CHLORALOSE POISONING

Alpha chloralose is a commonly used rodenticide and a pesticide for wood pigeons. It is a common cause of poisoning in small animals, especially in cats. Alpha chloralose acts to lower the metabolic rate (except in cats). Ataxia and coma are frequently sequelae. In cats, excitement, aggression, and convulsions are common. Toxicity can be manifested either by a hyperexcitable state or a comatose state. Pentobarbital sodium is indicated in the former state and doxapram in the latter, in which respiratory depression is evident. Evacuation of alpha chloralose by induced emesis and local gut neutralization should also be attempted. Osmotic diuresis is indicated to increase excretion of toxic products.

ETHYLENE GLYCOL POISONING

Commonly known and used as antifreeze, the seasonality of ethylene glycol toxicity outbreaks is usually in autumn or spring. Symptoms include depression, incoordination, polyuria/polydipsia, renal failure, convulsions, and coma. Formation of oxalate crystals may occur in the urine, kidney, or brain. Ethylene glycol constitutes 95% of most antifreeze preparations. Antifreeze poisoning occurs frequently in dogs and cats and is most common in autumn when car radiators are being drained. The sweet taste of ethylene glycol encourages consumption by dogs and cats.

Ethylene glycol and its metabolites are extremely toxic to animals. Ethylene glycol is metabolized in the liver by alcohol dehydrogenase to form oxalates. Because the same enzyme also metabolizes ethanol, ethylene glycol toxicity can be treated by administration of ethanol. The ethanol competes for the enzyme and decreases the amount of oxalate formed.

Activated charcoal and a saline cathartic should be given when animals are presented within 3 hours of ingestion. Fluid therapy (dextrose saline) is important in combating dehydration and in promoting urinary excretion of ethylene glycol. A classic treatment for many years has been the application of ethanol and bicarbonate. Ethanol competitively inhibits ethylene glycol metabolism, facilitating its excretion in the urine and reducing the development of acidosis. Sodium bicarbonate is used to correct the acidosis and enhance urinary excretion. Treatment is usually 5 ml 20% ethanol/kg and 8 ml sodium bicarbonate/kg intraperitoneally in saline. Intraperitoneal injection of 20% pure ethanol (5.5 mg/kg) and 5% sodium bicarbonate (8.8 mg/kg) every 6 hours for 2 to 3 days is an alternative to this combination.

Aggressive fluid therapy is required to compensate for osmotic diuresis induced by ethanol. Ethanol or 4-methylpyrazole can inhibit ethylene glycol metabolism, which facilitates its excretion in the urine and reduces development of acidosis. Repeated doses of 4-methylpyrazole inhibit the metabolism of ethylene glycol and prevent the appearance of plasma and urinary metabolites of ethylene glycol. In humans, 4-methylpyrazole is used as an antidote to ethylene glycol intoxication. The proposed dose regimen is 20 mg/kg/day orally or 7 mg/kg/day in an intravenous infusion of isotonic sodium chloride solution.

STRYCHNINE POISONING

This pesticide induces severe convulsions beginning 10 minutes to 2 hours after administration. Acting as a potent spinal convulsant, strychnine induces apprehension, stiffness, tetanic convulsions, intermittent opisthotonos, dyspnea, cyanosis, and extensor rigidity. Animals (dogs) are usually more hypersensitive to noise and external movements.

Strychnine, an indole alkaloid, antagonizes glycine, an inhibitory transmitter in the spinal cord and medulla. Reduced postsynaptic inhibition causes uncontrolled diffuse spinal reflex activity in tonic convulsions with predominant extensor rigidity. Treatment is largely symptomatic but can be relatively successful if initiated in the early stages. The remaining toxicant in the stomach must be evacuated by emesis or neutralized using 1:1000 potassium permanganate, strong tea, or 2% tannic acid in the form of gastric lavage. Activated charcoal (5 g/kg) can be used after lavage to prevent further absorption of the alkaloid. Although no specific antidote exists, convulsions may be controlled with intravenous diazepam (2 to 5 mg/kg), barbiturate, or intravenous methocarbamol (40 mg/kg) for muscle spasms. Diazepam possesses some muscle relaxant effects in addition to its antianxiety effects. Quietness, warm dark surroundings, and maintenance with intraperitoneal barbiturate are also desirable. Intravenous fluids and diuretics are indicated. Body temperature must be maintained and vital signs monitored.

IVERMECTIN IN COLLIES

Collies and Collie crosses are susceptible to ivermectin toxicity when given the drug at 200 µg/kg doses to treat ectoparasites or endoparasites. Toxicity in Collies can result from the extralabel use of ivermectin. Signs of toxicity in the Collie include ataxia, depression, tremors, recumbency, and mydriasis. The varied neurologic signs seen indicate that ivermectin can enter the central nervous system in the Collie and disrupt functioning of the neurotransmitter gamma-aminobutyric acid (GABA). In practically all species, ivermectin, being a large macrolide molecule, does not enter the central nervous system. The exception appears to be the Collie. Picrotoxin, a stimulant and antagonist of GABA, has been reportedly effective in treating ivermectin toxicity, administered by intravenous infusion at the rate of 1 mg/minute in a 0.1% dilution of isotonic dextrose. Picrotoxin, however, can induce violent clonic seizures, hence its general use for ivermectin toxicity is not recommended. Physostigmine at a dosage of 1 mg/kg intravenously is safer, more effective and more rationally indicated. Physostigmine should be accompanied by the use of activated charcoal and saline or osmotic purgatives. (Ivermectin is excreted primarily by the fecal route.) Current formulations of ivermectin are not licensed for use in dogs. The only formulation that can be used in Collies (with care) is the low dosage of 6 µg/kg monthly prophylactic tablet for heartworm infection. Thus there does appear to be a threshold dosage in Collies above which dose-toxicity effects can be noted.

ASPIRIN POISONING

This commonly used analgesic is particularly toxic to cats on account of its long half-life and tendency toward cumulation. Aspirin (acetylsalicylic acid) is probably the most widely used over-the-counter drug in small animals and also in humans. It has been prohibited in many countries in human medicine for use in young children because of its correlation with Reye's syndrome.

In animals, therapeutic doses for aspirin range from 10 to 20 mg/kg twice a day. Particular care must be taken in cats to prevent overdosage. Owing to the feline's deficiency in glucuronyl transferase, the half-life is longer in the cat, and hence cumulation to toxic levels is more likely to occur. Accordingly dosage in the cat (10 to 20 mg/kg) should be every 48 hours.

Aspirin overdosage is displayed by nausea, vomiting, central nervous system seizures, and coma. A respiratory alkalosis develops secondary to metabolic acidosis. In cats, the most susceptible species, toxicity is dose dependent and can be manifested by depression, anorexia, vomiting, gastric hemorrhage, bone marrow hypoplasia, and hyperpyrexia.

Emptying of the stomach contents is a prerequisite of treatment, and this should be followed by administration of activated charcoal and a cathartic (preferably saline). Owing to the effects on the gastric mucosa, antagonists, such as cimetidine, ranitidine, and omeprazole, can be used to minimize gastrointestinal irritation, ulceration, and hemorrhage. Sucralfate binds pepsin and bile salts and can be employed for gastric injury associated with aspirin use. Vitamin K_1, corrects hypoprothrombinemia. The usual metabolic acidosis is treated with slow intravenous infusion of sodium bicarbonate. Sodium bicarbonate also enhances renal excretion of acetylsalicylic acid and other acidic metabolites because the urine is alkaline. Emesis and gastric lavage should be attempted, glucose saline should be infused parenterally, and nikethamide should be employed as a respiratory stimulant. Broad-spectrum antibiotics and gastrointestinal tract protectants may also be warranted.

In cats and dogs, species and age differences play a significant role in the rates of elimination. In the dog, the plasma half-life is 8.6 hours; in the cat, it is 37.5 hours. Hepatic clearance is thus most prolonged in cats. Newborn animals are also deficient in microsomal enzymes necessary for biotransformation of salicylate and can decrease clearance of these drugs. Accordingly salicylates have longer half-lives in neonates.

PARACETAMOL (ACETAMINOPHEN) POISONING

In most species, paracetamol is conjugated, with glucuronide or sulfate, resulting in the production of nontoxic metabolites. In cats, detoxification involving conjugation with glucuronide is poor because the cat has a low level of glucuronyl transferase, which catalyzes the final step in the pathway. Methemoglobin is formed in toxicity states.

Sodium sulfate 1.6% (50 mg/kg) is given by slow intravenous injection every 4 hours on three occasions for conjugation. N-acetylcysteine also elevates plasma sulfate levels and so also acts by this mechanism. Methemoglobin is reduced to hemoglobin by administration of ascorbic acid (30 mg/kg) by slow intravenous injection every 4 hours on 3 occasions. Fluid therapy may be needed in severe cases either to replace hemoglobin (whole blood) or reverse acidosis (e.g., Ringer's lactate or fluid containing bicarbonate).

METALDEHYDE POISONING

Metaldehyde is a cyclic polymer of acetaldehyde widely used as a molluscacide. Its main use is as a slug and snail bait in gardening. In poisoning, the released acetaldehyde crosses the blood brain barrier, inhibits gamma aminobutyric acid and increases monoamino oxide. Metaldehyde is probably one of the most commonly used garden pellets for control of snails. Poisoning is common with the molluscacide, and a broad scatter of symptoms may be presented: hyperesthesia, salivation, hyperpnea, depression, vomiting, tremors, convulsions, opisthotonos, and nystagmus in cats. Severe acidosis develops.

No specific antidote is available. If seen early enough, gastric lavage or emesis may be of use. Barbiturates or diazepam intravenously to control the convulsions, nikethamide or doxapram for respiratory depression, and parenteral glucose saline are the general approaches to treatment. Fluids are used to reverse the acidosis induced by metaldehyde (fluids with sodium lactate or bicarbonate). Acetylpromazine has also been reported to be useful in treatment and does not appear to increase the incidence of convulsions. To reverse acidosis and prevent dehydration, intravenous fluid therapy is essential. Fluids such as Ringer's lactate or normal saline with bicarbonate supplementation are suitable.

FLUOROACETATE (1080)/FLUOROACETAMIDE (1081) POISONING

These rodenticides cause animal poisoning (in the form of convulsions) by blockade of the citric acid cycle. Secondary poisoning by ingestion of a poisoned rodent may also occur (in cats). The poisoned animal often attempts to vomit and defecate. Other signs include excitement convulsions (not precipitated by noise) and cardiac arrhythmias. Treatment is largely symptomatic: induction of emesis, gastric lavage, or both. Barbiturates are indicated for epileptiform convulsions; parenteral glucose or saline is usually indicated also. Antiarrhythmic drugs, e.g., lidocaine, procainamide, and quinidine, should also be used.

ALPHA-NAPHTHYLTHIOUREA (ANTU) POISONING

ANTU is a rodenticide that increases the permeability of lung capillaries, causing pleural effusion and pulmonary edema. Dyspnea, moist rales, coughing, tachycardia, cyanosis, and hypothermia represent fairly typical symptoms, although vomiting, diarrhea, and incoordination may also occur. Emetics, oxygen therapy, osmotics, diuretics (mannitol), and atropine sulfate must be given rapidly after ingestion of the poison if any success is to be hoped for. Steroids and sedatives may be useful also. Agents providing sulfhydryl groups, e.g., sodium thiosulfate 10%, can be beneficial.

WARFARIN AND COUMARIN DERIVATIVES

Warfarin, a coumarin derivative, is a rodenticide causing slow hemorrhaging in the affected rodent. Dogs and cats often pick up this palatable poison directly or through ingestion of a poisoned rodent. As an anticoagulant, warfarin competes with vitamin K, causing factor II, VII, IX, and X deficiencies. It reduces the conversion of prothrombin to thrombin. Symptoms of warfarin poisoning in dogs include blanched gums and mucous membranes; bleeding from the nose, rectum, and subcutaneous tissues; and painful joints with stiffness. Severe anaemia, depression, hemorrhage, and hypovolemic shock are the usual sequelae. Prolonged clotting and extended one-stage prothrombin time are typical.

For treatment, an emetic can be attempted if ingestion is recent. Bruising must be avoided at all costs. Whole blood transfusion (20 ml/kg) is normally indicated on account of the hemorrhaging and hypovolemic shock. This replaces the clotting factors as well as replacing blood loss through hemorrhage. Vitamin K_1 2.0 to 5.0 mg/kg intramuscularly or subcutaneously or 1 mg/kg (in 5% dextrose) intravenously for up to 2 weeks is indicated followed by oral treatment for a subsequent 4-week period. Phytomenadione, a vitamin K_1 analog available as tablets or injection, is the drug of choice and reverses low prothrombin levels in 30 minutes. Menadiol is a synthetic vitamin K_3 and is not as effective. Dosing is as follows: Fluids, plasma volume expanders, vitamin B_{12}, and hematinics may also be required in addition to general symptomatic therapy. Coagulation should be monitored weekly until normal values stabilize for 5 to 6 days after the end of treatment.

ORGANOPHOSPHATES AND CARBAMATES

These compounds of narrow safety index are used primarily as topical or systemic acaricides (insecticides) and sometimes as anthelmintics. Organophosphates and carbamates include such compounds as parathion, malathion, dichlorvos, diazinon, fenthion, ronnel, metrifonate, carbaryl, coumaphos, sebacil, and phosmet. AChE is involved in the removal of ACh, which is a neurotransmitter released at parasympathetic, nicotinic, cholinergic, and some central nervous system nerve endings. The clinical signs in acute toxicity are referable to overstimulation of these nerve endings. Occasionally a myopathy may develop after recovery, which is thought to be secondary to excessive ACh stimulation of muscle.

Acting as anticholinesterase compounds, organophosphates and carbomates induce in toxic doses cholinergic agonistic activity. ACh is released (1) at all ganglia, (2) at the parasympathetic neuroeffector junction, and (3) at the myoneural junction. Hence toxicity is manifested by muscarinic and nicotinic effects. In addition, organophosphates are lipid soluble and traverse the blood-brain barrier without undue difficulty, giving rise to inhibition of central nervous system neurohumeral transmitters and stimulation. Symptoms of toxicity are salivation, lacrimation, abdominal pains, gut hypermotility, vomiting, diarrhea, nausea, and convulsions. Death occurs from hypoxia owing to bronchoconstriction and excessive respiratory secretions.

An emetic or gastric lavage is indicated in the early stages as well as shampooing, rinsing, and drying the skin. Other cholinergic agonists (such as levamisole) can potentiate the toxicity of organophosphates. Atropine, 0.2 to 0.5 mg/kg intravenously is the treatment for reversal of the muscarinic effects. Atropine is given as needed for the next 24 hours. Pralidoxine (2 PAM), 20 to 50 mg/kg intramuscularly, can be used to reactivate the enzyme-organophosphate complex. The dose for small animals is 20 to 50 mg/kg intravenously or intramuscularly as a 10% solution. Activated charcoal (3 to 6 g/kg) adsorbs organophosphate and assists fecal elimination.

LEAD POISONING

Lead poisoning is more common in dogs than in cats. The lead may be derived from paint putty, linoleum, batteries, ointments (White lotion), or lead shot. After absorption, lead binds to red cell membranes (80%) and plasma albumin (19% in equilibrium). Less than 1% remains free. Some is bound in the liver and excreted in bile and some by way of the kidneys. Lead is trapped in bone, which acts as a "sink" and can store 90 to 98% of the body burden. This store does not operate in acute poisoning but is an important detoxification mechanism in chronic exposure, and toxicity may not be seen until this store becomes saturated. Symptoms in small animals include vomiting, abdominal pain, hysteria, blind-

ness, mania, and convulsions. For laboratory analysis, 5 to 10 ml of whole blood should be submitted in heparin (not EDTA) anticoagulants. Treatment requires chelating agents, such as EDTA, 75 mg/kg in divided doses slowly intravenously (1 ml 25% solution/10 ml glucose saline) for 3 to 5 days. Other chelators, such as oral penicillamine, 100 mg/kg/day or dimercaprol, 4 µg/kg four times a day, can also be given. Give oral penicillamine on an empty stomach, and if a 2-week course is required, give for 1 week, then 1 week off, then 1 week on. It also chelates copper so hypocupremia is possible. Parenteral fluids are normally indicated, as also are barbiturates or diazepam intravenously to control central stimulation convulsions and anxiety.

PHENOLS, CRESOLS, AND COALTAR PRODUCTS

These may be present in a variety of preparations—disinfectants, soaps, ointments, and wood preservatives. Cats are particularly susceptible to these agents. Symptoms include depression, profuse vomiting, incoordination, thirst convulsions, and coma. There is no specific antidote for phenol poisoning. Symptomatic treatment must be embarked on—emesis or gastric lavage, infusion of glucose saline, and central nervous system stimulants if necessary.

8.7 GENERAL THERAPY OF COMMON TOXICOSES

BARBITURATES (THIOPENTONE, PENTOBARBITAL, PHENOBARBITAL)

This well-established family of central nervous system depressants has wide-ranging, dose-dependent actions from general anesthetic, hypnotic sedative, to anticonvulsant effects. Treatment of barbiturate overdosage consists of reversal of the typical symptoms of depression, incoordination, pupillary dilatation, coma, and slow shallow breathing. Emesis is not recommended but rather the administration of respiratory stimulants, such as bemegride, 20 mg/kg intravenously every 15 minutes, or nikethamide, 250 to 750 mg for dogs, 250 to 500 mg for cats. Animals should be kept warm and vital signs closely monitored and supported. Doxapram is a useful respiratory stimulant in combination with dobutamine as a cardiac beta$_1$ agonist.

HEAVY METALS (OTHER THAN LEAD)

Heavy metals, such as arsenic, mercury, phosphorus, or thallium, are found under a wide range of commercial guises. They may be used as rodenticides (thallium, phosphorus); herbicides (arsenic, mercury); fireworks (phosphorus); or antiseptic, fungicidal, or dermatologic preparations. These agents usually give rise to severe gastroenteritis with vomiting, watery or bloody diarrhea, and intense abdominal pain. Treatment consists of (1) lavage or emesis if just ingested; (2) dimercaprol, 3 mg/kg intramuscularly every 4 hours; (3) 20% solution of sodium thiosulfate intravenously, 20 mg/kg; (4) dextrose saline; and (5) pethidine, 3 to 5 mg/kg intramuscularly.

WEED-KILLERS (2-4D; 2-4-5T McPA)

The toxicity of these plant hormone weed-killers varies with the compound. Depression, anorexia, weakness, vomiting, and convulsions are common signs. Treatment is largely symptomatic; emesis or gastric lavage may be necessary. Toxic contaminants of some of these are dioxins, which are carcinogenic and teratogenic and cause reproductive damage, and chloracne in man.

CHLORINATED HYDROCARBONS

These residually active stable insecticides have now been phased out of general use in many countries. Their biostability, accumulation in the food chain and body fat, soil stability, toxicity, and carcinogenicity in humans has led to their gradual withdrawal from the market. Chlorinated hydrocarbons, such as DDT, gamma BHC, dieldrin, aldrin, and bromocyclen, tend to be more toxic to cats. Symptoms of toxicity include central nervous system stimulation, muscle tremors (cranial-caudal), salivation, violent excitation, convulsions, and perhaps vomiting or diarrhea.

Treatment of poisoning is symptomatic, using emesis, gastric lavage, or the universal antidote to minimize further gut absorption. Skin contamination must be promptly washed off and dried. When convulsions occur, barbiturates slowly intravenously or diazepam to effect should be administered. Affected animals should preferably be kept in warm dark surroundings. Supportive care includes fluid therapy, dexamethasone or mannitol for cerebral edema, and calcium gluconate 10%.

PLANT POISONS

Brackens

Thiaminase is one of the five toxic factors of bracken (for nonruminants). The plant also contains a hematuria-producing factor, a carcinogen, an aplastic anemia factor, and a cyanogenetic glycoide. The toxic factors of bracken are as follows:

1. A carcinogen causing benign and malignant tumors in the wall of the bladder and esophagus following interaction with a papilloma virus; results in the signs seen in enzootic hematuria
2. An unidentified factor that leads to destruction of the rods, cones, and nuclear layer of the retina, causing bright blindness in sheep.
3. A thiaminase, which disrupts thiamine (vitamin B$_1$) so none is available for carboxylase production and a buildup of toxic pyruvate metabolite occurs. These metabolites cause central nervous system disturbances and cardiac and skeletal muscle dysfunction. The signs of bracken poisoning seen in horses and pigs are caused by thiaminase.

The toxic factor in bracken fern that causes poisoning in ruminants has not been identified. The toxin causes depression of bone marrow activity and capillary fragility. In the bone marrow, the myeloid cells are particularly affected, causing a reduction in platelets and granular leukocytes. In the terminal stages, the erythrocyte series is also affected. Bracken is carcinogenic and its intake over a longer period can give rise to carcinomas of the alimentary and urinary tracts. Bone marrow suppression gives rise to prostration, pyrexia, and hemorrhaging in cattle. In horses, ataxia, tremors, and convulsions are the usual manifestations of bracken intoxication.

Treatment requires the specific use of (1) thiamine (100 mg) in horses—(100 mg/kg thiamine twice daily (intravenously or intramuscularly) on first day, then 100 mg daily for 7 days or 200 mg if the condition is severe)—and also (2) Batyl alcohol in cattle. In cattle, blood transfusion and 10 ml of 1% protamine sulfate may be indicated.

Beet, Docks, and Rhubarb

The common feature of toxicity here is the formation of oxalate crystals. Symptoms include depression, anorexia, and dyspnea. The offending material must be removed and symptomatic therapy instituted.

Ergot

Derived from *Claviceps purpurea*, "St. Anthony's fire," as it was known in the Middle Ages, can give rise to severe gangrene on account of the potent effects at alpha receptors on vascular smooth muscle. Their dominant effect is one of vasoconstriction. Ergot alkaloids are widely used in humans for therapy of migraine (also as an ecbolic agent in small animals). Poisoning is most likely to be encountered after fungal contamination of moldy ryegrass. Symptoms include diarrhea, stiffness, lameness, and gangrene in extreme cases. No specific antidote exists, although vasodilators ($beta_2$ agonists), $alpha_1$ blockers, and removal of the ingested toxicant are general symptomatic avenues of approach.

Yew

Among the most hazardous of plants, the active principle in yew is the alkaloid taxine, which is cardiotoxic. Sudden death is the earliest suggestion of yew tree toxicity (especially following a storm). In less severe cases, tremors, dyspnea, and convulsions are observed. Therapy involves removal of the ingested yew (rumenotomy) and judi-

cious use of sedatives. Intravenous calcium borogluconate, tripelennamine, and purgatives are also indicated.

Kale and Rape

The Brassica family contain goitrogens and nitrites and can also cause photosensitization. The active principles induce anemia, ataxia, and hematuria. Treatment must include the use of hematinics, gastrointestinal tract protectants, blood transfusion, and attempted removal of the poison.

Laburnum

Clippings from laburnum contain copious amounts of the alkaloid cytisine. Symptoms include excitement, ataxia, and convulsions. Removal of the toxicant and symptomatic therapy are indicated.

Cherry Laurel

Ingestion can give rise to sudden death, ataxia, and convulsions on account of the active ingredient cyanide. Therapy involves a combination of 1% sodium nitrite, 25 mg/kg, followed by sodium thiosulfate, 1.25 g/kg intravenously.

Green Potatoes and Deadly and Woody Nightshades

Green potatoes are rich in solanine. Deadly nightshade possesses the active ingredient atropine. Poisoning causes irritation to the alimentary membranes. Depression, salivation, and diarrhea are associated with these anticholinergic agents. Hemolysis, hemaglobinuria, and central nervous system disturbances are sometimes seen also. Treatment is symptomatic and includes removal of the poison and purgatives followed by stimulants, pilocarpine, and physostigmine.

Ragwort

A common cause of poisoning, ragwort contains pyrrolizidine alkaloids, which are hepatotoxic. Ingestion over a long period results in cirrhosis with megalocytosis of the hepatic cells. Ingestion of ragwort is marked by tenesmus, depression, ataxia, and pressing. Therapy is symptomatic, including removal of the alkaloids or their neutralization if that is feasible. Further intake of toxic material must be prevented. Rations high in carbohydrate may be beneficial. Methionine in 10% dextrose intravenously is useful in horses.

Rhododendrons and Azaleas

These contain the glycoside andromedotoxin which possesses (1) a curare-type effect, (2) direct stimulatory then depressant effects on striated muscle, (3) inhibitory effects on the smooth muscle of the heart, and (4) depression of the central nervous system. Toxic effects following ingestion include vomiting and colic in cattle and salivation weakness and ataxia in horses. Symptomatic therapy and removal of the ingested toxicant are necessary. Treatment is generally supportive and symptomatic because there is no specific antidote for the toxin. Rumenotomy may be helpful in individual animals if ingestion is known to have occurred. Fluid therapy, when practicable, is used to counter hypotension. Bloat should be relieved by passing a stomach tube or by the use of trochar and cannula.

MYCOTOXINS

The term "mycotoxin" refers to a family of toxins that are produced by various species of molds (fungi). Many of these molds are ubiquitous in nature and can be found normally in stored foodstuffs. The molds themselves are not inherently toxic, but under inappropriate conditions of storage, they may proliferate rapidly, resulting in a marked deterioration in the quality of the feedstuff. The extent of spoilage of grain by fungi depends both on the prevailing environmental conditions and on the nature of the cereal, temperature and moisture content being especially critical factors. Although moldiness is not synonymous with toxin production, nevertheless under specific yet undefined conditions, some strains of fungi elaborate toxic substances (mycotoxins), which are deleterious to the health of humans and animals. Aflatoxins are specific mycotoxins produced by the mold *Aspergillus flavus*.

Many feedstuffs can support the growth of aflatoxin-producing molds. The highest levels and incidence of contamination with aflatoxin are found in tropical and semitropical regions, where climatic conditions favor the growth of aflatoxin-producing molds. Conditions of high humidity and temperature during harvesting, drying, transportation, and storage favor growth of the *Aspergillus* mold and production of its toxin. Accordingly aflatoxin-contaminated products present a problem particularly in the hot and humid parts of the world. A significant portion of the mycotoxin problem is associated with stored grain and other concentrate rations with high moisture content. Because of the involvement of stored feeds, mycotoxins are especially important in intensively housed animals, such as poultry, pigs, and cattle. Although many of the fungi such as *Aspergillus* are ubiquitous, however, only some strains are capable of producing the toxin, and the conditions under which aflatoxin production occurs are unknown. Aflatoxins are stable compounds and can survive heating and processing operations. They therefore persist in animal feeds long after their production.

Aflatoxins

Aflatoxin refers to a group of closely related toxins produced by *Aspergillus flavus*. The aflatoxins generally recognized are aflatoxin B_1 (most toxic), B_2, G_1, G_2, M_1, M_2, B_2A and G_2A. The "B" and "G" designation refers to a "blue" and "green" fluorescence that these aflatoxins emit during analytical tests in the laboratory. Aflatoxins M_1 and M_2 are excreted through the milk of dairy cows, following intake of aflatoxin B_1. This poses a great threat to the health of the human consumer.

Aflatoxins are highly toxic compounds, producing severe liver damage, and are among the most potent cancer-inducing agents known. They are highly dangerous compounds to humans, being active in only trace amounts (ppm). Because of their extreme toxicity, carcinogenicity, and widespread distribution, the control of aflatoxin residues in animal tissues intended for human consumption has assumed greater public health significance in recent years.

Aflatoxin Poisoning in Animals

Animal species vary in their susceptibility to aflatoxin poisoning. In general, poultry are most susceptible (aflatoxicosis was first identified in turkeys). The decreasing order of susceptibility across the species of domestic animals is ducklings (most susceptible), turkeys, chickens, pigs, dogs, calves, cows, and sheep. Young animals are usually more susceptible than older animals to the effects of aflatoxin. The adverse effects of aflatoxins on animals may assume one of three general forms depending on the level of intake:

1. Acute aflatoxicosis is due to severe liver damage. Death usually occurs following severe and extensive damage to the target organ, which for aflatoxins is the liver. All chemical signs and all postmortem changes are referable specifically to liver damage. Symptoms in acutely affected animals include hepatitis, jaundice, hemorrhaging, anemia, prolonged blood clotting time, and possibly convulsions.
2. Chronic aflatoxicosis is due to the effects of smaller amounts of aflatoxin over a prolonged period of time. In this form of the disease, the amount of liver damage is insufficient to cause immediate death, but owing to malfunctioning of the organ, marked unthriftiness and loss of production of the animals ensue. The chronic form is usually marked by weight loss, decreased feed efficiency, mild jaundice, and perhaps an increased susceptibility to infection caused by interference with the defense mechanisms (immune system) of the body.
3. Damage to the liver is the most outstanding pathologic change that occurs in animals poisoned by aflatoxins, and specific characteristic changes can be observed under the microscope in liver tissues taken from the dead animals. Insofar as the symptoms of the disease, and ultimately the cause of death, derive from the failure of liver function, a definitive diagnosis of death from aflatoxicosis can be made only by examination of the liver for characteristic aflatoxin-induced pathologic changes, coupled with the feed commensurate with toxicity or the induction of such lesions.

Reason for Tolerance Levels in Animal Feeds

Aflatoxins are notoriously toxic compounds to humans in trace amounts. As already stated, they are among the most potent carcinogens known. They bind to macromolecules, especially nucleic acids; they are antimitotic, mutagenic, immunosuppressive, and teratogenic. They are primarily hepatotoxins. They can persist in animal tissues for long periods and can be passed onto the consumer through the meat, or they could be excreted through the mammary gland and passed on to the consumer through the milk. About 2% of aflatoxin B_1 ingested by a cow appears in the milk as aflatoxin M_1. This M_1 is just as toxic and carcinogenic in humans as aflatoxin B_1. Most regulatory authorities are committed to the goal of maintaining the milk supply free of detectable aflatoxin residues (less than 0.1 ppb). This goal can be achieved only by limiting the aflatoxin level in animal feed to 20 ppb, and so the maximum permitted levels of aflatoxins in feedstuffs for cattle are set largely with a view to protecting the human consumer from unacceptable tissue residues in meat or milk because frequent intake of trace amounts in the food would present a serious health hazard to humans. Thus maximum aflatoxin levels of 10 to 20 ppb in animal feeds are designed with the consumer in mind; they are highly unlikely to produce toxic symptoms in animals at such low concentration in the diet.

In addition, most modern laboratory analytical techniques can now detect minute amounts of aflatoxins in feed (PPT, Charm II Test). Generally speaking, as these laboratory methods become more sensitive at detecting ever-decreasing amounts of aflatoxins, so in turn do national regulatory authorities tend to lower the acceptable threshold levels in feedstuffs. This is done with the aim of moving forward toward the ideal situation of "zero residues" in animal tissues for human consumption. Although modern laboratory analytical techniques can now detect aflatoxin at trace levels, it is

TABLE 8–9
SOME COMMON MOLDS

Genus	Species	Produces
Aspergillus	*flavus*	Aflatoxin
	parasiticus	Aflatoxin
	ochraceus	Ochratoxin
Penicillium	*notatum*	Antibiotic penicillin
	citrinum	Kidney toxin—citrinin
	roquefort	Blue cheese mold
Fusarium	*graminearum*	T_2 toxin/zearalenone
	moniliforme	6 severe toxins
	tricinctum	T_2 toxin

generally accepted scientifically that at this minute level, there may be a margin of error of ±50% in the analytical procedure, thus rendering the final figure subject to variation if repeat testing is carried out.

Another area of concern, from the point of view of public health, is the transfer of aflatoxins to the tissue of food animals and to the milk of cows consuming aflatoxin-containing feed. Residues of aflatoxin B_1 have been found in the liver and musculature of pigs given aflatoxin in the feed. Bacon pigs fed aflatoxin-contaminated feed contained sizable amounts of aflatoxin residue in their tissues on slaughter. The macroscopic appearance of these tissues and organs, however, was sufficiently good enough to allow them to pass meat inspection and thus be distributed for human consumption. Aflatoxin in dairy rations is transformed to an aflatoxin metabolite, aflatoxin M_1, in the cow's milk. This metabolite is as patent a carcinogen as the parent compound and produces local tumors on subcutaneous injection into rats.

Control

Mold inhibitors can be used to minimize the growth of *A. flavus* in the grain. 8–hydroxyquinoline (500 ppm); propionic acid (500–1500 ppm) and thiabendazole are useful mold suppressors. The main avenue of control is through correct grain storage and also routine aflatoxin feed (and residue) assays by sensitive tests, such as the CHARM II test.

Many other fungal species are capable of producing toxins having deleterious effects on animal tissues. Ochratoxin A is the major toxin of a group of related compounds produced by a species belonging to the *Aspergillus ochraceus* group of fungi. A number of the *Penicillium* species also produce the toxin. The occurrence of ochratoxin in naturally moldy substances is associated with the growth of *Penicillium viridicatum* and some other penicillin species. Some strains of *P. viridicatum* can produce both ochratoxin and also citrinim, another mycotoxin. In Denmark, a condition of porcine necropathy has been associated with feeds containing ochratoxin A and citrinin. Rats fed barley, experimentally contaminated with *P. viridicatum*, developed clinical and pathologic features similar to those seen with this mycotoxin, including hyaline degeneration and desquamation of the epithelial cells of the proximate convoluted tubules in the kidney. Nephrotoxicity in pigs associated with consumption of moldy barley has also been recognized. Ochratoxin A also has deleterious effects when fed to poultry. High mortality and morbidity, depression of body weight, and reduced egg production and feed efficiency have been recorded. Ochratoxin has been reported to cause embryotoxic effects in laboratory and domestic animals.

The rubratoxins are mycotoxins produced by the fungus *Penicillium rubrum* and *Penicillium purpurogenum*. They are potent hepatotoxic, hemorrhage-inducing mycotoxins that can frequently contaminate animal feeds. The fungus *Fusarium graminearum* produces a potent estrogenic substance called F-2 toxin or zearalenone.

There are many other fungi capable of producing potent mycotoxins, but because the list is expanding at an ever-increasing rate, it is not possible to mention them all. The major part of the mycotoxicosis problem remains obscure owing to the unspectacular nature of the effects of continuous low-level toxin consumption. Apart from the potential hazards to humans, the economic importance of chronic mycotoxin toxicity to the livestock industry of the United States is largely unknown. Thus for the veterinary practitioner, it might be a helpful reminder to reiterate useful diagnostic features that generally characterise outbreaks of mycotoxicoses: The toxicoses are not transmissible, drug or antibiotic treatments have little effects, outbreaks are often seasonal, the toxicosis is often associated with a specific food, and the suspected feed shows signs of fungal activity. Table 8–9 lists some common molds.

APPENDIX 8–1
CENTRAL NERVOUS SYSTEM EFFECTS

POISONS AND CENTRAL NERVOUS SYSTEM STIMULATION

Strychnine
Lead
Metaldehyde
Organophosphates and carbamates
Chlorinated hydrocarbons
Fluoroacetate (Monosodium)
Ethylene glycol
Phenols, rotenone, and various medicines in cats

POISONS AND CENTRAL NERVOUS SYSTEM DEPRESSION

Barbiturates
Valium/other sedatives
Alpha-chloralose
Ethylene glycol
Metaldehyde (?)
Paraquat
Selective weed-killers
Aspirin/paracetamol (cat)

SELECTED REFERENCES

Abdallah, A.H., and Tye, A.: A comparison of the efficacy of emetic drugs and stomach lavage. Am. J. Dis. Child., 113:571, 1967.

Abdelsalam, E.B.: Comparative effect of certain organophosphorus compounds and other chemicals on whole blood, plasma, and tissue cholinesterase activity in goats. Vet. Hum. Toxicol., 29:146, 1987.

Alden, C.L.: Japanese Yew poisoning in large domestic animals in the midwest. J. Am. Vet. Med. Assoc., 170:314, 1977.

Andrews, A.H.: Abnormal reactions and their frequency in cattle following the use of organophosphate warble fly dressings. Vet. Rec., 109:171, 1981.

Aphosian, H.V.: DMSA and DMPS. Water soluble antidotes for heavy metal poisoning. Ann. Rev. Pharmacol. Toxicol., 23:193, 1983.

Barton, J., and Oehme, F.W.: The incidence and characteristics of animal poisoning seen at Kansas State University from 1975 to 1980. Vet. Hum. Toxicol., 23:101, 1981.

Black, R.P.: Ethylene glycol intoxication. Feline Pract., 15:43, 1985.

Boehm, J.J., and Oppenheim, R.C.: An in vitro study of the absorption of various drugs, by activated charcoal. Aust. J. Pharm. Sci., 4:107, 1977.

Boermans, H.J.: Diagnosis of nitrate toxicosis in cattle using biological fluids and a rapid ion chromatographic method. Am. J. Vet. Res., 51:491, 1990.

Brown, S.A., Barsanti, J.A., and Cromwell, W.A.: Gentamicin associated acute renal failure in the dog. J. Am. Vet. Med. Assoc., 186:686, 1985.

Buck, W.B.: Bovine toxicology. Mod. Vet. Pract., 66:1001, 1985.

Buck, W.B.: Toxicology in bovine practice. Proceedings 13th World Congress on Diseases of Cattle. Durban, South Africa, 1984.

Buck, W.B., and Bratich, B.S.: Activated charcoal preventing unnecessary death by poisoning. Veterinary Medicine, 73, 1986.

Buck, W.B., and Bratich, P.M.: Experimental studies with activated charcoals and oils in preventing toxicoses. Am. Assn. Vet. Lab. Diag. 28th Ann. Proc., 1985.

Buck, W.B., et al.: Clinical and Diagnostic Veterinary Toxicology. 2nd ed. Dubuque, IA, Kendall/Hunt, 1976.

Carver, L.A., and Pfander, W.H.: Urea utilization by sheep in the presence of potassium nitrate. J. Am. Sci., 36:581, 1973.

Casteel, S.W., and Bailey, M.: Dealing with sudden death in cattle. Vet. Med., 78, 1986.

Casteel, S.W., and Carson, T.L.: Organophosphorous toxicosis in beef heifers. Mod. Vet. Pract., 81:945, 1984.

Casteel, S.W., and Cook, W.O.: Urea toxicosis in cattle. A dangerous and avoidable dietary problem. Vet. Med., 1523, 1984.

Cawley, G.D., and Collings, D.F.: Nitrate poisoning. Vet. Rec., 106:311, 1977.

Clemmons, R.M., Meyer, D.J., and Sundlof, S.F.: Correction of organophosphate-induced neuromuscular blockade by diphenhydramine. Am. J. Vet. Res., 45:2167, 1984.

Davis, L.E., and Westfall, B.A.: Species differences in biotransformation and excretion of salicylate. Am. J. Vet. Res., 33:1253, 1972.

Dial, S.M., Thrall, M.A., and Hamar, D.W.: 4-methylpyrazole as treatment for naturally acquired ethylene glycol intoxication in dogs. J. Am. Vet. Med. Assoc., 195:73, 1989.

Dougherty, R.W., Coburn, K.S., Cook, H.M., and Allison, M.J.: Preliminary study of appearance of endotoxin in circulatory system of sheep, and cattle after induced grain engorgment. Am. J. Vet. Res., 36:6, 1975.

Eckhoff, G.A.: Mechanisms of adverse drug reactions and interactions in veterinary medicine. J. Am. Vet. Med. Assoc., 176:1131, 1980.

El Bahri, L.: 4-Methyl pyrazole: An antidote for ethylene glycol intoxication in dogs. Comp. Cont. Educ. Vet. Pract., 13:1123, 1991.

Engelhardt, J.A., and Brown, S.A.: Drug related nephropathies. Part II. Commonly used drugs. Comp. Cont. Ed. Vet. Pract., 9:281, 1987.

Furr, A.A., and Carson, T.L.: Therapeutic measures used in the treatment of organophosphorous insecticide toxicosis in sheep. Vet. Toxicol., 17:121, 1975.

Grauer, G.F., Thrall, M.A., Henri, B.A., et al.: Early clinicopathologic findings in dogs ingesting ethylene glycol. Am. J. Vet. Res., 45:2599, 1984.

Greene, C.E.: Effects of aspirin and propranolol on feline platelet aggregation. Am. J. Vet. Res., 48:1820, 1985.

Gyrd Hansen, N., Rasmissen, F., and Smith, M.: Cardiovascular effects of intravenous administration of tetracycline in cattle. J. Vet. Pharmacol. Ther., 4:15, 1981.

Hewitt, G.R.: Vomiting and antiemetics in small animal practice. In Y. Ruckebush, P.C. Toutain, and C.D. Koritz. Veterinary Pharmacology and Toxicology. Boston, MTP Press, 1983.

Jenkins, W.L.: Pharmacological aspects of analgesic drugs in animals: An overview. J. Am. Vet. Med. Assoc., 191:1231, 1987.

Kaufman, G.: Aspirin-induced gastric mucosal injury: Lessons learned from animal models. Gastroenterology, 96:606, 1989.

Kyle, R., and Allen, W.M.: Accidental selenium poisoning of a flock of sheep. Vet. Rec., 126:601, 1990.

Lalonde, R.L., Deshponde, R., Hamilton, P.P., et al.: Acceleration of digoxin clearance by activated charcoal. Clin. Pharm. Ther., 37:367, 1985.

Levy, G.: Gastrointestinal clearance of drugs with activated charcoal. N. Engl. J. Med., 307:676, 1982.

Lloyd, W.E.: Chemical and Metabolic Aspects of Urea-Ammonia Toxicosis in Cattle and Sheep. Ph.D. Thesis, Iowa State University, Ames, 1970.

Maiti, S.K., Swarup, D., and Chandra, S.V.: Treatment of lead poisoning in goats with thiamine. Res. Vet. Sci., 48:377, 1990.

Malone, P.: Monensin sodium toxicity in cattle. Vet. Rec., *103*:21, 1978.

Meerdink, G.L.: Organophosphorus and carbamate insecticide poisoning in large animals. Vet. Clin. North Am. [Food Anim. Pract.] *5*:375, 1989.

Moncol, D.J., and Battle, E.G.: Cholinesterase activity in the normal blood of swine. Vet. Med. Small Anim. Clin., *59*:947, 1964.

Montgomery, R.D., and Pidgeon, G.L.: Levamisole toxicity in a dog. J. Am. Vet. Med. Assoc., *189*:684, 1986.

Muller, F.O., and Hundt, H.K.L.: Chronic organophosphate poisoning. S. African Med. J., *57*:344, 1980.

Ndiritu, C.G., and Enos, L.R.: Adverse reactions to drugs in a veterinary hospital. J. Am. Vet. Med. Assoc., *171*:335, 1977.

Neuvomen, P.J.: Clinical pharmacokinetics of oral activated charcoal in acute intoxications. Clin. Pharmacokinet., *7*:465, 1982.

Oehme, F.W.: *In* Current Veterinary Therapy VII. Small Animal Practice. Edited by R.W. Kirk. Philadelphia, W.B. Saunders, 1983.

Oehme, F.W.: Antifreeze ethylene glycol poisoning. *In* Current Veterinary Therapy VI. Edited by R.W. Kirk and F.W. Scott. Philadelphia, W.B. Saunders, 1977.

Osweiler, G.D.: Clinical and Diagnostic Veterinary Toxicology. 3rd ed. Dubuque, IA, Kendall Hunt, 1985.

Osweiler, G.D., and Ruhi, L.P.: Lead poisoning in feeder calves. J. Am. Vet. Med. Assoc., *172*:498, 1978.

Penumarthy, L., and Oehme, F.W.: Treatment of ethylene glycol toxicosis in cats. Am. J. Vet. Res., *36*:209, 1975.

Pierson, R.E.: Differential diagnosis of cattle exhibiting central nervous symptoms. Proceedings 14th Annual Meeting AABP, 1981.

Potter, E.L., Van Duyn, R.L., and Cooley, C.O.: Monensin toxicity in cattle. J. Anim. Sci., *58*:1499, 1984.

Rainsford, K.D.: Gastrointestinal damage from nonsteroidal antiinflammatory drugs. Toxicol. Pathol., *16*:251, 1988.

Rude, T.A.: Post vaccination type I hypersensitivity in cattle. Agric. Pract., *11*:29, 1990.

Ryhanen, R., Kajovaara, M., Harri, M. et al.: Physical exercise affects cholinesterases and organophosphate response. Gen. Pharmacol., *19*:815, 1988.

Slenning, B.P., Galey, F.D., and Anderson, M.: Forage related nitrate toxicosis possibly confounded by nonprotein nitrogen and monensin in the diet used at a commercial dairy heifer replacement operation. J. Am. Vet. Med. Assoc., *198*:867, 1991.

Stillman, M.T., Napier, J., and Blackshear, J.L.: Adverse effects of nonsteroidal antiinflammatory drugs on the kidney. Med. Clin. North Am., *86*:371, 1984.

Stowe, C.M.: Central nervous system intoxications other than lead. Vet. Clin. North Am. [Food Anim. Pract.], *3*:154, 1987.

Stowe, C.M.: Antimicrobial drug interactions. J. Am. Vet. Med. Assoc., *185*:1137, 1984.

Surber, E.: Common household toxicities in cats. Vet. Med. Small Anim. Clin., 535, 1983.

Vale, J.A., and Meredith, T.J.: Acute poisoning due to nonsteroidal antiinflammatory drugs. Clinical features and management. Med. Toxicol., *1*:12, 1966.

Vogt, M., Smith, A.D., and Fuenmayor, L.D.: Factors influencing the cholinesterases of cerebrospinal fluid in the anaesthetised cat. Neuroscience, *12*:979, 1984.

Wills, J.H.: The measurement and significance of changes in the cholinesterase activities of erythrocytes and plasma in man and animals. CRC Crit. Rev. Toxicol., *1*:153, 1972.

Yeary, R.A., and Brant, R.J.: Aspirin doses for the dog. J. Am. Vet. Med. Assoc., *167*:63, 1975.

Yeary, R.A., and Swanson, W.: Aspirin dosages for the cat. J. Am. Vet. Med. Assoc., *163*:1177, 1973.

9

BETA LACTAM ANTIBIOTICS

9.1 Introduction
9.2 Mechanism of Action
9.3 Beta-Lactamase Inhibition
9.4 Natural Penicillins
9.5 Extended-Spectrum Penicillins
9.6 Antipseudomonal Penicillins
9.7 Antistaphylococcal Penicillins
9.8 New Beta Lactams
9.9 Cephalosporins
9.10 First-Generation Cephalosporins
9.11 Second-Generation Cephalosporins
9.12 Third-Generation Cephalosporins
9.13 Kinetics
9.14 Cephalosporin Therapy

9.1 INTRODUCTION

The beta lactam antibiotics include penicillins, cephalosporins, monobactams, and carbapenems. All have a beta lactam ring, which is essential for antibacterial activity. In general, these agents have favorable ratios of therapeutic to toxic effects, and the newer agents have enhanced antibacterial spectrums or favorable pharmacokinetic characteristics. They are the most widely used antimicrobial drugs in veterinary practice.

The drugs in this class are chemically similar in that each contains a beta lactam ring, which is responsible for the antibacterial activity. Additions to or substitutions in the beta lactam compound change the disposition and spectrum of activity of individual drugs. The rapid development of resistance limits the spectrum of activity of some beta lactam antibiotics. All of these drugs are bactericidal against gram-positive microorganisms.

The discovery of penicillin nucleus (6-aminopenicillanic acid) ushered in the era of semisynthetic penicillin chemistry that has provided veterinary medicine with the isoxazolyl (e.g., cloxacillin) and aminopenicillins (e.g., ampicillin and amoxicillin). In the penicillins, the beta lactam ring is fused to a five-membered thiazolidine ring. Most of the newer penicillins are modifications of ampicillin. Substitution of a carboxy group for the amino group of ampicillin on the acyl side chain produced carbenicillin and ticarcillin. The substitution of this acidic side group in these compounds decreased binding to penicillin-binding proteins (PBPs) of *Streptococcus faecalis*, thereby decreasing activity against this organism. There was more activity, however, against gram-negative rods, including *Pseudomonas aeruginosa*, partly because of increased penetration of the drug through the bacterial cell wall. Substitution of ureido groups (-NH-C-O-N-R2) for the carboxy group produced the ureido penicillins—piperacillin, azlocillin, and mezlocillin—which maintained ampicillin's activity against *S. faecalis* and *Streptococcus faecium* and increased its activity against gram-negative bacilli and anaerobes by means of greater penetration through bacterial cell walls and greater affinity for penicillin receptors.

Many penicillins have been developed and are classified as natural penicillins, semisynthetic penicillins such as beta-lactamase-resistant penicillins, broad-spectrum penicillins (aminopenicillins), and antipseudomonal and extended-spectrum penicillins. Some of the newer extended-spectrum penicillins, which are derivatives of amipicillin, include piperacillin, azlocillin, and mezlocillin. These have increased activity against *Klebsiella, Pseudomonas aeruginosa,* and *Serratia*. The great expense of these agents, however, and lack of information on their pharmacokinetics argue against their use. Other semisynthetic penicillins have such therapeutic features as increased resistance to acid, less binding to serum protein, resistance to digestion by beta-lactamases, and a broad spectrum of antibacterial action.

The carboxy penicillins, carbenicillin and ticarcillin, and the ureido penicillins, piperacillin, mezlocillin, and azlocillin, are considered extended-spectrum penicillins because they inhibit a variety of aerobic gram-negative bacilli, including *P. aeruginosa*. Extended-spectrum penicillins are susceptible to staphylococcal beta-lactamases and are not reliable for treating staphylococcal disease. They are less active than penicillin and ampicillin against most gram-positive organisms except that the ureido penicillins inhibit enterococci to a degree comparable to that achieved with ampicillin.

Ticarcillin is two to four times more active than carbenicillin against *P. aeruginosa*. Piperacillin is more potent than ticarcillin against *P. aeruginosa* and *Klebsiella* but has activity similar to that of ticarcillin against most other gram-negative pathogens. Azlocillin is as active as piperacillin against *P. aeruginosa* but is less active against most other gram-negative organisms. Mezlocillin is similar to ticarcillin in regard to antimicrobial spectrum, but it has more activity against *Klebsiella*. Extended-spectrum penicillins are often more susceptible to beta-lactamases produced by gram-negative bacteria than are third-generation cephalosporins. All extended-spectrum penicillins are highly active against anaerobes.

9.2 MECHANISM OF ACTION

The beta lactam antibiotics, which include penicillins and cephalosporins, alone or combined with clavulanic acid or sulbactam, are bactericidal. They disrupt the bacterial cell wall by binding to a variety of proteins, which are responsible for cell wall synthesis. Interference with these proteins results in death and lysis of bacterial cells.

Beta-lactam antibiotics bind to and inactivate specific targets on the inner surface of the bacterial cell membrane, the PBPs. The PBPs are enzymes (transpeptidases, carboxypeptidases, and endopeptidases) that are involved in the terminal stages of assembling the bacterial cell wall and in reshaping the cell wall during growth and division. Beta-lactam compounds have different affinities for the various PBPs and, depending on the specific PBP bound, have different effects on bacteria. The inactivation of some PBPs causes bacterial cell death. Binding of PBPs causes inhibition of cell wall peptidoglycan synthesis and might activate bacterial autolytic enzymes. The peptidoglycan component of the cell wall is essential to the integrity of the bacterial envelope. It consists of alternating units of *N*-acetylglucosamine and *N*-acetylmuramic acid cross linked by short strands of peptides. As the peptidoglycan layer is synthesized, a series of long, threadlike molecules is assembled.

Cross linking of the threads to form a netlike protective structure (the transpeptidation reaction) significantly strengthens the peptidoglycan layer. The primary action of beta lactam antibiotics is to inhibit cross linking by binding to a set of PBPs responsible for transpeptidation. The cell wall subsequently weakens. As the bacteria continue to grow, they rupture because of high internal osmotic pressure. Because peptidoglycans are not a component of any other cell, these antimicrobial drugs are examples of selectively toxic drugs. Bacterial cell death is not due to direct action of these drugs but to lysis of drug-induced, defective cell walls of susceptible bacteria. They rupture because of their intracellular hypertonicity relative to that of the surrounding microenvironment. Treated, susceptible bacteria in an environment that is isotonic, relative to their intracellular osmotic pressure, continue to exist in the form of protoplasts or spheroplasts. Penicillins are structural analogs of D-alanyl-D-alanine and exert their action by binding with high affinity to PBPs in the bacterial cell membrane. Several of these proteins have been identified as enzymes (primarily transpeptidase) involved with the cross-linking process of cell wall formation. Because of the analogy of penicillins to D-alanyl-D-alanine, the transpeptidase enzyme is inactivated with subsequent failure of the cross-linkage reactions that it catalyzes. Some of the PBPs are important in the production and cross linking of the peptidoglycan layer (e.g., transpeptidases), functioning either to form the septum between dividing organisms or to elongate the cell walls during growth of the bacteria. Other PBPs act as beta-lactamases to cleave the beta lactam ring, thereby inactivating penicillins and cephalosporins.

The activity of each beta lactam antibiotic depends on its ability to bind to one of the PBPs that form or maintain cell wall structure while avoiding the destructive PBPs. The beta-lactamases are generally secreted extracellularly in large amounts by gram-positive bacteria, whereas relatively small quantities of beta-lactamases are strategically produced in the periplasmic space in gram-negative bacteria for optimal protection of the organisms. Although the genetic coding for beta-lactamases is located principally on plasmids of staphylococci and can be induced by substrates, the beta-lactamases found in gram-negative bacteria are encoded either in plasmids or chromosomes and may be constitutive or inducible. The plasmid-mediated beta-lactamases of gram-negative bacteria (e.g., *Escherichia coli, Enterobacter, Proteus, Shigella, P. aeruginosa, Haemophilus,* and *Klebsiella*) are effective in destroying both penicillins and cephalosporins, whereas the chromosomally mediated beta-lactamases, with the exception of *Klebsiella*, are specific for penicillins (*Proteus mirabilis* and *Proteus morganii*) or cephalosporins (*P. aeruginosa, Bacteroides fragilis,* indole-positive *Proteus, Escherichia coli,* and *Enterobacter*).

For a beta-lactam antibiotic to be effective against gram-negative organisms, it must first penetrate the lipopolysaccharide outer membrane of the cell wall. Penetration is often accomplished through porins. Once the antimicrobial is inside either a gram-negative or gram-positive organism, it must then combine with PBPs on the inner cell membranes, while avoiding destruction by enzymes known as beta-lactamases. These enzymes exist in the periplasmic space between the cell wall and the cell membrane and are capable of hydrolyzing and inactivating beta lactam antibiotics.

The activity of beta lactam antibiotics against gram-negative bacteria also relates to the rate at which the antibiotic is able to penetrate the outer membranes. Antibiotics that penetrate rapidly have greater antibacterial activity. The addition of an aminobenzyl side chain to penicillin to form ampicillin increases the penetration of ampicillin over penicillin G and improves the activity against gram-negative bacteria. The addition of a hydroxyl group to the aminobenzyl group to form amoxicillin permits even greater penetration through the outer layer. This results in the reported increased efficacy of amoxicillin over ampicillin for some gram-negative organisms.

Penetration is achieved more easily in gram-positive than in gram-negative bacterial cells. Gram-positive organisms have a thin outer layer exterior to the peptidoglycan layer, and beta lactam antibiotics rapidly enter to the site of antibacterial activity. The lipopolysaccharide and lipoprotein outer membranes of gram-negative bacteria present a more difficult barrier to entry by antibiotics. The production of an impermeable outer membrane is a major mechanism of resistance for some gram-negative bacteria, for example, *Pseudomonas*. Similarly, the success of certain beta lactam antibiotics lies in their ability to pass through the outer wall pore proteins and enter the bacterial periplasmic space.

Alterations in the binding characteristics of PBPs for beta lactam compounds may result in the development of resistance, and such changes have been demonstrated in *E. coli, S. faecium, Haemophilus influenzae, Streptococcus pneumoniae*, and methicillin-resistant *Staphylococcus aureus*. The most important mechanism of bacterial resistance to the beta lactam antibiotics is bacterial production of beta-lactamases, enzymes that hydrolyze the cyclic amide bond of the beta lactam ring and render it inactive. Beta-lactamases are made by many gram-positive and gram-negative organisms and are encoded either chromosomally or extrachromosomally by means of plasmids or transposons. The ease of transfer of the plasmids and transposons plays a leading part in the spread of antibiotic resistance from one bacterial strain to another.

9.3 BETA-LACTAMASE INHIBITION

Overcoming bacterial resistance caused by beta-lactamase production has taken two directions. One approach is to modify the beta lactam nucleus to produce an antibiotic that is stable in the presence of beta-lactamase, such as cloxacillin. Although this has been successful, the spectrum of activity has been sacrificed to produce a beta-lactamase-stable antibiotic. The alternate approach is to find a substance that can inhibit beta-lactamase enzymes, thereby protecting penicillin or cephalosporin from destruction by beta-lactamase. A number of inhibitors with therapeutic potential have been described: 6-halopenicillanic acid, 6-acetyl methylene penicillanic acid, penicillanic acid sulfone, and the naturally occurring compounds (clavulanic acid, olivanic acids, and thienzmycin). Beta-lactamase inhibitors, such as clavulanic acid and sulbactam, resemble penicillin structurally and enhance the in vitro activity of certain beta lactam antibiotics by protecting them from hydrolysis by beta-lactamases. They are termed "suicide inhibitors" because they bind to and inactivate bacterial beta-lactamases but are destroyed in the process.

The ideal beta-lactamase inhibitor should be active against a wide range of beta-lactamases; pharmacologically it should match closely its antibiotic partner, and enzyme inactivation should be irreversible. Clavulanic acid and sulbactam (penicillanic acid sulfone) have been evaluated and meet these criteria. Both possess beta lactam structure, have minimal antibacterial effects on their own, and are capable of inhibiting beta-lactamase enzymes. The beta lactam ring of clavulanic acid binds irreversibly with the beta-lactamase enzyme and prevents inactivation. Clavulanic acid is an ideal example of this group. It is a potent, irreversible inhibitor of beta-lactamase of staphylococci and many gram-negative bacteria. It closely matches its antibiotic partners, especially amoxicillin, and has little antibacterial activity of its own that might interfere with the action of the intended primary antibiotic. The minimum inhibitory concentration required for amoxicillin is markedly reduced when used with cloxacillin against beta-lactamase-producing isolates. Clavulanic acid's wide range of effectiveness makes it a useful potentiator of many penicillins.

Clavulanic acid is a fermentation product of the actinomycete *Streptomyces clavuligerus*. Although its chemical structure contains a beta lactam ring, it has scant inherent antibacterial activity. It does, however, possess a strong affinity for a broad range of beta-lactamases, including the enzymes active against amoxicillin. When beta-lactamase is encountered intracellularly or extracellularly, a chemical complex is formed, effectively preventing the beta-lactamase from destroying the accompanying amoxicillin. Clavulanic acid has little inherent antibacterial activity. The minimal inhibitory concentration (MIC) of amoxicillin for beta-lactamase-producing human isolates is markedly decreased in the presence of clavulanic acid, whereas the MIC of non-beta-lactamase-producing organisms is not. The same is true for beta-lactamase-producing veterinary isolates. The inhibitory spectrum of clavulanic acid is excellent, making it a useful potentiator of many penicillins. The enhanced antibacterial activity produced by this protective effect includes organisms that might have acquired their resistance and those that are historically resistant.

The use of two beta lactam antibiotics together might permit one antibiotic to bind to PBPs and injure bacteria, while the other is typing up beta-lactamase. Clavulanic acid, which is a noncompetitive inhibitor of many beta-lactamase enzymes, has been marketed in combination with amoxicillin (Synulox) and with ticarcillin to employ this strategy. Clavulanic acid effectively extends the spectrum of amoxicillin to include beta-lactamase-positive staphylococci and many gram-negative bacteria. One study showed that in 346 staphylococcal isolates from canine and feline clinical cases, 50% were resistant to amoxicillin, but 97.7% of the isolates were sensitive to amoxicillin combined with clavulanic acid. The combination is formulated in a ratio of 4:1 of amoxicillin to clavulate. Both agents share similar pharmacokinetic properties, and the concentration achieved in the serum for each drug

parallels the interstitial fluid concentration, maintaining an optimal ratio of antibacterial activity.

Clavulanic acid in a fixed combination with ticarcillin (Timentin, 3 g of ticarcillin and 100 mg of clavulanic acid) increases the activity of ticarcillin against 60 to 80% of ticarcillin-resistant strains of *Enterobacteriaceae*, beta-lactamase-producing strains of *H. influenzae* and *S. aureus*, and *Bacteroides*. No increased activity is provided against *P. aeruginosa*. The combination, given intravenously every 4 to 6 hours, is more useful than ticarcillin for treating infections in which *S. aureus*, beta-lactamase-producing, aerobic gram-negative bacilli are implicated.

Sulbactam is also an excellent example of this class of drugs because it is an irreversible beta-lactamase inhibitor yet provides no useful antibiotic activity. Its main difference when compared with clavulanic acid is the twofold to fivefold decrease in potency. Sulbactam is a semisynthetic beta-lactamase inhibitor with activity against a broad range of beta-lactamases, including those produced by *Bacteroides, Haemophilus, Klebsiella, E. coli*, and *Neisseria gonorrhoeae*. It is currently available as a parenteral preparation in combination with ampicillin. Similar to clavulanic acid, sulbactam alone has limited antibacterial activity; however, the combination of sulbactam and ampicillin is effective against bacteria that otherwise would be resistant. The recommended dose in cattle is 6.6 mg/kg (of the ampicillin) once daily. Susceptibility studies have proved Synergistin to be effective against ampicillin/penicillin-resistant *Pasteurella haemolytica, Pasteurella multocida*, and *S. aureus*.

Sulbactam shares many of the features of clavulanic acid: lack of clinically useful antibacterial activity, irreversible enzyme inhibition, and a similar inhibitory spectrum. Sulbactam, however, is considerably less potent, particularly in relation to the clinically important *E. coli* beta-lactamases. Combining ampicillin with sulbactam may help overcome infections caused by ampicillin-resistant *Pasteurella*.

9.4 NATURAL PENICILLINS

Natural penicillins (e.g., penicillin G, penicillin V, and phenethicillin) were some of the original penicillins produced. They have a limited range of activity and are highly susceptible to beta-lactamases, which are produced by many staphylococci and gram-negative bacteria. They are also inactivated by gastric acid. These are efficacious only against gram-positive bacteria.

Benzylpenicillin (penicillin G) remains the most commonly used beta lactam antibiotic for large and small animals. Giving penicillin G is confined to parenteral routes with procaine penicillin G (a poorly soluble aqueous suspension) or sodium and potassium penicillin G (highly soluble forms of crystalline penicillin). Penicillin G in either form is hydrolyzed rapidly in the acid of the stomach and the abomasum and should not be given orally. Sodium and potassium penicillins are the only forms given intravenously.

Procaine penicillin G prolongs the plasma concentrations of penicillin G over the sodium and potassium salts but at lower levels. Long-acting benzathine penicillin produces prolonged plasma concentrations because of its slow absorption; however, it produces low serum concentrations.

Penicillin G should not be administered orally because it is unstable in stomach acid. Parenteral formulations of sodium and potassium penicillin G are water soluble and achieve rapid but short-lived (half-life is 30 minutes) peak plasma concentrations.

Procaine and benzathine penicillins are repository preparations of penicillin G. They have low solubility and, following intramuscular or subcutaneous administration, attain plasma concentrations that persist for 24 hours (procaine penicillin) and 72 hours (benzathine penicillin). The concentrations achieved with benzathine penicillin are too low to result in therapeutic effectiveness for infections in small animals.

Penicillin V (phenoxymethyl penicillin) resists degradation by stomach acid and is available in various tablet formulations. Penicillin V is not routinely used in small animals because other beta lactams (e.g., ampicillin, amoxicillin) that have a broader spectrum have become popular.

Aqueous, crystalline penicillin G (K^+ or Na^+ penicillin G) should be used when a rapid effect and high plasma penicillin concentrations are required. High concentrations of short duration are achieved with intravenous administration. The intra-muscular route results in lower plasma concentrations of longer duration.

Procaine penicillin G is formulated only for intramuscular administration and relatively slow absorption. Serum concentrations must be maintained to ensure adequate extravascular diffusion. Benzathine penicillin G provides slower absorption from the intramuscular infection site and relatively low peak serum concentrations.

Beta lactam antibiotics are polar antibiotics and in general have volumes of distribution that are approximately equal to extracellular body water. They are able to achieve concentrations in tissue fluids (bone, bile, soft tissue, peritoneum) that are adequate to kill or inhibit susceptible bacteria. They are generally excluded from the prostate, cerebrospinal fluid, and aqueous humor. Because they do not readily enter cells, they are not effective for treating intracellular infections.

Distribution of penicillin antibiotics is limited to extracellular fluids, although inflammation may enhance their distribution into target tissues. Except for ampicillin, penicillins undergo minimal hepatic metabolism. Most are cleared from the plasma primarily by renal excretion. Both glomerular filtration and tubular secretion are important in their elimination.

Penicillins are actively transported in kidney, brain, and liver. Secretion of penicillins by the renal tubules results in high urine concentrations and rapid elimination from the body, so the soluble salts of benzylpenicillin (the most rapidly excreted of the group) maintain effective plasma levels for only 4 hours, hence the wide use of depot preparations, such as the insoluble procaine salt.

The penicillins all attain adequate plasma levels after injection. Following oral administration, benzyl penicillin G is largely inactivated in the gut and not absorbed. This is due to the action of gastric acid and beta-lactamase enzymes produced by microorganisms of the normal gut flora. The improved semisynthetic penicillins, ampicillin, cloxacillin, and phenoxymethyl penicillin, however, are stable to acid and in some cases also resist the action of beta-lactamase and so are better absorbed from the gut. Similar to most other antibiotics, penicillin diffuses freely from the capillaries so the effective concentration in the tissue fluid is similar to that in the plasma. It achieves effective concentrations at inflammatory foci, but it has limited ability to cross physiologic barriers. It does not for practical purposes diffuse well into brain tissue, into the internal structures of the eye, or across serous membranes, such as the pleura paritneum or joint capsules. Accordingly it is not of great use in the treatment of infections in these locations. In general, penicillin does not diffuse well, does not enter liver cells, is not metabolized, and is excreted unchanged in the urine. Penicillin is rapidly excreted by the kidney both by tubular secretion and by glomerular filtration. This accounts for its high concentration in urine and rapid elimination from the blood. In fact, the soluble salts of benzyl penicillin maintain effective plasma levels for only 4 hours, hence the widespread usage of depot preparations of the insoluble procaine salt. These maintain effective blood levels for 24 hours. With regard to dosage, because penicillin has little or no inherent toxicity for the animal and is relatively inexpensive, dosages are limited only by what the practitioner thinks is required. High plasma levels help the diffusion of penicillin into areas of difficult access by simple mass action, and high doses tend to delay the appearance of resistant forms of bacteria.

Another reason to administer high doses of penicillin is that penicillin generally crosses cell membranes poorly and may be difficult to get to the sites where its action is required. Thus there can be problems in attaining useful levels of penicillin in joint cavities, pleural and peritoneal cavities, and cerebrospinal fluid. It may be helpful under some circumstances, to administer penicillin directly into the affected area.

Because penicillin binds irreversibly to the PBP, the antibacterial action of penicillin persists for a period after plasma levels of the drug decline. For this reason, penicillin is one of the few antibiotics for which one can let blood levels drop below a MIC for a period during therapy safely. Although this practice is not recommended, it is helpful to know that one has this extra margin of safety with penicillin.

Penicillin G is generally active against both aerobic and anaerobic gram-positive organisms and, with few exceptions, is inactive against most gram-negative organisms in usual therapeutic concentrations. Penicillin G is active against most streptococci, although these bacteria rarely cause infections in dogs and cats with the frequency that they do in humans. Enteric streptococci generally develop resistance to penicillin, but a synergistic effect occurs with the combination of penicillin and an aminoglycoside (e.g., gentamicin, tobramycin, amikacin) or rifampin.

Penicillin has good activity against all anaerobic bacteria except beta-lactamase-producing strains of *Bacteroides*. Penicillin is not a good choice to treat staphylococcal infections because these bacteria commonly produce beta-lactamase.

Therapy with amoxicillin and ampicillin, the most commonly used beta lactams in practice, is indicated for a variety of gram-positive, gram-negative, and anaerobic organisms. Because the drugs are eliminated essentially unchanged in the urine, they are particularly useful in treating urinary tract infections. These drugs are also effective against infections of the respiratory tract and skin.

9.5 EXTENDED-SPECTRUM PENICILLINS

The isolation of the penicillin nucleus 6-amino penicillanic acid provided chemists with a substance that was to be the starting point for the synthesis of the large number of new penicillins, which, while maintaining the nontoxic advantage of penicillin, extended the range of antibacterial activity to cover both gram-positive and gram-negative activity. The new structures produced the following advantages:

1. Stability in acid media and improved oral absorption
2. Protection against the attack of beta-lactamase-producing staphylococci
3. Gram-negative activity against such organisms as *E. coli*, *Salmonella*, and *Proteus*, at relatively low levels
4. Activity against *P. aeruginosa*

A defect of penicillin G was its low degree of activity against many gram-negative organisms, such as *E. coli* and *Salmonella*. The development of ampicillin, then amoxicillin, revolutionized the position of penicillins in the field of antibiotic therapy. They became important members of the broad-spectrum group of drugs used for a wide range of therapy in humans and animals.

The broad-spectrum penicillins (e.g., ampicillin, amoxicillin, and hetacillin) are an important group of drugs owing to their activity against both gram-positive and some gram-negative organisms. They are, however, susceptible to beta-lactamase. This group is stable in gastric acid and therefore effective orally.

AMINOPENICILLINS

Aminopenicillins (ampicillin, amoxicillin, hetacillin) differ from penicillin G in that they can be absorbed orally and can penetrate the outer layer of gram-negative bacteria more readily, which increases the activity against many gram-negative pathogens. Their activity against susceptible gram-positive bacteria is essentially similar to that of penicillin G.

Amoxicillin and ampicillin have equal activity, but amoxicillin is absorbed better orally and has more rapid action. Hetacillin is inactive *per se*, it is a pro-drug, but is more stable in gastric acid than amoxicillin and ampicillin, and therefore it is absorbed best. After it enters the circulation, it is metabolized to ampicillin and becomes active. Amoxicillin and ampicillin are two of the most widely used penicillins because of their wide range of activity. Amoxicillin and ampicillin are classified as broad-spectrum antibiotics because they are effective against a variety of gram-positive and gram-negative organisms. They are also extremely effective against most anaerobic organisms except for *Bacteroides fragilis*, which produces beta-lactamases. Because aminopenicillins are sensitive to beta-lactamases, combining them with clavulanic acid or sulbactam markedly reduces their MICs for a number of microbial organisms.

Ampicillin was the first of the broad-spectrum penicillins. It is active against gram-positive and gram-negative bacteria. It is not active against beta-lactamase-producing staphylococci nor against *Pseudomonas*, *Klebsiella* and indole-positive *Proteus*. Ampicillin is stable to gastric acid. It was marketed in 1961 and has remained one of the most widely used semisynthetic penicillins. The forms of injectable ampicillin available are the trihydrate and sodium salts. Sodium ampicillin can be given intramuscularly or intravenously to achieve rapid plasma concentrations. The sodium salt of ampicillin is highly water soluble and is ideal for injection, but it must be reconstituted by the clinician before use and is not stable for long once it is made up. The aqueous suspension, ampicillin trihydrate, is poorly water soluble and cannot be given intravenously but has a prolonged shelf life once it is reconstituted. Ampicillin trihydrate is absorbed slowly from an intramuscular injection and produces prolonged plasma concentrations but at a lower peak.

When given intravenously, the sodium salt produces relatively high serum levels of short duration. When given intramuscularly, it produces much higher blood levels than the trihydrate salt but persists for a slightly shorter period. Sodium ampicillin has a half-life of 93 minutes after intravenous injection and 124 minutes after intramuscular injection in horses. At recommended doses, the serum concentration of sodium ampicillin peaks at 6.1 $\mu g/ml$ after intramuscular injection and 11.9 $\mu g/ml$ after intravenous injection. At a similar dosage, the peak serum concentration of ampicillin trihydrate may not exceed 1 $\mu g/ml$.

Intramuscular injection of ampicillin trihydrate in cattle at recommended levels results in peak blood levels within 1 hour. Blood levels are detectable for 24 hours. Ampicillin trihydrate produces local reactions at the site of intramuscular injection and lower serum ampicillin concentrations than does sodium ampicillin. The erratic absorption of ampicillin trihydrate may be related to the concentration of the injected product and site of injection. The relatively low serum concentrations of ampicillin produced by ampicillin trihydrate limit its usefulness against systemic infections. Ampicillin is primarily eliminated, and achieves very high concentrations, in urine. Therefore the trihydrate salt may be of value in the treatment of urinary tract infections caused by organisms that would be insusceptible if present in other tissues.

Most of the oral ampicillin available today is in the trihydrate form. About 35% of an oral dose is absorbed, with a half-life of

60 minutes in dogs. Most of the ampicillin is excreted in the urine, as with the other penicillins. Ampicillin is also excreted in the bile to a minor extent and undergoes enterohepatic circulation.

Because the absorption of oral ampicillin is not complete, one line of development has been preparation of ampicillin derivatives that are more readily absorbed and that can be metabolized to yield ampicillin. The first attempt in this direction was hetacillin, but it proved to be discouraging because its absorption was at best only equal to ampicillin. Hetacillin is produced by a reaction of ampicillin with acetone. The compound itself is inactive and must be hydrolyzed to ampicillin and acetone by the body.

Three esters of ampicillin are available: pivampicillin, becampicillin, and talampicillin. All three have greater absorption and produce higher blood levels than ampicillin.

Amoxicillin has an identical antibacterial spectrum to ampicillin. It, however, shows four significant advantages:

1. Amoxicillin can easily be made into a palatable oral tablet.
2. Amoxicillin gives 50 to 100% higher blood levels than ampicillin after oral administration.
3. Amoxicillin has a different and much faster bactericidal action.
4. There is evidence in humans that amoxicillin penetrates some tissues better than ampicillin, for example, sputum in chronic bronchitis.

Amoxicillin is formed by modifying ampicillin. Amoxicillin differs chemically from ampicillin by the addition of a hydroxyl group to the aminobenzyl side chain. Amoxicillin reportedly has increased activity against certain gram-negative bacteria: It also has the advantage of high bioavailability when given orally in preruminant calves, pigs, and small animals.

In contrast to the esters of ampicillin, amoxicillin is a biologically distinct, active compound and need not be converted in vivo to ampicillin. When given orally, amoxicillin is absorbed twice as well as ampicillin in dogs and reaches peak serum levels double those obtained with ampicillin. Amoxicillin trihydrate is available as an injectable formulation for use in most species,

and amoxicillin in combination with clavulanic acid is available for small animal patients. With few exceptions, however, amoxicillin, alone or in combination, is of limited application in horses. Food can impair absorption of ampicillin, but not amoxicillin. Equivalent doses of amoxicillin and ampicillin may yield up to twice the plasma drug concentration of amoxicillin compared with ampicillin. Hetacillin is a prodrug form of ampicillin. It was designed to enhance the availability of ampicillin because it is metabolized to ampicillin after oral administration.

Ampicillin, hetacillin, and amoxicillin have antibacterial activity against the gram-positive organisms sensitive to penicillin G. They are known as broad-spectrum penicillins owing to their additional activity against many gram-negative pathogens. The in vitro antibacterial spectrum of these three compounds essentially is the same, with almost complete cross resistance between them. Both in vivo and in vitro studies, however, have shown amoxicillin to have much more rapid and complete bactericidal activity.

Amoxicillin is slightly less active than penicillin against gram-positive bacteria but is more active against *S. faecalis*. Its outstanding property is activity four to eight times greater than that of penicillin against gram-negative bacilli.

The administration of aminopenicillins offers no advantage over penicillin G for treating staphylococci (except for oral absorption) because they are equally susceptible to beta-lactamase. If one is treating a nonenteric streptococcal infection, ampicillin and amoxicillin are excellent choices. Hetacillin is rapidly hydrolyzed to ampicillin and acetone after ingestion and should be considered equal to ampicillin.

Ampicillin and later amoxicillin have proved to be ideal broad-spectrum penicillins for treating the range of gram-positive and gram-negative organisms that attack both domestic and farm animals. As in human therapy, both ampicillin and amoxicillin have one disadvantage in that inactivation by beta-lactamase-producing *E. coli* and staphylococci can inhibit their effectiveness in certain disease problems. Because of the recognition of this problem, a continual search was made for inhibitors of the enzyme beta-lactamase.

9.6 ANTIPSEUDOMONAL PENICILLINS

Antipseudomonal penicillins are the so-called fourth generation of penicillins. They include dicarboxylic derivatives and ureidopenicillins. The dicarboxylic derivatives are carbenicillin and ticarcillin disodium. The ureidopenicillins are mezlocillin sodium, azlocillin sodium, and piperacillin sodium.

Antipseudomonal penicillins (e.g., carbenicillin and ticarcillin) are more active against *Pseudomonas* and some anaerobes. They are inactivated by beta-lactamases and gastric acid. Their activity is increased when aminoglycoside antibiotics are also given.

Extended-spectrum (antipseudomonal) penicillins, such as carbenicillin and ticarcillin, inhibit a greater variety of gram-negative organisms than the aminopenicillins (including *Pseudomonas*), but their gram-positive spectrum is limited. Ticarcillin is more effective than carbenicillin against *P. aeruginosa*. Both antibiotics are susceptible to beta-lactamases, but ticarcillin is available in combination with clavulanic acid. Their activity against *Pseudomonas* results from their ability to enter the so-called impenetrable cell wall of *Pseudomonas* and bind to PBPs in the periplasmic space. Carbenicillin and ticarcillin are not resistant to beta-lactamase enzymes and are less effective than penicillin G for killing susceptible gram-positive organisms.

The antipseudomonal penicillins are synergistic with aminoglycosides, and some practitioners give an aminoglycoside (e.g., gentamicin sulfate) concurrently with carbenicillin or ticarcillin.

CARBENICILLIN

Carbenicillin was introduced to human medicine 6 years after ampicillin was marketed. Carbenicillin offers a greater spectrum of activity against gram-negative organisms than ampicillin and has excellent activity against *Pseudomonas*. Although the MICs for carbenicillin against *Pseudomonas* are relatively high, its low toxicity allows administration of doses large enough to reach inhibitory levels. The proper dosage should be given to lessen development of resistant bacterial strains. Carbenicillin is available for intravenous or intramuscular use in humans as disodium salt.

After intramuscular administration, peak blood levels are obtained within 1 to 2 hours; the half-life is about 1 hour in humans. Because carbenicillin is not absorbed from the gastrointestinal tract, oral forms of the drug were developed. Carbenicillin indanyl sodium and the phenyl ester carfecillin are both well absorbed when given orally, resulting in high levels in the urine.

Oral carbenicillin is particularly suited for treatment of cystitis caused by *P. aeruginosa, E. coli, Proteus* (indole positive and negative, including ampicillin-resistant strains), *S. faecalis*, and *Enterobacter/Citrobacter*. It is not active against penicillinase-producing staphylococci or *Klebsiella*. Studies conducted in dogs indicate that oral carbenicillin may have limited application in systemic diseases other than urinary tract infections owing to the relatively low peak blood levels. Although carbenicillin is absorbed orally if given as the indanyl form, therapeutic drug concentrations may not be achieved.

Carbenicillin has an antibacterial spectrum similar to that of ampicillin with the addition of certain strains of *P. aeruginosa*, indole-positive *Proteus*, and *Enterobacter*. *Klebsiella* and penicillinase-producing *S. aureus* are not susceptible to carbenicillin. This drug should be reserved for infections caused by organisms that are resistant to other drugs. Concurrent use of gentamicin may be advocated in severe infections caused by *Pseudomonas*, but those two drugs should not be mixed in the same syringe.

Ticarcillin is similar to carbenicillin but has more activity against *P. aeruginosa*. Frequent administration may be necessary for the treatment of infections caused by *P. aeruginosa*. This extended-spectrum antibiotic is usually reserved for treatment of serious gram-negative infections (i.e., *Pseudomonas*); it is also available in combination with clavulanic acid.

Ticarcillin is not absorbed from the gastrointestinal tract and must be given intravenously or intramuscularly to obtain systemic levels. Peak serum concentrations of 46 μg/lb occur within 1 to 2 hours of intramuscular injection at 20 mg/lb in horses. As with carbenicillin, the MICs for many strains of *Pseudomonas* are relatively high, but ticarcillin's low toxicity allows the administration of doses large enough to reach inhibitory levels. As with the other penicillins, ticarcillin is eliminated by glomerular filtration and tubular secretion. It is not highly bound to serum protein (about 45% in humans) and is excreted unchanged in high concentrations in the urine.

Clinical research indicates that ticarcillin is effective against both gram-positive and gram-negative organisms causing equine endometritis, at a dose of 6 g by intrauterine infusion once daily for 3 days. Ticarcillin's spectrum is similar to that of carbenicillin but with much greater activity against *Pseudomonas*. Ticarcillin and an aminoglycoside, such as gentamicin or tobramycin, are synergistic and provide a broader spectrum of activity than either antibiotic alone. The MIC of each antibiotic against many strains of *Pseudomonas* may be reduced by a factor of four or more through concomitant use. These agents, however, must not be mixed in the same syringe because the ticarcillin gradually inactivates the aminoglycoside.

9.7 ANTISTAPHYLOCOCCAL PENICILLINS

Infections caused by beta-lactamase-producing (penicillinase) staphylococci are resistant to treatment with conventional penicillins. Beta-lactamase-resistant penicillins (e.g., methicillin, nafcillin, cloxacillin, dicloxacillin, and oxacillin) were developed by adding substituents onto the aromatic ring of penicillin to inhibit sterically beta-lactamases. Methicillin was the first semisynthetic penicillin developed but is poorly absorbed orally owing to gastric acid instability and is not potent. All of the later developed drugs in this group are well absorbed orally except for nafcillin. All of these are effective against gram-positive beta-lactamase-producing bacteria.

The following are synthetic derivatives of penicillin: methicillin sodium, nafcillin sodium, and isoxazolyl penicillins. The isoxazolyl penicillins include oxacillin sodium, cloxacillin sodium monohydrate, and dicloxacillin sodium. These synthetic derivatives had a modification in the molecule that has made them resistant to hydrolysis by staphylococcal beta-lactamase. Gram-

negative organisms generally are resistant to antistaphylococcal penicillins. These drugs cannot pass through the outer layers of a gram-negative cell wall easily, and there is low affinity for the PBPs of gram-negative bacteria.

Methicillin, oxacillin, nafcillin, cloxacillin, and dicloxacillin are semisynthetic penicillins that resist the action of beta lactamase because the acyl side chain of each drug creates steric hindrance of the enzyme. These drugs should be reserved for treatment of infections caused by bacteria that are susceptible only to these drugs. Their activity against streptococci is less than that of penicillin G. Oxacillin is primarily indicated for the treatment of infections caused by beta lactamase-producing *S. aureus*. Occasionally some strains of *S. aureus* are resistant to this group of drugs, but the resistance is not conveyed by production of beta lactamase. Methacillin is not acid stable and cannot be administered orally. Nafcillin is erratically and poorly absorbed. Cloxacillin and dicloxacillin are absorbed to a greater extent in comparison to oxacillin. Dicloxacillin is a narrow-spectrum, beta-lactamase-resistant antibiotic used to treat infections caused by *Staphylococcus*.

There is little rationale for using these drugs except when treating a beta-lactamase-positive staphylococcal infection. For treating infections resulting from nonpenicillinase-producing, gram-positive bacteria, penicillin G is a better choice. The isoxazolyl penicillins are similar in their antibacterial activity, with MIC values of 0.1 to 0.4 µg/ml.

Antistaphylococcal penicillins have no activity against anaerobes and poor activity against gram-negative bacteria. Their use should be restricted to treating staphylococcal infections. Temocillin is a beta lactamase-resistant penicillin that is active against almost all gram-negative bacteria except *Pseudomonas*. Because of this, it is effective in treating coliform infections, especially enteritis and mastitis. It is poorly absorbed orally, but when administered parenterally it has an unusually long half-life in humans.

9.8 NEW BETA LACTAMS

Carbapenems and monobactams are two classes of compounds with structures markedly different from those previously described. Carbapenems have a carbon instead of a sulfur on the five-membered ring attached to the beta lactam ring. The small size and compact structure of these agents allow them to pass easily through gram-negative bacterial cell walls. Imipenem, the only carbapenem currently available, has a hydroxyethyl side chain rather than the classic acylamino moiety of penicillin and cephalosporins. It has a broad spectrum of activity, including against such gram-negative aerobes and anaerobes as *Pseudomonas* and *Bacteroides*. It is resistant to beta-lactamase inactivation and so is effective for staphylococcal infections.

Monobactams are a novel group of compounds in which the bicyclic structure characteristic of the other beta lactams is absent. The core configuration is that of a beta lactam ring. This new class of antimicrobials is represented by the prototype aztreonam, which has a monocyclic ring instead of the standard bicyclic structure characteristic of the penicillins and cephalosporins. Their anticipated use is in treatment of Enterobacteriaceae infections.

9.9 CEPHALOSPORINS

Chemically cephalosporins and penicillins are closely related. Both contain a beta lactam ring and hence are collectively called beta lactam antibiotics. In general, the antibacterial actions of corresponding penicillins and cephalosporins are somewhat similar. Cephalosporins, however, seem to be more resistant to the action of beta-lactamase. Cephalosporins have antibacterial action similar to that of the other beta lactam antibiotics: the inhibition of cell wall synthesis. The popularity and usefulness of cephalosporins result from their resistance to many beta-lactamase enzymes, their wide spectrum of activity compared with penicillin G, and their wide safety margin.

Since the synthesis of the first cephalosporins from the fungus *Cephalosporium acremonium*, this class has expanded. The class is broadly divided into first, second, and third generations. They have been little used in food animal medicine until recently because of their relatively high cost. Cephalosporins differed from one another primarily with respect to their kinetic fate

rather than their antibacterial spectra. The newer cephalosporins have a broader range of activity.

As a group, these beta lactam antibiotics have pharmacologic features similar to those of penicillins. Their usual antibacterial spectra are comparable to those of broad-spectrum semisynthetic penicillins, but they are generally more active against *Pasteurella* strains and less effective against *Corynebacterium pyogenes*.

Although this group of compounds has been classified in several ways using a variety of criteria, the term "generation" was originally devised as a means of separating the cephalosporins based solely on the in vitro antibacterial potency and spectrum of activity. With the introduction of each cephalosporin generation, there has been a loss of gram-positive activity, an increase in gram-negative activity and spectrum, an increased resistance to beta-lactamase enzymes, and a marked increase in cost. These cephalosporins are even more active against many of the isolates of *P. aeruginosa*, often at the expense of diminished activity against gram-positive cocci, particularly *S. aureus*. Some third-generation cephalosporins have long half-lives in humans as well as good penetration of cerebrospinal fluid and peritoneal fluid. Clinically cephalosporins are usually assigned to one of three generations according to their relative in vitro antibacterial spectrum. The 7-aminocephalosporanic acid nucleus of the cephalosporins consists of a six-membered dihydrothiazine ring fused with a four-membered beta lactam ring; the beta lactam ring is essential for antibacterial activity. The chemical structure of 7-aminocephalosporanic acid is similar to that of the 6-aminopenicillanic acid nucleus of the penicillin group of antimicrobial agents. In both cases, the beta lactam ring and its adjacent atoms have a spatial configuration similar to that of the peptidoglycans used in the synthesis of bacterial cell walls. In the case of the cephalosporins, the dihydrothiazine ring confers a steric advantage to the beta lactam ring in terms of increased resistance to the action of extrachromosomally mediated staphylococcal beta-lactamases (penicillinases) such that the cephalosporins have an inherently broader spectrum of activity.

In gram-positive and gram-negative bacteria, one layer of the cell wall is comprised of the macromolecule peptidoglycan. A cross-linking reaction involving peptidoglycan induced by the bacterial enzyme transpeptidase gives the bacterial cell wall the structural strength to withstand the high intracellular osmotic pressure. The beta lactam ring covalently binds with the transpeptidase enzyme, preventing the cross-linking reaction, and the weakened cell wall eventually ruptures.

When the beta lactam ring is opened by hydrolysis, as it is by the beta-lactamase enzyme, the cephalosporins are no longer able to bind transpeptidase and become biologically inactive.

In cephalosporins, the beta lactam ring is attached to the six-membered dihydrothiazine ring. In contrast to the penicillin nucleus, the cephalosporin nucleus is inherently more resistant to beta-lactamases and is more active against beta-lactamase-producing (penicillin-resistant) bacteria, including *S. aureus* and *E. coli*. The cephalosporin molecule also provides more sites for potential manipulation. Therapeutically important modifications have been made at the sulfur atom.

A large number of cephalosporin antibiotics have become available through chemical modification of the basic nucleus. All of the marketed cephalosporins are semisynthetic; the basic cephalosporin nucleus is isolated from a fermentation broth, and the chemical substitutions are made. Technically because moxalactam has an oxygen replacing the sulfur atom at position 1 of the dihydrothiazine ring, it is not a true cephalosporin.

Changes in the antibacterial spectrum, pharmacokinetic behavior, and increases in resistance to the beta-lactamase enzymes have been obtained through various substitutions.

9.10 FIRST-GENERATION CEPHALOSPORINS

First-generation cephalosporins, introduced into human medicine in the 1960s and 1970s, are basically similar in antibacterial activity and differ mainly in their pharmacokinetic properties. These first-generation products, which include all of the currently available, orally active cephalosporins, are relatively susceptible to beta-lactamase, are active against most gram-positive bacteria, and have a limited spectrum of activity against gram-negative organisms.

First-generation cephalosporins are the main cephalosporins used to an extent in veterinary medicine and are effective alternatives to penicillin in treating staphylococcal and nonenterococcal streptococcal infections in patients allergic to penicillin. First-generation cephalosporins include cephalothin, cephapirin, cephalexin, cephradine, and cefadroxil. Cephalothin, cephapirin, and cefazolin are injectable solutions, and cefadroxil, cephalexin, and cephradine are oral formulations. Cephalexin is also an injectable.

Although many of these cephalosporins have varied effectiveness against gram-negative bacteria, cephalothin and cephalexin especially display useful broad-spectrum activity. First-generation cephalosporins are effective against a variety of gram-positive and gram-negative organisms, but they are sensitive to some beta-lactamases. Most isolates of *E. coli*, *Proteus mirabilis*, and *Klebsiella pneumoniae* are inhibited by first-generation cephalosporins. Compared with other first-generation cephalosporins, cefazolin has the greatest activity against *E. coli* and *Klebsiella*. First-generation cephalosporins are also effective against many anaerobic bacteria except for *Bacteroides* strains that produce beta-lactamase (e.g., *Bacteroides fragilis*). Cefadroxil is an oral cephalosporin that is absorbed rapidly from the gastrointestinal tract. It is approved for use in dogs, but its pharmacokinetic properties have been studied in horses. In dogs, cefadroxil has the advantage of a long plasma half-life. In horses, cefadroxil has rapid clearance from the serum and a short half-life (46 minutes), which necessitates frequent dosing.

Other first-generation cephalosporins used in veterinary medicine are cephalothin sodium, cephapirin sodium, and cefazolin sodium. They are almost identical in their spectrum of activity and are more resistant to staphylococcal beta-lactamase than other first-generation cephalosporins.

Cephalexin is a broad-spectrum, bactericidal cephalosporin antibiotic, active against a wide range of gram-positive and gram-negative bacteria. It is resistant to staphylococcal penicillinase and is therefore active against the strains of *S. aureus* that are insensitive to penicillin or related antibiotics, such as ampicillin or amoxicillin. Cephalexin is also active against the majority of ampicillin-resistant *E. coli*. Cephalexin is indicated for treating infections of the respiratory tract, urogenital tract, gastrointestinal tract, and skin as well as localized infections.

In trials, it has been shown to be successful in treating a variety of conditions, including respiratory infections, with effective penetration of the lungs, larynx, and trachea; gastroenteritis, with a 90% success rate in dogs; urinary tract infections, with up to 60 of the active ingredient remaining unchanged in the urine; renal/hepatic infections, with liver and kidney concentrations exceeding serum levels even after oral dosing; skin infections, with concentration in the skin well maintained; and muscle and bone infections.

Cefadroxil and cephalexin are the two oral cephalosporins with which veterinarians have had the most experience, and these two agents seem to be therapeutically equivalent. Dosage regimens have ranged from 10 to 30 mg/kg given orally two or three times daily for treatment of urinary tract, skin and soft tissue, and respiratory tract infections.

9.11 SECOND-GENERATION CEPHALOSPORINS

Second-generation cephalosporins offer no advantage over first-generation agents in terms of gram-positive spectrum and activity; in fact, their activity against some of these bacteria may actually be slightly less. They do offer expanded coverage against a few specific gram-negative bacteria. Second-generation cephalosporins, initially introduced in the late 1970s, tend to be more resistant to beta-lactamase and more active against a broader spectrum of gram-negative bacteria. Although their activity against gram-positive bacteria is often thought to be less than first-generation compounds, this is usually in reference to penicillin-resistant *S. aureus*.

Second-generation cephalosporins include the parenteral agents cefamandole, cefuroxime, cefonicid, cefoxitin, and cefotetan and the oral agent cefaclor. Compared with first-generation drugs, second-generation cephalosporins (e.g., cefoxitin) are more resistant to beta-lactamases and so are more effective against gram-negative organisms, particularly *E. coli* and *Klebsiella*, *Enterobacter*, and *Proteus*. Second-generation cephalosporins are less effective than first-generation cephalosporins against gram-positive organisms but are effective against some anaerobes. Cefoxitin, in particular, is effective against anaerobes. In vitro these agents are more effective than first-generation agents against *E. coli*, *Klebsiella*, and *P. mirabilis*. Individual members of this group of agents extend the antibiotic coverage of cephalosporins to include many strains of *Enterobacter*, *Serratia*, indole-positive *Proteus*, and *H. influenzae*.

Second-generation cephalosporins are used infrequently in veterinary medicine because of their expense. In general, they are less active against beta-lactamase-producing bacteria, especially *Staphylococcus*. Because of their ability to penetrate the outer envelope, they are more active against gram-negative bacteria than the first-generation cephalosporins.

9.12 THIRD-GENERATION CEPHALOSPORINS

Third-generation cephalosporins are no more effective against gram-positive bacteria than first-generation cephalosporins, and there is no reason for choosing these more expensive products over first-generation agents. Further, it is often observed that second-generation and third-generation cephalosporins are less active against gram-positive bacteria than first-generation cephalosporins.

Third-generation cephalosporins were developed in response to the needs of specialized situations, as in burn, cancer, and complicated surgery patients, in whom antibiotic-resistant, gram-negative infections are common and are difficult to treat safely. Although most of these agents have broad gram-positive and gram-negative antibacterial activity, their cost is often five to six times that of first-generation cephalosporins and for many patients may be prohibitive. These agents may be useful in patients with multiple-drug-resistant, gram-negative infections or in whom other effective antimicrobials carry unacceptable risks of serious toxicity. Gram-negative meningitis, which is unresponsive to other agents, may also be an indication for the use of these drugs.

Third-generation cephalosporins are effective primarily against gram-negative organisms. *Enterobacter, Serratia*, and *Pseudomonas* tend to be more resistant to cefotaxime than other gram-negative organisms. These agents may be divided into two groups: those with important activity against *P. aeruginosa* and those without such activity. The latter group consists of cefotaxime, ceftriaxone, ceftizoxime, and moxalactam. Ceftazidime and cefoperazone are in the former group.

Third-generation cephalosporins are reserved for infections resulting from resistant *Pseudomonas, Klebsiella*, or other highly resistant, gram-negative bacteria. The high cost of these cephalosporins makes their use prohibitive in large animals. Their activity against gram-positive organisms is lower than that of other cephalosporins. As with penicillins, commonly isolated anaerobic organisms are sensitive to cephalosporins, with the exception of *B. fragilis*, which might be resistant to all cephalosporins except cefoxitin and moxalactam. Moxalactam is an oxa-beta-lactam agent, not a true cephalosporin. Moxalactam, ceftizoxime, and ceftazidime also penetrate well into cerebrospinal fluid in the presence of inflamed meninges. Cefotaxime, ceftriaxone, and ceftazidime have proved to be effective in treating meningitis. In children, in whom *H. influenzae, Streptococcus pneumoniae*, and *Neisseria meningitidis* are leading etiologic agents, these drugs are as effective as a combination of ampicillin and chloramphenicol or of ampicillin and gentamicin. Cefotaxime, because of its resistance to beta-lactamases, provides a potent broad spectrum of activity against aerobic gram-negative bacteria that is markedly greater than that provided by first-generation and second-generation agents.

9.13 KINETICS

Many cephalosporins resist inactivation by staphylococcal beta-lactamase and have good affinity for the PBPs of gram-positive bacteria. Resistance is possible, however, among certain staphylococci that are related to altered PBPs (methicillin-resistant staphylococci), but fortunately the incidence is rare in veterinary medicine. The only streptococci of importance in veterinary medicine that have shown resistance to cephalosporins are the enterococci (e.g., *S. faecalis*).

The cephalosporins are relatively widely distributed throughout the body. In general, they penetrate well into pleural, pericardial, and synovial fluid and into most tissue spaces. Urine concentrations of active drug are extremely high, and bile levels are also high as long as no biliary obstruction exists. Cephalosporins penetrate poorly into prostatic tissue, ocular humor, and, with a few exceptions, cerebrospinal fluid. A unique feature of several of the more recent cephalosporins is that they are able to penetrate into cerebrospinal fluid in amounts that are adequate to treat certain bacterial infections of the central nervous system successfully.

Elimination half-lives are similar for all first-generation cephalosporins with the exception of cefadroxil, which has a longer half-life and a duration of therapeutic serum concentrations that varies from 2.5 to 6.5 hours and subsequently can be administered every 12 hours, instead of every 6 to 8 hours, as for most cephalosporins. Cefazolin differs from other parenteral first-generation cephalosporins because it achieves higher peak plasma concentrations in comparison to other cephalosporins following administration. Because it also produces less pain after intramuscular injection, it is often preferred over other first-generation cephalosporins for parenteral administration.

Similar to other beta lactam antibiotics, cephalosporins have a volume of distribution that is limited to the extracellular space. They achieve therapeutic concentrations for susceptible bacteria in most tissues. Concentrations achieved in bone are sufficient to account for their efficacy in treating osteomyelitis. For orally administered first-generation cephalosporins, systemic availability is good, ranging from 74 to 90%.

Although there may be subtle differences in MIC for bacteria among first-generation cephalosporins, when interpreting culture and sensitivity tests, all first-generation cephalosporins should be considered equal. Cephalothin is the drug of choice for measuring susceptibility for all first-generation agents.

Cephalosporins share pharmacokinetic characteristics with other beta lactam compounds in that they all have relatively short elimination half-lives and are excreted primarily by renal clearance. Cephalothin and cephapirin are metabolized in the liver to the less active desacetyl-cephalosporin products, which are subsequently excreted in the urine.

9.14 CEPHALOSPORIN THERAPY

In most cases, cephalosporins are not the preferred drug but rather are used in infections caused by organisms resistant to other antibiotics. There is a trend, however, to use cephalosporins for presurgical prophylaxis, especially in certain orthopedic procedures. Several of these cephalosporins distribute well into osseous tissue, synovial fluid, and peritoneal fluid of dogs. Some third-generation cephalosporins have the ability to penetrate the cerebrospinal fluid to a marked extent. Of first-generation cephalosporins, cefazolin has somewhat higher activity against E. coli and Klebsiella than either cephalothin or cephalexin. Second-generation cephalosporins, such as cefamandole, cefaclor, cefonicid, ceforanide, and cefuroxime and the cephamycin, cefoxitin, have enhanced activity over first-generation cephalosporins against Enterobacter, indole-positive Proteus, E. coli, and Klebsiella, particularly when these bacteria are resistant to cephalothin. These cephalosporins are less active against beta-lactamase-producing gram-positive bacteria, but are more effective against gram-negative bacteria because they can easily penetrate the outer membrane of gram-negative organisms. Third-generation cephalosporins (including cefoperazone, cefotaxime, ceftriaxone, ceftizoxime, and the oxa-beta-lactam moxalactam) have been targeted for serious gram-negative infections caused by pathogens such as P. aeruginosa, beta-lactamase-producing H. influenzae, Neisseria, Enterobacter, and Serratia infections. In general, larger concentrations of these drugs are required to inhibit bacteria such as Enterobacter, Serratia, Bacteroides, and Pseudomonas.

First-generation cephalosporins have been widely used for prophylaxis in cardiovascular, orthopedic, biliary, pelvic, and intra-abdominal surgery. They are preferable to second-generation or third-generation agents because they are as effective, they cost less, and they have a more narrow range of activity. Cefazolin, because it has a longer half-life than other first-generation agents, is viewed as the first-generation agent of choice for prophylaxis. Cefuroxime is effective in therapy of pneumonia in which ampicillin-resistant H. influenza is a possible etiologic agent.

Skin infections in the canine are invariably caused by coagulase-positive staphylococci, of which Staphylococcus intermedius is the most commonly isolated species. Agents that are usually active against this organism are penicillinase-resistant penicillins, amoxicillin clavulanate, cephalosporins, trimethoprim sulfonamide, erythromycin, and tetracycline; if the isolate is a non-beta-lactamase-producing Staphylococcus species, ampicillin and amoxicillin may also be expected to be effective in veterinary medicine. Cephalosporins have been used in the treatment of a variety of infectious processes caused by many different pathogens. Respiratory, urinary tract, skin, soft tissue, bone and joint, intra-abdominal, obstetric, and gynecologic infections caused by cephalosporin-susceptible bacteria have all been successfully treated with these agents. In addition, several third-generation cephalosporins have also been efficacious in treating central nervous system infections. Cephalosporins are also popular agents for surgical prophylaxis.

Cephalosporins are currently becoming widely used for the treatment and prevention of bovine mastitis. Cephalosporin antibiotics were first made available to veterinary surgeons in the 1970s for the treatment and prevention of bovine mastitis. A broad-spectrum antibiotic, cephalonium, was developed for administration to cows at drying off and was designed to treat existing infections and prevent new infections during the dry period. A broad-spectrum combination containing cephoxazole and penicillin was developed for treatment of clinical mastitis in the milking cow.

The increasing incidence of gram-negative infections in the milking cow strengthened the requirement for a bactericidal antibiotic with as wide a spectrum as possible for first-line, on farm treatment of bovine clinical mastitis. Cefuroxime, a semisynthetic cephalosporin antibiotic, was selected for development as a treatment for bovine clinical mastitis because it has a broad spectrum of activity against the majority of mastitis pathogens, has resistance to hydrolysis by beta-lactamase enzymes, is bactericidal in action, penetrates tissues well, and is rapidly excreted from the udder. Cefuroxime is a cephalosporin that combines activity against a wide range of bacteria together with resistance to hydrolysis by beta-lactamases produced by both gram-positive and gram-negative strains. Preliminary investigations suggested that cefuroxime would be effective for the treatment of mastitis.

Another cephalosporin used for mastitis is cephacetrile. Cephacetrile has a wide range of activity. It is active against *S. aureus* strains that are benzylpenicillin sensitive or benzylpenicillin resistant and strains with multiple antibiotic resistance. Cephacetrile concentrations of 4.0 μg/ml inhibit the growth of most mastitis strains of *E. coli*

tested. Cephacetrile is relatively stable to beta-lactamase degradation.

Cefoperazone is a third-generation cephalosporin that is resistant to the hydrolysis caused by the beta-lactamases produced not only by certain staphylococci, but also those produced by *E. coli* and other gram-negative organisms, including *P. aeruginosa*. Preliminary investigations on the pharmacokinetic properties of this antibiotic both in lactating mice and in dairy cows indicated that cefoperazone would be suitable to use as an intramammary product in the treatment of bovine mastitis. This is because of its demonstrated broad-spectrum activity, its nonirritant properties, and its persistence at a significant level in the treated quarter of a cow for three to four milkings after a single intramammary infusion of 250 mg in an oil base. Cefoperazone possesses activity against both gram-positive and gram-negative pathogens. Its broad spectrum includes activity against many strains that may be resistant to natural and synthetic penicillins, aminoglycosides, and other earlier generation cephalosporins.

Ceftiofur is a new cephalosporin for respiratory use in cattle. It displays excellent activity against *P. multocida*, *P. haemolytica* and *Haemophilus somnus*. Given at a dose of 1 mg/kg, it is indicated for parenteral injection in cases of bovine respiratory disease.

APPENDIX 9–1

CLASSES OF PENICILLINS

Natural Penicillins	*Broad-Spectrum Penicillins*
Penicillin G (aqueous, procaine, benzathine)	Ampicillin
Penicillin V	Amoxicillin
Phenethicillin	Hetacillin
Penicillinase-Resistant Penicillins	Carbenicillin
Methicillin	Ticarcillin
Nafcillin	Piperacillin
Oxacillin	Mezlocillin
Cloxacillin	Azlocillin
Dicloxacillin	

SENSITIVITY OF BACTERIA TO AMOXICILLIN

	Gram-Negative	Gram-Positive
Highly Sensitive	Pasteurella Brucella Fusobacterium Haemophilus Fusiformis	Bacillus anthracis Erysipelothri streptococcus D Staphylococcus Clostridium Streptococcus Corynebacterium
Very Sensitive	Proteus mirabilis Salmonella Treponema Moraxella	
Somewhat Sensitive	Bordetella Escherichia	
Highly Resistant	Pseudomonas Klebsiella Indole-positive Proteus	Penicillinase-producing Staphylococcus

SENSITIVITY OF BACTERIA TO AMPICILLIN

Highly Sensitive	Staphylococcus aureus (nonpenicillinase producing) Beta-hemolytic streptococcus Streptococcus equi Streptococcus pneumoniae Haemophilus influenzae
Sensitive	Streptococcus faecalis Proteus mirabilis Shigella sonnei Salmonella Escherichia coli Pasteurella
Resistant	Staphylococcus aureus (penicillinase producing) Proteus Klebsiella pneumoniae Pseudomonas aeruginosa

BETA-LACTAMASE-PRODUCING BACTERIA

Gram-Positive	Gram-Negative
Staphylococcus	Escherichia Haemophilus Klebsiella Pasteurella Proteus Pseudomonas Salmonella

DOSE INFORMATION FOR BETA-LACTAM ANTIBIOTICS IN HORSES AND CATTLE

Drug	Species	Recommended Dose	Dose Interval (hours)
Penicillin G	Horses	20,000–60,000 U/kg	8–24
	Cattle	20,000–50,000 U/kg	12–24
Ampicillin	Horses	2–7 mg/kg	6–12
	Cattle	15–20 mg/kg	12
Amoxicillin	Horses	10 mg/kg	12–24
	Cattle	6–10 mg/kg	12–24
Ticarcillin	Horses	44 mg/kg	5 (IV)
Carbenicillin	Horses	12–50 mg/kg	6
Cephalothin	Horses	10–25 mg/kg	4
	Cattle	20 mg/kg	6
Cefadroxil	Horses	25 mg/kg	4

CEPHALOSPORIN GENERATION CHARACTERISTICS

Generation	US Approval	In vitro activity		Susceptibility to Beta-Lactamase
		Gram-Positive	Gram-Negative	
First	1960s and 1970s	Good	Moderate	Relatively susceptible
Second	Late 1970s	Good	Good, broader spectrum	Resistant
Third	1980s	Moderate	Very good, broader spectrum (*Pseudomonas*)	Highly resistant

CLASSIFICATION OF CEPHALOSPORINS

First Generation
  Cephalothin
  Cephaloridine
  Cephapirin
  Cefazolin
  Cephalexin
  Cefaclor
  Cephradine
  Cefadroxil

Spectrum
Most aerobic gram-positive bacteria except enterococci and methicillin-resistant *Staphylococcus aureus*; most anaerobic gram-positive and gram-negative bacteria except *Bacteroides fragilis*, common aerobic gram-negative enterics

Second Generation
  Cefamandole
  Cefoxitin
  Cefotiam
  Cefuroxime
  Ceforanide

More aerobic gram-negative bacteria, such as indole-positive *Proteus* and *Bacteroides fragilis*

Third Generation
  Ceftriaxone
  Ceftizoxime
  Ceftazidime
  Cefsulodin
  Cefotaxime
  Cefoperazone
  Cefmenoxime
  Moxalactam

Some strains of *Pseudomonas aeruginosa* as well as some unusual *Enterobacteriaciae*. Less active against/gram-positive bacteria

SELECTED REFERENCES

Abramowiez, M.: Amoxicillin-clavulanic acid (augmentin). Med. Lett. Drugs Ther., *26*: 99, 1984.

Ambler, R.P.: The structure of B, lactamanes. Philos. Trans. R. Soc. Lond. Biol., *289*: 321, 1980.

Barriere, S.L.: Therapeutic considerations using combinations of newer beta lactam antibiotics. Clin. Pharm., *5*: 24, 1986.

Barriere, S.L., and Flaherty, J.F.: Third generation cephalosporins: A critical evaluation. Clin. Pharm., *3*: 351, 1984.

Birnbaum, J., Kahan, F.M., Kropp, H., and McDonald, J.S.: Carbopenems: A new class of beta lactam antibiotics: Discovery and development of imipenem/cilastatin. Am. J. Med., *78* (Suppl. 6A): 3, 1985.

Brown, M.P., Gronwell, R.R., and Martinez, D.S.: Pharmacokinetics of amikacin in pony foals after a single intramuscular injection. Am. J. Vet. Res., *47*: 453, 1986.

Bywater, R.J., Palmer, G.H., Buswell, J.F., et al.: Clavulanate-potentiated amoxicillin. Activity in vitro and bioavailability in the dog. Vet. Rec., *116*: 33, 1985.

Caprile, K.A.: The cephalosporin antimicrobial agents: A comprehensive review. J. Pharmacol. Ther., *11*: 1, 1988.

Chatfield, R.C., Gingerich, D.A., Rourke, J.E., and Strom, B.W.: Cedadroxil: A new orally effective cephalosporin antibiotic. Vet. Med., *79*: 339, 1984.

Cimarust, C.M., and Sykes, R.B.: Monobactams—novel antibiotics. Chem. Br., *19*: 302, 1983.

Donowitz, G.R., and Mandell, G.L.: Beta lactam antibiotics. Parts 1 and 2. N. Engl. J. Med., *318*: 419, 490, 1988.

Eagle, J., Fleishman, R., and Levy, M.: Discontinuous therapy with penicillin. N. Engl. J. Med., *248*: 481, 1953.

Eliopoulos, G.M.: Induction of beta lactamases. J. Antimicrob. Chemo., *22* (Suppl.): 34, 1988.

Girard, A.E.: Activity of beta lactamase inhibitor sulbactam plus ampicillin against animal isolates of Pasteurella, Haemophilus and Staphylococcus. Am. J. Vet. Res., *48*: 1678, 1987.

Girard, A.E.: Activity of B lactamase inhibition sulbactam plus ampicillin versus animal isolates of Pasteurella, Hemophilus, and Staphylococcus. Proc. 25th Int. Conf. Antimicrol. Agents, Chemother., 1985.

Goldberg, D.M.: The cephalosporins. Med. Clin. North Am., *71*: 1113, 1987.

Hilledge, C.J.: Erythromycin and rifampin in combination for treatment of R. Equi. lung abscesses in foals. In Proceedings of the Thirty-First Convention of the American Association of Equine Practitioners, 1985.

Indiveri, M.C., and Hirsh, D.C.: Clavulanic acid potentiated activity of amoxicillin against Bacteroides fragilis. Am. J. Vet. Res., *46*: 2207, 1985.

Jawetz, E.: Aminoglycosides and penicillins. In Basic and Clinical Pharmacology. 2nd ed. Edited by B.G. Katzung. Los Altos, CA, Lange Medical Publications, 1984.

Jawetz, E.: Penicillins and cephalosporins. In Basic and Clinical Pharmacology. 2nd ed. Edited by B.G. Katzung. Los Altos, CA, Lange Medical Publications, 1984.

Jawetz, E., Melnick, J.C., and Adelberg, E.A.: Cell Structure in Review of Medical Microbiology. 16th ed. Los Altos, CA, Lange Medical Publications, 1984.

Kilgore, W.R., Simmons, R.D., and Jackson, J.W.: B-Lactamase inhibition: A new approach in overcoming bacterial resistance. Comp. Cont. Educ. Pract. Vet., *8*: 325, 1986.

Ling, G.V., Rohrich, P.J., and Ruby, A.L.: Canine urinary tract infections. A comparison of in vitro antimicrobial susceptibility test results and response to oral therapy with ampicillin or with trimethogrina sulfa. J. Am. Vet. Med. Assoc., *185*: 277, 1984.

Neu, H.C.: Relation of structural properties of beta lactam antibiotics to antibacterial activity. Am. J. Med., *79* (Suppl. 2A), 1985.

New, H.C.: The new beta lactamase stable cephalosporins. Ann. Intern. Med., *97*: 408, 1982.

Nikaido, H., Rosenberg, E.Y., and Foulds, J.: Porin channels in E. coli: Studies with B lactams in intact cells. J. Bacteriol., *153*: 232, 1983.

Papich, M.G.: The B lactam antibiotics: Clinical pharmacology and recent developments. Comp. Con. Educ. Pract. Vet., *9*: 68, 1987.

Papich, M.G.: Clinical pharmacokinetics of cephalosporin antibiotics. J. Am. Vet. Med. Assoc., *184*: 344, 1984.

Powers, T.E., and Garg, R.C.: Pharmacotherapeutics of newer penicillins and cephalosporins. J. Am. Vet. Med. Assoc., *176*: 1054, 1980.

Simmons, R.D., and Keefe, T.J.: Penicillins an expanding spectrum. Mod. Vet. Pract., 49, 1983.

Slocombe, B., Beals, A.S., Boom, R.J., et al.: Antibacterial activity in vitro and in vivo of amoxicillin in the presence of clavulanic acid. Postgrad. Med., 29, 1984.

Sweeney, C.R., Soma, L.R., Beech, J., et al.: Pharmacokinetics of ticarcillin in the horse after intravenous and intramuscular administration. Am. J. Vet. Res., *45*: 1000, 1984.

Sykes, R.B.: The classification and terminology of enzymes that hydrolyse B-lactam antibiotics. J. Infect. Dis., *145*: 762, 1982.

Thompson, R.L., and Wright, A.J.: Cephalosporin antibiotics. Mayo Clin. Proc., *58*: 79, 1983.

Thompson, T.D., Quay, J.F., and Webber, J.A.: Cephalosporin group of antimicrobial drugs. J. Am. Vet. Med. Assoc., *185*: 1109, 1984.

Tipper, D.J.: Mode of action of beta lactam antibiotics. In Beta Lactam Antibiotics for Clinical Use. Edited by S.F. Queener, J.A. Webber, and S.W. Queener. New York, Marcel Dekker, 1986.

Turk, M.: Clinical Applications of the newer beta lactam antibiotics. J. Antimicrob. Chemother., *22* (Suppl.): 45, 1988.

Waxman, D.J., and Strominger, J.L.: Penicillin binding proteins and the mechanism of action of B lactam antibiotics. Ann. Rev. Biochem., *52*: 825, 1983.

Wishart, D.F.: Recent advances in antimicrobial drugs: The penicillins. J. Am. Vet. Med. Assoc., *185*: 1106, 1984.

Wright, A.J.: The penicillins. Mayo Clin. Proc., *58*: 183, 1983.

Wright, A.J., and Wilkowske, C.J.: The penicillins. Mayo Clin. Proc., *58*: 21, 1983.

10

C H A P T E R

AMINOGLYCOSIDES, MACROLIDES, AND LINCOSAMIDES

10.1 Aminoglycosides
10.2 Pharmacokinetics
10.3 Mechanism of Action
10.4 Resistance
10.5 Clinical Use
10.6 Specific Aminoglycosides
10.7 Aminoglycoside Toxicity
10.8 Macrolides and Lincosamides
10.9 Mechanism of Action
10.10 Resistance
10.11 Antibacterial Spectrum
10.12 Pharmacokinetics
10.13 Clinical Application
10.14 Toxicity of Macrolides

10.1 AMINOGLYCOSIDES

This class includes narrow-spectrum (e.g., streptomycin, dihydrostreptomycin), extended-spectrum (e.g., neomycin, kanamycin), and broad-spectrum, including *Pseudomonas* (e.g., gentamicin, amikacin, tobramycin, netilmicin) aminoglycosides as well as other aminocyclitols (e.g., spectinomycin, apramycin). Aminoglycoside (aminocyclitol) antibiotics are valuable therapeutic agents and among the oldest known antibiotics. In 1944, streptomycin was isolated from a species of *Streptomyces*. Since then, many other aminoglycosides have been isolated from soil microorganisms, such as neomycin (1949), kanamycin (1957), gentamicin (1963), and sisomicin (1967). Kanamycin was synthetically modified to produce tobramycin (1967) and amikacin (1972), and sisomicin has been synthetically modified to produce netilmicin (1973). The objective of modifying the naturally fermented aminoglycosides is to decrease the potential for toxicity yet maintain their broad-spectrum activity.

Despite the arrival of third-generation and fourth-generation broad-spectrum cephalosporins, aminoglycosides continue to be the only agents in many cases that can overcome serious gram-negative infections, especially those caused by *Pseudomonas aeruginosa*. Although they are efficacious for a variety of gram-negative infections, their use is often limited by their toxicity. Despite their potential for toxicity and nephrotoxicity, plus the need for laboratory monitoring of treated patients, this family of antimicrobials remains the standard for treatment of serous aerobic gram-negative rod infections outside the central nervous system.

Aminoglycoside (or aminocyclitol) antibiotics are polycations that are poorly absorbed from the gastrointestinal tract and that do not diffuse well into the cerebrospinal fluid. They are minimally bound to plasma proteins, are distributed primarily in the extracellular fluid, and are rapidly excreted unchanged by the normal kidney. All aminoglycoside antibiotics are relatively small, basic, water-soluble molecules that form stable salts.

Chemically aminoglycoside antibiotics are closely related: They are characterized by an aminocyclitol group and amino sugars attached to the aminocyclitol ring in glycosidic linkage. The amino groups contribute to the basic nature of this class of antibiotics, and the hydroxyl groups on the sugar moieties give high aqueous solubility and poor lipid solubility. If these hydroxyl groups are removed, antibiotic activity is markedly increased. Differences in the substitutions on the basic ring structures between the various aminoglycosides account for the relatively minor differences in antimicrobial spectra, patterns of resistance, and toxicity.

Aminoglycoside antibiotics have many similarities. Each is poorly absorbed from the gastrointestinal tract and thus must be given parenterally. Owing to their low lipid solubility, these drugs diffuse poorly, if at all, into the central nervous system and the eye. All of these agents are rapidly excreted unchanged in the urine by glomerular filtration.

Aminoglycosides are basic drugs and are much more active in alkaline (pH 8) than acidic environments. They localize well in the alkaline pH of the mammary gland. The efficacy of gentamicin and other aminoglycosides in cystitis can be increased by alkalinizing the urine. Aminoglycosides and other alkaline drugs can, however, be more rapidly eliminated by acidifying the urine. Rapidly multiplying bacteria are more sensitive to aminocyclitols than are more static populations.

Resistance to aminocyclitols may take a number of forms, such as ribosomal-binding mutants, aminoglycoside-modifying enzymes, and mutants defective in drug accumulation. Cross resistance is common. For all members of the group, the margin between therapeutic and toxic concentrations is not as great as with penicillins. All have some potential for toxicity to the kidney and the auditory or vestibular pathways of the eighth cranial nerve.

10.2 PHARMACOKINETICS

These drugs are poorly lipid soluble, highly polar, and must therefore be administered parenterally to achieve therapeutically adequate systemic concentrations. Because of their chemical makeup and mechanisms of action, these drugs are more effective at an alkaline pH and in an aerobic environment. They are of no value in an anaerobic environment.

Aminoglycosides are generally well absorbed after intramuscular injection and are distributed well into body fluids, including synovial, peritoneal, and pleural fluids. These agents distribute slowly in the bile, feces, prostate, and amniotic fluid. Owing to their low lipid solubility, they are distributed poorly in the central nervous system and the vitreous humor of the eye. Binding of serum proteins is less than 20% and is not considered to be important clinically. All of these agents are rapidly secreted unchanged in the urine by glomerular filtration.

Because aminoglycosides are positively charged at physiologic pH, their movement into cells of the body is limited to active transport processes. This distribution of aminoglycosides approximates that of extracellular fluid. Of particular relevance is their distribution into the mammary gland—many are used systemically for *E. coli* mastitis.

ABSORPTION

Aminoglycosides are poorly absorbed (about 10%) from the intact gastrointestinal tract. Enteritis and other pathologic changes, however, may allow significantly greater absorption to take place, and in cases of renal failure, toxic levels can accumulate. Absorption from intramuscular injection sites is rapid and nearly complete. Peak blood levels are usually achieved within 30 to 90 minutes after intramuscular administration. Absorption after subcutaneous injection may be protracted. Absorption after intraperitoneal administration can be rapid and substantial with a potential for producing serious side effects. Aminoglycosides can be administered by nebulization for treatment of upper respiratory infections with little absorption into the systemic circulation, especially in horses.

METABOLISM

Metabolism of aminoglycosides has not been reported. The serum clearance correlates highly with creatinine clearance, a clinical indicator of the glomerular filtration rate. Aminoglycoside antibiotics are eliminated unchanged in the urine, and 80 to 100% of administered drug is recoverable from the urine within 24 hours after intramuscular administration.

A variable fraction of filtered aminoglycoside is absorbed onto the brush border of the proximal tubule and loop of Henle cells. After binding, it is transported into the cell by pinocytosis and is then sequestered in lysosomes; subsequently redistribution into the cytosol occurs. Excessive accumulation leads to tubular cell necrosis characteristic of aminoglycoside nephrotoxicity.

The elimination of aminoglycosides depends on renal function, age, fever, and volume of distribution (V_d) of the drug in the body. Aminoglycosides have relatively short plasma half-lives of 1 to 2.5 hours. The elimination kinetics often follow those of a three-compartment model.

DISTRIBUTION

Aminoglycosides distribute into the extracellular fluid space with minimal penetration into most tissues except the kidney, where they accumulate in the renal cortex. The extracellular fluid compartment approximates 25% of body weight, but this volume can change substantially and significantly influence the concentration of an aminoglycoside. Contraction of the extracellular fluid volume occurs with dehydration from any cause and during gram-negative sepsis. An increase in antibiotic distribution volume can occur in patients with congestive heart failure or ascites.

Aminoglycosides attain therapeutic concentrations in pleural fluid, particularly if inflammation is present. Therapeutic levels are not reached in tracheobronchial secretions.

Aminoglycosides are not metabolized and are excreted unchanged by glomerular filtration. Accumulation in renal tubular epithelial cells results in prolonged tissue levels.

10.3 MECHANISM OF ACTION

The mechanism of action of all the aminoglycosides is believed to be the same. After oxygen-dependent active transport into the bacteria, aminoglycosides exert their activity by binding to a specific receptor protein on the 30S ribosomal subunit, thereby blocking the complexation of mRNA with formylmethionine and tRNA. This results in the improper translation of the tRNA, and the wrong amino acid is inserted into the protein being formed, rendering it nonfunctional. Additionally, aminoglycosides cause disruption of polysomes into monosomes incapable of protein synthesis. The intracellular site of action of the aminoglycosides is the ribosome, which has binding sites at both the 30S and 50S subunits.

Some variation exists between aminoglycosides with respect to their affinity and degree of binding. A number of steps in protein synthesis appear to be affected, but this varies among aminoglycosides: Spectinomycin lacks the capacity to produce misreading of the mRNA and often is not bactericidal in contrast to the other members. At low concentrations, however, all aminoglycosides may be only bacteriostatic.

Binding of the drug to the ribosome sufficiently alters the tRNA binding and distorts the codon-anticodon interaction with subsequent faulty protein production. Resistant organisms have an altered target protein on the 30S subunits. Membrane permeability (uptake) may be altered in some resistant organisms as well.

Because of the polarity of these aminoglycosides, a specialized transport process is required to enter the bacterium. The first concentration-dependent step requires binding of the aminoglycoside to anionic components in the cell membrane. The subsequent steps are energy dependent and involve the transport of the polar, highly charged aminoglycoside across the cytoplasmic membrane and then interaction with the ribosomes. The driving force for this transfer is probably the membrane potential. These processes are much more efficient if the energy used is aerobically generated. Several features of these mechanisms are of clinical significance:

1. The antibacterial activity of the aminoglycosides depends on an effective concentration of antibiotic outside the cell. They do not possess a residual effect (cf. penicillins).

2. Anaerobic bacteria and induced mutants are generally resistant because they lack appropriate transport systems.
3. With low oxygen tension, as in hypoxic tissues, transfer into bacteria is diminished.
4. Divalent cations, such as calcium and magnesium, are capable of antagonizing aminoglycoside transport into bacteria because they can combine with the specific anionic sites to the exclusion of the cationic aminoglycosides.
5. Transport of aminoglycosides across bacterial cell membranes is facilitated by an alkaline pH; a low pH may increase membrane resistance more than 100-fold.
6. Changes in osmolarity also can alter the uptake of aminoglycosides.
7. Some are transported more efficiently than others and thus tend to possess greater antibacterial activity.
8. Synergism is common when aminoglycosides and beta lactam antibiotics (penicillins or cephalosporins) are used in combination.

10.4 RESISTANCE

Resistance to aminoglycosides, which is often plasmid mediated, can develop rapidly. Bacteria acquire resistance to aminoglycosides by:

1. Mutation of the organisms, leading to altered ribosomes that no longer bind the drug
2. Reduced permeability of the bacterium to the drug
3. Bacterial enzymes that inactivate the drug

Resistance caused by ribosomal mutation is restricted to aminoglycosides of the streptomycin type. Ribosomal resistance to gentamicin and kanamycin has not been confirmed. Ribosomal resistance to streptomycin occurs by way of spontaneous mutation, resulting in a single amino acid change in one of the 21 proteins of the small ribosomal subunit. Such altered ribosomes are incapable of binding streptomycin.

The main mechanism of resistance to the aminoglycoside antibiotic may be plasmid mediated or due to mutation. Resistant strains can be obtained easily by laboratory habituation procedures; they do not transfer their resistance but characteristically exhibit extensive cross resistance with the aminoglycoside group, although not to other antibiotics. The mechanisms of resistance are the following:

1. **Impaired transport**. One mechanism of nonplasmid-mediated resistance is impaired transport across the cell membrane. Because the transport process is active and oxygen dependent, anaerobic bacteria and facultative anaerobes are more resistant to the aminoglycosides when in an anaerobic environment. Resistance owing to impaired transport can be induced by exposure to sublethal concentrations of these antibiotics. Bacterial resistance as a result of reduced permeability to aminoglycosides probably accounts for less than 20% of total clinical resistance.
2. **Impaired ribosomal binding**. Resistance owing to ribosomal mutation is restricted to aminoglycosides of the streptomycin type. A single mutation may be sufficient to alter the ribosomal-streptomycin binding sites.
3. **Amino-modifying enzymes**. The most common mode of resistance to aminoglycosides involves inactivation of the antibiotic by bacterial enzymes. The enzymes are encountered in both gram-negative and gram-positive bacteria.

Most resistance of gram-negative bacteria to aminoglycoside antibiotics is the result of drug-inactivating enzymes in the periplasmic space of the bacteria. Major inactivation mechanisms are acetylation of amino groups and phosphorylation or adenylation of hydroxyl groups. Some resistance is related to penetration of drug.

Enzymes responsible for aminoglycoside inactivation are coded by small, self-replicating, extrachromosomal loops of DNA (plasmids) known as R factors. The R factors often are able to transfer their genetic information to other bacteria by a process known as conjugation and are responsible for the spread of antibiotic resistance. The first case of inactivation of an aminoglycoside studied involved a kanamycin-resistant *Escherichia coli* isolate. Since this initial finding, other types of bacterial enzymatic inactivation of aminoglycosides have also been discovered.

10.5 CLINICAL USE

Aminoglycosides are important for initial treatment of life-threatening infections caused by gram-negative aerobes. The spectrum of activity of aminoglycosides includes many aerobic gram-negative bacteria, particularly *E. coli*, *Klebsiella pneumoniae*, *P. aeruginosa*, *Proteus*, and *Serratia*. Gentamicin is more effective than amikacin in killing most organisms except *Pseudomonas*, for which amikacin is more effective. Although *E. coli* and some *Pasteurella*, *Salmonella*, and *Brucella* species are susceptible to streptomycin and dihydrostreptomycin, applications of these drugs are limited. Aminoglycosides are not effective against most gram-positive organisms except for *Staphylococcus*. Because they require active transport and thus oxygen for bacterial cell uptake, they are ineffective against anaerobes.

Aminoglycosides in current clinical use include streptomycin, neomycin, kanamycin, gentamicin, amikacin, apramycin, and spectinomycin. Because of bacterial resistance to streptomycin, this drug is of limited use. Gentamicin is probably the drug of choice for initial therapy against *P. aeruginosa* infections. Gentamicin is inactivated by seven of the eight commonly recognized, bacterially produced enzymes that inactivate the aminoglycosides. Amikacin is the aminoglycoside of choice when resistance to gentamicin (or other aminoglycosides) is prevalent. Amikacin is inactivated by only two of the eight inactivating enzymes. Both gentamicin and amikacin are approved for intrauterine administration as indicated treatment against endometritis in mares.

Aminoglycosides in the kanamycin group are less potent in terms of efficacy and toxicity than those in the gentamicin group. Thus systemic bacterial infections that are considered susceptible to amikacin have minimum inhibitory concentrations (MICs) of 4 μg/ml or less, whereas for gentamicin the MIC of susceptible systemic infections is often 2 μg/ml. Aminoglycosides have relatively poor activity against *Strep-*

tococcus. Apramycin is of particular use not only against *E. coli,* but also *Salmonella* infections.

Streptomycin and dihydrostreptomycin have relatively narrow spectra. Bacterial resistance to streptomycin is becoming common. Gram-negative bacilli and some *Staphylococcus* are susceptible. Neomycin and kanamycin have much broader spectra, but their clinical use is mainly directed against gram-negative organisms. Gentamicin, tobramycin, amikacin, and netilmicin have somewhat extended spectra as compared with those agents previously mentioned. Resistance and cross resistance develop with continuous use. Anaerobic bacteria are not affected by aminocyclitol-aminoglycoside antibiotics.

10.6 SPECIFIC AMINOGLYCOSIDES

STREPTOMYCIN

Information about the pharmacokinetics of streptomycin is limited for animal species. In humans, it is known that after intramuscular administration peak plasma concentrations are attained within 1 to 2 hours. The plasma elimination half-life is usually 2 to 3 hours in adults with normal renal function and has been reported to range up to 110 hours in humans with severe renal impairment. In adults with normal renal function, 30 to 90% of a single intramuscular dose of streptomycin is excreted unchanged by glomerular filtration within 24 hours, with the greater part being excreted within the first 12 hours.

Streptomycin is widely used generally in combination with penicillin or other drugs. The usual regimen is 11 mg/kg of body weight given intramuscularly every 12 hours for 2 to 3 days. In dogs and cats, products containing streptomycin are commonly used in treatment of cellulitis, abscesses and other complications of wounds, upper respiratory tract infections, and tracheobronchitis. Streptomycin, in combination with penicillin, is used for treatment of cattle with shipping fever or after surgery or trauma.

Formulations containing streptomycin are indicated for treatment of infections caused by susceptible organisms, including *Corynebacterium pyogenes, Staphylococcus aureus, Klebsiella, Leptospira, Pasteurella, E. coli, Listeria,* and *Proteus.* Because many organisms are resistant to streptomycin, isolation and sensitivity testing are recommended when possible. Although streptomycin is not absorbed from the gastrointestinal tract, it can be used parenterally for treatment of susceptible systemic infections.

Streptomycin, in combination with penicillin, is most widely used in cattle for treatment of shipping fever, foot rot, mastitis, umbilical infections, wound infections, and other conditions caused by susceptible bacteria. Combinations containing streptomycin often are used prophylactically in cases of stress associated with shipping, surgery, or other trauma. The elimination kinetics of penicillin and streptomycin, however, are quite different.

GENTAMICIN

Gentamicin is active against nearly all strains of *Staphylococcus, Streptococcus, Pseudomonas, Proteus, E. coli, Klebsiella, Aerobacter,* and *Alcaligenes.* Gentamicin has been used in dogs and cats for treatment of cystitis, nephritis, upper respiratory infections, pneumonia, tracheobronchitis, pyodermatitis, and infected wounds. In addition, gentamicin is indicated in horses for control of bacterial infections of the uterus and as an aid to improving conception in mares. Gentamicin has been used parenterally for the treatment of colibacillosis and swine dysentery in piglets. Gentamicin has been used in cattle by intramammary infusion for treatment of mastitis, by intrauterine infusion for treatment of metritis, and parenterally for treatment of respiratory infections. A popular treatment regimen combines gentamicin and penicillin. These drugs should be delivered in separate syringes.

The recommended dosage level is 4.4 mg/kg twice the first day and once daily thereafter. Gentamicin is indicated in horses for control of bacterial infections of the uterus and as an aid to improving conception in mares. The dose is 2 g of gentamicin mixed with 200 ml of sterile saline solution infused into the uterus daily for 3 days. Gentamicin has been used systemically in stallions for treatment of genital tract infections owing to *Pseudomonas* at a dosage level of 4.4 mg/kg intramuscularly or intravenously every 12 hours for 10 days and in the treatment of horses with pneumonia, urinary tract infections, and infectious joint disease at 2.2 mg/kg every 8 hours for 6 days. In addition, gentamicin is indicated for treatment of pigs with colibacillosis or swine dysentery at a dose of 5 mg/kg intramuscularly or orally as well as administered in drinking water. It is also useful for osteomyelitis, particularly if staphylococcal infection is suspected. Gentamicin therapy for renal infections must always be accompanied by rigorous renal monitoring, especially in young animals.

AMIKACIN

Amikacin is a semisynthetic aminoglycoside derived from kanamycin. Amikacin is active against *Proteus, Pseudomonas, E. coli, Klebsiella*, and *Staphylococcus*, including some strains that are resistant to gentamicin, tobramycin, and kanamycin. Amikacin is indicated for treatment of genital tract infections in mares. The dose is 2 g of amikacin mixed with 200 ml of sterile saline solution infused into the uterus daily for 3 days.

Similar to other aminoglycosides, amikacin is potentially nephrotoxic and ototoxic and is not absorbed by the gastrointestinal tract. The recommended human dosage is 15 mg/kg divided into two or three equal doses. The usual duration of treatment is 7 to 10 days.

NEOMYCIN

Neomycin is also widely used in combination with other drugs. Neomycin has good activity against *Streptococcus, Staphylococcus, E. coli, Pseudomonas, Proteus*, and other organisms. Parenterally neomycin is nephrotoxic. Neomycin is most often used topically in infectious diseases of the eye and external ear and in contaminated wounds. Neomycin is also available alone or in combination with other drugs for treatment of enteric infections. Topical and oral formulations are available for companion and food animals.

KANAMYCIN

Kanamycin is active against many pathogenic bacteria, including *E. coli, Aerobacter, Salmonella, Proteus, Pasteurella*, and *Staphylococcus*. Kanamycin is not absorbed by the gastrointestinal tract but is frequently used for treatment of bacterial enteritis. Kanamycin is recommended for subcutaneous use at 5 mg/lb in divided doses at 12-hour intervals. In dogs, kanamycin has been used for treatment of cystitis, pyelonephritis, sinusitis, tracheitis, pneumonia, wound infections, osteomyelitis, and arthritis caused by susceptible organisms. Kanamycin has been used for treatment of bovine respiratory disease, mastitis, and other infectious conditions. A popular combination used in horses and cattle with respiratory conditions is kanamycin and penicillin G. These should not be delivered in the same syringe because excipients in the formulations may inactivate one or both drugs.

SPECTINOMYCIN

Spectinomycin is an aminocyclitol antibiotic rather than an aminoglycoside, and thus its action and toxicities differ substantially from those of a typical aminoglycoside. Spectinomycin, an aminocyclitol, is a tricyclic containing several oxygens, with amino and hydroxyl substitutes on the rings. It is similar to and has much in common with aminoglycosides, although its effect is bacteriostatic rather than bactericidal. It binds to the 30S ribosomal subunit but also appears to inhibit the translocation step. It does to perturbate codon recognition as do the aminoglycosides.

Spectinomycin is rapidly absorbed after intramuscular administration. Because it penetrates tissues poorly, its distribution is extracellular. Metabolic transformation of spectinomycin is limited: About 75% of the drug is eliminated by glomerular filtration in about 4 hours. Spectinomycin is also absorbed well after intramuscular use, and peak serum concentrations occur within 1 hour. With the highly water-soluble spectinomycin, serum concentrations can be readily and proportionately increased by increasing dosage.

Spectinomycin is available as a hydrochloride for parenteral or oral use; however, oral absorption is poor and is not accompanied by appreciable systemic activity. Lincomycin and spectinomycin are available in a 1:2 ratio as a water-soluble combination product intended for use in poultry and is now used also for swine dysentery. Spectinomycin is active against gram-negative coliforms and *Pasteurella* with MICs in the 15 to 20 μg/ml range. It is ineffective against anaerobes but active against mycoplasmae. The combination of lincomycin with spectinomycin has attained popularity for use in respiratory tract diseases of cattle. This combination appears to be of greatest value against *Mycoplasma* and perhaps *Pasteurella* secondarily.

Spectinomycin may be a particularly valuable antibiotic because of its low toxicity and usefulness against gram-negative coliforms. It can be used in high doses to compensate for low in vitro antibacterial activity. It is used in many countries for *E. coli* mastitis. The acute toxicity is of low order, with the LD_{50} (intravenous) in mice ranging up to 2000 mg/kg for spectinomycin. Protein binding is low to moderate, with spectinomycin less than 10%.

Spectinomycin resistance occurs by R factor transfer. An adenyltransferase-inactivating enzyme occurs that provides some cross resistance between spectinomycin and dihydrostreptomycin, but this is not an important clinical problem.

APRAMYCIN

Apramycin can be considered an aminoglycoside chemotherapeutic agent owing to its chemical structure. Use of this antibiotic is specifically aimed at mass therapy of colibacillosis and salmonellosis in veal calves and pigs.

Apramycin was discovered in 1968 as part of the fermentation product of *Streptomyces tenebrarius*. It is a member of the aminoglycoside group of antibiotics and is thus related to neomycin, kanamycin, gentamicin, spectinomycin, and streptomycin. Despite this close relationship, its chemical structure differs from the members of the group, and as a result it is stable in the presence of all but one of the enzymes produced by resistant bacteria.

Mode of Action

Apramycin is bacteriocidal in action. It has the property of inhibiting protein synthesis within the bacterial cell owing to the antibiotic altering the coding within the DNA of the cell nucleus, resulting in the formation of unacceptable proteins.

Resistance

One of the ways bacteria become resistant to antibiotics is by developing enzyme systems that inactivate the antibiotic. Although several enzymes exist that are effective against the majority of the aminoglycoside group, only one has been found that is effective against apramycin. Although transmissible drug resistance has been demonstrated in vitro, it is believed to be a rare occurrence in vivo.

When resistance does develop, it occurs in a stepwise manner so it builds up slowly. This resistance subsides when exposure to the antibiotic is removed. Cross resistance does occur within the aminoglycoside group, but it is not consistent. Thus apramycin-resistant organisms are not necessarily resistant to gentamicin or neomycin and vice versa. Apramycin is not inactivated by any of the known enzymes that confer resistance to aminocyclitol antibiotics.

Apramycin is a broad-spectrum antibiotic and is effective against gram-negative organisms, such as *E. coli, Salmonella, Bordetella, Pasteurella, Klebsiella,* and *Haemophilus pleuropneumoniae*. It is also shows activity against *Mycoplasma, Staphylococcus aureus,* and haemolytic streptococci. An organism with an in vitro MIC of less than 16 μg/ml is regarded as being sensitive to apramycin; however, in most cases the MIC is much lower, typical values for *Salmonella* and *E. coli* being below 8 μg/ml. An exception is *Salmonella* type 204C, in which some resistance has been reported.

Retention of the antibiotic within the bowel makes it especially suited to treatment of colibacillosis in pigs, and a choice of oral formulations in the form of a paste, soluble powder, and an in feed premix is available to provide for all ages and management practices. Accordingly its use in feed or water can be contemplated in the event of outbreaks of salmonellosis or coliform scours. The septicemic nature of salmonellosis in calves necessitates a parenteral approach to therapy with apramycin in view of its poor absorption after oral administration. An injectable formulation is thus preferred. Given intramuscularly at the recommended dosage rate of 20 mg/kg, peak plasma levels in the region of 21 μg/ml are achieved within an hour of administration. This is well above the MICs for susceptible bacteria. Effective levels are maintained for a period of 5 to 8 hours, but owing to the "postantibiotic" effect already referred to, it is usually unnecessary to repeat injection more than once every 24 hours. The optimum duration of treatment is considered to be 5 days, although in pigs the premix formulations may be administered for up to 28 days.

Advantages

The sensitivity pattern of apramycin is superior to two other commonly used antibiotics: neomycin and streptomycin, which, similar to apramycin, belong to the aminoglycoside group. Apramycin has a unique chemical structure that renders it stable in the presence of all but one of the bacterially produced enzymes (transferases) that form the basis for resistance to the group. The exception is acetyltransferase, which was first identified in 1987. Fortunately the onset of resistance if and when it occurs is "stepwise" rather than appearing suddenly, and field experience has shown that such resistance declines rapidly once the drug is withheld.

Apramycin is bacteriocidal, being a potent inhibitor of protein synthesis, its primary effect being on translocation. In common with the other members of the group, it has been shown to cause a degree of "misreading" of bacterial genes in vitro. It is well tolerated in the species for which it is intended with minimal toxic activity in target animals.

NEW AMINOGLYCOSIDES

Several new aminoglycosides are available for human use or are being developed for human and veterinary use, such as tobra-mycin, sisomicin, netilmicin, dibekacin, and habekacin.

Tobramycin is effective against *Proteus*, *Pseudomonas, E. coli, Klebsiella*, and *Staphylococcus*. The recommended human dosage is 1 mg/kg three times a day. Tobramycin, similar to other aminoglycosides, is not absorbed by the gastrointestinal tract and must be used cautiously in patients with decreased renal function.

The recommended human dosage level for tobramycin is 1 mg/kg every 8 hours, for netilmicin, to 3 mg/kg every 12 hours.

Sisomicin is a new aminoglycoside similar to gentamicin. Sisomicin, however, is protein bound to a lesser extent and is more potent in vivo. This drug is approved for human use in a number of countries (but not the United States) and is used in animals in France, Belgium, and other European countries. In dogs, sisomicin given once a day at 2 mg/lb is effective in cystitis and soft tissue infections caused by susceptible organisms.

Netilmicin is approved for human use in a number of countries. Netilmicin has a spectrum of activity similar to that of gentamicin and amikacin but is active against some organisms resistant to gentamicin, tobramycin, and kanamycin. Netilmicin is less nephrotoxic and ototoxic than gentamicin, tobramycin, and kanamycin.

10.7 AMINOGLYCOSIDE TOXICITY

The margin between therapeutic and toxic concentrations for all members of this group is not as great as that with the penicillins or macrolides. Toxic effects of aminoglycoside administration, ototoxicosis, and nephrotoxicosis are thought to be related to the drug given, the peak and trough concentrations in the blood, duration of therapy, state of hydration, and pretreatment renal function.

When used at therapeutic dosages, all aminoglycosides have a similar toxicologic profile. The kidney and the vestibular or auditory pathways of the eighth cranial nerve are the common targets of toxicity. Aminoglycosides also have a curarelike effect on neuromuscular junctions and have been associated with neuromuscular blockade. Anticholinesterase agents and Ca^+ preparations antagonize this effect.

Prolonged neuromuscular paralysis can occur when aminoglycosides are concurrently administered with other drugs that affect neuromuscular transmission, in particular anesthetics and skeletal muscle relaxants. Neurotoxicity manifests as a nondepolarizing, neuromuscular blockade with high drug concentrations or at lower concentrations in the presence of other drugs that alter neuromuscular function. The aminoglycosides inhibit the release of acetylcholine from motor end plates. They prevent binding of calcium to vascular smooth muscle preparations in vitro and are thought to act similarly at the presynaptic membrane.

All aminoglycosides are potentially toxic and should be used with caution in patients with impaired renal function. Aminoglycoside therapy is contraindicated after prolonged therapy with other similarly toxic compounds or other aminoglycosides. Use of aminoglycosides in animals undergoing anesthesia or in animals with rare hypersensitive reactions to other aminoglycosides is not recommended. Therapy should be discontinued if signs of auditory or vestibular impairment or depression occur. Elevations in blood urea nitrogen (BUN) or serum creatinine level, polyuria, or the presence of protein, casts, or cells in the urine may indicate nephrotoxicity. Aminoglycosides should be discontinued in such cases.

Cats are more susceptible to ototoxicities induced by aminoglycosides than dogs and are especially vulnerable when their renal function is impaired. Cats are exquisitely sensitive to the ototoxicity of aminoglycosides and are frequently used as animal models for human ototoxicity studies. Aminoglycoside antibiotics produce signs of vestibular toxicity, including vertigo, head tilt, ataxia, impaired righting reflex, and postrotatory righting reflex; signs of cochlear toxicity (nerve deafness in certain frequency ranges) can also occur. Amikacin causes primarily cochlear toxicity, whereas gentamicin causes predominantly vestibular toxicity. Netilmicin is twofold to fourfold less toxic to the eighth cranial nerve than gentamicin or tobramycin. Gentamicin causes more severe ototoxicity in cats than tobramycin, although amikacin may produce the most severe ototoxicity.

Streptomycin is more likely to damage the vestibular portion of the eighth nerve, whereas dihydrostreptomycin and kanamycin produce injury to the auditory portion. Other drugs in this class have the potential for damaging each portion of the eighth nerve.

Although all drugs of this class have nephrotoxic potential, gentamicin is probably the most and streptomycin the least nephrotoxic. Ototoxicity and nephrotoxicity caused by aminoglycosides are related to the drugs' ability to inhibit the incorporation of phosphate into phosphoinositides and blockade of calcium-binding sites.

It appears that all toxic side effects of aminoglycosides are due to blockade of the calcium-binding sites in tissues where the drugs accumulate. Nephrotoxicity is related to the number of amino groups present on the particular aminoglycoside. Toxicity of the clinically important aminoglycosides is, in order of greatest to least, neomycin, kanamycin, gentamicin, amikacin, and streptomycin or dihydrostreptomycin. In humans, gentamicin, amikacin, and tobramycin are considered equally nephrotoxic. A report of tobramycin use in cats, however, revealed that it may be more nephrotoxic to cats than gentamicin and amikacin; a single dose of 3 to 5 mg/kg can be nephrotoxic. The elimination of tobramycin in cats may be dose dependent (i.e., the rate of elimination decreases as the dose rises), which increases the risk of toxicity.

Nephrotoxicity is of major concern and is related to dosage and duration of treatment. Nephrotoxicity is uncommon when drugs are used for fewer than 7 days. Ototoxicity can occur but is rare in food animals. To avoid toxic effects, therapeutic doses of aminoglycosides should not be given for more than a week, and they should be given cautiously in animals with renal impairment. Failure of the kidneys to eliminate aminoglycosides results in high blood levels, even with therapeutic doses, that can cause further renal and vestibular damage. The oral administration of aminoglycosides is seldom dangerous when normal therapeutic doses are employed. Although it is remote, the possibility exists that animals with renal impairment and intestinal obstruction may become intoxicated.

Kanamycin is less nephrotoxic to dogs than neomycin, and it is less destructive to the auditory nerve than dihydrostreptomycin. In cats, kanamycin caused less vestibular damage than streptomycin. Gentamicin in cats is twice as toxic to the vestibular apparatus as streptomycin and more toxic to the cochlea than streptomycin or dihydrostreptomycin. Neomycin is more toxic than kanamycin, gentamicin, and streptomycin in both cats and dogs. Amikacin causes renal damage in dogs similar to other aminoglycosides. It also causes vestibular damage.

Aminoglycoside-induced acute renal proximal tubular nephrosis is due to their pinocytotic uptake by and accumulation inside renal proximal epithelial cells, primarily in lysosomes. Accumulation of aminoglycosides within these cells disrupts phospholipid metabolism and mitochondrial function. Histologically aminoglycosides cause typical morphologic changes associated with acute tubular necrosis; the proximal tubular epithelium shows evidence of hyaline degeneration, nuclear pyknosis and karyolysis, cellular desquamation, and intraluminal protein deposition and cast formation. Ultrastructural examination of renal proximal tubular epithelium from both dogs and cats reveals increases in the number of lysosomes, loss of tubular brush border, and myelin figures formation (also known as myelin figures). These ultrastructural changes occur during aminoglycoside treatment at clinical doses even without clinical signs of nephrotoxicity and may occur after only one dose of gentamicin in dogs.

The accumulation of drug into the proximal tubular cells and the consequent nephrotoxicity increase with the duration of therapy. Further, aminoglycosides decrease the renal production of vasodilatory prostaglandins, and replacement of these vasodilatory prostaglandins may diminish aminoglycoside nephrotoxicity. Neomycin is the most nephrotoxic of all the aminoglycosides, whereas streptomycin is the least nephrotoxic. The scale of nephrotoxicity of the other aminoglycosides, in order of decreasing nephrotoxicity, is gentamicin, tobramycin, kanamycin, and amikacin.

Several factors associated with a higher risk of nephrotoxicity include increasing age; compromised renal function; total dose; duration of treatment; and concurrent use of furosemide, methoxyflurane, or other potentially nephrotoxic drugs, such as cephalosporins. The new aminoglycosides are less nephrotoxic than the original ones, with netilmicin being the least nephrotoxic when compared with kanamycin, gentamicin, and tobramycin in dogs. In cats, aminoglycosides cause vestibular damage, with renal damage occurring a few days after, whereas the reverse is true in the dog, with the exception of streptomycin which causes vestibular damage before renal damage. Therapy should be discontinued if clinical signs of auditory or vestibular impairment or depression occur. Increases in BUN or serum creatinine; polyurea; or the presence of protein, casts, or cells in the urine may indicate nephrotoxicosis, and the use of aminoglycosides should be discontinued.

Nephrotoxicity of aminoglycosides can be minimized by:

1. Basing drug selection on culture and susceptibility results, thus ensuring that the drug used is effective against the target organisms
2. Using the proper dosing regimen
3. Using the least nephrotoxic drug (e.g., amikacin rather than gentamicin)
4. Maintaining the patient's hydration status
5. Using combination therapy with synergistic antibiotics (e.g., penicillins or quinolones) when the infection is serious or persistent
6. Monitoring the serum drug levels to ensure they are therapeutic (1 to 10 µg/ml gentamicin, 2.5 to 25 µg/ml amikacin) but not toxic.

10.8 MACROLIDES AND LINCOSAMIDES

In 1952, two closely similar antibiotics, erythromycin and carbomycin, were isolated from strains of *Streptomyces* from soil samples. Several other antibiotics with similar properties were isolated in the next few years, and two of these, spiramycin and oleandomycin, have been used clinically. All these antibiotics have a macrocyclic lactone ring, and the name "macrolides" has been suggested for them. They all have a complicated structure and a molecular weight of more than 700 and have unique nitrogen-containing sugars. They are weak bases, only slightly soluble in water but freely soluble in organic solvents. They form esters that are of clinical importance because they are better absorbed from the intestinal tract but may also be more toxic.

The macrolides are a large group of structurally related antibiotics. Only erythromycin and tilmilosin are clinically useful in cattle. Macrolides are weak bases with low aqueous solubility. They are unstable in both alkaline and acidic media. More stable ester forms are used in pharmaceutical preparations.

Macrolides are a group of antibiotics with a general structure containing a large lactone ring with 13 to 15 carbons, one amino sugar, and sometimes other sugar side chains. A number of antibiotics, including erythromycin, oleandomycin, triacetylo-leandomycin (troleandomycin), carbomycin, spiramycin, leucomycin, tylosin, and rosamicin (experimental drug), are members of this group.

Most macrolides and lincomycins are produced by *Streptomyces* bacteria. An exception is rosamicin, which is produced by *Micromonospora*. All of these antibiotics are basic compounds with a pH in the 6.6 to 8.8 range (tylosin, 7.1; lincomycin, 7.6; and erythromycin, 8.8). Macrolides are more effective as antibacterial agents in a slightly alkaline pH. Macrolides and lincomycins are of high lipid solubility.

Oleandomycin and erythromycin are similar, with the same basic 13-carbon lactone ring and side chain sugars. The compounds comprise a basic 15-carbon lactone ring with one or two side chain sugars, as represented by tylosin and rosamicin. At present, clinical use in the United States is restricted mainly to erythromycin and tylosin. Lincomycins, which are monoglycosides with an amino-acid-like side chain, are structurally dissimilar to macrolides, but they share many characteristics and are often included with them. Clindamycin has a chlorine replacing a hydroxyl in the seven position of lincomycin.

TYLOSIN (ELANCO)

This macrolide antibiotic was developed exclusively for veterinary use. Most of its therapeutic usage is directed against mycoplasmal diseases, particularly in poultry. It is also used as a growth promoter for pigs. Its spectrum of activity is typical of the macrolides, being basically gram-positive but also strongly active against *Mycoplasma*, particularly in the avian species.

Tylosin is well absorbed orally. The tartrate salt is used for water medication and the phosphate for feed. It is a safe antibiotic at recommended dosage rates, but intramuscular injection may cause some tissue irritation.

Tylosin has been obtained from soil isolates tentatively identified as strains of *Streptomyces fradiae*. It is markedly active in vitro against gram-positive bacteria, certain gram-negative bacteria, and mycoplasmae. It is well tolerated in animals and is effective in experimental mouse infections against gram-positive bacteria, *H. influenzae*, and meningopneumonitis virus. The pattern of induced resistance in *S. aureus* is similar to that with penicillin and erythromycin. Partial cross resistance with erythromycin is found, but no cross resistance with penicillin or tetracyclines has been demonstrated.

Tylosin is a fermentation product of *S. fradiae*, an actinomyces, that was isolated from a soil sample obtained in Thailand. The antibacterial spectrum is essentially against gram-positive bacteria. In addition, tylosin is widely recognized for its activity against *Mycoplasma*. Its toxicity is low, thus giving a high therapeutic index. Blood levels in cattle lasting beyond 24 hours from intramuscular administration of tylosin at various dosages have been reported.

Certain properties of tylosin indicate that it belongs to the macrolide class of antibiotics. The reported cross resistance of microorganisms to tylosin and erythromycin supports this view. The chemical and physical properties that lend support to this proposal are:

1. The identity of its sugars with those of magnamycin and spiramycin
2. The lactone ring as suggested by the infrared spectrum
3. Presence of a carbonyl group as suggested by the infrared spectrum
4. The high C-methyl content
5. The solubility properties of tylosin

An important feature of tylosin that is not shared by other macrolide antibiotics is the formation of desmycosin, a microbiologically active degradation product, by mild acid hydrolysis. Desmycosin exhibits physical, chemical, and antimicrobial properties that are similar to those of tylosin. Tylosin has been reported to inhibit the growth of spirochetes, protozoa, and mouse oxyurids and has been shown to be effective against mycoplasmae. When fed to animals, the antibiotic has been observed to stimulate growth.

ERYTHROMYCIN, LINCOMYCIN, AND CLINDAMYCIN

Erythromycin has been a popular antibiotic in human medicine for several years. It is usually the drug of choice for treatment of gram-positive infections in humans who are allergic to beta lactam antibiotics. Veterinarians have found erythromycin useful as well, although frequent gastrointestinal problems following administration of erythromycin have resulted in the use of lincomycin (Lincocin) and clindamycin (Antirobe) for infections that usually respond to erythromycin.

Erythromycin is the most active member of this group in vitro and is for most purposes the macrolide of choice. Oleandomycin is sometimes effective in treatment of infections resistant to erythromycin, but in most cases an unrelated antibiotic is preferable. Spiramycin is the least active of the three in vitro, but it gives the highest and best-sustained tissue levels and is unexpectedly active in vivo, especially for respiratory and mastitic infection.

These antibiotics, because of their poor solubility, are not easy to administer parenterally. Two salts of erythromycin are available for intravenous administration: the glucoheptonate and the lactobionate. Both must be injected slowly, over 5 to 10 minutes, and in a concentration of not more than 1 to 2%. Erythromycin lactobionate and erythromycin ethyl succinate dissolved in propylene glycol have been used for this purpose, but the injections are painful. The estolate is available for oral use.

LINCOSAMIDES

These drugs are not truly broad-spectrum antibiotics because their spectrum of activity includes gram-positive and anaerobic bacteria but not gram-negative bacteria. They act by binding bacterial ribosomes, thus inhibiting or impairing bacterial protein synthesis. Lincomycin and its semisynthetic derivative clindamycin (Antirobe, Upjohn) are lincosamides with a spectrum of activity that includes many gram-positive and *Mycoplasma* species. They are also highly effective against most anaerobic organisms, the major exceptions being some *Clostridium* species. Generally gram-negative organisms are resistant. Of the two drugs, clindamycin is the more effective. Clindamycin is active against gram-positive organisms, such as *Staphylococcus, Streptococcus, Actinomyces, Nocardia, Mycoplasma,* and *Toxoplasma*. Anaerobic bacteria, such as *B. fragilis, Fusobacterium, Peptostreptococcus,* and *Clostridium perfringens*, are susceptible to clindamycin. In suspected anaerobic infections, clindamycin is recommended for treatment until culture and susceptibility results are known. Lincomycin, used in cattle with systemic infections, is primarily bacteriostatic (inhibits protein synthesis) and has an antimicrobial spectrum that includes mainly gram-positive organisms.

10.9 MECHANISM OF ACTION

Macrolides interfere with bacterial protein synthesis at the ribosomal level. The effect is confined to rapidly dividing bacteria and mycoplasmae. They are bacteriostatic, but high concentrations may be bactericidal. Bacterial resistance can occur by inability to penetrate the microbe and by alteration of the receptor site on the ribosome. Cross resistance among macrolides is common. Macrolides are most active at a pH of 8.0.

Erythromycin and tylosin are bacteriostatic and act by binding to bacterial ribosomes and impairing protein synthesis in bacteria. Erythromycin is approved for use in cats, but tylosin is not. Chloramphenicol and lincosamides have similar mechanisms of action, so they should not be combined with erythromycin. All of these antibiotics are mainly bacteriostatic at the concentrations attainable in tissues with normal dosage.

The mechanism of action of erythromycin as a representative macrolide is inhibition of protein synthesis by way of interference with the translocation step. Erythromycin binds to the 50S ribosomal subunit at or near the donor or P site and, as a consequence, appears to produce strict inhibition of peptidyl transfer RNA binding to the donor site. The effect is inhibition of translocation of the developing peptide chain from the acceptor or A site to the donor or P site, which is required for elongation of the peptide chain as the ribosome moves along the mRNA strand. Small peptides may be formed but not highly polymerized peptide chains. The mode of action, although not identical, is probably of similar nature for all macrolide antibiotics. Lincomycins bind to a similar 50S ribosomal site and also inhibit methylation at or near the binding site. Decreased cellular penetration of the antibiotic also may be of importance in some instances and is perhaps partly the cause of the low activity against gram-negative organisms at physiologic pH.

Erythromycin and lincomycin inhibit protein synthesis in susceptible bacteria. Erythromycin is a macrolide antibiotic, and although lincomycin and clindamycin are unrelated in chemical structure, the mechanisms of action and spectrum of activity are similar, and the drugs are discussed together. Erythromycin binds to the 50S ribosomal subunit of the bacteria and interferes with the growth of the peptide chain. Because chloramphenicol, lincomycin, and clindamycin act at a similar site, these drugs may interact and should not be used together. It is often said that erythromycin is a bacteriostatic antibiotic. In reality, the "cidal" or static action is relative, depending on the bacteria and the antibiotic tissue concentrations achieved. Against sensitive organisms at full dose concentrations, erythromycin is bactericidal.

Lincomycin is bacteriostatic. Clindamycin is bactericidal to organisms that are particularly sensitive (e.g., *Streptococcus*) but may be bactericidal or only bacteriostatic to others (e.g., *S. aureus, B. fragilis*). Several *Actinomyces* and some *Nocardia* species are also sensitive to the lincosamides. Lincosamides are not effective against *Clostridium difficile*. Rapid colonic growth of *C. difficile* after administration of lincosamides has been implicated as a cause of serious and fatal diarrhea in several species.

10.10 RESISTANCE

Resistance may occur by stepwise mutation selection or plasmid R factor transfer. For macrolides, R factors are limited to *Staphylococcus*-resistance development. Fortunately the resistance problem appears to decline rapidly with discontinuance of erythromycin use. Erythromycin and oleandomycin can induce cross resistance to other macrolides and lincomycin but apparently not to chloramphenicol even though they all bind to a similar 50S ribosomal region. Cross resistance between erythromycin and other macrolides may occur, and consideration should be given to this factor when choosing alternative antibiotics. Resistance is associated primarily with decreased binding to the subunit active site. Resistance to erythromycin may be caused by decreased antibiotic entry into bacteria or an inability to bind to receptor sites. The activity of erythromycin is diminished in environments with acidic pH and in pus; therefore an in vitro susceptibility test may indicate sensitivity to erythromycin, but conditions at the site of infection may cause erythromycin to be ineffective. Conversely, the activity of erythromycin is greatly increased in an alkaline environment. At an alkaline pH, some gram-negative organisms are susceptible to erythromycin, but at a neutral or acidic pH, they are not. Organisms that are resistant to erythromycin may show cross resistance to lincomycin and clindamycin as well.

Bacterial resistance can occur by inability to penetrate the microbe and by alteration of the receptor site on the ribosome. Cross resistance among macrolides is common. Tylosin appears to have little involvement with side resistance compared with other macrolides. It is not involved in R factor transferable resistance with the *Enterobacteriaceae*.

10.11 ANTIBACTERIAL SPECTRUM

Macrolides are primarily active against gram-positive organisms, although some gram-negative bacteria, including *Pasteurella* and *Haemophilus*, may be sensitive. *Mycoplasma, Chlamydia, Rickettsia*, and *Actinomyces* are usually susceptible. Erythromycin's spectrum of activity includes gram-positive organisms, particularly *Staphylococcus* and *Streptococcus*, and those organisms resistant to penicillins. Therefore it may be used instead of penicillin for these organisms. Gram-negative organisms that are generally sensitive to erythromycin include *Pasteurella*. Although *Chlamydia* tend to be sensitive to erythromycin, *Mycoplasma* are often resistant.

The spectrum of activity for erythromycin and lincomycin include primarily gram-positive bacteria. Because they do not share the beta lactam structure, they resist inactivation by staphylococcal enzymes and are a good choice for the initial treatment of canine pyoderma. As mentioned earlier, resistance may develop with repeated use. Because these drugs are metabolized in the liver to inactive products before renal excretion, they do not achieve the high concentrations in urine that have been reported for other antibiotics. Consequently erythromycin, clindamycin, and lincomycin are not good choices for treating urinary tract infection.

The main use of erythromycin and lincomycin has been to treat staphylococcal infections in cases of penicillin resistance or to avoid penicillin-allergic reactions. Erythromycin is the most active macrolide against *Staphylococcus*, with the order of activity roughly as follows: erythromycin four times greater than oleandomycin, which is two to four times greater than carbomycin, which is four times greater than spiramycin. Lincomycins are effective mainly against gram-positive cocci; selected anaerobes, such as *Bacteroides* and *Fusobacterium*; and spirochetes, such as *Treponema*. Clindamycin is more efficient than lincomycin against most sensitive bacteria and anaerobes.

10.12 PHARMACOKINETICS

Macrolides diffuse well in tissues and body fluids, resulting in high concentrations in lung, liver, kidney, spleen, and reproductive tract but low levels in skeletal muscle. Macrolides and their metabolites are excreted mainly in bile. Urinary clearance is often slow and variable. Milk often has macrolide concentrations severalfold greater than in plasma.

These antibiotics are rapidly and widely distributed in the tissues and concentrated in the liver, spleen, and lungs. They are retained in the tissues for long periods after the levels in the blood have ceased to be detectable. Spiramycin gives higher and better-sustained tissue concentrations than any other member of the group. A large proportion of these antibiotics is excreted by way of the bile. Urinary levels are variable but tend to be low; only about 15% of the dose is recoverable in the urine.

Although lipid solubility of the macrolides and lincomycins is an important determinant of distribution, ion trapping of the basic compounds is also of considerable importance in tissues with a pH lower than blood, i.e., mammary gland and prostate gland (pH 6.8 to 7.0). The characteristic tissue accumulation of macrolides may allow for effective use of doses that appear to produce suboptimal serum concentrations. Respiratory tract infections may be effectively treated with doses actually producing serum concentrations lower than the MIC for the offending organisms because the lung-to-serum ratios are of the order of $3 \times$ to $5 \times$. The situation in other organs may be similar. With erythromycin and tylosin, peak serum concentration occurs 1 to 3 hours after intramuscular administration and 1 to 2 hours after oral use. After intramuscular administration, peak serum concentrations are maintained for several hours and then decline slowly. Tissue macrolide concentrations (peripheral compartment) are consistently larger than are serum (central) concentrations, and peak organ tissue concentrations may be as much as 5 to 10 times serum concentrations. Erythromycin is distributed well in most tissues. The volume of distribution exceeds extracellular water, and it achieves concentrations in certain tissues (e.g., lung) that are higher than corresponding plasma concentrations. Erythromycin also appears to concentrate in some tissue macrophages and leukocytes, which may account for its efficacy in treating intracellular infections, especially in the respiratory tract.

The pharmacokinetics of these antibiotics are best described by a two-compartment open model with at least two distinct body compartments. The elimination half-life and apparent V_d of the body for erythromycin in the cow are 190 minutes and 0.8 liter/kg of body weight, whereas in the dog, the half-life is about 60 minutes and the V_d is in excess of 2 liter/kg. The half-life and V_d for tylosin are 55 minutes and 1.7 liter/kg in the dog and 97 minutes and 1.1 liter/kg in the cow. The half-life for lincomycin is in excess of 3 hours, and the V_d is 1 liter/kg or more.

Erythromycin distributes widely in the body, including intracellular compartments. Erythromycin concentrations in tissues generally exceed those in serum. Erythromycin and tylosin are well distributed to most body tissues, including the skin and particularly the respiratory tract. The drugs are eliminated primarily unchanged in the bile. Erythromycin and tylosin are given intramuscularly. Pain and swelling may occur at the injection site.

Although tissue concentrations for tylosin appear to be sustained for long periods in cattle, the best clinical results are obtained using twice-daily administration or high-dose levels. Oral lincomycin produces peak blood concentrations within 2 hours, with absorption complete in 3 to 4 hours. Clindamycin is absorbed more rapidly orally and produces peak concentrations within an hour. After intramuscular use, peak serum concentrations of lincomycin or clindamycin occur at approximately 1 hour. Lincomycin and clindamycin should be administered at least twice daily for maximal benefit.

Studies that show erythromycin estolate to be absorbed to a greater degree than the other preparations have measured the total drug present in the plasma and not the concentration of the free, active base. It appears that no one oral preparation offers a significant advantage over another in terms of the attainable levels of free base in the plasma. Studies that have compared the efficacy of the various preparations have failed to show a difference. Erythromycin is painful when injected intramuscularly, and its use by way of this route is discouraged.

Only free erythromycin has antibacterial activity. Erythromycin stearate is absorbed as the base, following dissociation in the gastrointestinal tract. Erythromycin estolate and erythromycin ethylsuccinate are acid stable and absorbed as the ester, which is hydrolyzed in the body to a free base. Pharmacokinetic studies have measured the comparative absorption of the various preparations, but the results are difficult to interpret because the drug assays cannot distinguish between the inactive ester and the base.

The tylosin lung-to-serum ratios may be slightly higher, whereas milk concentrations are lower (lower pH). Spiramycin organ tissue-to-serum ratios, including milk, are considerably higher. Rosamicin prostatic tissue and secretion-to-serum ratios are about double those for erythromycin. Tissue concentrations of the lincomycins also often exceed serum concentrations. Lincomycin concentrations in skin appear to be equivalent to serum concentrations and bone, which usually contain low concentrations of antibiotic, and may have tissue-to-serum ratios in excess of 0.4 or 0.5. Most of the peripheral content appears to be in lung, liver, kidney, spleen, and reproductive tract, with relatively low concentrations in skeletal muscle. Care should be taken to prevent extravascular deposition of these drugs during intravenous administration. The lincomycins also may be slightly irritating by intramuscular administration. Both the lauryl sulfate ester or erythromycin (estolate) and troleandomycin have been associated with reversible hepatotoxicosis and icterus when used for prolonged periods in humans.

ORAL ADMINISTRATION

All macrolides are absorbed from the alimentary tract, but blood levels obtained after administration of the unprotected bases are low and variable. This is partly because their activity is reduced by gastric acid, and better levels are obtained by use of tablets coated with an acid-resistant material. It has also been shown that certain esters are better absorbed than the parent compounds; lauryl sulfate of propionyl erythromycin is both well absorbed and relatively acid resistant, but it is probably more toxic. Similarly, triacetyloleandomycin is better absorbed but more toxic than oleandomycin.

Veterinary macrolide preparations are limited to base forms of erythromycin and tylosin for oral and parenteral use. The base preparations of erythromycin for oral use are coated tablets to prevent acid degradation in the stomach. Absorption of all forms of these basic drugs occurs in the more favorable high pH of the small intestine. Maximal oral absorption occurs with the estolate preparation, which appears to be enhanced by the presence of ingesta in the intestinal tract. Effects of concurrent feeding on the absorption of other erythromycin preparations is variable, but to reduce the problem of emesis, administration after feeding may be required. Erythromycin is the most acid labile of the macrolides. Other members of the group are sufficiently acid stable to allow oral use without special preparations. Lincomycin is available as the hydrochloride in an injectable or tablet form. Because oral absorption is less than 50%, oral dosage is usually double the parenteral dosage. The drug should be given before feeding because the presence of ingesta reduces absorption and is not necessary to prevent emesis. Clindamycin is available as a hydrochloride, phosphate, or palmitate. The phosphate, which is less irritating, is used parenterally and orally, whereas the palmitate and hydrochloride forms are used orally. Oral absorption of clindamycin is high, and oral and parenteral dosages are similar. Clindamycin absorption is not affected by food. (Lincomycin and spectinomycin are available in a 1:2 ratio as a water-soluble combination product intended for use in poultry.)

Formulations of erythromycin are available as enteric-coated tablets, erythromycin stearate (salt), erythromycin ethylsuccinate (ester), or erythromycin estolate (salt of an ester). Because there are no published reports of studies that compare the systemic availability of erythromycin following oral administration in dogs or cats, information must be extrapolated from studies performed in humans. Erythromycin base is absorbed intact and usually shows good bioavailability, depending on the nature of the enteric coating. It is not known whether there are interspecies differences in absorption of enteric-coated tablets owing to the differences between gastrointestinal tracts in humans and small animals. Erythromycin is usually administered orally because intramuscular administration often causes pain at the injection site.

In humans, dogs, and cats, clindamycin is almost completely absorbed after oral administration. The presence of food in the gastrointestinal tract does not decrease absorption of the drug. Peak serum concentrations of clindamycin are attained within 75 minutes after dosing. The half-life of clindamycin is 5 hours, and therapeutic serum values can be maintained by oral dosing at 5.5 mg/kg every 12 hours.

In humans, dogs, and cats, clindamycin is widely distributed in many body fluids and tissues and penetrates well into respiratory secretions, pleural fluid, soft tissues, prostate gland, bones, and joints. Clindamycin is taken up rapidly by neutrophils, and the peak concentration in neutrophils is 40 times greater than the extracellular concentration. Antimicrobial activity is maintained within the neutrophil. Clindamycin readily crosses the placental barrier, but substantial concentrations are not attained in cerebrospinal fluid, even in human patients with meningitis. Most clindamycin is metabolized in the liver and excreted in the bile and urine as parent drug and active metabolites. The half-life of clindamycin may be prolonged in humans with impaired renal or hepatic function.

ELIMINATION

Both hepatic and renal routes of elimination of erythromycin are significant, and it undergoes enterohepatic circulation. Diarrhea is a potential side effect of erythromycin; however, this incidence seems to be acceptably low, and diarrhea resolves when the drug is stopped. It is not known whether the diarrhea is due to microfloral alteration or irritation of the gastrointestinal tract by the drug. Similarly, the relative contribution of the drug and the infecting organisms may not be obvious in some instances.

Elimination of macrolides and lincomycin occurs primarily through hepatic metabolism, which accounts for approximately 60% of an administered intravenous dose. The remainder is excreted in active form in the urine (20%) and bile (7%). With oral and intramuscular erythromycin and oral lincomycin administration, urinary excretion decreases to 10%, and biliary excretion and hepatic metabolism increase proportionately. Minor amounts are excreted in prostatic and pancreatic secretions, through the small intestinal mucosa, and in the milk (94%) of lactating animals. Although the total amount excreted through these minor pathways is low, the actual drug concentrations may be sufficient to provide adequate antibacterial activity. More hepatic metabolism with proportionately lower urinary and biliary excretion occurs with clindamycin as compared with lincomycin. Clearance of clindamycin depends on hepatic metabolism to both active and inactive metabolites. These are then cleared through biliary and renal elimination.

10.13 CLINICAL APPLICATION

Macrolides have been used as second-line antibiotics against gram-positive bacteria and mycoplasmae, and they may, under special conditions (such as pneumonia and mastitis), be of particular value because of their propensity to achieve high tissue concentrations. Serum concentrations are of value in predicting efficacy only as long as the tissue-to-serum ratios are kept in perspective. When used in an environment of alkaline pH (approximately 8), the efficacy for the macrolides against gram-negative bacteria can be markedly enhanced. This characteristic may be of particular value in urinary tract infections involving gram-negative bacteria and indicates that these drugs should not be used with urinary acidifiers. Tylosin may represent a first choice in some *Mycoplasma*-caused diseases. A new, experimental macrolide, rosamicin, may be of particular value because of its more favorable activity against gram-negative bacteria at lower pH values and its ability to achieve high concentrations in tissue, such as the prostate gland. Oleandomycin and its triacetyl derivative, troleandomycin, are less effective than erythromycin and hold no special advantages to recommend their use clinically. Macrolides may be effective for some problems in the horse, but gastrointestinal side effects limit clinical usefulness in this species. Lincomycins should not be used in the horse. Tilmycosin is a new macrolide for respiratory use in cattle.

Tylosin and lincomycins are effective against many *Mycoplasma* species of animal origin. Erythromycin effectiveness against *Leptospira* appears to be limited to *Leptospira pomona*, with a MIC of 5. The MIC against most of the other species is 20 or more and is probably much higher than is the antibiotic concentration normally attainable in tissues.

The macrolides are often combined with other antibiotics to increase effectiveness. This is not necessarily a recommended practice, but there are few combinations that are actually antagonistic or detrimental. Combinations of gentamicin with erythromycin against *E. coli* or with clindamycin against *E. coli*, *Klebsiella*, *Proteus*, or *Enterobacter* are reported to be synergistic or additive in some cases.

Erythromycin, clindamycin, and lincomycin are good choices for the initial treatment of mild to moderate staphylococcal infections. Because erythromycin has been frequently associated with gastrointestinal distress (e.g., vomiting, nausea, diarrhea), particularly in dogs, lincomycin has become a more popular choice among many veterinarians for oral administration to small animals. Clindamycin (Antirobe) has been approved for veterinary use and may show promise for treatment of infection caused by staphylococcal and anaerobic bacteria. Clindamycin appears to achieve adequate tissue concentrations that are effective against susceptible bacteria. Because these concentrations can be achieved in bone, clindamycin has been evaluated for treatment of experimentally induced osteomyelitis in dogs caused by *S. aureus*. The dose that was most efficacious was 11 mg/kg every 12 hours for 28 days. Lower doses or treatment for a shorter time was not as effective. It should be noted that the particular strain of *S. aureus* for these studies was selected for its sensitivity to clindamycin.

In dogs and cats, clindamycin has been used in treatment of wounds, abscesses, osteomyelitis, and periodontal diseases caused by gram-positive cocci or anaerobic bacteria. Clindamycin has also been used in the treatment of polymyositis caused by *Toxoplasma gondii* in a dog.

The combination of lincomycin with spectinomycin has attained recent popularity for use in respiratory tract diseases of cattle. This combination appears to be of greatest values against *Mycoplasma* and perhaps *Pasteurella* secondarily. The combination of lincomycin and spectinomycin may be expected to be at least additive or even synergistic because both appear to act on the translocation step but at different sites. In this respect, spectinomycin also may be useful in some situations in combination with a macrolide (*Pasteurella*) or chloramphenicol (*E. coli, Klebsiella,* or *Salmonella*). Unfortunately, the ratio of the preparation most commonly used, one part of lincomycin to two parts spectinomycin (1:2), may not represent the most effective ratio against all organisms. The dosage that is used against *Mycoplasma* may be too low when used against other organisms affected by only one of the drugs.

In the horse, because *Rhodococcus equi* exists intracellularly and elicits a pyogranulomatous inflammatory response, erythromycin was suggested as the drug of choice against that bacterium. Synergism was demonstrated in vitro against eight of nine strains of the organism with erythromycin (0.25 µg/ml) plus penicillin G (4.0 µg/ml) and against five of nine strains with erythromycin (0.25 µg/ml) plus rifampin (0.063 µg/ml). Penicillin does not readily penetrate into intracellular compartments. The popular use of erythromycin plus rifampin in the treatment of *R. equi* pneumonia is well known, but prospective clinical investigation of the synergistic combinations just described should be developed so the most beneficial and cost-effective use of drugs may be applied.

Lincomycin is well absorbed from intramuscular injection sites, with effective concentrations achieved in most tissues and fluids. Lincomycin is excreted mostly unchanged in bile, urine, and milk. It is given intramuscularly every 24 hours and only rarely causes side effects.

10.14 TOXICITY OF MACROLIDES

Gastrointestinal upsets are a common complication of oral therapy and occasionally may be severe. Apart from these, no serious side effects have been noted with the basic antibiotics, but jaundice and other signs of liver damage have been recorded in a few patients after administration of the esters propionyl, erythromycin, lauryl sulfate, and triacetyloleandomycin. This is a rare complication and occurs only after treatment has been continued for at least 12 days. No fatalities have been recorded, and in all cases the changes have been reversible. It has been suggested that the damage is a hypersensitivity phenomenon; allergic manifestations such as skin eruptions, which are rare with other forms of erythromycin, occur in approximately 0.5% of patients taking the propionyl ester.

Except for the gastrointestinal effects already mentioned, erythromycin, lincomycin, and clindamycin are safe antibiotics. Pseudomembranous colitis caused by an overgrowth of *C. difficile* is a significant complication in humans associated with lincomycin and clindamycin administration, but this has not been reported as a complication in dogs and cats. Hepatotoxicity has been described in humans associated with the administration of erythromycin estolate, but this complication has not been described in veterinary medicine. Inhibition of hepatic microsomal enzymes and subsequent decreased clearance of drugs coadministered with erythromycin have been described in humans (for example, decreased theophylline clearance), but the relevance of this observation has been controversial and is of doubtful importance in small animals.

Significant side effects have not been reported in small animals receiving lincomycin. Oral clindamycin is unpalatable, and its administration may cause excessive salivation. Clindamycin's side effects in humans and dogs include gastrointestinal upset characterized by vomiting and diarrhea, and these effects should probably also be expected in cats. Alterations in normal gastrointestinal microflora and overgrowth with *C. difficile* or other organisms are probably important in pathogenesis of diarrhea. A low incidence of skin disorders have been reported in dogs receiving clindamycin.

ADVERSE EFFECTS

Approximately 8 to 10% of human patients given clindamycin develop severe, possibly fatal, pseudomembranous colitis caused by a toxin secreted by clindamycin-resistant *C. difficile*. This suprainfection may be controlled with vancomycin or metronidazole, is not dose related, and may develop after oral or parenteral therapy. An antimicrobial-induced alteration of normal gastrointestinal bacterial flora, which is often fatal, may also develop in rabbits, guinea pigs, hamsters, or horses given lincomycin. Melena, hematochezia, and frequent defecation were reported in a dog with *T. gondii* infection and given clindamycin. These gastrointestinal signs resolved when clindamycin administration was discontinued.

Clindamycin has inherent neuromuscular-blocking properties and may potentiate effects of nondepolarizing neuromuscular blocking agents during anesthesia. The safety of clindamycin therapy in pregnant and breeding dogs has not been established.

All of these antibiotics are of a low order of toxicity. The main toxic manifestations of the macrolides and lincomycins are related to gastrointestinal dysfunction and to allergic manifestations. Erythromycin use may be accompanied by vomiting and occasionally by diarrhea, particularly when high doses are used. These problems are of lower frequency with tylosin use but may be seen with any of the macrolides. Horses seem to be sensitive to macrolide-induced gastrointestinal disturbances, and this factor has severely limited the use of erythromycin and perhaps even tylosin in horses. Lincomycin's use may also be associated with diarrhea; however, this is not the result of direct drug irritation but of preferential growth of certain toxin-producing bacteria. The problem is manifest by the development of pseudomembranous colitis, which occurs in humans, rabbits, and hamsters and which may be associated with elaboration of a clostridial enterotoxin. A similar problem may account for the purported effects in horses, which contraindicate the use of lincomycins in this species. Diarrhea has not been a problem in dogs given lincomycin even when given for months at large dosages. Anaphylaxis may occur after use of any of these antibiotics, but it is of low order of frequency. Bone marrow depression, ototoxicosis, or other central nervous system abnormalities have not been observed, even under conditions of prolonged high dosage in dogs or in cats with any of these antibiotics. The macrolides are directly irritating and may produce a marked inflammatory tissue reaction. For this reason, intramuscular administration should be used with some caution, and injections should be made deep into the largest muscle masses. Care should be taken to prevent perivascular deposition during intravenous administration as well. The lincomycins and spectinomycin also may be slightly irritating by intramuscular administration. Both the lauryl sulfate ester of erythromycin (estolate) and troleandomycin have been associated with reversible hepatotoxicosis and icterus when used for prolonged periods in humans. Erythromycin and the other macrolides appear to have little effect on polymorphonuclear granulocyte function until the concentrations are increased to 100 μg/ml, which is far beyond the concentrations attainable in body fluids with reasonable doses.

The overall toxicity of the macrolides and lincomycins is much higher in the newborn, possibly owing to lower hepatic metabolism, and the recent labeling of tylosin preparations includes recommendations for avoiding its use in the newborn. The lincomycins and spectinomycin are capable of producing neuromuscular blockade, although this is quite rare. Concurrent administration of anesthetics or other neuromuscular blocking relaxants may severely compound the problem, which is primarily manifested as respiratory paralysis. Macrolides should not be used concurrently with lincosamides. Acidic solutions depress macrolide activity. Erythromycin and tylosin are incompatible with many other drugs.

Tilmicosin ('Micotil') A new macrolide antibiotic, tilmicosin (Micotil), has been prepared by chemical modification of desmycosin. In vitro against selected animal bacterial pathogens, it inhibited growth of *Pasteurella multicida, Pasteurella haemolytica, Mycoplasma hyopneumoniae, Actinobacillus pleuropneumoniae, Streptococcus suis, Actinomyces pyogenes*, and certain other bacteria. The semisynthetic macrolide tilmicosin is an antibiotic with good in vitro activity against pasteurellae and mycoplasmae. A formulation has been developed that produces therapeutic levels in the lungs for 3 to 4 days.

A single subcutaneous injection of tilmicosin at 10 mg/kg body weight in cattle results in peak tilmicosin levels within 1 hour and detectable levels (0.07 mug/ml) in serum beyond 3 days. Lung concentrations of tilmicosin, however, in excess of the MIC of 3.12 µg/ml for *P. haemolytica* were observed in 95% of animals for at least 3 days following the single injection.

The pharmacokinetics of the antibiotic as formulated into propylene glycol at a high concentration of 300 mg/ml has allowed prolonged effectiveness from a single subcutaneous injection. Extensive safety studies in laboratory animals and cattle have shown that tilmicosin injection is safe to cattle and does not result in unsafe residues when used as directed on the labeling.

Tylosin, although an effective macrolide for bovine respiratory diseases, is primarily effective against mycoplasmae. Tilmicosin, the new semisynthetic derivative, retains this potent antimycoplasmal activity, but in addition the efficacy against *Pasteurella* is strengthened. Molecular modification has also resulted in higher lung concentrations being achieved and persistence of antimicrobial activity such that one subcutaneous injection provides antibiotic cover for 3 to 4 days.

In vitro more than 90% of the *P. haemolytica* and *P. multocida* isolates tested are sensitive to tilmicosin at a concentration of less than 6.25 µg/ml. Tilmicosin is also active in vitro against *Mycoplasma*, including bovine isolates. Levels four times the MIC are bactericidal for *Pasteurella*.

Micotil injection contains 300 mg tilmicosin per milliter and is administered as a single subcutaneous injection. Tilmicosin has an in vitro antibacterial spectrum that is predominantly gram positive with activity against certain gram-negative microorganisms and several *Mycoplasma* species as well. The antibacterial activity of tilmicosin led to its development for the treatment of bovine respiratory disease in cattle associated with *P. haemolytica* and *P. multocida* and other sensitive organisms. Tilmicosin was initially evaluated for treatment of bovine respiratory disease in newly weaned, recently shipped feedlot beef calves in Canadian and U.S. studies with very favorable results.

The tilmicosin formulation used is an aqueous solution contacting 300 mg tilmicosin activity in 25% propylene glycol.

Treatment consists of 10 mg/kg tilmicosin as a single injection administered subcutaneously in the neck. The use of a single injection, rather than several daily injections, is based on data that show that one injection of tilmicosin results in long-lived serum and tissue levels.

The effectiveness of tilmicosin in neonatal calves with pneumonia supports the continued evaluation of this compound in cattle especially as a treatment for the bovine respiratory disease complex (shipping fever) in feedlot cattle in which *P. haemolytica* is the most frequently involved bacterial pathogen.

The only adverse effect that may be noted in cattle with tilmicosin is transient swelling at the injection site. Hence not more than 25 ml of this concentrated solution should be injected at any one site. On account of its tardy kinetic excretory pattern, this drug is contraindicated for use in lactating animals. A withholding time of at least 56 days is recommended for meat. Of major significance is the fact that in contrast to other macrolides, tilmicosin is not safe for use in pigs. Fatalities in pigs may occur at doses as low as 20 mg/kg and in monkeys at 30 mg/kg. The drug is not intended for human use. The lethal dose for the primate is equivalent to a 6-ml injection in a 60-kg human. For this reason, accidental self-injection with tilmicosin would be especially dangerous, and the drug must never be used carelessly by the human operator.

SELECTED REFERENCES

Abramowiez, M.: Oral erythromycins. Med. Lett. Drugs Ther., *27*:1, 1985.

Adams, H.R.: Acute adverse effects of antibiotics. J. Am. Vet. Med. Assoc., *166*:983, 1975.

Baggot, J.D., Ling, G.V., and Chatfield, R.C. et al.: Clinical pharmacokinetics of Amikacin in dogs. Am. J. Vet. Res., *46*:1793, 1985.

Beech, J., Koln, C., and Leitch, M.: Therapeutic use of gentamicin in horses. Concentrations in serum urine, and synovial fluid, and evaluation of renal function. Am. J. Vet. Res., *38*:1085, 1977.

Benitz, A.M.: Future developments in the aminoglycoside group of antimicrobial drugs. J. Am. Vet. Med. Assoc., *185*:1118, 1984.

Braden, T.D., Johnson, C.A., and Wakenell, H.P.: Efficacy of clindamycin in the treatment of Staphylococcus aureus osteomyelitis in dogs. J. Am. Vet. Med. Assoc., *192*:1721, 1988.

Brewer, N.S.: The aminoglycosides: Streptomycin, kanamycin, gentamicin, tobramycin, amikacin, neomycin. Mayo Clin. Proc., *52*:675, 1976.

Brittain, D.C.: Erythromycin. Med. Clin. North Am., *71*:1147, 1987.

Brown, R.B., Barza, M., and Brush, J.L.: Pharmacokinetics of lincomycin and clindamycin phosphate in a canine model. J. Infect. Dis., *131*:252, 1975.

Brown, S.A., Dieringer, T.M., and Hunter, R.P. et al.: Oral clindamycin disposition after single and multiple doses in normal cats. J. Vet. Pharmacol. Ther., *12*:209, 1987.

Burrows, G.E.: Pharmacotherapeutics of macrolides, lincomycins and spectinomycin. J. Am. Vet. Med. Assoc., *176*:1072, 1980.

Burrows, G.E.: Gentamicin. J. Am. Vet. Med. Assoc., *175*:301, 1979.

Conzelman, G.M.: Pharmacotherapeutics of aminoglycoside antibiotics. J. Am. Vet. Med. Assoc., *176*:1078, 1980.

Dow, S.W.: Management of anaerobic infections. Vet. Clin. North Am., *18*:1867, 1988.

Dow, S.W.: Anaerobic bacterial infections and response to treatment in dogs and cats: 36 cases (1983–1985). J. Am. Vet. Med. Assoc., *189*:930, 1986.

Dow, S.W., and Jones, R.L.: Anaerobic infections. Part II. Diagnosis and treatment. Compend. Cont. Educ. Pract. Vet., *9*:827, 1987.

Engelhardt, J.A., and Brown, S.A.: Drug related nephropathies. Part II. Commonly used drugs. Compend. Cont. Ed. Pract. Vet., *9*:281, 1987.

George, W.L., Sutter, V.L., and Goldstein, E.J.C.: Aetiology of antimicrobial agent associated colitis. Lancet, *1*:802, 1978.

Gingerich, D.A., Baggot, J.D., and Kowolski, J.J.: Tylosin antimicrobial activity and pharmacokinetics in cows. Can. Vet. J., *18*:96, 1977.

Gingerich, D.A., Rourke, J.E., Chatfield, R.D., et al.: Amikacin: A new aminoglycoside for treating equine metivitis. Vet. Med. Small Anim. Clin., *78*:783, 1983.

Gourlay, L.H., Thomas, L.H., and Wyld, S.G.: Effects of a new macrolide antibiotic (tilmicosin) on pneumonia experimentally induced in calves by mycoplasma bovis and pasteurella haemolytica. Res. Vet. Sci., *47*:84, 1989.

Haddad, N.S., Ravis, W.R., Pedersoli, W.M. et al.: Pharmacokinetics of a single dose of gentamicin given by intramuscular and intravenous route to lactating cows. Am. J. Vet. Res., *47*:808, 1986.

Harari, J., and Lincoln, J.: Pharmacologic features of clindamycin in dogs and cats. J. Am. Vet. Med. Assoc., *195*:124, 1989.

Hardie, H.: Spectinomycin in veterinary practice. Vet. Rec., *92*:3, 1973.

Houdeshell, J.W., Lamendola, J.F., and McCracken, J.S.: Clinical pharmacology of aminoglycosides. Mod. Vet. Pract., *63*:619, 1982.

Huber, W.C.: Aminoglycosides, macrolides, lincosamides, polymyxins, chloramphenicol and other antibacterial drugs. *In* Veterinary Pharmacology and Therapeutics. 6th Ed. Edited by N.H. Booth and L.E. McDonald. Ames, Iowa State University Press, 1988.

Ihrke, P.J.: An overview of bacterial skin disease in the dog. Br. Vet. J., *143*:112, 1987.

Ihrke, P.J.: Therapeutic strategies involving antimicrobial treatment of the canine urinary tract. J. Am. Vet. Med. Assoc., *185*:1165, 1984.

Ihrke, P.J.: Halliwell, R.E.W., and Beubler, M.J.: Canine pyoderma. *In* Current Veterinary Therapy VI. Edited by R.W. Kirk. Philadelphia, W.B. Saunders, 1977.

Indiveri, I., and Hirsch, D.C.: Susceptibility of obligate anaerobes to trimethoprim-sulfamethoxazole. J. Am. Vet. Med. Assoc., *188*:46, 1986.

Jacobson, E.R.: Serum concentrations of gentamicin in cats. Am. J. Vet. Res., *46*:1356, 1985.

Jenkins, W.L.: Clinical pharmacology of antibacterials used in bacterial bronchopneumonia in cattle. Mod. Vet. Pract., *66*:264, 1985.

Jernigan, A.D.: Pharmacokinetics of amikacin in cats. Am. J. Vet. Res., *49*:355, 1988.

Kunkle, G.A.: New considerations for rational antibiotic therapy of cutaneous staphylococcal infection in the dog. Semin. Vet. Med. Surg. [Small Anim.], *2*:212, 1987.

Lees, G.E., and Rogers, K.S.: Treatment of urinary tract infections in dogs and cats. J. Am. Vet. Med. Assoc., *184*:648, 1986.

Ling, G.V.: Therapeutic strategies involving antimicrobial treatment of the canine urinary tract. J. Am. Vet. Med. Assoc., *185*:1162, 1984.

Prescott, J.F., and Baggot, J.D.: Aminoglycosides and aminocyclitols. *In* Antimicrobiol Therapy in Veterinary Medicine. Boston, Blackwell Scientific Publications, 1988.

Queener, S.F., Luft, F.C., and Hamel, F.G.: Effect of gentamicin treatment on adenylatecyclase and Na+, K+, ATPase activities in renal tissues of rats. Antimicrob. Agents Chemother. *24*:815, 1983.

Tobin, T.: Pharmacology review: Streptomycin, gentamicin and the aminoglycoside antibiotics. J. Equine Med. Surg., 206, 1977.

Wilkins, R.J., and Helland, D.R.: Antibacterial sensitivities of bacteria isolated from dogs with tracheobronchitis. J. Am. Vet. Med. Assoc., *162*:47, 1973.

Ziv, G., and Sulman, F.G.: Distribution of aminoglycoside antibiotics in blood and milk. Res. Vet. Sci., *17*:68, 1974.

CHAPTER

11

TETRACYCLINES, CHLORAMPHENICOL, AND QUINOLONES

11.1 Tetracyclines
11.2 Mode of Action
11.3 Kinetic Fate
11.4 Formulations
11.5 Side Effects and Toxicity
11.6 Doxycycline
11.7 Chloramphenicol
11.8 Kinetic Disposition
11.9 Adverse Effects
11.10 Chloramphenicol Analogs
11.11 Quinolones—Enrofloxacin
11.12 Spectrum of Activity
11.13 Mechanism of Action
11.14 Pharmacokinetics
11.15 Toxicity
11.16 Therapeutic Indications

11.1 TETRACYCLINES

A systematic search for new antibiotics in the late 1940s led to the discovery of the tetracycline group of antibiotics. The first was chlortetracycline (Aureomycin) in 1948, then oxytetracycline (Terramycin) in 1950, and finally the basic structure tetracycline in 1952. Tetracyclines have been available for human and veterinary medical use for more than 30 years.

The drugs in this group are effective against a variety of gram-negative, gram-positive, and anaerobic organisms as well as intracellular organisms, such as *Chlamydia, Mycoplasma*, and *Rickettsia*. Tetracyclines are also effective against *Actinomyces*. Their gram-negative spectrum includes *Escherichia coli, Pasteurella multocida, Klebsiella, Enterobacter, Brucella*, and some *Haemophilus* species. As with choloramphenicol, they act by binding to bacterial ribosomes and inhibiting or impairing bacterial protein synthesis.

Tetracyclines are all broad-spectrum antibacterial agents with additional activity against *Mycoplasma, Rickettsia* and *Chlamydia*. In vitro activity of members of this group is almost identical, but differences are seen in their stability absorption and binding characteristics, which cause significant differences in their activity in vivo. In addition, variation in physical properties governs suitability of various tetracyclines for parenteral, ocular, and intramammary use.

Tetracycline, oxytetracycline, and chlortetracycline are the only tetracyclines of route use in veterinary medicine. There are three naturally occurring tetracyclines (oxytetracycline, chlortetracycline, and demethylchlortetracycline) and several that are derived semisynthetically (tetracycline, rolitetracycline, methacycline, minocycline, doxycycline, lymecycline, and others).

Since the isolation of chlortetracycline from the fungus *Streptomyces aureofaciens* in 1948, several other tetracyclines of clinical value have been isolated from fungi or have resulted from the chemical manipulation of the basic tetracycline molecule. The objectives of these chemical manipulations have been to modify natural tetracyclines to improve gastrointestinal absorption, to enhance tissue distribution, to prolong reten-

tion in the body, and to enhance their antimicrobial activity. Minocycline and doxycycline are the most lipid soluble of the tetracyclines available clinically.

Tetracyclines exert antimicrobial activity against a range of gram-positive and gram-negative bacteria, *Rickettsia, Chlamydia, Actinomyces*, and *Protozoa*. The antimicrobial spectrum of the various tetracyclines is similar, although some quantitative and qualitative differences do exist. Minocycline and doxycycline are more active than other tetracyclines against anaerobic bacteria and several facultative gram-negative bacteria. Tetracyclines used in cattle (oxytetracycline, chlortetracycline, tetracycline) are similar.

The tetracyclines compose a group of antibiotics characterized by a common hydronaphtracene skeleton. Chlortetracycline was isolated from the fungus *S. aureofaciens* and oxytetracycline from *Streptomyces rimosus*. Although strains of *Streptomyces* are capable of producing tetracycline, this drug is produced commercially by hydrogenolysis of chlortetracycline. Demeclocycline is produced from a mutant strain of *S. aureofaciens*, whereas methacycline, doxycycline, and minocycline are produced semisynthetically.

The differences are small in terms of molecular structure. The halogenation of the tetracycline molecule with chlorine increases its affinity for chemical reactions, and hence it is less stable than the other tetracyclines in certain situations. Oxytetracycline is the only one of the three with acceptable tissue irritation and can be used parenterally.

Since the original three, other tetracyclines have been produced:

Demethylchlortetracycline
Methacycline
Doxycycline
Minocycline
Rolitetracycline

Tetracyclines are thermally unstable and active in either acidic or alkaline environments. Aqueous solutions are unstable. Tetracyclines chelate divalent and trivalent cations to form insoluble complexes. All of the tetracycline derivatives are crystalline, yellowish, amphoteric substances that in aqueous solution form salts with both acids and bases. They are characteristically fluorescent compounds. The most common salt form is the hydrochloride except for doxycycline, which is available as doxycycline hyclate. The tetracyclines are stable as dry powders but not in aqueous solution, particularly at high pH ranges (7.0 to 8.5). The base forms are relatively insoluble in water, but hydrochlorides are much more soluble. Aqueous solutions are unstable but tend to be more unstable at alkaline pH.

They all have an affinity for metallic ions, especially magnesium, calcium, aluminum, and iron, and should not be administered with milk or high calcium levels in feed unless an appropriate upward adjustment in dose is made. This metallic binding tendency precludes their use in milk fever solutions and other situations in which they are likely to come into contact with high concentrations or metallic ions.

Oxytetracycline is in common use in cattle, mainly because of its wide antibacterial spectrum. The half-life in serum is about 8 hours. This means that after an intramuscular injection of the highest recommended dose, 10 mg/kg body weight, a therapeutic serum concentration (>0.5 μg/ml) is maintained for about 24 hours. This long dosage interval is of value from a practical point of view, especially in the treatment of beef cattle.

SPECTRUM OF ACTIVITY AND MINIMAL INHIBITORY CONCENTRATIONS

Tetracyclines are broad-spectrum antibacterial agents with activity against a wide range of gram-positive and gram-negative bacteria, including obligate anaerobes. When their activity against *Chlamydia*, *Rickettsia*, and certain protozoa is considered, they have the widest range of activity of any antibiotics. As a general rule, it is accepted that the level of 0.5 μg/ml of any tetracycline antibiotic at the infection site should be accepted as a minimal inhibitory concentration (MIC).

Tetracyclines are active against *E. coli*, *Klebsiella*, *Enterobacter*, *Brucella*, and *P. multocida*, although many strains of these bacteria have acquired resistance to tetracyclines. *Proteus mirabilis* and *Pseudomonas aeruginosa* are resistant, but many strains of

Haemophilus have remained susceptible. Tetracyclines are also effective against some mycobacterias as well as many *Mycoplasma*, *Chlamydia*, and *Rickettsia*.

Tetracycline resistance in bacteria is caused by a decreased uptake of tetracycline into the bacterial cell and acquired ability of the bacteria to "excrete" the drug out of the cell. Most of the resistance to tetracyclines, transferred by R plasmids, increases in response to subinhibitory concentrations of tetracyclines.

11.2 MODE OF ACTION

Tetracyclines enter microorganisms partly by passive diffusion and partly by an energy-dependent process of active transport. As a result, susceptible cells concentrate the drug, so the intracellular drug concentration is much higher than the extracellular one. Once inside the cell, tetracyclines bind reversibly to receptors of the 30S subunit of the bacterial ribosome in a position that blocks the binding of the aminoacyl-tRNA to the acceptor site on the mRNA-ribosome complex. This effectively prevents the addition of new amino acids to the growing peptide chain, inhibiting protein synthesis. The selective inhibition of protein synthesis in microorganisms may be explained by the lack of concentration of tetracyclines in mammalian cells.

Tetracyclines must enter bacteria to inhibit protein synthesis. This uptake appears to depend on an active transport process. Resistance to tetracyclines seems to result from decreased uptake of drug in strains of bacteria carrying an R factor. It has been shown that R-factor-mediated resistance is accompanied by a decreased uptake of labeled tetracycline. Evidence suggests that R-factor-mediated resistance to tetracyclines results from the induced synthesis of an inhibitor of transport of these antibiotics.

Tetracyclines bind to the bacterial ribosome and mRNA, thereby inhibiting protein synthesis within the bacterial cell. The primary tetracycline-binding site is on the 30S ribosomal subunit. There is no competition between these agents and aminoglycosides, indicating that the binding sites are separate and distinct. When bound to that subunit, tetracyclines prevent binding of the aminoacyl-tRNA to the acceptor site. The selective toxicity for bacteria is due to tetracycline accumulation within bacterial cells; mammalian cells do not actively accumulate these compounds. The first part of the bacteria's two-part uptake system is a rapid uptake driven by the proton-motive force caused by the pH differential between the environment and the cytoplasm. The second uptake system is a slower energy-dependent uptake. In gram-negative bacteria, tetracyclines must pass through the outer membrane to reach the uptake systems.

It has been known for some time that the primary action is against prokaryotic protein synthesis and that this is mediated by prevention of the attachment of aminoacyl-tRNA to the A site of the ribosome.

A tetracycline molecule binds to a ribosome in such a way that the codon-anticodon interaction between the tRNA and the A site on the ribosome is disrupted. Tetracyclines are more effective against multiplying microorganisms and as a group tend to be more active in a pH range of 6.0 to 6.5.

Resistance is conferred by plasmid-mediated reduction in tetracycline uptake by the bacterium. Resistance develops by the bacterial cell wall becoming less permeable to the antibiotic. The two forms recognized are mutant strains and plasmid-mediated resistance. Resistance develops slowly in steps and is widespread today. Cross resistance among tetracyclines is common.

11.3 KINETIC FATE

Tetracyclines are absorbed irregularly from the small intestine; they suppress ruminal fermentation. The absorption of tetracyclines can be adversely affected by the presence of metals in the gastrointestinal tract. Tetracyclines react with divalent and trivalent metals, such as calcium, magnesium, aluminum, and iron, to form relatively insoluble chelates.

Antacids containing aluminum, magnesium, or calcium also adversely affect the absorption of tetracyclines. The simultaneous intake of sodium bicarbonate (2 g) results in a 50% reduction in serum concentrations after ingestion of 250 mg of tetracycline when the antibiotic is given in capsules. When tetracycline is dissolved before its administration, however, sodium bicarbonate does not depress absorption, indicating that the dissolution of the capsules is affected. Apparently a low pH is necessary for dissolution of tetracycline capsules.

Absorption occurs mainly in the upper small intestine and is best in the absence of food. It is impaired by chelation with divalent cations (Ca^{2+}, Mg^{2+}, Fe^{2+}) or with Al^{3+}, especially in milk and antacids, and by alkaline pH.

Peak plasma levels are achieved within 2 to 4 hours. Thus oral doses (if following oral administration) persist longer than any other oral antibiotics, and in this the tetracycline group is unique. There is, however, a threshold level for oral administration above which no further increase in blood and tissue levels results. This is a built-in safety factor but is unpredictable and varies from one species to another.

Tetracyclines are absorbed somewhat irregularly from the gastrointestinal tract. A portion of an orally administered dose of tetracycline remains in the gut lumen, modifies intestinal flora, and is excreted in the bile.

Tetracyclines are also eliminated in milk, attaining approximately 50 to 60% of the plasma concentration in most instances. The levels are often higher in mastitic milk. Peak concentrations occur in milk 6 hours after a parenteral dose, and traces are still present up to 48 hours.

Because of their excretion by way of the bile into the gastrointestinal tract, tetracyclines can disturb the normal intestinal flora, resulting in nausea, vomiting, and diarrhea. Further, because of the broad spectrum of activity, suprainfections with *Clostridium difficile* and *Candida albicans* have been reported after tetracycline administration. The water-soluble tetracyclines are eliminated principally by renal mechanisms.

Tetracyclines may induce a fever (as high as 106° F after 2 to 3 days of treatment), but it resolves when the drug is discontinued. Tetracyclines also can cause gastrointestinal upset characterized by anorexia, nausea, and vomiting. Anaphylactic reactions also have been reported to occur after receiving tetracyclines.

Because therapeutic concentrations of tetracyclines occur in the liver, kidney, and urine, these drugs work well for infections in these systems. Once absorbed, tetracyclines are well distributed throughout the body, with highest concentrations found in liver, spleen, kidney, and lung. They enter the fetal circulation in antibacterial concentrations but somewhat lower (50 to 70%) than the maternal circulation. Levels in bile are 5 to 15 times greater than in plasma, and the liver is an important source of excretion; also, relatively high levels can be achieved in the gastrointestinal tract after parenteral therapy. They diffuse relatively slowly into the aqueous humor and cerebrospinal fluid, and high concentrations by intravenous infusion appear to be indicated for good therapeutic results in diseases of these systems.

Levels in saliva, pleural fluids, and peritoneal fluids are somewhat lower than in serum. Tetracyclines are slowly excreted in urine, explaining their long persistence in blood. Higher concentrations persisting for up to 3 days after cessation of therapy can be achieved by long-term administration owing to a cumulative effect, and concentrations 100 to 300 µg/ml are feasible. This makes tetracyclines excellent agents for treatment of urinary tract infections. Also, because of the threshold on absorption, large oral doses maintain high concentrations in the gastrointestinal tract. Thus, in addition to their broad spectrum, their excellent gastrointestinal and tissue concentration over a long period as well as high concentrations in urine and bile make tetracycline excellent therapeutic agents in animals.

DISPOSITION IN NORMAL ANIMALS

Plasma-protein binding varies from 20 to 40% for oxytetracycline. Tetracyclines are distributed extensively through the body, with the highest concentrations found in the kidneys, liver, bile, spleen, and lungs. Most tetracyclines are only partially metabolized, with most being excreted in the urine and feces, although biliary elimination also occurs.

The plasma half-lives of tetracyclines in adult cattle vary from about 6 to 12 hours. The long-acting formulation of oxytetracycline, given intramuscularly, provides effective plasma concentrations for about 72 hours.

DISTRIBUTION

After absorption, tetracyclines enter the blood stream, where binding to plasma proteins occurs. Much variation has been reported for determinations made in humans, and this is reflected in the reactions. The binding of oxytetracycline is relatively small compared with other tetracyclines. This generalization appears to hold for studies made in dogs, cattle, and horses. In the blood, 20 to 80% of various tetracyclines is protein bound. With oral doses of 500 mg every 6 hours, tetracycline hydrochloride and oxytetracycline reach peak levels of 4 to 6 µg/ml. With doxycycline and minocycline, the peak levels are somewhat lower (2 to 4 µg/ml). Intravenously injected tetracyclines give somewhat higher levels only temporarily. The drugs are distributed widely to tissues and body fluids except for the cerebrospinal fluid, where concentrations are low. Minocycline is unique in reaching high concentrations in tears and saliva—a feature that permits it to eradicate the meningococcal carrier state. Tetracyclines cross the placenta to reach the fetus and are also excreted in milk. As a result of chelation with calcium, tetracyclines are excreted mainly in bile and urine. Concentrations in bile are 10 times higher than in serum; some of the drug excreted in bile is reabsorbed from the intestine (enterohepatic circulation) and contributes to maintenance of serum levels. Ten to 50% of various tetracyclines is excreted into the urine, mainly by glomerular filtration. The renal clearance of tetracyclines ranges from 10 to 90 ml/minute.

Oxytetracycline distributes into synovial and peritoneal fluids, lung bronchial fluid, and renal tissues and reaches high concentrations in urine of horses. It is distributed to the liver, is significantly eliminated in bile, and undergoes enterohepatic circulation. It is this route of elimination that probably causes the alteration of intestinal microflora.

All tetracyclines reach tissue concentrations in liver, kidney, and urine that exceed serum concentrations. The volume of distribution of minocycline is approximately 2 liters/kg, and serum clearance is 3.2 ml/kg/minute. This results in a serum half-life of approximately 7 hours. Biliary concentrations of active drug are high owing to active biliary transport of tetracyclines. Biliary concentrations of minocycline can exceed concurrent serum concentrations by 30-fold. Enterohepatic recirculation of the tetracyclines prevents biliary excretion from contributing a large amount to the elimination of these agents, and only 20 to 50% of tetracyclines are eliminated in the feces. Most tetracyclines are eliminated by glomerular filtration either as parent compound or as conjugated drug. Approximately 60 to 70% of the hydrophilic tetracyclines and 30% of lipophilic tetracyclines are eliminated by the kidneys. Mean urine tetracycline concentrations in dogs given 18 mg/kg orally every 8 hours were approximately 140 µg/ml.

11.4 FORMULATIONS

PARENTERAL ADMINISTRATION

Preparations for parenteral administration need to be carefully formulated, often in propylene glycol or polyvinylpyrrolidone with additional dispersing agents, to provide stable solutions for injection and to minimize pain and irritation. Tetracyclines form poorly soluble chelates with bivalent and trivalent cations.

Oxytetracycline, a broad-spectrum antibiotic, has been widely used for many years for disease treatment and control in human and animal medicine as well as an agent for improving productivity. As with other injectable preparations, repeated daily injections are necessary to maintain adequate blood levels for the control of disease. Over the years, some improvements have been made in drug concentration of parenteral oxytetracycline products, and different solvent systems have been used to minimize the pain associated with injection. Specially buffered tetracycline solutions can be administered intramuscularly or intravenously. Absorption of long-acting oxytetracycline from intramuscular sites may be substantially delayed. The necrosis resulting at intramuscular injection sites takes time to heal.

RECENT ADVANCES WITH OXYTETRACYCLINE

A great deal of sophisticated formulation technology goes into creating stable oxytetracycline solutions for injections. Propylene glycol has been used as a base but causes tissue irritation with pain and inflammation when given subcutaneously or intramuscularly. By the intravenous route, it can cause temporary recumbency unless given slowly. Lactamide base is an improvement on propylene glycol.

Polyvinylpyrrolidone is a more recent base that has allowed more concentrated solutions (100 mg oxytetracycline/ml) to be administered with less pain and tissue damage and additionally prolongs effective blood levels after a single administration. Thus 10 mg/kg intramuscularly using Terramycin 100 polyvinylpyrrolidone maintains plasma levels above 0.5 µg/ml for 40 hours, making 2-day intervals between administration feasible.

Complexing with P.V.P. a large molecular weight polymer surrounds the magnesium salt of oxytetracycline. This stable water-soluble complex transports the antibiotic away from the site of injection initially in the form of the complex. As a result, little or no irritation is seen at the site of injection.

The product containing polyvinylpyrrolidone as a vehicle causes much less tissue damage, and healing takes place more rapidly. The reason why it is so much less irritant cannot be explained at this stage. It has been suggested that the oxytetracycline may form a complex with polyvinylpyrrolidone and that this complex is less irritant.

All tetracycline antibiotics when administered intramuscularly may cause severe tissue damage, characterized by necrosis and polymorphonuclear infiltration. Oxytetracycline administered in a propylene glycol water solvent produced the least tissue damage. The clinical signs of pain and irritation after an intramuscular injection are well known.

Lesions may remain in the muscle tissue for a considerable period, and it is therefore preferable that injected animals should not be slaughtered within 30 days for human consumption. In an attempt to minimize this undesirable side effect, oxytetracycline was formulated by some manufacturers with polyvinylpyrrolidone incorporated as a vehicle.

An advance on this concept is a patented injectable formulation of Terramycin using 2-pyrollidone with an oxytetracycline concentration of 200 mg/ml. This has allowed even smaller dose volumes while not increasing tissue irritation and pain. More significant, however, is its action in prolonging blood levels. Thus a single injection of 20 mg/kg intramuscularly maintains a therapeutic blood level over a 3- to 4-day period, which should cover the length of therapy required in most acute infections with a single injection.

A depot formulation of oxytetracycline is now available. The product contains 200 mg/ml, and the solvent system is based on 2-pyrollidone. After intramuscular injection of 20 mg/kg body weight, therapeutic serum concentrations are said to be maintained for 3 to 5 days. The mode of action depends on a controlled precipitation of the drug at the injection site.

Despite the unprecedented high concentration of 200 mg/ml, the drug is not only well tolerated at site of injection, but also the residue profile indicates all tissues are clear of residue 28 days after injection. The maximum lesion at the injection site consists of a small amount of fibrous tissue, which does not necessitate trimming even when animals are slaughtered immediately at the end of the withdrawal period.

This product (Liquamycin LA-200) employs a unique patented solvent system based on 2-polyvinylpyrrolidone, the lactam of gamma-aminobutyric acid (GABA). It occurs in low concentration in a number of common foodstuffs, such as tomatoes and catsup. It has the advantage of being rapidly metabolized in the animal and poses no safety or residue problems. LA-200 was specifically formulated to produce, after a single intramuscular dose, both a high peak and a sustained blood antibiotic level extending over 3 to 4 days.

Basically oxytetracycline itself is an irritative compound; the higher and the longer the local oxytetracycline concentration, the more tissue irritation. The composition of the preparation may limit this irritation, or it may itself enhance the irritant effect. The solvent system for solubilizing the oxytetracycline complex contains as a rule an organic solvent with several additives (e.g., buffers, magnesium salts, antioxidants).

So-called long-acting formulations (20%) claim a long oxytetracycline persistence in plasma. This "retard effect" is related to the degree of irritation as well as to oxytetracycline persistence at the injection site. Thus this retard effect is not an exclusive finding with 20% formulations.

11.5 SIDE EFFECTS AND TOXICITY

Because of their excretion through the bile into the gastrointestinal tract, tetracyclines can disturb the normal intestinal flora, resulting in nausea, vomiting, and diarrhea. Further, because of the broad spectrum of activity, suprainfections with *C. difficile* and *C. albicans* have been reported after tetracycline administration.

Accidental and experimental production of fatal diarrhea in the horse after intravenous administration of oxytetracycline has been described. The dose of oxytetracycline was higher than the normal therapeutic dose, and the reaction was attributed to an enterotoxemia consequent on a marked increase in *Clostridium perfringens* in the gut. Overgrowth by *Salmonella* could have been responsible for many of these cases.

Oxytetracyclines have been frequently used in equine practice without adverse reactions ensuing. Based on antimicrobial sensitivity and most pharmacologic data, a tetracycline is often the drug of choice. The discomfort produced after intramuscular injection influences use of the intravenous route in tetracycline therapy. Careful consideration, however, must be given to the routine use of tetracyclines in the horse, and, in view of the known dangers and possible legal implications, tetracyclines should not be given to horses by any route unless infecting microorganisms are solely sensitive to them; the prophylactic use of this group of antibiotics should be resisted.

There is little doubt that at highest levels oxytetracycline is a gastrointestinal irritant, but when given by the parenteral route, these levels would not be reached by biliary excretion. Superinfection is a more likely sequela and cannot be ruled out. The cause(s) of colitis-X in horses have not been identified, and its onset has been linked with many agents, both natural and manmade. Also, most other antibiotics have been associated with the condition as well, including penicillia/streptomicin combinations. Because many practitioners use oxytetracycline injectables without side effects in horses, and in view of their value as therapeutic agents, evidence at this time would support their continued use in horses.

The adverse reactions to members of this group, in particular oxytetracycline, should be familiar to all equine clinicians. The more uncommon acute reaction observed during or shortly after intravenous oxytetracycline is characterized by shivering, ataxia, collapse, dyspnea, and recumbency lasting 5 to 45 minutes. This could be an anaphylactic reaction, possibly elicited by degradation products of the antibiotic, found even after proper storage for prolonged periods.

In humans, diarrhea can be induced directly by the irritant effect of oral tetracyclines and indirectly by the development of superinfections, particularly of salmonellae, regardless of the route of administration. Accidental and the experimental induction of severe diarrhea and death in horses after a single intravenous dose of 15 g (27 to 45 mg/kg) oxytetracycline has been described. The delayed reaction was attributed to toxemia following an increase in *Clostridium welchii* in the gut. Three horses developed severe diarrhea after general anesthesia and intravenous use of oxytetracycline at 4.4 mg/kg, two dying despite intensive fluid therapy. Further, local and systemic usage at half this dose rate produced fatal diarrhea in five horses after general anesthesia or transport. *Salmonella* overgrowth could have caused some of the reported cases because the biliary excretion of tetracyclines produces intestinal levels higher than the simultaneous plasma levels and greater than the MICs for many gram-negative organisms. The nondetection of *Salmonella* in most instances could be misleading because repeated sampling and selective culturing are essential to confirm negative results. Anaerobic culturing of intestinal contents must not be overlooked, however, because there is some evidence that enterotoxinlike substances, possibly produced by *Clostridium,* may play a role in the pathogenesis of antibiotic-induced colitis in other species.

There is a similarity between the oxytetracycline reactions and the colitis-X syndrome, and in many documented cases of the latter, a broad-spectrum antibiotic was given in high doses before the onset of diarrhea. Treatment of antibiotic-induced diarrheas should be based on vigorous body fluid replacement, intestinal protectants, good nursing, and immediate cessation of antimicrobial therapy.

OTHER GASTROINTESTINAL DISTURBANCES

As a rule, oral antibiotic therapy should be avoided in treatment of gastrointestinal conditions in the horse because alteration in bacterial flora may favor superinfection with pathogenic microorganisms, such as salmonellae or fungi. The principal effect occurs in the large intestine, where ultimately there is malabsorption of water and electrolytes followed by osmotic diarrhea. If antimicrobial drugs must be used in diarrhea, they should be given via parenteral routes; nevertheless, care must be taken with antibiotics, such as the tetracyclines, that are largely excreted in the bile and undergo an enterohepatic cycle, which enhances their deleterious effect on the resident bacterial population of the gut.

In the neonate, whether enteric disease is the sole presenting sign or part of septicemia, oral use of antibiotics has been advocated for treatment and prophylaxis. If antimicrobials are used, appropriate parenteral administration is preferred, even during the first week of life. It should be borne in mind that most infections and deaths in neonatal foals are associated with failure of colostral immunoglobulin transfer.

Tetracyclines can induce catabolism, causing acidosis and increased serum urea nitrogen, when administered to patients with renal dysfunction. This catabolic state may contribute to the hair loss in cats that have received tetracyclines. As with many antibiotics, low-grade febrile reactions have been observed in cats, probably related to the patient immune response to the foreign compound. Finally, administration of tetracycline to growing animals or to pregnant females results in brown discoloration of bones and teeth in the juvenile and neonate.

Tetracyclines chelate multivalent cations, thereby inactivating themselves. The tetracyclines also disturb neuromuscular transmission, particularly when they are administered in conjunction with other neuromuscular blocking agents and anesthetics. Co-administration of tetracyclines with methoxyflurane produces renal failure in humans, but concurrent administration of these agents has caused only polyuria in dogs. Chlortetracycline, owing to nonspecific inhibition of protein synthesis in the liver, may decrease the metabolism of biotransformed drugs. Finally, intravenous bolus administrations can cause collapse, especially if propylene glycol is the vehicle.

INTERACTIONS

The absorption of tetracyclines from the gastrointestinal tract is decreased by milk and milk products (less so for doxycycline and minocycline), antacids, kaolin, and iron preparations. Tetracyclines chelate calcium in teeth and bones and thereby become incorporated into these structures, inhibiting calcification and causing brown or yellowish discoloration. At extremely high concentrations, the healing processes in fractured bones are impaired.

Rapid intravenous injection of a tetracycline can produce hypotension and sudden collapse. This acute depression of cardiovascular function appears to be related to the ability of the tetracyclines to chelate ionized calcium, although a depressant effect by the propylene glycol carrier itself may also be involved. This effect can be avoided by slow infusion of the drug (>5 minutes) or by pretreatment with intravenous calcium gluconate. Intravenous administration of undiluted propylene-glycol-based preparations leads to intravascular hemolysis with hemoglobinuria and possibly other reactions, such as hypotension, ataxia, and central nervous system depression.

Tetracyclines interfere with protein synthesis even in host cells and therefore tend to be catabolic. An elevation in blood urea nitrogen (BUN) values can thus be expected. The combined use of glucocorticoids and tetracyclines often leads to a significant weight loss, particularly in anorexic animals.

Hepatoxic effects owing to large doses of tetracyclines have been reported in pregnant women and in other animals.

Tetracyclines are also potentially nephrotoxic and are contraindicated (except for doxycycline) in cases of renal insufficiency. Fatal cases of renal failure have been reported in cattle that have received high doses of oxytetracycline in the presence of septicemia and endotoxemia. The administration of expired tetracycline products may lead to acute tubular nephrosis.

Swelling, necrosis, and yellow discoloration at the injection site almost inevitably occur. Hypersensitivity reactions do occur; e.g., cats may show a "drug fever" reaction often accompanied by vomiting, diarrhea, depression, and inappetence.

Tetracyclines are capable of inhibiting leukocyte chemotaxis and phagocytosis when present in high concentrations at sites of infection. This clearly hinders normal host defense mechanisms. The addition of glucocorticoids to the therapeutics regimen would have impact even on the immunocompetence of the patient.

Large oral doses of tetracycline depress ruminal microfloral activity and produce ruminoreticular stasis. Intravenous administration of undiluted propylene-glycol-based preparations lead to intravascular hemolysis. Rapid intravenous injection may produce sudden collapse from acute hypotension. Tetracyclines chelate calcium in teeth and bones. They are antianabolic; use of a tetracycline with a corticosteroid can lead to pronounced weight loss. Tetracyclines may also cause hepatosis owing to fatty infiltration of the liver. Use of outdated tetracycline products may lead to acute renal tubular nephrosis. Excessive doses of oxytetracycline also produce nephrotoxicity.

POTENTIAL DRUG INTERACTIONS

Absorption of tetracyclines from the gastrointestinal tract is impaired by milk, antacids, kaolin, and iron preparations. Tetracyclines lose activity when diluted in infusion fluids and are chelated with divalent or trivalent cations when mixed with any other medication.

11.6 DOXYCYCLINE

Chlortetracycline was first isolated from *S. aureofaciens* in 1948. Tetracycline congeners that followed all had broad-spectrum antimicrobial activity and clinical efficacy and had relatively few side effects. These facts have resulted in tetracyclines becoming some of the most widely used antibiotics in human and veterinary medicine. Constant modification of the tetracycline ring structure resulted in oxytetracycline, tetracycline, demethylchlortetracycline, and methacycline as well as doxycycline and minocycline. Elimination times permit a further classification into short-acting (tetracycline, oxytetracycline, chlortetracycline), intermediate-acting (demethylchlortetracycline and methacycline), and long-acting (doxycycline and minocycline) agents.

Of these, doxycycline and minocycline appear to offer advantages that render them useful in certain situations in veterinary medicine. Their major advantage lies in their greater lipid solubility relative to other tetracyclines. This characteristic probably accounts for their enhanced antimicrobial effectiveness for some organisms, more efficient absorption after oral administration, and enhanced distribution in the body. The principal excretory organ for doxycycline is the intestine, where the drug diffuses through the intestinal mucosa into the intestinal tract. This unique characteristic makes this drug useful in cases of pre-existing renal dysfunction and may render this drug superior to other tetracyclines in treatment of intestinal infections. Doxycycline is used for respiratory tract and intestinal tract diseases.

Although the hydrophilic congeners, such as tetracycline and oxytetracycline, have been used extensively, the more lipid-soluble derivatives, doxycycline and minocycline, have recently become more widely used in veterinary medicine. A direct relationship exists between lipid solubility and biliary excretion as well as in the penetration of antibiotics across the blood-brain and blood-ocular barrier. The concentrations of minocycline and doxycycline are markedly higher than those of oxytetracycline and tetracycline in cerebrospinal, brain, and ocular fluids and aqueous and vitreous humor. Penetration of doxycycline into pulmonary tissue, bronchial wall, and bronchial secretions is good.

PHARMACOKINETICS

All tetracyclines except doxycycline and minocycline have similar pharmacodynamic and pharmacokinetic properties. Doxycycline and minocycline have the advantage of greater tissue penetration because of increased lipid solubility and an expanded antimicrobial spectrum. Pharmacokinetics of doxycycline differ greatly from that of older tetracyclines. Major differences include a five fold to ten fold increase in lipid solubility and more extensive protein binding. These properties enhance tissue penetration and prolong the biological half-life.

Minocycline and doxycycline are more lipid soluble than older tetracyclines, so they more easily cross cell membranes. Thus they are better able to penetrate tissues (e.g., the central nervous system and lungs) and to accumulate in secretions (e.g., bronchial secretions, tears, saliva, and bile) and are more effective against intracellular organisms. The lipid-soluble drugs are cleared primarily by hepatic metabolism and biliary elimination.

Absorption

Although the tetracyclines are generally well absorbed when administered orally, their absorption may be hindered in the digestive tract owing to binding by food, milk, or drugs that contain calcium, magnesium, or iron. Minocycline and doxycycline absorption is not as affected as that of the older tetracyclines, such as tetracycline, oxytetracycline, and chlortetracycline. The reason for milk having less effect on doxycycline absorption may be related to the fact that this drug has less affinity for calcium than do other tetracyclines.

Absorption of doxycycline is rapid and almost complete (93% from the upper portion of the gastrointestinal tract in humans). Peak serum concentrations occur between 2 and 3 hours after ingestion. Doxycycline absorption is much less affected by food or Ca^{2+} as compared with absorption of other tetracyclines. Although only 30% of chlortetracycline and 70 to 80% of tetracycline, oxytetracycline, and demedocycline is absorbed in the gut, absorption is 90 to 100% for doxycycline and minocycline. Doxycycline and minocycline are almost completely absorbed from the gut and are excreted more slowly, leading to persistent serum levels. Doxycycline does not require renal excretion and does not accumulate significantly in renal failure. Doxycycline and minocycline may be more extensively biotransformed than other tetracyclines (up to 40% of a given dose).

DISTRIBUTION

Plasma protein binding varies from 20 to 40% for oxytetracycline to approximately 90% for doxycycline and is proportional to the relative lipid solubility of the congener. Only lipid-soluble tetracyclines, such as minocycline and doxycycline, diffuse appreciably into the cerebrospinal fluid, even in the presence of meningeal inflammation. Minocycline and doxycycline penetrate lung, bronchial secretions, sputum, tears, and saliva. Cerebrospinal fluid levels reach up to 30% of the plasma doxycycline concentration.

Of all tetracyclines, only doxycycline and minocycline penetrate to any major extent into the central nervous system.

Doxycycline is distributed widely to most body tissues. After giving doxycycline at 10 mg/kg body weight orally in dogs, peak serum concentrations of 4 µg/ml are reached after 24 hours. The biologic half-life in dogs has been reported to be 10 hours and 12 hours. In dogs, the ratios of tissue-to-serum concentrations are as follows: heart, 2; lungs, 1.3; muscle, 1.4; liver, 2.8; and kidney, 3.8.

Other studies also have reported on the abilities of doxycycline in achieving greater tissue and tissue fluid concentrations than other tetracyclines in the prostate gland, saliva and tears, lungs, bronchial secretions, and milk. In cattle, absorption rates of several tetracyclines from the mammary gland correlate with their lipid solubility. Minocycline or doxycycline are absorbed much more rapidly than oxytetracycline or tetracycline. The persistence of doxycycline in milk is considerably greater than that of oxytetracycline after intramuscular injection of these antibiotics. Highly lipid-soluble tetracyclines concentrate in tissues to a greater extent than less lipid-soluble analogs. Doxycycline, being much more lipid soluble than oxytetracycline, attains a far greater degree of penetration in muscle for given free-drug concentrations in serum.

EXCRETION

The excretion of doxycycline is somewhat unique. In the dog, urinary, fecal, and biliary routes constitute 16 to 22%, 75%, and less than 5% of doxycycline's elimination. Although doxycycline attains high concentrations in the bile, biliary excretion accounts for a minor fraction of the drug's elimination. Small intestinal excretion constitutes the major route of elimination. An inverse relationship exists between lipid solubility and urinary excretion, presumably because of greater tubular reabsorption of doxycycline.

The disappearance of doxycycline and minocycline after intravenous injection generally is slower than that of other tetracyclines.

In humans, the renal clearance of doxycycline was shown to be considerably less than that of tetracycline throughout a wide range of urinary pH. This observation is consistent with expectations of greater tubular reabsorption of the more lipid-soluble doxycycline.

Doxycycline can safely be given to patients with impaired renal function without modification in dosage. Major modifications in dosage are required for all other tetracyclines if renal function is impaired.

ANTIBACTERIAL SPECTRUM

For entry of tetracyclines into the microbial cell, it appears as though this process is favored by the lipid solubility of the antibiotic. Tetracyclines show their greatest antimicrobial activity in vitro in an acidic pH range close to their isoelectric point. Moreover, the most lipid soluble of the tetracyclines, doxycycline and especially minocycline, have been shown to exert greater antimicrobial activity in vitro against several organisms than is the case for other members of this class of antibiotics.

The hydrophilic congeners pass through the pores of the outer membrane; the more lipid-soluble tetracycline derivatives diffuse through the lipid bilayer of the outer membrane. If the pores are not present, the lipophilic congeners may inhibit the bacteria, whereas the hydrophilic congeners may have no effect. Doxycycline and minocycline exhibit the greatest liposolubility and better penetration of bacteria, such as *Staphylococcus aureus*, than do the group as a whole.

The cell walls of staphylococci resistant to tetracyclines contain more lipid than susceptible staphylococci. Perhaps it may be speculated that minocycline and doxycycline, being much more lipophilic than tetracycline, are capable of entering the lipid-rich, resistant staphylococci cells by simple diffusion. Thus minocycline and doxycycline may be capable of circumventing the active transport process required for tetracycline.

The antimicrobial spectrum of doxycycline is similar to that of other tetracyclines. Doxycycline has broad-spectrum activity against gram-positive and gram-negative aerobic and anaerobic bacteria. In general, doxycycline is more active against most staphylococci, streptococci, and anaerobic bacteria. Doxycycline has good activity against *Mycoplasma, Ureaplasma, Chlamydia,* and the Rickettsiaceae.

Most members of the Enterobacteriaceae have variable sensitivity to doxycycline. Most strains of *P. mirabilis* and *P. aeruginosa* demonstrate resistance in vitro. Similar to tetracyclines, minocycline and doxycycline are more active than other tetracyclines against anaerobic bacteria and several facultative gram-negative bacteria. Minocycline is 4 to 64 times more active in vitro than are other tetracyclines against *Nocardia*. Perhaps most interesting is the observation that minocycline is markedly more active than are other tetracyclines against *S. aureus*. Further, minocycline is active against staphylococci that are resistant to other tetracyclines.

SIDE EFFECTS

Staining of teeth can occur in pups when tetracyclines are given to the bitch during the last 2 to 3 weeks of pregnancy or to pups during their first month of life. Doxycycline is reported to be less prone than other tetracyclines in producing this effect in children (presumably because doxycycline appears to be less susceptible to interactions with calcium). Doxycycline also disturbs the normal intestinal flora to a lesser extent than do the other tetracyclines.

Tetracyclines are included among those drugs for which major modifications in dosage must be made in patients with pre-existing renal dysfunction. Doxycycline represents an important exception to this generalization because the intestine, rather than the kidney, is the major excretory organ. Doxycycline has been used safely in humans with pre-existing renal dysfunction, without dosage modification.

Microsomal enzyme inducers, such as phenobarbital and phenytoin, shorten the plasma half-lives of minocycline and doxycycline. With the exception of minocycline and doxycycline, the presence of food can substantially delay the absorption of tetracyclines from the gastrointestinal tract.

Doxycycline may offer advantages over other tetracyclines in:

1. Treatment with a tetracycline in patients with renal dysfunction. The major excretory route for doxycycline is the gastrointestinal tract and not the kidney.
2. Treatment of tetracycline-sensitive intestinal infections. It is possible that the diffusion of doxycycline through the intestinal mucosa provided better distribution to the infecting organisms. It would seem worthwhile to evaluate the effectiveness of this drug for some of the tetracycline-sensitive gastrointestinal infections in domestic animals.
3. Less toxicity to horses and cats than other tetracyclines.

It has been reported that doxycycline has less effect on the normal intestinal flora of humans than do other tetracyclines.

CLINICAL USES

Doxycycline is a semisynthetic tetracycline derivative. It differs from traditional tetracyclines in terms of greater lipid solubility and an expanded antimicrobial spectrum. Doxycycline has a much longer elimination half-life than older tetracyclines, and adequate plasma concentrations are achieved by oral administration once daily. The combination of once-daily administration, excellent oral absorption with a high systemic availability, and broad-spectrum activity make it an attractive choice for antimicrobial therapy in dogs and cats.

In food animals, veal calves with *Mycoplasma* infection have responded well to doxycycline in feed. The broad-spectrum, good oral bioavailability (lipophilicity and absorption), not modified by feed characteristics, suggests a useful role in food animals. Pharmacokinetic studies, however, would suggest retarded excretion rates and the formation of persistent drug residues.

11.7 CHLORAMPHENICOL

Chloramphenicol, a highly active, broad-spectrum antibiotic with excellent pharmacokinetic properties, is one of the most discussed drugs. It has a broad spectrum of activity and good penetration of cells, most tissues, and secretions. Chloramphenicol is a non-ionized, highly lipid-soluble molecule that crosses cellular barriers to be widely distributed in body tissues and fluids. It also diffuses well in agar plates, and the wide zones of inhibition may lead to unduly optimistic views about its clinical efficacy. Two of the reasons for its popularity are:

- Antimicrobial activity—effective against a variety of infective pathogens, including staphylococci, salmonellae, *Pasteurella, Bordetella, Haemophilus*, coliform organisms, chlamydiae, and rickettsiae, many of which may be resistant to other antimicrobial agents
- Kinetic properties—allowing production and maintenance of effective therapeutic concentrations in body fluids and tissues, with a practicable dosage schedule in most species

Besides its advantages, chloramphenicol also has serious drawbacks: myelotoxicity, cardiotoxicity, allergic reactions, enzyme inhibitions. After its discovery, it was widely used (1947–1950); then, recognizing its toxicity (1950s), chloramphenicol was strongly overshadowed in the 1960s. The emergence of ampicillin-resistant *H. influenzae* and penicillin-resistant *Streptococcus pneumoniae* strains brought the renaissance of chloramphenicol. In the 1990s, when the third-generation cephalosporins offered new possibilities in antimicrobial therapy, the status of chloramphenicol was reassessed in human medicine.

Chloramphenicol usage has decreased owing to concerns about its potential danger to human health. In animals, after systemic administration of chloramphenicol, its residues persist in body tissues for several days. In the United States, the Food and Drug Administration (FDA) has not approved the use of chloramphenicol in food-producing animals.

Chloramphenicol is one of a few regulated animal drugs for which the Code of Federal Regulations prescribes a label bearing the statement: " . . . the product is not to be used in animals which are raised for food production. . . ."

MECHANISM OF ACTION

Chloramphenicol is bacteriostatic at therapeutic concentrations owing to its inhibition of bacterial protein synthesis. It binds to the 50S ribosomal subunit of the 70S ribosome, preventing peptide bond formation by interfering with the binding of the amino-acid-containing end of the tRNA to the 50S ribosomal subunit.

Protein synthesis is inhibited when one molecule of chloramphenicol binds per ribosome. Chloramphenicol distorts the region of the 50S subunit containing peptidyl transferase so the area of aminoacyl tRNA is wrongly oriented. It does not affect the codon-anticodon region.

SPECTRUM

The spectrum of activity of this bacteriostatic antibiotic includes a variety of gram-negative, gram-positive, and anaerobic organisms as well as *Chlamydia, Mycoplasma,* and *Rickettsia*. Chloramphenicol acts by binding to microbial ribosomes and inhibiting or impairing bacterial protein synthesis. Its activity is limited by the rapid development of resistance. It is particularly efficacious against *E. coli* and *Salmonella,* whereas *Enterobacter, Serratia,* and *Klebsiella* tend to be resistant.

Chloramphenicol is active against most anaerobic bacteria, including *Bacteroides fragilis.* In most instances, chloramphenicol reaches serum concentrations that are bacteriostatic against most bacteria, but it is bactericidal at therapeutic concentrations against *H. influenzae.* The minimum concentration considered therapeutic against susceptible bacteria is 5 µg/ml, although the minimum for urinary tract infections is approximately 126 µg/ml.

Although *P. aeruginosa* is resistant to this drug, the Enterobacteriaceae have variable sensitivities, with many previously sensitive organisms, including *E. coli, Klebsiella, Enterobacter,* and *Salmonella,* now showing significant patterns of plasmid-mediated resistance.

Enteric bacteria usually acquire resistance to chloramphenicol via transfer of R plasmids that contain the genetic coding for the production of chloramphenicol acetyltransferase. Three separate types of chloramphenicol acetyltransferase are determined by plasmids in gram-negative bacteria. Resistance can be transferred from resistant *E. coli* to sensitive *Salmonella,* thereby conferring resistance to *Salmonella.*

Resistance to chloramphenicol results from:

1. Plasmid-mediated bacterial production of chloramphenicol acetyl transferase
2. Reduced target sites on the ribosome
3. Reduced permeability of the bacteria to the drug

The first mechanism of resistance is probably the most common. Acetylated chloramphenicol does not bind with the 50S ribosomal subunit and is therefore biologically inactive. Because of plasmids that code for multiple resistance, antimicrobial drug susceptibility evaluation is important to the modification of therapeutic regimens against *Salmonella.*

11.8 KINETIC DISPOSITION

Chloramphenicol behaves as a non-ionizable, highly lipid-soluble compound and readily diffuses across biological membranes. Its bitter taste and poor water solubility, however, are undesirable features for oral and parenteral administrations. Chloramphenicol palmitate, being almost tasteless, is preferred for oral administration. The microbiologically inert ester is hydrolyzed by intestinal and pancreatic lipases to release the active chloramphenicol. The sodium salt of the succinate ester of chloramphenicol is freely soluble in water, and its aqueous solution is better tolerated by tissues than is chloramphenicol, which must be dissolved in solvents, such as propylene glycol, for parenteral administration. In the blood, chloramphenicol is bound to red blood cells and plasma proteins, producing almost similar concentrations in cells and plasma. Administration of its succinate ester provides comparable concentrations in whole blood but much higher concentrations in plasma because it does not bind with red blood cells, and it stays almost exclusively in plasma. Similar to palmitate, the inactive succinate ester also undergoes hydrolysis to release free chloramphenicol.

ABSORPTION

In most species, chloramphenicol is readily absorbed from the gastrointestinal tract. This route of administration provides antibiotic concentrations in blood comparable with or better than the intramuscular or the subcutaneous route. The only known exception to this fact is ruminants, in which chloramphenicol is destroyed by the rumen microflora, resulting in poor net absorption.

ADMINISTRATION ROUTES

The oral route is the most effective for dogs and cats. The required active blood concentration in these species, however, necessitates dosages per kilogram of body weight to be applied, which are significantly higher than the dosages used for humans: about 50 mg/kg/day every 8 to 12 hours. In pigs, 50 mg/kg/day by the oral route enables only 3.5 µg/ml to be reached. The same situation occurs in horses, in which 30 mg/kg does not permit 5 µg/ml to be reached. For ruminants, the oral route cannot be used, the drug being diluted in the upper stomach in young calves or destroyed by the rumen flora in adult ruminants.

Chloramphenicol, formulated as tablets or capsules, is well absorbed from the gut in dogs and cats, and plasma concentrations are similar to those following parenteral administration. The palmitate ester was originally developed for oral administration to children because it lacks the bitter taste of crystalline chloramphenicol. It is not antibacterial in itself but is hydrolyzed in the small intestine to release active chloramphenicol, which is then available for absorption into the circulation.

In cats, it has been shown that plasma concentrations of chloramphenicol after oral administration of the palmitate are lower than with chloramphenicol tablets, and the bioavailability from the palmitate formulation is particularly poor in fasted cats, although this difference was not observed in dogs. The poor bioavailability of chloramphenicol from the palmitate in fasted cats might be caused by reduced secretion of digestive enzymes and consequently impaired hydrolysis of the ester. Because most sick cats for which oral chloramphenicol therapy is intended are inappetent, it is suggested that tablets rather than palmitate suspension should be used.

The intramuscular route gives different levels of blood concentration according to species. Chloramphenicol sodium succinate is rapidly absorbed after intramuscular administration. The succinate ester, however, must be hydrolyzed in vivo to yield the parent compound. Studies have been made of the relative bioavailability of chloramphenicol from sodium succinate (a water-soluble ester) and aqueous suspension formulations.

Chloramphenicol sodium succinate is considered to be the better formulation because maximum plasma concentrations are significantly higher than with the aqueous suspensions and are attained about 30 minutes after intramuscular administration, compared with about 6 hours for the aqueous suspension. Further, the sodium succinate preparation is a solution that can be administered by any parenteral route, although there is no difference in the bioavailability of chloramphenicol in the cat whichever parenteral route of administration is used.

When chloramphenicol is administered parenterally, it rapidly enters the enterohepatic cycle to the extent that it ultimately affects chloramphenicol concentrations in the blood. This cycle is of significance because it prolongs the sojourn of the drug in the body and also provides high intraluminal levels of the drug in the small and upper large intestines.

Deposition of chloramphenicol residue in food animal tissues results from this prolongation of excretion. In diseased animals, CAP can be detected weeks after the initial administration. The high incidence of these stable residues, allied to their potential for idiosyncratic human toxicity, is the fundamental reason behind the FDA's prohibition of chloramphenicol usage in food animals. Because no acceptable residue level (MRL or tolerance) can be defined for chloramphenicol, the residue hazard is minimized by its abolition as a therapeutic tool in food animals.

DISTRIBUTION

Chloramphenicol has relatively high lipid solubility and distributes into the aqueous humor; central nervous system; and pleural, peritoneal, and synovial fluids. It attains therapeutic intracellular concentrations and is the second drug of choice for anaerobic bacterial infections. Its spectrum includes certain gram-positive and gram-negative bacteria and *Rickettsia*. This antibiotic diffuses into tissues remarkably well, with a volume of distribution of 2.4 liters/kg in cats. The highest drug concentrations are found in liver, bile, and kidneys. In most species, the drug is readily absorbed orally. Elimination depends on hepatic glucuronidation and renal excretion.

In domesticated animals, 30 to 46% of chloramphenicol in the circulation is bound to plasma proteins. A high proportion is therefore in the free, active form and can diffuse into extracellular tissue fluid through the fenestrated capillary walls. The capillaries in the eye and brain are not fenestrated, and drugs must cross an intact cell membrane to reach the internal structures of the eye or the cerebrospinal fluid. Because chloramphenicol is a non-ionized, highly lipid-soluble molecule, however, it readily penetrates cellular barriers to become widely distributed in the tissues.

For example, penetration into all parts of the eye has been demonstrated after systemic administration, and therapeutic concentrations were attained in the aqueous humor after local application of a 0.5% ophthalmic solution. Greater concentrations of chloramphenicol succinate is administered by subconjunctival injection. It is one of the few antibiotics that penetrates into the ocular fluids after systemic administration, and it is one of the best antibiotics in its ability to diffuse across the cornea after topical applications.

Many antibiotics cross the blood-brain barrier and attain antibacterial concentrations in the cerebrospinal fluid when the meninges are inflamed, but a few (chloramphenicol, doxycycline, trimethoprim, sulfadiazine) can do so in the absence of meningitis. Chloramphenicol attains higher concentrations in the cerebrospinal fluid than those of any other antibiotic: Concentrations of 30 to 50% of those in blood have been reported even in the absence of meningitis.

METABOLISM AND EXCRETION

Chloramphenicol is inactivated by hepatic biotransformation followed by biliary and urinary elimination. It undergoes enterohepatic circulation after biliary elimination.

Chloramphenicol is metabolized in the liver (and by the rumen microflora), and a large proportion of a dose is excreted as inactive metabolites in the urine. Consequently it is not indicated in treatment of urinary tract infections. Cats are relatively deficient in chloramphenicol-metabolizing enzymes, and about 25% of a dose is excreted unchanged in the urine compared with 6% in dogs.

A large portion of inactive metabolized drug is excreted in the bile of dogs as aromatic amines derived from chloramphenicol by nitro reduction. Because cats do not form glucuronide conjugates efficiently, elimination of chloramphenicol from the blood stream is prolonged in the cat (half-life of 5.1 hours) compared with the dog (half-life of 4.2 hours). Young animals of all species are similarly ill-equipped with me-

tabolizing enzymes and so in these and in adults with liver disease, there is a danger that repeated dosing may lead to cumulation and toxicity.

11.9 ADVERSE EFFECTS

Biologically chloramphenicol can cause two types of toxic manifestations in bone marrow. One is the more commonly encountered bone marrow depression, which is reversible and dose related and which occurs concurrently during administration of the antibiotic. It is characterized by normal cellularity to hypocellularity of the marrow, maturation arrest, vacuolation of early erythroid and myeloid cells, reticulocytopenia, depressed erythropoiesis, and occasionally neutropenia and thrombocytopenia. The other type is the bone marrow aplasia, which is irreversible and often fatal and which occurs sometimes (often weeks and months) after administration of the antibiotic has been discontinued. There is no evidence of any linkage between these two types of syndromes. Either of them can occur in humans, whereas only bone marrow suppression has been reported in domestic animals.

One effect of chloramphenicol in the eukaryotic cell is inhibition of mitochondrial protein synthesis. Mitochondria contain ribosomes composed of 50S and 30S subunits, which are responsible for synthesis of protein involved in the electron transport system that is necessary for the synthesis of adenosine triphosphate (ATP). Because ATP is necessary for protein synthesis, chloramphenicol indirectly inhibits mitochondrial nicotinamide-adenine dinucleotide (NADH) oxidation, thereby inhibiting respiration in eukaryotic cells. It further inhibits hepatic microsomal enzymes necessary for drug biotransformation.

The most prevalent toxic effects observed after administration of chloramphenicol to humans are explicable in terms of the demonstrated inhibitions of mitochondrial function and protein synthesis. Toxic effects include bone marrow suppression characterized by decreased erythropoiesis; a perturbation of the immune response; interference with the metabolism of exogenous compounds normally accomplished by hepatic microsomal enzymes; gray syndrome, an often fatal condition characterized by circulatory collapse and observed in infants and possibly others who have a defective capacity for conjugating and excreting chloramphenicol; teratogenicity (in rats); and anorexia, depression, and behavioral modifications, such as lethargy and loss of recent memory. The toxic properties described are dose dependent, are observed at doses considerably higher than those that would be expected in residues after use of the drug in food-producing animals, and (with the exception of the reported teratogenicity) are readily reversible on withdrawal of the drug.

This effect of chloramphenicol is most likely due to inhibition of protein synthesis that occurs within the mammalian mitochondria, which is remarkably similar to the protein synthesis machinery of bacteria. Chloramphenicol is immunosuppressive, and vaccination may not be as effective when administered during chloramphenicol therapy.

Because it is a protein-synthesis inhibitor, chloramphenicol can interfere with synthesis of immunoglobulins, and multiplying cells are the most adversely affected. This would account for the exhaustion and aplasia seen in humans and certain other animals. In rats, chloramphenicol caused an adverse effect on the structures and functions of the gonads in both males and females. Chloramphenicol also has the potential to enhance the action of 3-methylcholanthrene as a carcinogen. Chloramphenicol also is well recognized now as a microsomal enzyme inhibitor and thus must be carefully used in conjunction with general anesthetics that involve the use of pentobarbital because of the prolonged recovery times and with digoxin because of delayed elimination of glycoside.

MYELOID TOXICITY

In humans, chloramphenicol can cause two different, potentially lethal toxic effects, but neither of these appears to have been reported in domesticated animals. The gray syndrome in infants is characterized by circulatory collapse with flaccidity, ashen color, and hypothermia. It is caused by the administration of a large dose of chloramphenicol, which, because of the immature metabolism and excretion mechanisms, results in abnormally high plasma concentration of the drug. The second potentially lethal effect is a non-dose-dependent and irreversible depression of the bone marrow, which may be delayed in onset and follow even the smallest dose. There is some evidence that such patients could have a preexisting marrow deficiency of genetic or environmental origin.

REVERSIBLE ANEMIC SYNDROME

This syndrome is characterized by marked cytopenia mainly involving red blood cells with interaction on other types of cells and results in agranulocytosis. It arises soon after the start of treatment; appears to be related to dosage; and is found in humans as well as animals, with cats exhibiting special dose sensitivity. It is well established that this syndrome is reversible and related to the inhibition of protein synthesis in the mitochondrial system.

APLASTIC ANEMIA

Aplastic anemia is a severe, often fatal, pancytopenia related with hypoplasia or aplasia of types of bone marrow cells (sharp decrease or complete suppression of stem cells producing the types of blood cells in the bone marrow). It occurs with a long interval of about 2 months or more elapsing between the last dose and the first symptoms. Survival is rare when latency exceeds 2 months.

Aplastic anemia occurs only in humans, as a spontaneous disease, not related to the dosage of chloramphenicol. It is not described in animals except on a model, the calf, when using high dosages at the limit of acute toxicity, 25 to 100 mg/kg body weight. The risk of aplastic anemia, estimated by epidemiologic surveys, is in the range of 1 in 10,000 to 1 in 40,000 of treatments identified.

The biochemical mechanism of inducing aplastic anemia is not completely known. There is a correlation, however, with the genetic capacity of some individuals to produce nitroso chloramphenicol by enzymatic transformation of the nitrobenzene radical present in the chloramphenicol.

In contrast to the common type of bone marrow depression caused by chloramphenicol, which is generally accepted as a consequence of mitochondrial injury and decreased erythropoiesis, the mechanisms of aplastic anemia caused by the drug is uncertain. Bone marrow stem cells are almost certainly involved. In several reports, it is postulated that there is formation of a nitroso reduction product.

The same nitroso chloramphenicol has been shown to induce aplastic anemia by the intravenous route in calves with 1 or 2% of the nitroso chloramphenicol dosage used on the model (or 0.25 to 1 mg/kg body weight).

Some cases of apparent racial sensitivity have been reported in black populations. Family sensitivity to blood dyscrasia has also been reported on parents of patients suffering from the disease.

Nitroso chloramphenicol and Para nitrobenzaldehyde are known to be irreversibly toxic for DNA synthesis in bone marrow cells at a concentration of $1.6 \times 10^{-5}/M$ in human or rat cells, whereas chloramphenicol alone requires concentrations above $3 \times 10^{-4}/M$ marrow cells. More recently, evidence that the nitro group is implicated as a source of intermediates, which react with DNA and which could be the basis of the changes leading to aplastic anemia, has been established from the study of synthetically made nitroso derivatives and other reduced intermediates of chloramphenicol.

TOXICITY IN ANIMALS

Chloramphenicol is perceived as a highly toxic antimicrobial agent. In domestic animals, however, it has minimal toxicity. In dogs and cats, chloramphenicol produces a dose-related leukopenia, and aplastic anemia of immunologic origin has been observed in dogs. Cats appear to be especially susceptible to chloramphenicol toxicity.

Despite its reputation as a highly toxic antimicrobial substance, it has proved to have a low order of toxicity in domestic animals. Chloramphenicol produces dose-related leukopenia in dogs, cats, and neonatal animals of all species. Aplastic anemia, which apparently is a form of hypersensitivity, has been observed in dogs. Chloramphenicol may suppress the immune response, so it would be prudent not to vaccinate animals while they are being treated with the antibiotics.

More commonly, chloramphenicol almost inevitably causes in humans a reversible dose-dependent bone marrow depression, and similar effects have been described in cats. Cats dosed with 60 mg/kg daily for 21 days become depressed and dehydrated; reversible marrow hypoplasia and a decrease in the numbers of neutrophils, lymphocytes, reticulocytes, and platelets occur. The drug has caused death in young calves from kidney damage. Chloramphenicol inhibits liver enzymes, which metabolize pentobarbitone and thus prolong its duration of action.

Chloramphenicol is metabolized mainly by reduction of the nitroso group and glucoronidation. Because newborn animals are generally deficient in metabolizing enzymes, the animals retain the drug for longer duration; therefore the dosage regimen must be reduced accordingly to prevent cumulation and toxicosis by the drug. Cats appear to be deficient in the ability to form glucuronide. This reduces the capacity of cats to metabolize chloramphenicol and renders them more prone to its toxicity than other species. Cats appear to be more sensitive than dogs to these toxic effects, which may reflect the feline liver's reduced ability to metabolize the drug.

Because chloramphenicol tends to cause anemia, prescribing it for cats should be avoided. When it cannot be avoided, the cat should be given a dose lower than that used in the dog, and the treatment should last for no more than 7 to 10 days. Chloramphenicol is a potent inhibitor of phase I drug metabolism, so it must be used cautiously in conjunction with any other drug that is metabolized by the liver.

Chloramphenicol can produce several dose-dependent toxic effects for which "no effect" levels can be defined. Unfortunately, a toxic effect may occur in human patients that is not dose dependent. This toxic effect is irreversible, idiosyncratic aplastic anemia; it is not possible to determine a no effect level. Therefore any level must be assumed to be potentially toxic.

With improvements in analytical technology, such as radioimmunoassay, it has been possible to detect residues of chloramphenicol following withholding periods three to four times longer than the withdrawal period recommended on chloramphenicol products labeled for food animal use. A further concern that has emerged regarding chloramphenicol usage is the potential hazard to individuals administering this drug to animals. These individuals could conceivably have a genetic predisposition to this irreversible toxic effect of chloramphenicol. Thus exposure to a small amount of chloramphenicol while administering the drug to an animal could trigger the occurrence of idiosyncratic aplastic anemia.

The last observation, together with the fact that the irreversible anemia has not been definitively demonstrated to occur in any animal other than humans, precludes the establishment of a safe level of chloramphenicol residues in animal-derived food through the use of the FDA's usual guidelines for approval of a new drug for use in a food animal. Hence because no tolerance is acceptable for chloramphenicol residue levels, its use in food animals is prohibited. The United States Department of Agriculture (USDA) surveillance program constantly monitors for chloramphenicol residues.

Any solace derived from the small percentages of animals with residues of chloramphenicol, however, is mitigated by the high concentrations of residues in these animals and by the fact that the USDA's method of analysis detects only residues of chloramphenicol itself. The glucuronide derivative of the drug, a major metabolite in several species (and a compound that is changed back to chloramphenicol in the human gastrointestinal tract), and the nitro-reduced metabolites discussed previously as possibly being involved in the development of aplastic anemia are not detected by the USDA assay. In addition, considerable concern has been voiced over the extralabel use of chloramphenicol in animals.

11.10 CHLORAMPHENICOL ANALOGS

Chloramphenicol has been reported to cause reversible, dose-related bone marrow suppression in humans by a mechanism involving inhibition of mitochondrial protein synthesis. It also causes irreversible non-dose-related aplastic anemia in humans by a mechanism that is not well understood. This aplastic anemia caused by chloramphenicol is the major factor that led to the FDA's ban on its use in food-producing animals. The absolute ban on the use of chloramphenicol in food-producing animals in the United States and Canada has accentuated the need for effective broad-spectrum antibiotics for use in food animal medicine.

Progress is being made in the development and evaluation of chloramphenicol analogs, which may prove valuable in veterinary medicine. Thiamphenicol is a broad-spectrum antibiotic with a range of activity similar to that of chloramphenicol. Its different structure confers distinct properties in metabolism and toxicity on the two molecules.

Thiamphenicol is a chloramphenicol analog that is formed by replacing the *p*-nitro group of chloramphenicol with a methylsulfonyl group. The *p*-nitro group is believed to play a role in producing aplastic anemia. The molecular modification appears to preserve the antibacterial properties, markedly decrease metabolism by the liver, enhance kidney excretion, and eliminate the occurrence of idiosyncratic aplastic anemia. It is now widely accepted that chloramphenicol can cause two types of hematologic toxicity. The first is dose related, relatively common, and reversible on drug withdrawal, and it consists essentially in erythropoietic slow-down. Because of the long life span of erythrocytes and their easy replacement by packed-cell transfusion, this disorder is not clinically serious. The second is not dose related, it has a delayed onset, and it is rare but clinically serious because it consists of progressive pancytopenia with frequently lethal outcome.

Thiamphenicol possesses the first type of toxicity, but it has proved free of the second type. Reversible, dose-dependent bone marrow suppression caused by inhibition of mitochondrial protein synthesis is also a side effect of thiamphenicol. With in excess of 65 million people in Europe, Japan, and South America having been treated with thiamphenicol, however, there has been no incidence of aplastic anemia associated with its use.

Thiamphenicol has been used in Europe since 1961 in human medicine. During the period 1980 through 1982, 16,000,000 patient treatments with thiamphenicol resulted in occurrence of no cases of non-dose-related, irreversible aplastic anemia. Experimental evaluation of thiamphenicol on *Pasteurella* pneumonia in cattle has provided encouraging results.

Florfenicol, a structural analog of thiamphenicol, is perhaps more promising than thiamphenicol. Florfenicol differs from thiamphenicol in that the hydroxyl group of the number three carbon of thiamphenicol has been replaced by fluorine to maintain the same spatial conformation. Florfenicol does not possess the *p*-nitro group that has been associated with irreversible aplastic anemia in humans. Florfenicol is also effective against some organisms that are resistant to chloramphenicol. Florfenicol has shown greater in vitro activity against pathogenic bacteria than either of its structural analogs, thiamphenicol or chloramphenicol. It also has activity against some bacteria that are resistant to chloramphenicol.

Fluorinated analogs of chloramphenicol and thiamphenicol present remarkable improved antibacterial activities against bacterial strains, particularly of enteric bacteria that are resistant to chloramphenicol and thiamphenicol by an enzymatic mechanism. Florfenicol is being developed for use in veterinary medicine. Although not used in human medicine, it is assumed that the structural modifications of florfenicol preclude its being associated with idiosyncratic aplastic anemia. Initial development efforts are being directed toward food-producing animal uses, but the drug is expected to be useful for other species. In veal calves, the bioavailability after oral administration (92%) indicates that the drug can be used therapeutically by this route of administration. Florfenicol shows promise to be a viable substitute for chloramphenicol in veterinary medicine, especially in food animal practice. Although approved in some countries for use in fish, florfenicol has been shown to be very effective for bovine respiratory disease (shipping fever).

11.11 QUINOLONES—ENROFLOXACIN

Nalidixic and oxolinic acids were the first antimicrobials based on the 4-quinolone ring. They are active in vitro only against gram-negative bacteria and show no activity against *P. aeruginosa*. In vivo their volume of distribution is limited.

Over the last decade, research on 4-quinolone-3-carboxylates has led to the discovery of a family of 6-fluoro-7-peperazinyl-4-quinolones active against gram-negative and gram-positive bacteria in vitro as well as intracellular pathogens and trimethoprim-sulfonamide-resistant microbes; in addition, these antimicrobials are active against mycoplasmas. Collectively these compounds are called "fluoroquinolones." All fluoroquinolones are bactericidal, and all act on the same bacterial target: the bacterial DNA gyrase.

Nalidixic acid was the first of a new class of 1,8-naphthyridine antimicrobial agents. Nalidixic acid and older quinolones, such as oxolinic acid, are active in vitro against a wide range of gram-negative bacilli (with the exception of *P. aeruginosa*) but are essentially inactive against gram-positive organisms. In addition to the restricted spectrum of activity of quinolones, their application has been limited because their clinical use often is accompanied by the rapid emergence of resistant mutants.

Older quinolones and naphthyridines also induced numerous gastrointestinal and dermatologic side effects, including nausea, vomiting, diarrhea, drug eruptions, and photosensitivity dermatitis. Cartilage damage also has been induced in Beagle pups. In humans, clinical use of these agents has been associated with various central nervous system complaints, including headache, drowsiness, sensory changes, toxic psychosis, and occasional grand mal seizures. Therefore these problems stimulated investigation into the development of new quinolone antimicrobial agents. Several new fluoroquinolone antimicrobial agents have been developed, i.e., norfloxacin, enoxacin, ciprofloxacin, ofloxacin, and pefloxacin.

Of these, norfloxacin, ciprofloxacin, and ofloxacin have been approved for human use in the United States. Quinolones are orally absorbed, are potent in vitro against a broad spectrum of bacterial species, and have favorable pharmacokinetic properties.

Pharmaceutical scientists had been searching for active derivatives of nalidixic acid since the early 1960s. This substance from the quinolones group had been used since then to treat bacterial infections of the urinary tract. Nalidixic acid did, however, have a number of disadvantages, the most important of which was that the bacteria against which it was used became resistant to the drug within a short time. Scientists therefore hoped to find a more effective substance in the same class. Over the following 10 years, more than 10,000 derivatives of nalidixic acid were synthesized all over the world, but none of them proved to be what the scientists were looking for.

CHEMISTRY

Enrofloxacin (I), I-Cyclopropyl-7-(4-ethyl-1-piperazinyl)-6-fluoro-1,4-dihydro-4-oxo-3-quinolone carboxylic acid, belongs to a series of chemical compounds of the nalidixic acid type where, as a result of gradual changes of the molecule—substitution of the nitrogen atom in the A ring by CH, introduction of the fluorine atom in position 6, substitution of the methyl group in the A ring by piperazinyl and, finally, variation of the substituent on the nitrogen atom of the B ring—the antimicrobial properties of the basic molecule are considerably increased and its adverse effects reduced. New substitutions further increased the antibacterial activity. This last-mentioned class of compounds comprises enrofloxacin which was developed exclusively for use in animals ('Baytril').

The quinolones are related to nalidixic acid, but have fewer toxic effects. Adding a fluorine group to quinolones had improved their tissue distribution as well as their spectrum of activity.

These newer 4-quinolones are quinoline carboxylic acids with efficacy and toxicity profiles different from those of nalidixic acid.

This newer class of antibiotics promises to be useful in treating both gram-positive and gram-negative infections, especially infections caused by virulent or resistant gram-negative bacteria. Of the various classes of quinolones, the fluorinated products, norfloxacin, ciprofloxacin, and enrofloxacin, have received the most attention in veterinary medicine.

Baytril (enrofloxacin), a chemotherapeutic agent from a group of new quinolone carboxylic acid derivatives developed by the Bayer research division, was selected for clinical trials in animals primarily because of the following properties:

1. Its broad antibacterial activity spectrum against gram-negative and gram-positive bacteria as well as mycoplasmas
2. Bactericidal and mycoplasmacidal activity at low concentrations, which in most cases are only twice as high as the MICs
3. Efficacy even against organisms that are resistant or multiresistant against beta lactam antibiotics, aminoglycosides, tetracyclines, folic acid antagonists, and other antibacterial substances
4. Absorption after parenteral and oral application with high bioavailability in body fluids and organs
5. Good tolerance in all species

Another aspect of great clinical importance is the fact that Baytril is equally well absorbed after parenteral and after oral application, is distributed rapidly throughout the organs and body fluids, and produces levels of active ingredient that justify intervals of as much as 24 hours between treatments from a pharmacokinetic point of view. The activity concentrations in most organs and body fluids are even higher than in the serum.

Another quinolone carboxylic acid derivative in veterinary medicine is flumequine. This drug, too, was directly compared with Baytril in tests on several representative microorganisms. The mean MIC values measured for flumequine, however, are on average three to five stages higher than those of Baytril; flumequine is not as effective against streptococci and mycoplasmas as enrofloxacin.

11.12 SPECTRUM OF ACTIVITY

Fluoroquinolones are active against enteric gram-negative bacilli and cocci and also against *P. aeruginosa*, *Aeromonas hydrophila*, and *Haemophilus*. These drugs have excellent activity against bacterial pathogens of the gastrointestinal tract, including *E. coli, Salmonella, Shigella, Yersinia enterocolitica, Campylobacter jejuni*, and *Vibrio*. Enrofloxacin generally is 16 to 64 times more active than the parent compound nalidixic acid and has a wider spectrum that includes *Pseudomonas* and staphylococci. Norfloxacin has activity against *P. aeruginosa* isolates that is superior to that of gentamicin, carbenicillin, ticarcillin, and cephalosporins and is similar to that of tobramycin.

Fluoroquinolones have variable activity against streptococci, with ciprofloxacin being the preferred drug. These compounds have little activity against anaerobic cocci, clostridia, and bacteroides. With the exception of MIC for anaerobes, MIC of fluoroquinolones for bacteria tend to be little affected by inoculum size, type of medium, or presence of serum. Combinations of fluoroquinolones with other antimicrobial agents rarely have shown synergy or antagonism.

The in vitro activity of enrofloxacin (Baytril) is particularly pronounced in gram-negative bacteria (e.g., *E. coli, Salmonella, Pasteurella, Haemophilus*) and mycoplasmas and also extends to gram-positive organisms (e.g., *Staphylococcus, Erysipelothrix*). The substance is rapidly absorbed even after oral administration. High concentrations of active ingredient are quickly achieved in body fluids and organs. Administration of the product in the drinking water presents little problem because it is highly soluble.

The quinolones are extremely active against gram-negative infections, particularly *E. coli, Klebsiella, Enterobacter cloacae, P. mirabilis*, indole-positive *Proteus, P. aeruginosa, Citrobacter freundii*, and *S. marcescens*; the activity persists even after resistance has developed to aminoglycosides, antipseudomonal penicillins, and third-generation cephalosporins. Norfloxacin was superior to aminoglycosides, tetracyclines, and chloramphenicol against several species of gram-negative bacteria in vitro, although its activity against *P. aeruginosa* was intermediate between amikacin and gentamicin. The combination of norfloxacin plus aminoglycosides is synergistic in vitro against many gram-negative bacteria isolated from human urinary tracts.

The spectrum of activity of the quinolones depends on the individual drug but includes most gram-negative organisms, particularly *E. coli, Klebsiella, Pasteurella, Enterobacter, Proteus, Pseudomonas, Citrobacter*, and *Serratia*. The spectrum of norfloxacin (a human product) is not as great as enrofloxacin. Ciprofloxacin has been used in human medicine for organisms resistant to norfloxacin. Most organisms sensitive to ciprofloxacin are also sensitive to enrofloxacin.

The quinolones' gram-positive spectrum is not as impressive as their gram-negative spectrum. Most *Staphylococcus* and some *Corynebacterium* are sensitive to enrofloxacin and other quinolones, although MICs for these organisms tend to be higher than for gram-negative organisms. *Streptococcus* tend to be resistant to quinolones. Quinolones that are more effective against gram-positive organisms are being developed. Quinolones are also effective in treating *Chlamydia* and *Mycoplasma* infections but are ineffective against most anaerobes.

The efficacy of quinolones toward gram-negative organisms is pH dependent. They are less active in acidic pH (<7.0) and more active in alkaline pH (>7.4). This may be clinically relevant when treating abscesses or urinary tract infections, or when organisms are located within phagocytic cells (i.e., neutrophils and macrophages). Quinolones penetrate intracellularly into phagocytic cells, and enrofloxacin reaches a concentration in neutrophils seven times higher than the extracellular concentration, therefore allowing it to be effective in intracellular killing of bacteria.

11.13 MECHANISM OF ACTION

The quinolones inhibit bacterial DNA synthesis by three mechanisms. First, the ATP-dependent enzyme DNA gyrase, which supercoils the DNA helix, is blocked. Second, relaxation of the supercoiled DNA is inhibited. Finally, the double-stranded DNA becomes more susceptible to breakage. Because quinolones block DNA synthesis, they are bactericidal.

The primary target of nalidixic acid, oxolinic acid, and probably all fluoroquinolones is DNA gyrase. These drugs are thought specifically to inhibit the A subunit

DNA gyrase, a type II topoisomerase, which appears to be essential for DNA replication. Fluoroquinolone antimicrobial agents in general and enrofloxacin in particular are bactericidal. Quinolones characteristically kill bacteria rapidly, with as much as a thousandfold decrease in the number of viable organisms within 1 to 2 hours of drug exposure at one to four times the MIC.

The DNA thread is about 1.3 mm long and consists of two coiled parallel strands ("double helix") that fit in a bacterial shell that is only one thousandth of a millimeter wide and high and two thousandths of a millimeter long.

The DNA thread is wound around twice. The first winding results in 65 "supercoil areas," each having a length of 20 thousandths of a millimeter and linked to a nucleus of the DNA matrix RNA. Each of these supercoils is wound once more in the opposite direction of the windings of the DNA double helix—in 400 super-supercoils ("supertwists") each. To make this countercurrent winding possible, the DNA double helix has to be opened and then closed again after the supertwist. This is accomplished by an enzyme, DNA gyrase. The miracle of accommodating the DNA thread in such a tiny space is performed with the help of this enzyme.

The fluoroquinolones inhibit replication of bacteria by an action on the functioning of the DNA gyrase. This enzyme is a type II topoisomerase and plays a crucial role in the unwinding, cutting, and consecutive resealing of DNA. The inhibition of the resealing leads to the liberation of fragments that are subsequently destroyed by the bacterial exonucleases.

As a result, the information stored in the DNA can no longer be optimally read, which of course causes the death of the bacterium. It is a swift death.

The quinolones are bactericidal. Susceptible organisms are killed within 30 minutes of exposure to effective concentrations. Although quinolones are effective at low MICs when compared with other antimicrobials, their efficacy is also characterized by a biphasic pattern. That is, they lose their effectiveness against susceptible organisms at concentrations both above and below the MIC. This characteristic is less pronounced

with ciprofloxacin and enrofloxacin. The quinolones also exhibit a postantibiotic effect, inhibiting bacterial growth for 4 to 8 hours after they have been eliminated from the body. Quinolones act by inhibiting the bacterium's production of gyrase, a microbial enzyme necessary for packaging cellular DNA into a tight coil so the organism can reproduce. Failure of DNA to be packaged renders it susceptible to destructive enzymes.

Even in the tiniest doses, the gyrase inhibitor kills 99.99% of many bacteria within 3 hours. By virtue of this unusual method of attack, the drug is successful against multiresistant strains of gram-positive as well as gram-negative bacteria. In large-scale studies with more than 20,000 different bacterial strains, 98.3% proved sensitive to the new drug. Only 0.6% were completely "immune" to it.

The efficacy of the quinolones is enhanced by the fact that resistance to them is not plasmid mediated but is currently limited to chromosomal mutation. Therefore resistance develops slowly and is usually accompanied by changes that weaken the bacterial cell.

Microorganisms have at their disposal more varied means of circumventing the defense mechanisms of the host's skin and mucous membranes, thus permitting more rapid colonization and infection. New pathogens emerge, and previously known organisms become resistant to older antibiotics. This phenomenon of resistance is a source of increasing concern to physicians. Anti-infective drugs that were highly effective yesterday may prove helpless against some bacteria today. Almost overnight the microscopically sized disease-causing agents become "immune" to a drug.

Being a quinolone carboxylic acid derivative, the antibacterial mode of action of Baytril is fundamentally different from that of other antibiotics/chemotherapeutic drugs, such as beta-lactam, aminoglycoside, tetracycline, and macrolide antibiotics or even sulfonamides and trimethoprim. This accounts for another noteworthy feature: Pathogens that are resistant to the aforementioned commonly used antibacterial substances are sensitive to Baytril. Compared with other quinolone carboxylic acid derivatives used in veterinary medicine (flumequine), Baytril is distinguished by considerably lower MIC values (factor 20 to 50) and the additional advantage of its efficacy against pseudomonads, streptococci, and mycoplasmas. In addition to a higher potency, there are also differences with regard to mode of action. As was to be expected, resistance selections emerged in subculture procedures under the influence of Baytril, but these follow the "multiple step type." They are thus slower than is the case with a number of other active substances.

Little is known about mechanisms of bacterial resistance to fluoroquinolones, but plasmid-mediated resistance to quinolones has not been detected. Resistance does develop to the quinolones, especially in *P. aeruginosa, K. pneumoniae, Acinetobacter*, and enterococci. The quinolones are not affected by transferable plasmid-mediated antibiotic resistance, and in fact R plasmids may increase bacterial sensitivity to these agents. Thus the only way bacteria can resist the 4-quinolones is by mutation. Bacterial isolates that are resistant to nalidixic acid are not necessarily resistant to newer quinolones. Campylobacter species have reportedly shown resistance to enrofloxacin.

One of the outstanding features of the quinolone carboxylic acid derivatives is their special mechanism of action. Although penicillins, cephalosporins, and bacitracin attack the cell wall; colistin and polymyxin act on the cytoplasmic membrane; and aminoglycosides, chloramphenicol, tetracyclines, and macrolides interfere with the protein synthesis, the quinolone carboxylic acid derivatives impair the bacterial gyrase, an enzyme that plays a major role in the replication of DNA. Inhibition of this enzyme leads to functional disturbances with blockage of certain stages in the synthesis, resulting in the death of the bacterium.

Attention has been drawn to the existence of further mechanisms, at least in some representatives of this group, which are additionally directed against the cell wall and the cytoplasmic membrane. This special mechanism of action rules out parallel resistance with well-known antibacterial agents that are commonly used in veterinary medicine, such as beta-lactam antibiotics, tetracyclines, aminoglycosides, macrolides, chloramphenicol, and folic acid antagonists (sulfonamides), which possess a different mode of action. Thus enrofloxacin possesses high antibacterial activity against strains that are resistant or even multiresistant to the aforementioned antibacterial agents.

11.14 PHARMACOKINETICS

The oral absorption of the fluoroquinolones is generally fast and substantial in humans, in monogastric species, and in preruminant calves: Up to 80% of the ingested dose is absorbed into the systemic circulation. The serum concentration peak is reached rapidly. Enrofloxacin is absorbed readily and quickly both after oral and after parenteral application. Maximum concentrations are reached within 0.5 to 2 hours.

As a rule, when quinolones are given orally, they are absorbed rapidly and almost completely, although food in the digestive tract may delay absorption. Food in the gastrointestinal tract does not significantly alter peak plasma concentrations, but it does delay the time of peak concentration. Delayed absorption does not seem to be clinically significant, so it is probably not necessary to administer quinolones between feedings. In fact, giving the drug with food may prevent gastrointestinal upset.

The Baytril serum levels after oral application in calves, pigs, and poultry are equivalent in amount to those after parenteral application at the same dosage, which suggests a good absorption of the active ingredient in the intestine. The special kinetic status of the growing ruminant after oral administration with reference to the development of the forestomachs must also be taken into consideration here. The activity levels and the onset of maximum concentrations to a particular degree depend on age, method of application, formulation of the active ingredient, and the animals' nutritional status.

In general, the 4-quinolones are active when administered orally, with 30 to 40% systemic availability. Food inhibits their oral absorption, so they should be dosed an hour before or 2 hours after a meal.

After absorption or intravenous injection, enrofloxacin is dispersed over all organs and tissues. The distribution pattern is similar in all studied species. The highest concentrations are observed almost without exception in the liver and the kidneys, the lowest in the brain. In the pig, conspicuously high activity levels are found in the lungs, the nasal mucosa, and the lymphatic tissue. The excellent tissue penetration is also evidenced by the fact that the organs often contain substantially higher microbiologic activates than the serum. Because infections tend to occur primarily in organs and tissues, this fact is a major advantage in the therapeutic use of the product. In this aspect, enrofloxacin differs from many other chemotherapeutic agents, including flumequine, another quinolone carboxylic acid derivative used in veterinary medicine.

DISTRIBUTION

One of the most attractive pharmacokinetic characteristics of the fluoroquinolones is their large volume of distribution. Additionally, their binding to plasma proteins is low: 10 to 40% in humans; in contrast, 90% of nalidixic acids bound. Pefloxacin administered to dogs resulted in concentrations higher in all tissues assayed except the central nervous system than in the plasma. This characteristic, associated with the wide spectrum of activity, makes the fluoroquinolones first-choice antimicrobials for treatment of deep tissue infections and pyoderma. Particularly high concentrations are achieved in the liver and urinary tract; consequently, they are widely used to treat the infections of the genitourinary system in humans.

These fluoroquinolones share a great availability in all monogastric species, a large volume of distribution, and a low binding to plasma proteins that allows them to cross membranes and reach the most remote parts of the body at concentrations above the MICs of most pathogens. Tissue and sites demonstrating high concentrations after systemic administration include the kidney, liver, and bile plus the prostate, female genital tract, bone, and inflammatory fluids. They are eliminated for the most part in the urine and reach levels 100 to 300 times more concentrated in the urine than in the serum. All the fluoroquinolones exhibit distributional and antimicrobial properties that make them potentially useful in veterinary medicine.

The volume of distribution of ciprofloxacin in humans was 1.8 liters/kg. The ratio of serum-to-tissue enrofloxacin concentrations ranges from 2:1 for brain to 1:4 for liver. Concentrations in urine and bile are from 8-fold to 20-fold higher than concurrent serum concentrations for at least 12 hours after drug administration in mammals. Therapeutic concentrations of ciprofloxacin (and most likely other 4-quinolone antibacterial agents) are achieved in the prostate, and they are expected to be present in large quantities in milk.

In dogs, the recommended oral dose of norfloxacin of 2.2 mg/kg every 12 hours produces peak serum concentrations of 2.6 μg/ml. The recommended dosage of enrofloxacin for dogs and cats is 2.5 mg/kg every 12 hours.

Bactericidal drug concentrations can be reached within 15 minutes of oral administration. The drugs, including enrofloxacin, are distributed well into tissues. The gastrointestinal absorption in mammals is rapid and substantial, the duration of action is long, and excretion is mainly through the kidney.

The liver, bile, and kidney develop the highest drug concentrations, but concentrations in essentially all tissues, including the skeletal and central nervous systems, reach therapeutic levels.

The mechanism of elimination of the quinolones depends on the individual drug. Enrofloxacin is partially metabolized in the liver to both active (e.g., ciprofloxacin) and inactive metabolites; however, a portion is eliminated in the kidney unchanged.

Pharmacokinetic properties of fluoroquinolones include rapid oral absorption, urinary drug concentrations substantially in excess of the MIC for virtually all susceptible bacterial pathogens, attainable serum and tissue concentrations above the MIC for most gram-negative and many gram-positive organisms, and relatively long half-lives in serum, allowing dose intervals of 8 to 12 hours or more. In humans with normal renal function, the half-life of fluoroquinolones is 3.1 hours.

Fluoroquinolones are partially metabolized in the liver and excreted in urine and bile as high concentrations of active drug (unchanged drug or active metabolites). In humans, urinary recovery 24 hours after a single dose was 30% for norfloxacin, 71% for enoxacin, 70% for ofloxacin, 30% for ciprofloxacin, and 5% for pefloxacin. The liver appears to be the primary site of norfloxacin metabolism. The elimination of the substance proceeds by different routes, depending on the species, primarily via the kidneys and to some extent via the bile, as can be deduced from the concentrations of active ingredient in urine and bile.

The high activity concentrations in the serum encountered in all species, and particularly the even higher tissue concentrations, the very low MIC, and minimum bactericidal concentration (MBC) values of most gram-negative and gram-positive bacteria, including mycoplasmas; a low therapeutic dose; and the absence of cross resistance to conventional chemotherapeutic agents used in veterinary medicine suggest that enrofloxacin may constitute a major step forward in the treatment of infectious diseases in animals. In the meantime, the excellent efficacy could be proved by many investigators in various countries.

11.15 TOXICITY

The quinolones can cause hypersensitivity reactions in patients and are contraindicated in patients who have shown hypersensitivity to nalidixic acid or to other quinolones. The quinolones can produce crystalluria in dogs owing to their limited solubility in acidic aqueous solutions. For this reason, adequate patient hydration is mandatory. Other more frequent adverse reactions include dizziness and gastrointestinal signs, such as nausea, vomiting, and diarrhea. The quinolones should not be administered to pregnant animals because premature embryonic loss and maternotoxicity (vomiting and anorexia) have occurred in monkeys at doses producing therapeutic serum concentrations. In immature animals, quinolones are associated with arthropathies and cartilage deterioration. Administration to dogs of less than one year is not recommended.

With few exceptions, the adverse effects of the fluoroquinolones are not of severe consequence when compared with the beneficial features they exhibit. The target tissues are the juvenile cartilage, central nervous system, urinary tract, and digestive tract. Some skin eruptions have also been seen in humans.

Lesions of the weight-bearing cartilage of juvenile rats and Beagle puppies have been observed after experimental exposure to nalidixic acid or fluoroquinolones, causing lameness and pain severe enough to impose humanitarian euthanasia. Their adverse effects are not severe when compared with the beneficial features fluoroquinolones exhibit. The target tissues for adverse effects are the juvenile cartilage, central nervous system, urinary tract, and digestive tract. In the United States, approved use is thus far limited to dogs; approval for use in food animals is currently being sought for several fluoroquinolones. Enrofloxacin is available in Europe for use in cattle, pigs, and poultry. In young dogs, lameness was noticed within 2 days after treatment was started, although it typically resolved within 8 weeks. In young dogs, these clinical signs developed as a result of erosion of the articular cartilage. Therefore use of these antimicrobial agents in immature animals cannot be recommended.

Three to 4-week-old whelps (Beagle) tolerated 15 mg/kg body weight administered orally for 14 days without suffering any harm. The highest tested dose (25 mg/kg) was equally safe in $1\frac{1}{2}$- to $2\frac{1}{2}$-week-old whelps (Beagle) treated orally for 30 days. Only dose rates for 30 to 60 mg/kg administered for 14 days led to primary degenerative damage of the cartilage in the weight-bearing joints, the characteristic lesions that this class of compounds is known to cause in growing animals. In fast-growing, large breeds, however, overdosage for prolonged treatment periods are not sufficiently safe with regard to potential cartilage damage of joints in the period of growth which led to the exclusion of dogs in the growing age (as a rule up to approximately 1 year) from the recommendation for use of Baytril, as a precaution, for the time being. Administration to horses is not recommended.

There are few toxicities associated with administering quinolones. At high doses, central nervous system signs have been noted in dogs. Gastrointestinal upset, which is probably the most common side effect in dogs and calves, may also occur in cats. Although earlier studies suggested that the quinolones might be embryocidal, more recent studies suggest that they can be administered safely to pregnant animals.

EMBRYOTOXICITY AND TERATOGENICITY

Trials in rats that were treated daily from the 6th to the 15th day of gestation produced no evidence of a teratogenic effect of enrofloxacin, including the highest dosage group (875 mg/kg body weight). Maternal toxic effects after 210 and 975 mg/kg, however, resulted in slightly reduced fetal weights and, in the top dosage group, in smaller litter sizes. A dose of 50 mg/kg body weight was tolerated without any adverse effect on dams and offspring.

MUTAGENICITY

The point mutagenic effect of enrofloxacin was studied in the Salmonella Microsome Test (Ames-Test) and in ovarian cells of the Chinese hamster (CHO-HGPRT forward mutation assay). The Unscheduled DNA Synthesis Test was performed to check for damage to the DNA. These test systems produce no evidence of a mutagenic effect.

The use of norfloxacin has been studied in dogs but not in cats. Before enrofloxacin became available, however, the canine dosage of norfloxacin was used (22 mg/kg orally twice a day) for feline patients with no apparent adverse effects. Practitioners have also used ciprofloxacin in cats, but there is concern about possible adverse reactions to the drug (e.g., malaise, inappetence). Because ciprofloxacin is a metabolite of enrofloxacin, there is little justification for its use in cats, dogs, and calves.

In humans, side effects have not been serious. Primary problems have been referable to the gastrointestinal tract (nausea, vomiting, anorexia) and central nervous system (lightheadedness, headache, drowsiness). Overall, adverse events with norfloxacin occurred in 1 to 3%, with nausea (2.8%), headache (2.7%), and dizziness (1.8%) being the most common.

11.16 THERAPEUTIC INDICATIONS

Because they can penetrate all body tissues, quinolones are indicated for infection in any tissue caused by any gram-negative and selected gram-positive bacteria. These drugs, however, should be reserved for serious infections or those that have failed to respond to other antibiotic therapy. Quinolones are especially useful for treating serious antibiotic-resistant bacterial infections of the respiratory tract or the genitourinary tract (particularly chronic urinary tract infections resistant to other drugs). They also work well in treating deep pyodermas, osteomyelitis, and gram-negative septicemias. Although specific studies have not been performed, quinolones should effectively treat gram-negative cholangiohepatitis. They are also good alternatives to aminoglycosides in animals with renal disease.

In humans, clinical uses of fluoroquinolones would include the following: (1) urinary tract infections, especially those caused by *P. aeruginosa*; (2) prostatitis; (3) severe bacterial gastroenteritis; (4) pneumonia caused by gram-negative bacilli; (5) selective decolonization of the gastrointestinal tract in granulocytopenic patients; (6) treatment of upper respiratory tract colonization by methicillin-resistant *S. aureus*; and (7) gram-negative bacillary osteomyelitis.

In human medicine, the preparation is used to treat infections of the respiratory tract; the kidneys and urinary tract; the sexual organs; the gastrointestinal tract and bile ducts; the skin and soft tissue; the bones and joints; and the middle ear, sinuses, and eyes.

VETERINARY USE

Enrofloxacin is an anti-infective agent from a group of new quinolone carboxylic acid derivatives that was developed for sole use in animals. It was selected because of its broad antibacterial spectrum, bactericidal and mycoplasmacidal activity at low concentrations, efficacy against multiresistant organisms, good absorption after parenteral as well as oral application, and low toxicity. These advantages have been demonstrated in extensive clinical studies in poultry, calves, pigs, dogs, and cats. Efficacy and tolerance in rabbits and fish are currently being evaluated.

Enrofloxacin was selected for clinical trials in animals because of the following properties:

1. Its broad spectrum of activity against gram-negative and gram-positive bacteria and mycoplasmas
2. Bactericidal and mycoplasmacidal activity at low concentrations
3. Efficacy against organisms that are resistant or multiresistant to beta-lactam antibiotics, aminoglycosides, tetracyclines, folic acid antagonists, and other antibacterial substances
4. Good absorption and bioavailability after either parenteral or oral administration
5. Good tolerance in target animal species
6. Compatibility with important agents in mass medication

Potential uses for Baytril, based on the microbiologic studies and the results of the clinical tests, are all infections involving the following gram-negative and gram-positive bacteria and mycoplasmas, either in a primary or a secondary capacity: *E. coli, Salmonella, Klebsiella, Proteus, Yersinia, Haemophilus, Pasteurella, Actinobacillus, Pseudomonas, Brucella, Moraxella, Campylobacter, Staphylococcus, Streptococcus* (except enterococci)*, Erysipelothrix, Bacteroides,* and *Mycoplasma.*

Poultry

The clinical efficacy of Baytril in poultry is documented in numerous experimental studies and field trails. The therapeutic efficacy of Baytril 10% solution in chicks of the layer type after experimental infection with *Mycoplasma gallisepticum* and *E. coli* was studied. The product was administered at concentrations of 50 and 100 mg of active ingredient/liter (ppm) for periods of 3 and 5 days in the drinking water. With reference to all tested parameters (mortality, pathomorphologic lesions, re-isolation rate, and development of body weight), Baytril proved superior to the substances tylosin and tiamulin, whose activity extends to mycoplasmas only. Better results were achieved even at the low dosage (50 ppm,

3 days): reduced mortality, fewer pathomorphologic lesions, and better body weight development. Attempts at re-isolation of *M. gallisepticum* failed in all birds treated with Baytril or tiamulin.

A similar pattern to that seen in the results of the pathoanatomic studies emerged with regard to the weight development of all groups treated with Baytril: This was distinctly better than in the controls treated with the reference products, and at the 100 ppm dosage, it was equivalent to that of the noninfected control group. The results described confirm the good therapeutic activity of Baytril in simultaneous experimental infections with *M. gallisepticum* and *E. coli.* The prevention of most of the specific pathomorphologic lesions and the good weight development in particular are undoubtedly to a large extent attributable to the simultaneous mycoplasmacidal activity of Baytril and its potency against *E. coli.* This advantage was demonstrated to be equally beneficial under field conditions because the major complicating factor in *Mycoplasma* infections of poultry is often infections with *E. coli.*

Calves, Pigs, and Small Animals

Depending on the species and the mode of administration, the same dosage produced different maximum concentrations after 0.5 to 2 hours; e.g., at a dosage of 2.5 mg/kg body weight, these were approximately 0.5 μg/ml serum in poultry and approximately 1.0 μg/ml serum in the studied mammals. The half-life periods of elimination from the serum, again depending on species and administration, were calculated as being 2 to 6 hours.

The concentrations of active ingredient measured in all organs and tissues were often substantially higher than those observed at the equivalent times in the serum. A good correlation was found to exist between serum and tissue levels and the dosage rate. An accumulation of active ingredient did not occur, even if the intervals between applications were short.

Potential uses for Baytril, based on the microbiologic studies and the results of the clinical tests available thus far, are systemic and local infections with primary or secondary involvement of the following gram-negative and gram-positive bacteria and mycoplasmas: *E. coli, Salmonella, Klebsiella, Proteus, Yersinia, Haemophilus, Pasteurella, Actinobacillus, Pseudomonas, Brucella, Moraxella, Campylobacter, Staphylococcus, Streptococcus,* (except enterococci), *Erysipelothrix, Bacteroides,* and *Mycoplasma.*

Baytril covers the following indications in pigs:

- Diarrhea of suckling piglets
- *E. coli* diarrhea and *E. coli* enterotoxemia of weaners and fatteners
- Bronchopneumonia, enzootic pneumonia
- Salmonellosis
- MMA syndrome

Baytril covers the following indications in calves:

- *E. coli* diarrhea, *E. coli* sepsis, and diarrhea of nonbacterial origin for prevention of intercurrent bacterial infections
- Bronchopneumonia due to primary bacterial infection and secondary bacterial infections of the respiratory organs in complex diseases, such as enzootic pneumonia
- Salmonellosis

The results of the clinical studies, in conjunction with the microbiologic and species-related pharmacokinetic studies suggest that for calves and pigs a dosage of 2.5 mg/ kg/day can be recommended both for parenteral and for oral application. The length of treatment is determined by the nature, degree, and course of the infection and can be shorter for treatment of diarrhea.

The high efficacy of Baytril has also been established for the complex of respiratory tract infections. In simultaneous experimental infection of calves with *Pasteurella haemolytica* and *Mycoplasma bovis*, the substance proved to be highly effective administered three to five times by the oral or parenteral route at dosage rates from 2.5 mg/kg body weight.

One of Baytril's current major applications outside of salmonellosis in cattle is treatment of respiratory disease. Its high solubility, rapidity of absorption regardless of route, high lung and serum concentration (2:1), potential to enter intracellularly, unique mechanism of action and hence lack of cross resistance, and finally very broad spectrum (including *Mycoplasma, Pasteu-*

rella, E. coli, Haemophilus, Pseudomonas, and *Chlamydia*) has to date rendered Baytril a useful product for therapy of bovine respiratory disease.

Dogs and Cats

Baytril is currently sold in the United States for use in small animal medicine. The recommended daily dose for dogs is 5 mg/kg given in one or two administrations. One dose of 5 mg/kg orally results in a peak plasma level of 1.66 μg/ml of serum. The same dose has been used in cats. Clinical and experimental trials have shown positive results of infections of the respiratory, digestive, and genitourinary tracts and the bone and skin in dogs and cats.

A new fluoroquinolone, danofloxacin, is currently under development and is expected to be launched soon for the treatment of bovine respiratory disease.

SELECTED REFERENCES

Ames, T.R., Larson, V.L., and Stowe, C.M.: Oxytetracycline concentrations in plasma and lung of healthy and diseased calves. Am. J. Vet. Res., *44*:1354, 1983.

Ames, T.R., Larson, V.R., and Stowe, C.M.: Oxytetracycline levels in healthy and diseased calves. Bov. Proc., *15*:136, 1983.

Aronson, A.L.: Pharmacotherapeutics of newer tetracyclines. J. Am. Vet. Med. Assoc., *176*:1061, 1980.

Barza, M., Brown, R.B., and Shanks, C.: Relation between lipophilicity and pharmacological behaviour of minocycline, doxycycline, tetracycline and oxytetracycline in dogs. Antimicrob. Agent Chemother., *8*:713, 1975.

Bauditz, R.: Results of clinical studies with Baytril in calves and pigs. Vet. Med. Rev., *2*:122, 1987.

Bauditz, R.: Results of clinical studies with Baytril in dogs and cats. Vet. Med. Rev., *2*:137, 1987.

Bauditz, R.: Results of clinical studies with Baytril in poultry. Vet. Med. Rev., *2*:130, 1987.

Black, W.D., Claxton, J., and Robinson, G.A.: Study of serum drug levels in calves following intramuscular administration of three tetracycline drug preparations. Can. Vet. J., *23*:296, 1982.

Blogg, J.R.: Chloramphenicol 4. Responsible use in opthalmology. Austral. Vet. J., *68*:7, 1991.

Booth, N.H., and McDonald, L.E. (eds.): Tetracyclines. *In* Veterinary Pharmacology and Therapeutics. 6th ed. Ames, Iowa State University Press, 1988.

Bretzlaff, K.N., Otts, R.S., Koritz, G.D., et al.: Distribution of oxytetracycline in genital tract tissues of post partum cows given the drug by intravenous and intrauterine routes. Am. J. Vet. Res., *44*:764, 1983.

Chloramphenicol therapy in large animals. J. Am. Vet. Med. Assoc., *178*:309, 1981.

Cornwell, R.L.: Long acting oxytetracycline therapy. Bov. Pract., 2:16, 1981.

Epstein, R.L., et al.: Influence of heat and cure preservatives on the residues of sulfamethaline, chloramphenicol and cyromazine in muscle tissues. J. Agric. Food Chem., *36*:1009, 1988.

Espinasse, J., Delac, B., Silmi, A.: Essai D'une Nouvelle quinolone Bay Vp 2674 (Baytril) dans le salmonellose experimentale des veaux, a Salmonella typhimurium. Proc. World Congr. Dis. Cattle, Dublin, Ireland. World Assoc. Buiat. Monaghan, M. Fac. Vet. Med., Dublin, 1986.

Flack, A.J.: Fatal aplastic anaemia following topical administration of ophthalmic chloramphenicol. Am. J. Ophthalmol., *94*:420, 1982.

Ford, R.B.: Enrofloxacin: A new antimicrobial strategy in small animal practice. *In* Quinolones: A New Class of Antimicrobial Agents for Use in Veterinary Medicine. Proc. Symp. Western Vet. Conf. Las Vegas. Shaunee, KS, Mobay Corporation, Animal Health Division, 1988.

Garnes, H.A.: Doxycycline levels in serum and prostatic tissue in man. Urology *1*:205, 1973.

Giles, C.J., Grimshaw, W.T., Shanks, D.J., and Smith, D.G.: Efficacy of danofloxocin in the therapy of bacterial pneumonia in housed beef cattle. Vet. Rec., *128*:296.

Gross, B.J., Branchflower, R.V., Burke, T.R., et al.: Bone marrow toxicity in vitro of chloramphenicol and its metabolites. Tox. Appl. Pharmacol., *64*:557, 1982.

Guest, G.B.: Use of chloramphenicol in the United States. Ann. Rech. Vet., *16*:161, 1985.

Hird, J.F., and Knifton, A.: Chloramphenicol in veterinary medicine. Vet. Rec., *119*:248, 1986.

Hooper, D.C., and Wolfson, J.F.: Fluoroquinoline antimicrobial agents. N. Engl. J. Med., *324*:384, 1991.

Hooper, E., and Wolfson, J.: The fluoroquinolous pharmacology, clinical uses and toxicities in horses. Antimicrob. Agents Chemother., *28*:716, 1985.

Immelman, A., Botha, W.S., and Grib, D.: Muscle irritation caused by different products containing oxytetracycline. J. S. African Vet. Assoc., *49*:103, 1978.

Jenkins, W., and Friedlander, L.: The pharmacology of quinolone antibacterial agents. *In* Quinolones: A New Class of Antimicrobial Agents for Use in Veterinary Medicine. Proc. West Vet. Conf. Las Vegas. Shawnee, KS, Mobay Corporation, Animal Health Division, 1988.

Jonas, M., et al.: Tetracyclines. *In* Antimicrobial Therapy. Edited by A.M. Ristuccin and B.A. Cunha. New York, Raven Press, 1984.

Kuttler, K.L., Young, M.F., and Simpson, J.E.: Use of an experimental long acting oxytetracycline (Terramycin L.A.) in the treatment of acute anaplasmosis. Vet. Med. Small Anim. Clin., 187, 1978.

Laceym, R.W.: Does the use of chloramphenicol in animals jeopardize the treatment of human infections. Vet. Rec., *114*:6, 1984.

Lekeux, P., and Art, T.: Effect of enrofloxacin therapy on shipping fever pneumonia in feedlot cattle. Vet. Rec., *123*:205, 1988.

Lery, N., Descoted, J., and Evreux, J.L.: A review of chloramphenicol-induced blood disorders. Vet. Hum. Toxicol., *20*:177, 1979.

Luthman, J., and Jacobsson, S.O.: A comparison of two oxytetracycline formulations in cattle. Acta Vet. Scand., *23*:147, 1982.

McGonigle, R.A., McManus, R.F., Davey, L.A.: Terramycin L.A. for the control of bovine respiratory disease. The Netherlands, 12th World Congress, Diseases of Cattle. 1982, p. 99.

Moellering, R.C.: Norfloxacin: A fluoroquinolene carboxylic acid antimicrobial agent. Am. J. Med., *82*:1, 1987.

Najean, Y.: Toxic etiology of aplastic anaemia. The Cooperative Study Group for Aplastic and Refractor Anaemias. International Symposium on Thiamphenicol and Sexually Transmitted Diseases. Edited by R. Franceschinis. Vol. 11. 1984.

Neer, T.M.: Clinical pharmacological features of the fluoroquinolone antimicrobial drugs. J. Am. Vet. Med. Assoc., *193*:577, 1988.

Neumann, M.: Clinical pharmacokinetics of the newer antibacterial 4-quinolones. Clin. Pharmacokin., *14*:96, 1988.

Nouns, J.F.: Tolerance and detection of antimicrobial residues in slaughtered animals. Arch. Lebensmittel Hyg., *32*:97, 1981.

Nouws, J.F.M.: Irritation, bioavailability and residue aspects of ten oxytetracycline formulations administered intramuscularly to pigs. Vet. Quart., *6*:80, 1984.

Page, S.W.: Chloramphenicol 1. Hazards of use and current regulatory environment. Austral. Vet. J., *68*:1, 1991.

Page, S.W.: Chloramphenicol 3. Clinical pharmacology of systemic use in the horse. Austral. Vet. J., *68*:5, 1991.

Prescott, J.F., and Baggott, J.D.: Chloramphenicol and thiamphenicol. *In* Antimicrobial Therapy in Veterinary Medicine. Blackwell Scientific Publications, 1988.

Protecting your practice and the food animal industry. J. Am. Vet. Med. Assoc., *190*:32, 1987.

Rasmussen, F.: Tissue damage at the injection site after intramuscular injection of drugs. Vet. Sci. Commun., *2*:173, 1978.

Scheer, M.: Concentrations of active ingredients in the serum and in tissues after oral and parenteral administration of Baytril. Vet. Med. Rev., *2*:104, 1987.

Scheer, M., Bauditz, R., and Linke, H.: Baytril—antibacterial activity as well as serum and tissue levels in pigs. Proc. 9th Cong. Int. Pig Vet. Soc. Barcelona, 1986.

Setlepani, J.S.: The hazard of using chloramphenicol in food animals. J. Am. Vet. Med. Assoc., *184*:930, 1984.

Shaw, D.H., and Rubin, S.I.: Pharmacologic activity of doxycycline. J. Am. Vet. Med. Assoc., *189*:801, 1986.

Smith, J.T.: The mode of action of 4 quinolones and possible mechanisms of resistance. J. Antimicrob. Chemother., *18*:(suppl. D):21, 1986.

The hazard of using chloramphenicol in food animals. J. Am. Vet. Med. Assoc., *184*:930, 1984.

Vancutsem, P.M., Babish, J.G., and Schwark, W.S.: The fluoroquinolone antimicrobiols: Structure, antimicrobial activity, pharmacokinetics, clinical use in domestic animals and toxicity. Cornell Vet., *80*:173, 1990.

Varma, K.J., Lamendola, J.F., Powers, T.E., and Adams, P.E.: Pharmacokinetics of florfenical in veal calves. Proc. Conf. Res. Workers Animals Diseases Abstract. No. 86, 1985.

Varma, K.J., Powers, T.E., Lobell, R.D., and Lichenvalner, D.M.: Pharmacology of a new broad spectrum antibiotic florfenicol in cattle and its antimicrobial spectrum. International Cattle Congress, Majorca, 1988.

Vincent, P.C.: Drug induced aplastic anaemia and agranulocytosis incidence and mechanisms. Drugs, *31*:52, 1986.

Watson, A.D.J.: Chloramphenicol 2. Clinical pharmacology in dogs and cats. Austral. Vet. J., *68*:2, 1991.

Wolfson, J.S., and Hooper, D.C.: The fluoroquinolous: Structure mechanics of action and resistance. Res. Clin. Forum, 1985, *28*:581, 1985.

Xia, W., Nielsen, P., and Gyrd-Hansen, N.: Oxytetracyclines in cattle. A comparison between a conventional and a long acting preparation. Acta Vet. Scand., *24*:20, 1983.

Yunis, A.A.: Chloramphenicol relation to structure to activity and toxicity. Am. Rev. Pharm. Toxicol., *83*:28, 1988.

Ziv, G.: Intramuscular bioavailability serum drug levels, and local irritation of several oxytetracycline veterinary injectables in cows. *In* Trends in Veterinary Pharmacology and Toxicology. Edited by A.S.J. Van Miert, J. Frens, and F.W. Van der Kreck. Amsterdam, Elsevier, 1980.

12

SULFONAMIDES

12.1 Drugs from Dyes: An Historical Perspective
12.2 Pharmacokinetics
12.3 Dihydrofolate Reductase Inhibitors
12.4 Potentiated Sulfonamides
12.5 Therapy with Sulfonamides
12.6 Therapy with Potentiated Sulfonamides
12.7 Side Effects and Toxicity
12.8 Sulfonamide Residues

12.1 DRUGS FROM DYES: AN HISTORICAL PERSPECTIVE

Pharmaceuticals are developed to achieve specific aims with the help of chemistry. The first step in this direction was the discovery, almost by chance, of the pain-relieving effects of certain compounds, such as phenacetin, which was a waste product in dye production. The compounds acted on the symptoms, however, rather than the causes. The next was the systematic development of medicines purposefully to combat a pathogen, e.g., bacteria. Koch made a major contribution to their discovery by staining bacteria with aniline dyes and thus making them visible. At the turn of the century, a young German physician, Ehrlich, researched behavior of disease-carrying bacteria. To be able to distinguish them from others, he stained the pathogen using the method developed by Koch. It soon occurred to him that the dyes could be used for purposes other than the marking of specific bacteria:

> If certain dyes have a certain tendency to stain specific types of cells and not to stain others, there must be a relation between dye and cell. If one found a dye that would stain certain bacteria and spare the remaining cells, could one not perhaps kill the pathogen with a poison coupled to the dye or even with the dye itself without damaging the other tissue?

Ehrlich started on a laborious search for "mysterious magic bullets that are directed exclusively toward the pathogenic organism and do not affect the body." After several years, his persistence paid off. On December 29, 1910, he was able to present the first chemotherapeutic agent in medical history to the Meeting of German Scientists and Physicians in Konigsberg. After numerous experiments with dyes, he had found that trypan red (arsenobenzene) was active against the causative agent of syphilis, a disease the whole world dreaded.

Ehrlich, with whom the Bayer chemist Roehl worked for 3 years, is generally regarded as the founder of chemotherapy. Ehrlich defined its aim as follows:

> In order to successfully practice chemotherapy, we must find substances in which the relation and killing power dominate in such a way that parasites are killed without significant damage to the organism. In other words we want to hit the parasites first, if possible in isolation, and that means learning to take aim, learning to take aim chemically.

Some of Ehrlich's pupils experimented further with other azo dyes and ultimately introduced a urea derivative under the trade name Germanin. A short time later, highly effective agents against different tropical diseases appeared—all based on dyes.

Domagk, who was working with the dyestuffs company I.G. Farben Fabriken in Leverkusen, Cologne, came across a curious brick red azo dyestuff during this research. Although thousands of azo dyestuffs had been evaluated, the preparation D 4145 proved to be superior to all the others. It was not until February 15, 1935, after many animal experiments and the first promising clinical trials, that Domagk published the results of his work on the active substance, which was later to make medical history under the trade name Prontosil. The publication, titled "On the Behaviour of Prontosil in Mice," started a revolution in the fight against dangerous infectious diseases.

Domagk correctly assumed that if azo dyestuffs containing sulfonamide groups selectively dye bacteria, they must be able to damage them. In the case of Prontosil, although it was inactive antibacterially in vitro, the active moiety sulfanilamide was released in the animal body. Thus Prontosil was the classic example of a pro-drug. It soon became clear that sulfonamides could cure not only acute streptococcal infections, but also those caused by pneumococci (pneumonia), gonococci (gonorrhea), meningococci (meningitis), and many other bacteria. In 1936, the son of President Franklin D. Roosevelt developed a severe purulent inflammation of the lymph nodes in his neck. One of his physicians obtained Prontosil, which he had read about in the medical journals and which was being used in clinical trials in the United States. The President's son recovered. From then on, the success of the first ever synthetic antibacterial agent was unstoppable.

In 1937, Prontosil was awarded the Grand Prix at the World Exhibition in Paris. Two years later, Domagk's achievements were honored with the Nobel Prize for Medicine. The prize, however, was conferred in absentia because Hitler had prohibited all Germans to receive Nobel Prizes. Domagk did not receive his medal and certificate until 1947.

Historically, in fact, sulfonamides originated as far back as 1908, when Gelmo first synthesized sulfanilamide for the dye industry. A quarter century was to pass, however, before it was used on human bacterial infections. In 1909, Hoerlein and co-workers at the I.G. Farbenindustrie, synthesized the first azo dyestuffs containing sulfonamide and substituted sulfonamides and noted them to be superior in color fastness. The firm combination that the complex azo dyes formed with proteins of wool and silk suggested that these agents might react with bacterial protoplasm. In 1913, Eisenberg discovered that the azo compounds chrysoidine and pyridium possessed antibacterial activity in vitro but were useless in vivo. In the years immediately following, scarlet red, another azo dye, came into prominence. In 1919, Heidelberger and Jacobs noted that certain azo-sulfonamide compounds containing the para-aminobenzenesulfonamide structure combined with hydrocupreine were bactericidal in vitro. The same investigators also prepared para-aminobenzenesulfonamide according to the method of Gelmo and suggested that this substance is liberated in the tissues by the breakdown of sulfonamide-chrysoidine. In 1930, Serenium, another azo compound, was introduced as a urinary antiseptic.

Domagk (1935) working at the German I.G. Farben Industrie, announced the discovery of Protonsil and observed that mice with streptococcal and other infections could be protected by the administration of this compound. Foerster (1933) reported the first clinical case responding to Prontosil; he obtained a spectacular result after treating a 10-month-old infant suffering from staphylococcal septicemia with the dye compound.

In France, Trefouels, Nitti, and Bovet, working at the Pasteur Institute in Paris, then announced the important finding that the chemotherapeutic effects of Prontosil were not due to its dye character but to the fact that in the tissues the azo linkage was split, so an active metabolite, para-aminobenzenesulfonamide (sulfanilamide) was released Fig. 12–1.

Fournea and associates then prepared this compound (sulfanilamide) and showed it to be as equally efficacious as Prontosil in curing experimental infections. Colebrook and Kenny and Buttle and co-workers reported their favorable findings with sulfanilamide and Prontosil in puerperal sepsis and meningococcal infections. In the United States, Long and Bliss pointed out that sulfanilamide was the effective radical of the Prontosil molecule and that it exerted a bacteriostatic rather than a bactericidal effect.

Woods (1940), made the important discovery that para-aminobenzoic acid (PABA) nullified the effects of sulfanilamide, and Fildes (1950) observed that a general approach to problems in chemotherapy might evolve from antimetabolite studies because PABA was an essential nutrient for many bacteria.

Close on the publication of the structure of folic acid, it was suggested that this molecule is formed by the condensation of pteridine with PABA and glutamate and that the effects of sulfanilamide were to be regarded primarily as competition in this condensation because the sulfonamide was structurally similar to PABA. The elucidation of the PABA-sulfanilamide relationship thus made it possible to approach chemotherapy on a mechanistic basis and to design or manipulate chemical molecules that would produce specific biochemical lesions and to use such biochemical blocks for selectively toxic effects because folic acid is synthesized in microorganisms, rather than required preformed, as in the mammalian cell.

The role of PABA was obscure in the beginning, but it had been suggested that it was to be regarded as an intermediate in the biosynthesis of some metabolite essential for the higher species. A number of findings pointed to the still unisolated folic acid as this metabolite. This view was supported by the nature of the secondary reversing agents of sulfonamide inhibition, such as purines and thymine, at least some of which appeared to be end products of a system in which folic acid was assumed to play a coenzymic role. Moreover, a number of microorganisms were able to use PABA and folic acid as alternative essential growth factors. The growth of certain organisms was seen to be inhibited by sulfonamides competitively in media containing PABA, but folic acid gave a noncompetitive (bypass) type of reversal of the inhibition, strongly suggesting that it was a product of the inhibited reaction.

12.2 PHARMACOKINETICS

For high clinical efficacy, an antimicrobial compound must exhibit good antimicrobial activity and favorable pharmacokinetic disposition to reach the infecting organisms in vivo with least toxicity to the host. Sulfonamides exhibit antimicrobial activity primarily against gram-positive bacteria, some gram-negative organisms, and certain protozoa.

Different sulfonamides may show quantitative differences in activity, but qualitatively they are all bacteriostatic. Since their discovery, sulfonamides have been important to veterinary practice. The various sulfa preparations do not differ significantly in their antibacterial spectra. They do differ, however, with regard to protein binding and pharmacokinetics. This is important because pharmacokinetic data are needed to design adequate administration schedules and to establish withdrawal times to avoid unwanted residues.

Sulfonamides inhibit gram-positive and gram-negative bacteria, *Rickettsia*, *Nocardia*, *Actinomyces*, and some protozoa. More active sulfonamides may include streptococci, staphylococci, *Escherichia coli*, *Salmonella*, *Pasteurella*, *Pseudomonas*, or *Proteus*. As a group, they are all bacteriostatic and are broad-spectrum agents. All sulfonamides are white crystalline powders, and most are relatively insoluble in water. Their sodium salts, however, are readily soluble.

Sulfonamides are given orally or intravenously, although sulfamethazine sodium and buffered sulfonamide solutions may be given by other parenteral routes. Slow-release oral boluses are also used in cattle. Sulfonamides can be given orally because they are rapidly absorbed from the stomach and small intestine, reaching therapeutic blood levels in 1 to 4 hours. Rapid renal excretion of most of the sulfas, however, necessitates at least twice-daily therapy to maintain inhibitory drug levels in the blood. These levels are assumed by most researchers to be 5 mg/dl blood.

For optimum clinical effect, sulfas should be administered in a way that provides an almost constant inhibitory level in the blood. This is a function of dose and frequency of administration. In ruminants, particularly calves, the practitioner often cannot give sulfas once or twice daily for 3 to 5 days because of economics. Therefore the sustained-release form has provided levels of sulfonamide for several days with a single dose (e.g., Albon slow-release bolus).

The solubility of sulfonamides in water is generally low but increases with alkalinity. Most soluble sulfonamides are sodium salts. Sulfisoxazole, sulfamethoxazole, sulfadiazine, sulfamerazine, sulfamethazine, and sulfathiazole are absorbed and excreted rapidly. Sulfamethoxypyridazine and sulfadimethoxine are classed as being rapidly absorbed and slowly excreted, owing to enterohepatic recycling. Some of these long-acting sulfas are used clinically for foot rot in cattle and coccidiosis in sheep. Poorly absorbed sulfonamides, including succinylsulfathiazole and phthalylsulfathiazole, are used for treatment of enteric infections. Special use sulfonamides include sulfacetamide, used in ophthalmic infections; sulfisoxazole, used in urinary infections; and salicylazosulfapyridine, used in therapy of ulcerative colitis in small animals.

The sodium salt of most sulfonamides is used for intravenous preparations. Such solutions tend to be unstable and may precipitate if mixed with polyenic electrolytes, such as lactate-chloride-carbonate solutions. Other parenteral routes of administration should be avoided because of irritation at the injection site. These sulfonamide solutions are highly alkaline and not stable.

Sulfonamides generally are more soluble at an alkaline pH than at an acid pH. In a mixture of sulfonamide drugs, each component drug exhibits its own solubility. Therefore a mixture, such as a triple sulfa combination, may be much more soluble than an equivalent amount of any of the constituent sulfas alone.

The absorption, distribution, metabolism, and elimination of antibacterials are subject to the same physiologic processes as other compounds, and within the limits of individual animal variations, the pharmacokinetic behavior of compounds can be defined for each target species. In drugs with direct pharmacodynamic effects on the host, such as circulatory stimulants and sedatives, pharmacokinetic properties can form the basis of decisions on dose levels and frequency of administration, but with antimicrobials the relationship between concentrations in body fluids and activity at the site of infection is much less direct and is subject to many variable factors. It is consequently difficult with antimicrobials to derive optimal dose schedule from pharmacokinetic properties and in vitro observations on minimum inhibitory concentrations (MIC).

The primary antibacterial activity of all sulfonamides is linked to their free para-amino group. There are some sulfonamides (e.g., phthalylsulfathiazole) in which the hydrogen atom in the amino group has been substituted, and these do not recover their activity until these radicals are hydrolized in the body. The inactivation of sulfonamides by acetylation is due to similar substitution. The substitution of the amino group by a large range of radicals is responsible for the differences in the effects of various sulfa drugs. The dissociating power of the radical determines both diffusibility through the cell walls and intensity of the response, whereas its chemical structure is responsible for any additional effects. Although sulfonamides have basically the same mechanism of action, their potency is subject to wide variation depending on the properties of the N_1 radical, which determines the degree to which the particular sulfonamide can replace PABA. In evaluating the therapeutic usefulness of a sulfonamide, the acetylation rate, the protein-binding effect, the relative solubility, and the PABA replacement's activity of the free form and the rate of diffusion through tissues must all be taken into consideration.

Many sulfonamide molecules, e.g., phthalylsulfathiazole, have been chemically substituted to prolong absorption from the gut. These compounds have been used to treat enteric infections and reduce the bacterial population of the gut before bowel surgery. Others have been made less toxic or blood levels have been extended by chemical manipulation.

Therapeutic blood levels may be extended in several ways. Altering the sulfa chemically to slow renal clearance of the drug may produce extended blood levels. Sulfadimethoxine has an extended blood level of up to 48 hours in calves when given once daily.

ABSORPTION AND EXCRETION

Most sulfonamides are absorbed from the gastrointestinal tract (except for the so-called enteric drugs). Absorption can take place from many sites, including the uterus and the mammary gland. Assuming that a sulfonamide is absorbed from the gastrointestinal tract, there is little difference between the blood level profiles given orally or parenterally after the first 2 hours. Distribution into all body fluids takes place by passive diffusion. Thus sulfonamides may be given orally; by intramammary infusion; by intrauterine route and by intramuscular, intraperitoneal, and intravenous injection as well as topically.

In blood, most sulfonamides are highly bound to plasma proteins. The majority of their N_4-acetyl derivatives (usual metabolites) and a few of the parent sulfonamides appear to be excreted mostly by renal tubular secretion.

Following the administration of any sulfonamide, a certain proportion of the dose is inactivated by N_4-acetylation. This takes place chiefly in the liver. This is undesirable because it inactivates the sulfonamide, and the acetylated portion tends to increase steadily and becomes bound to plasma proteins more readily than the free form. In addition, this acetylated form is more easily excreted with the urine than the free form. Acetylation, however, is an irreversible process, and some de-acetylation ensures that a balance is maintained between the inactive and the free form in the blood.

The free unacetylated form can be absorbed onto the surface of plasma proteins, especially albumin. As the drug concentration in the blood increases, the amount of sulfonamide bound to plasma proteins also increases but at a slower rate, and the relative percentage bound to free sulfonamide falls. Only the unbound drug can leave the blood vessels and enter the tissue to exert its antibacterial effect.

It is generally thought that only non-protein-bound sulfas are bacteriostatically active. Plasma protein binding may range from 20 to 90% depending on the sulfonamides administered.

The degree to which sulfonamide binds with protein varies from one species of animal to another. Moreover, the acetylation process varies from species to species, and dogs, rabbits, mice, and humans can reverse this process. Certain disease states can affect the acetylation rate. With ketosis in cows, their capacity to acetylate sulfonamides is reduced. Acetylation does not take place in dogs.

To illustrate the effects that the physical and chemical properties have on the various forms of sulfonamide, sulfadiazine is probably one of the most active sulfonamides and is still used in human medicine. It has excellent diffusion through all tissue fluids and is excreted slowly with a half-life of 8 hours. It has low solubility in the urine, however, and has a high potential for renal toxicity unless the situation is well managed. Sulfadimidine is 80% protein bound with 40% acetylation and is less well distributed in tissue fluids. It is shorter acting, but its urinary solubility is high, and therefore it is much safer than sulfadiazine. The third example is sulfamethoxypyridazine, which has good absorption, lower acetylation, and long action but poor protein-binding characteristics (90%).

Drugs with high binding to plasma proteins compete for the binding site with most sulfonamides. This displaces one or both compounds from the proteins and increases the concentration of their active (free) molecules in blood. This interaction, however, is not expected to be a frequent occurrence except in the case of some extremely active drugs, such as phenylbutazone.

Excretion is via the kidneys in the urine except for the enteric sulfas, which have radicals attached to the basic sulfonamide ring that make them too large to be absorbed from the gut. These are excreted through the feces. After absorption into the blood stream, the total blood level is made up of three components:

1. The fraction generally dissolved in the aqueous phase
2. The fraction bound to plasma albumins
3. The fraction bound to erythrocytes

12.3 DIHYDROFOLATE REDUCTASE INHIBITORS

Sulfonamides are important in the armamentarium of chemotherapeutic agents used in combatting bacterial disease in animals and in humans. The possibility has existed for many years that their efficacy might be improved through their conjoint use with inhibitors of bacterial dihydrofolate reductases.

Folic acid plays a vital role in the body principally as a coenzyme specifically concerned with transfer and use of single carbon moieties. This specific coenzymatic function leads to synthesis of purines and of the methylated pyrimidine thymine, which are indispensable components of DNA and thus of cellular reproduction.

Accordingly in states of folate deficiency or maluse, tissues with a high cellular turnover, such as hematopoietic tissues, are primarily affected—the effect generally manifested as megaloblastic anemia. Another aspect of folate metabolism is the development of the antifolate group of compounds, substances that can inhibit folate synthesis in bacterial or mammalian tissue cells, leading to arrest of their replication. This type of action is used in many of today's chemotherapeutic, antineoplastic, and antimalarial drugs.

The conversion of folic acid to folinic acid involves hydrogenation first to dihydrofolic acid and then to tetrahydrofolic acid. A formyl grouping is then introduced into the tetrahydrofolic acid molecule, and the resultant reduced formulated compound is folinic acid. The conversion to folinic acid is apparently accomplished by enzyme systems, and in humans, it occurs primarily in the liver and bone marrow. The reduction of the pteridine moiety of folate or dihydrofolate to tetrahydrofolate is catalyzed by reductase enzymes both in microorganisms and in mammalian tissue cells.

The diaminopyrimidines are a group of chemical agents that inhibit dihydrofolate reductase in bacteria and protozoa. Although this enzyme is common to higher forms of life (e.g., mammals), the diaminopyrimidines used as antimicrobial drugs display a greater selectivity and affinity for the microbial enzyme than for the corresponding mammalian host enzymes. Used alone, these inhibitory substances are not effective against bacteria, but when combined with sulfonamides, a synergistic double blockade of folic acid biosynthesis occurs. Useful inhibitors of dihydrofolate reductase include trimethoprim, ormethoprim, methoprim, and pyrimethamine. A novel addition to the list includes baquiloprim, a new pyrimidine developed solely for veterinary use.

In the selection of an inhibitor of dihydrofolate reductase, key essentials include:

1. High selectivity for the bacterial enzyme
2. Half-life comparable with the accompanying sulfonamide
3. Stability in the rumen

The inhibitory effect on the folic acid metabolism of 2,4-diaminopyrimidines and similar compounds has been known for more than 30 years. Blocking of the dihydrofolate reductase by pyrimethamine (Daraprim) together with competitive inhibition by sulfonamide in the incorporation of the PABA necessary for dihydrofolate formation has been used in the control of toxoplasmosis. The relatively severe side effects of pyrimethamine on erythropoiesis and leukopoiesis as well as its phytotoxic and teratogenic effects have militated against widespread application of this combination. The search has therefore been directed toward a substance of the same group that would have a special affinity for bacterial dihydrofolate reductases but not for that of animals, so as largely to exclude the harmful effects on the enzyme of mammals owing to folinic acid deficiency.

TRIMETHOPRIM

One of the first dihydrofolate reductase inhibitors to be used was trimethoprim (2,4 diamino-5[3,4,5,-trimethoxybenzyl] pyrimidine). Trimethoprim has been used alone as an antibacterial agent, but combination with sulfonamides offers many advantages. It should be remembered that sulfonamides act by competing with PABA for the enzyme that converts this essential bacterial metabolite to folic acid, thus inhibiting one of the first steps in the metabolic synthesis of nucleic acids. Trimethoprim acts in a sim-

ilar way but blocks a later state in this metabolic pathway.

Sulfonamide Block
$$\downarrow\downarrow$$
PABA →   dihydrofolic acid →

         Trimethoprim Block
         $\downarrow\downarrow$
         tetrahydrofolic acid

The effect of this sequential blockade of metabolism is a marked potentiation of activity with extension of chemotherapeutic effectiveness to include organisms that show only borderline sensitivities to the individual drugs. The combination of the two compounds also has a bactericidal effect as opposed to the mainly bacteriostatic effect of either sulfonamides or trimethoprim when acting alone. The drug combinations are also less vulnerable than the individual drugs to the development of resistant strains and have a wider therapeutic index.

Animals, including humans, do not synthesis folate, and therefore in contrast to bacteria, they are not directly concerned with metabolism involving PABA. Consequently, folate metabolism in animals is not directly affected by sulfonamide therapy, but because animals need to reduce exogenous folic acid to folinic acid, they are at least theoretically vulnerable to the action of trimethoprim. The results from trimethoprim use in humans would seem to bear this out, in which measurable effects on folate metabolism have been observed.

Trimethoprim affects a pathway common to both mammalian and bacterial cells, the selective chemotherapeutic effect being due to the greater affinity that trimethoprim has for the bacterial dihydrofolate reductase. It is widely held that this drug combination does not interfere with the mammalian metabolism of folic acid. Interference with folate metabolism in humans, however, has been reported in some patients receiving trimethoprim. Neutropenia and thrombocytopenia have also been observed as well as megaloblastic anemia.

In subchronic and chronic toxicity tests, doses considerably higher than therapeutic doses lead to the effect on hematopoiesis in dogs, cats, and monkeys, with and without the combination of sulfonamides. Disturbances in the folate metabolism in pregnant animals caused by high trimethoprim doses can result in fetal resorption and malformation. Simultaneous folinic acid administration has been found to reduce these harmful effects considerably.

The chemical structure of trimethoprim (an aromatic amine) and its mode of action (affecting bacterial DNA synthesis) suggest that it would give positive results in some mutagenicity assays. It was mutagenic in several Ames tests using *Salmonella typhimurium* TA 98 and TA 1538, and the incidence of micronuclei was significantly increased in the bone marrow of humans administered trimethoprim. Trimethoprim, however, was not mutagenic in a rat dominant lethal assay, and no chromosome effects above the spontaneous level were detected in human patients administered trimethoprim, and the substance did not induce chromosomal damage in human lymphocytes in vitro. No oncogenicity studies with trimethoprim have been reported, so the significance of the positive mutagenicity assays is not clear. No evidence of any preneoplastic effects, however, was evident from the short-term studies, and the use of trimethoprim in human medicine has not been associated with any carcinogenic effect.

In humans, trimethoprim has been reported to cause gastrointestinal disturbances (nausea, vomiting), pruritus, rashes, and depression of hematopoiesis. It may predispose to folate deficiency and is contraindicated in pregnancy, neonates, and renal impairment.

In long-term therapy, which might become necessary, particularly in chronic lung, kidney, or urinary tract disease, blood tests should be obtained because of reports of toxicity in the literature. The hematopoietic system and all tissues with high nuclear division rate are especially sensitive to the folinic acid deficiency occasionally induced by high doses. In longer periods of treatment with the dosage stated, blood tests that were carried out after 3 or 5 weeks showed no deviations from the normal red and white blood picture. Giving the drug to young animals during the first weeks of life should, however, be avoided. Pregnant animals are also better not treated because the risk of malformation cannot be excluded.

ORMETOPRIM

Ormetoprim is another reductase inhibitor, which tends to display a longer half-life than trimethoprim in most species. (Trimethoprim, it should be remembered, possesses an exceedingly short half-life in all domestic animals.) Because of its relatively longer half-life, ormetoprim is often combined with the long-acting sulfa, sulfadimethoxine. (Primor)

In adult ruminants, most of the diaminopyrimidines are substantially degraded by the ruminal microflora. Hence the oral administration of potentiated sulfonamides to ruminants is not a practicable proposition on account of:

1. Degradation of certain dihydrofolate reductase inhibitors by the ruminal microflora (e.g., trimethoprim)
2. Suppression of the gut flora leading to superinfection or diarrhea (or both)

In the adult ruminant, trimethoprim is virtually undetectable in plasma after oral administration, and, although dilution in the ruminal contents may be responsible for this, evidence also suggests that first-pass hepatic metabolism may be important in preventing the significant accumulation of trimethoprim in plasma in older ruminants after oral administration.

BAQUILOPRIM AND ADITOPRIM

A new reductase inhibitor, baquiloprim possesses a number of novel properties rendering it particularly useful in veterinary therapy:

1. It is not degraded by ruminal microflora.
2. It possesses a longer half-life (10 hours in cattle).
3. It can be incorporated in bolus form with sulfonamide to provide extended release over a 2-day period in ruminants.

One of the recently developed dihydrofolate reductase inhibitors is aditoprim. In pigs, the elimination half-life of this drug is 8.0 to 9.3 hours, in contrast to trimethoprim, which has a shorter half-life of 2.1 to 3.5 hours in this species. The in vitro antimicrobial activity of both compounds against common pathogens has been suggested to be similar.

12.4 POTENTIATED SULFONAMIDES

A major breakthrough in sulfonamide therapy has come about with the discovery of trimethoprim, a diaminopyrimidine. The compound is an antimetabolite of folic acid and has antimicrobial properties of its own. It prevents conversion of folic acid into folinic acid by inhibiting the enzyme dihydrofolate reductase. The mechanism of antimicrobial action differs from that of sulfonamides, which, owing to their structural similarity, compete with PABA in folic acid synthesis. Sulfonamides interfere with the synthesis, whereas trimethoprim blocks the use of folic acid by the organisms. The double-barrel attack by the combination (sulfonamide and trimethoprim) synergistically produces "thymineless death" of the organism. The antibacterial efficacy of the combination has been widely acclaimed and is favorably compared with various antibiotics.

Sulfonamide
Block
PABA→   ↓   Dihydrofolic Acid→

Trimethoprim
Block
                  ↓   Tetrahydrofolic Acid

The fact that trimethoprim and sulfonamides are highly synergistic can be demonstrated in several ways, and the enhanced susceptibility of many bacteria has been convincingly shown. Potentiation may be demonstrated in vitro by the disc diffusion method. Discs impregnated with trimethoprim and a sulfonamide, singly and in combination, are applied to plates seeded with the test organisms. Enhanced susceptibility is seen when the zone of inhibition around the combination disc is larger than the zones around either of the single component discus. In general, the greater the difference in zone sizes, the greater the degree of potentiation. An extended zone in inhibition develops between two single component discs placed adjacently to each other.

The marked mutual potentiation of in vitro activity of trimethoprim and sulfonamides against bacterial pathogens has been well established, and clinical trial results in large numbers of cattle and pigs indicated that the two drugs when used together gave superior results to sulfonamide alone. Potentiation, as measured by a reduction of the MIC of each individual drug, has been demonstrated by many investigators for both human and veterinary strains.

Sulfonamides are weak organic acids, whereas trimethoprim is a weak organic base. Sulfonamides partition between body fluid compartments in a different way than trimethoprim. The respective half-lives of each component are also quite dissimilar. Choice of the sulfonamide that "best fits" the pharmacokinetic patterns of trimethoprim has been more difficult in veterinary medicine than in human medicine.

Each animal species does not excrete these drugs at the same rate, and therefore matching cannot be simply attained with a single sulfonamide. Favorable results have been obtained with sulfadoxine, a long-acting sulfonamide, when combined with trimethoprim in an injectable form in treatment of various infections of farm animals. Trimethoprim and sulfadiazine, a relatively short-acting sulfonamide, is effective in oral tablets for treating cats and dogs. The superior clinical effects of the combination sulfadoxine plus trimethoprim, when compared with that of sulfadoxine alone, permits not only a considerable reduction of the initial dose, but also increases the therapeutic effect. Ormetoprim is usually paired with sulfadimethoxine (both long acting), and baquiloprim is combined with sulfamezathine for use in ruminants. An oral bolus of this long-acting combination is available for enteric and respiratory therapy in ruminants because baquiloprim is not degraded in the rumen.

Contrary to the widely held view, however, the pharmacokinetic matching of the components and the ratio at which they are administered are seldom important. Because the elimination rates differ and they are administered in a ratio of 5:1, it is impossible to determine the duration of an optimal synergistic concentration for each drug at the site of infection. Studies showed that trimethoprim persists longer in tissues than in plasma following drug administration, which suggests that the slow release of trimethoprim from tissues compensates for the short half-life in comparison to the sulfonamide component of the formulation.

TABLE 12–1
SULFAS USED IN VETERINARY MEDICINE

Drug	Species	Route
Sulfathiazole	Swine, calves	PO
Sulfamethazine	Cattle, swine	PO, IV
Sulfamerazine	Cattle, swine	PO, IV
Sulfadiazine	Cattle, swine, dogs	PO
Sulfabromomethazine	Cattle	PO
Sulfadimethoxine/Methoprim/(Primor)	Dogs, cats, cattle, horses	PO, IV, SC
Sulfachlorpyridazine	Swine, calves	SC, IV
Sulfadiazine-trimethoprim	Dogs	PO, SC
Sulfamethoxypyridazine	Cattle	PO, IV
Sulfadiazine/Trimethoprim (Tribrissin)	Dogs, Cats	IV, PO
Trimethoprim (Di-Trim)		
Sulfamethoxazole (Bactrim)	Dogs, cats	PO PO

PO, Oral; IV, intravenous; SC, subcutaneous.

In contrast to the sulfonamides, the concentration of trimethoprim in tissues is higher than that in plasma owing to its higher lipophilicity. Trimethoprim and sulfadiazine readily crossed into synovial and peritoneal fluid when 15 mg/kg of combined product was administered intravenously. The trimethoprim and sulfonamide penetrate the blood-brain barrier when meningitis is present and achieve therapeutic concentrations in the cerebrospinal fluid. The distribution and elimination of trimethoprim take place independently of those of the sulfonamide.

The high tissue concentrations of trimethoprim are predictable from the high apparent volume of distribution (V_d) following intravenous injection (a V_d of 1.5 liters/kg in the pig). The accumulation of trimethoprim in extravascular fluid compartments is explicable by the physical properties of trimethoprim, which is a weak base with pKa 7.3. It is considered that diffusion of drugs across membranes between fluid compartments takes place only in the un-ionized form. In contrast to those of the sulfonamides, the concentrations of trimethoprim in tissues is higher than in plasma, and trimethoprim is excreted, mainly unaltered, in the urine.

12.5 THERAPY WITH SULFONAMIDES

Sulfonamides are effective only against proliferating microorganisms. Growth can resume when sulfonamide concentrations become low. Therefore host defense mechanisms are critical for successful sulfonamide therapy.

Sulfonamides are most effective when given early in the course of a disease. In severe infections, the initial dose should be given intravenously and should be greater than maintenance doses. Urine output should be monitored and drinking water provided at all times. Treatment should not exceed 7 days and should be continued for 48 hours after remission (Table 12–1).

Treatment should be initiated as early as possible in the course of the disease. A sufficiently high initial dose should be given to

TABLE 12–2
SULFOMAMIDE DOSAGE THERAPY—CATTLE

Sulfonamide	Priming	Maintenance	Treatment Interval
Sulfamethazine, USP	1 1/2 g/lb	3/4–1 g/lb	24 hours
Sulfamerazine	1 1/2 g/lb	1/2 g/lb	12 hours
Sulfapyridine	1 g/lb	1/2 g/lb	12 hours
Sulfathiazole	1 1/2 g/lb	1/2 g/lb	6–8 hours
Sulfachlorpyridiazine (Vetisulid)	30–40 mg/lb	15–23 mg/lb	12 hours
Sulfadimethoxine (Albon)	25 mg/lb (IV, IM)	12.5 mg/lb	24 hours
Sulfadimethoxine bolus (Albon-SR)	62.5 mg/lb		4 days
Sulfamethazine bolus (Spanbolet II)	1 bolus/150 lbs		5 days
Sulfamethazine bolus (Hava-Span)	1 bolus/200 lbs		3 1/2 days
Sulfadimethoxine/ormetoprim (Primor)	55 mg/kg	27.5 mg/kg	24 hours

IV, Intravenous; IM, intramuscular.

ensure adequate levels of the free dissolved fraction at the site of the infection. The size of the maintenance doses and intervals between should be adapted to the properties of the preparation used (follow manufacturer's recommendations closely). Fluid intake should not be restricted during treatment. If the sulfonamides fail to elicit a response within a reasonable time, the treatment schedule should be subjected to a careful reappraisal.

Indications for sulfonamides are wide owing to the wide spectrum of activity of sulfonamides and cover infectious diseases of the digestive and respiratory tracts, septicemia, secondary infections, peritonitis, mastitis, and metritis. More specifically, sulfonamides are particularly suitable for the following indications:

Cattle: foot rot, coccidiosis, actinomycosis, scours, calf diphtheria, polyarthritis, navel ill, respiratory infection (Table 12–2)
Horses: strangles and secondary infections of the upper respiratory tract; polyarthritis and navel ill in foals
Sheep: coccidiosis, foot abscess, enteritis
Pigs: pneumonia, rhinitis, scours
Dogs and cats: urinary tract infections, skin infections, respiratory infections
Rabbits: coccidiosis

For many modern sulfonamides, it is necessary for them to achieve a total blood concentration of 5 mg/100 ml to ensure an adequate level of free dissolved fraction. This results in much higher loading doses of sulfonamide than is the case with antibiotics.

Several sulfonamides are sometimes combined in one preparation to ensure a wider range of activity, to enhance the therapeutic effect, and to reduce toxicity. Thus, by employing lower doses of each sulfonamide to build up a higher total serum level, an increased bacteriostatic effect can be achieved. An enhanced effect can also be achieved by combining sulfonamides endowed with different properties regarding absorption, diffusion, and excretion. Despite their close chemical relationship to one another, sulfonamides do not give rise to additive side effects when administered in combined preparations.

Because of their general pharmacokinetic properties, sulfonamides have been major drugs in veterinary antimicrobial therapeutics. Various structural modifications can alter both the partitioning characteristics and the antibacterial potency of the individual compounds.

Sulfonamides as a group possess similar pharmacologic properties qualitatively but often exhibit quantitative differences in the protein binding, passage across biological membranes, and renal excretion, owing to their inherent physicochemical properties, e.g., pKa and solubility. Poorly soluble and therefore poorly absorbed sulfonamides, e.g., sulfaguanidine, succinylsulfathiazole, phthalylsulfacetamide, and phthalylsulfathiazole, stay mostly in the gastrointestinal tract after oral administration and hence are used against enteric infections.

In vitro sulfanilamide appears to be the least active and sulfathiazole the most active, with sulfapyrimidines close behind. Because of their physicochemical and pharmacokinetic properties, however, sulfapyrimidines have been found to be more useful than sulfathiazole. Among sulfapyrimidines, sulfadiazine has become more popular in human medicine. In animals, however, because of its more reliable absorption from the gastrointestinal tract, sulfamerazine is preferred over sulfadiazine. The antibacterial activity of sulfamethazine in vitro is probably a bit lower than sulfadiazine and sulfamerazine, but it has a longer sojourn in the body and is one of the most widely used sulfonamides in veterinary medicine. Sulfonamides vary somewhat with respect to their kinetic fate and toxicity.

The inherent activity of sulfonamide drugs is due to the various groups attached to the basic sulfonamide nucleus, and thus each sulfa drug exhibits its own blood level, antibacterial efficiency, length of action, acetylation, tissue distribution, protein binding, and toxicity. Dosages and dosage intervals recommended by manufacturers of different sulfa drugs are adjusted so they are about equally effective when used at these doses.

Drugs with a long sojourn in the body often allow a reduction in the size of dose and frequency of administration. Sulfadimethoxine, sulfamethoxypyridazine, sulfametopyrazine, sulfamethylphenazole, sulfamethoxazole, sulfasomizole, and sulfasymazine are some long-acting systemic sulfonamides. They usually are absorbed readily from the gastrointestinal tract, bound highly to plasma proteins, and excreted slowly. They are popular in sheep and cattle on account of their longevity of effectiveness.

Another approach to obtain extended effect of sulfonamides has been via sustained-release preparations. Following oral administration, these release the active drug slowly in the gastrointestinal tract for absorption over prolonged periods. Such repository forms, however, provide considerably lower levels of drugs in the body than normal preparations.

Sulfadimethoxine and sulfamonomethoxine are two long-acting sulfonamides formulated in bolus form. Protein binding, plasma half-life, and residue depletion studies for these two drugs illustrate their longevity in the animal body. It must be pointed out that in establishing withdrawal times, it should be taken into consideration that the data usually published are obtained from healthy animals. In diseased animals, there may be deviations of elimination half-life and distribution pattern.

Sulfamonomethoxine is a bacteriostatic substance, which exerts a selective toxic effect on bacteria during the multiplication phase. The antibacterial activity of sulfamonomethoxine is due to the sulfanilamide radical, which is a structural analog of PABA.

As one of the long-acting sulfonamides, sulfadimethoxine has been widely applied to clinical treatment of various bacterial infections. Sulfadimethoxine and sulfamethoxypyridazine are useful in control of coccidiosis and cholera in poultry. Several workers have reported on the pharmacologic properties of these compounds in cattle, sheep, and pigs, especially for enteric and respiratory infections (shipping fever-pasteurellosis in feedlot cattle).

Sulfadimethoxine is a low-dose, rapidly absorbed, long-acting sulfonamide that is effective in the treatment of bacterial infections commonly associated with shipping fever complex, bacterial pneumonia, calf diphtheria, and foot rot in cattle. The drug is well tolerated, has a low degree of toxicity, and at the recommended doses does not produce undesirable effects. Coccidiosis in ruminants is another key indication.

Sulfamerazine is a bacteriostatic agent, which has been employed for treatment of infectious diseases of cattle for some 30 years. The drug has been found to be of value in treating bovine mastitis, metritis, pneumonia, bacterial enteritis, and foot rot.

The effectiveness of sulfadimidine has been frequently demonstrated in treatment of pneumonia in cattle as well as treatment of foot rot. Within 24 hours of treatment, a marked improvement in condition is apparent, and by 72 hours, swelling disappears and a good recovery takes place.

For treatment or prevention of coccidiosis, sulfonamides continue to be effective drugs. Among established drugs in ruminants, sulfaquinoxaline, sulfadimethoxine, sulfamethylphenazole, and sulfamethoxypyridazine are the most useful coccidiostats. Sulfadimethoxine, sulfachloropyrazine, and sulfamonomethoxine, however, also have been reported to be highly effective. Other coccidiostats, e.g., amprolium, diaveridine, pyrimethamine, and adjuvants such as ethopabate and chlortetracycline, are often combined with sulfonamides for synergistic effects in poultry.

12.6 THERAPY WITH POTENTIATED SULFONAMIDES

Although the half-life of trimethoprim is short in most species, nonetheless when combined with sulfonamides (usually sulfadiazine, sulfadoxine, or sulfadimidine), a marked clinical synergy is evident. Enteritis (*E. coli*, salmonellosis), respiratory infections, and urogenital infections respond particularly well to potentiated sulfonamides. Ormetoprim is combined usually with sulfadimethoxine (Primor, Roche), and baquiloprim with sulfadimidine on account of better matching half-lives.

The in vitro antibacterial activity of trimethoprim/sulfonamide combinations is extensive and covers the majority of gram-positive and gram-negative bacteria that cause diseases in animals and birds. Potentiated sulfonamides are effective against many gram-positive and gram-negative organisms. In addition, *Chlamydia* and *Actinomyces* are sensitive to them, as are *Nocardia* at high drug doses. *Pseudomonas* and *Mycoplasma* tend to be resistant. The efficacy of potentiated sulfonamides against anaerobic organisms is questionable. Pathogenic bacteria sensitive to potentiated sulfonamides, which may cause disease in animals and birds and against which it is accepted practice in veterinary medicine to instigate treatment, include:

Actinomyces
Actinobacillus
Aeromonas
Bordetella
Brucella
Corynebacterium
E. coli
Fusiformis
Klebsiella
Listeria monocytogenes
Moraxella bovis
Mycobacterium
Neisseria
Nocardia
Pasteurella
Proteus
Salmonella
Shigella
Staphylococci (including penicillinase-producing strains)
Streptococci (including enterococci and diplococci)
Vibrio (campylobacter)

Trimethoprim/sulfonamide combinations have become valuable antimicrobials for therapy of a broad spectrum of microbial infections in human and veterinary medicine. Their usefulness lies in their wide spectrum of activity, good tissue distribution, and desirable pharmacokinetic properties.

Trimethoprim/sulfonamide combinations are widely distributed throughout the body's tissues and readily penetrate into pleural, peritoneal, synovial, ocular, and cerebrospinal fluids. Trimethoprim/sulfonamide combinations are effective against bacteria that would otherwise be resistant to either agent alone. Similarly, each agent alone may be bacteriostatic; together they are bactericidal.

The commercial product is formulated in a ratio of 5:1, sulfonamide:trimethoprim. Although a ratio of 20:1 is reported as optimal for antibacterial activity, synergy occurs over a wide ratio of drug concentrations—1:1 to 1:40. Baquiloprim: sulfadimidine is in a ratio of 9:1.

Clinical experience in humans has shown, however, that the ration of 1 part trimethoprim to 5 parts of sulfonamide is probably superior to the 1:10 ratio and therefore to the 1:20. This difference between the optimum ratios for in vitro and in vivo activities is at least partly explained by trimethoprim passing more readily from the blood into the tissues. Usually the injection contains 4% w/v trimethoprim and 20% w/v sulfadoxine in an organic solvent: equivalent to 40 mg trimethoprim and 200 mg sulfadoxine per milliliter.

The injection is recommended for treatment and control of a wide range of bacterial diseases and certain protozoal diseases in dogs and of bacterial diseases in farm animals, especially young stock. The recommended routes of administration are:

• Cattle and sheep, intramuscular injection, preferably into the neck
• Pigs, intramuscular injection at the usual site behind the ears.
• Horses and dogs, slow intravenous injection only

The recommended dose is 15 to 24 mg/kg body weight combined active ingredients (trimethoprim and sulfadoxine) daily: equivalent to 1 ml/16 kg body weight, which may be increased in severe infections to 1 ml/10 kg body weight, daily. A single treatment may be sufficient in some cases, but in severe infections the dose should be repeated daily for 5 days or until 2 days after the symptoms have subsided. In vitro activity of trimethoprim/sulfonamide combination is widely documented, from early work in development of the human oral product septrin.

The long-acting sulfonamide, sulfadoxine, is highly satisfactory as the companion sulfonamide when the combination is administered intramuscularly once daily to large animals; the relatively short-acting sulfonamide, sulfadiazine, whose half-life matches more closely that of trimethoprim, has apparently proved equally satisfactory when given orally with trimethoprim twice daily to small animals.

Sulfadoxine/trimethoprim is used as a potentiated sulfa drug, chiefly for cattle and pigs, in veterinary practice. Potentiation by trimethoprim substantially enhances the effect of sulfadoxine, which could be used to reduce the dosage to less than one half the sulfadoxine dose and about one tenth of the dose of conventional sulfa drugs, such as sulfadimethoxine. This lower dosage, and the fact that the antibacterial efficacy remains stable, has the additional advantage of easier handling of the solution of injection (smaller injection volume) and less stress on the tissues from exposure to foreign substances.

With the exception of *Pseudomonas*, *Erysipelothrix*, *Leptospira*, and *Mycobacterium tuberculosis*, most of the common bacterial pathogens are susceptible to its bactericidal effects.

The in vitro antibacterial spectrum of trimethoprim resembles that of sulfadiazine, which has a relatively brief effect. Trimethoprim on its own, however, is effective against streptococci and a number of gram-negative bacteria but has a relatively slight effect on *Pseudomonas aeruginosa* and *Clostridium perfringens*.

The half-life of sulfadiazine is also somewhat similar to that of trimethoprim. Combination of the two substances therefore seems theoretically practicable but does require at least two oral administrations over 24 hours.

The absorption of orally administered potentiated sulfonamides in small animals is generally good. Once absorbed, these combination drugs are well distributed to most body tissues. Their elimination depends on hepatic metabolism and renal elimination. Although there are differences in the disposition of the sulfonamide and trimethoprim components, these differences do not appear to alter the clinical efficacy of the combined product. Trimethoprim is available in combination with sulfadiazine (Tribrissen, Coopers; Di-Trim, Syntex) or sulfamethoxazole (Bactrim, Roche). Trimethoprim/sulfonamide is a common choice for treating pyoderma, urinary tract infection, and soft tissue infections caused by gram-positive bacteria. Many physicians and veterinarians consider trimethoprim/sulfonamide to be the drug of choice against methicillin-resistant staphylococci. Trimethoprim/sulfonamide is highly effective for treatment of urinary tract infection. Resistance to sulfonamides is frequently seen, and the best-documented mechanism of resistance of bacteria to sulfonamides is an alteration in the cell receptors to which the drug and PABA are bound.

RESISTANCE

Microorganisms that do not synthesize folic acid are naturally resistant, but fortunately most of these are nonpathogenic. Resistance development is not uncommon with sulfonamide therapy and is encouraged by exposing susceptible organisms to suboptimal concentrations of the active drug. This can occur by underdosing; intermittent dosing; presence of chronic inflammation; presence of large depots of PABA, e.g., pus; and presence of other inflammatory exudates. Sulfonamides should never be used sparingly in a therapeutic situation.

12.7 SIDE EFFECTS AND TOXICITY

Sulfonamides may give rise to a number of potential side effects:

1. Following oral medication, some symptoms of gastrointestinal intolerance may be seen.
2. Allergic reactions have been noted.
3. Large doses over a long period may give rise to a hemorrhagic syndrome.
4. Signs of shock in young animals may occur. This may be liable to occur in the first few weeks of life, when the animal's liver and kidneys are not yet functioning properly, and blood protein levels are still below normal.
5. Potassium salts of sulfonamides used to increase solubility need to be used cautiously if heart damage is suspected, and the intravenous route should be avoided because cardiac arrest may be precipitated by the potassium.

Therapeutic doses are relatively nontoxic, but agranulocytosis, hemolytic anemia and avitaminosis K have been reported following prolonged administration. Prolonged treatment with sulfas should be avoided, especially in young stock. Sulfonamides occasionally cause crystalluria, particularly when urinary pH is low. Ensure adequate water intake during treatment, and take particular care in animals suffering from renal damage. To minimize the risk of occasional local tissue reaction when administering potentiated sulfonamides by subcutaneous injection, the dose should be divided and administered at several sites and the sites well massaged.

Acute toxic reactions may follow rapid intravenous injection. Hypersensitivity reactions have been reported. Crystalluria, with hematuria, is rare in cattle. Sulfonamides transiently depress normal cellulolytic function in the ruminoreticulum.

Rapid intravenous injections of sulfonamides have occasionally resulted in acute neurologic signs with emesis, ataxia, muscular weakness, spastic paresis, and convulsions. Dairy cows injected with sulfaquinoxaline have developed severe muscular weakness and visual disturbances, with acute deaths in some cows.

Combinations of trimethoprim and a sulfonamide have been widely used in treatment of various infections in humans and in animals. Injury to muscle tissue at the site of injection has occurred after intramuscular administration of such combinations to animals.

Adverse reactions to rapidly injected intravenous trimethoprim have been reported in horses. Such reactions to potentiated sulfonamides injected intravenously have occasionally led to collapse. In the adult horse, administration of trimethoprim-sulfonamide combinations has been associated, albeit rarely, with transient neutropenia, acute toxic enteritis, transient ataxia, and sudden death.

With sulfonamide therapy, renal toxicity is the main cause of concern. The drug is concentrated 50-fold by the glomerulus, then as water is reabsorbed by the tubules, the pH falls, reducing solubility of the sulfonamide, and the proportion of the acetylated form is increased. This is a process by which sulfonamides are crystallized out in the kidney. Crystalluria is the most common toxic manifestation in sulfonamide therapy. This is primarily because the acetylated forms of most sulfonamides are less soluble than the parent compounds.

With more modern compounds, this danger is minimal because, with their greater effectiveness and longer duration of action, a therapeutic response is achieved with lower dose rates administered at longer intervals. In addition, the degree of acetylation has been reduced, with the acetylated form sometimes being even more readily soluble than the free form. These characteristics are highly desirable in searching for new sulfonamides.

Well-established sulfonamides, such as sulfadimidine, sulfamethoxazole, sulfafurazole, sulfisoxazole, and sulfachlorpyridazine, are highly soluble compounds. They are readily excreted in the urine but, owing to their high solubility even in acidic urine, pose little danger of crystalluria and are therefore suitable for urinary tract infections.

It is often forgotten that sulfonamides are oxidizing agents and that the erythrocytes of newborn foals are reported to be quite sensitive to their oxidative effects, with resulting hemolysis and methemoglobinemia. Sulfonamides may also displace drugs and endogenous substances from their binding sites on albumin, resulting in higher serum concentrations of free (active) drug or other substances, such as bilirubin. This interaction has resulted in kernicterus in premature and newborn human infants and could potentially be of importance when dealing with premature newborn foals.

The hematopoietic system has been reported to be susceptible to sulfonamide toxicity. Such adverse effects caused by sulfonamides are either dose-dependent or hypersensitivity reactions. Acute hemolytic anemia, with resultant nausea, fever, icterus, hemoglobinuric nephrosis, and shock, has been reported to be caused by sulfonamides in humans. Other reported blood dyscrasias are agranulocytosis, aplastic anemia, thrombocytopenia, and eosinophilia.

Mild hemolytic anemias in calves have occurred with sulfonamide treatment. Hemorrhagic diathesis has been observed in calves and chickens owing to the well-known suppression of gut flora responsible for the natural synthesis of vitamin K. Sulfaquinoxaline has also been the cause of a complete disappearance of granulocyte precursors in the marrow of 10-week-old pullets and 32-week-old hens. Anorexia, severe anemia, agranulocytosis, hypoprothrombinemia, and hydropericardium have also been reported as sequelae to sulfaquinoxaline therapy. Most of the disorders relating to effects on the gut flora can be remedied by the use of vitamin K supplementation in the rations.

Hypersensitivity reactions caused by sulfonamides include systemic lupus erythematosus and skin and mucous membrane manifestations, such as purpuric and petechial rashes. Exfoliative dermatitis, photosensitization, anaphylactoid reactions, hepatitis, and drug fever have also been reported. Manifestations of hypersensitivity to sulfonamides have been reported to occur in approximately 20% of human patients with previous sulfonamide therapy.

Long-term studies have demonstrated other effects by sulfonamides. The oral administration of 500 mg/kg/day to chickens of a variety of sulfonamide drugs resulted in an increased incidence of neuropathy. The mildest changes consisted of demyelinization of cord and brain tissue, with chromatolysis of nerve cells and fragmentation of their axons. Higher concentrations of the drugs were found in the sciatic nerve than in the blood, suggesting some preferential attraction or binding to nerve tissue.

Few side effects are associated with potentiated sulfonamides when used in cats. Megaloblastic anemia may occur when high doses of the drugs are given over the long term. Treatment with folic acid (2.5 mg/kg/day) counteracts this side effect in cats receiving the drug longer than 2 weeks. Dogs have developed skin reactions, which are presumably a result of drug hypersensitivity, but similar reactions have not been documented in cats. Keratoconjunctivitis sicca occasionally occurs in dogs receiving sulfonamides but has not been reported in cats.

The most important adverse effect of trimethoprim/sulfonamide therapy that is seen in dogs is drug-induced keratoconjunctivitis sicca resulting from a toxic effect of the sulfonamide component on the lacrimal gland. Drug exposure does not necessarily have to be prolonged, and drug-induced keratoconjunctivitis sicca is not always reversible when the sulfonamide is discontinued. This is associated with carbonic anhydrase inhibition.

Goitrogenic effects of sulfonamides have given rise to concern. Rat studies have revealed evidence of a carcinogenic effect on the thyroid tissue. The goitrogenic action of sulfonamides in the rat is not believed to be a direct effect on the thyroid but an indirect effect mediated by the excessive release of pituitary thyrotropin response to a deficiency of circulating thyroid hormone. This hormonal effect has not been observed in primates, thus signalling some species specificity to this effect. This carcinogenicity (albeit by a secondary mechanism) is now the subject of intense investigation by the Food and Drug Administration (FDA) with respect to the potential epigenetic or secondary mechanisms of sulfonamides on the development of tumors of the thyroid gland.

Residues of sulfonamides in edible tissues have been problems for regulatory officials, animal feeders, and feed companies. The residues have occurred most frequently in porcine liver and kidney and to a lesser extent in avian tissues. Sulfamethazine, sulfaquinoxaline, and sulfadimethoxine have been most frequently detected (in order of frequency).

12.8 SULFONAMIDE RESIDUES

Sulfonamides play an important role as effective chemotherapy of bacterial and protozoal diseases in veterinary medicine. They are frequently administered in combination with dihydrofolate reductase inhibitors of the group of diaminopyrimidines. In food-producing animals, residues are formed on administration, which deplete with widely variable velocity depending on many factors, such as the nature of the compound, its formulation and route of administration, the treated animal species, and genotypes.

Decline of drug residues in body tissues and fluids to permissible limits (<0.1 ppm in edible products) differs for each sulfonamide and depends on the dose, route of administration, and species. It also appears that sulfonamide residues disappear much earlier from most organs, e.g., liver and kidney, and fluids, e.g., milk, than from muscles and fat. Withdrawal periods to attain the permissible residues in meat or milk therefore differ for each sulfonamide.

Sulfamethazine has been widely used as an antibacterial drug additive in feeds for swine. It is also used for chicken and cattle and for companion animals to treat and prevent respiratory and gastrointestinal diseases.

The current safe residue level for swine is set at 0.1 ppm using older data. This level includes a 1000-fold safety factor, so a consumer exposed to levels slightly over the 0.1 ppm level does not suffer ill effects.

The National Center for Toxicological Research (NCTR) conducted a long-term bioassay study in mice with moderate to high levels of sulfamethazine. A draft NCTR report to the Center for Veterinary Medicine (CVM) concluded that the drug produced tumors in the thyroid gland of male and female mice at the dose levels used. It was shown that mice receiving the highest levels of sulfamethazine revealed evidence of neoplastic lesions, and there was some evidence of thyroid hyperplasia. There was also an increase in the incidence of adenomas in the thyroid gland of mice that received the highest dose: 4800 ppm. The results of a 2-year rat study illustrated similar findings. Rats were fed diets including sulfamethazine at levels between 10 and 2400 ppm and were sacrificed at 3, 12, 18, and 24 months to assess tumor development. The conclusions of the rat study showed that neoplasia occurred in the thyroid gland only late in the study, that thyroid hyperplasia was related to sulfamethazine, and that there was an inverse dose response on mortality.

Sulfonamide-induced tumors of the thyroid gland in mice and rats may occur by a secondary mechanism of oncogenesis. It has been postulated that sulfonamides produce thyroid hyperplasia and tumor development by inhibiting thyroid hormone synthesis and eliciting, as a result, a stimulation of thyroid-stimulating hormone secretion. This rather than any direct genotoxic or mutagenic effect may well be the cause of the anatomic changes that sulfonamides induce.

The FAO/WHO Joint Expert Committee on Food Additives established maximum residue levels of 100 ppb for meat and 25 ppb for milk for parent sulfamethazine. Current US tolerances for the drug are 100 ppb for meat and 10 ppb for milk.

If US drug sponsors can establish that the carcinogenic effect of sulfamethazine results from a secondary mechanism rather than a direct process, the FDA could regulate the drug based on a "no observed effect level" (NOEL).

This indication that the US agency would be prepared to consider this as an alternative to regulating the drug under the Delaney Clause based on NCTR data could have significance not only for the sulfonamides in general, but also for future FDA policy regarding the regulation of secondary carcinogens.

If the secondary mechanism theory can be proven, however, the FDA could establish a safe level based on the lowest NOEL in the most sensitive species. Those conducting the AHI study believe that the high concentration of sulfamethazine serves as a triggering mechanism, causing release of thyroid-stimulating hormone that, in turn, is the actual agent that promotes the tumor formation observed in the NCTR study. New data also indicate that there is a no-effect concentration at which sulfamethazine can be fed and have no effect on thyroid-stimulating hormone release. Another aspect of the cooperative study that has been initiated is an attempt to demonstrate that tumors do not develop when primates are fed diets containing high concentrations of sulfamethazine.

Time becomes an extremely important consideration, given the FDA-CVM's announced intent of lowering sulfamethazine tolerance in less than 1 ppb in food animal tissue. The presently accepted tolerance is 0.1 ppm. Most experts agree that a tolerance of 1 ppb or less would virtually eliminate the use of sulfamethazine as a feed additive or therapeutic drug. Because of the ubiquitous nature of the sulfamethazine and its presence in minute amounts in water, feeds and bedding, it may even be possible to produce pork that is free of sulfamethazine at a tolerance of 1 ppb. It is hoped that the FDA will hold its proposed tolerance in abeyance until the AHI studies are complete and appropriate data are presented that would allow the current tolerance to be continued.

The United States Department of Agriculture (USDA) (whose subagencies are responsible for monitoring the use of animal drugs, whereas the FDA sets guidelines as to how they should be used) has meanwhile responded to the sulfamethazine affair with a four-part action plan designed to eliminate violative residues. The Department's Food Safety and Inspection Service notes in a document outlining the plan that although a decade of agency efforts to counter violative levels as high as 13% have significantly reduced the violative percentage, around 5% of swine tested still exceed the FDA-stipulated maximum tolerance of 0.1 ppm.

Stage one of the plan is to see rapid implementation of a comprehensive swine identification program devised jointly by the FSIS and its sister agency, the Animal and Plant Health Inspection Service (APHIS). The joint FSIS/APHIS scheme addresses what is described in the plan of action as a persistent problem in enforcement of safe residues: the inability to identify the source of hog carcasses during processing.

The second element in the FSIS plan is a program designed to intensify the action taken by the agency to prevent violative residues. Scheduled action is to hinge on a in-plant rapid sulfamethazine test, called the "sulfa-on-site" (SOS) test, which permits swift identification of animals with high residue levels.

Recognizing that the prevention of residues during the production process is the best if not the only way to achieve residue control, the agency will continue to encourage approved veterinarians, producers, and others to perform the SOS test on animals before marketing.

Stage four of the FSIS policy, providing for rapid development and verification of new or improved effective test methods, seems already to have been realized in part, with news from the agency that a new enzyme-linked immunosorbent assay (ELISA) card test is available, which has the ability to detect smaller amounts of sulfamethazine than the SOS system. Being simple both to operate and to interpret, the new test is said to offer the potential for use in testing live animals by the producer.

Results for fiscal 1992 indicate that the incidence of violative residues of sulfamethazine is below 1% in the United States. Contributing to this decline has been the action by the National Pork Producers Council and farmer groups. Many producers have stopped using the drug, and the tighter controls on producers have exerted an effect.

The agency's SOS testing program is also cited as a contributing factor. In the year to October 5th, 1989, 121,905 SOS tests were run on urine samples in the 100 largest plants. Of these, 905 were sent for confirmatory laboratory analyses, with 364 confirmed violations being recorded.

The agency's program of testing six samples per day in each of the 100 plants is continuing, and the possibility of expanding the sampling to smaller plants is under review. Consideration is being given as to whether to propose a regulation to implement phase II of the program. This would involve lot testing in all plants, with one of the 10 lots being SOS tested per day. The size of a lot would probably comprise six pigs.

Although the level of illegal sulfamethazine residue should be considered reasonable compared with other drugs, no violative levels will ever be acceptable to the FSIS, whose goal is to reach zero residues. Sulfamethazine is currently under review at the FDA, and decisions relating to the future regulation of the drug could mean that it will eventually be withdrawn from the market if the tolerance level set is so low as to make it impractical.

The AHI contends that animal drugs that are secondary carcinogens should be recognized as such and not be subjected to the Delaney "anticancer" clause. The industry organization is collating information that supports adoption by the FDA of a policy recognizing the role of secondary mechanisms of action and the need to set tolerances on this basis, according to the AHI.

It notes that in calculating a tolerance for sulfamethazine, the Joint Expert Committee on Food Additives of the WHO and FAO (JECFA) used the principle of secondary mechanism. The 0.1 ppm level recommended by JECFA is the same as the currently approved US FDA tolerance for tissue.

The CVM has indicated that based on the NCTR rodent study results, a tolerance for sulfamethazine would be set in the low parts per billion range, or even sub-part per billion. Such a reduction would have the same effect as an outright ban because the withdrawal time would have to be lengthened impracticably. The 100-fold tolerance reduction, however, would depend on the absence of evidence that sulfamethazine is a secondary carcinogen.

Commenting on the safety concerns raised by residues of sulfamethazine above the tolerance level of 0.1 ppm in edible tissues of swine, the CVM has pointed out that high levels can cause an effect on the thyroid and kidneys in laboratory animals and may result in allergic reactions in man. If illegal residues of the drug are not reduced to a satisfactory level, the CVM has to ban the use of sulfamethazine in swine feeds.

In the carcinogenicity study in mice, thyroid follicular cell adenomas occurred in male and female mice at a dietary level of 48,000 ppm. In the carcinogenicity study in rats, thyroid follicular cell adenomas and adenocarcinomas occurred in females at a dietary level of 2400 ppm and in males at a dietary level of 1200 to 2400 ppm.

The toxicologic conclusions have been that the thyroid tumors observed in mice and rats were most likely the result of perturbation of the thyroid-hypothalamus-pituitary axis and that humans would not be at carcinogenic risk if the exposure to sulfamethazine was below the NOEL for a sensitive parameter of thyroid function.

Because the class of sulfonamides includes a vast number of old compounds, no toxicologic database meeting modern requirements of testing exists for any particular member. From the overall picture, however, it is clear that the number of effects that are not always related to dose and may be limited to predisposed humans include allergic reactions. No adequate experimental data relating to potential mutagenic or carcinogenic effects are available.

Having regard to the available toxicologic data and current practices in veterinary therapy, the international opinion has recommended that an analytical procedure for monitoring the observance of appropriate withdrawal times for sulfonamide compounds sensitive to at least 100 µg/kg of the original drug substance should be used.

Residues of sulfonamides can be routinely monitored at and below the above-required limits using, for example, high-performance liquid chromatography. Reliable confirmatory or reference methods should be based on known procedures using gas chromatography mass spectrometry. See also Chapters 14 and 23. Hypersensitive reactions to sulfonamides appear to be highly dose related.

SELECTED REFERENCES

Ahlers von, D., and Andresen, P.: Therapie-Versuch mit Trimethoprim/S bei fieberhaften Mastitiden, Puerperalstorungen und Sauglingskrankheiten des Rindes (Vorlaufige Mitteilung). Dtsch. Tierarztl. Wschr., 78:201, 1971.

Alexander, F., and Collett, R.A.: Trimethoprim in the horse. Eq. Vet. J., 4:203, 1975.

Appelgate, J.: Clinical pharmacology of sulfonamides. Mod. Vet. Pract., 667, 1983.

Barell, J.H., Garrod, L.P., and Waterworth, P.M.: Trimethoprim: Laboratory and clinical studies. J. Clin. Pathol., *21*:202, 1968.

Barnett, M., and Bushby, S.R.M.: Trimethoprim and the sulphonamides. Vet. Rec., *87*:43, 1970.

Bohni, E.: Experimental data on the antibacterial effects of the sulphadoxine trimethoprim combination. Berl. Mich. Tierazrliche Wschr., *84*:87, 1971.

Bohni, E.: Sensitivity testing and outcome of therapy with the combination trimethoprim sulfamethoxazole in patients with urinary tract infections. Proc. 6th Int. Congr. Chemother., *1*:975, 1970.

Bohni, E.: Uber antibacterielle Eigenschaftern der Kombination Trimethoprim/Sulphamethoxazol in Vergleich mit Antibiotika. Schweiz. Med. Wschr., *99*:1505, 1969.

Brown, M.P., Kelly, R.H., and Stover, S.M.: Trimethoprim-sulfadiazine in the horse: Serum synovial, peritoneal and urine concentrations after single dose intravenous administration. Am. J. Vet. Res., *44*:540, 1983.

Burchall, J.J.: Mechanism of action of trimethoprim sulfamethoxazole. J. Infect. Dis., *128* (Suppl.):437, 1973.

Bushby, S.R.M.: Sulfonamide and trimethoprim combinations. J. Am. Vet. Med. Assoc., *176*:1049, 1980.

Bushby, S.R.M.: Combined antibacterial action in vitro of trimethoprim and sulphonamides. The in vitro nature of synergy. Postgrad. Med. J., *45* (Suppl.):10, 1969.

Bushby, S.R.M., and Barnett, M.: Trimethoprim-sulphamethoxazole tetracycline and the penicillins in vitro. Proc. 6th Int. Congr. Chemother., *1*:1008, 1969.

Bushby, S.R.M., and Hitchings, G.H.: Trimethoprim, a sulphonamide potentiator. Br. J. Pharmacol. Chemother., *33*:72, 1968.

Collins, B.K.: Sulfonamide associated keratoconjunctivitis sicca and corneal ulceration in dysuric dogs. J. Am. Vet. Med. Assoc., *189*:926, 1986.

Craig, G.R.: The place of potentiated trimethoprim in the therapy of diseases of the skin in dogs and cats. J. Small Anim. Pract., *13*:65, 1972.

Craig, G.R., and White, G.: Studies in dogs and cats dosed with trimethoprim and sulfadiazine. Vet. Rec., *98*:82, 1976.

Foltzer, M.A., and Reese, R.E.: Trimethoprim-sulfamethoxazole and other sulfonamides. Med. Clin. North Am., *71*:1177, 1987.

Giger, U., Werner, L.L., and Millichamp, N.J.: Sulfadiazine induced allergy in six Doberman Pinschers. J. Am. Vet. Med. Assoc., *186*:479, 1985.

Hamza, B., and Rehm, W.F.: Report on the use of a combination of sulphadoxine and trimethoprim in 10,063 cases in veterinary practice (scientific report). The Blue Book, *23*:36, 1973.

Hitchings, G.H.: Mechanism of action of trimethoprim sulfamethoxazole. J. Infect. Dis., *128* (Suppl.):433, 1973.

Hitchings, G.H.: Species differences among dihydrofolate reductase as a basis for chemotherapy. Postgrad. Med. J., *45* (Suppl.):7, 1969.

Indiveri, I., and Hirsch, D.C.: Susceptibility of obligate anaerobes to trimethoprim-sulfamethoxazole. J. Am. Vet. Med. Assoc., *188*:46, 1986.

Koritz, G., Bourne, D., Dittert, L., and Bevill, R.F.: Disposition of sulfonamides in food producing animals: Pharmacokinetics of sulfamerazine in cattle. J. Vet. Pharm. Ther., *1*:285, 1978.

Markiewicz, K., Kuleta, Z., and Borzemski, J.: Sulphonamide preparation trivetrin in treatment of certain diseases of animals. Weterynaria, *2*:57, 1974.

Mengelers, M.J., Van Klingeren, B., Van Miert, J.P.: In vitro susceptibility of some porcine pathogens to aditoprim, trimethoprim, sulfadimethoxine, sulfamethoxazole combination of these agents. Am. J. Vet. Res., *51*:1860, 1990.

Neilson, R., and Rasmussen, F.: Trimethoprim and sulfadoxine in swine. Zbl. Vet. Med. A., *22*:564, 1975.

Piercy, D.W.T.: Distribution of trimethoprim sulfadiazine in plasma tissue and synovial fluids. Vet. Rec., *102*:523, 1978.

Prescott, J.F., and Baggott, J.D.: Sulfonamides, trimethoprim and their combination. *In* Antimicrobial Therapy in Veterinary Medicine. New York, Blackwell Scientific 1988.

Rail, W., and Kaller, H.: A contribution from practice on the effectiveness of the trimethoprim/sulfonamide principle, in Bavarian cattle holdings with bacterial problems in rearing. Der Praktische Tierarzt., *52*:8, 1971.

Rasmussen, F.: In vitro antibacterial activity of trimethoprim and sulphonamides on bacteria causing bovine mastitis. Acta Vet. Scand., *12*:131, 1971.

Rehm, W.F.: Evaluation of the optimal initial dose of sulfadoxine compared with a combination containing sulfadoxine and trimethoprim. Proc. 6th Int. Cong. Chemother., *3*:382, 1970.

Rehm, W.F., and White, G.: A field trial with trimethoprim and sulfadoxine in bacterial diseases of cattle and pigs. Vet. Rec., *87*:39, 1970.

Vitali, E., and Stefanon, G.: The use of the trimethoprim-sulphadoxine combination in the treatment of bovine actinogranulomatosis. Proc. Italian Soc. Vet. Sci., *25*:162, 1971.

Waterworth, P.M.: Practical aspects of testing sensitivity to trimethoprim and sulphonamide. Postgrad. Med. J., *45*:21, 1969.

White, G., and Withnell, C.G.: Chemotherapeutic evaluation of trimethoprim and sulphonamides in experimental salmonellosis of sheep. Res. Vet. Sci., *14*:245, 1973.

Zeljko, M.: Assessing the value of Trivetrin and Tribrissen in various infections in pigs, calves and fowl in practice. Vet. Glas., *26*:351, 1972.

13

PUBLIC HEALTH CONCERNS OF VETERINARY DRUG RESIDUES

13.1 Introduction
13.2 Formation of Drug Residues
13.3 Carcinogenicity
13.4 Mutagenicity
13.5 Teratogenicity
13.6 Residues of Antibacterial Drugs
13.7 Resistance Induction
13.8 Drug Allergy
13.9 Miscellaneous Effects
13.10 Residue Analysis and Evaluation

13.1 INTRODUCTION

With the rapid expansion of the world population, the problem of satisfying the global demand for edible protein is becoming more intense. The challenge of producing wholesome food of animal origin necessitates a continual search for new means of improving productivity and efficiency in animal husbandry. The use of drugs in food-producing animals is an accepted and well-established practice on a worldwide basis. Animal production systems are becoming more dependent on pharmacologically and toxicologically potent substances that confer economic benefits both to the producer and to the consumer. Inherent in this widespread use of drugs, however, is the problem associated with drug residues, which may remain in the tissues of the medicated animals and which may ultimately become a part of the human diet. If most veterinary drugs were not systemically absorbed or if they were extensively metabolized to biologically inactive end products, no consumer risk would exist. This idealistic situation is biologically unrealistic and unattainable in most veterinary products now in use. Accordingly the advantages of enhanced food production arising from pharmacologic intervention must be weighed against the attendant disadvantages of residue formation in edible tissues. The most important basis for regulatory authorization of drug use in animals is the establishment of drug safety. This requires adequate toxicologic evaluation of residues in tissues and organs likely to be eaten by humans.

The advent of modern antibiotics, anthelmintics, and growth-promoting substances has facilitated the development of intensivism in animal production systems. This is most apparent in poultry, swine, veal, and beef industries, where minimal disease programs attain high priority. The pharmaceutical industry is constantly researching new areas for the development of safer, more efficacious animal health products. Mass medication systems of drug delivery through feedstuffs or drinking water have become a significant area in feedlots because of their convenience, ease, and efficiency. These routes of administration, however, possess the highest potential for creating problems owing to the presence of residues of these drugs in foodstuffs and in the environment.

A high percentage of livestock are exposed for a significant portion of their life span to exogenous chemical substances for prophylactic, therapeutic, growth-promoting or management-aid purposes. Growth promoters, antibiotics, antibacterials, parasiticides, and coccidiostats, for example, are administered to many animals for prolonged periods, during times of peak production, or near to slaughter, giving rise to the potential for residue formation in edible tissues, such as milk, eggs, or meat. Antibiotic therapy is most commonly performed under veterinary supervision or against the authority of a veterinarian's prescription, and usually if the specified withdrawal time of the drug is rigidly observed, unacceptable antibacterial tissue residues do not occur in the human food supply. Emergency slaughter of antibiotic-treated animals is undoubtedly a significant residue hazard, and in such cases, tissue monitoring for drug residues is of especial importance.

Since the 1950s, it has been common practice in many countries to include antibacterial drugs in animal feeds to improve growth efficiency. International policy differences exist with respect to the type of antibiotics that may be used for growth promotion. Other agents for growth-promoting purposes, with a propensity toward residue formation when incorrectly employed, are the anabolic hormonal-type substances. Such drugs are extensively used in beef production, and in the United States, large numbers of feedlot cattle are treated with both hormonal and nonhormonal (ionophore) growth promoters. Most countries have prohibited the use of synthetic estrogenic stilbenes, such as diethylstilbestral (DES), on the grounds of carcinogenicity. Estradiol, progesterone, testosterone, zeranol, and trenbolone are permitted for use in beef cattle in the United States.

None of these agents may be used as growth promoters on food animals in European Community states. Residues of hormonal-type substances have always given rise to some consumer fears (not always scientifically based), and it is clear that scientific findings must be clearly communicated to consumer groups if confusion is to be avoided. If criteria other than scientific criteria were to be applied to the animal health products market internationally, one could envisage insurmountable problems in the future with disastrous consequences for the world livestock industry. The animal health industry must always be regulated on the issues of safety and efficacy alone.

Other potent drugs, such as prostaglandins (and their analogs), corticosteroids, and sex hormones, are widely employed in the control of reproduction in ruminants and pigs. In many cases, they are used as abortifacients or to control timing of parturition. Residues of these veterinary drugs may arise from emergency slaughter of treated animals or from the entry of these drugs into milk at parturition. A different type of hazard is presented by tranquilizers, neuroleptics, and stress-alleviating drugs that are administered shortly before slaughter. These types of drugs as well as a number of beta-blocking agents indicated for prevention of transportation stress can pose definite consumer hazards on account of the high levels of active agent present in the tissues immediately before slaughter.

Apart from the risks associated with the correct uses of drugs in animals, illegal use of prohibited substances is perhaps the most sinister and insidious hazard. A number of veterinary compounds no longer permitted for use in animals possess carcinogenic, mutagenic, or allergenic properties. The illegal use of DES and related stilbenes in veal calves and of chloramphenicol in lactating cattle and laying hens is a constant problem in some countries where restrictive legislation coupled with inadequate enforcement and residue monitoring has led to the spawning of a lucrative black market. It is axiomatic that international cooperation and legislative concordance are essential to harmonize international trade and to set agreed standards and tolerances for residue avoidance programs. Good regulatory evaluation and clearance of veterinary drugs is a prerequisite for safe use of quality drugs in animals. It is also an assurance that unacceptable residues will not arise in food when the drug is used according to the directions on the registered label. Beta agonists such as clenbuterol are also causing international consumer hazards.

Toxicologic evaluation of animal drug residues requires a multidisciplinary approach involving the chemist and pharmacokineticist, who relate not only the type of residue, but also its projected persistence. From this information, the toxicologist must endeavor to define the hazard(s) that this residue poses once it enters the food chain.

Initially information is needed concerning the nature and amount of residue in the major edible tissues of treated animals, so probable human exposure can be determined. Studies must identify and characterize residues as to whether they consist of parent compound or compounds derived from the parent drug, including metabolites, conjugates, or fractions bound to macromolecules.

Toxicity tests are conducted to identify the type of effect produced and to ascertain the exposure concentrations that would be expected not to produce this effect. Such data provide the basis for defining the acceptable daily intake for drug residues, and this is then used to establish a tolerance. Tolerances, in addition to being safe, must be no higher than necessary to provide for the effective use of the drug under conditions of use that are reasonably likely to be adhered to in practice. Tolerances are calculated based on safety data obtained in toxicity trials and acceptable daily intake by percentage of meat consumed in the diet. The withdrawal time established subsequently permits the residues to deplete below the tolerance level before animals are slaughtered for use as food.

From the public standpoint, residue levels in excess of the legal tolerance may result in possible toxic effects in the consumer. Adequate protection of the consumer requires that no allergenic, teratogenic, or carcinogenic effects result from ingestion of residue-contaminated foodstuffs.

The Federal Food, Drug, and Cosmetic Act (1938) governs the marketing of animal drugs in the United States. Under the act, marketing authorization of a new animal drug depends on the approval of a New Animal Drug Application (NADA), which is submitted to the Food and Drug Administration (FDA) by a pharmaceutical company. For approval of a NADA, two basic criteria must be met:

1. The drug must be effective and safe for the animal when used as recommended.

2. For a drug for use in food animals, edible products from treated animals must be safe for human consumption.

Registration of products for use in food-producing animals requires submission of considerable data on the analysis of edible tissues for drug residues. For food animals, the FDA places high priority on drug residue studies in target animals, metabolism studies, and data related to human toxicity potential.

SAFETY OF VETERINARY DRUGS

Safety of the veterinary drug should be demonstrated for:

1. The animal for which the drug is intended
2. The users of veterinary drugs
3. The environment
4. The consumers likely to be exposed to residues of veterinary drugs in food of animal origin
5. The industrial processing of the food

Safety for Treated Animal

Thorough tests, which may be performed with clinical trials, should allow the accurate assessment of the safety of the veterinary drugs in the treated animals. These tolerance studies should take into consideration all the physiopathologic and zootechnical effects. Because the clinical tests performed to put together a file for approval remain necessarily limited, it is essential to continue to control the safety of the registered veterinary drug by means of an appropriate system of pharmacovigilance.

Safety for Users of Veterinary Drugs

When necessary, the precautions that should be taken so the users may handle the drugs without risk are indicated as well as the procedures to follow in case of an accident.

Safety for Environment

If necessary, adequate information should be furnished to ensure the absence of any undesirable effect of the veterinary drugs on the environment or to prevent undesirable effects by providing the appropriate instructions for their use.

13.2 FORMATION OF DRUG RESIDUES

The compound administered to a food-producing animal is not necessarily the substance present in the edible product from that animal. The rate and extent of absorption, the rate and extent of metabolism of the parent compound, and the rate of excretion of the parent compound and its various metabolites govern both the relative and absolute amount of each part of the residue.

The total drug residue in treated animals therefore consists of parent compound, free metabolites, and metabolites covalently bound to macromolecules. Different toxicologic significances can be associated with these individual fractions of the total residue burden. The concentrations and persistance of the dissimilar residue components are a function of the dosage of drug and the time following the last administration of the drug to the animal.

The amount of drug deposited as a residue in tissues varies with time, and elimination or depletion from the animal body may vary from a period of minutes to the entire life span of the animal. Quantitatively residue formation directly relates to the basic metabolic profile of each individual compound. The quantity of residues formed depends on the pharmacokinetic parameters. Depending on the type of formulation used and the absorption rate from the site of application, residues can be present in edible animal tissues over an extended period from depot suspensions, implantation of slow-release devices, or controlled-release delivery systems. The ability of the treated animal to detoxify and eliminate the drug has a significant bearing on the amount of drug residue likely to remain in its tissues.

Basically two key pharmacologic principles underpin any discussion of veterinary drug residues:

1. What is the pharmacokinetic disposition profile of the drug in the animal body?
2. What are the known or postulated pharmacodynamic effects of the drug?

In other words, it is necessary to establish quantitatively and qualitatively where drug residues are likely to be laid down in the animal's tissues and also what is the biological significance of such residues. It should be remembered that pharmacokinetics refers to what the body does to the drug (absorption, distribution, biotransformation, tissue sequestration, elimination), and pharmacodynamics refers to what the drug may do to the body (biological activity, mechanism of action, molecular activity).

In short, residue studies are concerned with:

1. Metabolism of drugs in the body
2. Analysis and measurement of the residue burden
3. Toxicologic hazards associated with tissue residues
4. Tolerance and threshold assessment

BIOTRANSFORMATION

The major site of drug metabolism is the liver, where the smooth endoplasmic reticulum is probably the most important site of biotransformation. Most drugs and foreign chemicals are metabolized by a nicotinamide-adenine dinucleotide phosphate (NADPH)-dependent microsomal enzyme system (cytochrome P-450). The function of the enzyme system is to convert lipophilic drugs into water-soluble compounds, which are more readily excreted. The rate of elimination of lipophilic drugs is determined by the activity of this hepatic microsomal P-450 mixed-function oxidase system. Any alteration in the activity of these enzymes can result in a modification of drug effect. Many compounds possess the capability of altering the activity of these drug-metabolizing enzymes by way of enzyme induction (increased concentration of a particular enzyme) or enzyme inhibition (reduced concentration of a particular enzyme).

The biotransformation of xenobiotics can be categorized into two major classes: phase I reactions, in which the drug substrate is inherently altered, and phase II, in which a specific group is conjugated to the substrate, resulting in the formation of a metabolite of increased polarity or hydrophilicity to hasten elimination. The liver possesses the greatest capacity for biotransformation, but lung, liver, kidney, gastrointestinal, epithelium, and intestinal bacterial flora are also involved (Table 13–1). Many factors influence both the rate and the extent of biotransformation of xenobiotic compounds and therefore the pharmacologic or toxicologic activity of the parent compound or of their metabolites:

1. Species differences
2. Sex differences
3. Inherent activity of metabolic biotransformation pathways

Neonatal animals of most species are relatively deficient in their capacity to detoxify many foreign compounds, particularly those pathways mediated via liver microsomal enzymes. Other contributory factors to the body processes include:

1. The drug used on the animal, the site and route of administration, formulation, dosage, duration of treatment period
2. The pharmacokinetic properties of the drug in the body, nature of the biotransformation processes, metabolites produced (active or inactive), tissue depletion rates, excretory pathways
3. The type of exposure, disease state, dietary factors (Table 13–2)

Biotransformation proceeds by conversion of a relatively nonpolar substance into one that is more polar by an oxidative reductive or hydrolytic process by conjugation with a highly polar substance. This frequently results in one or a combination of three situations:

1. A change in the chemical configuration of the substance may alter its affinity for specific receptor sites.
2. The decreased lipid solubility normally attendant on an increase in polarity makes passage of the substance through lipoidal cell membranes more difficult, and therefore distribution of the drug to its site of action is restricted.
3. The biotransformed substance may be more readily excreted either because the polar, less lipid-soluble form is less readily absorbed or because the highly polar form is more susceptible to active secretory mechanisms.

TABLE 13-1
DRUG METABOLIZING PATHWAYS

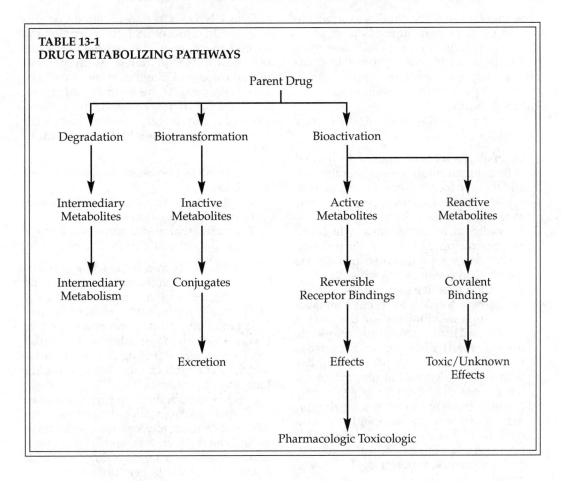

TABLE 13-2
FACTORS AFFECTING BIOTRANSFORMATION

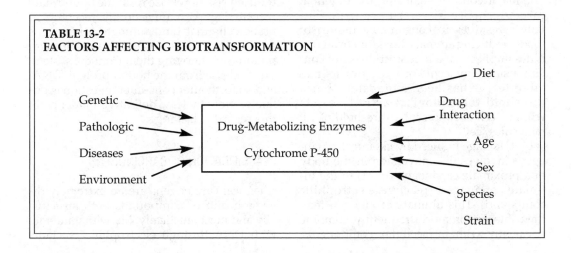

Thus the term "detoxication" was coined to describe this overall diminution in pharmacologic activity. In many cases, however, biotransformation of xenobiotic compounds may give rise to the appearance in the body of substances with increased biological activity.

Three primary classes of products may appear:

1. Compounds that are similar to normal substrates of endogenous metabolism and that are then subjected to normal enzymatic processes. This occurs for a wide range of veterinary drugs.
2. Degradation to metabolites, which are pharmacologically inactive. Such detoxicated drugs are eliminated usually via the urine in conjugated form.
3. Formation of active metabolites. This involves bioactivation to reactive metabolites. Such metabolites (or the parent compound) may undergo reversible noncovalent binding to receptors through hydrogen bonds, or Van der Waals forces. Reversible pharmacologic hazard potential because of frequently covalent binding can arise after the formation of a reactive metabolite or "ultimate toxin." Such electrophilic metabolites possess high biological reactivity and bind to macromolecules, DNA, and protein. These are of particular toxicologic significance.

13.3 CARCINOGENICITY

The major concern regarding the potential carcinogenicity of veterinary drugs involves residues in consumable tissues of food-producing animals. Freedom from residues implies that a foodstuff does not contain a single molecule of a drug or its metabolites. It has been suggested that a threshold for biological activity exists within a cell at a molecular threshold of 10^4 molecules/cell.

Cell damage induced by chemical carcinogens involves the conversion in the body of a proximate carcinogen (inert) to the ultimate carcinogen (reactive electrophilic compound). This ultimate carcinogen may then interact or more frequently combine covalently with intracellular components,

such as DNA, RNA, phospholipids, or glutathione. In terms of molecular activity, the precise mechanism of carcinogenesis has not been fully elucidated. Many general mechanisms underlie induction of carcinogenic changes. Alone or in combination, these may initiate neoplastic alterations. Chemical carcinogens that interact with DNA differ from other biological toxins in that:

1. The effect is persistent, cumulative, and delayed.
2. Divided doses are usually more deleterious than single doses.
3. The individual mechanisms of action are quite distinct and variable.

Formation of chemically reactive metabolites or ultimate carcinogens may occur by a complicated, varied process of biological mechanisms. A number of metabolites may exist in the free radical form or the epoxide form, which then complex with cellular macromolecules initiating structural, functional, or chemical change, especially in informational proteins.

Reactive metabolites can give rise to various types of toxicity, including carcinogenesis, mutagenesis, teratogenesis, cellular necrosis, blood dyscrasias, and immunologic effects. Mechanisms underlying these toxic manifestations are largely unknown.

The persistence of covalent bound residues in food animal tissues poses many problems from the standpoint of both analytical detection and safety assessment. It may be that such bound residues pose little real hazard to the consumer because of the reduced risk of release from the bound state reoccurring. Also, nucleophilic receptors in tissue cells that bind ultimate carcinogens act in many ways to deactivate the compounds by removing them from the system: Thus release from the bound protein, DNA, and so forth after consumer ingestion is unlikely. Nonetheless, definitive evidence in this regard is lacking.

CLASSIFICATION OF CARCINOGENS

Chemical carcinogens are an extremely diverse group of compounds both structurally and mechanistically. Many that interact with DNA through electrophilic reactants

TABLE 13–3
DNA-REACTIVE GENOTOXIC
CARCINOGENS

Procarcinogens (Activation Dependent)

Polycyclic aromatic hydrocarbons
Aromatic and heterocyclic amines
Nitrofurans
AZO compounds
N-Nitroso compounds
Carbamates
Mycotoxins (aflatoxin)

Direct-Acting Carcinogens (Activation Independent)

Mustards
Active halogens
Alkylene epoxide
Small ring lactones
Nitrosamides

TABLE 13-5
MECHANISM OF CARCINOGENESIS

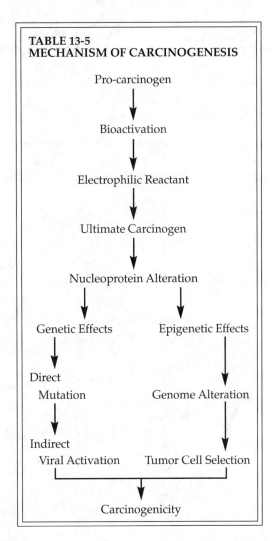

are also mutagenic. Carcinogens can be subdivided into major types: (1) genotoxic and (2) epigenetic (Table 13–3).

Genotoxic carcinogens are compounds that either in their parent form or after metabolism in the body possess direct biological capability to damage DNA. Genetic toxicity tests reveal such carcinogens. These pose a major hazard because they can be effective after a single exposure. Direct-acting and activation-dependent carcinogens are included in this class.

Epigenetic carcinogens do not directly damage DNA. These operate indirectly by a variety of mechanisms, including hormonal effects, immunosuppression, and co-carcinogenic effects. Carcinogenic effects occur with high or sustained levels of exposure, which in turn can lead to physiologic imbalances, hormonal dysfunction, or tissue injury. Included in this category are promotional agents, cytotoxic agents, hormone modifiers, and immunosuppressors. Many hormonal substances act as promoters (Tables 13–4 and 13–5).

TABLE 13–4
EPIGENETIC CARCINOGENS

Immunosuppressors
±
Modifers
  Promoters/hormonally active
    compounds
  Co-carcinogens

Promoters
Agents that facilitate growth of a latent neoplastic cell into a tumor, possibly by interference of tissue growth proliferation mechanisms, e.g., organochlorine pesticides, saccharin, sex hormones

Co-carcinogens
Agents that enhance the carcinogenic process initiated by a genotoxic carcinogen

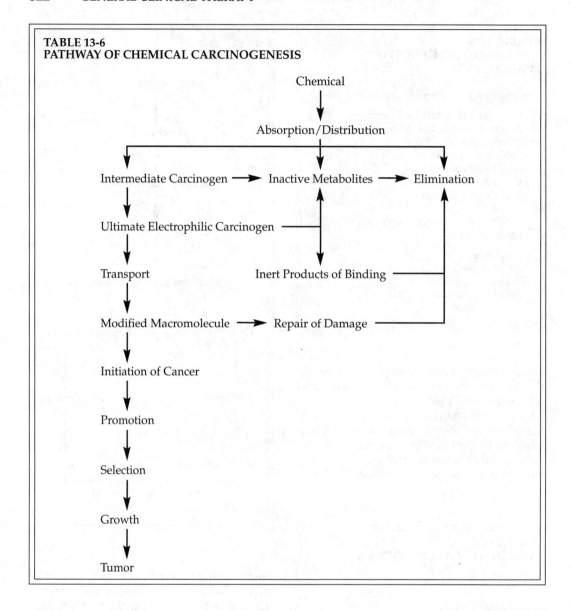

TABLE 13-6
PATHWAY OF CHEMICAL CARCINOGENESIS

MECHANISMS OF ACTION

The exact mechanisms through which any carcinogen exerts its cancer-causing effects are not known; however, initiation of the cancer process is widely postulated to involve structural changes in DNA. When the DNA is damaged, repair systems exist that can eliminate the lesion caused by the carcinogen. The efficacy of these major processes and their ability to determine thresholds for low doses are known (Table 13–6).

As part of enzymatic biotransformation pathways, many carcinogens undergo acti-

vation to the reactive ultimate carcinogen. (This is not always a prerequisite; some carcinogens are active in the parent form.) Steps involved are as follows:

1. Transport of the agent from its site of application and, if necessary, its subsequent metabolic activation
2. The interaction of the ultimate carcinogen with DNA in the cells of a target organ
3. Processing of the initial damage by DNA repair and replication enzymes in the tumor progenitor cell

TABLE 13–7
GENERAL MECHANISM OF TUMOR FORMATION

Biotransformation to Electrophilic Ultimate Carcinogen
↓
Covalent Bonding with Cellular Macromolecules (DNA)
↓
Fixation of Carcinogen Damage
↓
Multiplication of Altered Tissue Cells
↓
Formation of Preneoplastic Lesions
↓
Progression/Promotion to Neoplasm Formation

4. Progressive development, possibly owing to alterations in cell behavior and ultimately to cancer formation

The ultimate carcinogen, which is electrophilic, interacts covalently with many cellular macromolecules, including DNA. Sometimes the damaged DNA is subject to repair processes, and the altered macromolecule may be removed. Cell recovery from carcinogen exposure can thus take place (Table 13–7).

Frequently after the initial fixing of the carcinogen and induction of DNA damage, the cell replicates, and so the genome alterations can be perpetuated. Mispairing of bases, point mutations, frame shift mutations, and altered sequences leading to oncogene formation may result. Interaction with the mitotic apparatus can generate a permanently altered cell.

Multiplication of the altered cells, if not fully neoplastic, may give rise to preneoplastic lesions. At this stage, further errors and DNA alterations may amplify the abnormality of the resultant cells. Growth to fully neoplastic cells progresses by a developmental procedure known as promotion.

When carcinogenic activation mechanisms occur, the end product is referred to as the "ultimate carcinogen." Such agents have the capacity to inactivate some essential enzymes or to change the regulatory function of a nucleic acid, thereby initiating an irreversible process leading to a condition of uncontrolled growth. Although hydrolysis of ester sites in many compounds yields water-soluble acids and alcohols that

are not cytotoxic, in other cases of xenobiotic biotransformation, dehydration processes may occur, resulting in the production of highly reactive metabolites that can react as potent alkylating agents toward nucleophilic groups as amines, thiols, and hydroxyl groups of essential macromolecules.

Many aromatic compounds or compounds containing activated double bonds produce highly reactive alkylating agents in the body. Bromobenzene is known to cause centrilobular necrosis for example. Many of its metabolites are formed from epoxide intermediates. When the epoxide is free to react with essential cellular components, their inactivation can lead to irreversible cell damage. Many bioactivation reactions are mediated by the liver microsomal drug-metabolizing enzyme systems. These are concentrated in the centrilobular proteins of the liver, and so it is here that tissue damage first appears.

TOXICOLOGIC STUDIES

Lengthy toxicologic studies are required when carcinogenicity is suspected because of the compound's chemical similarity to known carcinogens or mutagens. When compounds are used for lifetime feeding to target animals, there is a higher potential for drug residues as well as exposure to the operator. Carcinogenicity studies are therefore required. The procedure is to treat animals for their life span and to determine the differences between control and treated groups with regard to tumor formation—

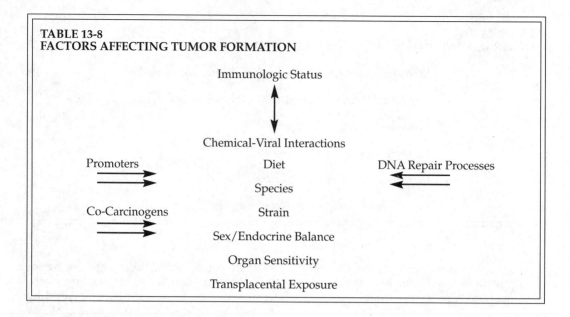

TABLE 13-8
FACTORS AFFECTING TUMOR FORMATION

Immunologic Status

Chemical-Viral Interactions

Promoters   Diet   DNA Repair Processes

Species

Co-Carcinogens   Strain

Sex/Endocrine Balance

Organ Sensitivity

Transplacental Exposure

time of appearance, number, type. Differences in susceptibility to carcinogens, however, can be seen between different strains of laboratory animals. For example, Fischer rats are relatively resistant to the induction of extrahepatic neoplasms by aromatic amines, whereas these compounds can cause increased occurrence of mammary tumors in Sprague-Dawley rats. Other known carcinogens in humans may not necessarily act as carcinogens in rats.

Susceptibility of animals to carcinogens is influenced not only by the potency or toxicity of the chemical agent, but also by many additional factors, including diet, species, period of exposure, strain, organ sensitivity, transplacental exposure, sex, endocrine balance, stress, disease, and exposure to secondary compounds that suppress or induce drug-metabolizing enzymes (Tables 13–8 and 13–9).

Exposure to minute amounts of carcinogens raises many difficult questions. This is important to regulatory agencies that must decide whether any degree of exposure to a carcinogen can be permitted. One particular viewpoint, the so-called single event hypothesis, presumes that carcinogenesis may be described as an irreversible phenomenon, whereby damage to cellular DNA occurs after interaction and complexation between one molecule of carcinogen and a sensitive receptor in one cell. An alternative perspective propounds that complex metabolic pathways may minimize real hazards from many carcinogens and that consequently thresholds or no-effect concentrations can occur. With advances in molecular pharmacology and genetic toxicology, it is hoped that adequate validated scientific data can become available to enable calculation of a safe degree of exposure to potential carcinogens. Resolution of this complex issue is clouded by the persistence of covalently bound carcinogens that remain in the body for lengthy periods after cessation of treatment.

Covalently bound intermediates have been implicated in kidney, liver, and lung toxicity as well as in mutagenesis and carcinogenesis. The effective irreversibility of the covalent associations mentioned here suggests that bound residues are chemically stable. It also implies that the toxicity of this type of residue would be low or negligible to consumers. Many studies have shown that the bioavailability of bound residues is generally low. This has been found to be true for cambendazole, trenbolone acetate, carbofuran, and carbaril.

The biologic reactivity of ultimate carcinogens is nonetheless causing increased concern. Induced conformational changes in DNA can affect replication transcription and translation processes within the cell. In many cases, the lag period for carcinogenesis can be 20 years in humans, and so it is extremely difficult not only to design effective toxicity tests for drugs whose residues have carcinogenic potential, but also to interpret mechanisms of activation and to define interpretive and predictive criteria. The rodent is used in assessment for carcinogenic potential of drugs or chemicals because its life span (2 to 3.5 years) is shorter than that of humans.

Accumulation of DNA damage over a period of years can contribute to carcinogenesis by way of somatic mutagenesis. Many mutagens are also carcinogens, for example, polycyclic hydrocarbons, and naturally occurring compounds, such as aflatoxins. In the body, these are activated to reactive nucleophilic agents that bind to cellular macromolecules. Manifestation of carcinogenesis can depend not only on the type and extent of cellular injury, but also on the rate and efficiency of their repair processes.

Mammalian cells possess an enzymatic mechanism for the removal of certain carcinogens bound to DNA. Not only is repair a natural process, but also spontaneous depurination of DNA is a naturally occurring phenomenon, albeit at a low rate constant.

Exposure to carcinogens (e.g., alkylating agents) can increase the rate of depurination with a significant increase in the number of apurinic sites. This creates vast capability for miscoding potential, especially if DNA repair is not complete. DNA repair errors induced by chemical exposure is another mechanism of action of carcinogens leading to mutations or carcinogenesis.

SCREENING FOR CARCINOGENS

FDA guidelines use a decision-tree approach to determine whether a new compound should be viewed and evaluated as a potential carcinogen. The decision-tree approach incorporates five distinct steps in the evaluation of the potential carcinogenicity of the chemical:

1. Structure of chemical
2. In vitro short-term tests
   a. Hepatocyte DNA repair
   b. Bacterial mutagenesis
   c. Mammalian cell mutagenesis
   d. Mammalian cell chromosome effect
   e. Mammalian cell transformation
3. In vivo bioassay
   a. Induction of altered foci in rat liver
   b. Skin tumor induction in mice
   c. Lung tumor induction in mice
   d. Breast cancer induction in rats
   e. Promoting effects
4. Chronic bioassay
5. Final evaluation

Chemicals are classified initially in accordance with their chemical structure, data from short-term genetic toxicity tests, ancillary biological or pharmacologic data, and data from subchronic or chronic feeding studies. The decision-tree approach system not only provides a stepwise framework for minimizing necessary testing, but also contributes toward an understanding of the mechanism of action of the test substance.

1. Structure of Chemical

With certain structural classes, reasonable predictions can be made as to the potential for electrophilic metabolites. Thus structure activity assessment is important. Substituents that block carcinogenicity have been identified.

2. In Vitro Short-Term Tests

A battery of tests is required because no single test details genotoxic carcinogens. A basic screening test is the *Salmonella*/microsome test (Ames test) as prediction for possible carcinogenicity. Similar to bacterial mutagenesis, mammalian cell mutagenicity testing is also carried out, for example, in the mouse lymphoma cell. Tests for DNA damage provide direct evidence that the drug can alter genetic material. Sensitive end point indicators include DNA binding, DNA fragmentation, inhibition of DNA synthesis, and DNA repair. DNA repair tests produce an end point of high specificity and biological significance.

Isolated hepatocytes offer a useful test system because they contain cell metabolism together with a broad capacity for biotransformation (Williams DNA repair test). Chromosomal tests are included to detect effects at the highest level of genetic organization.

Cell transformation effects correlate with potential carcinogenic effects, but this type of complicated assay is resorted to only if the preceding test battery indicated further investigation. If the results of the battery of short-term tests provide no tangible evidence of genotoxicity, the decision for further testing depends on (1) the structure and known physiologic properties of the compound, e.g., hormone, and (2) the potential human exposure.

Positive results from two in vivo bioassays are considered a clear indication of carcinogenicity. A positive result in only one in vitro test and one in vivo bioassay is considered equivocal.

Positive results in reliable tests for DNA reactivity are highly predictive of carcinogenicity, probably because DNA damage is the basis for the carcinogenicity of some chemicals. It is now recognized, however, that carcinogens may be of at least two types: genotoxic or DNA reaction carcinogens that damage DNA and epigenetic carcinogens that do not damage DNA but produce neoplasia through another biological effect. Thus DNA damage and repair tests do not detect epigenetic carcinogens.

The distinction between different types of carcinogens is extremely important in the area of food toxicology. The characteristics of genotoxic carcinogens make them qualitative hazards, whereas with epigenetic agents, a safe threshold of exposure may be delineated.

DNA reactive chemicals represent significant health hazards. They have the potential to produce toxicity, birth defects, genetic disease, and cancer. Thus short-term tests that measure DNA reactivity are an important component of the toxicologic assessment of a chemical, particularly agents that occur in or enter the food supply. DNA reactivity can be measured directly using a variety of biochemical or biophysical techniques. In addition, the production of DNA damage can be assessed indirectly by the measurement of DNA repair.

To establish whether or not a carcinogen, or for that matter any other chemical, has genotoxic activity, a battery of tests devised to give the maximum genotoxic information about the chemical must be used. Such a battery cannot be specified with confidence based on present knowledge, but the inclusion of eukaryotic (as well as prokaryotic) and of in vivo (as well as in vitro) test systems deserves systematic investigation. Also warranting further study is the extent to which certain carcinogens that do not interact directly with DNA may exert genotoxic effects indirectly, through the production of the free radicals. Epigenetic carcinogens are tentatively identified based on promotional effects.

Longterm bioassay procedures are used as a final definitive evaluation procedure, in which preceding tests generating equivocal results suggest the need for further investigation on the basis that extensive exposure is likely and in which epigenetic mechanisms may be involved. In the absence of convincing evidence for genotoxicity of a chemical, but the presence of definitive carcinogenicity in animal bioassays, it is likely that the compound under test functions as an epigenetic carcinogen. These types of chemicals may pose the greater hazard to humans in quantitative terms. Their mechanisms of action, although different from direct-acting genotoxins, may involve diverse pathways in the body, including chronic tissue injury, immunosuppressive effects, hormone imbalances, stimulation of cell proliferation, or unknown processes. A drug that is not genotoxic in hepatocyte cultures in vitro but that does induce this effect in vivo is suggestive of epigenetic mechanisms of activity by conversion to electrophilic metabolites in the body.

DES, which has been used as a feed additive growth promoter, possesses a stilbene double bond and therefore has been suggested to be capable of interacting with DNA through formation of a reactive species. With chronic exposure in adult mice, DES produces tumors only in mice carrying the mammary tumor virus. Thus its effect is a promotional type. Similarly, after high exposure to DES in neonates, tissue changes are induced in the hormonally sensitive target tissues, such as the vagina. Neoplasia occurs later in life only when endocrine changes occur in the female reproductive system. DES then would be mechanistically classed as an epigenetic carcinogen and therefore requires a different evaluation from "straightforward" genotoxic in vitro carcinogens. This classification, however, is currently under review. DES may be a genotoxic carcinogen.

Quinoxaline compounds are commonly used agents for growth promotion or enteric disease therapy in swine. Therefore two closely related veterinary compounds, carbadox and olaquindox, were evaluated in the *Salmonella*/microsome test (Ames test) and the hepatocyte/DNA repair test (Williams test). Both were positive. Thus not only are they potentially genotoxic and mutagenic, but also should be considered potential carcinogens. Not only do they share a common structural similarity, but also they are deemed to be a hazard at any level of exposure because of their in vitro genotoxic activity.

In short, nongenotoxic or epigenetic carcinogens (such as certain stable organochlorines) may represent only quantitative human hazards because of their dependence on mammalian activation systems of variable intensities. Thus safe levels of exposures of these types of agents could be at least theoretically defined. Conversely, human exposure to direct genotoxic carcinogenic veterinary drugs must be minimized.

In vivo bioassays are performed based on limited or inconclusive evidence of genotoxicity. In this type of system approach, although positive results are definitely significant, negative results cannot be overlooked. Accordingly interpretation and decision making are difficult. These in vivo tests are geared to provide definitive evidence of carcinogenicity, co-carcinogenicity, or promotion. Among the assays employed in this approach are the following:

1. Altered foci induction in rat livers. The basis of this test is the fact that the hepatic lesions, altered foci, and hyperplastic nodules frequently precede development of hepatocellular carcinomas. Sensitivity of these tests can be enhanced by subsequent administration of a tumor promoter, such as phenobarbital.
2. Skin tumor induction in mice. Certain carcinogens can be revealed by continuous application of the test compound to the skin of mice producing papillomas and carcinomas.
3. Pulmonary tumor induction in mice. Certain strains of young mice are partic-

ularly susceptible to induction of lung tumors by drugs and chemicals. Young rodents are invariably used to avoid the overlying complications of the occurrence of spontaneous tumors in adult mice.
4. Breast cancer induction in Sprague-Dawley rats. Mammary tumors in young female Sprague-Dawley rats are rapidly induced by certain neoplastic agents. The number of induced tumors is taken as an additional indicator of carcinogen potency.
5. Assays for promoters. This approach involves the initial administration for small doses of a known genotoxic carcinogen followed by administration of the test substance. The carcinogenic promotional effect of the latter is then evaluated.

Thresholds for carcinogenic compounds are extremely difficult to determine from analysis of standard animal carcinogenicity tests. Animals with short life spans develop a higher rate of cellular DNA mutation after exposure to carcinogens than do long-lived species. As DNA mutations accumulate over years, within cells, and attain a threshold concentration, carcinogenesis is triggered. Covalently bound residues present a hazard in terms of assessment of safety. Although it may be unlikely that these will present a hazard, data to support this are unavailable.

The problem for estimating human health risks stems from lack of general agreement among toxicologists as to the mathematical method of extrapolation of the estimated risk. It has been suggested that, based on their putative mechanisms of action, a distinction should be made between those carcinogens that, with or without metabolic activation, interact with cellular DNA and thus cause morphologic or functional alterations in the genetic expression of cells and those that do not. The distinction between genotoxic and epigenetic carcinogens appears to be reasonable also from the regulatory viewpoint.

The FDA has chosen to define "no residue" operationally based on quantitative carcinogenicity testing of residues and the extrapolation of animal test data to arrive at a concentration of residue that presents an insignificant risk to humans. The virtually safe level of exposure will be determined by this linear-extrapolation model for each test compound, expressed as a fraction of the total diet fed to the test animal, calculated for a maximum lifetime risk that is essentially zero but never expected to exceed 1 in 1 million. The lowest of all calculated acceptable levels for the parent drug or its metabolites will be designated as the required sensitivity of the method for the tissue assay.

The 1 in 1 million level of risk used in the guidelines does not mean that 1 in 1 million people will develop cancer as a result of the regulation of an animal drug carcinogen. Rather it represents a 1 in 1 million increase of risk over the normal risk of death and also represents a lifetime—not annual—risk.

The number of chemicals, however, that have been shown to be carcinogenic in animals has increased enormously over the past decade. They represent a wide spectrum of unrelated chemical structures, including many that are apparently nongenotoxic in most test systems.

13.4 MUTAGENICITY

Mutagenesis is the induction of changes in the genetic component of the cell. In many cases, mutagens also cause cancer in laboratory animals. Because of this, an added benefit of mutagenicity studies is to provide short-term predictive tests of carcinogenicity potential. A close correlation also exists between mutagenicity and mutagenic tests in early pregnancy may indicate teratogenic potential.

Many carcinogens are mutagenic in bacteria and bacteriophages, and therefore mutagenic effects are frequently interpreted as an indirect measure of carcinogenic potential. Mutagenic compounds may react with a base in DNA and modify it chemically. At the next replication, the modified base may pair with a new base partner. Subsequent replication ensures completion of the mutational process. The sequence of base pairs in DNA determines the corresponding sequence of base pairs in DNA, which determines the corresponding sequence of bases in RNA. When DNA base pairings are changed by mutational mechanisms, during replication and transcription, because a new genetic code has now been established, formation of a different amino acid may be specified. This may be quite deleterious to cellular function. Replication of genetic information in ensured by the mechanism of base pairing in the double-stranded DNA helix in which purines are paired against pyrimidines. The hydrogen bonding arrangements across the double helix ensure that spatially a purine can always match with a pyrimidine base and vice versa. If a pyrimidine paired with a pyrimidine, the gap in the double helix would mean a purine could not pair with a purine. The structural integrity of the double helix would therefore collapse. The hydrogen bonding relationships are optimal for pairing of adenine to thymine and guanosine to cytosine. There are many of these hydrogen-bonded base pairs of purine-pyrimidine in the long DNA molecule chain.

Mutations can take a number of forms:

1. Base pair transformation. A mutational process operating through this mechanism could result in (a) a specific purine being replaced by a different purine, (b) a specific pyrimidine being replaced by a different pyrimidine, (c) a purine being replaced by a pyrimidine, or (d) a pyrimidine being replaced by a purine.
2. Deletion or addition of a base pair. This is conventionally referred to as a frameshift mutation. If a base pair partnership disappears or if an additional base pair is inserted across the double helix, the ordered sequencing of the chain is severely disturbed. The DNA code is then put totally out of phase.
3. Deletions. This involves a breakage followed by attempted reconstitution of the molecular fragments, which may or may not be successful.
4. Nondisjunction. Occurring at mitosis or meiosis, an unequal partitioning of chromosomes between the daughter cells at cell division results from disruption of the formation and function of the spindle fibers. The so-called spindle poisons have been implicated in this phenomenon of metaphase inactivation.

SCREENING FOR MUTAGENICITY

An initial approach usually entails an examination of the structure of the drug or chemical to ascertain whether any similarities exist with other compounds of known mutagenic potential. As in the case of many pharmacologic agents, however, slight structural modifications can profoundly alter biological reactivity, and so undue reliance cannot automatically be placed on structural similarities.

Mutagenicity testing identifies the capacity of the compound (and its residues) to interact with DNA of genes or to affect chromosomal numbers or structure. Many different mechanisms of mutagenicity exist, and it is not possible to devise a single definitive test that can take account of all the variable molecular interaction. Assays for genetic damage may be directed toward specific gene activity or specific chromosomal activity. In vitro techniques are inexpensive tests of short duration but are more limited in their potential for interpretation of the hazards to humans. In vivo study systems tend to be more laborious but may be more reflective of the mammalian system. Quite often a parent drug compound is not in itself mutagenic, but mammalian biotransformation gives rise to the production of the ultimate mutagen (i.e., the activated electrophilic metabolite), which then binds to genetic material. To simulate this metabolic function, in vitro tests may incorporate enzymatic activation systems, or alternatively animal testing may be required as a further assessment step.

Mutagenicity Tests

A battery of tests is desirable:

Test 1: A test designed to demonstrate the induction of point mutations (base pair change and frame shift mutations) in established bacterial test systems, such as *Salmonella typhimurium*, *Escherichia coli*, or *Bacillus subtilis*. The test should be conducted with and without the use of appropriate metabolic activation systems.

Test 2: A test designed to demonstrate the production of chromosome damage in appropriate mammalian cells grown in vitro with and without the use of appropriate metabolic activation systems.

Test 3: The induction of mutations in mammalian cells grown in vitro or tests designed to induce recessive lethals in *Drosophila melanogaster*.

Test 4: A test designed to demonstrate the induction of chromosomal damage in the intact animal using either the micronucleus test or preferably the metaphase analysis of bone marrow or other proliferative cell or the induction of germ cell damage as demonstrated by the dominant lethal test in the rat or mouse (Table 13–9).

In vitro tests using bacteria are routine baseline assays for examining gene mutation, and if such toxicologic studies reveal drug-induced genetic damage, there obviously is profound significance for the use of the drug in animals and humans. Difficulty in interpretation of these bacterial mutagenicity tests arise because DNA structure differs between bacterial and mammalian systems and because mechanisms of repair are not identical between humans and lower organisms.

The Ames test is a short test for the detection of carcinogens using mutagenicity in bacteria as an end point. By the use of liver homogenate, the test takes into account mammalian metabolism of the carcinogen. A high, but not complete, correlation has been found between carcinogenicity in animals and mutagenicity in the Ames test. The question arises whether the Ames test is the appropriate tool to investigate mutagenicity of anabolic drugs. Although steroids are proven carcinogens in several animal models, they are not mutagenic in the bacterial test system.

The *Salmonella*/microsome assay (referred to as the Ames test) is currently the most widely used short-term assay for mutagenic compounds. These strains of *S. typhimurium* contain a mutation requirement for the amino acid histidine in their growth. The test organisms cannot synthesize the amino acid histidine. The assay is performed on a selective growth medium, which does not contain enough histidine for growth. Unless a reverse mutation occurs, they do not survive on culture, and this

TABLE 13-9
MUTAGENICITY TESTS

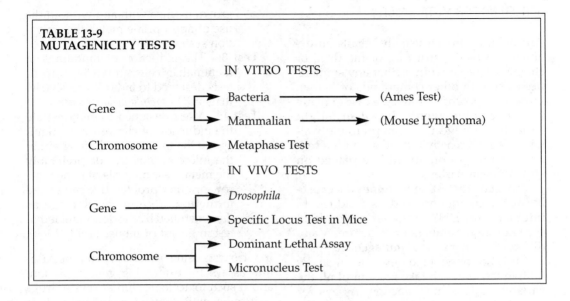

IN VITRO TESTS

Gene ──────┬──→ Bacteria ──────────→ (Ames Test)
           └──→ Mammalian ─────────→ (Mouse Lymphoma)

Chromosome ──────→ Metaphase Test

IN VIVO TESTS

Gene ──────┬──→ *Drosophila*
           └──→ Specific Locus Test in Mice

Chromosome ──────┬──→ Dominant Lethal Assay
                 └──→ Micronucleus Test

forms the basis of testing of drugs and chemicals for their ability to induce mutation. After a suitable incubation time in the presence of the test substance, the number of revertant colonies are counted. Such revertant colonies are derived from an organism, which, in response to the chemical, mutated by reversion back to a form with an ability to synthesize histidine. The strains of *S. typhimurium* used in the assay are artificial stains rendered highly sensitive to the effects of mutagens by removal of their lipopolysaccharide coat and by a reduction in their capability to repair damage to DNA. Although the Ames test possesses good routine predictive value, it is often criticized on grounds of selectivity of chemicals tested, the occurrence of false-negative results (e.g., for spindle poisons, such as DES), and for various chemicals that are inherently toxic to bacteria. In addition, such an artificially created bacterial in vitro system does not truly mimic the mammalian system as exemplified by humans or animals. Despite these limitations, the Ames/ *Salmonella*/Microsome test, although controversial, still remains one of the primary assay systems for quick screening and detection of possible mutagens and is of importance as a predictive test for carcinogens. A positive but not perfect correlation of results between the Ames test and carcinogenicity exists.

Considerable effort has been devoted to improving the sensitivity and reliability of this particular test system. For example, additional mutations have been introduced into the test strains to increase sensitivity. Supplementation by additional strains with different specificities has also been undertaken. A major disadvantage of the test system has been the failure to detect mutagenicity attributable to drug or chemical metabolites. Incorporation of a mammalian metabolic activation system or various microsomal tissues facilitates increased reliability by detecting mutagenic effects induced by metabolites. Without this addition, the performance of the Ames test would be limited exclusively to direct-acting agents that do not require metabolic activation.

Because most carcinogens are not carcinogenic themselves but are active only after metabolism, the compounds are tested in the Ames test in the presence of a mammalian metabolizing system as well as directly. A supernatant fraction of liver homogenate from rats treated with Aroclor 1254 and NADPH-generating system has been shown to be favorable for activation. The liver represents the most important organ for metabolism of foreign compounds, and several drug-metabolizing enzymes are induced by Aroclor.

The Ames test is a reversion assay test. One of the greatest mutagenic hazards to humans is gene deletion, and this type of change is detectable only in forward mutation tests. In vitro systems using cultured mammalian cells are used for this particular type of assay. Similar in many respects to the Ames test, a mammalian activation system is incorporated in the form of liver microsome fractions (to simulate mammalian metabolism), and both forward and reverse mutations can be detected. Choice of cell type, culture medium, duration of exposure, and end-point criteria are crucial for the decision-making process to assess suitable cytotoxicity tests.

Macrophage cells play a crucial role in the immune response of the body, and such cell lines can enable screening of a range of unknown chemicals for this effect on the immune system. Epidermal culture for production of skin irritation, the Draize test for assessing cutaneous toxicity, and enzyme leakage tests have been focused on with increasing attention as alternate methods for risk assessment of drugs with potential for general cytotoxicity.

The *Salmonella*/microsome test performance is a function of the chemical class. Inadequacy of the metabolic activation or the existence of nonmutational mechanisms for carcinogenesis may be contributing factors to its overall limitation. Damage to DNA may be converted to specific mutational events by repair system variations and not by direct interaction of the chemical or its metabolite with DNA. Assays that rely on covalent binding to DNA may not be effective in assessing mutagenic potential.

The Ames test rests on two types of bacterial DNA alterations: base-pair substitution and frame-shift mutations induced by deletion, insertion, or biochemical modification of base. The principle of this test has been extended to other species, i.e., yeasts for antibiotic studies and mammalian cultured cells. Tests on whole animals are restricted to somatic mutations in a few well-known species (e.g., *Drosophila*, mice, hamsters), to chromosomal anomalies (micronucleus test, sister chromatid exchange test), and less often to whole effects (dominant lethal test).

As part of the toxicologic evaluation of any compound, the ability to induce un-scheduled DNA synthesis in primary rat hepatocytes after in vitro treatment is tested. In the assessment of chromosomal damage, in vitro tests are based on cultural lymphocytes of mammalian systems, which following addition of the substance, are arrested in metaphase and then studied for abnormalities. Cytogenetic studies pay particular attention to inversion, translocation gaps, and chromosomal breakages. Such metaphase tests are time-consuming and laborious. A more rapid approach involves identification of micronuclei or Howell-Jolly bodies. There are fragments of chromosomes that are ejected after drug-induced chromosomal damage. Although similar to metaphase analysis in principle, it is a quicker test for assessment of mutagenicity.

One important in vivo test for gene damage is called the dominant lethal assay. Oriented to germinative cell damage, the test involves treating male mice at high dosage levels and mating with females over a span that covers the entire spermatogenic development period. Metaphase examination can also be carried out in vivo by collecting and culturing bone marrow cells after chemical exposure.

Micronucleus Test. The mutagenic potential of a substance can be tested by the micronucleus test, using bone marrow cells in mice. Any toxic effects of the test substance on immature nucleated cells may lead to a reduction in cell division, thus causing cell death. This in turn leads to a reduction in cell volume, and to compensate for this, peripheral blood is shunted into the bone marrow. If the ratio of the normochromatic to the polychromatic erythrocytes is scored and found to be significantly different from the control value, this is taken as indicative of toxicity.

At least 1000 polychromatic erythrocytes from the animal are evaluated for the presence of micronuclei; the observed number of micronucleated normochromatic erythrocytes is also recorded. The ratio of polychromatic to normochromatic erythrocytes after counting 1000 is determined.

For additional study of gene damage, the fly *Drosophila* is used as an in vivo test method. *Drosophila* has a classic genetic system, which has been thoroughly and extensively characterized. Enzymatic metabolizing pathways similar to humans are also present. Many genetic aberrations are detectable in recessive lethal tests in this species.

Test Limitations

General problems associated with current mutagenicity testing procedures relate to the difficulty in extrapolating the results from highly artificial in vitro and in vivo studies to humans with respect to human risk assessment. Although chromosomal tests appear to be less sensitive than bacterial tests, false-negative or false positive results can occur, rendering criteria for further experimentation difficult.

There is also a need for development of further test systems that would detect substances that depend for their mutagenic activity on tissue or cell type metabolic activation system (other than the liver microsomal enzyme systems). Human epithelial cells may have a role to play here, and second-order tests would require methods for maintenance of a range of differentiated tissue cells or target cells incorporating a number of the tissue-specific properties that could affect toxicity.

Mutagenic potential is assessed in tests on microorganisms and mammalian somatic cell lines. As in all toxicologic experiments, the results of laboratory testing are influenced by a number of parameters: the dose selected; mode of administration; cell lines; experimental conditions; pharmacokinetic, pharmacodynamic, and metabolic patterns of the drug in the test species; enzyme induction; enzyme inhibition; criteria of end-point assessment; and extrapolation of data to humans. Negative findings cannot be uncritically accepted as evidence of nontoxicity.

Mutagenicity Test Battery

The battery of mutagenicity tests is summarized as follows:

1. Bacterial point mutation assay, such as the Ames test, with and without activation
2. Mammalian point-mutation assay using mouse lymphoma, Chinese hamster ovary, or hamster V.79 cells, or sex-linked recessive lethal test in *Drosophila*
3. Unscheduled DNA repair in mammalian cells in culture

13.5 TERATOGENICITY

A teratogen is a chemical agent that can affect the somatic cells of a developing fetus such that defective development of organ systems occurs. Teratology is the study of developmental abnormalities produced by a drug or during the critical period of organogenesis. These effects can range from fetal death and resorption to malformation and growth retardation effects. For teratogenic effects to occur, all that is required is transient exposure to a potentially embryotoxic agent during a critical period of early pregnancy.

ORGANOGENESIS

Organogenesis begins early in gestation, and this is followed by finer biochemical and morphologic differentiation during the second trimester. Fetal development involves rapid and extensive cellular proliferation, differentiation, migration, and then organogenesis in a programed fashion. Accompanying early morphologic development and biochemical development is the translation and transcription of genetic messages. During the embryonic stages, organogenesis is taking place, and at this stage the conceptus is particularly sensitive to the toxic effects of drugs. Because the rate of cellular turnover is high in the first trimester of gestation, agents that interfere with the cellular proliferation can be embryotoxic, giving rise to a variety of developmental abnormalities. Teratogenesis is a unique, complex process, the finer points of which have yet to be clarified.

CRITICAL PERIODS

During early fetal development, there are critical or sensitive periods when malformations are most likely to be induced. These critical periods are short windows of time during the phase of organogenesis.

Teratologic calendars have been drawn up for humans, laboratory animals, and target animals identifying the critical time periods. Teratogenicity is essentially a "one hit" phenomenon; that is, it is really a form of acute toxicity, and it can appear after only a single exposure to the drug or chemical. Most teratogens do not affect the dam but display a selective toxic effect for the fetus. Level of exposure and dosage are important because although certain fetal concentrations may be teratogenic, higher levels may actually kill a fetus and are not necessarily teratogenic for the survivors. At the early developmental stages, some teratogens display an all-or-none effect: Either no malformation is induced and the fetus is killed, or it survives with normal organ systems. Exposure later on in pregnancy is unlikely to result in malformations because by that stage organ systems have completed their development. Thus there is just a single critical time span during the early developmental stage when teratogenic potential is at its maximum.

Drug effects on a fetus are of two major types: Early in gestation, the major risk is one of morphologic abnormality (congenital anomalies), whereas later in pregnancy, functional considerations are of greater importance. Among the overlying key factors complicating the process of embryotoxicity are:

1. The manner in which drugs are absorbed, metabolized, and excreted during pregnancy
2. The nature of the placental barrier
3. Whether or not the drug reaches the conceptus, in what form, and in what concentration
4. The mechanism of action of the drug
5. The stage of organogenesis

PLACENTAL TRANSFER OF DRUGS

The placenta is a unique membrane system in that it separates two individuals possessing differing genetic makeup, physiologic systems, and susceptibilities to drugs. From this placenta, the fetus obtains its nourishment and eliminates its own metabolic waste products in the absence of a developed fetal excretory system. The dependence on placental function, however, also places the fetus at risk for transfer of potentially embryotoxic substances that may appear in the maternal blood stream.

Most xenobiotics absorbed by pregnant females rapidly traverse the placental barrier. The permeability of the placental barrier is a function of several characteristics, including:

1. The drug substance—its lipophilicity, dissociation constant, and plasma protein binding
2. The mechanism of transfer to the fetus—passive diffusion along a concentration gradient, facilitated diffusion, active transport, or pinocytosis
3. Placental structure and fetal and maternal blood supply

Despite species differences in placental structure, many drugs permeate this barrier with relative ease.

The placenta of primates (including humans) and of rodents is of the hemochorial type in which the maternal blood bathes the chorion directly. Here it is exposed to the fetal membranes, and xenobiotics need only to cross the fetal trophoblast basement membrane and endothelium to enter the fetal circulation. In pigs and horses, the epitheliochorial-type placenta possesses the maximum six tissue layers separating the maternal and fetal blood stream. Drugs and chemicals are transported from the placenta to the fetal liver by the umbilical vein, and approximately 50% of this blood flow is distributed to the fetal liver. Although many distinct types of biotransformation enzymes are present along the placenta, this does not pose a major barrier to placental transfer.

FETAL EXPOSURE

Once a drug or its metabolites are presented to the developing fetus, morphologic or biochemical processes may be impaired if blockade of DNA synthesis, RNA synthesis, or general protein synthesis occurs. This may result in teratogenic effects if exposure occurs at an early critical period and if the fetus as a whole survives.

Many agents that are mutagenic and carcinogenic also display teratogenic activity.

Induction of mutational or chromosomal abnormality can cause abnormal fetal development. Teratogenicity and congenital abnormalities, however, are not necessarily associated with obvious chromosomal abnormalities, and so the malformations are not heritable. This is in contrast to mutagens and carcinogens, in which a heritable alteration in a cell line is a prerequisite. Nonetheless, genetic factors, in the form of an increased susceptibility to embryotoxic effects, may play a role in teratogenesis. In other words, any developmental deficiency that has an inherent genetic basis may be greatly amplified and openly manifested by exposure to a teratogenic agent.

Many agents known to interfere with cellular proliferation are embryotoxic by causing excessive cell death in specific target organs, which are then destined to become malformed. Cytotoxic agents, for example, can induce selective necrosis at critical periods or organogenesis. Other teratogens exert their effects by altering hormonal status in the developmental stage. Alteration in the thyroid status may produce teratogenic effects. Compounds with similar structures to thyroxine (T_4) thyroid-stimulating hormone may lower maternal and T_4 levels as well as the T_4 level in the fetus. This may be associated with cardiac abnormalities. Antithyroid agents, such as methyluracil, can potentiate the teratogenic effects of vitamin A.

Frequently fetal abnormalities can be produced by nutritional deficiencies (especially vitamins); hormonal deficiencies and excesses may also prove to be teratogenic. Hormonal substances themselves may potentiate the effects of other teratogens. In laboratory animals, teratogenic effects have been demonstrated for antithyroid substances, alkylating agents, heavy metals, vitamin antagonists, antifolate agents, hormonal excesses, and some antibacterial sulfonamides.

TERATOGENS IN HUMAN MEDICINE

In human medicine, it has long been established that mutational deficiencies, intrauterine infections, and environmental influences can result in fetal abnormalities. Historically one of the most dramatic outbreaks of congenital malformations was first associated with rubella virus infection during the 1940s. Different defects were noted in the offspring depending on the timing of uterine exposure. Heart and eye defects predominated when rubella occurred during the first and second months; deafness was more marked when infection occurred in the third month. Other infectious agents, such as *Toxoplasma*, cause teratogenicity by direct invasion of the fetal tissue cells.

Drug-associated congenital abnormalities were identified with the widespread use of the abortifacient drug aminopterin when failure to induce abortion resulted in congenital anomalies in surviving offspring. Of all drugs, perhaps thalidomide illustrated more than any other agent the necessity for adequate and thorough screening for teratogenicity before marketing of a compound and its introduction as a medicine. Thalidomide was a tranquilizer and hypnotic drug used in the late 1950s as an effective, nontoxic therapeutic agent in women. A disastrous outbreak of congenital abnormalities was observed in the offspring of women who had taken thalidomide during the third and eighth weeks of pregnancy, which was retrospectively identified as the critical period. Typical abnormalities in the offspring included either amelia (absence of limbs) or phocomelia (reduction of long bones of limbs). The thalidomide outbreak led to the establishment of a routine practice for improved screening procedures for all new drugs.

Potential embryotoxicity is now revealed in screening procedures either by short-term feeding tests in pregnant animals or during multigeneration feeding studies. In the former, the drug is administered only during the critical phase of organ development. The laboratory species most commonly used are mice, rats, and especially rabbits because of the latter species' high susceptibility to teratogenicity.

One of the current problems in such testing procedures in species specificity. In rats, for instance, congenital defects cannot be induced by thalidomide. Mice, rabbits, monkeys, dogs, and humans are susceptible, however. Teratogenicity testing is difficult, time-consuming, and expensive and not always clear-cut. Teratogens constitute a diverse body of known and unknown chemicals with no clear structural similarities. In the evaluation of test compounds, timing of drug administration is crucial to identifying the critical susceptible period, and so the precise time of conception must be known.

One of the great difficulties in teratogenicity testing techniques is the idiosyncrasies of the test species used. Different structures and functions of the test species' placentae; the varying sites, rates, and extent of biotransformation; the different metabolites consequently formed; and the different rates and patterns of embryologic development render the predictive value of such tests variable. Variations in the rate and extent of biotransformation and the production of "ultimate teratogens" is a possible cause of species variation in such screening procedures.

Thalidomide is known to be extensively metabolized, and it is probable that a metabolite rather than a parent compound is in fact this "ultimate teratogen." Surprisingly, however, early laboratory studies on pregnant animals demonstrated that administration of these metabolites did not bring about teratogenic effects in experimental animals. The reason was that the metabolites were unable to pass from the maternal circulation into the fetus. In the specific case of thalidomide, biotransformation to the ultimate teratogen occurs on the fetal site of the placenta after transplacental diffusion of the parent molecule. Permeation of the placental barrier is therefore of critical importance. Trapping of highly polar metabolites on the fetal side is responsible for the circulation of these teratogenic substances in the fetal tissues. Another major teratogen for humans is diphenylhydantoin. As in the case of thalidomide, the embryotoxic effect is attributable to the formation of a reactive metabolite in the body. In mice, diphenylhydantoin is teratogenic, but its metabolites are not. An increase in embryotoxicity is observed when the parent compound is combined with an inhibitor of the enzyme epoxide hydrase. This indicates that the ultimate teratogen is an electrophilic arene-oxide. Another important teratogen in human medicine is the antiepileptic drug valproic acid. Pregnant women taking such medication have up to 2% risk of producing a child with spina bifidia.

Many pollutants to which people may be exposed in the environment are teratogens in animal tests. These include dioxin (a potent mutagen and carcinogen also), 245 T, captan, organic mercurials, and lead.

ANIMAL TERATOGENS

For veterinary drugs, the same basic principles of teratogenicity potential apply, i.e., fetus selectivity, species sensitivity, critical period of exposure, pharmacokinetic and biotransformational effects, types of ultimate teratogens, placental transfer dosage effects, and mechanism of embryotoxic action. Many of the benzimidazole parasiticides exhibit teratogenic properties. This was first recorded with parbendazole, which is teratogenic in sheep and rats but not in pigs, cattle, or rabbits. Species sensitivities can thus be quite dissimilar. Oxfendazole is teratogenic in sheep but not in cattle.

In the well-documented case of parbendazole in sheep, dosing of the pregnant ewe is associated with congenital abnormalities in the offspring. The anomalies are primarily those of the bones and joints affecting the pelvis, long bones, and digits. Exposure at different times of early pregnancy give rise to different manifestations of abnormality, for example, day 12—exencephaly, day 16—fused vertebrae, day 24—arthrogryposis. Albendazole administered on day 12 in sheep causes exencephaly and on day 17 causes skeletal abnormalities. In sheep, head and face abnormalities tend to occur following exposure from day 12 to 17, spinal column defects from day 16 to 21, and limb distortion from day 22 to 25. A number of organophosphate and carbamate insecticides possess teratogenic effects also, and certain corticosteroids are teratogenic in a number of laboratory animals.

During the later stages of pregnancy, the urogenital system is susceptible to the action of steroid hormones. Progesterone and progestagens given to the dam can produce masculinization of female fetuses; androgens and anabolic steroids may induce female pseudohermaphroditism. In the bitch, dexamethasone may result in birth of pups with deformed limbs.

Griseofulvin is teratogenic (cleft palate, skeletal abnormalities) in cats but not in dogs. Depending on the species, parbendazole, mebendazole, albendazole, oxfendazole, cambendazole, and febantel can be teratogenic in the parent form or indirectly from metabolite formation. Oxibendazole and fenbendazole in parent form are not teratogenic, although one of the metabolites of fenbendazole, a sulfoxide found in the milk of cows treated with fenbendazole, is teratogenic in the rat and sheep. Albendazole displays similar biotransformation pathways in cattle as it does in sheep, yet the bovine animal is refractory to its teratogenic effect at normal dosage rates. With many of the benzimidazoles, not only is the critical exposure time span of early pregnancy important, but also the dosage rate. Many label instructions accompanying these parasiticides draw attention of the necessity to avoid supratherapeutic dosages in early pregnancy.

The general pharmacologic principles for species variation in the metabolism of drugs in the liver (and to a lesser extent in the placenta) may be an important underlying factor in explaining this refractoriness of some species to teratogenic drugs. For instance, thalidomide is active in rabbits, dogs, pigs, and humans but not in rats. The mechanism of teratogenic activity of this compound involves the microsomal creation of an arene-oxide reactive metabolite. This metabolite is not found in rat livers. Even when identical active metabolites for teratogenic drugs are present in different species, other factors, such as placental transfer, ion trapping in fetal tissues, mechanism of action, the critical exposure period, and the different rates and patterns of organogenesis and morphologic differentiation, may determine the presence or absence of a congenital abnormality effect.

TESTING FOR REPRODUCTIVE AND FETAL TOXICITY

Reproductive and teratology studies should be carried out on either chemicals with structures closely related to known reproductive toxins/teratogens or substances that have demonstrated an ability to affect the gonads adversely, e.g., a chemical that caused some degree of testicular atrophy during a 90-day (or 280-day) study would be a candidate for testing in a reproductive study.

The most commonly used species are the rat, hamster, mouse, and rabbit, but the rat and rabbit are preferred. Approximately 20 pregnant animals per dose level are used except for the rabbit, in which groups of 12 are considered sufficient. Pregnant animals are dosed throughout the period of organogenesis: days 6 to 15 for rat and mouse; 6 to 14 for hamster; and 6 to 18 for the rabbit, with day 0 being the day on which a vaginal plug or sperm is detected (unless mating was observed or artificial insemination was used, when the times listed should be adjusted by adding 1 day).

Dams should be observed for signs of maternal toxicity (which may influence the offspring). At sacrifice of death, the uterus should be removed and examined for the number of live fetuses and the incidence of embryonic or fetal deaths. Sex and weights of fetuses should be noted. Rats, mice, and hamsters should be examined for visceral defects (one third to one half of litter) and skeletal defects (remainder), whereas each rabbit fetus should be prepared and examined for both visceral and skeletal defects. All fetuses in all species should be examined externally. The distinction between maternotoxicity and teratogenicity must always be recognized.

POTENTIAL HAZARDS

The greatest problem from the human health safety point of view is inadvertent or accidental exposure to possible teratogens. This "invisible" or "unrecognized" exposure poses the greatest risk, especially in the context of drug residues from food animals. Most of the newer second-generation benzimidazoles have long half-lives, are slowly depleted from the tissues, and are excreted through the milk in metabolite form.

Although volitional medication during human pregnancy is best avoided, any medication to a woman of child-bearing age must always be weighed against the possibility of pregnancy occurring during the course of therapy. This does not, however, take account of the risks inherent from the possible intake of teratogenic compounds in foodstuffs during pregnancy. One of the dilemmas of this accidental human exposure to teratogens is knowing whether pregnancy can be recognized early enough so exposure can be avoided.

Experiments for teratogenic effects in laboratory animals are conducted under highly artificial conditions in the sense that the precise time of mating is established, and so the crucial dates of early pregnancy are known and identified. This obviously does not mirror the human situation. For a woman with irregular cycles, it takes longer for a missed cycle to be noted and therefore for the woman to consider herself pregnant. By that time, however, drug effects on the developing fetus through inadvertent exposure to a possible teratogen may already be taking place. Potentially a large population of women of child-bearing age could unknowingly expose their embryos to the risks of malformation before pregnancy has in fact been recognized.

13.6 RESIDUES OF ANTIBACTERIAL DRUGS

The use of antibiotic drugs and other antibacterial drugs, e.g., sulfonamides and nitrofurans, has been extensive in livestock and poultry destined for human consumption. In the United States, antibacterial drugs are used professionally by veterinarians and nonprofessionally by laymen for therapeutic and nontherapeutic purposes at low concentrations, i.e., less than 100 ppm in attempts to increase the daily rate of growth and to improve feed efficiency. Adherence to withdrawal times can be cumbersome, inconvenient, and an additional expense for the livestock and poultry producer. The use of nonmedicated feed during the withdrawal time is essential if the consumer is to receive unadulterated safe meat.

Antibacterial drug residues may have a twofold effect on human health. Drug residues in contaminated foodstuffs can produce direct toxic effects. The impact may range from sensitizing reactions to drug-induced organ damage, in which metabolites, degradation products, or both may act as

intoxicants to the liver, hematopoeitic system, kidney, and so forth.

In addition to direct toxic effects, microorganisms of the enteric flora could acquire antimicrobial resistance as a result of selection pressure by ingestion of trace amounts of antibiotics. As little as 2 ppm daily intake of antibiotic can give rise to development of drug-resistant gram-negative organisms. With antibiotic residues that are stable to cooking processes, this could pose a serious hazard. Population shifts may occur under pressure of the selection process.

Antibiotic residues in food constitute a variety of health hazards to humans. These hazards depend on the frequency and degree of exposure. Continuous exposure is more probable when a side or quarter of a food animal is purchased for deep-freeze use.

The most serious objections to the presence of antibiotics and their metabolites in food intended for human consumption arise as a consequence of human health considerations. The potential for a toxic risk to humans from the presence of antibiotics or their residues in milk or meat products, raw or cooked, is limited. A few reports in the literature suggest that prolonged ingestion of tetracyclines from any source, including food, has detrimental effects on teeth and bones in growing children, whereas reactivation of signs of chloramphenicol toxicity have been reported after consumption of meat, milk, or eggs containing chloramphenicol residues. The quantities that could be ingested by such means, however, scarcely approach the therapeutic range and do not reach the levels ordinarily required to produce toxicity, which are usually 100 times the therapeutic dose.

The two main risks relate (1) to hypersensitivity reactions, which may be induced in the allergic individual, and (2) to the acquisition by pathogenic microorganisms of resistance to certain antibiotics.

Nonpathogenic *E. coli* in the human gut flora have the ability to acquire drug resistance and to transfer this resistance to sensitive pathogenic salmonellae. These latter organisms may then become refractory to a range of antibiotic compounds without ever contacting them directly.

Of primary significance is the fact that pathogenic bacteria may acquire resistance

---

TABLE 13–10
PENICILLIN SENSITIZATION

Penicillin
↓
Cleavage (Beta-Lactamase)
↓
Penicilloic Acid (Hapten)
↓
+ Protein
↓
Antigen
↓
T Lymphocytes/B Lymphocytes
↓
Antibody

---

as a result of their continual exposure to minute amounts of antibiotic residues in foodstuffs. Some antibacterial drugs and their metabolites of degradation products are potent sensitizing agents, e.g., penicillin. Humans may become sensitized to drugs by a number of means; however, consumption of food containing drug residues resulting from administration of antibiotic drugs to domestic animals and poultry represents a potential but unquantifiable problem (Table 13–10).

Except for some tetracyclines, most therapeutic antibiotics are relatively heat stable and resist both pasteurization and cooking processes. The microbiologically inactive breakdown products of tetracyclines may themselves possess some toxic potential.

Drug sensitization can be acquired by consuming any one of the many antibacterial drugs, their metabolites, or degradation products. Resistance to antibacterial drugs can be acquired by bacteria through a variety of modes. Tolerance may appear because of mutational changes. In other instances, the selective pressure exerted by the continuous presence of antibacterial substances in animal feed inhibiting or killing off the sensitive organisms results in the emergence of a predominantly resistant bacterial population.

So-called natural resistance is a characteristic of all species that are homogeneously resistant to a particular antibiotic. In these species, usually the target for an antimicrobial agent is missing. This form of resistance may even be a species-specific characteristic, e.g., the resistance of gram-negative organisms or *Pseudomonas* to penicillin G.

Chromosomal resistance is based on the selection of mutants from a mostly sensitive population. This kind of resistance is inherited clonally.

The third type of resistance is based on the acquisition of additional genetic elements. It is localized on so-called plasmids outside the chromosome and may be transferred from one bacterium to another. When resistance genes are carried by a plasmid, they are called R factors.

Infectious or transferable drug resistance can develop at a much faster rate than the foregoing. By this process, bacteria are enabled to become resistant to several drugs without being exposed to even one antibiotic. Transfer of resistance in this form takes place through conjugation, during which there is transfer of extrachromosomal particles of DNA plasmids that replicate within bacterial cells outside the control of the cells' chromosomes. By means of this independent transfer, plasmids carrying R factor rapidly induce infectious resistance throughout a bacterial population.

A further hazard is the possibility that the absorption of drug residues may in some instances result in an untoward response owing to direct effects on specific physiologic functions, particularly in individuals receiving medication with the unrelated drugs. In the case of emergency slaughtered animals, bacteriostatic antibiotic residue levels may militate against the detection of pathogenic bacteria, such as salmonellae, at slaughter, with the result that such infected carcases may be released into the consumer market.

Additionally, such meat has the potential either to serve as an allergen or to initiate antibiotic resistance in the bacterial flora of food handlers and consumers as well as being a source of R+ enterobacteria.

13.7 RESISTANCE INDUCTION

Bacterial resistance to drugs has been known as long as chemotherapeutic agents have been in use. Antibiotic resistance in microorganisms harbored by animals and poultry could present a hazard to humans in two ways:

1. Emergence of resistant strains of organisms of animal origin could directly cause illness in humans.
2. The genes encoding for resistance in animal microorganisms could become incorporated into commensals or pathogens of humans. Subsequent disease in the human patient would become refractory to antibiotic therapy.

If animals or their products (milk, meat, eggs) contain traces of antibiotics when eaten by humans, the effect of these antibiotic residues on the consumer is presumably that of the equivalent dose of antibiotic given directly. The consumption by humans of antibiotic residues could produce harmful effects from direct toxicity or from allergic reactions in persons who have been previously sensitized. Such residues could also provoke sensitization and so expose the consumer to the future risk of allergic reaction to the antibiotic. Antibiotic residues could also lead to the emergence of resistant strains of organisms in humans.

Although the emergence of resistant strains of microorganisms usually follows the prolonged use of chemotherapeutic agents in human medicine, during hospitalization, or in veterinary practice, the role of extremely minute levels of these drugs in the development of resistance is not clearly understood. Any discussion dealing with residues of antimicrobial agents in food must always address itself to the possibility of induced antibiotic resistance in the consumer. In other words, does the continued trace ingestion of antimicrobial agents through food of animal origin pose a real danger to human health? This potential danger could arise through the exertion of a selection pressure on the human intestinal flora, thus favoring the growth of microorganisms with natural or acquired resistance. Alternatively, the possibilities of giving rise directly or indirectly to the development of acquired resistance in the pathogenic enterobacteria cannot be ignored.

It is difficult to establish the minimal exposure time or the minimum antibiotic concentration in the human digestive tract. For this possibility to arise, there is undoubtedly a considerable degree of variation between the susceptibility of individual consumers to such induced bacterial resistance following residue intake.

The current approach to antibiotic residue control is based on in vitro experimentation and analysis. Its underlying philosophy is that no residue levels exerting antimicrobial activity are tolerable in edible tissues of animal origin. For such in vitro determination, test organisms are used. Such organisms are chosen on account of their high sensitivity to the widest possible range of antibiotics. The successful growth of the organisms in the presence of animal tissue extracts is conventionally interpreted as an indication of no detectable antimicrobial residue. Tolerance levels can be established in accordance with the level of residue ceasing to inhibit bacterial growth.

Although microbiologic in vitro assays are the currently accepted international detection methods, many problems surround their usefulness. Test strains of microorganisms differ widely, as also does their susceptibility to antimicrobial inhibition. A negative result generated from one particular assay technique may yield a positive result when a different test organism is used. The predictive value of such microbiologic tests is also open to question. Assay strains are nonpathogenic test organisms, many of which bear little relevance to pathogenic strains of relevance in human health. Many false-negative results can therefore occur.

The appropriateness of any microbiologic assay, if it is to be of real relevance to human health hazard potential, must establish tolerance levels based on minimum inhibitory concentrations (MICs) of target microorganisms of the human flora. This is because the primary resistance-inducing potential of ingested antibiotic residues is most probably oriented to the human gut flora. Strains of enterobacteria (*E. coli*) as representatives of the normal gut flora are being increasingly used as test organisms in microbiologic assay systems. This approach has the advantage of taking into account the relevance of antibiotic residues to organisms of direct significance in human health.

RESISTANCE IN MICROORGANISMS

The types of resistance that bacteria may develop to the action of antibiotics involve two distinct mechanisms—mutation and inheritance. The problem is widely regarded as manmade and is cited as yet another example of man's culpability in fouling his environment. The false conclusion is commonly drawn that humans, through the discovery of antibiotics, created the phenomenon of resistance. This is not so: Soon after the discovery of penicillin, resistant strains were isolated in cultures of bacteria that had been laid down in the preantibiotic era, and since then, resistant isolates have been obtained from sources of great antiquity.

Since the first emergence of life on earth, its lower forms have been involved in a continual form of biochemical warfare, as each species seeks to defend and extend its ecologic niche. When molds came into conflict with bacteria—a common feature of the constant competition for the recycling of biological matter—there were strong evolutionary pressures for the molds to develop antibacterial techniques and for the bacteria to defend themselves. Antibiotic resistance in bacteria is not a fixed characteristic, and the degree of resistance detectable in the laboratory probably bears little relationship to the resistance of the organism when growing in the intestinal tract of animals.

MUTATIONS

These affect DNA sequences and result in the synthesis of a protein or macromolecule by the bacterial chromosome that differs sufficiently from the original chemical entity to interfere with the antibiotic activity. Because an antibiotic inhibits a bacterium only after it has entered or crossed the cell wall and is bound to a target site, resistance can develop directly if the mutation has so altered the characteristics of the protein or macromolecule that the cell wall, transport mechanism, or receptor site is no longer "congenial" to the antibiotic. Resistance can also develop indirectly if the altered protein blocks a biochemical pathway that uses the antibiotics. In the simplest terms, a sensitive population of bacteria can be changed into a resistant population by the selection pressure created by the presence of an antibiotic.

Resistance can derive from mutation of a single pre-exiting gene.

Resistance to antibiotics arises from new genetic forms (mutants or variants) that may appear during multiplication. Their incidence is low, usually about 1 per 100,000 to 1000 million organisms. Mutants remain unrecognized until the sensitive organisms are eliminated. This occurs when antibiotic is present in excess of the MIC. Hence, it is the therapeutic use of antibiotics (high concentrations) and not the growth promotion use (low concentrations) that exerts selection pressure in favor of the mutants. Selection pressure can thus occur both in human and in veterinary medicine. In human medicine, selection pressure is at its most intense in hospitals, where antibiotics are extensively used.

The major cause of problems of antimicrobial resistance in humans arises from overuse of antimicrobials at therapeutic levels in humans. It is generally accepted that drug resistance that develops in a bacterium as a result of mutation is only of importance with the *individual* host and a single bacterial strain. Because the determinant is chromosomal, the resistance cannot be transferred between different bacterial species and genera. In addition, the mutationally resistant microorganism is not usually as viable as the "wild" ones; hence once the selective antibiotic is removed from the environment, the proportions of the mutant decrease. If exposure to the antibiotic continues, however, the mutants can become life-threatening to the patient.

It should be understood that the antibiotic does not induce the mutation. The mutant simply takes advantage of its fortuitous spontaneous appearance to flourish in the presence of a selected antibiotic.

INHERITANCE

The element by which the development of resistance by inheritance is achieved is the resistance plasmid (R factor). Plasmids are of varying size and have been identified in most bacteria. Although outside the bacterial chromosome, there is little to distinguish between the plasmids and the chromosomes because the former also are collections of DNA, genes capable of coding and inducing the manufacture of new proteins in the bacterial cell. In this fashion, the plasmid is important in bacterial evolution, functioning as it does in replication, fertility, resistance to toxins, antibiotics and bacteriophage, metabolism, and relationships to the local environment (e.g., adhesiveness) and indeed providing the cell with often novel biochemical capabilities and therefore with a greater chance of survival and propagation.

A number of characteristics of plasmids are significant in relation to the development of bacterial resistance. These include the encoding of resistance capability for as many as six unrelated antibiotics in the same DNA particles; the capacity to transfer from one cell to another, resulting in wide dissemination of the resistance; and the mobilization whereby ordinarily nontransferable gene fragments can be transferred by the plasmid from one bacterial cell to others.

Many different R plasmids have been identified in various gram-negative and gram-positive bacteria, and the majority carry resistance determinants for two or more antibiotics not of the same chemical class. It appears that two identical plasmids cannot coexist in the one cell, but plasmids of different groups can—increasing even further the possibilities for resistance spread. The transfer or acquisition of other plasmid-mediated characteristics, such as virulence and enterotoxin production, in gram-negative bacteria is facilitated by the presence of resistance plasmids.

TRANSFER OF RESISTANCE

The transfer of resistance material can be achieved by:

1. Conjugation (i.e., physically through cytoplasmic bridges between individual cells, particularly belonging to the same strain but often to other gram-negative microorganisms). This mechanism is limited almost entirely to gram-negative organisms, although it has been identified also in streptococci.
2. Transduction (whereby R plasmids are carried between species). The quantity and size are limited by the phage head structure, and transduction is therefore most effective in passage of smaller plasmid DNAs. This mechanism is used by gram-negative organisms and by staphylococci.
3. Transformation (direct DNA transfer, such as might occur in vivo with plasmid DNA lysed bacteria). This transfer also occurs between bacterial genera as well as intragenerically. The transformation of genetic material is used in recombinant DNA technology.

There is also a phenomenon of transposition whereby resistance determinants pass from one plasmid to another or to a chromosome or to a bacteriophage, thus allowing the construction of new R plasmids under pressure of new antibiotic exposure. The mobilization effect is significant in the transfer of plasmids, which are ordinarily not transferable, and is found most commonly in *Pseudomonas*; again the passage may be between genera.

INHERITED RESISTANCE

Inherited resistance in bacteria is accepted as the most important type from the standpoint of the community and the environment. Studies of isolated microorganisms of animal and human origin have demonstrated that plasmids from both sorts of isolates are practically identical. In terms of the dissemination of resistance determinants of R factors, one must regard the problem as involving both humans and animals as vectors. The dissemination may occur as clonal distribution, by transfer or transportation to various microorganisms with a gradual buildup in their population carrying one or several R plasmids. The presence of a large reservoir of antibiotic-resistant organisms in animals has been shown by investigation in the United States.

R-PLASMID-MEDIATED RESISTANCE

R-plasmid-mediated resistance is almost invariably associated with cross resistance to a number of related and unrelated antibiotics. The reasons for the association lie in the resistance mechanism to related compounds that have been coded, the usual presence of more than one R determinant in the same plasmid, and the frequent coexistence of several different plasmids in the same bacterial cell. As a result, the use of any antibiotic usually leads to the development of resistance to itself and to other related and unrelated antibiotics; e.g., if a plasmid is encoded for resistance to ampicillin, tetracycline, sulfonamide, and streptomycin, the exposure to any of these antibiotics results in resistance to all the others, whereas the use of a beta-lactamase-containing strain results in resistance to other members of this group.

The transmission of antibiotic resistance was first demonstrated in 1958 and involved the transmission of the capacity to produce pencillinase by a bacteriophage to a penicillin-sensitive staphylococcus. The first discovery of R factors was made in 1963, and by 1967 it had been demonstrated that R transfer from gram-negative organisms could occur in the intestines of animals and humans and probably in the upper respiratory tracts and in the urinary tract.

If resistant organisms are selected owing to the use of an antibiotic, they do not only show resistance to this particular substance, but also resistance to many other antimicrobial agents. This principle became even clearer when molecular biologists and geneticists examined the structure of R factors in more detail. They found a further fundamental component of the "infectious antibiotic resistance," the transposons, or "jumping genes." A characteristic of transposons is that they are capable of jumping from one DNA molecule to the other (e.g., from plasmid to plasmid, plasmid to chromosome, plasmid to bacteriophage, and vice versa) giving rise to another effective mode for the spreading of resistance genes.

In short, the spreading of R factors and transposons as a consequence of the uptake of antimicrobial agents represents the main risks for human health. In turn, this spreading results in the development and an increasing incidence of organisms not accessible to therapy. Organisms so far known to be involved include *Salmonella* (*S. typhi* and *S. typhimurium*) *E. coli, Campylobacter, Vibrio cholerae, Yersinia pestis, Shigella, Proteus,* and *Pseudomonas aeruginosa.* These include the causative agents of such diseases as typhoid fever, infantile gastroenteritis, pyelitis, plague, and cholera. A number of different reports have been published that show an alarming rise in the incidence of organisms resistant to the usual antibiotics.

FACTORS AFFECTING RESISTANCE

At present, it is not possible to determine all the factors that are involved in the spread of microorganismal resistances. In addition to the selective pressure of the use of an antibiotic in one situation, there is the influence of the quantities and types of antibiotics generally used in the community, the type of usage, the movement of persons, hygiene in animals and humans, climate, methods of food handling, and methods of animal slaughter.

Experimental techniques are now available that allow determination of resistance phenotypes in microorganismal strains and their tracing through animals and humans. If a collection of plasmids from an environment belong to the same compatibility type, there is strong suggestive evidence for transfer, and increasing sophistication permits the tracing of the route of transfer.

With these data taken together, it can be concluded that according to the present state of knowledge and also in the near future, it is probably not possible to define no-effect levels for residues of antimicrobial agents. A number of studies, however, has indicated also that amounts far below the MIC of a substance may have effects on the cells, their growth characteristics, and resistance genes. Therefore the MIC range, as proposed as a limit, would certainly mean too high amounts of residues.

In this connection, the MIC value for the most sensitive bacterial species of the human intestinal flora may normally serve as a criterion. In some cases, however, the MIC value for the bacterium that is the primary target of the active substance should be the basis for evaluation.

It is well known that MIC is determined under specific experimental conditions and that its determination depends closely on the experimental conditions of an antibiotic. In any case, even leaving aside these major difficulties, the MIC can at most allow evaluation of the active antibiotic concentrations in the intestine, but not, or at least not directly, the tolerable concentrations of antibiotic residues in food. To do this, it is necessary to take into account:

- The degree of resorption of the antibiotic in the digestive tract, which may be compensated to a greater or lesser degree by biliary excretion
- The degree of degradation in the digestive tract
- The dilution of the bolus in the proximal part of the intestine
- The concentration of the bolus in the distal part of the intestine

The MIC is the minimum concentration that can inhibit growth of the test organism. What is perhaps of more significance is the sub-MIC level. Many authors have shown already that at antibiotic concentrations below the MIC, dramatic changes of the bacteria and their resistance may occur.

Beneficial effects of sub-MIC levels of antibiotics include:

- Changes in bacterial morphology
- Reduction of bacterial growth
- Inhibition of enzyme or toxin production
- Loss of adhesive properties

Within ranges of $\frac{1}{8}$ to $\frac{1}{32}$ of the MIC, changes in the cell wall, the generation periods, and the agglutination properties of *E. coli* occurred.

To provide for adequate consumer protection and to preclude resistance development, residues of antibiotics and thus their tolerance levels should be well below the MIC as deduced from in vitro microbiologic assays. At best, the MIC, particularly for enteric organisms, is a rough estimate of the susceptibility of the bacterium under the artificial conditions in which the organism was tested. When using laboratory methods, it is essential to challenge a bacterial population with a lethal or inhibitory concentration of antibiotic to select the organisms that can resist the challenge. In practical terms, the use of a sublethal or a subinhibitory antibiotic concentration is therefore unable to select resistant strains from a bacterial population.

13.8 DRUG ALLERGY

For a drug to produce an allergic reaction, a prior sensitizing contact is required either with the same drug or with one closely related. Exposure to the drug, which is the primary eliciting contact, results in an antigen-antibody interaction that provokes the typical manifestation of allergy. Such manifestations can range from minor skin lesions to anaphylactic shock. In humans, involvement of the skin is most common, whereas in guinea pigs, bronchiolar constriction leading to asphyxia is the more usual response. Penicillin allergy, for instance, frequently elicits urticaria and pruritus. When animal drug residues lead to detrimental hypersensitivity in the consumer, penicillins tend to be most commonly implicated. This antibiotic is well known for its allergenic properties in human clinical medicine. Cephalosporins, sulfonamides, and nitrofurans are also implicated in human drug allergy.

The marked differences in the pathways and rates of metabolism among the various species of target animals introduce many variables into the complex problems of the likelihood of an allergic drug reaction. Practically all commonly used veterinary drugs could act as antigens, provided that they possess the appropriate molecular structure. For small molecules to become immunologic, they must be able to form covalent bonds with macromolecules, such as proteins, or polysaccharides and polynucleolides.

Activation of T lymphocytes and B lymphocytes synthesize antibodies in response to the haptenogenic stimulus. Binding to T lymphocytes produces specifically sensitized lymphocytes, which are responsible for cell-mediated immunity. When B lymphocytes are exposed to the original antigen, humeral antibodies are produced.

The reactive antigenic fraction for many veterinary drugs consists a cleavage metabolite, which forms hapten conjugates by covalent binding to protein. In humans, several haptenic derivatives are formed from benzyl penicillin. The major reactive product is the pencilloyl moiety, which forms more than 95% of the penicillin hapten conjugates. This determinant can combine with a carrier protein through the opening of the beta lactam ring. All penicillins contain the 6-amino-penicillinic nucleus and are therefore cross allergenic.

Many individuals treated with penicillin undergo an immune reaction to the penicilloyl group. The structural integrity of 6-amino-penicillinic acid nucleus is essential for the antibacterial activity of the molecule. If the beta lactam ring is cleaved by bacterial beta-lactamase (penicillinase), the resulting compound penicilloic acid is devoid of antibacterial activity. It carries an antigenic determinant of the penicillins, however, and acts as a sensitizing agent. In positive reactions to skin tests, the incidence of penicillin reaction is high and is associated with cell-bound IgE antibodies. About 10 to 15% of persons with a history of a penicillin reaction have an allergic reaction when given penicillin again.

After the antigen has been formed and T lymphocytes have undergone activation, IgE, IgM, IgA, and IgG are synthesized by the B lymphocytes. IgE becomes fixed to the mast cells, and the immunoglobulins generally modulate the immune response to antigen. Sensitivity to penicillin G also implies sensitivity to other penicillins and semisynthetic penicillins. All penicillins share the basic 6-amino-penicillinic acid nucleus, which can form the benzyl pencilloyl metabolite following opening of the beta lactam ring. This haptenic derivative is responsible for the cross allergenicity demonstrated to the semisynthetic penicillins, such as carbenicillin or ampicillin.

Although primary sensitization occurs most commonly by parenteral penicillin therapy, in sensitized persons the oral route can be just as hazardous. The situation from the penicillin residue standpoints is confusing because of the propensity of humans to develop allergic sensitivity to milk proteins, by the variable nature and extent of penicillin allergy, and perhaps also by the likely exposure to penicillinlike molecules in molds in the environment.

Antibiotic allergy in humans is a complex subject. Generally antibiotics have a low molecular weight and are immunogens or haptens. To initiate an immune response, the antigenic determinants must combine with a carrier protein or form dimers, oligomers, or polymers. Antibiotics that undergo spontaneous or metabolic degradation to present potential antigenic determinants are those most probable to cause hypersensitivity.

Animal drug residues are unlikely to play a role as sensitizing agents but could trigger an allergic response in sensitized persons. Because of the paucity of valid predictive tests for assessing the allergenic potential of veterinary drug residues, it is difficult to evaluate this commodity in premarket evaluation and screening. For drugs for which high allergenic potential is likely, the lowest practical tolerance levels must be set. For penicillins, 10 IU of benzyl penicillin has been regarded as safe on oral ingestion in sensitized individuals. Microbiologic assays capable of detecting 0.005 ppm of this antibiotic should accordingly be adequate to guard against the likely induction of allergy in sensitized individuals. Nonetheless, some extremely sensitive individuals may experience adverse reactions to lower levels of penicillin, even levels undetectable by standard assay methods. Because of the limitations of current knowledge on the role of low drug concentrations in hypersensitivity reactions, there is little clinical, experimental, or epidemiologic data from which to estimate the risk to humans from consumption of food products containing antibiotic residues.

Adverse drug reactions, typified by hemolytic anemia, thrombocytopenia, and agranulocytosis, can be mediated through immune mechanisms. The drug hapten may induce antibody formation in the blood stream, and the antigen-antibody complex is then adsorbed onto the cell membrane. Lysis occurs when complement is activated. Agranulocytosis is a serious drug allergy that is of much greater significance and occurrence in humans than in animals. (Direct cytotoxic drug effects may also elicit this response.) Immunologic effects on the stem cells in the bone marrow may underline the manifestation of this form of adverse drug reaction.

Chloramphenicol is one of a few regulated animal drugs for which the Code of Federal Regulations prescribes a label bearing the statement: "the product is not to be used in animals which are raised for food production." The toxicity of chloramphenicol has been studied widely since the drug's introduction into human medicine in the 1940s and its widespread use as a broad-spectrum antibiotic in the 1950s. The primary toxic effects associated with chloramphenicol therapy derive from the drug's principal action on inhibiting protein synthesis. Chloramphenicol blocks mitochondrial protein synthesis in mammals. Toxic effects include bone marrow suppression characterized by decreased erythropoiesis, modification of the immune response, and interference with the hepatic microsomal enzymatic system; the gray baby syndrome in infants; and teratogenicity in rats. Such toxic properties are dose dependent and are reversible on withdrawal of the drug. They are observed at dose levels considerably higher than could be attained in food animal tissues following residue formation. Because it is a general protein synthesis inhibitor, chloramphenicol can interfere with synthesis of immunoglobulins.

The more serious manifestation of chloramphenicol toxicity is quite distinct from the dose-related toxicity. The severe curtailment of its usage by physicians in human medicine is because of association between the antibiotic and the development of a usually irreversible type of bone marrow depression (aplastic anemia). This is an idiosyncratic reaction; it is fatal in almost 70% of cases, it is characterized by pancytopenia, and a high incidence of leukemia is experienced in those patients who recover. Its appearance does not appear to be related to the frequency of level of exposure. Thus the establishment of a safe level of chloramphenicol-residue exposure from food animal tissues is precluded.

The mechanism of chloramphenicol-induced aplastic anemia is uncertain. Bone marrow stem cells are believed to be involved. Formation of a nitroso reduction product of the *p*-nitro group of chloramphenicol can irreversibly inhibit growth of bone marrow precursor cells. This has been verified in vitro. Thiamphenicol, an analog of chloramphenicol, devoid of the p-nitro group, although sharing many of the clinical antibacterial and toxicologic properties of chloramphenicol, has not been implicated to date in the aplastic anemia syndrome. Considerable controversy still exists as to whether chloramphenicol-associated bone marrow depression is a toxigenic or allergenic effect.

The frequency of drug allergy in humans depends on the nature of the drug, the route of administration, the genetic predisposition of those who receive the drug, and the extent of prior exposure and of cross reactivity to the same or related drugs. Drug allergy may be induced by any route of administration but not with equal efficiency. The oral route appears to be associated with a lower incidence of allergenic sensitization than any other, whereas topical application of drugs to the skin is especially prone to sensitize. Only the phenomenon of immediate hypersensitivity has been linked to the presence of animal drug residues in edible products of food-producing animals.

Streptomycin sensitizes readily, and skin sensitivity is not unusual. Neomycin displays cross sensitization with streptomycin. The perplexing question is one of unraveling the relationship between dose and hypersensitivity reactions. Allergic reactions cannot be anticipated and are not dose related.

A fairly common allergic drug reaction not only in humans and animals, but also in veterinarians handling drugs, is contact dermatitis. Here the drug acts as a hapten that combines with skin proteins.

Almost any substance to which humans are exposed is potentially capable of inducing an allergic response in some individuals. If the opportunity for contact with an allergen is increased, its potential for inducing allergic reactions is correspondingly increased, and the potential for the reactions to become more severe is also increased. For this reason, exposure of individuals to antibiotics via their food as well as through medical therapy increases significantly the frequency of hypersensitivity to antibiotics.

Manifestation of hypersensitivity reactions can range from benign skin rashes to more serious presentations, such as urticaria, anaphylactic shock, serum sickness arthropathy, lymphadenopathy, nephropathy, gastroenteritis, encephalitis, hepatitis, and blood dyscrasias. Fatalities can occur. Cross reactivity occurs between related antibiotics, for example, all penicillins, including ampicillin, and cephalosporins, erythromycin, and spiramycin.

Numerous published and unpublished studies have been carried out using both the general population and patients attending hospital clinics. Based on these reports, it is estimated that the incidence of antibiotic allergies in the population is as follows:

Penicillins including ampicillin	10%
Cephalosporins	5%
Erythromycin	0.5%
Sulfonamides	13%
Tetracyclines	5%
Trimethoprim	3%

Apart from the direct consequences of an illness attributable to antibiotic allergy, a more serious effect may be the resultant deletion of that antibiotic from the choice of effective antimicrobial agents with which a physician may choose to combat infectious disease in that individual. Human allergy restricts the options for antibiotic therapy.

13.9 MISCELLANEOUS EFFECTS

It is important to be aware that many other residue hazards are still inadequately investigated. From in vivo and in vitro studies, it is known that many residues affect enzyme systems. This may involve either induction or inhibition of hepatic microsomal enzyme systems. Although it is difficult to assess whether this phenomenon will have any practical bearing on the health of humans, the possibility cannot be excluded.

Animals and humans have an apparent unlimited capacity to adapt to contact with new substances, provided that this contact is on a low scale. Such adaptation depends on the detoxification and sequestration mechanisms inherent in the individual's metabolic system. Degradation and elimination of many toxins are a fundamental capacity of the biosystem, provided that the toxins are presented in relatively small doses. At certain points of the individual's life span, however, this potential for detoxification may be insufficient. This is especially true of the fetus in utero, the neonate, the elderly patient, or the individual with dysfunction of the liver or kidney. In such instances, severe toxic effects to the intake of drugs and chemicals can be manifested in a most severe fashion. Such groups are also at most risk from residue ingestion of xenobiotic agents. What may be an acceptable risk for a healthy adult may not be so

for the neonate with underdeveloped drug-metabolizing enzyme capacity. It is incumbent to decide whether the benefits accruing from the use of a particular substance in food animals is likely to outweigh the risks entailed to the consumer. A substance with an established lack of safety presents no problem and obviously should not be used. A substance with a potential for human health hazard presents a different problem and must be assessed under the circumstances of its use and its toxicologic potential.

Imprinting or programming of enzyme activity is a form of permanent modulation of enzyme activity that results for neonatal exposure to hormones or hormonally active agents. Exposure of newborn rats to hormones alters their response later in life to carcinogens that are biotransformed in the liver. Prenatal or neonatal exposure of animals to hormonal substances, generally such that chronic estrogenic stimulation is induced, can render such animals more susceptible to carcinogenic effects later in life. Many carcinogens are active transplacentally and in the neonatal period. Such compounds are usually of the type that damage DNA and hence are referred to as genotoxic. Although DNA damage can be repaired, if it is not and the cell replicates using the damaged DNA as a template, permanent alterations in DNA result. This genetic alteration can lead to neoplastic conversion of the cell.

DES is genotoxic, but restriction of its carcinogenic effects to hormonally responsive tissues indicates the hormonal mechanisms underlying its carcinogenicity. The subsequent appearance of DES tumors at puberty suggests the development of neoplasia by the process of imprinting of enzymatic systems during in utero exposure.

Enzyme induction involves an adaptive change and increase in the number of drug-metabolizing enzymes in response to an enzyme-inducing agent. Major drug-metabolizing enzymatic systems (such as cytochrome P-450 in the liver microsomal system) can increase (or decrease) after exposure to lipophilic drugs of relatively long biological half-lives that possess an ability to bind to cytochrome P-450 enzymes.

Significant changes in drug-metabolizing activities can be detected by pharmacokinetic studies, which indicate an increased ability to stimulate the metabolism of differing substrates by a variety of biotransformation pathways. Relative changes in the amounts of multiple forms of cytochrome P-450 can be induced by exogenous or endogenous factors, such as disease states, drug intake, and perhaps drug intake in food. Polycyclic aromatic hydrocarbon produced from steroids in meat when cooked over charcoal can exert a selective inductive effect.

Enzymes responsible for the bioactivation of drugs to chemically reactive metabolites constitute the microsomal P-450 mixed function enzymes. Induction of such enzymes by secondary drugs may play a critical role, albeit an indeterminate one, in the final establishment of the ultimate toxicity of the metabolite to the body system. In this context, hepatitis is an occasional hazard accompanying halothane anesthesia, especially following repeated exposure.

A number of substances that are enzyme inducers are also carcinogens (e.g., polycyclic hydrocarbon). Establishing a correlation between the two properties is a vexed question. The possibility remains, however, that enzyme induction may influence both the initiation and the promotion of experimentally induced carcinogenesis. Commonly used veterinary drugs are known enzyme inducers: chloral hydrate, phenobarbital, phenylbutazone, griseofulvin, phenytoin, and halogenated anesthetics. In experimental work in mice, phenobarbital and griseofulvin have been observed to increase the incidence of hepatic neoplasms.

The sequelae of enzymatic induction are numerous:

1. Tolerance, or diminished biological effect in response to increased biotransformation activity, may result.
2. Drug interaction can arise after the concomitant administration of two or more drugs, either or both of which may be enzyme inducers.
3. Increased toxicologic effects whereby the endogenous production of chemically reactive electrophilic metabolites can trigger a range of toxic activities by reacting covalently with essentially cellular components is another significant possibility.

Enzyme inhibition mediated via suicide enzyme inactivators and suicide enzyme inhibitors is another critical dimension of toxicologic potential of drugs. This phenomenon may induce side effects or drug interactions.

Impairment of microsomal drug-metabolizing capacity can lead to reduced clearance and elevated plasma levels of other drugs or metabolites. Interactions with oral hypoglycemic agents, such as tolbutamide, can precipitate a hypoglycemic crisis from the co-administration of chloramphenicol, a known microsomal enzyme inhibitor. Chloramphenicol increases the duration of pentobarbital anesthesia significantly in dogs and cats. Other inhibitors include organophosphate insecticides, piperonyl butoxide, and carbon tetrachloride. Steroid metabolism is impaired by drug-metabolizing enzyme inhibitors.

Enzyme induction refers to the increase in activity of enzymes of xenobiotic transformation that occurs on exposure of animals to various chemical agents. Pretreatment of animals with drugs can greatly enhance the toxicity of compounds that are activated by enzymes to toxic forms, such as bromobenzene or carbon tetrachloride. A number of environmental toxicants are effective inducers of the liver microsomal system: Among these are the polychlorinated biphenyls and the chlorinated insecticides, both of which are now widespread pollutants in the environment.

13.10 RESIDUE ANALYSIS AND EVALUATION

One of the most important requirements for development of new animal drugs is to have an assay procedure that is a reliable indicator of the possible drug residues in tissues of treated animals. The application of such a procedure is twofold. The first is during product development, when quantifiable residue data must be generated. The second is after product approval, when it is used by the regulatory agency for monitoring the safe use of the new veterinary products. Current analytical procedures are forced to operate at or near the limits of their performance when applied on an ap-

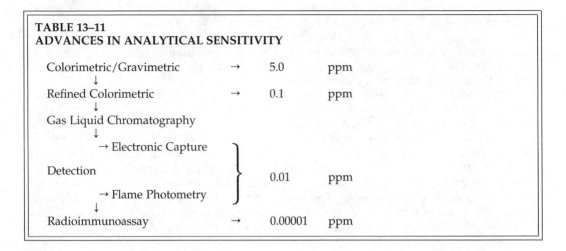

TABLE 13–11
ADVANCES IN ANALYTICAL SENSITIVITY

Colorimetric/Gravimetric	→	5.0	ppm
↓			
Refined Colorimetric	→	0.1	ppm
↓			
Gas Liquid Chromatography			
↓			
→ Electronic Capture			
Detection		0.01	ppm
→ Flame Photometry			
↓			
Radioimmunoassay	→	0.00001	ppm

proved finite tolerance or negligible tolerance basis.

With each advance in analytical ability, "zero" has become smaller. Therefore the FDA had to redefine this "no-residue" level operationally (Table 13–11).

Methods of analysis are essential not only for the determination of residues of veterinary drugs in food, but also for the ultimate safety evaluation of these drugs. To facilitate the use of uniform methods for the verification of the presence of drug residues, analytical methods must fulfill a number of performance criteria. In general, methods of sampling must be well defined with regard to the point of sampling, type of tissue, and sample size. Methods of analysis should be cost-efficient, be of adequate sensitivity, and comply with designated performance characteristics as verified by collaborative testing procedures.

METABOLISM STUDIES

The primary objective in metabolism studies in target animals is to identify and quantitate the drug-derived residue in the edible tissues of target animals. Target animals are dosed at the maximum use level of the drug and sacrificed when tissue residues are likely to be highest, and the total residue content is then assayed. Procedures for extraction, separation, and isolation of metabolites are employed to provide metabolic profiles for each tissue and to facilitate comparison with the metabolic profiles derived from laboratory studies.

The following aspects must be addressed in these metabolic studies:

1. The levels of drug-derived residue in edible tissues after a normal but maximal treatment program
2. The structural identification or characterization of the metabolites
3. The number of metabolites present in the tissues and their relative amounts
4. Identification of the most abundant tissue metabolites
5. Identification of the most appropriate metabolite as an indicator for routine assay procedures
6. Persistence of the metabolites and their decline after withdrawal of drug treatment
7. The extractability of the total residue in each edible tissue
8. The presence of covalently bound residues

RADIOTRACER TISSUE RESIDUE STUDIES

Originally the term "residue" was accepted to mean the parent drug compound and its related metabolites from which the parent drug could be regenerated. With advancements in the field of metabolite studies, the definition of residue now includes all drug-derived chemical compounds in the body burden.

The primary objective of tissue metabolite studies is to identify and quantitate the drug-derived residue. This identification and quantification does not in any way assess the toxicologic hazard. That requires a separate series of evaluations.

Total residue depletion studies involve the measurement of the depletion of the total drug-related residue in the edible tissues of the target animals after the last administration of the drug compound. For large animals, the edible tissues are muscle, liver, and kidney (and milk). For poultry, the edible tissues are muscle, liver, and eggs. Fatty tissue consumption is important, as also is the rate of depletion of the drug from its injection site.

"Drug residue" incorporates all drug-derived residue in the body, and so radiotracer methodology is currently the most useful technique for determining total drug-related tissue metabolites. Radiolabeled drugs are administered to the animals, and the amount of radioactivity is measured in the tissues. The radiochemical purity of the drug should be as high as possible because even a trace amount of a radiolabeled impurity retained in a specific tissue could result in an artifact, giving the appearance of persistent drug residues. Another concern of drug radiolabeling is the precise location of the radiolabel on the molecule, where it is not readily removed through metabolic conversions. Incorrect positioning of the radiolabel could result in the following:

1. Easy metabolism of the label from the drug in the body, with the result that metabolites likely to be of toxicologic concern would become nonlabeled and pass undetected
2. Entry of the radioactive fragment into the general metabolic pool, deposition into tissues giving the appearance of drug-related residue

DEPLETION STUDIES

Total residue depletion studies are performed by administering radiolabeled drug to a sufficient number of animals at intervals after the last treatment. The metabolism of the compound varies according to species, sex, age, dose, and duration of treatment. Neonatal animals are included in many of these studies on account of their underdeveloped hepatic biotransformation capacities. The total residue of the compound consists of parent compound, free metabolites, and metabolites that are covalently bound to macromolecules. The relative and absolute amount of each residue tends to vary in accordance with time after the last drug treatment. Because different components of the residue can possess dissimilar toxicologic potential, information is necessary on the amount, persistence, and chemical nature of the total residue in the edible products of treated target animals.

14C is the most used isotope for radiotracer studies because there is usually little problem with the intermolecular exchange of the label. Residue values are assayed by measuring total radioactivity. The residues are a combination of unchanged parent drug and its degradation products. More specific methods are available, e.g., radioimmunoassay, but the more specific the assay method, the more metabolic degradation products are ignored. Specific assay of only the parent compound could indicate very low residues, although in fact metabolite residues could be quite high.

Other isotopes such as 3H, 32P, and 35S are appropriate for some assays. Because the radiolabel attached to the drug molecule can be incorporated into endogenous metabolism, erroneous conclusions as to residue levels can easily be drawn. For this reason, a chemical or, in the case of antibiotic compounds, a microbiologic assay specific to quantitate only the exogenous or drug-related residue is required. Information from such chemical studies, not just from the radioactive residue data, is used by regulatory agencies in the final clearance of drug products. Nonetheless, correlation between both methods is necessary to validate the accuracy of the chemical assay method.

COVALENTLY BOUND RESIDUES

Many radioactive residues are nonextractable. This slowly depleting radioactivity may be drug related, or it may be from radioactivity that has been metabolized and incorporated into normal tissue components. Covalently bound residues derived from the reaction between a metabolite of the compound and cellular macromolecules present a difficult problem in residue assessment.

Residues can be present in five forms: the parent molecule or molecules; bioactive metabolites (nonnatural), inactive metabolites (nonnatural), material arising from the metabolism of the xenobiotic substance that also occur naturally, and bound metabolites. The nature of these residues can be determined only after almost complete breakage, particularly of proteins (e.g., enzymatic or acid hydrolysis): It may, or may not, be related to that of the initial molecule. In fact, this fraction is found to contain:

1. Endogenous compounds—natural, resulting from incorporation of the degradation products of the parent compound at the intermediate stage of metabolism (e.g., amino acids)
2. New compounds—resulting from covalent binding of the parent drug or metabolites to endogenous macromolecules.

The covalent, so-called irreversible binding of toxic substances to endogenous products is currently much studied. It accounts for many deleterious effects from necrosis to chemical carcinogenesis. These mechanisms are not easily demonstrated because in most cases the initial compound must be converted in the body to chemically reactive metabolite. The ultimate toxic metabolite is hardly ever isolated, but it is indirectly suspected by the demonstration mainly of a covalent binding to endogenous components, i.e., of bound residues.

The "nonextractable residues" are obtained by subtracting the extractable residues from the total residues and compromise:

1. Residues of the drug incorporated through normal metabolic pathways into endogenous compounds (e.g., amino acids, proteins, nucleic acid). These residues are of no toxicologic concern.
2. Chemically bound residues derived by the interaction of residues of the parent drug or its metabolites with macromolecules. These residues may be of toxicologic concern.

The following assays may be used to measure and to differentiate between these various forms. Radiochemical assays measure the total product-derived residue; bound metabolites can be measured as the difference between the total and extractable residue. Biological assays measure the parent molecule and its bioactive metabolites, e.g., microbiologic assay. Immunologic assays measure the parent molecule and closely chemically related metabolites, depending on their cross reactivity, e.g., radioimmunoassays.

In assessing the safety of the residues of xenobiotic compounds, the form in which the residues are present has to be taken into account. Available information on the chemical structure of tissue-bound residues of veterinary drugs is scarce. There is an undoubted need for the further characterization of their potential adverse effects in humans after ingestion of food products of animal origin. Concern arises because of their long persistence in organs. Carcinogenic potential has been linked to covalent binding in tissue, but whether these bound residues are less hazardous than free residues is not known. A significant factor is their bioavailability.

Bioavailability of the components of a residue varies from component to component. More particularly, there are marked differences between the free and the bound fraction. In vitro residual radioactivity of the bound fraction can be eliminated only by drastic procedures: It is obvious that its bioavailability may be low, as it has been demonstrated by few relay bioavailability studies. In the case of anabolic agents, such as trenbolone acetate, it has been shown that the bioavailability of the radioactive fraction in the rat liver (the tissue containing the highest level of radioactivity) is small.

The significance of covalently bound residues is usually concerned with a number of critical questions:

1. Are bound residues likely to be bioavailable?
2. If they are bioavailable, will they be rapidly cleared from the body by excretory processes?
3. If the reactive portion of the drug molecule is already involved in a covalent

linkage, is it likely that further metabolic activation to a toxic metabolite will occur in the body?

4. Is there a clear correlation between co-valently bound residues and carcinogenicity?
5. Is the bound metabolite itself more toxic and more biologically potent than the parent compound?

Because of these difficulties in assessment and evaluation, alternative indirect methods are employed to gain further insight into their toxicologic potential.

RELAY TOXICITY

In cases in which it is not possible to characterize the exact nature of the tissue residues, safety can be assessed by the method of relay toxicity. This procedure provides a useful means of equating test animals and human exposure. Target tissue from farm animals receiving the drug is mixed with normal feed and fed to laboratory animals for varying periods. The animals are then sacrificed and observed for signs of toxicity. The technique is attractive because it experimentally simulates exposure of humans to tissue residues by ensuring that the test animal, i.e., the rat, is exposed to the same mixture of metabolites as humans. It is a relatively inexpensive test because it is not necessary to characterize the residues that are present in the target animal's tissues. The residue containing parent drug and metabolites is present in the proportions to which humans might be exposed. Any positive response in relay toxicity test is indicative of a serious toxicologic residue hazard that cannot be ignored.

RELAY BIOAVAILABILITY

This method endeavors to provide information about the degree of absorption of residues by establishing a ratio between the absorbed and unabsorbed fractions. The "bioavailable residues" are the residues that can be shown, by means of an appropriate method, to be absorbed when fed to laboratory animals. Once generated, bio-

availability data can be used to assess the toxicologic significance of residues.

In target animals, certain metabolites are produced that may be different for the metabolites arising from biotransformation processes in laboratory animal testing. Using standard chronic toxicologic procedures in the rat, these metabolites are not evaluated, simply because the rat may not produce these metabolites. It must be remembered, however, that humans who consume meat from the treated animals may be exposed to these "untested" metabolites, which may be present as residues in meat. This problem may be handled as follows:

1. Use a species for chronic toxicology study that metabolizes the drug in the same way as the target animal species.
2. Identify and characterize the major metabolites in the target species, synthesize the metabolites, and use these in the chronic rodent toxicology study.
3. Use relay toxicity techniques. This involves feeding residue-containing tissues from treated target animals to rodents. These target animal tissues contain the metabolites to which humans are exposed.

Relay bioavailability can be carried out by feeding freeze-dried tissues from target animals treated with radiolabeled drug to laboratory animals. After sacrificing the animals, the radioactivity of the liver and kidney is measured. An approximate estimate of the proportion of radioactivity absorbed can be made by summing the radioactivity found in the bile and urine.

The main parameter for the efficacy of reactive metabolites is their electrophilicity. These unstable reactive metabolites are produced by "suicide enzymes" and bound to their site of production. The question is whether bound metabolites in animal tissues, ingested by the human consumer, can be reactivated to produce second-generation metabolites in humans. It is also possible that the potential hazard in bound residues is abolished once they are firmly bound to animal tissues. A logical deduction from this latter statement would be that the most electrophilic and most reactive metabolite in the target animal is safest for the human consumer.

SELECTED REFERENCES

Acros, J.C.: Criteria for delecting chemical compounds for carcinogenicity testing: An essay. J. Environ. Pathol. Toxicol., 1:433, 1978.

Adamson, R.H., and Sieber, S.M.: Chemically induced leukemia in humans. Environ. Health Perspect., 39:93, 1981.

Ames, B.N., Lee, F.D., and Durston, W.E.: Carcinogens and mutagens: A simple test combining liver homogenates for activation and bacteria for detection. Proc. Natl. Acad. Sci., 70:2281, 1973.

Ames, B.N., McCann, J., and Yamasaki, E.: Methods for detecting carcinogens and mutagens with the Salmonella/mammalian-microsome mutagenicity test. Mutat. Res., 31:347, 1975.

Baer, J.E., Jacob, T.A., and Wolf, F.J.: Cambendazole and nondrug molecules in tissue residues. J. Toxicol. Environ. Health, 2:895, 1977.

Beauchene, R.E., Bales, C.W., Bragg, C.S., et al.: Effect of age of initiation of feed restriction on growth, body composition, and longevity of rates. J. Gerontol., 41:13, 1986.

Bishop, J.M.: Viral oncogenes. Cell, 42:23, 1985.

Bochner, B.R., Huang, H.C., Schieven, G.L., and Ames, B.N.: Positive selection for loss of tetracycline resistance. J. Bacteriol., 143:926, 1980.

Brookes, P. (ed.): Chemical Carcinogenesis. Br. Med. Bull., 36, 1980.

Brown, J.P., and Bietrich, P.S.: Mutagenicity of selected sulfonated azo dyes in the Salmonella/microsome assay: Use of aerobic and anaerobic activation procedures. Mutat. Res., 116:305, 1983.

Burgat, V., Delatour, P., Benard, P., et al.: Metabolism and residues toxicity of benzimidazole drugs. Communication to the World Veterinary Congress, 1983.

Burgat-Sacaze, V., Delatour, P., and Rico, A.: Bound residues of veterinary drugs: Bioavailability and toxicological implications. Annales de Rechercher Veterinaires, 13:277, 1981.

Codex Alimentarium Commission: Report of the Third Session of the Codex Committee on Residues of Veterinary Drugs in Foods. Washington, D.C., Food and Agriculture Organization of the United Nations, 1988 (unpublished FAO document, ALINORM 89/31A; available from FAO or WHO).

Corpet, D.: Antibiotic residues and R plasmid selection. Are in vitro methods good models? Zbl. Bakt. Hyg., 264:178, 1987.

Delage, C., and Irey, N.S.P.: Anaphylactic deaths. A clinicopathologic study of 43 cases. J. Forensic Sci., 17:525, 1972.

Delatour, P.: Some aspects of the teratogenicity of veterinary drugs. Paper presented at the International Conference on Veterinary Pharmacology, Toxicology and Therapy, Cambridge, 1980.

Delatour, P., Dams, R., and Favre-Tissot, M.: Thalidomide: Embryopathies chez le chien. Therapie, 20:573, 1965.

Dinman, B.D.: "Non concept" of "No threshold." Chemicals in the environment. Science, 175:495, 1972.

Federal Food, Drug and Cosmetic Act, 21 U.S.C., Section 512, 1983.

Federal Register, 47, 4972–4977, 1982.

Federal Register, 44, 17070–17114, 1979.

Fry, J.R., and Bridges, J.W.: Use of primary hepatocyte cultures in biochemical toxicology. Rev. Biochem. Toxicol., 1:201, 1979.

Gallo-Torres, H.E.: Methodology for the determination of bioavailability of labelled residues. J. Toxicol. Environ. Health, 2:827, 1977.

Gaylor, D.W., and Kodell, R.L.: Linear interpolation algorithm for low dose risk assessment of toxic substances. J. Environ. Pathol. Toxicol., 4:305, 1980.

Glatt, H.R., Metzler, M., and Oersch, F.: Diethylstilbestrol and 11 derivatives: A mutagenicity study with Salmonella typhimurium. Mutation Res., 69:113, 1979.

Goldberg, H.S., Goodman, R.N., Logue, J.T., and Handler, F.P.: Long-term, low-level antibiotics and the emergence of antibiotic-resistant bacteria in human volunteers. Antimicrob. Agents Chemother., 80, 1961.

Gordon, G.B., Spielberg, S.P., Blake, D.A., et al.: Thalidomide teratogenesis: Evidence for a toxic arene oxide metabolite. Proc. Natl. Acad. Sci. USA, 78:2545, 1981.

Grundin, R., Moldeus, P., Vadi, H., et al.: Drug metabolism is isolated rat liver cells. Adv. Exp. Med. Biol., 58:251, 1975.

Gyrd-Hansen, N., Rasmussen, F., and Smith, M.: Cardiovascular effects on intravenous administration of tetracycline in cattle. J. Vet. Pharmacol. Ther., 4:15, 1981.

Huseby, R.A.: Demonstration of a direct carcinogenic effect of estradiol on Leydig cells of the mouse. Cancer Res., 40:1006, .

IARC Monographs on the Evaluation of Carcinogenic Risk of Chemicals to Humans. Overall Evaluations of Carcinogenicity: An Update of IARC Monographs, volumes 1–42, Suppl. 7. Lyon, International Agency for Research on Cancer, 1987.

Idsoe, O., Guthe, T., Willcos, R.R., et al.: Nature and extent of penicillin side-reactions, with particular reference to fatalities from anaphylactic shock. Bull. WHO, 38:159, 1968.

Ivett, J.L., and Tice, R.R.: Cytogenetic effects of diethylbestrol-diphosphate in murine bone marrow. Environ. Mutagen., 1:184 (abstr.), 1979.

Jenson, E., and De Sombre, E.R.: Estrogen-receptor interaction. Science, 182:126, 1973.

Klein, M.F., and Beale, J.R.: Griseofulvin: A teratogenic study. Science, 175:1483, 1972.

Knothe, H.: Darmflora und antibiotics. Archiv. Hyg. Bakt., 149:642, 1965.

Krishna, G., and Bonanomi, L.: Covalent binding of chloramphenicol as a biochemical basis for chloramphenicol induced bone marrow damage. *In* Drug Interactions. Edited by P.L. Morselli, S. Garattini, and S.N. Cohen. New York, Raven Press, 1974.

Lairns, J.: The origin of human cancers. Nature, *289*:353, 1981.

Lebek, G., and Egger, R.: R selection of sub-bacteriostatic tetracycline concentrations. Zbl. Bakt. Hyg., *255*:340, 1983.

Lebrun, A., et al.: Antimicrobial agents and chemotherapy. 2093, 1992.

Lemon, H.M.: Experimental basis for multiple primary carcinogenesis by sex hormones. Cancer, *40*:1825, 1977.

Lijinsky, W., Reuber, M.D., and Blackwell, B.N.: Liver tumors induced in rats by oral administration of the antihistaminic drug methapyrilene hydrochloride. Science, *209*:817, 1980.

Lorian, V.: Antibiotic sensitivity patterns of human pathogens in American hospitals. J. Anim. Sci., *62* (Suppl.):49, 1986.

Lorian, V.: Some effects of subinhibitory concentrations of antibiotics on bacteria. Bull. N.Y. Acad. Med., *51*:1046, 1975.

Lutz, W.K.: In vivo covalent binding of organic chemicals to DNA as a quantitative indicator in the process of chemical carcinogenesis. Mutat. Res., *65*:289, 1970.

Magee, P.H., and Barnes, J.M.: Carcinogenic nitroso compounds. Adv. Cancer Res., *10*:103, 1967.

Mantel, N., Bohidar, N.R., Brown, C.C., et al.: An improved Mantel-Bryan procedure for safety testing of carcinogens. Cancer Res., *35*:865, 1975.

Marshall, T.C., and Dorough, H.W.: Bioavailability in rats of bound and conjugated plant carbamate insecticide residues. J. Agric. Food Chem., *25*:1003, 1977.

Metzler, M.: Metabolic activation of carcinogenic diethylstilbestrol in rodents and humans. J. Toxicol. Environ. Health, *1* (Suppl.):21, 1976.

Metzler, M., and McLachlan, J.A.: Diethylstilbestrol metabolic transformation in relation to organ specific tumor manifestation. Arch. Toxicol., (Suppl. 2):275, 1979.

Michalopoulos, G., Sattler, G.L., O'Connor, L., et al.: Unscheduled DNA synthesis induced by procarcinogens in suspensions and primary cultures of hepatocytes on collagen membranes. Cancer Res., *38*:1866, 1978.

Middleton, M.D., Plant, J.W., Walker, C.E., et al.: The effects of methyl 5(6)-butyl-2-benzimidazole carbamate (parbendazole) on reproduction in sheep and other animals: Teratological studies in ewes in Australia. Cornell Vet., *64* (Suppl.):56, 1974.

Mitchell, I. de G.: Microbial assays for mutagenicity: A modified liquid culture method compared with the agar plate system for precision and sensitivity. Mutat. Res., *54*:1, 1978.

Montesano, R., Bartsch, H., and Tomatis, L.: Long term and short term screening assays for carcinogens: A critical appraisal. IARC Supplement 2, 1980.

Mori, T., et al.: Long-term effect of neonatal steroid exposure on mammary gland development and tumorigenesis in mice. J. Natl. Cancer Inst., *57*:1057, 1976.

National Cancer Advisory Board: General criteria for assessing the evidence for carcinogenicity of chemical substances: Report of the Subcommittee on Environmental Carcinogenesis. J. Natl. Cancer Inst., *58*:461, 1977.

Parker, C.W.: Allergic reactions in man. Pharmacol. Rev., *34*:85, 1982.

Piercy, D.W.T., Reynolds, J., and Brown, P.R.M.: Reproductive safety studies on oxfendazole in sheep and cattle. Br. Vet. J., *135*:405, 1979.

Rapport du groupe d'expert sur les residus de medicaments vétérinares dans les denrées alimentaires d'origine animals. Conseil de l'Europe. Accord partiel dans le domaine social et de la santé publique. 1986.

Residues of veterinary drugs in foods. Report of a Joint FAO/WHO Expert Consultation. FAO Food and Nutrition Paper, No. 32, 1985.

Rodgers, W.H., Jr.: Benefits, costs and risks: Oversight of health and environmental decision making. Harvard Environmental Law Review, *4*:191, 1980.

Ryan, J.L., and Hoffmann, B.: Trenbolone acetate: Experiences with bound residues in cattle tissues. Journal of the Association of Official Analytical Chemists, *61*:1274, 1978.

Sanders, L.Z., Shone, D.K., Philip, J.R., et al.: The effects of methyl 5(6)-butyl-2-benzimidazole carbamate (parbendazole) on reproduction in sheep and other animals: Malformation in newborn lambs. Cornell Vet., *64* (Suppl.):7, 1974.

Sirica, A.E., and Pitot, H.C.: Drug metabolism and effects of carcinogens in cultured hepatic cells. Pharmacol. Rev., *31*:205, 1980.

Stich, H.F., and San, R.H.C. (eds.): Short-Term Tests for Chemical Carcinogens. New York, Springer-Verlag, 1981.

Swarm, R.L., Roberts, G.K.S., Levy, A.C., and Hines, L.R.: Observation on the thyroid gland in rate following the administration of sulfomethoxaxole and trimethoprim. Toxicol. Appl. Pharmacol., *24*:351, 1973.

Symposium on Risk/Benefit Decisions and the Public Health. Proceedings of the 3rd FDA Science Symposium, Colorado Springs, CO, 1978.

Tancrede, C.: Ecological impact of low doses of oxytetracycline on human intestinal microflore. Seminar on Rationale View of Antimicrobial Residues. An Assessment of Human Safety. Zurich 1987.

Tomich, P.K., An, F.Y., and Clewell, D.B.: Properties of erythromycin inducible transposon Tn 917 in Streptococcus faecalis. J. Bacteriol., *141*:1366, 1980.

Tucker, M.J.: Carcinogenic action of quinoxaline 1,4-dioxide in rats. J. Natl. Cancer Inst., *55*:137, 1975.

Voogd, C.E., Van der Stel, J.J., and Jacobs, J.J.: The mutagenic action of quindoxin carbodox, olaquindox and some other N-oxides on bacteria and yeast. Mutat. Res., *78*:233, 1980.

Weiner, M., and Newberne, J.W.: Drug metabolites in the toxicologic evaluation of drug safety. Toxicol. Appl. Pharmacol., *41*:231, 1977.

Weisburger, J.H., and Williams, G.M.: Carcinogen testing. Current problems and new approaches. Science, *214*:401, 1981.

Weisburger, J.H., and Williams, G.M.: Chemical carcinogens. *In* Toxicology: The Basic Science of Poisons. 2nd ed. Edited by J. Doul, C.D. Klaasen, and M.O. Amdur. New York, Macmillan 1980.

Williams, G.M., and Weisburger, J.H.: Risk assessment of dietary carcinogens and tumor promoters. *In* Diet, Nutrition and Cancer: From Basic Research to Policy Implications. Edited by T.C. Campbell and D. Schottenfeld. New York, Alan R. Liss, Inc., 1983.

CURRENT RESIDUE CONCERNS AND TOLERANCES

14.1 Veterinary Drug Residues in Food

14.2 Maximum Residue Limits and Tolerances

14.3 Food Safety and Inspection Service Residue Testing System

14.4 Rapid Tests

14.5 Work of Codex Alimentarius Committee on Residues of Veterinary Drugs

14.6 Specific Drug Residue Concerns

14.7 Joint Expert Committee on Food Additives Evaluation of Priority List of Veterinary Drugs

14.1 VETERINARY DRUG RESIDUES IN FOOD

POTENTIAL PUBLIC HEALTH CONCERNS

Consumer confidence in the safety of food has become a priority issue for all those involved in the food supply chain. Manufacturers of veterinary medicinal products, livestock producers, and regulatory authorities all have responsibility to ensure that human health is not placed at risk by the presence of hazardous residues in food.

No veterinary drug may be marketed in a country before having received the approval of the competent national authority. Specific and exceptional circumstances, however, may lead the competent national authority to authorize the use of an unregistered drug, especially in the case of clinical tests aimed at demonstrating the efficacy of the drug and performed according to protocol determined in advance.

The costs involved in generating data to meet ever-increasing regulatory requirements could mean that many smaller volume products will disappear from veterinary use.

The potential dangers that could arise from residues of veterinary drugs in food can be classified as follows.

Toxicologic Aspects

The major toxicologic effects of concern are:

1. Genotoxicity
2. Carcinogenicity
3. Teratogenicity
4. Effects on reproduction
5. Immunopathologic effects (allergic reactions)

Resistance Phenomena

The incorporation of antibiotics in animal feed at low concentrations may give rise to resistant populations of microorganisms. There are two possible areas of concern for human health: Resistant bacteria may be selected in the gut flora of treated animals and subsequently spread to humans (this is subject to much debate), or consumption of antimicrobial residues in food might lead to the development of resistance in the gut flora of the consumer.

The following two definitions were adopted by the Codex Committee of Residues of Veterinary Drugs in Foods:

A *veterinary drug* is "any substance applied or administered to any food-producing animal, such as meat-producing or milk-producing animals, poultry, fish, or bees, whether used for therapeutic, prophylactic, or diagnostic purposes or for modification of physiologic functions or behavior."

Residues of veterinary drugs include "the parent compounds, their metabolites, or both in any edible portion of the animal product and residues of associated impurities of the veterinary drug concerned."

The use of veterinary drugs in food-producing animals can result in residues that are neither extractable from tissues nor readily characterized. Because some compounds—trenbolone acetate, albendazole, and 5-nitroimidazoles—produce nonextractable residues, the question arises of how one should evaluate the safety of such veterinary drugs.

The "total residues" of a drug in animal-derived food consist of the parent drug, together with all the metabolites and drug-based products that remain in the food after the administration of the drug to food-producing animals. The amount of total residues is generally determined by means of study using the radiolabeled drug and is expressed as the parent drug equivalent in milligrams per kilogram of the food. Also of concern would be a drug whose presence in food could result in a pharmacologic effect in the consumer in the absence of conventional toxicologic effects.

Modern livestock and poultry farming methods involve use of many different veterinary drugs, for both therapeutic and prophylactic purposes. Animals given such products contain drug residues in their tissues and body fluids for a period of time after treatment. Such residues may be ingested by people consuming food derived from treated animals.

Laying birds pose special problems, which have not yet been resolved. Residues of systemically acting drugs may appear in eggs, and the time over which such residues may occur may vary from days to several weeks.

If lactating cows are given drugs, residues may occur in milk. In particular, the use of intramammary antibiotics, either during lactation or in the dry period, may lead to residues in milk. Apart from public health concerns, the presence of these compounds in milk also has important consequences for the processing industry.

Aquaculture is now being studied by other international organizations, including the Food and Agriculture Organization (FAO) (i.e., question of the use of veterinary drugs in fish).

Veterinary drug residues should not be considered in isolation because they form only part of the group of chemical residues that are found in foodstuffs. Unfortunately, the consumer perception of residues is one of health hazard without differentiation. This perception is completely out of proportion to the significance of residues. There have been specific instances, however, in which residues have led to problems in the past. Use of penicillin in mastitis therapy has led to problems of human health, but this is now resolved to a greater degree. More recently, there have been cases in which residues of diethylstilbestrol gave rise to side effects in children who had a high intake of veal.

At present, the main implication for residues is as a barrier to trade. The situation exists in which a single positive sample from a consignment can jeopardize trade in that commodity for a significant period of time. In such situations, human operator error should be considered.

In the control of residues, it is necessary to have a good internal system of regulatory control of drugs. It is also necessary to have a good residue monitoring operation at national levels. Cooperation between the bodies operating these schemes is vital to the evolution of a policy that serves the producer, the consumer, and the pharmaceutical industry. There should be no incentive to livestock owners to misuse drugs—as a growth promotant, as a preventive in disease situations, or in therapy of diseases.

The Food Safety and Inspection Service (FSIS) is involved in four areas:

1. Inspection—on-line process and slaughter inspection
2. Technical services—new inspector procedure evaluation and the evaluation of new methods

3. Monitoring—for import and export of food products
4. Science program—technical support for inspection operations, including pathology, microbiology, and chemistry

RESIDUE MONITORING

Monitoring of residues of substances used in animal production is conducted to protect the consumer from exposure to unacceptable levels of certain compounds. Residue detection can be used to monitor usage of approved substances, to ensure that recommendations concerning dosages and withdrawal times are being followed. In the case of illegal compounds, monitoring is carried out both to detect and to deter unauthorized usage.

Residue testing of animals slaughtered in the United States is subdivided into two major activities: monitoring and surveillance.

Monitoring is designed to provide information on the occurrence of residue violations in meat and meat products on an annual, national basis. Monitoring information is obtained through a statistically based selection of random samples from healthy-appearing animals.

In addition to profile information, the monitoring program provides a basis for further action. In particular, the results are used to identify producers marketing animals with violative levels of residues. When such violations occur, the animals are subjected to surveillance sampling and testing until compliance is demonstrated. Other uses of data are to indicate incidences and levels of residue occurrence, to evaluate residue trends, and to identify problems within the industry for which educational or other corrective measures may be needed. Because of occasional laboratory limitations, some animals containing violative residues could pass into the food chain. The consequences to human health, however, are minimal as long as the violative rate is low.

Surveillance is designed to investigate and control the movement of potentially adulterated products. The sampling is biased to regional areas and is directed to particular carcasses or products in response to information from monitoring or other sources or from observations during antemortem or postmortem inspection.

The Environmental Protection Agency (EPA) and the Food and Drug Administration (FDA) establish the acceptable levels of residues (tolerances, maximum residue limits [MRLs]) for these compounds and the approved methods of use to ensure that tolerances are not exceeded. If formal tolerances are not established, the FDA and EPA recommend action levels to FSIS on request. A two-tiered system for compound assessment is used for monitoring residues. This system is based on the inherent toxicity of the compound and potential exposure in humans to residues.

PRACTICAL ASPECTS OF MONITORING AND SURVEILLANCE OF CHEMICAL RESIDUES

When examining the effect of residues, it is necessary to consider both short-term and longterm effects. The metabolic profile of the active metabolite under investigation must be available, all important metabolites should be listed, and depletion times from various tissues are required. Extralabel use of drugs can lead to residue problems. There is undoubtedly a need for guidelines to encourage good agricultural practice at the farm level and to highlight the problems that can result from misuse of medicines in animal production.

Overall a number of points must be borne in mind in any practical approach to the monitoring and surveillance of residues:

1. Establishment of withdrawal times
2. Establishment of MRLs
3. Validation of analytical methods
4. Laboratory quality assurance program and monitoring of analysts
5. Criteria used for evaluation of a compound specified
6. Statistical design criteria clearly stated
7. Establishment of education program that embodies preventive approaches
8. Preparation of detailed residue enforcement programs

14.2 MAXIMUM RESIDUE LIMITS AND TOLERANCES

Advances in analytical techniques have contributed to heightened awareness and concern about residues. Drugs can now be detected at extremely low concentrations—1000 or more times less than was possible 20 years ago. This has lead to a re-evaluation of the concept of "no detectable residues" in food. MRL is the maximum concentration of residue resulting from the use of a veterinary drug (expressed in milligrams or micrograms per kilogram on a fresh weight basis) that is recommended by the Codex Alimentarius Commission to be legally permitted or recognized as acceptable in or on a food.

The European Community definition of a maximum residue limit is virtually the same as that adopted by the FAO/World Health Organization (WHO) Codex Alimentarium Committee for Residues of Veterinary Drugs in Foods. Further, the overall approach to the safety evaluation of residues of veterinary medicinal products within the Community is similar to that employed by the Joint FAO/WHO Expert Committee on Food Additives (JECFA), which undertakes the safety evaluation of residues of veterinary medicines on behalf of the Codex Alimentarium.

The approach is based on the type and amount of residue considered to be without any toxicologic hazard for human health as expressed by the acceptable daily intake (ADI) or on a temporary ADI that uses an additional safety factor. It also takes into account other relevant public health risks as well as food technologic aspects and estimated food intakes.

When establishing a MRL, consideration is also given to residues that occur in food of plant origin or in the environment. Further, the MRL may be reduced to be consistent with good practices in use of veterinary drugs and to the extent that practical analytical methods are available.

MRLs must be proposed for the various edible tissues and produce in which residues of the substance concerned could occur. Proposals for MRLs should be based on the ADI of the substance established from safety studies. This evaluation of safety covers not only toxicologic properties, but also pharmacologic properties; possible allergenic potential; and, for antimicrobial substances, the possible effect of residues on the human gut flora. The ADI is defined as the quantity of residue that can be ingested daily over a lifetime without appreciable health risk. It is derived from the no observed effect level (NOEL) for the most sensitive parameter in the most sensitive appropriate test species:

ADI (mg/day) =

$$\frac{\text{NOEL (mg/kg body weight)} \times \text{Standard Human Weight (kg)}}{\text{Safety Factor}}$$

The MRLs set for individual tissues should reflect the relative distribution of residue between the tissues observed in residue studies, so practical withdrawal times can be set for products containing the active substance concerned. This is an important point that distinguishes the approach used to set MRLs in the European Community from the approach used by the US FDA to set residue tolerances. The FDA uses food consumption data and food factors in conjunction with the ADI to set safe concentrations of residues in edible tissues. This "safe concentration" or residue can be considered equivalent to a MRL.

TABLE 14–1 FOOD FACTOR BREAKDOWN OF A 1500-g DIET	
Edible Product	Food Factor
Cattle	
Milk	3
Muscle	1
Liver	$\frac{1}{2}$
Kidney	$\frac{1}{3}$
Fat	$\frac{1}{4}$
Swine	
Muscle	1
Liver	$\frac{1}{3}$
Kidney	$\frac{1}{4}$
Fat	$\frac{1}{4}$
Sheep	
Muscle	1
Liver	$\frac{1}{5}$
Kidney	$\frac{1}{5}$
Fat	$\frac{1}{5}$
Poultry	
Eggs	1
Muscle	1
Liver	$\frac{1}{3}$
Fat/skin	$\frac{1}{2}$

FDA METHOD—TOLERANCES

Food Factors

The FDA assumes that, at a maximum, muscle or eggs constitute 500 g of a 1500-g diet and that organ meats are consumed in lesser quantities. The FDA also assumes that milk may constitute the total diet of some individuals. These factors are summarized in Table 14–1.

Establishing Tolerance

The tolerance establishes the concentration of marker residue permitted in the target tissue of a treated animal. The target tissue and marker residue are selected so the absence of marker residue above a designated concentration confirms that each edible tissue has a concentration of total residue at or below its safe concentration. The FDA calculates the safe concentration for each edible tissue using the ADI, the weight in kilograms of an average adult (60 kg), the amount of the product eaten per day, and

the food consumption factor for the particular edible product. The ADI is obtained by dividing the NOEL from the results of toxicologic studies in the most sensitive species by an appropriate safety factor.

Safe Concentration =

$$\frac{\text{ADI } (\mu\text{g/kg/day}) \times 60 \text{ kg}}{\text{Food Factor} \times 500 \text{ g/day}}$$

Example of FDA Method

1. Calculation of ADI:
   NOEL: 0.25 mg/kg body weight
   Safety factor: 100
   ADI: 150 μg per person per day

2. FDA determination of safe concentration of total residue in cattle tissues:

	FOOD FACTOR	SAFE CONCENTRATION
Muscle	1.0	0.3 ppm
Liver	0.5	0.6 ppm
Kidney	0.33	0.9 ppm
Fat	0.25	1.2 ppm
Milk	3.0	0.1 ppm

Legal Limits

Violative residue levels are those that exceed the legal limits of tolerances for residues as set by the FDA and EPA. "Action levels" recommended by the FDA and EPA, although not supported by law, are used by the FDA in a discretionary manner to determine the safety of food when no tolerance exists for a compound.

Most limits for residues are set at the parts per million or parts per billion level. To date, any violative residue results have usually been near these limits. Residue limits are set with a margin of safety that is usually thousands of times more conservative than the point at which human health would be affected. One should not be complacent about a single violation, however, because there can be no certainty of the cumulative long-term health risks of longterm consumption of low levels of residues. The weight of the evidence suggests the risks are small, but they cannot be entirely ruled out.

EUROPEAN COMMUNITY SYSTEM—TOLERANCES

Elaboration of Proposed Maximum Residue Limits

1. Establish ADI.
2. To protect all segments of the population, intake data at the upper limit of the range for individual edible tissues and animal products should be used. The European Community has therefore used the following daily intake values: 300 g of meat (as muscle tissue), 100 g of liver, 50 g of kidney, 50 g of tissue fat, 100 g of egg, and 1.5 g of milk.
3. Establish kinetic parameters from aforementioned tissues.
4. Establish time interval from administration of drug until tissue residue levels are depleted to the ADI.
5. Add a safety span factor to take account of kinetic variables: e.g., age, sex, disease, status.

This safety factor usually has a value of 100 in the case of a NOEL derived from a longterm animal study, on the assumption that humans are 10 times as sensitive as the test animal used and that there is a tenfold range of sensitivity within the human population. There are times, however, when a safety factor of 100 is considered insufficient. Thus higher safety factors may be required when the data are incomplete; when the study in which the NOEL was established was inadequate (e.g., too few animals, no individual animal results); or when irreversible, especially teratogenic and carcinogenic, effects have been seen.

Because the ADI is related to body weight, a 60-kg average body weight has been internationally accepted. In addition, because any tolerance level for residues in various edible tissues is a function of the amount of food items consumed, an average daily consumption must be fixed. This has been agreed as 300 g meat, 100 g liver, 50 g kidney, 50 g fat, 2 eggs, and 1.5 liters of milk. A single ADI should be contained in these added items. Once an ADI has been established for a veterinary drug, it must be translated into tolerance levels. Any tolerance level for residues in various edible tissues is a function of the amount of food items consumed.

The MRLs for residues in various edible tissues and products are a function of the amount of food items consumed. Because data based on scientifically reliable surveys are difficult, if not impossible, to acquire, the arbitrary daily consumptions listed in Table 14–2 should be applied.

The individual MRLs in different tissues should also reflect the kinetics of the depletion of the residues to be consistent with the established withdrawal times. MRLs should be proposed in such a way that the total amount of residues ingested with 500 g meat *or* 500 g poultry *or* 300 g fish, *plus* 1500 g milk, *plus* 100 g egg, *plus* 20 g honey does not exceed the ADI.

The "withdrawal time," as usually defined by national licensing authorities, is the interval between the time of the last administration of a veterinary drug and the time when the animal can be safely slaughtered for food, or the milk or eggs can be safely consumed. After the MRL has been established for a named marker residue, the corresponding withdrawal time must be calculated such that the concentration of this residue in the target tissue falls with reasonable statistical certainty below it.

TABLE 14–2
DAILY FOOD CONSUMPTIONS

Large Animals		Poultry		Fish	
Muscle	300 g	Muscle	300 g	Muscle and skin in natural proportions	300 g
Liver	100 g	Liver	100 g		
Kidney	50 g	Kidney	10 g		
Fat	50 g*	Fat and skin in natural proportions	90 g		
	500 g				
Milk	1500 g	Egg	100 g		
Honey	20 g				

---

*For pigs, 50 g of fat and skin in natural proportions.

For residue monitoring purposes, it is essential to define a tolerance for a particular marker residue in a particular target tissue. In this way, the tolerance establishes the concentration of marker residue permitted in the target tissue. Although the ADI is related to any residue of toxicologic concern, the marker metabolite represents the preferable analyte for a residue assay method. A residue above the tolerance is deemed a "violative residue."

The target tissue is the edible tissue selected to monitor for the total residue in the target animal. The target tissue is usually, but not necessarily, the tissue with the slowest depletion rate of the residues. When a compound is to be used in lactating animals or laying birds, milk or eggs are target tissues in addition to the target tissue selected for residue monitoring in the edible carcass.

For residue monitoring purposes, it is frequently useful to define MRLs for a particular marker residue. A "marker residue" is a residue whose level decreases in a known relationship to the level of total residues in tissues, eggs, or milk. A specific quantitative analytical method for measuring the concentration of the residue with the required sensitivity must be available.

The MRL establishes the concentration of marker residue permitted in the target tissue. Marker residue and target tissue are selected in such a way that total residues in each edible tissue are at or below its safe concentration if the marker residue is at or below the MRLs. For milk or eggs, it may be necessary to select a marker residue that is different from the marker residue selected for the target tissue representing the edible carcass.

Withdrawal times should take into account not only the ADI and tolerance, but also pharmacokinetic data plus a safety factor to ensure tissue residue levels are well below the ADI or other appropriate safe figures. The question of drug metabolites and bound residues also arises in the context of tolerance establishment. Pharmacokinetics must be taken into account to calculate withdrawal times that will not allow the tissue tolerance level to be exceeded.

Problems of determining ADIs can readily be identified for allergenic drugs in sensitive persons (e.g., penicillins), if there also is a lack of data for other older drugs, and in the case of carcinogenic compounds. Dietary intake studies and tissue residue concentrations are critical for ADI and tolerance establishment.

14.3 FOOD SAFETY AND INSPECTION SERVICE RESIDUE TESTING SYSTEM

FSIS conducts three different types of residue testing programs.

ROUTINE MONITORING

The core of the current testing program is routine, nationwide sampling and analysis in FSIS or accredited laboratories. In 1990, only 0.3% of more than 41,000 samples analyzed in the routine monitoring program showed illegal residue levels. Statistically that means fewer than 1 out of each 100 animals marketed contained illegal residues and perhaps as few as 1 in 1000 animals.

The routine monitoring program provides the most meaningful residue statistics, first because the samples for analysis are randomly selected according to a statistical plan and second because they are nationwide.

The results from routine testing highlight potential problems, for which intensive testing may be necessary to protect the public. They also provide a good basis for long-term planning, helping the agencies to implement a total coordinated approach to residue control and prevention.

ENFORCEMENT OR SURVEILLANCE OF RESIDUE MONITORING

In the enforcement phase of testing, animals may be kept out of the food supply until regulatory test results confirm that they can be marketed or should be condemned, in whole or in part. Surveillance testing is biased toward resolving a specific problem. Surveillance testing, however, is not nationwide in scope; it is not random; and the amount of sampling and testing is determined pragmatically, not necessarily statistically.

Enforcement testing can be small-scale or widespread. It can be as isolated as one inspector noticing an injection blemish and holding the animal carcass until laboratory results verify the presence or absence of illegal residues. In such cases, inspection findings trigger enforcement testing.

Surveillance sampling can be as broad in scope as the U.S. nationwide program for sulfa compounds, in place since 1988 in the 100 largest hog-slaughtering plants. Monitoring results have helped to trigger this program, showing chronically unacceptable levels of sulfamethazine residues in swine over time. The FDA's changing view of the safety of sulfamethazine also intensified the need for strong regulatory action to deter violators, as did international concerns about sulfa that threatened US exports. See Chapters 12 and also 23.

COMPOUND EVALUATION SYSTEM

The compound evaluation system (CES) provides FSIS with a systematic approach for categorizing compounds with respect to the likelihood of their occurrence in meat and poultry and their potential impact on public health. In the United States, a hierarchical system of compound evaluation is used to rank a compound, and in this system, a number of points have to be considered:

1. The amount of actual or probable use of the compound
2. The conditions under which the compound will be used
3. The potential for misuse of the compound
4. Its metabolic pattern in animals and in the environment, including bioavailability
5. The acute and chronic toxicity data available

In ranking a compound for residue control stringency, the degree of hazard and period or duration of exposure are both considered (Table 14–3).

The CES addresses the risk of residues based on hazard (adverse effects that may be produced by a given compound) and exposure (residue level; factors affecting the residue level, such as withdrawal times; duration of or frequency of consumption of products containing residues of concern). The proposed system is a hierarchical system that classifies a given pesticide, animal drug, or contaminant in any of 16 categories. Compounds of greater concern carry a designation of "A1" (high health hazard potential, high likelihood residue occurrence); those compounds of least concern are designated "D4" (negligible health hazard potential, negligible likelihood of residue occurrence). The letter "Z" is used to indicate an element of the two value systems lacking the information needed for classification. Compound evaluation and ranking is a dynamic process. Additional compounds have to be considered in the system, and additional research on a compound's toxicity and its potential for leaving harmful residues may affect previous rankings.

TABLE 14–3
COMPOUND EVALUATION SYSTEM RANKING

Exposure is expressed on a *scale 1–4*
Hazard is expressed on a *scale A–D*

Grid Ranking

Hazard	Exposure			
	1	2	3	4
A	A1	A2	A3	A4
B	B1	B2	B3	B4
C	C1	C2	C3	C4
D	D1	D2	D3	D4

On this table, an *A1* classification would require *very* detailed assessment, whereas *D4* would be regarded as *not* requiring any great degree of scrutiny.

The assignment of a specific ranking is based on review of information entered into a comprehensive system of CES worksheets prepared for each compound evaluated. These worksheets provide a permanent record and chronology of the nature and extent of the technical and scientific data that were considered.

The selection of compounds for monitoring is based on the compound ranking assigned, whether a practical test method is available and is suitable for regulatory use, whether the compound is measurable in a multiresidue method, and whether monitoring or other experience shows that adulterated residues are present.

Monitoring triggers surveillance within 14 days. When an injection site is seen postmortem, an inspector-generated sample is taken. The carcass is retained. If chloramphenicol violations are found on monitoring, all the meat products are recalled. Pretesting of animals is carried out if surveillance indicates that violations are occurring. In cattle, pretesting of tissue is carried out (e.g., fat biopsy), whereas in poultry, a random tissue sample selected by the inspector is taken.

EXPLORATORY PROJECTS

Exploratory testing may be conducted for many reasons directed at strengthening the residue regulatory program as a whole. For example, exploratory testing may gather more information about:

1. The prevalence of a residue for which no safe limits have yet been established (such as trace metals)
2. A residue being considered for inclusion in the monitoring plan
3. The usefulness of new methods and approaches to monitoring

Currently data from exploratory testing are not used to take regulatory action. Exploratory projects are also conducted on a limited scale to provide information on studying the occurrence of residues for which no safe limits have been established or for evaluating new methods and approaches to monitoring.

When an animal leaves its farm of origin, it may be sold through a dealer to a producer group and then again to another factory supplier. FSIS now requires all slaughter plants to maintain records of the ownership of animals for a 30-day period immediately preceding slaughter. (In poultry, only 5 to 10% of residue violations are untraceable.)

FOOD SAFETY AND INSPECTION SERVICE RESIDUE CAPABILITY

A minimum of three laboratories is needed to verify the method used in residue analysis. (EPA methods do not require multilaboratory validation). Research is constantly conducted for new methods, and the CES forms the basis for this research. Methods are described in terms of levels of use:

Level 1: These are assays with the highest level of credibility. They determine both the concentration and the identity of the analyte.

Level 2: These assays are used to determine the qualitative concentration of an analyte or information on the structural formulation.

Level 3: These are screening methods carried out in plants and are semiquantitative positive-negative-type assays.

Contract laboratories supplement the analytical capabilities when this is deemed appropriate.

The field service laboratory division of FSIS is involved in the monitoring program. For surveillance analysis, accredited laboratories may be used. In the accredited laboratory program, there are 300 nonfederal laboratories. Of these, 225 are accredited for food chemistry analysis, e.g., for moisture, protein, fat, and salt, whereas 75 are accredited for residues, e.g., chlorinated hydrocarbons, polychlorinated biphenols, arsenicals, sulfonamides, and nitrosamines. These laboratories must meet standards of quality assurance.

For food chemistry inspection, the processing plant pays the accredited laboratory. This ensures a quicker result. Samples may also be sent to the federal laboratories at no expense, but this takes longer. Laboratories are reappraised to check on staff, equipment, and technical expertise regularly. They must demonstrate proficiency using blind samples, and check samples are used to monitor the accredited laboratories against the federal laboratories. A bimonthly check of laboratories involved in residues is done for each of the specific residues for which accreditation is given. Such laboratories are accredited each year. If a problem occurs, however, the accreditation is lost, and proficiency must be redemonstrated.

14.4 RAPID TESTS

The advent of rapid, easy-to-use screening tests has revolutionized surveillance programs and is in large measure responsible for the dramatic downturn in sulfa violations. A new emphasis has been placed on rapid screening tests. These take place in the slaughter plant. The carcass may be retained pending results of a qualitative test.

Among the rapid tests used are the following:

1. **Swab Test On Premises (STOP)**. This test is carried out on kidney samples and is conducted overnight. It is a microbial inhibition assay.
2. **Calf Antibiotic and Sulfa Test (CAST)**. This is an overnight kidney test using different media in agar.
3. **Live Animal Swab Test (LAST)**. This test is carried out on the urine of live animals and is a microbial-type test.
4. **Sulfa-On-Site (SOS) test**. This test detects sulfonamides using animal urine or blood. Urine is preferred because it requires no preparation, whereas blood serum must be separated from red blood cells and proteins. Urine concentrations are approximately 12 times those of muscle and 4 times those of liver and kidneys for sulfonamides. This test can be completed in 30 to 40 minutes.
5. **Card test for chloramphenicol**. This is an immunologic-based test sensitive to 5 ppb (μg/kg) in tissue and urine. It is used in conjunction with chemical assays at present.

The first rapid test, STOP, was developed and introduced in 1980. It screens for the presence of antibiotics in a swab sample from the kidney of an animal carcass. Originally used only for "cull" dairy cows, STOP is now used with all species. Since 1985, well over 200,000 in-plant STOP analyses have been conducted, leading to laboratory confirmation of more than 8000 violations and subsequent condemnation of carcasses or tissues. Antibiotics are a persistent, continuing concern, particularly in bob veal calves and cull dairy cows. In 1989, 85,083 samples were analyzed using STOP, and 2937 violations were confirmed in the laboratory.

CAST is a rapid test designed for in-plant use with bob veal calves (those weighing less than 150 pounds under 3 weeks of age). Uniquely, positive CAST results support immediate condemnation decisions. CAST was first implemented in 1984. In 1989,

175,427 CAST analyses were performed, and 4599 violations were confirmed based on those tests.

The (SOS) test (a thin-layer chromotography test) screens for the presence of sulfa compounds in urine. Laboratory confirmation in muscle tissue is required for condemnation, but SOS enables FSIS inspectors to screen large numbers of samples in the plant. In 1989, 116,726 samples were analyzed using SOS; 318 violations were confirmed in the laboratory. In recent years using SOS, sulfa violations have come down to an all-time low (from 13 to 1%).

Rapid tests have helped to extend analytical capability dramatically over the last 10 years. In 1979, FSIS could test for only about 55 different compounds; in 1989, tests were available for 120 compounds; and in 1990, tests were available for 133 compounds. Since 1985, FSIS inspectors have conducted well over 1 million analyses using in-plant rapid tests.

The rapid tests and certain laboratory tests are multiresidue tests that detect or rule out several compounds at once. This means that although the domestic regulatory program included 428,000 samples, those samples actually represented about 1.5 million analyses. If residue results for imports were included, the total would be even higher.

A tremendous amount of scientific analysis, time, money, and labor goes into the development and validation of any new method. Also, some drugs are easier to test for than others.

In addition, types of detection methods are always evolving. Gene probes, for instance, hold great promise for residue methods development. It is unlikely that one will find a perfect regulatory test that is rugged, practical, simple, rapid, and cheap; at the moment, however, there are several that meet many of those criteria.

Of critical importance, however, is the fact that even though there are many compounds to which an animal may theoretically be exposed, many of those compounds are known to be of little hazard to public health, or they simply do not leave a residue that can be detected in animal tissue. Tests must be prioritized to look for compounds that would be of significant public health concern if a residue occurred, and this is done based on usual risk assessment procedures.

Antimicrobial properties become the determining factor in safety evaluation when the toxicity of the substances to be considered (e.g., tetracyclines, beta lactam antibiotics) is so low that their residues in food could, from the toxicologic viewpoint, be tolerated even at the height of therapeutically effective tissue concentrations, i.e., without any withdrawal period.

At the microbiologic level, concern for food safety is centered on the question of whether or not residues of antimicrobial agents ingested by way of food of animal origin pose a danger to human health by exerting a selective pressure on the intestinal flora and thus favoring the growth of microorganisms with natural or acquired resistance.

Finally one must remember that testing is not the whole story of residue control. It is an important regulatory aid in a comprehensive control and prevention program, but it is only an aid. Judicious use of pesticides and animal drugs, industry accountability for residue control systems, research, and education are other important ancillary aids.

SOME ANTIMICROBIAL ASSAY TESTS

Antibacterial Residues

The SOS test is a thin-layer chromatography (TLC) method. Samples and standard solutions are spotted onto a plate coated with absorbent material. The plate is placed in a shallow depth of solvent that migrates up the plate. Compounds are visualized, after drying the plate, by spraying with a fluorescent compound, fluorescamine. After 15 to 20 minutes of development in the dark, sulfonamides are seen as fluorescent spots when viewed under ultraviolet light.

Microbiologic Methods

A number of microbiologic methods are available, which rely on the fact that in the presence of antibiotic bacterial growth is inhibited. Such assay methods therefore detect only active antibiotic residues but not inactive metabolites. The most common format is an indicator system that monitors how well the test sample inhibits the growth of an organism.

Diffusion tests include the following:

LAST—*Bacillus subtilis*
STOP—*B. subtilis*
CAST—*Bacillus megaterium*
Sulfonamide swab test (SST)

The colorimetric test is used by dairies to test milk received for antibiotic residues. This test uses *Streptococcus thermophilus var. calidolactis* (DELVO P and DELVO S test). This is a standard diffusion test designed to detect antibiotic residues in milk. It measures the growth inhibition of *Bacillus stearothemophilus var. calidolactis* in a solid medium. For penicillin, the reported detection limits are 0.003 to 0.005 IU/ml. Addition of beta-lactamase or para-aminobenzoic acid identifies penicillins or sulfonamides.

Immunologic Tests and Binding Assays

SPOT Test for Antibiotics in milk. One type of binding test, which uses monoclonal antibodies bound to latex particles for detection of antibiotics in milk, is the SPOT test. The end point is agglutination of the latex particles. The test gives results in 6 minutes and is sufficiently sensitive to detect low levels of antibiotics. It is suitable for use on the farm or in the dairy.

Binding Assays. Assays based on competition for a limited number of binding sites, between the substance to be measured in a sample and a labeled compound, have been used in clinical medicine for more than 20 years. The label used may be an enzyme, for example, in enzyme-linked immunosorbent assays (ELISAs). Such types of assays offer the advantages of sensitivity, specificity, and high sample throughput. Immunoassay technology has gained rapid acceptance in veterinary and human medicine owing to its high performance capabilities and versatility in applications, such as the diagnosis of disease, the assessment of immune status, the detection of contaminants and residues, and the monitoring of reproductive status.

First, reactants in the test sample and the assay must be brought together so the an-

tigen-antibody reactions can occur. In addition, one component of the assay must have an enzyme attached to provide a marker for the extent of the antigen-antibody reaction. Finally, a substrate chromogen system suitable for the particular enzyme must be provided to allow quantification of the extent of the antigen-antibody reaction.

E-Z Screen Card Tests (Quik-Cards). The E-Z Screen Card tests, from Enzyme Diagnostics, Inc. are simple, on-farm tests based on ELISA techniques. Tests for a number of compounds, including penicillin, chloramphenicol, neomycin, gentamicin, tylosin, sulfadimethoxime, and sulfamethazine, have been developed. The tests are performed on a small card, the Quik-Card, which is impregnated with the appropriate antibody. A control port is included, so the operator can check that the test has been properly performed. The tests are rapid; results are obtained in less than 10 minutes.

Beta Lactam LacTek. This test is based on the immunobinding principles of an ELISA system.

Receptor Assays

Charm Test. Charm assays are quantitative, accommodate any requirement easily, and detect eight families of antibiotics as well as aflatoxins. Additionally, Charm Systems perform the multipurpose Charm ABC (Activity Bacteria Count) for microbial counts in raw milk (8 minutes), shelf-life prediction (18 to 27-hour incubation, 8 minute assay), and hygiene monitoring of surfaces and containers (2 minutes). Other Charm assays include the 4-minute Charm Alkaline Phosphatase Test and the Charm Pesticide Test for multiple families of pesticides (15 minutes).

An assay for beta lactam antibiotics in milk, using the principle of binding to microbial receptor sites, which can give results in 6 minutes, has been developed (Charm I). Charm tests can accurately measure residues to the MRL. The FDA's Center for Veterinary Medicine is to carry out a limited evaluation of the Charm II test for sulfonamide residues in raw milk. The evaluation will be conducted at the same time as, but independent of, a method trial of a multiresidue high-pressure-liquid-chromatography (HPLC)-based method of analysis for eight sulfa drugs: sulfadiazine, sulfamethazine, sulfathiazole, sulfadimethoxine, sulfaquinoxaline, sulfamerazine, sulfachloropyridazine, and sulfapyridine.

Charm Farm Assay. According to the manufacturer of the assay, the lower limits of detection for this assay are 2.5 to 100 ppb for beta lactam antibiotics, 20 to 150 ppb for tetracycline, 50 to 1000 ppb for aminoglycosides, 50 to 200 ppb for macrolides, and 30 to 150 ppb for sulfonamides.

Beta Lactam CITE Probe. This assay system is based on binding of the beta lactam antibiotic by a penicillin-binding protein on a membrane matrix. According to the manufacturer, the assay detects beta lactam antibiotic residues in milk at varying levels: 5 ppb for penicillin, 10 ppb for ampicillin, 100 ppb for cloxacillin, 5 ppb for cephapirin, 10 ppb for ceftiofur, and 10 ppb for amoxicillin. The beta lactam CITE Probe system employs a penicillin-binding protein on a membrane matrix, whereas the tetracycline CITE Probe test kit uses a tetracycline-binding antibody on a membrane matrix.

Enzyme Assays

The Penzym Parlor Mate Test is a kinetic enzyme test that can be completed in 20 minutes. Bacterial cell wall enzymes, which are inhibited by the presence of beta lactam antibiotics, are used. The test is a qualitative screening test for all beta lactam antibiotics. The end point of the test is a color change, yellow indicating the presence of antibiotics and orange/pink their absence.

14.5 WORK OF CODEX ALIMENTARIUS COMMITTEE ON RESIDUES OF VETERINARY DRUGS

The Codex Alimentarium Commission was established by the FAO and WHO to develop international standards for foods of animal origin, to oversee and protect the health of the consumer, to ensure fair practices in international trade, and to harmonize requirements facilitating trade.

The Codex Committee on Residues of Veterinary Drugs in Foods (CCRVDF) is the most recently established Codex committee. It held its first session in 1986 and is hosted annually by the United States. The CCRVDF was established on the recommendation of a Codex Joint Expert Consultation, set up to examine the question of veterinary residues in food. The Joint Expert Consultation concluded that this was a complex, worldwide question that causes significant public health and consumer concern. It recommended that a committee be set up to consider the question of residues of veterinary drugs in food and specifically to address the following issues:

1. To examine the problems associated with residues in foods arising from the use of veterinary drugs and other chemicals in food-producing animals
2. To advise the Codex Alimentarium commission on how to consider these problems
3. To examine the ways and means of regulating control
4. To suggest priority criteria for substances to be considered
5. To establish international guidelines regarding the use of drugs in food animals, acceptable residue levels, and principles of regulatory clearance.

The new committee establishes a list of drugs for priority review, recommends MRLs, develops codes of practice, and looks into analytical methods used in the control of veterinary drug residues. It liaises with a number of other, longer established Codex committees with which it has areas of common interest. These include the committees on food additives, analysis and sampling, and food hygiene. For the purpose outlined, the term "veterinary drug" was defined as any substance applied or administered to food-producing animals, including meat-producing or milk-producing animals, poultry, or fish, whether used for therapeutic, prophylactic, or diagnostic purposes or for the modification of physiologic function or behavior.

The growing challenge to secure wholesome food of animal origin in quantities sufficient to feed the increasing world population leads to the compelling need to search for new means of enhancing productivity in animal husbandry systems. This often involves the use of pharmacologically and toxicologically potent substances. Many drugs are administered to increasingly large herds or flocks during a significant portion of their life span (coccidiostats) or at the height of milk production (anthelmintics), during growth phases (antibiotics, anabolic agents), or shortly before slaughter (tranquilizers, antibiotics, beta blockers). Public concern over the presence of drug residues in edible products of food-producing animals has reached unprecedented heights. In many countries, product licensing and approval for products for use in food animals has been a high priority, and legislation restricting or prohibiting the use and application of certain substances has been introduced. At present, neither the principles nor the actual process of safety evaluation of animal drugs or their residues has been scientifically clearly defined or internationally accepted. Hence certain countries have banned the use of specific compounds, whereas other countries on the basis of scientific criteria have permitted the continued use of similar products (e.g., growth promoters are banned in the European Community and permitted in the United States and Australia).

The most certain way to avoid any potential deleterious health effects of residues would be the avoidance of residues themselves, and many countries have adopted the stance of "zero residue" concepts. This concept, however, is scientifically untenable insofar as detection of residues is a function of the sensitivity of the analytical method used. Production of food free of residues is a practical impossibility, and this objective could be achieved only by abandoning the use of therapeutic agents altogether. The alternative is to attempt to define acceptable residue levels in foodstuffs based on their pharmacologic, toxicologic, microbiologic, and immunopathologic hazard potential.

Analytical methods currently used for many of these residues are expensive HPLC methods. Recent developments include ELISA-based quick-card tests. These are quick economic screening tests for use in meat, milk, and eggs, and greater emphasis should be placed on developing ELISA methods for residues of other compounds. Substances for which suitable analytical methods have not been developed should be withdrawn from use in food animals. The availability of reliable analytical methods for screening, identification, and quantification is urgently needed. Common reagents and standard reference materials containing residue concentrations of given drugs at or near the agreed MRLs should be made available. New data on residues of veterinary drugs and training of analysts should receive high priority.

METHODS OF ANALYSIS AND SAMPLING

The Codex committee is also concerned with standardizing analytical methods dealing with the development of criteria, elaborating methods of analysis and sampling, and identifying useful analytical methods. This obviously relates to commercial test kits for information regarding performance characteristics of such procedures, commercial availability of necessary reagents, and the role of standard reference materials for the validation of analytical methods for compounds of priority interest. There is considerable international agreement that publishing methods of analysis for compounds of interest is an important consideration in the Codex committee's activities, to minimize drug residues in food animals.

Classes of analytical methods have been drawn up as follows:

- Methods suitable for routing use in enforcement of tolerances
- Nonroutine methods suitable for enforcement
- Methods suitable for enforcement only at residue levels above the tolerance
- Methods for which additional analysis is required to support regulatory action
- Nonroutine methods suitable for determining whether or not a residue problem exists

Screening and quantitative methods are identified as two further categories.

SCREENING METHODS

The most important aspect of performance is that the incidence of false-negative results at the level of interest must be minimal.

CONFIRMATORY METHODS

Specificity

As far as possible, confirmatory methods must provide unambiguous information on the chemical structure of the analyte. Quality control factors are essential in any laboratory procedure to ensure features such as (1) accuracy, (2) specificity, (3) precision, (4) sensitivity, and (5) limit of decision.

Radioimmunoassay (RIA) is used as the optimum method for screening of samples for hormonal or other residues of antibiotics. Advantages are high specificity, which allows direct measurement of the antigen in the presence of much higher concentrations of accompanying substances, e.g., serum proteins, and high sensitivity, which allows levels of f- 10-5gr of a substance to be detected. RIA and ELISA are similar methods that have a useful scope in meat analysis.

HPLC and TLC are used particularly for:

1. Analysis of pellet material
2. Residues of sulfonamides in porcine urine
3. As a cleanup step in analysis of injection sites for hormone cocktails.

Analytical Criteria

Methods of analysis should be specified. These are needed to detect, quantify, and identify positively residues of veterinary drugs; support toxicologic, drug metabolism, and pharmacokinetic studies; support residue studies of compounds to be evaluated; and satisfy the needs of public health agencies. The performance of analytical methods should be assessed, as appropriate, according to some or all of the following criteria:

1. **Assay sensitivity**. Any assay procedure must be sufficiently sensitive to monitor a component or components of the total drug residue down to a level at which the safety of edible products for human consumption is assured. This is a measure of the ability of a method to discriminate between small differences in analyte content.
2. **Accuracy**. The accuracy procedure must be highly selective or specific for the designated compound. Specificity is the ability of a given method to respond only to the substance being measured.
3. **Specificity**. The assay procedure must be highly selective or specific for the designated compound. Specificity is the ability of a given method to respond only to the substance being measured. The incidence of false-negative and false-positive results should be minimal.
4. **Reliability**. Any assay procedure must give reasonably reproducible results when performed by different analysts in different laboratories. The repeatability of the measurement denotes the closeness with which the measurement approaches the average during a series of measurements made under similar conditions. Repetitive measurements must ensure analytical precision and reproducible results both within a laboratory and from different laboratories.
5. **Practicability and ruggedness**. Reagents and instrumentation used for the assay procedure should be readily available. The method's performance must not be adversely affected by minor deviations from the well-described procedural assay steps.
6. **Validation**. Positive results require further examination by validated quantitative methods. Confirmatory techniques are used to provide unequivocal proof of the presence of the suspected drug residue.
7. **Precision**. This is the closeness of agreement between the results obtained by applying the experimental procedure several times under prescribed conditions.
8. **Repeatability**. This is the closeness of agreement between mutually independent test results obtained under repeatability conditions.
9. **Reproducibility**. This is the closeness of agreement between mutually indepen-

dent test results obtained under reproducibility conditions, i.e., with the same
method on identical test material in different laboratories with different operators using different equipment.
10. **Limit of detection**. The smallest measured content from which it is possible
to deduce the presence of the analyte
with reasonable statistical certainty is
the limit of detection. This is the lowest
analyte content for which the method
has been validated with specified degrees of accuracy and repeatability.
11. **Susceptibility to interference**. For all
experimental conditions that could in
practice be subject to fluctuation (e.g.,
stability of reagents, composition of the
sample, pH, temperature), any variations that could affect the analytical result should be indicated.

The typical approach to development of
suitable residue assay methods involves extraction, purification, and measurement
procedures. Purification systems include
liquid extraction, column chromatography,
and TLC. Measurement systems include gas
liquid chromatography, HPLC, fluorome-
try, spectrophotometry, and RIA. Microbiologic assays are used for routine measurement of antimicrobial drug residues.
Structures of metabolites can be determined
by mass spectrometry.

With reference to analyses and tolerances, the Codex committee has agreed that
any acceptable international format should
include:

1. Name of the veterinary drug
2. ADI for the drug
3. Commodity, e.g., beef muscle
4. Definition of the residue on which the
tolerance was set
5. Recommended method of analysis

CODE OF PRACTICE FOR USE OF VETERINARY DRUGS

The Codex committee has also introduced
a code of practice for use of veterinary
drugs that is directed to farmers. If necessary, a second part of the code specifically
advising veterinarians will be elaborated.
The Codex code covers all aspects relating
to good animal husbandry and veterinary

practice geared to minimize residues. The
code encourages:

- Proper use of veterinary drugs
- Limitation of the use of drugs in animals
to the necessary extent to minimize residue formation
- Reduction of unavoidable residues to safe
and, if appropriate, the lowest possible
levels

During the Second Session of the
CCRVDF, in October 1987, it was decided
that it would be useful to establish a code
of practice for approval of veterinary drugs
to guarantee, in particular, that the established MRLs not be exceeded. The preparation of this code of practice is based on:

- A procedure of approval of veterinary
drugs intended to evaluate objectively the
technical and scientific data relative to the
quality, efficacy, and safety of the veterinary drugs. Likewise, it should allow the
determination of the MRLs that should be
respected at the time of the authorized use
of veterinary drugs.
- A procedure for authorization of manufacturing that ensures that manufacturing
is carried out according to the rules of
good manufacturing practices.

Good practice in the use of veterinary
drugs, as defined by the CCRVDF, is the
official recommended or authorized usage,
including withdrawal periods, approved by
national authorities, of veterinary drugs under practical conditions. The MRL for veterinary drugs may be reduced to be consistent with good practice in use of veterinary
drugs. The MRL for veterinary drugs is
based on the type and amount of residue
considered to be without toxicologic hazard
for human health while taking into account
other relevant public health risks as well as
food technologic aspects. Veterinary products (including premixes for manufacture of
medicated feeding stuffs) used in food-producing animals should be administered (or
incorporated into feed) in compliance with
the relevant product information approved
by national authorities or in accordance
with a prescription or instruction issued by
a qualified veterinarian.

In addition to the specifics already outlined, the Codex committee is addressing
the following major issues:

1. Use of veterinary drugs for prophylactic and therapeutic purposes
2. Use for growth promotion
3. Safety evaluation of residues: bound residues and problems in evaluation of residues
4. Analytical methods for veterinary drug residues
5. Regulatory control of residues

GUIDELINES FOR ESTABLISHMENT OF A REGULATORY CONTROL PROGRAM

The Codex is agreed that such guidelines would be beneficial to countries with the ultimate objective of establishing food control programs. The basic elements of the current US philosophy are as follows:

- The country must have a basic food law for residue control and regulatory controls regarding production, distribution, and use of veterinary drugs.
- The country must demonstrate a capacity for regulatory enforcement.
- Proper surveillance and monitoring programs must be established.
- The residue control program must have analytical capacity and proficiency to detect compounds at or below prescribed tolerance levels using reliable analytical techniques.
- Tolerance levels must be determined from the ADI rather than on the limit of the sensitivity of the analytical techniques.
- Tolerances must be established in accordance with international trading conditions.

As regards mutually acceptable analytical methods, there is an urgent need to make available reliable analytical techniques for screening, identification, and quantification. Common reagents and standard reference materials containing residue concentrations of given drugs at or near the agreed MRLs must be made available if international harmonization is to be achieved.

OTHER IMPORTANT CONCERNS FOR CODEX

The use of fixed-dosage combination products should be examined from the veterinary viewpoint and from the viewpoint of clearance and residue toxicology (potentiation). Further attention should be paid to interactions between veterinary drugs and other components present in feed, drinking water, or both (e.g., sulfonamides, tetracyclines, and nitrite).

In various countries, different safety evaluation procedures are applied concerning the teratogenic, carcinogenic, and mutagenic properties of substances. In some countries, a distinction is made between tumor-promoting and genotoxic compounds (i.e., epigenetic or genotoxic). An international forum is needed to identify these problems and establish a philosophy for use or nonuse in food animals.

Because the residues of many commonly used drugs (e.g., nitrofurans, benzimidazoles, nitroimidazoles) in edible products are covalently bound and therefore persistently present after medication has stopped, attention should be paid to the toxicologic significance of covalently bound material with respect to the human consumption of edible products.

International harmonization is required on the criteria on the basis of which residue tolerance levels can be set. Starting points are toxicity of the parent compound and metabolites, good agricultural and veterinary practice, and availability of analytical detection methods. Enforcement of these tolerance levels should be performed by supervising the observance of withdrawal times (administrative) and by detecting residues in practice.

More methods for the analysis of residues of veterinary drugs are needed. Although the routine meat inspection test for residues of antibiotics is performed through the Microbiological Sarcina Lutea Test, in other countries more extensive microbiologic testing systems are applied to improve the sensitivity as well as the scope of the method.

For chemotherapeutic agents, however, it is essential to develop chemical-analytical methods to detect those drugs and metabolites for which the microbiologic test is not applicable or not sensitive enough. Other chemical methods can be used for specific (confirmatory) analysis of antibiotics or chemotherapeutic agents. Groups of substances for which the microbiologic analysis is not effective are nitrofurans, nitroimidazoles, chloramphenicol, benzimidazoles, polyether antibiotics, and tetracyclines (<50 µg/kg). In poultry meat, this also applies to coccidiostats, although there seems to be no suitable microbiologic methods for the detection of these drugs in eggs.

When monitoring residues, it is important that the correct target organ or the correct body fluid is examined. In this target sample, the residue concentration is highest, and the observance of withdrawal periods can be controlled most effectively. If the relation between the concentrations in the various body fluids and tissues is known, the presence of residues in edible parts may be predicted. Further, it is essential to monitor the proper target compound. From the viewpoint of efficiency, groups of substances should be examined rather than each individual compound. In this way, the costs of testing are kept as low as possible, and a wide range of compounds may be monitored. Therefore multiple methods need to be developed at a low sensitivity level (1 to 100 µg/kg) for residues of veterinary drugs and the important metabolites.

The ongoing work of Codex relates to a number of key areas, including the following:

1. Survey of intake studies of drugs on agreed priority list (to establish ADI)
2. Report of working groups reviewing current methods of analysis and sampling
3. Report of working groups on definitions for good practice in the use of veterinary drugs
4. Report of working groups on glossary of terms and definitions on all areas relating to residues
5. Consideration of data pertaining to acceptable residue levels, for old and new compounds

Committee meetings will be held annually, and regular reports will be produced. Drugs given priority will be reviewed by a scientific committee (JECFA), and formal recommendations will be put to the following Codex committee meeting. Although problem drugs constitute the principal area of the committee's business, Codex hopes to involve itself nonetheless in other areas, such as the eventual develop-

ment of an international drug registration system, the adoption of internationally acceptable scientific guidelines, and lists of approved international drugs for use in food animals. Although member countries are not obliged to adopt the Codex committee's recommendations at a national level, it is hoped that they will. Hence the findings of the committee on the initial priority list (e.g., hormones, chloramphenicol) may impinge on legislation within approach to drug residue avoidance and believes that all matters relating to veterinary drug regulatory clearance, withdrawal times, ADIs, and tolerances must always be based solely on impeccable scientific criteria.

14.6 SPECIFIC DRUG RESIDUE CONCERNS

In 1986, the United States recommended that priority consideration by the First Session of the CCRVDF should be given to the use of anabolic agents for meat production. The ban, implemented in January 1988 by the European Economic Community on use of hormones as growth promotants, would create a serious nontariff trade barrier to the European Community's importation of US meat and meat products derived from animals treated with these products. The United States recommended that, in addition to hormones, priority consideration at the First Session of the CCRVDF be given to additional animal drugs because each has unresolved safety concerns that could become trade barriers to exports or imports. The first Codex priority list was drawn up to include the following compounds:

Sulfonamides
Nitrofurans
Nitroimidazoles (dimetridazole, metronidazole, ronidazole)
Quinoxalines (carbadox, olaquindox)
Trypanocides
Benzimidazoles (albendazole)
Oxytetracycline
Beta lactam antibiotics
Ivermectin

This list has received considerable attention from Codex regarding MRLs and whether certain of these drugs should continue in use. Establishing a list of compounds that should not be licensed for use in veterinary medicine has been considered. Such a list could include, for instance, stilbenes and chlorinated hydrocarbons. It is important to arrive on a worldwide agreement, especially for substances that have an environmental impact. Teratogenic and carcinogenic compounds could be in this list as well. Although it might be difficult to enforce this listing on a worldwide basis because conditions vary in different countries, requiring an accurate risk/benefit analysis, nonetheless as an interim measure a list of banned or restricted drugs from individual countries has been circulated to members of the Codex Alimentarium.

ALBENDAZOLE

Albendazole was selected as a priority drug for evaluation because:

1. Use of the drug may give rise to residues in meat or offal.
2. Concern has been raised about the possible carcinogenicity of this drug.
3. International trade could be affected.
4. The manufacturers were prepared to present an extensive toxicology data package to JECFA.

QUINOXALINES: CARBADOX

Although used in Europe and many other countries for *Escherichia coli* scour in pigs and for swine dysentry, taking account of the number of alternative drugs available, there is hardly any necessity of application of carbadox as therapeutic agent.

Toxicity

Prolonged administration of carbadox to rats causes toxic effects in the liver. Carbadox induces mutagenic effects in various strains of microorganisms, *Drosophila*, and mice. Metabolites have a much lower toxic potency than the parent compound. Although relay-toxicity studies in rats (three generations) did not show any harmful effects, formation of dust during the production of premixes and complete feeds should be avoided.

Methods of Analysis

For carbadox, the situation is similar to furazolidone; the parent compound apparently is no criterion for the residue profile, owing to the short half-life. Analytical methods for carbadox and the final metabolite quinoxaline acid in meat have been described.

The United States considers carbadox to be a suspect carcinogen and a 70 day withdrawal time has been applied, with a zero tolerance. It has not been banned in the United States, but was banned in 1986 in the United Kingdom, and is still permissible under the European Community Feed Additive Directive. The United Kingdom has reintroduced carbadox but with strict label directions to avoid contact with this mutagen. Withdrawal times for this drug in Europe are long to minimize consumer hazard.

NITROFURANS: FURAZOLIDONE AND FURALTADONE

Application

Gram-positive and gram-negative bacteria, some fungi, and protozoa are sensitive to nitrofurans, particularly furazolidone and furaltadone. *Pseudomonas* are noted for their resistance. These substances are predominantly used for enteritis, especially salmonellosis. These agents may well be phased out over the next few years—they are old drugs, and a paucity of toxicologic data exists.

Nitrofurans are carcinogenic and mutagenic compounds. If furazolidone is applied, the parent compound is metabolized relatively fast and eliminated, whereas covalent residues of furazolidone metabolites can remain present in edible products for a long time. Therefore the use of this group of substances in food-producing animals should perhaps be reconsidered. Nitrofurans are now being prohibited except for topical use.

Methods of Analysis

For furazolidone, a FAST-LC screening method is available for milk, meat, and eggs with a sensitivity of 10 µg/kg. Further, confirmatory methods for positive screening samples exist. Research of the metabolism of furazolidone in pigs is being carried out simultaneously with the development of analytical methods for the determination of metabolites. These analytical methods can be applied for other nitrofurans, with a somewhat lower sensitivity for furaltadone.

Many 5-nitrofurans exhibit mutagenic activity in a variety of bacterial and eukaryotic test systems. In bacteria, reduction of the 5-nitro group is essential for the mutagenicity of these substances. The relative mutagenic properties of individual members depend largely on the nature of the substituent at the 2-position of the furan ring. Several nitrofurans have been investigated for their carcinogenic potential in chronic bioassays. From the results of such studies, it was concluded that nitrofurans can produce tumors in experimental animals and must be assumed as potential human carcinogens.

The available toxicologic data do not allow a threshold level to be established without carcinogenic risk, and residues of intact nitro-group-containing substances should be tolerated only at the lowest possible level. The FDA's has decided to withdraw existing NADAs for nitrofurans. The FDA ban does not extend to furazolidone-based or nitrofurazone-based products that are administered topically.

From in vivo studies, it can be concluded that furazolidone is rapidly and almost completely metabolized on oral administration to piglets. A major part of the residual 14C proved to be nonextractable from the tissues. This nonextractable 14C is probably not the result of endogenous incorporation of 14C in natural compounds but more likely the result of covalent binding of reaction intermediate(s) of furazolidone to macromolecules. From in vitro studies using swine liver microsomes, evidence has been obtained showing that the open chain acrylonitrile plays a central role in the reductive biotransformation of furazolidone.

As previously mentioned, the FDA's decision to withdraw approval of furazolidone, nitrofurazone, and other nitrofurans in food-producing animals does not affect topical preparations. Other approved nitrofuran products labeled for topical use in companion animals and for intrauterine use in horses are specifically excluded from extralabel use. The storage or use on dairy farms of any nitrofuran drug except the approved cattle topicals constitutes a violation of the regulations.

Regulatory authorities worldwide recommend that the pharmaceutical industry be required to develop validated analytical methods sensitive to residue levels at or below 1 μg/kg and to provide a complete review of toxicologic data. Thereafter a reassessment of the use of nitrofurans in veterinary medicine should be undertaken. At present, methods with sensitivity of less than 5 ppb must be used. The decision of future licensing of furazolidone will be based on the recommendations of the WHO/FAO JECFA.

ANTIBIOTICS—GENERAL CONSIDERATIONS

The necessity of application of antibiotics, based on therapeutic considerations, can be absolute (no alternative) and relative (the substance is more effective than its alternative). The necessity of treatment of infections exists in view of public health and animal disease control. The necessity of nontreatment exists if the occurrence of harmful residues, as a result of the treatment, is inevitable.

CHLORAMPHENICOL

This agent is banned in the United States for use in food animals but is permitted in other countries (for bone marrow damage or aplastic anemia).

Application

Gram-positive bacteria, rickettsiae, and the viruses of the psittacosis-lymphogranuloma group are sensitive to this drug. It is specifically used for infections with staphylococci, streptococci, shigellae, *Pseudomonas*, *Pasteurella*, *E. coli*, and salmonellae.

Chloramphenicol is still approved in some countries for use in food animals to treat persistent bacterial infections. It is not approved for use in food animals in the United States because this country believes there are insufficient data to determine safe conditions of use and to establish an acceptable tolerance for residues of the drug.

In 1985, the US swine industry severely criticized the US Department of Agriculture for allowing the importation of Canadian live hogs and pork products and suggested banning imports from any country where the drug is approved for food animals. Although the Canadian government subsequently withdrew the drug for use in food animals, it is still approved in many other countries and still poses potential trade problems.

Methods of Analysis

Chemical methods are available for the analysis of chloramphenicol in meat, milk, and eggs. These HPLC methods are expensive. Recent developments include the detection of chloramphenicol with a Quick-Card kit. This is an ELISA-based rapid, relatively economic screening method, the application of which is currently being tested in meat and eggs. Further, an automatic HPLC method (FAST-LC) is being developed to screen milk and eggs for the presence of chloramphenicol. All methods are carried out at a 10-μg/kg level. Microbiologic detection is possible from only 1 mg/kg. No tolerance of chloramphenicol is acceptable. Sensitivity methods of 1 μcg/kg in milk, and 5–10 μcg/kg in meat are used.

NITROIMIDAZOLES

Uses for two nitroimidazoles, ipronidazole and dimetridazole, are limited to turkeys in the United States but are approved for use in both turkeys and swine in other countries. The United States considers nitroimidazoles to be suspect carcinogens. US swine producers in the past have requested a ban on imported pork from hogs treated with dimetridazole. In 1987, the U.S. withdrew DMD from veterinary use.

Nitroimidazoles (dimetridazole, metronidazole, ipronidazole):

1. Possess capability of residue formation in food animals
2. Are potentially mutagenic and carcinogenic
3. Have residues that could affect international trade

Dimetridazole is a veterinary medicinal product traditionally used for prevention and treatment of histomoniasis in turkeys, treatment of trichomoniasis in pigeons, treatment of genital trichomoniasis in cattle, and prevention and treatment of hemorrhagic enteritis in pigs. Dimetridazole has shown mutagenic activity in all bacterial tests carried out. It has been proved, however, that this activity was linked to the enzyme activity of the nitroreductases of the bacteria used in the tests. Dimetridazole did not show any mutagenic activity in any of the numerous other tests carried out. It was inferred that dimetridazole was not a genotoxic compound.

The information available, even though it has been obtained from previous studies carried out using insufficiently sensitive methods of analysis, indicates nevertheless considerable metabolization of dimetridazole and rapid elimination of the metabolites produced. In the European community, based on available information, a provisional tolerance of 10 μg/kg is proposed for extractable residues, including dimetridazole and metabolites that retain the nitroimidazole structure.

RONIDAZOLE

Ronidazole is a veterinary medicinal product traditionally used for prevention and treatment of histomoniasis in turkeys, treatment of trichomoniasis in pigeons, treatment of trichomoniasis in cattle, and prevention and treatment of hemorrhagic enteritis in pigs. Ronidazole has shown mutagenic activity in all bacterial tests carried out. Although such an effect might, as in the case of dimetridazole, be due to the enzyme activity of bacterial nitroreductase, this has not yet been proved. Ronidazole increases the incidence of various types of benign tumor in laboratory animals: mammary fibroadenoma in rats and lung tumors in mice.

A provisional tolerance of 2 μg/kg has been proposed for extractable residues, including ronidazole and metabolites that retain the nitroimidazole structure.

BETA LACTAM ANTIBIOTICS: PENICILLIN G, AMPICILLIN, AND CEPHALONIUM

Beta lactam antibiotics are included because it is believed that low concentrations of residues could give rise to immunologic problems in humans.

SULFONAMIDES (See also Chapters 13 and 23.)

Application

Organisms that depend on their folic acid synthesis, such as a number of gram-positive and gram-negative bacteria and coccidia, are sensitive. Sulfonamides are predominantly used to treat infections of the respiratory tract, gastrointestinal tract, and urinary tract. Owing to the wide range of activity, sulfonamides can be considered a first-line chemotherapeutic agent, which can be applied before the sensitivity test has been completed.

Toxicity

Sulfonamides are used on a large scale, in particular in pig farming. Hitherto toxicology information on sulfonamides was limited. A carcinogenic study involving sulfamethazine was concluded in the United States; the results depicting thyroid gland effects gave cause for concern. In the United States and many other countries, a tolerance level of 0.1 mg/kg has been established for sulfa residues in meat; this tolerance level is based on semichronic toxicity data from rat studies.

In the European Community, a tolerance level of 0.1 mg/kg for the parent compound has been suggested. In the United States, problems have been encountered with sulfamethazine contamination of so-called sulfa-free animal feed. Concentrations of 2 mg of sulfamethazine/kg feedstuff can result in residue levels in meat that exceed 0.1 mg/kg.

Sulfamethazine is widely used around the world. The residue includes parent drug and metabolites; however, the regulatory method measures only parent drug. Use of this drug requires special care and management controls to prevent residues above tolerance levels. The results of new studies could alter the regulatory status of sulfamethazine in many countries, including the United States, resulting in restrictions on imports and exports.

Methods of Analysis

Detection of sulfamethazine together with the main metabolite (N_4-acetyl-sulfamethazine) in milk, meat, and eggs is possible with FAST-LC. In milk and meat, sulfamethazine can also be detected by TLC or HPLC. Trimethoprim, which is often administered in combination with sulfamethazine, can also be analyzed with the FAST-LC method; the limit of detection, however, needs to be lowered. For sulfamethazine and N_4-acetyl-sulfamethazine, 100 µg/kg can easily be detected. The analytical methods mentioned here can also be applied for other sulfonamides. The European Community has a current tolerance of 100 ppb.

AMPROLIUM

Application

Coccidia are especially sensitive to amprolium. Amprolium is predominantly used in poultry and sheep. The necessity of application is great because of changing resistance patterns with respect to other coccidiostats and the effectiveness of amprolium, often in combination with ethopabate.

Methods of Analysis

Information of residue methods for amprolium is limited. It is therefore useful to develop residue methods for meat and eggs because the use of amprolium is considerable.

TETRACYCLINES (POTENTIAL HEPATOTOXINS): TETRACYCLINE, OXYTETRACYCLINE, CHLORTETRACYCLINE

Application

Streptococci, clostridia, *Brucella*, *Haemophilus*, *Klebsiella*, and many gram-negative bacteria, such as *E. coli* and *Salmonella*, are sensitive to tetracycline. Owing to their wide range of activity, tetracyclines are generally applicable antibiotics. The necessity of application, however, is relative.

Toxicity

Tetracyclines may alter the liver function (fat accumulation, glycogen decrease, degeneration) and kidney function. Further, complex formation of tetracyclines with metal ions may interfere with the bioavailability and metabolism of essential trace metal ions. Findings indicate immunomodulated hemolytic effects. There are indications for an increased occurrence of subcutaneous tumors in rats after oral administration of oxytetracycline. Results of a carcinogenicity study currently being carried out in the United States (NTP) are not yet available. Little is known of the metabolism of tetracyclines and the toxicity of metabolites.

Analytical methods currently used for many of these are expensive HPLC methods. Recent developments include ELISA-based quick-card tests. These are quick, economic, screening tests for use in meat, milk, and eggs, and greater emphasis should be placed on developing ELISA methods for residues of other compounds. Substances for which suitable analytical methods have not been developed should be withdrawn from use in food animals.

14.7 JOINT EXPERT COMMITTEE ON FOOD ADDITIVES EVALUATION OF PRIORITY LIST OF VETERINARY DRUGS

In order that the Codex committees can obtain objective, expert advice on specific topics, expert committees are set up, composed of recognized experts in specialist areas. These experts are appointed in an individual capacity, by the Directors General of the FAO and WHO. They can therefore report in an impartial manner. The JECFA supports the CCRVD.

Lists of drugs for priority evaluation have been drawn up by Codex. These are dealt with on a priority basis by JECFA on a year-by-year basis. For example:

1. Substances scheduled for JECFA evaluation *1990* were:
   a. Benzyl penicillin
   b. Carbadox
   c. Closantel
   d. Ivermectin
   e. Levamisole
   f. Olaquindox
   g. Oxytetracycline
2. Substances proposed for evaluation at the JECFA meeting devoted to veterinary drug residues in *1991* were:
   a. Febantel
   b. Fenbendazole
   c. Oxfendazole
   d. Carazolol
   e. Spiramycin
   f. Sulfadimidine
3. Substances considered for evaluation at the JECFA meeting devoted to veterinary drug residues in *1992* were:
   a. Closantel Triclabendazole
   b. Furazolidone
   c. Nitrofurazone
   d. Flubendazole
   e. Ivermectin
   f. Bovine somatotropin
4. Substances of potential interest that may not currently meet all criteria selection include:
   a. Ractopamine (beta-agonist; repartitioning agent)
   b. Porcine somatropin
5. Substances not yet scheduled for evaluation include:
   a. Tetracycline
   b. Chlortetracycline
   c. Phenothiazines (acetylpromazine, promazine)

APPENDIX A*

JECFA 1988: RECOMMENDATIONS ON COMPOUNDS ON THE AGENDA*

Substance	ADI for Humans	Acceptable Residue Level
Antimicrobial agent		
Chloramphenicol	Not allocated	Not allocated
Growth promoters		
Endogenous		
Estradiol-17β	Unnecessary	Unnecessary
Progesterone	Unnecessary	Unnecessary
Testosterone	Unnecessary	Unnecessary
Xenobiotic		
Trenbolone acetate	0–0.01 µg/kg of body weight	1.4 µg/kg (bovine tissue) for beta-trenbolone 14 µg/kg (bovine liver and kidney) for alpha-trenbolone
Zeranol	0–0.5 µg/kg of body weight	10 µg/kg (bovine liver) 2 µg/kg (bovine muscle)

JECFA 1989: RECOMMENDATIONS ON COMPOUNDS ON THE AGENDA

Substance	ADI for Humans	Recommended MRL
Anthelminthic drug		
Albendazole	0–0.05 mg/kg of body weight	Muscle, fat, and milk: 0.1 mg/kg Liver and kidney: 5 mg/kg
Antiprotozoal drugs		
Dimetridazole	Not allocated	No MRLs allocated
Ipronidazole	Not allocated	No MRLs allocated
Metronidazole	Not evaluated	No MRLs allocated
Ronidazole	0–0.025 mg/kg of body weight	No MRLs allocated
Antimicrobial sulfonamides		
Sulfadimidine	0–0.004 mg/kg of body weight	Meat, liver, kidney, and fat: 0.3 mg/kg as total residue; 0.1 mg/kg as sulfadimidine Milk: 0.05 mg/kg as total residue; 0.025 mg/kg as sulfadimidine
Sulfathiazole	Not allocated	No MRLs allocated
Growth promoter		
Trenbolone acetate	0–0.02 µg/kg of body weight	Muscle: 2 µg/kg as beta-trenbolone Liver: 10 µg/kg as alpha-trenbolone
Trypanocides		
Diminazene	Not allocated	No MRLs allocated
Isometamidium	Not allocated	No MRLs allocated

*From JECFA/FAO/WHO report, Evaluation of Certain Veterinary Food Residues. Geneva, WHO, 1988.

JECFA 1990: RECOMMENDED ADIs AND MRLs FOR SIX VETERINARY DRUGS

Compound/ADI	MRLs

Closantel
0–0.03 mg/kg
	Sheep: 1.15 mg/kg
	Bovine:
	    Muscle, 0.5 mg/kg*
	    Kidney, 2 mg/kg*
	    Liver, 1 mg/kg*

Ivermectin
0–0.0002 mg/kg
	All species:
	    Liver, 0.015 mg/kg
	    Fat, 0.02 mg/kg

Levamisole 0–0.003 mg/kg*	Tissues and milk, 0.01 mg/kg*

Benzyl penicillin
0.03 mg/person/day
	All species:
	    Liver, 0.05 mg/kg
	    Kidney, 0.05 mg/kg
	    Muscle, 0.05 mg/kg
	    Milk, 0.004 mg/kg

Oxytetracycline
0–0.003 mg/kg
	All species:
	    Muscle, 0.1 mg/kg
	    Liver, 0.3 mg/kg
	    Kidney, 0.6 mg/kg
	    Fat, 0.01 mg/kg
	    Milk, 0.1 mg/kg
	    Eggs, 0.2 mg/kg

Carbadox (Insufficient
data for ADI)
	Swine:
	    Liver, 0.03 mg/kg
	    Muscle, 0.005 mg/kg

*Temporary levels.

JECFA 1991: RECOMMENDED ADIs AND MRLs FOR 10 VETERINARY DRUGS

Substance	ADI (per kg body weight)	MRL (per kg)

Carazolol	0.1 μg	Cattle and pigs:
		    Muscle, 5 μg
		    Fat, 5 μg
		    Liver, 30 μg
		    Kidney, 30 μg

Febantel
Fenbendazole
Oxfendazole
	10 μg
	25 μg
	4 μg
		Cattle, sheep, pigs:
		    Muscle, 100 μg
		    Fat, 100 μg
		    Kidney, 100 μg
		    Liver, 500 μg
		Cattle*:
		    Milk, 150 μg/liter

Spiramycin	5 μg	Cattle and pigs:
		    Muscle, 50 μg
		    Liver, 300 μg
		    Kidney, 200 μg

Sulfadimidine	4 μg	Cattle: Milk, 150 μg/liter

JECFA 1992: RECOMMENDATIONS FOR ADIs AND MRLs FOR 10 VETERINARY COMPOUNDS, INCLUDING BOVINE SOMATOTROPINS*

Substance	ADI (per kg body weight) and Other Toxicologic Recommendations	Recommended MRL
Anthelmintic agents		
Closantel	Not evaluated	Muscle and kidney (sheep): 1500 μg/kg Liver (sheep): 5000 μg/kg Fat (sheep): 2000 μg/kg Muscle and liver (cattle): 1000 μg/kg Kidney and fat (cattle): 3000 μg/kg
Flubendazole	0.12 μg	Muscle and liver (pigs): 10 μg/kg Muscle (poultry): 200 μg/kg Liver (poultry): 500 μg/kg Eggs: 400 μg/kg
Ivermectin	0.1 μg	Liver (cattle): 100 μg/kg Fat (cattle): 40 μg/kg
Thiabendazole	0.1 μg	Edible tissues (cattle, pigs, goats and sheep) and milk (cattle and goats): 100 μg/kg
Triclabendazole	0.3 μg	Muscle (cattle): 200 μg/kg Liver and kidney (cattle): 300 μg/kg Fat (cattle): 100 μg/kg Edible tissues (sheep): 100 μg/kg
Antimicrobial agents		
Furazolidone	Not allocated	No MRLs allocated
Nitrofurazone	Not allocated	No MRLs allocated

*From JECFA/FAO/WHO report, Evaluation of Certain Veterinary Food Residues. Geneva, WHO, 1988.

Priority list for evaluation by JECFA 1993:

Rafoxanide
Chloramphenicol
Olaquindox
Ronidazole
Sulfadimidine
Isometamidium
Dexamethasone
Enrofloxacin
Flumequine
Apramycin
Spectinomycin

Priority list for evaluation by JECFA in 1994:

Levamisole
Oxolinic acid
Dihydrostreptomycin
Gentamicin
Imidocarb
Kanamycin
Neomycin
Streptomycin
Chlortetracycline
Tetracycline
Carazolol

SELECTED REFERENCES

Codex Alimentarius Commission. F.A.O./W.H.O. Joint FAO/WHO Food Standards Programme. Codex Committee on Residues of Veterinary Drugs in Food. (C.C.R.V.D.F.) Reports Nos. 1, 2, 3, 4, 5, 6. 1986–1991, Washington, D.C.

Compound Evaluation and Analytical Capability National Residue Program Plan 1991. United States Depart. Agriculture.

Egan, J., and Meaney, W.J.: The inhibitory effect of mastitic milk and colostrum on test methods used for antibiotic detection. Ir. J. Food. Sci. Technol., *8*:115, 1984.

Evaluation of Certain Veterinary Drug Residues in Food. 32nd Report of Joint FAO/WHO Expert Commission on Food Additives.

Herrick, J.B.: Milk quality assurance and dairy practitioners. J. Am. Vet. Med. Assoc., *199*:1268, 1991.

Reports of Joint FAO/WHO Expert Committee on Food Additives W.H.O. Geneva, 1990, 1991, 1992.

Residues of Veterinary Drugs in Food. Report of a Joint FAO/WHO Expert Consultation. No. 32 November, 1984. Rome.

Salton, M.R.J.: Action of lysozyme on gram-positive bacteria and the structure of cell walls. Expo. Annu. Biochem. med., *27*:35, 1966.

Thirty-fourth Report of Joint FAO/WHO Expert Committee on Food Additives. W.H.O. Geneva, 1989.

Vakil, J.R., et al.: Susceptibility of several microorganisms to milk lysozymes. J. Dairy Sci., *52*:1192, 1969.

CHAPTER

15

DRUG DISTRIBUTION, PHARMACOKINETICS, AND RESIDUES

15.1 Binding of Drugs to Plasma Proteins
15.2 Passage of Drugs Across Biological Membranes
15.3 Influence of pH
15.4 Specialized Transport Processes
15.5 Modern Concepts of Pharmacokinetics
15.6 Pharmacokinetic Considerations and Withdrawal Times

15.1 BINDING OF DRUGS TO PLASMA PROTEINS

Drug action is often explained with a lock and key analogy, whereby the drug is the key and the lock is the ultimate site of action, known as the receptor. Receptors are reactive chemical groupings situated on the surface of the cell or within the cell itself. When a drug reacts with a receptor, it does so through the formation of weak chemical bonds, which are usually reversible. These are forces that bind the compound onto the receptor site. The union of drug and receptor yields the drug-receptor complex, which is then responsible for the initiation of pharmacologic activity.

The effects of a drug in the body can be viewed as the ultimate consequences of interaction between the drug and its receptor, once the drug has diffused across the various biological membranes in the body and reached the vicinity of the receptor at its site of action. When one administers a drug therefore, the objective is to achieve an adequate concentration of the drug at its site of action and to maintain this concentration for a desired period of time. The concentration attained at the receptor site depends on a number of factors, which include the extent and rate of absorption, distribution, metabolism, and elimination. Generally only a small proportion of the total drug in the body is at any particular time present at its site of action, complexing with the receptor, and producing a pharmacologic effect. This is because the bulk of the drug may bind with other tissues. Although this latter portion of the drug is not involved directly in the production of the pharmacologic effect, it does have an important role to play in that it governs the kinetics of redistribution and the ultimate disappearance of the drug from the body.

Most drugs are carried from the site of absorption to the site of action and elimination by the circulating blood. From the blood stream, the drug must traverse the various biological membranes and fluid compartments before its molecules can reach intracellular receptor sites. Some drugs cannot pass all types of membranes and therefore are restricted in their distribution and in their potential effect, whereas others pass through all membranes and become distributed throughout the various fluid compartments. In addition, some drugs may accumulate in various areas as a result of binding, dissolving in fat, or an active transport mechanism. The accumulation can be at the site of action or, more often, in some other location. In the latter situation, the site of accumulation may serve as a storage depot for the drug. Although it is in itself pharmacologically inactive, the drug in the storage depot is in equilibrium with the free drug and thereby maintains an effective concentration of the drug at its site of action. Binding of drugs to proteins and other macromolecules is known to occur in almost every tissue of the body. It has been demonstrated with albumin, globulins, hemoglobin, mucopolysaccharides, nucleoproteins, phospholipids, and additional substances. Binding is generally a reversible process because nearly all drugs eventually disappear from the body. The majority of drugs appear to be held to binding sites by weak chemical bonds of the Van der Waals, hydrogen, or ionic types. The reversible binding of drugs to various intracellular and extracellular substances is important in determining how long a drug remains in the body. Without these storage pools, many drugs would be metabolized and excreted so rapidly that they would hardly have time to exert their pharmacologic action.

An important factor in the distribution of drugs is their binding to proteins. Because most drugs are carried from their site of absorption to their sites of action and elimination by the circulating blood, any binding that occurs within the blood stream profoundly alters the distribution and pharmacologic activity of a particular drug. Once a drug has gained access to the blood stream, binding to plasma protein almost invariably occurs. For the majority of drugs, binding to plasma albumin is quantitatively the most important and often accounts for almost all the drug binding in plasma, although globulins have been shown to have a high affinity for corticosteroids. Albumin binding influences the fate of drugs in the body because only the unbound or free drug diffuses through capillary walls, reaches the site of drug action, and is subject to elimination from the body. As a rule, most drugs are reversibly bound to plasma

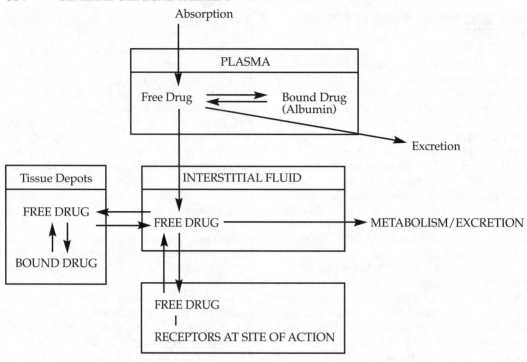

FIG. 15–1. Factors affecting the concentration of a drug at its site of action.

albumin by weak chemical forces. The reversible nature of the binding is necessary because an equilibrium exists between the bound and unbound (free) drug fractions. The albumin-drug complex serves as a circulating drug reservoir that releases more drug to restore the equilibrium as the free drug diffuses out from the capillaries. It is in this way that the plasma concentration of even highly bound drugs falls to low levels and eventually disappears (Fig. 15–1).

The fate of many drugs in the body is influenced by their binding to serum albumin. Whatever the route of administration, almost all therapeutic agents reach their sites of action through the systemic circulation. Only the fraction of the drug in the blood stream that does not bind to albumin can leave the circulation, become distributed throughout the body, and reach the sites of action. Because the equilibrium between bound and free drug is constantly maintained, some of the drug-albumin complex continuously dissociates out of the blood through capillary membranes. Once drug distribution is complete, the free drug concentration throughout extracellular water equals that in serum water. It is not the total

but rather the free drug concentration in serum that correlates with the concentration at the sites of action. For highly bound drugs, the free drug concentration in serum is only a small percentage of the total amount present. The exact fraction that is protein bound depends on the specific drug, species, drug and albumin concentrations, and any interference with binding by other drugs. Table 15–1 shows the extent of protein binding undergone by some commonly used drugs.

Binding is a function of the concentration of the free drug; with increasing drug concentration, the plasma protein gradually approaches saturation. If the plasma level of the total drug (bound and unbound) is gradually increased, the concentration of the free drug tends to rise slowly at first, but later as the protein-binding sites become saturated, the concentration rises sharply.

The influence of protein binding on the distribution of a drug between plasma and a relatively protein-free fluid, such as synovial fluid, is illustrated in Fig. 15–2. An unequal distribution of drug across the cell membrane can exist at equilibrium if there is a difference in the extent of protein bind-

TABLE 15–1
PROTEIN BINDING OF SOME COMMONLY USED DRUGS IN VARIOUS SPECIES

Drug	Species	Percent Bound
Phenylbutazone	Horse	96
Oxyphenbutazone	Horse	87
Chloramphenicol	Dog	40
Sulfamethazine	Cow	65
Digitoxin	Dog	88
Cloxacillin	Human	95
Chlorpromazine	Human	96
Benzylpenicillin	Human	64
Ampicillin	Human	22

sites of biotransformation in the liver. The greater the extent of albumin binding, the less drug is available at any one time at the site of hepatic biotransformation. Consequently, extensive binding to plasma proteins can reduce the rate of elimination of drugs and also their metabolism or biotransformation. Because albumin slows the elimination of drugs that are removed from serum by glomerular filtration or by diffusion to the hepatic biotransformation site, it increases the duration of action of a single dose of such drugs. The duration of action of some diuretics, sulfonamides, and tetracyclines tends to correlate with their degree of protein binding. Differences in the drug-binding capacity of plasma proteins exist among mammalian species. Variation in the plasma protein binding of a drug may contribute to species differences in tissue levels of the drug, in toxicity, and in overall kinetics, particularly if the binding is extensive (approximately 90%).

One of the most important practical aspects of protein binding is the fact that drugs of similar or markedly dissimilar structure may compete for the same binding sites on the protein. Multidrug therapy may lead to alterations in the plasma concentration and the rate of elimination of drugs because of competition for plasma protein binding sites. Many drugs can partially displace one another from albumin, and this may lead to an intensification of pharmacologic action. It is only when substances are extensively bound in plasma that displacement from binding sites would release amounts of drug that on distribution

ing on each side of the membrane. Protein-bound drug molecules cannot permeate cellular membranes. Thus at equilibrium, there is a larger total amount of drug on the side of the membrane where the greater extent of binding occurs.

The kidneys remove drugs and their metabolites from the blood by glomerular filtration or by tubular excretion. Because albumin does not appreciably pass through the glomerular membrane, neither does drug bound to albumin. If excretion by filtration is the major mode of elimination of a drug, protein binding can decrease the rate of elimination to an important extent. Also, because protein binding decreases the amount of diffusible drug, a reduced concentration of free drug usually exists at the

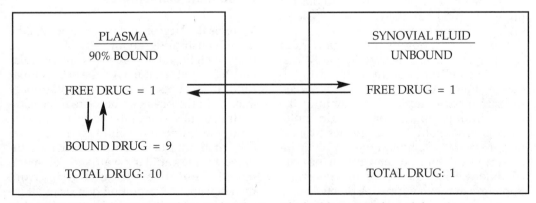

FIG. 15–2. Effect of protein binding on distribution of a highly protein-bound drug (e.g., phenylbutazone) between blood plasma and a relatively protein-free fluid (e.g., synovial fluid).

into other parts of the body would significantly increase the concentration in the tissue. For example, displacement from albumin of 1% of a 99% bound drug doubles the percentage of free drug. This free drug is then available for distribution to the tissues. This could result in a sufficiently large increase in concentration at its site of action to intensify the drug's activity or toxicity in a clinically important fashion.

Drugs with higher affinities for plasma albumin can also displace drugs with lower ones. For example, sulfonamides are bound to plasma proteins, but if phenylbutazone, which has a greater affinity for the binding sites, is administered, it increases the concentration of free sulfonamides in the plasma by displacement.

Potentiation of a drug's pharmacologic action is not the only consequence of its partial displacement from albumin. An increase in the concentration of unbound drug in the serum also makes more drug available for glomerular filtration as well as for diffusion into hepatic cells and its subsequent biotransformation. Thus the immediate consequences of displacement of most albumin-bound drugs are an increase in free drug concentration in the blood; a redistribution of drug from the circulation into the rest of the body; and an increase in drug concentration at the site of action, an enhanced pharmacologic effect, and a more rapid elimination from the body (owing to enhanced biotransformation and glomerular filtration). The extent to which these effects are seen depends largely on the amount of protein binding before displacement and the amount of displacement. Only drugs that are extensively bound to plasma protein (>90%) are likely to be displaced, giving a clinical effect.

The concentration or the properties of serum albumin are altered in many diseases. Such changes decrease the drug albumin interaction. In other words, when the serum concentration of albumin or the drug-binding capacity of albumin molecules is abnormally low, a smaller proportion of a potential albumin-binding drug interacts with albumin than under normal conditions. Thus the free drug concentration is greater than normal. A practical consequence of this is that the toxicity of drugs that are normally highly bound is greatly increased by hypoproteinemia (assuming that the dosage is not reduced).

Overall, there are a number of important consequences of protein binding:

1. The distribution of the drug becomes strongly modified because any drug that is bound to plasma protein is retained within the vascular compartment.
2. Cumulation is more likely to occur with drugs that are highly bound to plasma protein. For example, the difference between the two cardiac drugs digitoxin and ouabain can be cited. Digitoxin is rather strongly bound to plasma proteins and therefore eliminated slowly, whereas ouabain is practically unbound, thus clearing the body rapidly.
3. Only the free fraction of the drug is in equilibrium with the drug at the site of action. If the drug is strongly bound in the plasma, estimates of the plasma concentration can be meaningless for the calculation of the concentration of the active drug at the site of action; e.g., for phenylbutazone (strongly bound), the plasma concentration might be 100 mg/liter, but at this level, the concentration of free drug is only about 2 mg/liter. This is then the concentration available for distribution into the tissues, i.e., at the site of action.
4. Binding may be modified in disease states, e.g., hypoalbuminemia in liver diseases, or by the concomitant administration of other drugs.

15.2 PASSAGE OF DRUGS ACROSS BIOLOGICAL MEMBRANES

Water is the largest single constituent of the body, constituting about 70% of the total body weight. Fifty percent is intracellular and 20% is extracellular. Of the extracellular fluid, 15% is present in the interstitial space and 5% in the plasma. There are three compartments of water in the body: the plasma fluid, the extracellular fluid, and the intracellular fluid. These compartments are divided by the capillary wall and cell membrane. The absorption, distribution, metabolism, and excretion of a drug all involve its passage across these cell membranes, and in fact, the systemic usefulness of a drug largely depends on its ability to cross the various barriers that could prevent its diffusing throughout the entire body water and thus reaching its site of action.

The endothelium of the capillaries is generally freely permeable to small molecules, and most drugs gain access to the extracellular fluid in a short time. If, however, a drug is reversibly bound to plasma albumin, it does not under normal circumstances leave the circulation because the molecular size of the protein exceeds the size of the endothelial pores. The plasma membranes of the tissue cells constitute barriers to penetration of drugs quite different from the capillary membranes. A drug that diffuses readily through capillary membranes into the extracellular fluid may penetrate cellular membranes slowly or scarcely at all. Thus an understanding of the nature of cell membranes and how they are penetrated by drugs is necessary to appreciate how drugs may be distributed in the body.

NATURE OF CELL MEMBRANES

Electron microscopic studies suggest that all cell membranes in the body are composed of a fundamental structure called the plasma membrane. This boundary, which is about 70–80Å thick, surrounds single cells, such as epithelial cells. More complex membranes, such as the intestinal epithelium and the skin, are composed of multiples of the fundamental structure. Overton first suggested that the rate at which various substances enter cells is proportional to the distribution of the substance between lipid and water, the lipid-soluble substances entering the cell more readily. This implies that the cell is surrounded by a membrane of a lipid nature, which Danielli and Davson in 1937 visualized as a bimolecular layer of lipid molecules with a monolayer of protein adsorbed into each surface. With the use of the electron microscope, the membrane structure is now seen to be essentially identical with the model suggested by these workers. The cell membrane is known also to be interspersed with small aqueous channels or pores. The diameter of these pores in the tissue cell membranes is calculated to be from 4 to 5 degrees A,

whereas those of the capillary endothelial cells are larger (40 to 100° A) in diameter. Consequently, large molecules can pass outward from the capillaries into the extracellular fluid, whereas only much smaller water-soluble substances can pass through the smaller pores of the cell membranes into the tissue cells. The membrane pores may be protein line channels through the lipid layer or simply spaces between the lipid molecules. In membranes composed of many cells, the spaces between the cells may constitute another kind of membrane pore. Lipid-soluble substances penetrate the membrane by dissolving in the lipid phase, whereas lipid-insoluble substances penetrate only if they are small enough to pass through the pores. Cell membranes, however, also possess specialized active transport systems that facilitate entry of certain large lipid-insoluble molecules, such as sugars and amino acids, into the cell against a concentration gradient. The protein component of the cell membrane may be responsible in part for this process.

PROCESSES BY WHICH DRUGS CROSS CELL MEMBRANES

The various ways in which drugs move across biological membranes can be grouped under two headings: passive transfer processes and specialized transport processes.

PASSIVE PROCESSES

Many drugs penetrate cell membranes by a process of simple diffusion; that is, their rate of transfer is directly proportional to their concentration gradient across the membrane, resulting in a net movement of particles from the higher to the lower concentration. The membrane is not involved in the passive transfer process, and the drug molecules penetrate either by passage through aqueous pores or by dissolving in the membrane substance itself. Lipid-soluble substances move across the predominantly lipid cell membrane by passive diffusion, the relative speed of passage being determined by the lipid solubility or, more precisely, the lipid to water partition coefficient of the substance. The greater the partition coefficient (or lipid solubility), the higher is the concentration of drug in the membrane and the faster its diffusion. Many lipid-insoluble compounds of small molecular size, however, can also diffuse rapidly across the cell membrane. Water should not be able to pass readily through the lipid membrane, yet it permeates membranes with extreme rapidity. Such behavior can be understood only if it is assumed that the lipid layer of the membrane is not continuous but contains pores, as mentioned earlier, that permit the passage of water, urea, small water-soluble particles, and many inorganic ions. Passage through the pores is a passive process called filtration because it involves bulk flow of water as a result of a hydrostatic or osmotic difference across the membranes. The bulk flow of water through the pores drags with it any soluble molecules whose dimensions are less than the pores. Most inorganic ions are sufficiently small to penetrate the pores in the membrane, but commonly active transport mechanisms are involved in which movement against an electrochemical gradient is involved (i.e., sodium and potassium ions).

15.3 INFLUENCE OF pH

In considering diffusion, it is necessary to bear in mind that most drugs are either weak acids (i.e., barbiturates) or weak bases (i.e., caffeine), which exist in solution as a mixture of the ionized and un-ionized forms. These compounds are more lipid soluble than water soluble in the non-ionized form but highly water soluble and less lipid soluble when ionized. Consequently, the non-ionized form permeates readily across cell membranes, whereas the ionized form does not. Ionized substances penetrate into cells poorly. First, ionized substances tend to be less lipid soluble and more water soluble and so cannot diffuse across the lipid phase of the cell membrane. Second, many ionized drugs are unable to be filtered through the aqueous pores of the membrane because of their own size, or they may also attract molecules of water (i.e., become hydrated), becoming more bulky and unable to traverse the pores. Third, ionized

molecules may be repelled from the surface of the cell by groups with like charge, or they may be attracted to it and held there by unlike charges. Thus only the non-ionized form is lipid soluble and able to permeate rapidly across cell membranes. The process is known as passive non-ionic diffusion. The ratio of ionized to un-ionized drug in any given tissue of the body is therefore important and depends on the pKa of the compound (known as the dissociation constant) and the pH of the medium. The pKa in effect is the pH at which 50% of the drug is in the un-ionized form and 50% is in the ionized form. The relationship is given by the Henderson-Hasselbach equation, which for a weak acid is:

$$pH - pKa = Log \frac{(Concentration\ of\ Ionized\ Acid)}{(Concentration\ of\ Un\text{-}ionized\ Acid)}$$

For a weak base:

$$pH - pKa = Log \frac{(Concentration\ of\ Un\text{-}ionized\ Base)}{(Concentration\ of\ Ionized\ Base)}$$

For drugs that ionize, it is possible under certain conditions to find at equilibrium unequal concentrations of the total drug (i.e., ionized plus un-ionized) on either side of the membrane. Only the un-ionized molecules readily cross this lipid barrier and achieve the same equilibrium concentration on both sides of the membrane; the ionized molecules are virtually excluded from transmembrane diffusion ("ion-trapping"). If a pH difference exists across a biological membrane, the drug ionizes to a different extent on each side of the membrane, and as a result there is an unequal total concentration (ionized plus un-ionized) of the drug on each side of the membrane. The partitioning of a weak acid pKa 4.4 between plasma (pH 7.4) and gastric juice (pH 1.4) is depicted in Fig. 15–3. It is assumed that the gastric mucous membrane behaves as a simple lipoid barrier permeable only to the lipid-soluble un-ionized form of drug. The ratio of un-ionized to ionized drug at each

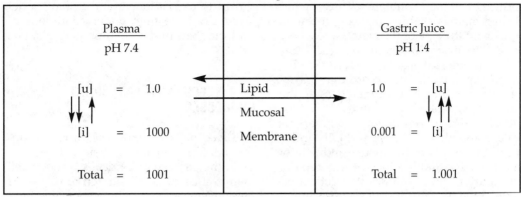

FIG. 15–3. Influence of pH on distribution of a weak acid between plasma and gastric juice. Note 1000-fold difference in total drug concentration across both sides of the pH gradient. u, un-ionized; i, ionized.

pH can be calculated from the Henderson-Hasselbach equation for a weak acid:

$$Ph - pKa =$$

$$\frac{Log\ Concentration\ Ionized\ Drug}{Concentration\ Un\text{-}ionized\ Drug}$$

Therefore in plasma:

$$7.4 - 4.4 =$$

$$\frac{Log\ Concentration\ Ionized\ Drug\ (i)}{Concentration\ Un\text{-}ionized\ Drug\ (u)}$$

$$3 = Log\ \frac{[i]}{[u]}$$

therefore $1000 = \dfrac{[i]}{[u]}$

1000:1 = Ionized: Un-ionized Drug

Thus in plasma, the ratio of un-ionized to ionized drug is 1.0:1000; in gastric juice, the ratio is 1.0:0.001. The total (ionized plus un-ionized) drug concentration ratio between the plasma and gastric juice sides of the barrier is 1000:1. For a weak base with a pKa of 4.4, the ratio would be reversed (Fig. 15–4). An unequal distribution of drug across the cell membrane can also exist at equilibrium if there is a difference in the extent of protein binding on each side of the membrane because protein-bound drug mole-

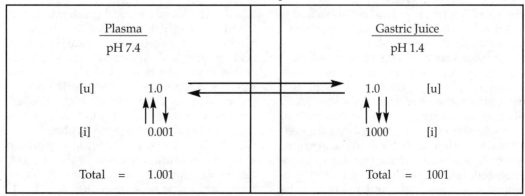

FIG. 15–4. Influence of pH on distribution of a weak base between plasma and gastric juice. Note in this case that the direction of the concentration gradient of the total drug is reversed.

cules, similar to ionized molecules, cannot permeate cellular membranes. Thus at equilibrium there is a larger total concentration of drug on the side of the membrane where the greater extent of binding occurs.

Because most drugs have pKa value between 3 and 11, they are, accordingly, partly ionized and partly un-ionized over the range of physiologic pH values. Their distribution and concentration in the various tissues are consequently markedly influenced by the pH of the tissues and pKa of the drug. The implications of this type of distribution have significant practical effects on the passage of drugs across any of the membranes of the body where a pH gradient may exist, e.g., across the mammary gland epithelium; the renal tubular epithelium; the salivary gland epithelium; and the ruminal, gastric, or intestinal epithelium. The more striking effects are seen when a large pH difference exists, e.g., between plasma and gastric juice or between plasma and urine. Sulfonamides, which are weak organic acids, pass from plasma to milk by a process of passive diffusion in the form of lipid-soluble, non-ionized molecules. A high milk pH tends to increase the excretion into milk. This is of practical importance in treating mastitis, in which the mastitic secretion is of an alkaline nature.

The significance of urinary pH in eliminating drugs from the body is also of practical significance in that when the tubular urine becomes alkaline, basic drugs tend to exist largely in the un-ionized form. Thus the drug is more lipid soluble and is able to back-diffuse through the lipid cell membrane of the renal tubular epithelium into the blood and so increase its persistence in the body. Acidic drugs tend to ionize under conditions of alkaline pH and so are unable to permeate the renal tubular epithelium. Being more water soluble, the ionized form is preferentially excreted. The converse situation applies to conditions of acidic urinary pH. In this way, variations in urinary pH may favor the excretion or retention of drugs in the body. This has been demonstrated experimentally for many drugs; e.g., amphetamine and quinine (weak bases) are excreted more rapidly in acidic urine, whereas salicyclic acid and phenobarbital (weak acids) are excreted more rapidly in alkaline urine. In the horse, phenylbutazone (weak organic acid pKa = 4.6) has been shown to persist longer and to have a delayed clearance time under conditions of aciduria than under conditions of alkaline urine.

15.4 SPECIALIZED TRANSPORT PROCESSES

The two passive processes already described, filtration and diffusion, do not explain the passage of all drugs through cell membranes. Specialized active transport mechanisms appear to be responsible for a rapid cellular transfer of certain large lipid-insoluble molecules and ionized molecules. Not only is the transfer process rapid, but also in most cases the substances can move across membranes in an uphill direction, i.e., from a solution of low concentration to that of a high concentration. It is assumed that their transport is facilitated by something in the membrane known as a "carrier," with which they combine temporarily. The carrier combines with a solute at one surface of the membrane, the carrier-solute complex moves across the membrane, the solute is released, and the carrier then returns to the original surface, where it can combine with another molecule of solute. This hypothetical carrier is available only in limited amounts in the cell membrane and is capable of displaying a high degree of structural specificity with the molecules that can complex with it. Two main types of carrier-mediated transport are recognized: active transport and facilitated diffusion.

If the process transports a substance against an electrochemical gradient (uphill transport) and is blocked by metabolic inhibitors, it is called active transport; ions such as Na^+ and K^+, amino acids, certain strong acids and bases, and ionized forms of weak electrolytes are transported across the renal tubule, choroid plexus, gastrointestinal tract, and liver cells in this way. Facilitated diffusion is the term applied to carrier-mediated transport, which operates along a concentration gradient (i.e., from a higher to a lower concentration). This is a more rapid type of simple diffusion. Facilitated diffusion has been shown to operate for the movement of sugars into erythrocytes and for sugars, amino acids, and nucleosides in various other cells and tissues.

Two other forms of specialized transport, pinocytosis and phagocytosis, may account for the transmembrane movement of proteins and other macromolecules. In these complex processes, the cell engulfs a droplet of extracellular fluid or a particle of solid material, such as a bacterium. The droplet or particle is completely surrounded by a portion of the cell membrane, and the resulting vesicle then becomes detached and moves into the cell cytoplasm. Pinocytosis is believed to be responsible for the transmembrane transport of large molecules and possibly the intestinal absorption of some protein molecules.

15.5 MODERN CONCEPTS OF PHARMACOKINETICS

Pharmacokinetics may be defined as the mathematical description of concentration changes of drugs within the body. Pharmacokinetics study the duration and persistance of drugs and metabolite concentrations in the body and as a result develop mathematical models and concepts to describe absorption, distribution, biotransformation, and excretion processes. Knowledge of these various patterns and processes for a particular drug enables predictions of dosage regimens to be made.

Usually in the study of pharmacokinetics, the body is depicted as comprising a number of compartments. These compartments have no real physiologic basis—they are simply mathematical entities useful in describing the movement of drugs. The body may be referred to as a "one-compartment open model" or a "two-compartment open model." The one-compartment open model is arbitrarily defined as one in which the drug entering the body is distributed instantly into the available space.

The two-compartment open model is taken as comprising both a central and a peripheral component. The central compartment refers to the blood plasma; the intestinal fluid, and vascular, well-perfused tissues and organs, such as the liver and kidney. The peripheral compartment refers to less well-perfused tissues, such as the skin, muscle, and body fat. The two-compartment model is based on the assumption that any drug entering the body distributes instantaneously into the central compartment and then much more slowly into the peripheral compartment. All drug elimination is taken to occur exclusively from the central compartment. The distribution and elimination processes are assumed to follow first-order kinetics; i.e., the rate of elimination is proportional to the amount of drug in the body (i.e., constant fraction excreted).

The starting point for pharmacokinetic study is to administer a drug intravenously and then to measure the concentration of the drug in the plasma over a period of time. Plotting these data on concentration versus time gives a curve the slope of which reflects the rate at which plasma concentration falls. This exponential or first-order curve can be converted to a straight line when the drug concentration is expressed logarithmically instead of arithmetically (i.e., a semi-log curve). This then shows that a constant fraction of drug is lost per unit time. Quite commonly this semi-log expression has an obvious kink in it and is then known as a bi-exponential curve. The initial steep fall in concentration, called the alpha phase, represents principally the rapid rate of drug loss from the plasma out into the other body-water compartments—the phase of equilibrium. The second, flatter portion of the curve, known as the beta phase, represents the balance of those events that occurs more slowly after the drug has diffused to equilibrium. This consists principally of metabolic and excretory processes. In turn, these two components can yield the distribution rate constant for the rapid initial process and the elimination rate constant for the second slower process. When plasma concentration versus time data are well fitted by a bi-exponential relationship, the body is said to be behaving as if it were a two-compartment open system.

The alpha phase, i.e., the distribution phase, has a slope of $-\alpha/2.303$, and the beta phase has a slope of $-\beta/2.303$. The value Ke represents the elimination rate constant and K12 and K21 the distribution constants between the central and peripheral compartments.

The same type of exponential curve also allows calculation of the apparent volume of distribution to be made. This can be defined as the volume of fluid that would be required to contain the amount of drug in the body if it were uniformly distributed at a concentration equal to that in the plasma. The assumption is made that the body acts as a single homogeneous compartment with respect to the drug. Extrapolation of the elimination phase curve back to the concentration axis gives an initial concentration of drug in the serum (B), assuming instantaneous distribution. The value (VD) can then be obtained from expression:

$$VD \text{ (liters)} = \frac{Dose \text{ (mg)}}{B \text{ (mg/liter) (Serum Concentration)}}$$

The extrapolation to the concentration axis gives a value, CPO, which is taken to be the maximum concentration of drug in all those compartments of body water it could enter if the distribution phase had been instantaneous and therefore no elimination had occurred.

The apparent volume of distribution of a drug is called apparent because it is recognized that all tissues in which the drug is distributed may not have the same concentration of drug. A large apparent volume of distribution implies wide distribution, extensive tissue binding, or both. Lipid-soluble organic bases are widely distributed in the body fluids and tissues and in some cases exceed the actual volume of the body (>1 liter/kg). The low lipid solubility of the aminoglycoside antibiotics restricts the distribution of these organic bases (VD <0.3 liter/kg).

A large volume of distribution suggests tissue storage. Many acidic drugs, such as sulfonamides, phenylbutazone, salicylates, and penicillins, are highly protein bound or too hydrophilic to diffuse across cell membranes and enter cellular water and adipose tissue in significant amounts. These drugs have low volumes of distribution (0.2 to 0.4 liter/kg) in monogastric animals. Basic drugs tend to be widely distributed and to have particularly large apparent volumes of distribution in ruminant animals because these drugs diffuse into the rumen and become trapped by ionization of ruminal liquor.

Another useful parameter that can be calculated from such a curve is the plasma half-life or biological half-life of the drug. The half-life may be defined as the time taken for the plasma concentration to be reduced by one half or as the time required for the body to eliminate one half of the drug it contains. The half-life of a drug is independent of the plasma drug concentration when first-order (i.e., constant rate) kinetics are operating. The half-life is found by measuring the time required for a given plasma level of drug to decline by one half during the terminal exponential phase of the curve (beta). It can also be calculated from the expression:

$$\frac{T}{2} = \frac{0.693 \text{ (Volume of Distribution)}}{Clearance}$$

Beta represents the negative value of the slope of the first-order curve for a one-compartment model or the slope of the terminal portion of the curve for a two-compartment model. Beta is the overall elimination rate constant, and a large value of beta corresponding to a short half-life indicates rapid elimination. The half-life of a first-order process is independent of the route of administration and the dose. Knowledge of the half-life of a drug can be useful in a predictive sense, especially with respect to the design of rational dosage regimens. Many factors can affect the half-life value, i.e., age, liver or kidney function, interaction with other drugs, and urinary pH. On the premise that distribution and elimination processes follow first-order kinetics, multiples of the half-life give a crude estimate of the fraction of the original amount of drug remaining in the body at intervals after administration of a single dose. When four half-lives have elapsed, 93.75% of a total dose has been eliminated. Hence repeat dosing within this time span means that the second dose is added to the drug remaining in the body from the previous dose with possible risk of cumulation and toxicity.

The clearance of a drug is defined as the volume of blood plasma cleared of drug by metabolism and excretion per unit time. By definition, this is also the number of milliliters of the volume of distribution (VD) cleared per unit time and therefore equal to beta × VD. Appropriately beta VD is termed the total body clearance, i.e.:

$$\text{Beta} \times \text{VD} = \text{VD} \times \frac{0.693}{\text{Half-life}}$$

or

$$\frac{\text{Elimination}}{\text{Serum Drug Concentration}}$$

For example, the half-life and body clearance of a barbituate in the pony can be calculated from values of the overall elimination rate constant (Beta = 0.46/hour) and the apparent specific volume of distribution (VD = 0.8 liter/kg):

$$\text{Half-life} = \frac{0.693}{\text{Beta}} = \frac{0.693}{0.46} = 1.5 \text{ hours}$$

and body clearance:

$$\text{Beta} \times \text{VD} = 0.46 \times 0.8 =$$

$$0.368 \text{ liter/kg/hour}$$

All of these various parameters can be used in pharmacokinetic studies to predict dose size and dosing frequency. Knowing the initial plasma concentration and the elimination, it is possible to calculate the time required for plasma concentration to fall to minimum levels. On this basis, dosing intervals can be recommended. When the desired concentration is known, the body weight, and the apparent specific volume of distribution, the dose of drug required to produce that desired plasma concentration can be calculated from the equation:

$$\text{Dose} = \text{VD} \times \text{BW} \times \text{CPD}$$

It is usually possible to identify a plasma concentration below which no drug effect is seen. This concentration is often described as the active threshold. In the case of an antibiotic, this is the minimum inhibitory concentration times an appropriate safety factor.

When circumstances necessitate drug therapy, it is usually desirable to establish an effective concentration of drug in the body fluids as soon as possible and to maintain this concentration for an adequate period of time. To achieve this objective, the dosage regimen often consists of an initial priming or loading dose followed by lower maintenance doses, which are administered at fixed time intervals. Inappropriate choice of the maintenance dose or the dosing interval leads to inadequate therapy or to accumulation of drugs with signs of attendant toxicity. Cumulation is not a property of the drug itself but rather a consequence of the dosage regimen. When the steady-state level of drug has been achieved, each maintenance dose replaces the amount lost during the preceding interval. The dosage regimen for a drug is determined by its biological half-life and the range of plasma levels that is considered therapeutic. Initiation of therapy with a priming dose and careful selection of the dosing interval are particularly important for drugs with long half-life values.

When the maintenance dose is given at intervals equal to the biological half-life of the drug, 50% fluctuation is obtained in plasma levels during the steady state. It is characteristic of first-order kinetics that the fraction of the drug in the body eliminated during any time span is constant. Thus as the concentration of drug in the body rises, so does the absolute amount excreted during the same time span. A situation occurs therefore in which a constant amount of drug is being added to the body with each dose, but an increasing amount is being excreted during the interval between each dose. The plateau concentration represents the point of stabilization in this progression at which the amount of drug absorbed per dose interval equates the amount of drug eliminated during the same interval. Changing either the dose or frequency causes the plateau concentration to shift. Drugs are often studies for convenience of administration at intervals equal to their half-lives. Employing this interval, one achieves about 96% of the theoretical plateau concentration after four half-lives, and the mean plateau concentration is almost 1.5 times peak concentration after the initial dose. To overcome the delay of four half-lives in achieving the plateau, the initial dose can be increased. Drugs with short half-lives quickly accumulate to the desired plateau concentration, those with long half-lives may be slow in achieving an effective concentration. Calculation of the loading dose (D+) is as follows if the maintenance dose is known:

$$D+ = \frac{D}{Ke \times T}$$

D = Maintenance Dose

T = Dosing Interval

Ke = Elimination Rate Constant

15.6 PHARMACOKINETIC CONSIDERATIONS AND WITHDRAWAL TIMES

Of importance to the practical concerns of the veterinary practitioner, is the half-life which is a function of two pharmacologically relevant parameters, the drug's volume of distribution and its clearances, shown by the equation:

Half-life =

$$\frac{(0.693)\ (Volume\ of\ Distribution)}{(Clearance)}$$

Drugs possessing a large volume of distribution have low serum concentrations for a given dose of drug owing to extensive tissue distribution (e.g., tetracycline). A compound with a small volume of distribution would have higher serum concentrations for similar dosages. Some widely used drugs have prolonged withdrawal times because of a large volume of distribution. Drugs that distribute only through extracellular fluid have a relatively small volume of distribution compared with more lipid-soluble compounds that achieve significant intracellular concentrations. The other major variable affecting volume of distribution is the extent of plasma protein binding, which tends to retain drug in the plasma compartment and diminish the calculated volume of distribution. Thus volumes of distribution should be interpreted in light of the degree of protein binding.

If a renal disease process results in a 50% reduction in renal function, evidenced by a clearance one half of normal or a serum creatinine or serum urea nitrogen level elevated two times normal, half-life would be doubled, necessitating a prolongation of withdrawal times. Both very young and very old animals have renal clearances less than normal adults. If compounds are eliminated primarily by hepatic metabolism, factors that decrease the liver's ability to biotransform drugs (e.g., decreased hepatic blood flow, reduced enzyme activity owing to toxicity, or inhibition) may prolong drug half-life.

Half-lives and other pharmacokinetic parameters are tabulated in various pharmacology texts and in handbook form and are accessible through the Food Animal Residue Avoidance Databank (FARAD) supported by US Department of Agriculture (USDA).

Drugs such as the aminoglycosides (streptomycin, neomycin, and gentamicin) drop to below therapeutic levels within a few hours of being administered to livestock, but infinitesimal levels of residues may persist for periods of 30 days or longer. Generally the practitioner should calculate that it takes approximately 10 half-lives for an aminoglycoside drug to disappear from food animal tissues or be below the level of 0.0097 ppm. A half-life is the period of time that it takes for half of the drug administered to be excreted by the animal. Ordinarily doubling the dose necessitates the addition of another half-life to the withdrawal time. In the diseased, dehydrated, or otherwise compromised animal, the withdrawal time of 10 half-lives should probably be doubled. In the case of drugs administered in delayed absorption vehicles, such as benzathine penicillin or long-acting oxytetracycline, it may be necessary to more than double the withdrawal time if the dosage is doubled.

When using drugs in an extralabel manner, it is wise to remember that doubling the drug dose adds at least one half-life to the withdrawal time. It takes seven half-lives to eliminate 99% of an administered dose. Usually the veterinarian should calculate a minimum withdrawal time of five half-lives (97% elimination from body) times two (as a safety factor). For example, if a drug usually has a half-life of 24 hours, the veterinarian could recommend a withdrawal time of at least 10 days. The problem facing veterinarians is that most pharmacokinetic parameters have been determined in healthy animals, yet diseased animals would be expected to have altered physiology.

A tolerance for the pharmacologically active ingredient in tissues is established by the USDA-Food Safety and Inspection Service (FSIS) or the Food and Drug Administration (FDA)-Center for Veterinary Medicine (CVM), based on human safety and analytic considerations. The tolerance is the tissue level below which drug concentrations must fall before an animal's tissues are considered safe for human consumption. A manufacturer then establishes a withdrawal time for a specific formulation at the approved dose in the intended species.

Using this concept, one may estimate half-life from the official withdrawal time. A conservative estimate is that in 10 half-lives, 99.9% of drug is eliminated, and a drug with an initial concentration of 10 ppm would deplete to 0.0097 or 0.01 ppm. Therefore if the withdrawal time is 30 days, as for a number of sulfonamide, tetracycline, and procaine penicillin G products, the half-life would be 3 days.

All of the drugs implicated as causing residues have already long half-lives, attributable to their molecular structure (sulfamethazine), long-acting formulations (penicillin and oxytetracycline), or the tendency of aminoglycosides to sequester in the renal tissue (streptomycin, neomycin). Sulfamethazine, a putative thyroid carcinogen in a mouse bioassay, is a long-acting sulfonamide with an elimination half-life longer than many other sulfonamides. In general, it would not be unreasonable to assume that disease prolongs the half-life by up to six times.

APPENDIX I

FSIS of the USDA is responsible for ensuring that USDA-inspected meat and poultry products are safe, wholesome, free of adulterating residues, and accurately labeled. FSIS conducts the National Residue Program (NRP) to help prevent the marketing of animals containing unacceptable (violative) residues from pesticides, animal drugs, or potentially hazardous chemicals. Violations are determined by reference to residue limits (tolerances or action levels) established for pesticides by the Environmental Protection Agency (EPA) and for animal drugs and environmental contaminants by the FDA. Monitoring is designed to provide information on the occurrence of residue violations in specified animal populations on an annual, national basis.

Surveillance is designed to investigate and control the movement of potentially adulterated products. The sampling may be purposely biased, i.e., directed at particular carcasses or products in response to information indicating that adulterating levels of residues may be present. This information may be derived from monitoring.

Violative tissue residues are most frequently found to be associated with drugs having the following pharmacologic or pharmacokinetic features: long-activity formulation penicillin and oxytetracycline tend to sequester in the renal tissue (streptomycin, neomycin, and gentamicin) and have relatively long half-lives attributable to their molecular structure. The most common cause of residue violations is a failure to adhere to the withdrawal time. Other causes include cross contamination carryover in feed milling operations usually located on the farm, poor husbandry practices, and passage of colostrum with residues.

In 1991, the FSIS monitoring program sampled and tested for 13 classes of animal drug and pesticide compounds, composing more than 60 residues. Of the 42,056 monitoring samples, 0.26% showed violative levels of illegal residues, down from 0.3% in 1990. Almost all violations detected in monitoring were from illegal levels of approved animal drugs, particularly sulfonamide and antibiotic compounds used to treat bacterial infections. Most antibiotic and sulfa residue violations are confined to a relatively small percentage of livestock that make up the meat supply. The recurring reason for drug residue violations in livestock (and poultry, in past years) is failure to allow adequate time for the drugs to clear the animal's system. Consequently detected illegal residues are usually concentrated in kidney, liver, or fat rather than muscle meat.

Sulfonamide drugs (except approved use of sulfadimethoxine, sulfabromomethazine, and sulfaethoxypyridazine) are prohibited from use in lactating dairy cattle according to the FDA's extralabel use compliance policy guide. The following drugs are prohibited from use in any species of food-producing animal:

- Chloramphenicol
- Clenbuterol
- Diethylstilbestrol
- Furazolidone (except for approved topical use)
- Nitrofurazone (except for approved topical use)
- Dimetridazole
- Ipronidazole
- Other nitroimidazoles

APPENDIX-IIA

1990: INCIDENCE BY ANIMAL TYPE IN TISSUE RESIDUE

Animal Type	Sample
• Cows	2895/(47)%
Veal	2443/(40)%
• Barrows and gilts	401/(7)%
• Steers	90/(1.5)%
• Sows	80/(1.3)%
• Heifers	77/(1.3)%
• Formula-fed veal	31/(0.5)%
• Bulls/stags	29/(0.5)%
• Heavy calves	23/(0.4)%
• Boars/stags	23/(0.4)%
• Horse	23/(0.4)%
• Other	56/(1)%
Total	6171

Source: Center for Veterinary Medicine, 1990.

APPENDIX-IIB

1991: INCIDENCE BY ANIMAL TYPE IN TISSUE RESIDUE

Animal type	Sample
• Cows	2338/(54)%
Veal	1293/(30)%
• Barrows/gilts	293/(7)%
• Steers	65/(2)%
• Heifers	59/(1)%
• Sows	54/(1)%
• Other calves	46/(1)%
• Horses	31/(0.7)%
• Formula-fed veal	30/(0.7)%
• Lambs and yearling	30/(0.7)%
• Other	100/(2)%
Total	4339

APPENDIX-IIC

IDENTIFIABLE POOR MANAGEMENT TRAITS

Trait
- Failure to adhere to withdrawal time, 46%
- Unapproved uses, 3%
- Passage of colostrum with residue, 3%
- Cross contamination, 3%
- Other, 45%

Source: Center for Veterinary Medicine, Annual Report Compliance Program (7371.06) Fiscal Year '90/'91. *A retrospective analysis of FDA inspectional investigations of drugs in edible animal tissues reported during fiscal years 1990–1991.*

SELECTED REFERENCES

Affrime, M., and Reidenberg, M.M.: The protein binding of some drugs in plasma from patients with alcoholic liver disease. Eur. J. Clin. Pharmacol., *8*: 267, 1975.

Baggot, J.D.: Principles of Drug Disposition in Domestic Animals: The Basis of Veterinary Clinical Pharmacology. Philadelphia, W.B. Saunders, 1977.

Bischoff, K.B., and Brown, R.G.: Drug distribution in mammals. Chem. Eng. Progr. Symp. Ser., *62*: 32, 1966.

Button, C., Gross, D.R., Johnston, J.T., et al.: Pharmacokinetics, bioavailability, and dosage regimens of digoxin in dogs. Am. J. Vet. Res., *41*: 1230, 1980.

Chronic Toxicity and Carcinogenesis Study of Sulfamethazine in B6C3F1 mice. Jefferson, AR, National Center for Toxicological Research, 1988.

Coffey, J.J.: Effect of protein binding of drugs on areas under plasma concentration time curves. J. Pharm. Sci., *61*: 138, 1972.

Davis, B.D.: The binding of sulfonamide drugs by plasma proteins: A factor in determining the distribution of drugs in the body. J. Clin. Invest., *22*: 752, 1943.

Gibaldi, M., Nagashima, R., and Levy, G.: Relationship between drug concentration in plasma or serum and amount of drug in the body. J. Pharm. Sci., *58*: 193, 1969.

Gibaldi, M., and Weintraub, H.: Some considerations as to the determination and significance of biologic half-life. J. Pharm. Sci., *60*: 624, 1971.

Goldstein, A., et al.: Principles of Drug Action. New York, John Wiley & Sons, 1974.

Holford, N.H.G., and Sheiner, L.B.: Understanding the dose-effect relationship: Clinical application of pharmacokinetic-pharmacodynamic models. Clin. Pharmacokinet., *6*: 429, 1981.

Kaplan, S.A., Weinfeld, R.E., Cotler, S., et al.: Pharmacokinetic profile of trimethoprim in dog and man. J. Pharm. Sci., *59*: 358, 1970.

Koritz, G.D.: Practical aspects of pharmacokinetics for the large animal practitioner. Compend. Cont. Educ. Pract. Vet., *11*: 201, 1989.

Kunin, C.M.: Clinical pharmacology of the new penicilins. 1. The importance of serum protein binding in determining antimicrobial activity and concentration in serum. Clin. Pharm. Ther., *7*: 166, 1966.

Martin, B.K.: Potential effect of the plasma proteins on drug distribution. Nature, *207*: 274, 1965.

Mercer, H.D.: Residue avoidance: Withdrawal times for drugs not labelled for food animals. *In* The Use of Drugs in Food Animal Medicine. Proceedings of the 10th Annual Food Animal Medicine Conference. Edited by J.D. Powers and T.E. Powers. Columbus, Ohio State University Press, 1984.

Mercer, H.D., Baggot, J.D., and Sams, R.A.: Application of pharmacokinetic methods to the drug residue profile. J. Toxicol. Environ. Health, *2*: 787, 1977.

Meyer, M.C., and Guttman, D.E.: The binding of drugs by plasma proteins. J. Pharm. Sci., *57*: 895, 1968.

Neff, C.A., Davis, L.E., and Baggot, J.D.: A comparative study of the pharmacokinetics of quinidine. Am. J. Vet. Res., *33*: 1521, 1972.

Notari, R.E.: Pharmacokinetics and molecular modification: Implications in drug design and evaluation. J. Pharm. Sci., *62*: 865, 1973.

Notari, R.E., et al.: Biopharmaceutics and Pharmacokinetics. New York, Marcel Dekker, 1975.

Piloud, M.: Pharmacokinetics, plasma protein binding and dosage of oxytetracycline in cattle and horses. Res. Vet. Sci., *15*: 224, 1973.

Program Report—Sulfamethazine (SMZ) Control Program, Part I. Washington, D.C., USDA Food Safety and Inspection Service, Science and Technology Program, 1988.

Riviere, J.E.: Veterinary clinical pharmacokinetics. Part I: Fundamental concepts. Compend. Cont. Educ. Pract. Vet., *10*: 24, 1988.

Riviere, J.E.: Veterinary clinical pharmacokinetics. Part II: Modelling. Compend. Cont. Educ. Pract. Vet., *10*: 314, 1988.

Riviere, J.E.: The value and limitations of pharmacokinetics in predicting dosage regimens: Effects of systemic disease. *In* Determination of Doses of Veterinary Pharmaceuticals. Edited by T.E. Powers and J.D. Powers. Columbus, Ohio State University Press, 1984.

Riviere, J.E., Craigmill, A.L., and Sundlof, S.F.: Handbook of Comparative Pharmacokinetics and Residues of Veterinary Antimicrobials. Boca Raton, FL, CRC Press, 1990.

Riviere, J.E., Craigmill, A.L., and Sundlof, S.F.: Food animal residue avoidance databank (FARAD): An automated pharmacologic databank for drug and chemical residue avoidance. J. Food Protect., *49*: 826, 1986.

Sellers, E.M., and Koch-Weser, J.: Kinetics and clinical importance of displacement of warfarin from albumin by acidic drugs. Ann. N.Y. Acad. Sci., *170*: 213, 1971.

Sundlof, S.F., Riviere, J.E., Craigmill, A.L., and Buck, W.B.: Computerized food animal residue avoidance databank for veterinarians. J. Am. Vet. Med. Assoc., *188*: 73, 1986.

Sundlof, S.F., Riviere, J.E., and Craigmill, A.L.: A Comprehensive Compendium of Food Animal Drugs. The Food Animal Residues Avoidance Databank Tradename File. 3rd Ed. Gainesville, University of Florida, 1989.

Teorell, T.: Kinetics of distribution of substances administered to the body. Arch. Inter. Pharmacodyn. Ther., *57*: 205, 1937.

Van Dresser, W.R., and Wilcke, J.R.: Drug residues in food animals. J. Am. Vet. Med. Assoc., *194*: 1700, 1989.

Wagner, J.G., and Nelson, E.: The kinetic analysis of blood levels and urinary excretion in the absorptive phase after single doses of drug. J. Pharm. Sci., *53*: 1392, 1964.

Ziv, G., Shani, J., and Sulman, F.G.: Pharmacokinetic evaluation of penicillin and cephalosporin derivatives in serum and milk of lactating cows and ewes. Am. J. Vet. Res., *34*: 1561, 1973.

Ziv, G., and Sulman, F.G.: Analysis of pharmacokinetic properties of nine tetracycline analogues in dairy cows and ewes. Am. J. Vet. Res., *35*: 1197, 1974.

PART II

THERAPEUTICS

Section A

EQUINE

16
CHAPTER

DRUG THERAPY OF EQUINE COLIC

16.1 Introduction
16.2 Types of Colic
16.3 Principles of Treatment
16.4 Analgesics
16.5 Nonsteroidal Anti-Inflammatory Drugs
16.6 Sedatives / Tranquilizers
16.7 Verminous Arteritis and Thromboembolic Colic
16.8 Shock
16.9 Fluid Therapy
16.10 Spasmodic Colic and Spasmolytic Agents
16.11 Colonic Impaction
16.12 Flatulent Colic
16.13 Miscellaneous Drugs

16.1 INTRODUCTION

Colic is the largest single cause of patient mortality in equine practice. *Colic and laminitis are medical emergencies.* The symptoms of acute colic can be attributed to distention of the bowel, whether this be the result of increased or decreased bowel motility. The attendant symptoms of colic—anxiety, sweating, glancing at the abdomen, foot stamping, teeth grinding, rolling, with increased pulse and respiratory rate—are well recognized by the clinician. Hyperactivity exhibited by the affected horse in lying down and rolling can lead to organ displacement and subsequent development of complicated colic. In colic, the pulse rate is elevated as a result of pain. It may also be raised, however, as a result of inflammation and circulating inflammatory mediators. Impaired gut function resulting in impaired fluid and electrolyte balance progressively affects the pulse rate when blood volume contracts (hypovolemic) as more fluid becomes trapped in the bowel lumen. Ultimately the electrolyte balance and blood volume are the most significant factors in determining the course of the disease.

Conditions associated with abdominal pain are usually multifactorial. Pain may be associated with distention of a hollow viscus accompanied by ischemia and peritonitis or smooth muscle spasm. Distention of a viscus directly stimulates receptors that are responsive to alterations in tension, pressure, or shape. When distention is severe, blood supply to the gut wall can be contracted to the point of ischemia. If the integrity of the epithelial lining of the intestine is damaged, passage of irritating substances, such as bacterial endotoxins, into the peritoneal cavity occurs, and initiation of pain mechanisms follows. A horse's response to abdominal pain is symptomatic of underlying causes and lesions and necessitates prompt clinical treatment.

16.2 TYPES OF COLIC

Types of colic are as follows:

1. Spasmodic
2. Tympanitic
3. Ischemic
4. Obstructive
5. Impactive
6. Idiopathic
7. Enteritis and peritonitis

SPASMODIC COLIC

This is probably the most common form and is associated with increased bowel motor activity. Intestinal ischemia plays an important role in the pathology of the disease. Ischemia is highly painful and causes hyperperistalsis in other segments of the bowel. It is mostly associated with migratory strongylus larvae and verminous arteritis.

TYMPANITIC OR FLATULENT COLIC

Distention of the smooth muscle of the gut wall by gas causes intense pain. Failure to eliminate gas and distention of the gut wall lead to compression of intravascular blood vessels and ultimately an ischemic state.

ISCHEMIC GUT DISEASE

Thromboembolism from intravascular residence of the *Strongylus vulgaris* larvae has long been thought to be the prime mover of ischemic bowel disease. Local intravascular coagulation and vasoconstriction following endotoxin absorption with prostaglandin and thromboxane formation is now established as a major factor in the cause of ischemic bowel disease.

Loss of motility and functional ileus compromises the blood supply to the bowel because of bowel distention. Other bowel segments then become hypermotile, increasing the risk of intussusception, torsion, volvulus, or incarceration.

OBSTRUCTIVE COLIC AND ILEUS

The intestine may become functionally or physically obstructed. Paralytic ileus results from decreased intestinal motility. Obstruction is most likely to occur at narrow junctions, e.g., junction of the right dorsal colon and small colon and the pelvic flexure. Obstruction leads to impaction. Fluid sequestration in the gut lumen following ileus compounds the clinical problem, leading to severe dehydration.

ENTERITIS

The most important type of enteritis associated with colic is salmonellosis. Hospitalized horses (deemed asymptomatic) but subject to stress (e.g., transport, surgery, hospitalization) can suddenly experience flareups into severe clinical diseases. Salmonellosis is primarily a problem of hospitalized animals subjected to various stresses, which may not have received antimicrobial therapy.

PERITONITIS

Peritonitis occurs when massive inflammatory reaction occurs in the body cavity as a result of absorption of injurious substances (bacteria, endotoxins) from the bowel. Peritonitis is manifested clinically by severe pain, intestinal hypermotility, and wasting.

IDIOPATHIC COLIC

Many cases of colic recover spontaneously, and so the true cause may never be determined. Transient bowel ischemia may be an explanation for the temporary nature of these colic syndromes because in many cases a collateral blood supply develops, which re-establishes vascular nutrition of the gut wall.

PATHOPHYSIOLOGY OF EQUINE COLIC

Cases of equine colic are frequent in occurrence, are invariably serious, and, if untreated, are fatal. Among the species of domestic animals, the horse most commonly suffers from colic. The anatomy of the horse's digestive tract and the labile nature of the vegetative system are contributing factors. The digestive tract is 30 to 40 m long with marked variation in lumen diameter. A narrow lumen can join a part of the diges-

tive tract with a wide lumen or vice versa. This occurs when the narrow ileum joins the wide caecum at the ileocecal junction or when the caecum joins the colon at the cecocolic junction, which causes a considerable constriction of the digestive tract at this point; at the pelvic flexure, where the dorsal and ventral portions of the colon meet; or at the stomachlike dilation at the wide-narrow junction of the small colon. The horse is particularly predisposed to colic as a result of (1) the specific anatomic configuration of the equine gastrointestinal tracts, (2) parasitic vascular or nervous phenomena, (3) incorrect feeding, and (4) infectious diseases. The major anatomical considerations include:

1. The mobility and numerous circumvolutions of the small intestine and floating colon
2. The curvatures of the colon
3. The method of attachment of certain segments
4. The alternating smooth and nonsmooth regions of the bowel leading to invagination of the smooth ileum into the base of the caecum, the apex of the caecum into the body of the caecum, and the descending of floating colon into the rectum

Dislocations easily lead to gut stasis or herniations. The various vascular phenomena can be related to infestation with strongylus larvae leading to arteritis, ischemia, and infarction; nervous phenomena leading to vagotonia; and incorrect feeding leading to impaction, obstruction, or microbial imbalance. Inflammation and obstruction of the mesenteric arteries owing to migrating *S. vulgaris* larvae result in local pain with small necrosis of the affected portion of the intestine, leading to symptoms of sudden violent colic and peristaltic intestinal spasm. In cecal impaction, the attacks of colic may be accompanied by only slight pain recurring at intervals of hours or days.

Gaseous distention of the intestine may occur in ileus, in prolonged impaction, or in the course of peritonitis when peristalsis is arrested. The animal often dies of circulatory collapse unless the distended abdominal loops are punctured and the pain alleviated. The intestine may be physically (mechanical ileus) or functionally (paralytic ileus) obstructed. The term "ileus" is used to describe this state but does not necessarily imply that the affected portion is the ileum. Mechanical ileus may result from lumen obstruction or topographic alterations or extraluminal compression (intestinal strangulation obstruction), whereas paralytic ileus results from decreased intestinal motility. Decreased flatus elimination (oral or anal) or increased fermentation leads to tympanitic colic. Again pain is probably the result of localized ischemia as distention of the bowel wall causes compression of intramural blood vessels. More often than not, the condition is self-limiting, but in a few cases rupture of a viscus can occur. In cases of impaction, gradual excessive accumulations occur in certain portions of the bowel, the primary form of which is caused by overfeeding; the secondary form is caused by dental defects, senile atony, lameness, or mechanical obstruction.

Because pain is the principal accompaniment to attacks of colic, drugs that alleviate pain by removing the cause or altering the animal's perception of pain are indicated. Experimental studies have revealed that the pelvic flexure acts as a pacemaker for colonic motility, generating propulsive movement of small particles to the rectum and retropulsive movement of larger particles back into the caecum and large colon to delay their passage and facilitate more complete digestion. Impairment of the neural or vascular supply to this important region (e.g., in *S. vulgaris* infestation) might therefore render it insensitive to distensive stimuli, leading to impaction. The role of *S. vulgaris* as a major cause of equine colic is, of course, well established. Recurrent mild or persistent colic is often attributed to episodes of bowel ischemia associated with repeated arterial thromboembolism and subsequent recanalization or establishment of a collateral circulation.

Although severe thromboembolism with bowel infarction progresses rapidly and is diagnosed either at surgery or necropsy, diagnostic difficulty is often experienced in recurrent mild cases. "Thromboembolic colic" is the term applied to intestinal disease produced by thrombosis or thromboembolism. The popular use of the term thromboembolic colic encompasses several diseases, including verminous arteritis, ver-minous colic, and focal or diffuse intestinal infarction. The cause of these conditions is thought to be the presence of migrating *S. vulgaris* larvae within the arterial system supplying the intestinal tract. The thrombotic reaction to the parasitic larvae has been recorded in many cases of horses on which necropsy has been performed and has been incriminated in 90% of all episodes of equine colic.

It is likely that ischemic bowel disease is mediated at the mural vessel level. Simultaneous, complete thromboembolism of all the mural vessels of a segment of gut with debris from a parasitic lesion in the craniomesenteric artery is unlikely. It is suggested that either a local intravascular coagulation or vasoconstriction occurs, and this might well be a hypersensitivity response to migrating fourth-stage *S. vulgaris* larvae. Subsequent loss of motility and functional ileus further compromise the blood supply because the bowel becomes distended. Ischemic bowel disease primarily affects the small intestine and, to a lesser extent, the caecum and colon, further supporting the hypothesis that migrating fourth-stage larvae are the etiologic link. Pain in suspected cases of verminous arteritis can be treated with a variety of analgesic agents. Nonsteroidal anti-inflammatory drugs (NSAIDs) have worked well to date. If the production of prostaglandins is one of the features of this disease, NSAIDs should be helpful in managing the disease by reducing platelet activity. An important adverse effect of some, especially flunixin meglumine, is the masking of pain and shock—signs associated with diseases that require surgical correction.

Colic-associated intestinal ischemia may result from vascular compression caused by intestinal distention; reduced cardiac output during hypovolemia and endotoxemia; mediator-induced vasoconstriction during shock and endotoxemia; therapeutic and anesthetic drugs; parasite-induced vascular damage; and vascular occlusion caused by intestinal torsion, volvulus, or displacement. Successful management of patients with decreased intestinal motility depends largely on differentiation of obstructive and nonobstructive diseases. Treatment of ileus includes nasogastric decompression, analgesics, and fluid and electrolyte replacement. Pharmacologic alteration of motility may be considered in cases of ileus. Hyoscine is one useful motility modifier. The most important consideration in colic resulting from all causes is relief of pain. Eighty percent of colics are simple and resolve spontaneously. The humane consideration to relieve pain fast and effectively is therefore the only necessary treatment in such cases. The cause in such cases is often unknown, although most are probably spasmodic colic. Spasmolytic preparations, frequently in combination with other drugs, are effective and often analgesic. The prolonged ocular side effects of atropine precludes its use in the horse, but hyoscine is effective as an alternative agent. Treatment of intestinal infarction resulting from thrombosis or thromboembolism is more difficult. The goal of the therapy is to preserve intestinal viability and the horse's life, and treating the arteritis becomes a secondary concern. Problems that must be treated include pain, shock, ileus, and possibly peritonitis.

The features of equine colic include:

1. Pain
2. Anxiety
3. Spasm
4. Impaction
5. Distention
6. Flatulence
7. Ischemia
8. Thromboembolic shock
9. Dehydration
10. Arteritis
11. Peritonitis

COLIC, PAIN, AND INTESTINAL SPASM

Intestinal spasm is the most common cause of abdominal pain in most forms of equine colic. In spasmodic colic, the peristaltic waves take place more frequently and with increased intensity, and the resting tonus of the intestines is also increased, which leads to the development of slight spasms of the intestine at rest. Atony of the intestinal wall develops only after the spasm subsides, especially in impaction of the caecum and colon. Spasmodic colic is the most common form of colic, usually occurring at points where there is an anatomic or pathologic

narrowing of the intestines. The most frequently affected sections of the bowel are the end of the ileum, the head of the blind gut, the left ventral longitudinal sections, the pelvic flexure, and the stomachlike dilatation of the large colon. When the wall of the intestine is stretched through the stasis of the ingesta, a reflex contraction of the smooth muscle occurs. As a result, fluid is squeezed out of the pulpy food and the feces become harder because of the resorptive activity of the intestinal mucosa. Treatment in such cases must always address the relief of intestinal pain.

Hyperperistalsis (an increase in the tonus and rhythm of the peristaltic wave) can increase to the point of chronic intestinal pain. This too results in spasmodic colic or intestinal spasm syndrome. The intestinal lumen then becomes narrowed or is completely occluded, which results in stasis of intestinal contents. Simultaneously with symptoms of spasm, the opposite state, atony of the intestinal wall, may occur elsewhere in the intestine. Spasmodic peristalsis means an excessive increase in muscle tone with a marked acceleration of its rhythm so intestinal movements become violent in nature. Tonic intestinal spasm is a prolonged, locally limited, excessive increase in tone of the intestinal musculature that can lead to complete spastic occlusion of the intestinal lumen. This prolonged tonus of the resting intestine may become so severe that the passage of a peristaltic wave is no longer possible. The intestinal pain caused by violent spasmodic peristalsis leads to the violent symptoms of colic. Defective intestinal movements and stasis of the contents can in turn progress to intestinal displacements, and the resultant torsions, rotations, and flexions occur most frequently in the large intestine and in the ascending colon in particular.

In spasmodic colic, there are episodes of powerful smooth muscular contractions that alternate with pain-free periods, and these painful spasms are associated with bursts of nervous activity (mainly parasympathetic). Drugs that block the effects of parasympathetic stimulation are indicated. In horses with severe visceral pain, analgesia may be required to quiet the animal sufficiently to perform an examination. Abdominal pain contributes to a high sympathetic nervous system tone, which reflexly inhibits intestinal motility. Control of pain with analgesics aids the return of normal motility. The intestinal musculature is subject to the antagonistic effects of the sympathetic and parasympathetic nervous system with the former inhibiting intestinal activity and the latter stimulating it. Intestinal motor activity is based on the autonomy mediated through the ganglion cells arranged between the annular and longitudinal musculature. Spasmolytic drugs are specific for treatment of spasmodic colic in which pain is due to increased muscular activity and spasm of intestinal muscle. Inhibition of gut motility extends from stomach to colon, although the degree of blockade may not be uniform, and the total inhibition of excessive motility may be incomplete because of the role of other mediators in stimulating smooth muscle, e.g., 5-hydroxytryptamine, histamine, and prostaglandin. Because intestinal spasm is the primary cause of various types of colic, in therapy peristalsis must be regulated and the local autonomic equilibrium restored to normal.

EQUINE ABDOMINAL PAIN

Abdominal pain in the horse is conveniently classified as visceral pain and parietal pain. Visceral pain is associated with the typical signs of colic, in which horses exhibit uncontrollable physical activity. External palpation, when possible, is usually not painful, unless the troubled viscus is contracted. Parietal pain differs: The horse tends to remain immobile, and palpation of the abdomen causes considerable pain. Abdominal pain in any species apparently develops in a limited number of ways. Pain-sensitive fibers in the abdominal viscera respond most readily to distention of the intestinal wall (tympanites), spasm of intestinal smooth muscle, intestinal ischemia, tension or stretching of the mesenteric supporting structure, and chemical irritation of the visceral or parietal peritoneum (peritonitis). These cause widespread stimulation of pain fibers and result in abdominal pain; however, such widespread excitation of nerve endings in a viscus results in poorly localized pain perception.

A horse's response to abdominal pain can be one of the only signs predicting lesions that require rapid, thorough treatment. Conditions associated with abdominal pain is most species often are multifactorial—pain cannot be attributed to only one of the mechanisms listed. More frequently, distention of a hollow viscus is accompanied by ischemia, peritonitis, or both. In less severe and often undiagnosed occurrences of colic, pain might be attributable to smooth muscle spasm. Distention of a viscus directly stimulates receptors that are responsive to alterations in tension, pressure, or shape. If distention is severe and intraluminal pressure rises, the blood supply in the intestinal wall can be compromised to the point of ischemia. Similarly, with localized loss of tissue perfusion or complete luminal obstruction, intestinal distention develops, and pain is increased by stretching of the viscus. When the integrity of the intestinal wall is violated, transmural movement of irritating substances (e.g., bacteria and bacterial endotoxins) into the peritoneal cavity occurs and initiates parietal pain mechanisms. Disturbances of gastrointestinal motility are sometimes associated with gastrointestinal diseases that result in diarrhea and colic in horses. Intestinal ischemia, intestinal obstruction, parasitic infection, inflammation of the intestinal serosa, and endotoxemia alter intestinal motility.

Abdominal problems are related to difficulties with the rapid progression of abundant digesta in organs of relatively limited volumes: stomach and small intestine. The large intestine, a much larger and more important digestive organ than in other domestic animals, is also vulnerable. To fit into the abdominal cavity, this voluminous intestinal tube is multifolded, its diameter is alternately dilated and narrowed, and the structure of its wall varies considerably from segment to segment. Accordingly, changes in the gastrointestinal transit and motility of feedings are more marked than in other species. The morphologic characteristics favor impaction, volvulus, and intussusception.

Problems in gastrointestinal motor functions lead to (1) interruption of the internal circulation of fluid and electrolytes, exsorption exceeding insorption; (2) perturbation of the enzymatic and bacterial digestive processes; and (3) intermittent or continuous visceral (sympathetic tract mediated) or parietal (somatic tract mediated) abdominal pain.

Treatment of equine colic and endotoxemia presently seems to center on the use of drugs that inhibit cyclooxygenase activity. These agents, NSAIDs, act to modify either temporarily or permanently the cyclooxygenase enzymes. Phenylbutazone, which is one of the best-known NSAID in equine practice, is an enolic acid that has been proposed to bind irreversibly to the enzyme. Other drugs used in treating colic and endotoxemia include ketoprofen, flunixin, meclofenamic acid, and (less frequently) aspirin. Theoretically all NSAIDs should act identically by inhibiting cyclooxygenase and preventing the generation of the arachidonic acid metabolites.

NSAIDs can be classified according to chemical structure: salicylates (e.g., aspirin); indoles (e.g., indomethacin); propionic acids (e.g., ibuprofen and naproxen); fenamates (e.g., meclofenamic acid and flunixin meglumine); and pyrazolones (e.g., phenylbutazone and dipyrone). Their analgesic, antipyretic, and anti-inflammatory properties no doubt result from the same mechanism of action: inhibition of prostaglandin formation. Prostaglandins and the related leukotrienes are eicosanoids that are formed in situ in cells. The chain of events that form these eicosanoids begins with a stimulus (such as mechanical, chemical, or thermal damage) or an immune-mediated or hormonal signal. This stimulus or signal perturbs the cell membrane and activates phospholipases (particularly A_2 and C), which hydrolyze cell membrane phospholipids, releasing fatty acids into the cell. The most important of these fatty acids is arachidonic acid. When released, arachidonic acid moves into the cell, where it serves as a substrate for lipoxygenases and cyclooxygenases to build the final eicosanoid product.

In colic, if the intestinal wall becomes inadequately perfused, bacterial endotoxin, lipopolysaccharide (LPS) passes transmurally into the peritoneal cavity and into the general circulation. The lipid nature of endotoxin evidently allows this substance to cross the intestinal wall much more quickly than intact bacteria do. This sequence of events has been demonstrated in several animal species, and endotoxin has been detected in plasma from horses with intestinal ischemia. The presence of endotoxin in the circulation initiates a series of circulatory, hormonal, hematologic, and metabolic changes that signal the need for therapy. In horses (as in other species studied to date), endotoxemia results in damage to the vascular endothelium. Specifically endotoxemia causes endothelial cells to separate from each other and to slough from the underlying basal lamina. This damage has been demonstrated in equine pulmonary arteries, pulmonary veins, and endocardial surface by scanning electron microscopy.

The alterations in the vascular endothelium serve as a focal point for involvement of vasoactive substances. When the cell membranes are damaged, the fatty acid components of the phospholipids are cleaved by specific phospholipase enzymes. One of the fatty acids, arachidonic acid, serves as the substrate for at least two enzyme systems: cyclooxygenase and lipoxygenase. Cyclooxygenase converts arachidonic acid to the unstable endoperoxide intermediates, which may be modified further to form the classic prostaglandins, prostacyclin, or thromboxane. These endogenous substances have profound effects on the local circulation, pain receptors, and thermoregulatory center. Prostaglandins, especially of the E series, are important eicosanoids in the process of inflammation and pain perception. By inhibition of the cyclooxygenase enzyme system, prostaglandin synthesis is blocked by NSAIDs. In the absence of these local prostaglandins, substances such as histamine and bradykinin can no longer activate the nociceptor. Pyrexia is associated with central synthesis of prostaglandins in the hypothalamus following activation by pyrogens. This then sets the temperature sensor at a higher than normal value.

16.3 PRINCIPLES OF TREATMENT

Therapy of equine colic can be subdivided into two major approaches: (1) general supportive therapy (Table 16–1), which is independent of the etiologic diagnosis, and

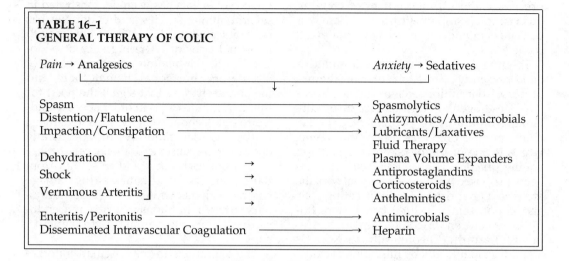

TABLE 16–1
GENERAL THERAPY OF COLIC

Pain → Analgesics   *Anxiety* → Sedatives

Spasm ————————————————————→ Spasmolytics
Distention/Flatulence ——————————————→ Antizymotics/Antimicrobials
Impaction/Constipation ——————————————→ Lubricants/Laxatives
                                                       Fluid Therapy
Dehydration ⎤   →   Plasma Volume Expanders
Shock   ⎬   →   Antiprostaglandins
Verminous Arteritis ⎦   →   Corticosteroids
                                  →   Anthelmintics
Enteritis/Peritonitis ——————————————→ Antimicrobials
Disseminated Intravascular Coagulation ————→ Heparin

(2) specific therapy necessitated by specific colic problems (verminous arteritis, colonic obstruction).

Supportive therapy is oriented toward relief of pain; prevention of treatment of gastrointestinal rupture; therapy of bacterial septicemia, endotoxemia, or peritonitis; and maintenance of peripheral perfusion, hydration, acid-base, and electrolyte balances. Types of drugs used in colic therapy include:

1. Narcotic analgesics
2. NSAIDs
3. Sedatives
4. Lubricants/purgatives
5. Fluids
6. Plasma volume expanders
7. Corticosteroids
8. Spasmolytics
9. Anthelmintics

In the treatment of pain, the classes of drugs that can be considered include (1) NSAIDs, (2) sedatives/analgesics, (3) narcotic analgesics, and (4) alpha$_2$ agonists.

Specific therapy treats:

1. Impactive colic—to promote evacuation of the luminal obstruction
2. Verminous arteritis—to treat migratory stages of *S. vulgaris*

Treatment of specific types of colic necessitates a definite, specific diagnosis of verminous arteritis (anthelmintics), bacterial enteritis (antibiotics), or impactions of the large bowel (laxatives).

16.4 ANALGESICS

The most important consideration in colic regardless of the specific type is relief of pain. Although approximately 80% of colics are simple and resolve spontaneously, nonetheless this condition is still the largest single cause of death in the horse. Because 20% of cases are therefore serious or potentially fatal if correct treatment is not provided, it is axiomatic that such cases should be recognized, diagnosed, and appropriately treated as quickly and as accurately as possible.

Horses with severe colic require analgesics to facilitate their proper and complete evaluation and initial therapy. Effective analgesia is of critical importance in horses experiencing acute abdominal pain to prevent self-inflicted trauma and intestinal displacement. An ideal analgesic agent for the horse with colic should act rapidly and should not mask signs suggesting the need for surgery.

CENTRALLY ACTING ANALGESICS: OPIATES AND OPIOIDS

These potent, centrally acting compounds provide deep analgesia with variable degrees of sedation. It is essential to provide analgesia for horses suffering from severe visceral pain owing to gastrointestinal tract disturbances. The centrally acting narcotic analgesics raise the pain threshold, produce euphoria and drowsiness, and modify the

TABLE 16–2
OPIOIDS

	Dose	
Meperidine hydrochloride	2.2–3.0	mg/kg IM, IV
Methadone	0.1	mg/kg IV, IM
Pentazocine lactate	0.4–0.6	mg/kg IV, IM
Butorphanol lactate	0.04–0.22	mg/kg IV, IM

IM, Intramuscular; IV, intravenous.

perception and interpretation of pain. Although opioids may be considered the most effective analgesic therapy for relief of visceral pain, an overall effect of morphine and related opiates in the digestive tract is the delayed passage of ingesta and constipation. These effects must be carefully considered when administering narcotics to the horse with colic.

The opiates and opioids are the major group of drugs used for analgesia in equine colic (Table 16–2). Receptors for these drugs in the brain and spinal cord are acted on by the body's endogenous morphine-type substances—the endorphins and enkephalins. Many types and classes of opioid receptors exist, each of which when stimulated produces specific effects (mu, kappa, sigma). One type of receptor produces the desirable effects, such as analgesia and sedation. Two other major receptor types produce generally undesired effects, such as cardiopulmonary depression, decreased gastrointestinal motility, and behavioral changes such as excitement and addiction.

These narcotic agents act through central nervous system receptors to raise the pain threshold and increase tolerance to pain. They act in a similar fashion to the body's endogenous opioids. Most opioidal compounds display a depressant effect on the intestinal musculature, inducing constipation with delayed passage of ingesta and enhanced reabsorption of water.

Opiates possess agonist and antagonistic properties. Cardiovascular and intestinal side effects occur in response to narcotics. Narcotics increase regional contraction of the gut, causing intestinal transit to be prolonged.

Because morphine causes excitement and gastrointestinal side effects, the synthetic opiate agonists-antagonists are preferable for clinical use. The most commonly used opioids include pentazocine lactate, meperidine hydrochloride, oxymorphone hydrochloride, and butorphanol lactate.

In the horse, increased locomotor activity (dopaminergic action) and central nervous system stimulation are commonly observed side effects with opioid drugs. Of particular legal significance to the practicing veterinarian is the fact that many of these morphine-type narcotics are subject to federal narcotics legislation. Many opioids are contraindicated if small intestinal obstruction is suspected because all of the morphine family have the potential to produce powerful smooth muscle contractions in the distended small intestine.

Meperidine

This is a potent analgesic with activity in the horse for approximately 4 hours. The synthetic opioid meperidine (pethidine) is approximately one tenth as potent as morphine in the horse and is rapidly cleared by the kidneys, its clinical effects lasting less than 1 hour. Similar to many opioids, this narcotic analgesic may cause central nervous system excitement in horses when given intravenously and may also worsen ileus. The amount of analgesia and duration of action are variable when given intramuscularly at a dose of 2.2 to 3 mg/kg. Its sedative effects can be reversed by naloxone (10 to 22 μg/kg). Meperidine is short acting; its effects persist for approximately 60 minutes.

The maximum recommended dose of meperidine is 2 mg/kg, and higher doses can cause central nervous system excitement, convulsions, and stimulation of the spinal cord. These signs are also seen after intravenous administration; thus the drug should be given only by the intramuscular route, at doses not higher than 2 mg/kg. Meperidine is relatively inexpensive and widely used in the horse. Its local spasmogenic effect on the gut musculature is considerably less than that of morphine.

Methadone

This can be used as an alternative to morphine. It is more potent than morphine and less likely to cause excitement. It is active for 4 to 6 hours, producing profound analgesia at a dosage rate of 0.1 mg/kg, intravenously or intramuscularly.

Pentazocine

This is a narcotic analgesic with potency of about a quarter that of morphine, providing analgesia for 30 minutes at a dosage rate of 0.15 mg/lb intravenously or intramuscularly. After intramuscular injection, relief lasts for two to six hours.

A synthetic narcotic agonist, pentazocine has less tendency to produce excitement and reduce gastrointestinal motility than the other pure narcotic agonists. A reasonable degree of analgesia can be expected with pentazocine that does not mask clinical signs of strangulatory obstruction. Pentazocine is a less potent analgesic than butorphanol or morphine because of its ratio of receptor agonist to antagonist properties.

Butorphanol

Butorphanol is a centrally acting opiate with mixed agonist-antagonist properties. It causes minimal sedation, and at a dose of 0.1 mg/kg, the duration of visceral analgesia is three to four hours. It does not tend to mask the early cardiovascular effects associated with endotoxemia and hence can be used to control pain without interfering with specific diagnosis.

Butorphanol tartrate (Torbugesic, Bristol) is a centrally acting morphine derivative possessing four times the analgesic potency of morphine and 30 times the potency of pentazocine. It is classified as a narcotic agonist-antagonist. The drug does not produce profound respiratory depression or cardiovascular changes.

This unique opioid possesses agonistic and antagonistic actions, stimulating the receptors responsible for analgesia and sedation, while antagonizing receptors responsible for the generally undesirable side effects. This produces minimal excitement at clinically useful dosage rates and little or no effect on bowel motility. As an analgesic, butorphanol is four times more potent than morphine and 40 times more potent than meperidine. Additionally, there is no significant depression to cardiopulmonary function, which renders butorphanol ideal for many colic cases regardless of the presence of circulatory shock. The profound, reliable and analgesic effect coupled with its mild sedative action makes butorphanol the drug of choice for either shocked or sound horses.

Butorphanol is a synthetic morphine derivative with narcotic agonist-antagonist properties producing minimal cardiopulmonary effects at analgesic doses (0.05 to 0.2 mg/kg). Doses exceeding 0.2 mg/kg may produce ataxia and excitement.

It is more effective than pentazocine, meperidine, or flunixin in alleviating visceral pain. The combination of butorphanol with a sedative minimizes excitatory side effects.

The combination of xylazine and butorphanol tartrate produces a synergistic analgesic effect that provides a useful level of analgesia and restraint (Tables 16–3 and 16–4).

Narcotic drugs cause constipation by decreasing propulsive motility and increasing segmental contractions.

Butorphanol has minimal untoward effects in this regard and is one of the best of the narcotics when ileus is present.

Naloxone

This is an opioid receptor antagonist. This drug reverses the effects of narcotic agonists on the gastrointestinal tract and cardiovascular system (dose 10 to 22 μg/kg intravenously).

Naloxone is an opiate receptor antagonist whose action has been shown to reverse the fall in arterial pressure following endotoxin administration.

TABLE 16–3
SEDATIVES

Sedatives	Dose	
Xylazine hydrochloride	0.2–1.0	mg/kg IV, IM
Detomidine	20–40	μg/kg IV, IM
Chloral hydrate	30.0	g/orally in water
	40.0	mg/kg IV, IM
Acetyl promazine	0.05–0.1	mg/kg IV, IM

Sedative-Analgesic Combinations	Dose	
Xylazine hydrochloride + butorphanol tartrate	0.3 mg/kg + 0.1	mg/kg
Xylazine hydrochloride + fentanyl citrate	1.1 mg/kg + 0.055	mg/kg
Xylazine hydrochloride + meperidine hydrochloride	1.1 mg/kg + 2.2	mg/kg
Xylazine hydrochloride + oxymorphone hydrochloride	1.1 mg/kg + 0.0165	mg/kg

16.5 NONSTEROIDAL ANTI-INFLAMMATORY DRUGS

These agents modify enzyme systems that produce prostaglandins. Members of this group, such as flunixin, phenylbutazone, ketoprofen, and dipyrone (metamizole), have been used with increasing frequency in many cases of equine colic. The pharmacologic activity of NSAIDs is based on their capacity to inhibit cyclooxygenase enzymes (prostaglandin synthetase) (Table 16–5). This enzymatic inhibition acts to prevent biosynthesis of prostaglandins and thromboxanes, and the ensuing analgesia is due to inhibition of prostaglandin formation. There are no inhibitory effects on prostaglandins and other local mediators of inflammation already preformed in the tissues. Prostaglandins sensitize receptors to the effects of mechanical stimulation and vasoactive substances, such as histamine and bradykinin.

When cell membranes are damaged, prostaglandin synthesis and release occur. These prostaglandins, through their vasoactive properties, increase vascular permeability, lower the threshold of pain, and produce fever. NSAIDs prevent the synthesis and release of prostaglandins in inflammation and thus prevent this sensitization of pain receptors. These drugs do not appear to be clinically effective until prostaglandins formed before administration are reduced. Thus a lag phase of up to 12 hours may occur until relief is seen. The analgesic effect is secondary to the anti-inflammatory effect, and the effects of NSAIDs outlast the high levels of the drug in the blood stream.

Locally produced prostaglandins are important in the generation of pain and fever associated with most inflammatory processes; therefore NSAIDs provide analgesia by inhibiting local inflammation through peripheral action.

NSAIDs act as cyclooxygenase inhibitors and may redirect arachidonic acid metabolism through the lipoxygenase pathway, resulting in production of leukotrienes, which are vasoactive and chemoattractant. Flunixin meglumine (0.25 mg/kg) suppresses plasma thromboxane levels via cyclooxygenase inhibition, thus reducing the clinical effects of endotoxins.

In colic, careful clinical assessment is necessary, especially when dealing with intestinal ischemia, in which the masking of clinical signs could lead to a fatal delay in surgical intervention.

Following endotoxin absorption, phenylbutazone, another anti-inflammatory and prostaglandin inhibitor, has been found to reduce hemoconcentration. Although drugs in this class interrupt a similar biochemical pathway (cyclooxygenase enzymes in different tissues and their sensitivity to inhibition by each drug), differences in drug potency may also be attributable to the type of enzymatic inhibitions, which may be reversible competitive, reversible noncompetitive, or irreversible.

TABLE 16–4
ANALGESIC PRODUCTS FOR COLIC THERAPY

Drug	Trade Name	Manufacturer
Butorphanol tartrate	Torbugesic	Bristol Laboratories
Flunixin meglumine	Banamine	Schering
Ketoprofen	Ketofen	Fort Dodge
Meperidine	Demerol	Winthrop
Oxymorphone	Numorphan	Dupont
Pentacozine	Talwin V	Winthrop
Phenylbutazone	Phenylzone	Luitpold
Xylazine	Rompun	Haver

Flunixin meglumine, ketoprofen, and dipyrone are the most popular drugs for control of abdominal pain in horses. Dipyrone is less potent than flunixin but tends to have stronger antipyretic effects.

Side effects of NSAIDs include gastric ulceration and kidney damage. Side effects can be heightened when these drugs are given concurrently with aminoglycosides or to hypovolemic/endotoxic patients.

Phenylbutazone and meclofenamic acid are excellent for treating pain associated with the locomotor system, whereas flunixin and ketoprofen are by far the most effective in treating colic. Dipyrone, phenylbutazone, and flunixin meglumine do not adversely affect cardiovascular status or gastrointestinal motility. Flunixin meglumine and phenylbutazone improve hemodynamics in horses with endotoxemia. Toxicity of NSAIDs varies, although all of these drugs possess the capability to induce acute renal disease and gastrointestinal tract ulceration, subsequent to local vasoconstriction, hypoxia, and necrosis.

FLUNIXIN MEGLUMINE

This NSAID reduces pain and inflammation in the colicky patient. Flunixin meglumine can be given with good effect intravenously as an analgesic at a dosage rate of 1.1 mg/kg every 12 hours to horses with severe pain. At lower doses (0.25 mg/kg), it counteracts shock.

This aminonicotinic acid derivative is one of the most potent of the currently available NSAIDs and is the most effective NSAID for treatment of visceral pain in the horse. Clinical effects are seen within 10 minutes of intravenous administration, and analgesia persists for up to 8 hours. Because of the drug's ability to mask endotoxin-induced cardiovascular derangements, it must be used judiciously in horses with colic or at the lower dose level 0.25 mg/kg. If used indiscriminately, flunixin can mask the signs of intestinal ischemia/endotoxemia, thereby delaying life-saving surgical intervention.

TABLE 16–5
NONSTEROIDAL ANTI-INFLAMMATORY DRUGS

Drug	Dose	
Flunixin meglumine	1.1–2.2	mg/kg IV, IM
Dipyrone	10.0–22.0	mg/kg IV, IM
Phenylbutazone	2.2–4.4	mg/kg IV; 2–4 g PO
Meclofenamic acid	2.2	mg/kg PO
Ketoprofen	2.2	mg/kg IV

IV, Intravenous; IM, intramuscular; PO, oral.

Flunixin is a powerful antiprotaglandin drug. The symptoms of endotoxic shock (blue-red tinge to mucous membranes, prolonged capillary refill time, increasing heart rate, hemoconcentration) as a result of intestinal strangulation, however, can be totally masked by this drug. Flunixin is also an excellent analgesic for severe abdominal pain. Thus colic patients requiring immediate surgery could be subjected to critical delays because their vital signs mislead the clinician into thinking that a conservative approach is appropriate when it is not.

A related but less potent NSAID is dipyrone, which by virtue of its local anti-inflammatory action alleviates the pain of spasm associated with contraction of gastrointestinal tract musculature. Dipyrone is frequently combined with spasmolytic compounds, such as methindizate, in commercial parenteral formulations.

This enolic acid derivative of aminopyrine is similar to phenylbutazone in structure. It possesses antipyretic and analgesic effects and antagonizes bradykinin-induced intestinal spasm. It provides short-term relief up to 1 hour in mild cases of colic (11 mg/kg) caused by tympany, intestinal spasm, or colonic impaction. It is not highly effective for most cases of colic when used alone.

PHENYLBUTAZONE

This is an enolic acid that has highly effective anti-inflammatory properties for most equine musculoskeletal disorders. The drug is preferentially indicated in the therapy of acute or chronic laminitis. Although not effective for soft tissue (visceral) pain in colic, it is effective in general treatment in which laminitis may be apparent as a sequela to the infarction-peritonitis sequence in the affected horse.

Phenylbutazone is given intravenously at 2 to 4 mg/kg and may be repeated every 12 hours. Phenylbutazone is associated with many toxic side effects, including anorexia, depression, gastrointestinal ulceration, protein-losing enteropathy, edema, and nephrotoxicity. Owing to its irritant nature, it may cause thrombophlebitis after injection. Horses receiving long-term therapy should be monitored closely for evidence of gas-trointestinal or renal disease. The dose should not exceed 4.4 mg/kg twice a day for more than 3 days.

KETOPROFEN

Ketoprofen is a potent, nonnarcotic NSAID. A member of the propionic acid class, ketoprofen inhibits both the cyclooxygenase and the lipoxygenase branches of the arachidonic acid cascade, resulting in potent analgesic and antipyretic activity. The cyclooxygenase branch is ultimately responsible for the myriad of prostaglandins and thromboxanes that serve as inflammatory mediators. The lipoxygenase branch produces a variety of leukotrienes and hydroxyeicosatetraenoic acids. These mediators are involved in leukocyte migration, activation, and control as well as the release of other inflammatory mediators. It is interesting to note that at therapeutic doses most other NSAIDs do not inhibit the lipoxygenase portion of the arachidonic cascade.

In contrast to other NSAIDs, which work by blocking the cyclooxygenase pathway and thereby preventing prostaglandin and thromboxane synthesis, ketoprofen blocks the lipoxygenase pathway (i.e., the synthesis of leukotrienes). The activity of bradykinin, a powerful mediator of the vascular phase of inflammation and pain, is also inhibited by ketoprofen.

Further, NSAIDs that work only on the cyclooxygenase pathway are known to divert the metabolism of arachidonic acid toward the lipoxygenase pathway. An innovative NSAID of the propionic acid class, ketofen inhibits not just one but both branches of the arachidonic acid cascade, which results in the anti-inflammatory, analgesic, and antipyretic actions. So it blocks the source of inflammation and pain effectively.

For use in equine colic, the recommended dose is 2.2 mg/kg (1 ml/45 kg) body weight, given by intravenous injection for immediate effect. A second injection may be given if the colic returns. Ketoprofen has a short half-life and is quickly eliminated in the horse.

16.6 SEDATIVES / TRANQUILIZERS

Sedatives are useful for the colic patient not only because they calm the affected horse, but also because the subsequent clinical examination can be performed more thoroughly. A number of sedatives possess useful additional properties, such as analgesia and spasmolytic action. Many mild cases of spasmodic colic resolve themselves. When it is desirable to reduce bowel motility in such cases, a suitable spasmolytic drug may be employed.

ACEPROMAZINE

Acepromazine is quite useful in the initial stages as an aid to decreasing motor activity of the bowel without adversely affecting fluid transportation. An additional useful feature of acepromazine is that it possesses tranquilizing effects, which can be considered desirable in colic. Although most spasmodic colics are simple and do not display evidence of marked impairment to the circulatory system, care must be taken in computing the dosage of acepromazine. This is because of the adrenoceptor blocking action of acepromazine. Such activity could give rise to hypotension, which would be especially serious in shocked animals, especially if surgery or anesthesia is to follow. For this reason, the maximum recommended dosage of acepromazine is 0.05 mg/kg intravenously.

Acepromazine possesses a spasmolytic effect in spasmodic colics, but it is important to remember that the drug has alpha$_1$-blocking effects, resulting in hypotension as well as flaccid smooth muscles in the small intestines. A patient in endotoxic shock that is attempting to maintain stable cardiovascular parameters by vasoconstriction could face difficulty if acepromazine-induced vasodilation occurred.

ALPHA$_2$ ADRENERGICS

This group includes xylazine and detomidine, which both provide a dose-dependent degree of sedation. The sedative duration of xylazine (mediated via central alpha$_2$ receptors) is shorter than that of detomidine.

Both produce bradycardia, an initial increase then a decrease in blood pressure, and some degree of analgesia, especially in the viscera. The analgesic effect in the viscera outlasts the sedative effect.

A reduced dose of xylazine (0.2 to 0.4 mg/kg intravenously) can be given to horses with colic in an attempt to avoid cardiovascular and gastrointestinal side effects. Xylazine produces sedation, muscle relaxation, and more profound visceral analgesia of longer duration than does butorphanol, pentazocine, or meperidine. It has been suggested that xylazine should not be used in horses with impaction colic because of the inhibiting atonic effect of xylazine on the gut musculature.

At doses of 1.1 mg/kg intravenously or 2.2 mg/kg intramuscularly, the visceral analgesia of xylazine approaches that of some opioids. It possesses good analgesic properties and a marked depression in gut motility (ileus).

The cardiovascular effects of xylazine include bradycardia, decreased cardiac output, and transient hypertension followed by hypotension. Increased vascular resistance may reduce organ blood flow, thus compromising the patient, which already has volume depletion and lowered vascular supply to the intestine. Inhibition of intestinal motility is mediated through stimulation of the alpha$_2$ adrenoceptors.

Low doses should be used in horses with colic or poor peripheral perfusion. The duration of analgesia provided by this lowered dose is shorter (30 to 40 minutes) and facilitates evaluation of the patient's status. Xylazine, although a reasonably potent analgesic agent, possesses a relatively short duration of action. Improved analgesia and less cardiovascular depression may be obtained with lower doses of xylazine when combined with butorphanol meperidine or fentanyl. Xylazine suppresses intestinal motility (especially colonic activity), which may be contraindicated in many cases.

When ileus is present, administration of drugs that inhibit intestinal motility should be avoided to prevent potentiation of ileus. Xylazine suppresses propulsive colonic and jejunal motility and hence is best avoided in these cases.

DETOMIDINE

This is another sedative that possesses analgesic properties: sedation at lower dosages, analgesia at higher dosages. It is classified as an alpha$_2$ adrenoceptor agonist. Its dose dependent effects of sedation and analgesia are longer acting than xylazine's. Doses of 20–40 mcg/kg iv/im provide effects for 0.5–1 hour; doses of 80–150 mcg/kg iv/im provide sedation and analgesia for two to six hours.

CHLORAL HYDRATE

This centrally acting sedative hypnotic has no major analgesic properties but reduces the response to painful stimuli. In therapeutic doses (22 to 40 mg/kg) chloral hydrate has minimal effects on respiration and blood pressure and does not mask signs of strangulatory obstructions. Although not really an analgesic, it can bring about a useful hypnotic state for purposes of restraint. It has minimal effects on the gastrointestinal tract and cardiovascular system and so is useful in cases of impaction or thromboembolic colic.

16.7 VERMINOUS ARTERITIS AND THROMBOEMBOLIC COLIC

The migration of *S. vulgaris* larvae through the cranial mesenteric artery and its branches supplying the intestine is frequently implicated in many equine colic syndromes. The thrombotic reaction to the presence of migratory *S. vulgaris* larvae has been observed in up to 90% of horses on which necropsy was performed and has been incriminated in 90% of all episodes of equine colic. Migration to and in the cranial mesenteric artery is associated with typical signs of colic. The presence of larvae induces an intraluminal inflammatory reaction, disrupting the intimal surface and normal endothelial cell lining. The thrombus can fill the lumen and reduce intestinal blood flow by up to 50%. Infarction and ischemia of the intestine follow. Vasoactive substances, such as thromboxane, formed during the coagulation process may be responsible for this ischemia. Resultant vasoconstriction or alternatively pressure on the celiac plexus produced by the arterial lesion has been incriminated as the cause of pain. Thromboembolism of the large thrombus or a part of the thrombus can cause capillary obstruction distally with diffuse or focal infarction of the bowel. The pathogenesis of verminous arteritis involves vascular occlusion, ischemia, increased mucosal or peritoneal permeability, endotoxin absorption, prostaglandin and thromboxane production, thromboembolic colic, fever, ileus, fluid sequestration, gut distention, pain, and hypovolemic shock.

Therapy for thromboembolic colic necessitates specific treatment of the arteritis. This encompasses (1) use of an anthelmintic effective against migratory strongylus larvae and (2) use of a potent NSAID to lessen the inflammatory response in the affected artery. Certain anthelmintics are effective against the migratory stages of *S. vulgaris*:

1. Thiabendazole is effective in killing early fourth-stage larvae at a dosage level of 440 mg/kg orally for 2 consecutive days.
2. Oral administration of fenbendazole, 10 mg/kg daily for 5 consecutive days, is effective in killing early and late fourth-stage larvae of *S. vulgaris*, thereby alleviating many of the symptoms likely to arise as a consequence of thromboembolism.
3. Oxfendazole, 10 mg/kg orally given twice at 48-hour intervals, is also effective.
4. Ivermectin is the most popular choice of anthelmintic for verminous arteritis. At the normal therapeutic dose, 0.2 mg/kg orally, ivermectin possesses potent larvicidal effect against migratory strongyli and used together with dextran 70 as an antithrombotic agent provides useful relief (Table 16–6).

Pain in suspected cases of verminous arteritis can be treated using the NSAID flunixin meglumine. One potential adverse effect of flunixin is the masking of pain and shock. A positive clinical response to the NSAID could conceivably postpone the perceived necessity for surgical intervention.

TABLE 16–6
LARVICIDAL ANTHELMINTICS FOR MIGRATORY STRONGYLUS LARVAE

Agent	Dosage
Invermectin	200 μg/kg
Fenbendazole	50 mg/kg orally 3 consecutive days/10 mg/kg 5 consecutive days
Oxfendazole	10 mg/kg twice at 48-hour intervals
Thiabendazole	440 mg/kg orally 2 consecutive days

16.8 SHOCK

In colic, various causes, such as overfeeding, abrupt changes in diet, strangulation or obstruction, and impactions, may compromise hemostasis. Hemostasis can be compromised by gas accumulation, which presses the intestinal wall against the blood vessels and occludes blood flow.

Decreased blood flow can lead to ischemia and necrosis and favors local accumulation of coagulation factors. Local accumulation of coagulation factors and impaired blood flow may lead to thrombus formation, which further impedes blood flow. Ischemic necrosis of the intestinal wall may increase absorption of endotoxins, which are protein lipo/polysaccharides from gram-negative bacteria in the gastrointestinal tract.

Horses are profoundly susceptible to the effects of endotoxin, resulting in marked leukopenia, followed by leukocytosis. In addition to changes in white blood cell counts, both the extensive and the intensive coagulation pathways can be rapidly activated to result in thrombus formation.

Endotoxin refers to part of the cell wall or envelope of gram-negative bacteria. At times referred to as LPS, it is synonymous with the 0 antigen or somatic antigen of these bacteria.

To be toxic, endotoxins must gain access to the circulation. They are usually nontoxic when given orally to an animal with a normal gastrointestinal tract, although large doses can cause diarrhea.

If the bowel mucosa is damaged or compromised via infarction, however, ischemia endotoxins can gain access to the systemic circulation. Most of the severe reactions they cause systemically are associated with cascades of local inflammatory hormones and mediators.

White cells respond to endotoxins by secretory increased amounts of opsin, interferon, prostaglandins, lymphocyte-activating factor, and interleukins. Platelets react by releasing bioactive substances, such as histamine and serotonin. These substances in turn cause the release of epinephrine and norepinephrine and enhance smooth muscle contractions.

Release of interleukin I causes release of local prostaglandins. Disseminated intravascular coagulation initiates microcirculatory disturbances, including construction of arterioles, dilatation of venules, release of thromboxane A_2, and increased permeability of capillary and venule walls. Systemic acidosis and anaerobic glycolysis result from the impaired local circulation and oxygenation. Low-dose heparin (40 iu/kg subcutaneously twice a day) is the standard therapy for disseminated intravascular coagulation. Heparin has a half-life of 8 to 12 hours in most species when injected subcutaneously and shorter if given intravenously.

Circulatory shock, in essence, means insufficient perfusion of the tissues. In many cases of equine colic, shock occurs as a result of intestinal ischemia (thromboembolism, small intestinal volvulus, or colonic torsion) following damage to the integrity of the intestinal mucosa. This damage facilitates the transmural movement of intraluminal substances, which then enter the general circulation (Table 16–7). Many studies have documented the significance of bacterial lipopolysaccharide (endotoxin) in the pathologic progression of colic. Endo-

TABLE 16–7
SHOCK IN EQUINE COLIC

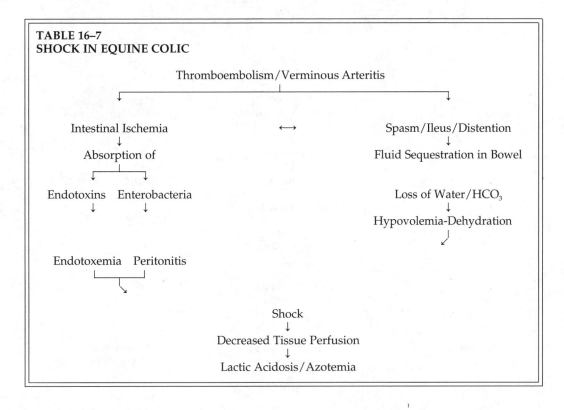

Thromboembolism/Verminous Arteritis

Intestinal Ischemia ⟷ Spasm/Ileus/Distention

Absorption of → Fluid Sequestration in Bowel

Endotoxins   Enterobacteria   Loss of Water/HCO_3

→ Hypovolemia-Dehydration

Endotoxemia   Peritonitis

Shock
↓
Decreased Tissue Perfusion
↓
Lactic Acidosis/Azotemia

toxin is a structural component of the outer surface of certain enteric gram-negative bacteria. Under normal circumstances, the mucosal surface of the intestine together with its epithelial lining, complete with chemical and immunologic mechanisms and its resident bacterial flora, impedes the inward passage of endotoxin from the gut lumen. Loss of integrity of this mucosal barrier by way of inadequate perfusion facilitates absorption of the lipid endotoxin into the general circulation. Once absorbed, endotoxins trigger the release of a cascade of vasoactive substances (prostaglandins, histamine, catecholamines), which dramatically alter vascular permeability and result in decreased circulatory plasma volume. Specifically damage to the vascular endothelium occurs, and this cellular damage by the endotoxin activates cleavage of phospholipids by phospholipase enzymes releasing arachidonic acid, which then serves as the substrate for at least two enzyme systems, cyclooxygenase and lipoxygenase (Table 16–8).

Cyclooxygenase converts arachidonic acid to the unstable endoperoxide interme-

diates, which may be further modified to form the classic prostaglandins, prostacyclin, or thromboxane. All of these endogenous, locally produced substances have profound effects on the local circulation and on pain receptors, as evidenced by the pain, fever, and altered tissue perfusion in equine colic.

Thromboxane A_2 mediates intense vasoconstriction and platelet aggregation. The sudden biosynthesis and release of this autocoid is undoubtedly responsible for the appearance of dyspnea, tachypnea, and pulmonary hypertension. Prostacyclin metabolites are associated with abdominal pain, systemic hypotension, and increased capillary refill time. Prostaglandin E_2 is associated with vasodilatation, fever, and a lowered pain threshold.

Contraction of plasma volume gives rise to hemoconcentration, dehydration, and reduced tissue perfusion (hypovolemia). Hypovolemia can directly result from sequestration of large volumes of fluid in the intestinal lumen. If small intestinal lesions predominate, functional reabsorptive failure occurs. Such failure means that the large

TABLE 16–8

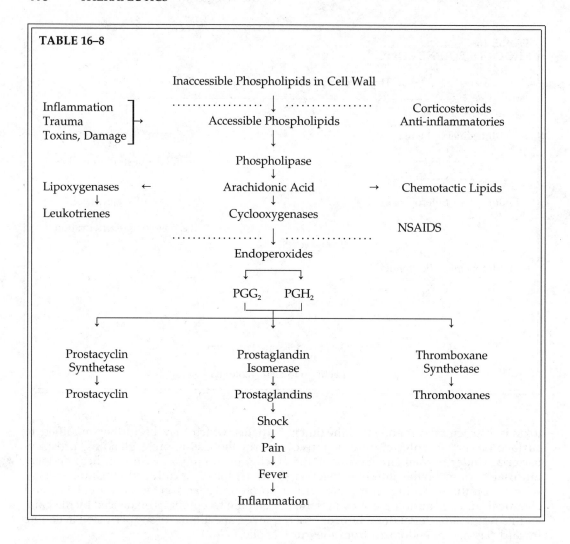

Inaccessible Phospholipids in Cell Wall

Inflammation
Trauma   →   Accessible Phospholipids   Corticosteroids
Toxins, Damage   Anti-inflammatories

Phospholipase

Lipoxygenases   ←   Arachidonic Acid   →   Chemotactic Lipids

Leukotrienes   Cyclooxygenases

NSAIDS

Endoperoxides

PGG$_2$ PGH$_2$

Prostacyclin   Prostaglandin   Thromboxane
Synthetase   Isomerase   Synthetase

Prostacyclin   Prostaglandins   Thromboxanes

Shock

Pain

Fever

Inflammation

volumes of fluid secreted into the upper small intestine remain "pooled" or trapped in the lumen, with a consequent hypovolemia occurring. Endotoxemia in the presence of gut sequestration compounds the problem of hypovolemia and leads to more rapid circulatory shutdown.

Therapy of equine colic and the accompanying endotoxemia centers on the use of drugs that inhibit cyclooxygenase activity. This has been based on a number of research findings indicating:

1. Exposure to endotoxin results in a dramatic increase in plasma levels of prostaglandin or thromboxane.
2. Increases in these substances can be correlated with chemical or hemodynamic responses.

3. NSAIDs (at low dose levels) significantly reduce production of arachidonic acid metabolites and improve survival times of affected animals.

Other general aspects of endotoxic shock treatment are as follows:

1. Antimicrobial drugs specifically useful against gram-negative organisms are indicated.
2. Vigorous intravenous fluid therapy with polyionic fluids is necessary. Ringer's solution with lactate acetate or bicarbonate is essential to help maintain blood volume as well as counteracting acidosis. Plasma administration also helps to restore blood volume and oncotic pressure. Immunoglobulins and complement con-

tained in the plasma infusion are also beneficial.

3. Glucose must always be supplied to animals in endotoxic shock, preferably in combination with the intravenous fluid (Table 16–9).

When considering treatment for endotoxemia it must be remembered that this is not a primary disease process but rather a secondary complication.

Antimicrobials do not neutralize the chemically stable lipopolysaccharides in the circulation. It has been claimed, however, that polymyxins possess some benefit by binding to and inactivating the endotoxin.

Active and passive immunization techniques are now available directed against the common core antigens. Passive immunity especially involves using serum that is rich in antibodies obtained from donors that are immunized against endotoxin.

Of the vasoactive prostaglandins, low-dose flunixin meglumine has been used extensively (0.25 mg/kg) in clinical cases of intestinal ischemia and endotoxemia. Flunixin therapy can have a "masking effect" to the ultimate detriment of the affected horse at normal analgesic doses. Thus although this NSAID has a valuable role in therapy for the relief of pain and endotoxemia, this should be viewed primarily as a short-term relief measure while a more thorough assessment of the case is being made.

NSAIDs act as cyclooxygenase inhibitors and may redirect arachidonic acid metabolism through the lipoxygenase pathway, resulting in the production of leukotrienes, which are vasoactive and chemoattractant.

It is highly likely, and supported by in vitro studies of equine cells, that inhibition of cyclooxygenase activity in the face of endotoxemia redirects the metabolism of arachidonic acid to the leukotrienes. The various effects of these substances include promoting chemotaxis, altering vascular tone, and enhancing microvascular permeability. Furthermore there is ample evidence that other inflammatory mediators (platelet-activating factor, procoagulant activity, tumor necrosis factor, and angiotensin II) interact with the cyclooxygenase-derived and lipoxygenase-derived metabolites of arachidonic acid.

After therapy with NSAIDs lipoxygenase products and chemotactic lipids may be unaffected or increased. Current evidence suggests that leukotrienes, such as the slow-reacting substance of anaphylaxis, may be important in inflammation.

The main mediators of inflammation are derived from arachidonic acid: the prostaglandins and thromboxanes and the leukotrienes. The higher in the cascade of arachidonic metabolism that an anti-inflammatory works, the more complete is its action. Corticosteroids act high up in the cascade.

Anticoagulants are indicated in some cases of endotoxemia because of the propensity toward red blood cell sludging and the intravascular stimulation of coagulation caused by endotoxins. The anticoagulant heparin (to 40 iu/kg three times a day) should be considered in patients with suspected endotoxemia.

16.9 FLUID THERAPY

Fluid therapy is important in the management of the patient. Endotoxin leads to splanchnic pooling, reducing the effective circulatory volume and resulting in hypovolemia. Endotoxins also act to increase the permeability of the gastrointestinal endothelium and capillaries, resulting in a net movement of fluid out of the intravascular space. Thromboxane and prostaglandin I_2 are released: Thromboxane produces vasoconstriction, tissue ischemia, and thrombosis owing to platelet aggregation. Prostacyclin has an opposing action, is mainly produced in endothelial cells, and has a short-lived potent vasodilative and antiaggregative effect on platelets.

Balanced polyenic solutions given intravenously are best during early cases. Acidosis frequently accompanies hypovolemia and shock associated with severe gastrointestinal tract disease. Sodium bicarbonate may be added to the intravenous fluids in cases in which marked acidosis is suspected. One liter of 5% sodium bicarbonate may be administered to an adult horse (Table 6–10).

Fluid therapy is an essential part of any therapy in the managing the colic patient. Fluid therapy is necessary:

TABLE 16–9
ENDOTOXIC SHOCK TREATMENT

Agent	Dose
Lactated Ringer's/Hartmann's fluid	30–50 liters IV
4.2% Sodium bicarbonate	2 ml/kg IV
Dextran	2.5–3.0 liters IV
Gelatin polymer	IV
Flunixin meglumine	0.25 mg/kg IV
Dexamethasone/betamethasone	250 mg IV
Ketoprofen	2.2 mg/kg IV
Dimethyl sulfoxide	60–200 mg/kg IV

1. To correct acid-base and electrolyte imbalances
2. To rectify fluid depletion from inadequate intake, shock, or bowel sequestration
3. To expand the plasma volume and to correct shock
4. To ensure adequate perfusion and oxygenation of tissues to maintain renal function and promote diuresis

The type and volume of fluid to be supplied to the affected horse is a function of the cause, severity, and site of the underlying fluid deficit problem.

Oral fluids are not indicated in the presence of obstructive gastrointestinal disease. When oral fluids are used they should be isotonic.

Clinical examination should provide some evidence as to the origin of the colic—whether it has originated from small intestinal or colonic obstruction. The site of the obstruction can give a useful idea of the type of metabolic disturbance to be expected. Normal secretions in the bowel remain unabsorbed proximal to the obstruction. This pooling of fluid secretion in the bowel lumen results in extensive losses of water, hydrogen ions, sodium, and chloride when the obstruction is high up the gastrointestinal tract. Lower down the tract, obstruction is associated with loss of water bicarbonate and potassium. Continuing fluid loss into the bowel lumen eventually precipitates dehydration, contraction of plasma volume, hypovolemic shock, and acidosis.

Most horses in shock have metabolic acidosis from bicarbonate loss, inadequate tissue perfusion, renal dysfunction (and accumulation of hydrogen ions), anaerobic metabolism, and lactic acid production. The horse often attempts to hyperventilate to correct the imbalance. Horses in shock need large volumes of replacement fluids. Therapy must be directed toward fluid volume

TABLE 16–10
CLINICAL ASSESSMENT OF FLUID REQUIREMENTS

Degree of Dehydration	Clinical Signs	Liters Lost/500 kg Horse
Mild (7%)	Loss of skin elasticity Pale mucous membranes	≈35
Moderate (10%)	Cold extremities Sunken eyes Weakness	≈50
Severe (12%)	Recumbent Hypothermic	≈60

deficits, acid-base and electrolyte imbalances, and vascular endothelial damage.

Immediate fluid replacement requirements in an adult horse can exceed 10 to 15 liters (approximately 50% of the patient's circulatory plasma volume can require replacement). Plasma volume in a healthy horse is estimated at 5% of body weight, or 22.5 liters for a 454-kg animal. Such a horse would require an immediate replacement of at least 6 liters.

The degree of dehydration is estimated by clinical examination of the patient with reference to skin elasticity, mucous membrane appearance, and temperature.

The required fluid volume in liters is calculated by multiplying the percentage of dehydration by body weight in kilograms.

Volume replacement with Ringer's solution or lactated Ringer's solution is usually sufficient. If acidosis is severe, bicarbonate and electrolytes must be supplied. If bicarbonate is added directly to Ringer's solution, some of the bicarbonate is lost as precipitated sodium bicarbonate. To control bicarbonate replacement adequately, a sterile 5% solution should be administered.

Alkalinizing fluid electrolyte solutions must be administered when an acidotic state accompanies dehydration. Lactate is a commonly used bicarbonate source in such solutions. Proper liver function, however, is necessary to convert lactate to bicarbonate. This cannot be relied on in a severely dehydrated or shocked horse, and so bicarbonate-containing solutions are preferable. Approximately 6 liters of 1.25% bicarbonate (containing 10 to 20 mEq potassium per liter) is required.

Plasma volume expanders (dextran 70) are indicated in severe shock to augment the cardiovascular osmotic skeleton and ensure adequate oncotic pressure and osmotic retention of the administered fluid within the vascular compartment to combat hypovolemia.

In case of dehydration and toxic shock, massive doses of corticosteroids could also be considered (250 mg dexamethasone or betamethasone).

Corticosteroids can be indicated in the management of endotoxemia because of their action in stabilizing cellular and subcellular membranes. There is considerable controversy involving the effectiveness of corticosteroids in treating endotoxemia. In addition, their use must be considered in the light of their potential side effects in horses, which include laminitis, immunosuppression, and adrenal atrophy.

Corticosteroids, if given before or immediately after exposure to endotoxin, act on macrophages to block interleukin 1. Steroids, generally by their inhibition of phospholipase, stabilize cell membranes and hence help curtail the sequence of events associated with shock.

NSAIDs do not hinder bacterial clearance, are less immunosuppressive, and possess potent antiprostaglandin activity. They have been shown to be beneficial in alleviating the effects of endotoxin-induced shock, especially in horses, at doses lower than the analgesic dose (flunixin meglumine, 0.25 mg/kg intravenously).

Support of the cardiovascular system with dopamine or dobutamine can be beneficial when the potential for circulatory collapse exists. When combined with appropriate fluid administration, these agents may be used to increase cardiac output and renal, mesenteric, and coronary perfusion.

16.10 SPASMODIC COLIC AND SPASMOLYTIC AGENTS

Many cases of spasmodic colic resolve themselves. When intense visceral pain is associated with increased muscular activity and spasm of intestinal muscle, however, a spasmolytic agent is indicated. Spasmolytic drugs (often combined with NSAIDs) are effective in reducing the spasmodic contraction of smooth muscle. Reduction of pain intensity associated with spasm follows the use of these spasmolytic drugs, although they are not classic pharmacologic analgesic agents. If hypomotility is suspected (e.g., impaction), however, such drugs are contraindicated.

Parasympatholytic agents have been used as antispasmodic agents on account of their muscarinic blocking effects at the level of the small intestine (Table 16–11). Atropine, although potent, has too many systemic side effects, especially its prolonged ocular side effects, to be recommended in the horse. Other spasmolytics, such as hyoscine, methindizate, and proquamezine,

TABLE 16–11
SPASMOLYTICS
(SPASM/HYPERMOTILITY)

	Dose
Hyoscine	20–30 ml IV
Methindizate	25–40 mg IV, IM
Proquamerazine	10–30 ml IV
Dipyrone and Hyoscine	20–30 ml IV, IM

IV, Intravenous; IM, intramuscular.

have proved more effective. By antagonizing the tonic effects of parasympathetic nerves to the gut, the anticholinergic group of drugs inhibits intestinal motility. Anticholinergic drugs are used to produce relaxation of gastrointestinal tract smooth muscle, with reduction in tone, amplitude, and frequency of peristaltic contractions. Intestinal secretions may also be blocked.

Although anticholinergics are used frequently in horses suffering from colic, caution should be exercised because intestinal stasis may be the fundamental problem in many instances. The main naturally occurring compounds in this class are atropine and hyoscine, but owing to their widespread activity throughout the body, inhibition of peristaltic activity is accompanied by many other effects. Secretions in the mouth and respiratory and gastrointestinal tracts are blocked; tachycardia owing to vagal blockage and disturbance of ocular accommodation with mydriasis occur. Methyl hyoscine is a slightly less potent alkaloid than hyoscine, and its major distinguishing feature is that owing to a quaternary nitrogen it does not cross the blood-brain barrier and produce that central excitement seen with other alkaloids. Hyoscine-*n*-butyl bromide is another quaternary antispasmodic with increased gut specificity of antimuscarinic effect. Commonly used antimuscarinic/spasmolytic agents include atropine (D.L. Hyoscyamine); scopolamine (hyoscine), methscopolamine, isopropramide, and benzethimide.

Popular spasmolytic preparations usually combine an anticholinergic agent, such as hyoscine, with dipyrone (e.g., Buscopan Compositum) (a NSAID) or metamizole with methindizate.

16.11 COLONIC IMPACTION

Impactions of ingesta in the horse commonly arise at the pelvic flexure or right dorsal colon. Other types of impaction (e.g., sand and gravel) usually involve the ventral colon. Such impactions are common causes of colic, and for the most part they respond to judicious medical treatment. Therapy is usually directed toward fluid supplementation, oral lubricants, and fecal softening agents. This should result in the expulsion of colonic impactions within 2 to 4 days.

Many refractory cases of colonic impaction are a result of incorrect initial therapy usually with opiates or spasmolytics and often with insufficient doses of laxative agents. Strong purgatives and augmenters of intestinal motility must be used with great care. They are contraindicated in cases of intestinal obstruction because rupture of the bowel is a likely occurrence. Pain may also be caused by their violent contractile action.

Laxatives are contraindicated in horses with surgically correctable disease because stimulation of intestinal motility may worsen pain and intestinal distention. Laxatives are usually used for impactions of the large colon. Hydration of the impaction by oral or parenteral fluids is a good alternative to a laxative, although a combination of both measures should be considered.

With severe impactions of the large colon, laxatives should be used carefully because drugs increasing intestinal water content cause further distention and pain (Table 16–12).

Liquid petrolatum (mineral oil) is the most commonly used laxative in equine

TABLE 16–12
CONSTIPATION/IMPACTION

Agent	Dose
Liquid paraffin	2–8 liters orally
Magnesium sulfate	250 g orally
Dioctyl sodium sulfosuccinate	10–30 mg/kg (5–30 g orally)
Psyllium	0.25 kg in 8 liters water

practice. Acting as a lubricant, its effects are safe, mild, and predictable. A dose of 2 to 6 liters in 2 to 4 liters of warm water once or twice daily by nasogastric tube for a maximum of 5 days may assist passage of ingesta. It is one of the safest lubricants, but prolonged oral intake of mineral oil can impede absorption of fat-soluble vitamins.

The anionic surfactant dioctyl sodium sulfosuccinate (DSS) is an alternative compound for promoting softening and passage of colonic impactions. The normal dose is 10 to 20 mg/kg given in 1 or 2 liters of warm water through a nasogastric tube. By reducing surface tension, DSS allows water to penetrate a mass of ingesta. Large doses (≥1.0 g) can cause damage to the gut wall and severe dehydration. DSS must not be administered concurrently with mineral oil. Bulk-forming laxatives increase fecal water content and rate of transit of ingesta in the colon. They absorb water from the body and increase the fluid and ion content of the gut, usually by an osmotic process.

Wheat bran and psyllium-type products are used as bulk-forming laxatives in equine practice. For impactions caused by sand ingestion, psyllium is given by nasogastric tube (0.25 kg in 8 liters of warm water). This mucilaginous compound forms a gelatinous mass in the intestine that physically drives intraluminal contents distally. Magnesium sulfate is a saline cathartic that draws water osmotically into the intestinal lumen. For impactions of the colon, doses of 0.5 mg/kg in 2 to 4 liters of warm water can be given. Because the osmotic action of magnesium sulfate can produce severe dehydration, this type of osmotic laxative should be used only in well-hydrated horses or at least in combination with intravenous fluids.

GASTROINTESTINAL TRACT STIMULANTS

Although anthraquinone cathartics and parasympathomimetic agents have theoretical indications for augmenting gastrointestinal motility, they should not be used in horses with colic because of their drastic effects, potential side actions, and doubtful benefit. Analgesic drugs that do not depress colonic activity, e.g., phenylbutazone (intravenously maximum two doses over 24

hours) or flunixin combined with large doses of laxatives (6 liters of liquid paraffin over 24 hours for a 500-kg horse), are preferred for the management of this impactive colic.

16.12 FLATULENT COLIC

Pain and gut distention can be caused by the fermentative activity of intestinal bacteria in cases of flatulent colic. Oral neomycin has been the drug of choice to suppress the activity of the bacterial flora and thereby the amount of gas production and gut distention. Chloral hydrate (30 g), turpentine (20 to 30 ml), and formalin (30 ml) are also antizymotic agents that have been extensively used by veterinarians. They are often given with 500 ml of raw linseed oil (Table 16–13).

Antimicrobial drugs may play a role in colic therapy in which invasion of the blood or peritoneal cavity by intestinal organisms is suspected (Tables 16–14 and 16–15). Penicillins and aminoglycosides are the antibiotics of choice to reduce the severity of bacteremia and other bacterial complications. Many other antibiotics, especially the tetracyclines, are strictly contraindicated because of their reputed adverse effects on the bowel. Aminoglycosides must be used with care because of their potential nephrotoxicity—impaired renal function can occur in colic. Thus horses that are in shock or dehydrated should be subjected only to low doses of aminoglycosides, and accompanying renal function must be carefully monitored. Penicillin is effective against gram-positive organisms and most anaerobes (except *Bacteroides fragilis*). If peritonitis is established or suspected, particularly after contamination at surgery, anaerobic

TABLE 16–13 FERMENTATION/FLATULENCE	
Antizymotics	Dose
Neomycin	4–8 g orally
Chloral hydrate	10–30 g orally
Oil of turpentine	30–60 ml orally

TABLE 16–14
ANTIMICROBIAL DRUGS USEFUL IN COLIC

Drug	Dose
Procaine penicillin G	22000 μ/kg
Potassium pencillin G	22000–50000 μg/kg
Sodium ampicillin	10–15 mg/kg
Ticarcillin	40 mg/kg
Neomycin	4–8 g
Gentamicin	2.2 mg/kg
Amikacin	6.6 mg/kg
Cephalexin	15–22 mg/kg
Sulfonamide/trimethoprim	15–30 mg/kg
Metronidazole	10–15 mg/kg

bacteria are involved. Metronidazole is the antibacterial agent of choice for such anaerobic infections.

Broad-spectrum antimicrobial therapy is associated with many deleterious side effects in horses. Oxytetracycline is the classic example; this antibiotic is known to precipitate acute colitis in stressed horses. Oral broad-spectrum therapy is also prone to cause problems of superinfection and resultant diarrhea and in some cases to trigger outbreaks of salmonellosis.

Horses hospitalized with colic are more likely to develop salmonellosis than other hospitalized cases, and in judicious antimi-

crobial therapy, the presence of stress may be an additional risk factor. Acute colitis in horses is not always due to salmonellosis infection but to imbalance of the bacterial flora. Clostridial overgrowth is perhaps one of the most common etiologic factors in the development of equine diarrhea.

PREVENTION OF GASTRIC DISTENTION

Of paramount importance in the management of colic is the relief of pain and the prevention of gastric rupture. Many colic cases result in gastric distention, and so na-

TABLE 16–15
ANTIMICROBIAL DRUGS FOR GRAM-NEGATIVE SEPSIS

Bacteria	Antimicrobial Drug
Escherichia coli	Gentamicin, amikacin, cephalothin, trimethoprim/sulpha
Enterobacter	Gentamicin, Trimethoprim/sulfa
Haemophilus	Penicillin, ampicillin
Actinobacillus	Ampicillin, gentamicin, trimethoprim/sulfa
Bacteroides fragilis	Metronidazole, penicillin, trimethoprim/sulfa
Salmonella	Trimethoprim/sulfa, gentamicin, amikacin
Klebsiella pneumoniae	Amikacin, cephalothin, trimethoprim/sulfa, gentamicin
Pasteurella	Penicillin, gentamicin, erythromycin, cephalothin, trimethoprim/sulfa
Proteus	Gentamicin, amikacin, carbenicillin
Fusobacterium	Metronidazole, penicillin, trimethoprim/sulfa

sogastric intubation should be performed on all horses to identify the presence of sequestered fluid. Nasogastric reflux of more than 8 liters is a possible indication of small intestinal obstruction or proximal enteritis. Colonic problems (obstruction or colitis) may give rise to ileus, which is severe enough to cause nasogastric reflux. Nasogastric intubation can be discontinued only when pain has disappeared and reflux is no longer present.

16.13 MISCELLANEOUS DRUGS

HEPARIN

In horses with colic or suspected endotoxemia, low-dosage heparin therapy (80 μ/kg subcutaneously twice a day) has been used to reduce the incidence of laminitis, thrombogenesis, and disseminated intravascular coagulation. Apart from its anticoagulant effects, heparin acts also as a nonspecific stimulant of phagocytic activity in the reticuloendothelial system. This property may assist in the removal of intravascular debris. Some horses develop anemia as a side effect of heparin therapy within a week of beginning treatment.

Complications of colic, such a laminitis, endotoxemia, and disseminated intravascular coagulation, can be treated by judicious use of heparin. The use of heparin prevents the formation of microthrombi. Dosage of heparin is 80 to 100 IU/kg every 4 to 6 hours. Heparin can be used in these patients to prevent disseminated intravascular coagulation. Overdoses of heparin may be by the antidotes protamine sulfate, polybrene (hexa dimethrine bromide), and toluidine blue or by infusion of whole blood. Protamine sulfate can be given by slow intravenous drip at a rate not exceeding 50 mg in a 10-minute period.

ASPIRIN

Aggregation of platelets is important in the causation of arterial thrombosis and is implicated in the pathophysiology of thromboembolism, laminitis, and other sequelae of endotoxemia. Biosynthesis of thromboxane is reduced by the activity of aspirin, which inhibits platelet cyclooxygenase enzymes and subsequent platelet clumping. Thromboembolic diseases, such as laminitis, may be treated with aspirin at a dose of 17–20 mg/kg orally owing to the inhibitory effect on thromboxane production. No clinically useful analgesic effect, however, is attained at this dosage rate.

FLUNIXIN MEGLUMINE

This NSAID decreases thromboxane A_2 production during endotoxemia at doses below the analgesic dosage. Thromboxane causes platelet aggregation and vasoconstriction, both of which have been implicated in the pathogenesis of laminitis and endotoxin-induced coagulopathy. Doses of 0.25 mg/kg three times a day suppress thromboxane production. Analgesics such as flunixin meglumine that have been shown to have no adverse effects on intestinal motility may be preferable.

DIMETHYL SULFOXIDE

Dimethyl sulfoxide (DMSO), an organic solvent, possesses anti-inflammatory analgesic and diuretic properties. During the inflammatory process, cytotoxic oxygen free radicals are released by neutrophils. DMSO prevents free-radical-mediated prostaglandin formation and hence mitigates the symptoms of laminitis and other endotoxin-mediated sequelae. Low doses of DMSO (60 to 200 mg/kg in 15 to 20% solution) are useful in treating horses with suspected endotoxemia or incipient laminitis. Higher doses, 1 g/kg (IV) have also been recommended.

DMSO has been used by many veterinarians for treatment of gastrointestinal disease in horses on account of its wide scatter of pharmacologic effects, including improved perfusion of ischemic bowel. Care must be taken when using DMSO intravenously at high doses (i.e., greater than 1 g/kg) to avoid hemolysis.

APPENDIX 1

DRUGS AND COLIC THERAPY

Drug	Indication	Dose and Route
Butorphanol	Pain	0.1 mg/kg IV/IM
Methadone	Pain	0.1 mg/kg IV
Pethidine	Pain	2 mg/kg IV
Pentazocine	Inflammation	0.6 mg/kg IV
Phenylbutazone	Inflammation	2.2–4.4 mg/kg IV
DiPyrone	Inflammation	10–22 mg/kg IV/IM
Flunixin	Inflammation	1 mg/kg IV
Ketoprofen	Inflammation	2.3 mg/kg
Acetylpromazine	Sedation	0.1 mg/kg IV or IM
Detomidine	Sedation	20–80 mcg/kg IV/IM
Xylazine	Sedation	1 mg/kg IV
Hyoscine	Hypermotility/spasm	20–30 ml iv
Methindizate		10–30 ml IV
Neomycin	Flatulence	4–8 orally
Liquid paraffin	Impaction	4–8 liters orally by stomach
Magnesium sulfate	Impaction	250 g orally
Dihydroxyanthroquinone	Impaction	10–20 g
Hartmann's solution	Shock	10–40 liters IV
Lactated Ringer's solution	Shock	10–40 liters IV
Betamethasone	Shock	250 mg IV
Dexamethasone	Shock	250 mg IV
Dextran	Shock	20 ml/kg
DMSO	Shock	60–200 mg/kg in 15–20% solution
Flunixin	Shock	0.25 mg/kg IV
Heparin	D.I.C.	40 u/kg, IV

IV, Intravenous, IM, intramuscular.

SELECTED REFERENCES

Alsup, E.M.: Dimethyl sulfoxide. J. Am. Vet. Med. Assoc., *185*:1011, 1984.

Brayton, C.F.: Dimethyl sulfoxide (DMSO). A review. Cornell Vet., *76*:61, 1986.

Davies, J.V., and Gerring, E.L.: Effects of spasmolytic analgesic drugs on the motility patterns of the equine small intestine. Res. Vet. Sci., *34*:334, 1983.

Duncan, S.G., and Reed, S.M.: Heparin anticoagulant therapy in equine colic. Mod. Vet. Pract., *65*:601, 1984.

Dunkle, N.J., Bottoms, G.D., et al. Effects of flunixin meglumine on blood pressure and fluid compartment volume changes in ponies given endotoxin. Am. J. Vet. Res., *46*:1540, 1985.

Gerring, E.L., and Davies, J.V.: Spasmolytic drugs and small intestinal functions in the horse. Proceedings from the 2nd European Association for Veterinary Pharmacology and Toxicology, Toulouse, 1982. Edited by Ruckebusch, Y., Toutain, P.L., and Koritz, G.D. UK, MTP Press, 1983.

Gingerich, D., Rourke, B.S., Chatfield, R.C. et al.: Butorphanol tartrate: A new analgesic to relieve the pain of equine colic. Vet. Med., *80*:72, 1985.

Holaday, J.W., and Faden, A.I.: Naloxone reversal of endotoxin hypotension suggests role of endorphins in shock. Nature, *275*:450, 1978.

Kalpravidh, M.: Analgesic effects of butorphanol in horses. Dose response studies. Am. J. Vet. Res., *45*:211, 1984.

Keller, H.: Diagnosis, therapy and prognosis in the conservative treatment of equine colic. Tierarztl Umschau *33*:71, 135, 1978.

Lees, P., and Higgins, A.J.: Clinical pharmacology and therapeutic uses of non steroidal anti-inflammatory drugs in the horse. Eq. Vet. J., *17*:83, 1985.

Lowe, J.E.: Xylazine, pentazocine, meperidine and dipyrone for relief of balloon induced equine colic. A double blind comparative evaluation. J. Eq. Med. Surg., *2*:286, 1978.

Lowe, J.E., Hintz, H.F., and Schrigver, H.F.: A new technique for long term caecal fistulation in ponies. Am. J. Vet. Res., *13*:1109, 1970.

Moore, J.N.: Management of pain and shock in equine colic. Compend. Cont. Educ. Pract. Vet., 7:S169, 1985.

Morris, D.D.: Antiendotoxin serum: Therapeutic rationale and clinical perspectives. Compend. Cont. Educ. Pract. Vet., *11*:1096, 1989.

Muir, W.W., and Robertson, J.T.: Visceral analgesia: Effects of xylazine, butorphanol, meperidine, and pentozocine in horses. Am. J. Vet. Res., *46*:2081, 1985.

Pippi, M.E., and Lumb, W.V.: Objective tests of analgesic drugs in ponies. Am. J. Vet. Res., *40*:1082, 1979.

Rose, J., and Rose, E.: Initial treatment of colic. Vet. Clin. North Am. [Eq. Pract.], *4*:35, 1988.

Sellers, A.F., and Lowe, J.E.: Review of large intestinal motility and mechanisms of impaction in the horse. Eq. Vet. J., *18*:261, 1986.

Semrad, S.D.: Flunixin meglumine given in small doses. Pharmacokinetics and prostaglandin inhibition in healthy horses. Am. J. Vet. Res., *46*:2474, 1985.

Smith, B.P.: Understanding the role of endotoxins in gram negative septicemia. Vet. Med., *81*:1148, 1986.

Trent, A.M.: What to do when your clinic cannot accommodate the colic patient. Vet. Med., 715, 1988.

Turek, J., Templeton, C., and Buttons, G.: Flunixin meglumine attenuation of endotoxin induced damage to the cardiopulmonary vascular endothelium of the pony. Am. J. Vet. Res., *46*:591, 1985.

Uytewael, C., and Strikkers, W.: Evaluation of Visceral Pain Suppression in the Horse. University of Utrecht, Clinic for Internal Medicine in Large Animals, 1987.

White, N.A.: Thromboembolic colic in horses. Comp. Cont. Educ. Pract. Vet., 7:156, 1985.

White, N.A., and Moore, J.N.: Diagnosis and management of the equine acute abdomen. In Proceedings of the American Association of Equine Practitioners, 1984.

17

THERAPY OF PARASITISM IN HORSES

17.1 Introduction
17.2 Large Strongylus Infection
17.3 *Gasterophilus* Infection
17.4 *Parascaris equorum* Infection
17.5 *Oxyuris equi* Infection
17.6 Small Strongylus Infection
17.7 *Trichostrongylus* Infection
17.8 *Strongyloides westeri* Infection
17.9 Tapeworm Infection
17.10 *Habronema* Infection and *Onchocerca* Infection
17.11 Lungworm Infection
17.12 Management of Equine Parasitic Problems
17.13 Anthelmintic Usage
17.14 Anthelmintic Resistance
17.15 Control Programs
17.16 Environmental Impact

17.1 INTRODUCTION

Horses are parasitized by many nematodes, but of these the most important are the strongylus worms and, wherever foals are kept, *Parascaris equorum*, the large roundworm of the small intestine. Other nematodes, such as *Strongyloides westeri*, *Oxyuris equi*, and *Dictyocaulus arnfieldi*, are only of sporadic importance.

Internal parasite control is one of the most important and most frequently administered health care measures for horses. Horse owners consider it essential for prevention of colic, maintenance of body weight and condition, and achievement of optimal growth and performance. The key elements in the success of an equine parasite control program are the choice of the appropriate anthelmintics and the proper timing of administration.

Anthelmintic wastage may be significant in horses insofar as horses are usually treated quite frequently. Also, many populations of cyathostomes (small strongyli) have now become resistant to several chemically related anthelmintics. Continued use of drugs to which a population of worms is resistant further intensifies selection and reduces the heterogeneity of the population.

Parasites of the equine gastrointestinal tract are responsible for acute clinical problems as well as chronic wasting and debilitation. Pathologic processes are represented by aneurysms, infarctions, blood loss, ulceration, and chronic irritation. These processes may result in death, acute colic, growth retardation, poor appearance, and suboptimal performance.

Control programs are designed principally toward preventing the deleterious effects of the most important group of parasites, the strongyli. *Strongylus* affect animals of all ages. The common large strongyli are *S. vulgaris* and *S. edentatus*. The small strongyli, referred to as the cyathostomes (trichonema) consist of more than 30 species, although only a proportion of these cause problems in horses. Other important parasites that require special control measures include *P. equorum* (especially in foals and young horses), *Gasterophilus* (stomach bots), *S. westeri* (threadworms), and *O. equi* (pinworms). *Habronema muscae* and *Draschia megastoma* in the stomach, *Trichostrongylus axei* in the stomach and small intestine, lungworms (*D. arnfieldi*), and tapeworms (*Anoplocephala*) merit specific control measures.

Although strongyli, ascarides and bots require most attention in a parasite control program, horses are occasionally subjected to problems caused by lungworms, pinworms, stomach worms, tapeworms, threadworms, summer sores, and cutaneous onchocerciasis. These are best treated as needs demand rather than being an integral part of a parasite control program.

Control measures are chiefly designed to prevent the deleterious effects of the most important group of equine parasites, the strongylus family. Although strongyli can affect horses of all ages, control strategies also take account of *P. equorum*, which is a serious parasitologic problem in foals and young horses.

In contrast to the situation in ruminant animals, seasonal outbreaks of parasitism with obvious clinical signs and some deaths are not frequently encountered in horses. Because the foal is capable of acquiring during the first few weeks of life a mixed burden of parasites, clinical signs of infestation usually affect individual animals, especially those under 3 years of age. Significant parasite burdens in horses, although giving rise only to subclinical infections, can have a major negative impact on the animal, reducing food conversion efficiency and lowering competitive performance. Many parasitic infections are subclinical, and when clinical signs develop, they often do so gradually. The signs vary widely and may include anorexia, varying degrees of dullness, colic, anemia, unthriftiness, reduced weight gain in young horses, progressive emaciation, poor performance, and diarrhea. Death occurs in some cases. Young horses usually suffer more than older horses. Older horses, although possibly not showing any signs of disease, may harbor a sufficient number of parasites to contaminate the pasture with worm eggs and thus serve as a dangerous source of infection for foals and young horses. Younger animals can be severely affected with worms because they have not developed any innate resistance to infection. With some species, e.g., *P. equorum*, foals are the principal source of infection for succeeding generations of foals.

In the majority of worm infections, horses become infected with worms by ingesting the larval worms with the grass while grazing or in some cases by ingesting infective worm eggs. The worms then develop into adult worms and lay numerous eggs, which pass out in the horses' feces. On the pasture, development of the egg and the worm larva is necessary before it is infective to another horse.

Worm parasites of horses do not multiply within the animal's body, so the level of infection in a susceptible animal depends on the number of parasites that the animal ingests with the grass. Because disease results from heavy infection, the aim should be to keep the level of infection on the pasture as low as possible. This can be achieved in a number of ways, and the method of choice varies according to local circumstances, such as the age of the horses, the number of horses, and the amount of land available.

All benzimidazoles and probenzimidazoles licensed for use in the horse are effective against *P. equorum*, *O. equi*, adult cyathostomes, and adult large strongyli, although thiabendazole must be given at an increased dosage rate for *P. equorum*. Thiabendazole, oxibendazole, and fenbendazole are effective against *S. westeri* if given at an increased dose, and fenbendazole and oxfendazole are effective against migrating cyathostome larvae and larvae of the large strongyli, although fenbendazole must be given at a much higher dosage rate. Fenbendazole and oxfendazole are effective against *D. arnfieldi* and *T. axei* when given at the standard doses, and mebendazole is effective against both of these parasites.

Ivermectin for horses was originally labeled only for intramuscular injection (Eqvalan, MSDAGVET) in the cervical area; however, oral administration of the injectable product began to gain popularity, particularly after some studies indicated almost identical efficacy using this route, and in June, 1984, an oral paste form (Eqvalan Paste, MSDAGVET) appeared on the market. Other studies found only minor differences between the two routes of administration, with one study showing lower efficacy for adult and larval stages of *Cyathostome* (usually classed as a small strongylus) with oral administration. Another investigator found increased activity against

O. equi: 93% effective as an injectable and 100% effective as a paste. There may, however, be a longer duration of effect with intramuscular administration. In a study comparing administration of the micelle formulation of ivermectin parenterally and orally, the fecal egg-per-gram (EPG) counts of horses given the injection remained near 100% through 8 weeks after treatment, or about 2 weeks longer than horses given the drug orally.

Ivermectin administered to mares at foaling protects the foals against *S. westeri* infection received through the mares' milk. Trichlorfon is an organophosphate compound that has been included in many animal health formulations. It is used to control or treat the mouth or stomach stage of bots (*Gasterophilus*), mature ascarids (*P. equorum*), and adult pinworms in horses and foals. If doses are carefully calculated, trichlorfon can be used alone or in combination with other anthelmintics that do not inhibit cholinesterase. At rates of 80 mg/kg, liquid trichlorfon given concurrently with febantal does not cause significant toxicosis.

Pinworms (*O. equi*) can be controlled by most drugs used in a routine worming program. Horses grazed with donkeys are often exposed to lungworms (*D. arnfieldi*). This responds to ivermectin at the usual treatment dose of 200 µg/kg. Pyrantel pamoate at two to three times the normal dosage has high efficacy against the common tapeworm (*Anophocephala perfoliata*). Problems due to *Habronema*, *Draschia*, *Trichostrongylus*, or *Onchocerca* respond to ivermectin. It is important to use anthelmintics in a preventive manner when a large number of horses are kept. All horses and donkeys, which harbor adult worms, should be treated. The particular anthelmintics and the timing, number, and frequency of treatments vary according to the species of worm, the ages of the horses, methods of management and other factors (Tables 17–1 and 17–2).

17.2 LARGE STRONGYLUS INFECTION

The three major species of large strongyli (redworms) are *S. vulgaris*, *S. edentatus*, and *S. equinus*. The predilection site of the adult parasites is the large intestine, where they

TABLE 17–1
PARASITICIDES FOR EQUINE USE

Parasite	Predilection Site	Parasiticide

Large strongyli
  S. vulgaris
  S. edentatus
	Caecum/colon	Ivermectin, pyrantel, oxibendazole, oxfendazole, fenbendazole, mebendazole, thiabendazole

Migratory strongyli	Intestinal arteries	Ivermectin, oxfendazole, fenbendazole*
Small strongyli Cyathostomum	Caecum/colon	Ivermectin, pyrantel, oxibendazole, febantel, oxfendazole, fenbendazole, mebendazole, thiabendazole, piperazine, dichlorvos
Roundworms P. equorum (foals)	Small intestine	Ivermectin, pyrantel, thiabendazole,† fenbendazole,† oxfendazole, oxibendazole
Bots Gasterophilus	Stomach	Ivermectin, dichlorvos, haloxan, trichlorfon
Threadworms S. westeri (foals)	Small intestine	Ivermectin, thiabendazole, oxibendazol, fenbendazole†
Pinworms O. equi	Colon/rectum	Thiabendazole, mebendazole, fenbendazole, oxfendazole, febantel, oxibendazole, pyrantel, ivermectin
Lungworms D. arnfieldi	Bronchi	Ivermectin, fenbendazole,† mebendazole, thiabendazole†
Tapeworms A. perfoliata	Ileum/caecum	Niclosamide, pyrantel,† mebendazole*

*Requires daily dosing for 5 days.
†Requires higher dosage rate.

feed on the intestinal mucosa. Infection is acquired by ingestion of the infective third-stage larva during grazing. Warm moist conditions favor development of infective larvae on pasture. Extensive migration of larvae occurs after ingestion before they finally settle and develop to maturity in the large intestine. The prepatent period is 6 to 12 months. In *S. vulgaris*, larvae migrate within the intestinal arterial system to the cranial mesenteric artery and its branches, where they may cause verminous arteritis and thrombosis.

Of the three main species of large strongyli that affect the horse, *S. vulgaris* is undoubtedly more important than *S. equinus* or *S. edentatus*.

S. vulgaris is the most pathogenic of all equine helminths and is capable of causing colic or death. Although the adult parasites do suck blood in the large intestine, the association with arteritis is a more significant effect pathologically. Verminous aneurysms, enlargement of arteries (usually the cranial mesenteric), thickening of walls with accumulation of fibrotic deposits, and

partial or complete occlusion of arteries are common sequelae resulting in colic and death. Migration of *S. vulgaris* is associated with signs of recurring colic.

Larvae of *S. edentatus* migrate to the liver and from there to their predilection site on the subperitoneal tissues of the flanks. Animals remain susceptible to strongylus infection throughout their lives. Minimizing exposure to infective strongylus larvae necessitates removal of the adult egg-laying parasites from the intestine by means of anthelmintic therapy. Repeat treatments are necessary to minimize this exposure to infective larvae.

Adult strongyli possess large buccal capsules, and their blood-sucking activities lead to anemias of varying severity. Weakness, emaciation, and diarrhea commonly occur. Colic is probably the most common clinical sign of strongylus infection, and the incidence of colic is sometimes taken as a useful index of the effectiveness of any strongylus control program. Gangrenous enteritis, intestinal stasis, torsion, intussusception, and rupture are other possible con-

TABLE 17–2
SPECTRUM OF ACTION OF EQUINE PARASITICIDES

Parasiticide	Usual dosage	Bots: *Gasterophilus*	Roundworms: *P. equorum*	Large strongyli: *Strongylus*	Small strongyli: *Trichonema/ Triodontophorus*	Pinworms: *O. equi*	Threadworms: *S. westeri*	Method
Thiabendazole	44–88 mg/kg	–	+ (2×)	+	+	+	+	Suspension, paste, powder
Mebendazole	8.8 mg/kg	–	+	+	+	+	–	Suspension, paste, powder
Fenbendazole	5–10 mg/kg	–	+	+	+	+	+ (4×)	Suspension, paste, powder
Oxfendazole	10 mg/kg	–	++	++	++	++	+	Pellets, powder
Oxibendazole	10–15 mg/kg	–	++	++	++	++	+ (2×)	Paste, suspension
Febantel	6 mg/kg	–	++	++	++	++	– NT	Paste, suspension
Pyrantel*	6.6 mg/kg	–	+	++	+	±	–	Pellets, suspension, paste
Dichlorvos	35 mg/kg	+	+	++	+	+++	CD in foals	Pellets
Trichlorfon	40 mg/kg	++	++	–	–	+++	CD in foals	Paste, liquid
Ivermectin	200 µg/kg	++	++	++	++	±+	+	Paste
Piperazine	88 mg/kg	–	+	++	++	±+	–	Powder, liquid
Levamisole/ piperazine	8 mg/kg (levamisole) 88 mg/kg (piperazine)	–	+		+	+	–	Oral solution

+ = Highly effective; ± = poorly effective; – = not effective; CD = contraindicated; NT = not tested.
*Pyrantel is also highly effective at elevated dosages against equine tapeworm (*A. perfoliata*).
(See text for proper dosages against specific or problem parasites.)

sequences of thromboembolism and impaired blood supply to the intestine. Suboptimal competitive performance and sometimes diarrhea are direct results of strongylosis. Foals can be particularly susceptible to *S. vulgaris*.

Strongylus control programs are based on the principle of minimizing the level of pasture contamination and exposure to infective larvae. Many anthelmintics are effective against *S. vulgaris*:

1. Ivermectin
2. Benzimidazoles: fenbendazole, mebendazole, oxfendazole, oxibendazole, and thiabendazole
3. Probenzimidazoles: febantel
4. Dichlorvos pellets
5. Pyrantel pamoate
6. Levamisole

Horses may remain infected with large numbers of gastrointestinal parasites throughout their lives, and so control is based on prophylactic control measures necessitating repeated treatment. Grazing animals of all ages may acquire heavy infections of *Strongylus*. The control of strongylosis in the horse is based on the regular use of broad-spectrum anthelmintics, which at routine dosage rates are efficient against adult and lumen-dwelling larval stages of intestinal parasites. Dosing at intervals of 4 weeks keeps the fecal egg count extremely low throughout the year. When treatment intervals are extended to 6 weeks, fecal egg counts tend to increase over the summer months.

Most currently available anthelmintics are broad spectrum in efficacy and safe when given at recommended dosage levels. Repeat treatment is usually necessary after 4 to 6 weeks after the initial dosing to attack the second generation of adult parasites that has developed from larval maturation.

Often routine treatment at 1- to 2-month intervals is necessary. This, however, depends on prevailing management and pasture conditions. Anthelmintic medication must never be regarded as the complete answer to equine parasitic problems; good sanitation, pasture management, and separation of foals from older stock are important features of control that cannot be overemphasized.

TABLE 17–3
EQUINE STRONGYLOSIS (Tissue Stages)

Drug	Dosage
Oxfendazole	10 mg/kg (2 doses 48 hours apart)
Fenbendazole	30–60 mg/kg (single dose) 7.5–10.0 mg/kg (5 consecutive days)
Ivermectin	0.2 mg/kg
Thiabendazole	440 mg/kg (2 days)

Parasite control programs are based on the premise that grazing horses harbor some level of infection. Drugs must be used at intervals, which should be the period after treatment during which time fecal strongylus eggs are negligible in number. For drugs with little effect against migratory larvae, the minimum interval is 4 weeks because this is the time required for larvae remaining after treatment to reach maturity and begin egg laying. For drugs with larvicidal activity (e.g., ivermectin), this interval can be extended to 8 weeks.

In the control of strongylosis, no untreated animal should be allowed access to pasture grazed by treated horses until that animal has been dosed and isolated for a few days. If animals are kept in intensively stocked permanent paddocks, rapid pasture infectivity can build up from accumulated fecal deposits. Removal of deposits from pasture on a weekly basis can help in such situations.

Although there are many compounds effective against adult and larval parasites in the intestinal lumen of horses, only a few have been shown to possess effects against tissue-dwelling strongylus larvae: ivermectin, fenbendazole, oxfendazole (and thiabendazole) (Table 17–3).

Thiabendazole, at a dosage rate of 440 mg/kg, provides larvicidal activity against migratory strongyli, and a single treatment of fenbendazole (30 to 60 mg/kg) or oxfendazole (10 to 50 mg/kg) also reduces the number of migratory larvae of *S. vulgaris* and *S. edentatus*. Fenbendazole at the normal dosage rate (7.5 mg/kg) but continuing administration for a period of 5 days is an alternative but equally effective regimen.

The normal dosage of ivermectin (200 µg/kg) is effective against migratory *S. vulgaris* larvae. At a standard dose of 200 µg/kg body weight, ivermectin is effective against fourth-stage larvae. It has prevented vascular damage after experimental infection and reduced the size of cranial mesenteric artery aneurysm, resulting in increased circulation to arteries distal to the aneurysm within 6 weeks of injection. Oxfendazole, at 10 mg/kg for 2 days (48 hours interval); fenbendazole, at 7.5 to 10 mg/kg for 5 days; and thiabendazole, at 440 mg/kg for 2 consecutive days, are also effective against these stages. Colic caused by arterial lesions has been successfully treated with large doses of thiabendazole and normal dosages of ivermectin.

17.3 *GASTEROPHILUS* INFECTION

Bots of the equine stomach are the larvae of botflies, *Gasterophilus* species. These are active during warm summer months and lay eggs on hairs of the legs, shoulder, and neck. Larvae hatch in approximately 7 days (*Gasterophilus intestinalis*). Eggs of *Gasterophilus haemorrhoidalis* (the nose or lip bot) are attached to the hairs of the lip, and larvae merge after 2 or 3 days. *Gastrophilus nasalis* (the throat bot) lays its eggs on the hairs of the submaxillary region; hatching occurs after about a week.

Hatching frequently occurs as a result of self-grooming, and larvae enter the mouth, where they remain for about a month. Development and maturity occur in the stomach, where they attach themselves to the cardiac or pyloric regions. After a period of 8 to 10 months, they are eliminated in the feces in springtime. The pupation period is about 3 to 5 weeks in the soil, and the adult fly emerges after approximately 1 month, thus completing the cycle.

Adult botflies cause great annoyance to horses during the process of egg deposition. Larvae attach to the stomach by oral hooks, inducing local gastric erosion, ulceration, and hyperplasia. Most bots are present in the stomach of horses from the end of the summer. A single treatment between late fall and early winter (November to January)

has been the traditional treatment to break the life cycle. This is usually adequate. Effective anthelmintics provide protection for the entire season.

Dichlorvos, trichlorfon, and ivermectin are the drugs of choice for bot treatment. Although it is impossible to protect horses from botfly attack, routine treatment strategies reduce the number of larvae pupae and adults.

17.4 *PARASCARIS EQUORUM* INFECTION

Infection with this ascarid parasite is most common in foals. Adult animals harbor few worms, and the main source of infection for foals is contamination of paddocks with ascarid eggs from foals of the previous season. *P. equorum* parasitizes the small intestine, and heavy infestations can produce respiratory signs, peritonitis (migratory larvae), unthriftiness, reduced weight gain, colic, or, rarely, rupture of the small intestine. Mature female worms produce thousands of eggs, which causes heavy, persistent environmental contamination. Foals can become infected shortly after birth and can harbor appreciable burdens of mature parasites at 4 to 5 months of age. Ascarid control programs should begin when foals are 2 months of age, and regular treatment at 8-week intervals should take place until they are yearlings. Modern broad-spectrum benzimidazoles are effective against *P. equorum* and the horse strongyli, and so ascarids are readily controllable in a routine worm control program.

Thiabendazole must be given at twice the normal dosage (88 mg/kg) to attack *P. equorum* successfully. Piperazine or piperazine-thiabendazole is effective against adult and immature stages also. Numerous practitioners have questioned ivermectin's efficacy against roundworms based on clinical impression of foals and visual response to treatment compared with other agents. Work in the field has reconfirmed ivermectin's efficacy against adult roundworms. No effect, however, has occurred on migrating phases of the parasites through liver and lung. The manufacturer recommends deworming as usual with ivermectin but following with a piperazine product in 4 weeks in areas of high infection. Migrating phases of ascarids may return to the bowel rapidly and then be susceptible to products efficacious against adults.

17.5 *OXYURIS EQUI* INFECTION

This infection is common, and signs of perineal irritation accompany the egg-laying activities of the adult female worm. *Oxyuris* infections are primarily within the large intestine (colon), but they are of little pathologic significance at this site. Migration from the colon to the anus causes local pruritus and rubbing of the tail and anal regions, with loss of hair and bare patches appearing around the tail and buttocks. *Oxyuris* is susceptible to most modern broad-spectrum anthelmintics and is controlled by regular strongylus control programs.

17.6 SMALL STRONGYLUS INFECTION

The small strongyli consist of numerous small parasites, only a small proportion of which cause problems under field conditions. Small strongyli are found in the large intestine, principally the caecum and colon, where they feed on the mucosal lining of the gut. Nodular enlargements frequently arise at the mucosal feeding sites. Completion of the life cycle takes place within the gut lumen, without any extraintestinal migration. The shallow buccal capsules of the cyathostomes facilitate the mucosal feeding patterns of these parasites within the wall of the large intestine. Veterinarians often think of *S. vulgaris* as the only parasite of major importance as a cause of verminous colic. Cyathostomes can cause colic, however, and serious pathologic changes and signs of colic mainly occur when large numbers of fourth-stage larvae emerge from the cecal and colonic mucosa. For the most part, few anthelmintics are effective against encysted cyathostomes at the normal dosages. It is only after encysted larvae have emerged that anthelmintics are effective. (*Triodontophorus tenuicollis* is almost as large as some of the large strongyli. This is a nonmigratory parasite sometimes classed as a large strongylus).

Heavy infection with small strongyli can contribute significantly to the severity of clinical parasitism in the horse. Attendant signs, such as diarrhea, can occur in young animals sometimes associated with the mass emergence of larvae from their mucosal feeding sites.

The small strongyli (cyathostomes) do not undergo larval migration outside the intestine but only onto the mucosa and submucosal tissues of the intestines. Larvae of cyathostomes in the encysted state can remain inhibited or hypobiotic for months or years. Diarrhea and weight loss can be associated with sudden emergence of many L4 larvae from their inhibited state.

Most drugs that are effective against large strongyli are also effective against small strongyli.

A major problem in treating cyathostomes, however, is the emergence of resistance. This resistance currently extends to the benzimidazoles, febantel, and phenothiazine. Oxibendazole is an exception, and curiously it usually retains efficacy in the presence of benzimidazole resistance (i.e., no side resistance). Of the nonbenzimidazoles, ivermectin, pyrantel, dichlorvos, and piperazine display activity against benzimidazole-resistant species.

Numerous reports, including work done on resistant small strongyli, have indicated ivermectin to be extremely effective against these strains. This would be expected considering its unique mode of action compared with any other anthelmintics. Additionally, supportive evidence for effects of hypobiosed L4 strongyli in the wall of the bowel has been noted.

17.7 *TRICHOSTRONGYLUS* INFECTION

Larvae of the small stomach worm *T. axei* can penetrate the gastric mucosa, causing catarrhal gastritis and weight loss. Nodule formation, erosions, and ulcerations occur primarily in the glandular portion of the stomach. Treatment is often difficult because of their relative inaccessibility owing to the surrounding heavy mucous exudate. Ivermectin and the benzimidazoles are the drugs of choice in therapy.

17.8 *STRONGYLOIDES WESTERI* INFECTION

S. westeri is found in the small intestine and is one of the first parasites to which the susceptible young foal may be exposed. Infection may occur through larvae in the mare's milk or by skin penetration of third-stage larvae from the environment. Diarrhea caused by *S. westeri* infection can be seen as early as 10 days in severe cases. High fecal egg counts associated with persistent diarrhea are seen at up to 4 months of age; by 6 months, foals are usually relatively resistant to infection.

S. westeri infections are self-limiting and typically disappear by the time foals are several months old. Horses more than 1 year old do not have mature *S. westeri* parasites present in the intestine. The life cycle of *S. westeri* is unique in the sense that transmammary transmission can occur. Foals can be affected by ingesting larvae in mare's milk. Infections from the environment are acquired by ingestion of larvae through the skin.

Thiabendazole, oxibendazole, fenbendazole, and ivermectin are all highly effective against enteric *S. westeri* in foals. Foals should be dewormed at 6 weeks of age. In mares, ivermectin possesses some activity against the tissue stages of the parasite and thus can lock, or reduce, transmammary transmission to foals.

Because these threadworms can be transmitted to foals through the mare's milk, mares should be treated at foaling with ivermectin. Foals can be given one or two treatments of ivermectin, oxibendazole, fenbendazole, or thiabendazole.

A single treatment of ivermectin at normal dosage given to mares on the day of foaling provides protection of foals against milk-borne transmission of *S. westeri* responsible for parasitic foal diarrhea.

Thiabendazole and ivermectin at normal dosages, oxibendazole at twice the normal dosage, and fenbendazole at 6 times the normal dosage are effective against *S. westeri* infections.

17.9 TAPEWORM INFECTION

Anoplocephala magna, *A. perfoliata*, and *Paranoplocephala mamillana* are the three major species of tapeworms found in horses.

Heavy infections give rise to anemia, unthriftiness, and digestive disturbances. The small intestine and sometimes the stomach are the predilection sites for *A. magna* and *P. mammillana*, *A perfoliata* being more commonly found in the caecum. Attachment of the scolex to the mucosa can cause some degree of local ulceration, especially at the site of attachment of *A. perfoliata*.

Although it is difficult to establish that *A. perfoliata* can cause significant detrimental effects and deaths in horses, some of the pathologic effects that this parasite can cause, mainly at the site of attachment, are ulceration, inflammation, edema, and production of a diphtheritic membrane.

In the past few years, there have been many clinical reports of a direct association between tapeworm infestations and intestinal disease of the horse, particularly intussusceptions. The worldwide prevalence of *A. perfoliata* infestations in horses at autopsy has shown a wide variation. It has been suggested that the prevalence of *A. perfoliata* infestation is highest in young horses.

There does appear to be a seasonal variation, with the greatest prevalence seen during the winter months, both in the northern and southern hemispheres. This results from the animals' greater exposure to the intermediate horse (mite) while at pasture in the summer, which includes two to four months for the intermediate stage to develop in the oribatid mite and six to ten weeks for development in the horse.

It has been suggested that the widespread use of ivermectin may, by removing other internal parasites, allow tapeworms to flourish because they are inherently insensitive to this drug. Many of the commonly used equine parasiticides are not labeled for use against tapeworms. The common equine tapeworm *A. perfoliata* is susceptible to pyrantel pamoate 13.2 mg/kg (2 times normal dosage rate), niclosamide (200 to 300 mg/kg), and mebendazole (20 mg/kg) for 5 consecutive days.

Even though the therapeutic dose of pyrantel embonate against tapeworms is double that for nematodes, field trials have suggested that when the drug is used at the nematode dosage rate, it may have some activity against tapeworms. The therapeutic dose rate for pyrantal pamoate against nematodes (6.6 mg/kg) does possess activity against *A. perfoliata*. Up to three times this dosage rate, 19.8 mg base/kg, has been effective in removing this parasite from equids in a number of tests, as has pyrantel embonate (38 mg/kg).

17.10 *HABRONEMA* INFECTION AND *ONCHOCERCA* INFECTION

Horses acquire infection with these stomach parasites (*H. muscae, Habronema microstoma,* and *Draschia (Habronema megastoma)* by ingesting flies containing infective larvae or by direct contact with larvae that emerge from the insects as they feed around the lips. Severe infection with *Draschia* results in gastritis. Occasionally large lesions are formed in the stomach, and these nodular-like enlargements are filled with necrotic material and encapsulated parasites. As eggs are laid by the enclosed worms, a small opening in the lesion allows their passage through the apparently intact epithelium. Larvae of *Draschia* and *Habronema* are sometimes found in pulmonary tissues, especially in foals, in which they can be associated with *Rhodococcus equi* infections.

Rupture of granulomatosis lesions rarely causes peritonitis, although mechanical obstruction is a risk associated with gross nodular enlargements. A limited number of studies have reported up to 80% success rate in treating *Habronema* granulomas with one injection of ivermectin and followed by topical lindane repellent. Rapid reinfection occurs with *Habronema* larvae in wounds exposed to the environment and may complicate therapy. Those with difficulty in resolution following ivermectin and repellent may need debridement and local injection of a corticosteroid to effect complete healing. This alternate therapy, by itself, may be responsible for favorable results with or without ivermectin.

Ivermectin is the most suitable anthelmintic for field use, and it has proved highly effective against cutaneous habronemiasis, "summer sores" in horses.

ONCHOCERA DERMATITIS

Ivermectin at a standard dose has been shown to be highly effective against *Onchocerca* microfilaria; however, it does not ap-

pear to kill adult *Onchocerca*. Resolution of clinical cases of *Onchocerca* dermatitis occurred within 2 to 3 weeks postinjection. Indeed a failure of a suspected case of *Onchocerca* dermatitis to respond to ivermectin would warrant consideration of an alternate diagnosis. A percentage of horses develop a facial and ventral midline edema posttreatment. The use of a corticosteroid for 48 to 72 hours has clinically seemed to reduce this occurrence. Ivermectin is extensively used in man for onchocerca infection in the tropics (Mectizan MSD).

17.11 LUNGWORM INFECTION

D. arnfieldi is a commonly reported cause of respiratory problems in donkeys. Cross infection with horses may occur when donkeys are mixed with horses. Infected horses must be isolated from donkeys or suspected contaminated pastures.

In treatment of lungworm infection, two doses of thiabendazole at 440 mg/kg with 24 hours between treatments and fenbendazole at doses of 15 to 30 mg/kg have been recommended. Mebendazole at a dosage rate of 20 mg/kg daily for 5 days is 75 to 100% effective against these parasites in the lungs. Ivermectin at the normal dosage (200 mg/kg) rate is effective against *D. arnfieldi* also.

17.12 MANAGEMENT OF EQUINE PARASITIC PROBLEMS

Because horses are susceptible to infection by parasites, often regardless of age, they must be routinely examined for parasites and treated prophylactically for them. Compounds used in modern treatment are broad spectrum in efficacy and safe when given at the recommended dosage levels. Separation of foals from adult stock, good sanitation, and pasture management are important complementary measures to anthelmintic control programs.

The number and timing of treatments vary according to local conditions, management practices, environmental factors, and availability of drugs. The principles of parasitic control are based fundamentally on the objective of reducing environmental contamination.

The interval between dosing depends on the type of anthelmintic used and the length of time feces are kept free of eggs. A time interval of 4 to 8 weeks is the most usual, but monitoring the fecal egg counts is necessary to devise a complete control program properly.

All horses must receive treatment, and animals that share the same paddock or pasture must be treated at the same time. Particular attention must be paid to new arrivals or boarding horses. These must be treated on arrival at the farm or stud.

If animals are housed in clean, dry surroundings, this reduces the likelihood of *P. equorum*, *S. westeri*, and *O. equi* infections. Separation of younger from older animals; removal of feces from pasture; mixed grazing or rotational grazing of paddocks; isolation of treated animals for 48 hours; and ploughing, reseeding, and chain harrowing of pastures are useful ancillary measures.

17.13 ANTHELMINTIC USAGE

One of the major drawbacks of most equine anthelmintics has been the lack of activity against migratory and tissue-dwelling larval stages of the horse strongyli. Although many parasiticides are effective against adult and larval parasites in the intestinal lumen of the horse, only oxfendazole, fenbendazole, and ivermectin are effective against tissue-dwelling strongylus larvae. Ivermectin and oxfendazole may be used at normal dosage rates; fenbendazole can be given either as a single dose or in a divided daily dose regimen. These drugs possess useful activity against *S. edentatus* larvae in the flanks and *S. vulgaris* L4 (fourth-stage larva) in the intestinal arteries. They are therefore the drugs of choice in the treatment of disease resulting from heavy larval infections when prophylactic measures have failed.

Paste formulations are convenient and easy to use and avoid the handling and labor problems of stomach tubing. In-feed preparations are also useful, but total consumption of the medicated diet is necessary to ensure that the animal receives the entire dose. Most prophylactic measures are designed to control the majority of major gastrointestinal parasites, with the exception of *S. westeri* in foals and stomach bots. When dichlorvos and ivermectin are used routinely, these anthelmintics also suffice for bot control. If, however, the routine program is based on the use of benzimidazoles or pyrantel, a separate winter treatment for bots is necessary with ivermectin, dichlorvos, or trichlorfon (metrifonate). Most of the commonly used drugs are effective mainly against adult worms or mature larvae in the intestinal lumen and not against larval trichonemes in the mucosa or migratory large strongylus larvae.

If parasite control measures are adequate, however, specific therapy against these stages should be unnecessary. Special precautions are necessary when using organophosphates (dichlorvos, trichlorfon). Concurrent use of other organophosphates or phenothiazine compounds (tranquilizers) must be avoided because of undesirable drug interactions. Clinical cases of parasitism respond well to larvicidal anthelmintics, such as ivermectin, fenbendazole, and oxfendazole. The aim of a control program, however, is to prevent clinical outbreaks, and thus prophylactic use of anthelmintics is the basis of parasite control.

17.14 ANTHELMINTIC RESISTANCE

Anthelmintic resistance is becoming an increasing problem worldwide, and some of the small strongyli especially have developed resistance to benzimidazoles. This is undoubtedly due to continual intensive use of similar types of anthelmintics exerting selection pressure on parasite populations. It is advisable to alter drugs in a control program each season and to rotate between chemically distinct classes of anthelmintics that possess dissimilar mechanisms of action, i.e., ivermectin, dichlorvos, pyrantel, and benzimidazoles.

Small strongyli are particularly prone to develop resistance. Resistance in thoroughbreds to thiabendazole, mebendazole, and oxfendazole was originally reported almost 30 years ago. Resistance of cyathostomes to fenbendazole has also been reported. Occasionally the efficacy of fenbendazole can be improved when it is combined with piperazine in treatment of horses infected with benzimidazole-resistant small strongyli. The efficacy of other benzimidazoles also, including mebendazole, can be enhanced by combination with piperazine.

Control programs should change over to a chemically unrelated compound every 12 months or so to minimize possible problems with resistance. The choice or rotation is limited usually to four distinct types: a benzimidazole, pyrantel, organophosphate, or ivermectin. Small strongyli have a tendency to acquire resistance relatively rapidly, although this problem has been overcome in many cases by the administration of piperazine with a benzimidazole.

Most control strategies are geared toward treating horses every 6 to 8 weeks throughout the year. Such treatment, however, can be too infrequent to keep pasture contamination low, and often fecal egg counts return to pretreatment levels 6 weeks after treatment. Shortening the treatment interval to 1 month may improve the situation, but accompanying this frequency of treatment is the risk of acquired anthelmintic resistance arising from intense selection pressure.

Adaptation by worms has diminished the effects of many control programs. It is believed that the incidence of *S. vulgaris* has been diminished by the intensive use of the benzimidazoles, the nonbenzimidazoles, and especially ivermectin, which offered the possibility of the complete eradication of the parasite. Before the benzimidazole era, the prevalence of large strongyli and especially of the arterial stages was high, and it was estimated that 90% of colics were due to the arterial stages of *S. vulgaris*. A relative decline in the number of cases of verminous arteritis was noted in the 1980s with the advent of avermectins, which displayed larvicidal effects in the mesenteric arteries against migratory strongyli.

Another feature of significance in recent years is the adaptation of parasites resulting in significant incidences of benzimidazole resistance by a number of species of cyathostomes. This was first reported on thoroughbred farms in 1965 where thiabendazole had been intensively used. Cross resistance commonly occurs between most benzimidazole drugs, including thiabendazole, albendazole, cambendazole, meben-

dazole, fenbendazole, oxfendazole, and the pro-drug febantel. Oxibendazole is the only benzimidazole drug with high efficacy against benzimidazole-resistant parasites for unknown reasons.

Since the development of cyathostome resistance to benzimidazole drugs and the decline of *S. vulgaris*, cyathostomes have made an even greater contribution to pasture contamination and pasture infectivity. It is likely that hypobiotic cyathostomes are primarily responsible for the spring and summer rises in fecal egg counts in horses, supplemented by recently ingested cyathostomes in the summer.

The nonsusceptibility of encysted cyathostomes to anthelmintics can be a major problem. This is true especially of young horses and yearlings, in which not only the cyathostome worm burden may be heavier, but also intensity of treatment may lead to more intense selection pressure and ensuing anthelmintic resistance.

17.15 CONTROL PROGRAMS

Bimonthly treatment of horses was the standard treatment in the benzimidazole era, with a variety of rotation systems being used that often failed to discriminate between benzimidazoles and nonbenzimidazole drugs. The advent of organophosphates (dichlorvos, metrifonate) and tetrahydropyrimidines (pyrantel) in the 1970s and avermectins (ivermectin) in the 1980s offered new choices of nonbenzimidazole drugs.

Because of different climatic conditions, seasonal control strategies vary between northern and southern climates. The general aim is to prevent a buildup of pasture infection in the summer and autumn in the north and avoid autumn and winter peaks in the south. In southern climates, prophylactic treatments in autumn and winter are indicated to prevent a buildup in pasture larvae toward spring, using ivermectin at 8-week intervals or other wormers at 4-week intervals. Spring and summer treatment is suitable for northern latitudes in the northern United States and Europe. Treatment during spring and summer reduces overall pasture contamination and infectivity and prevents buildup of large and small strongyli on pasture. This should prevent clinical signs of parasitism during the season.

Suitable benzimidazole anthelmintics can be given every month from spring until autumn, reducing fecal egg counts during the intervals between treatment. The longer lasting and residual effects of ivermectin allow for extension of the treatment intervals to 8 weeks because of its more prolonged suppression of egg counts (7 to 10 weeks). With other anthelmintics, treatment should be repeated at 4-week intervals throughout spring and summer because they suppress fecal egg counts for 4 to 5 weeks.

When ivermectin is used, bots are also controlled, but when using other drugs, a bot treatment in the autumn with ivermectin trichlorfon or dichlorvos is desirable. Chemically unrelated anthelmintics should be rotated annually, and no single drug should be used year after year. Such strategy suppresses spring and summer peaks of worm egg output and significantly reduces pasture infectivity. A treatment for bots in the fall completes the prophylactic program.

Horses in northern latitudes show a seasonal rise in strongylus output, with peak counts occurring in spring and summer. The spring rise leads to massive increases in pasture larvae in summer and fall. Once pastures become infected heavily, many larvae survive until the following spring. In these conditions, treatment does not prevent reinfections, and horses may exhibit a loss of performance, ill thrift, colic diarrhea, and anorexia.

Prophylactic treatments of adult horses in spring and summer ensure that pastures remain safe the rest of the year. Ivermectin could be used successfully in three treatments at 8-week intervals in April, June, and August for adult horses because of its prolonged suppression of egg counts for 8 to 10 weeks.

Although spring and summer treatments prevent the buildup of pasture larvae in summer and autumn, they do not usually eliminate all pasture contamination or stop worm egg output in autumn and winter. This can be an advantage because it ensures sufficient worm transmission to provoke some immunity to large and strong strongyli, while protecting against serious worm exposure.

In southern latitudes, treatments in autumn and winter are more important. Treatment with ivermectin every 8 weeks or with benzimidazoles every 4 weeks is suitable to contain egg production and pasture infectivity.

Too-frequent dosing with anthelmintics, especially with ivermectin, at short intervals possesses some inherent risks. Apart from the danger of inducing resistance to anthelmintics, complete suppression of egg production and pasture infectivity is undesirable. This is because some degree of exposure of young stock to low levels of infection is necessary if they are to acquire some degree of natural protection against parasite infection later on in life.

In breeding establishments, the majority of problems arise from the continual trafficking of horses into and out of the premises, new arrivals, and the particular susceptibility of young horses and foals to strongylus and ascarid infections. A structured control program must be instituted in such breeding farms, incorporating at least some of the following measures.

Mares and new arrivals should be treated with preferably a nonbenzimidazole anthelmintic or oxibendazole at least 48 hours before being put out to grass. Mares must also be treated immediately after foaling. Foals over 2 months old should receive anthelmintic treatment every month or every 2 months depending on the individual situation. Particular attention to dosing is necessary when weanlings enter paddocks. Removal of feces once or twice weekly from paddocks may be necessary to minimize sudden exposure to pasture infectivity by young susceptible animals. Regular treatment of all animals at 4- to 8-week intervals is necessary throughout the first year. Such regular treatment suppresses worm egg output, reduces parasite population on pasture to low levels, and accordingly reduces the likelihood of clinical parasitism. In northern latitudes, mares and foals should be treated throughout the grazing season with either ivermectin every 8 weeks or with other parasiticides every 4 weeks. In warmer southern latitudes, this schedule should be continued throughout the winter.

When horses are removed from pasture in autumn, a larvicidal anthelmintic dose reduces the number of developing strongyli. A similar dose is necessary at turnout in springtime to prevent any carryover of infection onto the pasture. For bot control, all horses, should receive treatment with ivermectin, dichlorvos, or trichlorfon in autumn or winter.

To avoid the development of anthelmintic resistance, drugs should be rotated over a 1- to 2-year period. If benzimidazole resistance is suspected or established, ivermectin, dichlorvos, pyrantel, piperazine, or oxibendazole may be employed as alternatives. The success of any treatment program must be carefully monitored by regular fecal egg count examinations. Quantitative assessment of egg counts can be performed simply by using the modified McMaster technique. Such laboratory aids facilitate evaluation of the progress of the treatment strategy employed and indicate any incipient problem of anthelmintic resistance.

17.16 ENVIRONMENTAL IMPACT

The ecologic and environmental consequences of anthelmintic use is an area that is rightly receiving much greater attention, especially from regulatory authorities. Residues and metabolites of phenothiazine, dichlorvos ruelene, and piperazine excreted in bovine feces possess deleterious effects on dung beetles of importance to the pasture ecosystem. Phenothiazine is known to have adverse effects via its excreted metabolites on pasture growth clover content and nitrification rate.

Horse excreta containing high concentrations of dichlorvos (usually from slow-release pellets) tends to remain insect free and longer on the ground because of the high insecticidal activity for 10 days or so after treatment. Dung contains a vast number of beneficial insects to the ecosystem. They aid in the degradation of dung, soil aeration, humus-content-enhanced water percolation, and posture productivity. Reduction in pasture fouling by degradation of dung by the dung beetles increases the zone of pasture available and reduces the foci for fly breeding. Dung beetles can reduce the number of infective nematode larvae and strongylus larvae that emerge from the feces.

Ivermectin, now widely used as the primary anthelmintic in horses, deserves special attention in this regard. This drug displays potent insecticidal activity and is almost wholly excreted in the feces. Dung from ivermectin-treated cattle can remain almost sterile for prolonged periods of time (up to 3 months), and the ivermectin excreted in the feces can adversely affect many beneficial dung-degrading beetles. This results in increased pasture fouling.

APPENDIX 1
EQUINE PARASITICIDES: PRECAUTIONS AND ADDITIONAL USES

Drug	Safety Index	Comments	Additional Uses
Thiabendazole	27	Very safe. Can be given to pregnant mares, foals, and in heavy infections	*S. vulgaris* larvae, 440 mg/kg for 2 consecutive days
Mebendazole	45	Doses of 400 mg/kg necessary to produce signs of toxicity (mild diarrhea)	*D. arnfieldi*, 15.2 to 20 mg/kg for 5 consecutive days
Fenbendazole	200	Up to 1000 mg/kg has been administered without adverse effects. Hypersensitivity can develop from deaths of large numbers of larvae killed by fenbendazole	*P. equorum*, 10 mg/kg Migratory strongyli, 10 mg/kg for 5 days; 50 mg/kg for 3 days; 60 mg/kg single dose *S. westeri* 4 times therapeutic dose
Oxfendazole	10	Mild diarrhea can occur after dose in excess of 100 mg/kg. Oxfendazole should not be given to severely debilitated animals	Migratory strongyli, 10 mg/kg 48 hours apart
Oxibendazole	60	Doses up to 600 mg/kg are tolerated without adverse effects. Do not use in animals suffering from colic or severe debilitation	*S. westeri*, 2 times therapeutic dose (−20 mg/kg) Effective against benzimidazole-resistant small strongyli
Febantel	33	Wide safety margin	Pro-benzimidazole
Pyrantel	Tartrate salt—6 Pamoate salt—20	The tartrate salt of pyrantel is soluble, and toxicity may be seen at doses at 55 mg/kg. The less soluble pamoate salt requires higher doses (132 mg/kg) for toxic symptoms to arise. Pyrantel preparations should not be given to severely debilitated animals	Tapeworms, 13.2 mg/kg (2 times therapeutic dose) Pamoate salt
Dichlorvos	3	Dichlorvos resin pellets must not be used in suckling foals or in animals suffering from diarrhea, constipation, colic, or pulmonary disease. Similar to all organophosphates, dichlorvos should not be used simultaneously or within a week of treatment with other cholinesterase inhibitors. Doses of 105 mg/kg are associated with signs of toxicity, and debilitated or severely parasitized animals should receive a reduced dosage of dichlorvos. Pellets passed out in feces are toxic to poultry and wildfowl. Water should be withheld before and after dosing for bots	
Trichlorfon	1	Trichlorfon can be toxic at doses near the therapeutic dose levels, inducing typical signs of diarrhea, colic, sweating. It is contraindicated in animals suffering from pulmonary disease, intestinal problems, or severe *P. equorum* infections. It must not be used simultaneously or within a few days of treatment with other cholinesterase inhibitors. Withholding of food before treatment increases risk of toxicity	

APPENDIX 1 (continued)

Drug	Safety Index	Comments	Additional Uses
Ivermectin	10	At 10 times the therapeutic dose (-2 mg/kg), visual impairment, ataxia, and depression have been reported. Although adverse effects are uncommon with the paste formulation, hypersensitivity and ventral midline edema can be seen as a result of death of *Onchocerca* larvae. Extralabel use of injectable ivermectin for cattle has been implicated in a number of local and systemic adverse effects. Ivermectin paste should be used with care in young foals	Effective also against *Onchocerca* microfilaria; migratory strongyli; Gastric/cutaneous stages of *Habronema* and *Draschia*; Adult/larvae of *D. arnfieldi, S. westeri*
Piperazine	17	Doses of 1500 mg/kg have been used without untoward effects other than slight softening of feces in the horse. Rupture or obstruction of the bowel is a risk if piperazine is given to treat massive *P. equorum* infections	Reduced dosage of 55 mg/kg in combination with benzimidazole in therapy of benzimidazole-resistant small strongyli
Levamisole	2–3	Sweating, lacrimation, ataxia, and incoordination have been observed with 30 mg/kg doses of levamisole. Because of its potent rapid action on parasites, sudden deaths of massive numbers of *P. equorum* may cause rupture or obstruction in the bowel. Deaths of *Onchocerca* larvae can precipitate hypersensitive reactions and ventral midline edema	

APPENDIX 2
PROPRIETARY EQUINE PARASITICIDES

Generic Name	Trade Name	Manufacturer
Febantel	Rintal	Haver/Diamond Scientific
Febantel/trichlorfon	Combotel Paste	Haver
Fenbendazole	Panacur	Hoechst-Roussel
Ivermectin	Eqvalan	MSD AgVet
Levamisole/piperazine	Ripercol piperazine	SmithKline Beecham
Mebendazole	Telmin	Pitman-Moore
Oxfendazole	Benzelmin	Syntex
Oxfendazole/trichlorfon	Benzelmin Plus	Syntex
Oxibendazole	Anthelcide	SmithKline Beecham
	Equipar	Coopers
Pyrantel pamoate	Strongid	Pfizer
Thiabendazole	Equizole	MSD AgVet
Thiabendazole/piperazine	Equizole A	MSD AgVet
Trichlorfon	Combot	Haver
Trichlorfon/phenothazine/piperazine	Dyrex T F	Fort Dodge
Dichlorvos	Equigard	Squibb

SELECTED REFERENCES

Anderson, R.A.: The use of ivermectin in horses. Research and clinical observations. Comp. Cont. Educ. Pract. Vet., *6*:S516, 1984.

Barragry, T.B.: Therapy of parasitic infestations. Irish Veterinary News, *14*:9, 1992.

Barragry, T.B.: Parasitism therapy in horses. Vet. Update, 29, 1989.

Bennett, D.G.: Clinical pharmacology of ivermectin. J. Am. Vet. Med. Assoc., *189*:100, 1986.

Blackwell, J.J.: Colitis in horses associated with strongyle larvae. Vet. Rec. 93:401, 1973.

Blagbum, B.L., Hendrix, C.M., Lindsay, D.S., and Schmacher, J.: Pathogenesis, treatment and control of gastric parasites in horses. Comp. Cont. Educ. Pract. Vet., *13*:850, 1991.

Blogburn, B.L., Linsay, D.S., and Hendux, C.M.: Pathogenesis, treatment and control of gastric parasites in horses. Comp. Cont. Educ. Pract. Vet., *13*:850, 1991.

Bogan, J.A., and Duncan, J.L.: Anthelmintics for dogs, cats and horses. Br. Vet. J., *140*:361, 1984.

Bridges, E. R.: The use of ivermectin to treat genital cutaneous habromemiasis in a stallion. Comp. Cont. Educ. Pract. Vet., *72*:S94, 1985.

Britt, D.P., and Clarkson, M.J.: Experimental chemotherapy in horses infected with benzimidazole resistant small strongyles. Vet. Rec., *123*:219, 1988.

Campbell, W.C.: Ivermectin: An update. Parasitol. Today, *1*:10, 1985.

Campbell, W.C., and Benz, G.W.: Ivermectin a review of efficacy and safety. J. Vet. Pharmacol. Ther., 7:1, 1984.

Campbell, W.C., Fischer, M.M., Stapley, E.O., et al.: Ivermectin a potent new antiparasitic agent. Science, *221*:823, 1983.

Church, S., Kelly, D.F., and Oburolo, M.J.: Diagnosis and successful treatment of diarrhoea in horses caused by immature small strongyle apparently unsusceptible to anthelmintics. Eq. Vet. J., *18*:401, 1986.

DiPietro, J.A., and Todd, K.S.: Anthelmintics used in treatment of parasitic infections of horses. Vet. Clin. North. Am. Equine Pract., 3:1014, 1987.

DiPietro, J.A., and Todd, K.S.: Control of internal parasites in the horse. Mod. Vet. Pract., *65*:B3, 1984.

Drudge, J.H.: Strongyles—an update. Eq. Pract., *11*:43, 1989.

Drudge, J.H. and Lyons, E.T.: Introduction: Strongyles, *Strongyloides*. Internal Parasites of Equines with Emphasis on Treatment and Control. Somerville, NJ, Hoechst-Roussel Aggravate Co., 1989.

Drudge, J.H., and Lyons, E.T.:Internal Parasites of Equines with Emphasis on Treatment and Control. Somerville, NJ, Hoechst Roussel, 1986.

Drudge, J.H., and Lyons, E.T.: Large strongyles: Recent advances. Vet. Clin. North. Am. (Equine Pract.), 2: 263, 1986.

Drudge, J.H., and Lyons, E.T.: Critical tests of a resin pellet formulation of dichlorous against internal parasites of the horse. Am. J. Vet. Res., *33*:1386, 1972.

Drudge, J.H., Lyons, E.T., and Tolliver, S.C.: Parasite control in the horse: A review of contemporary drugs. Vet. Med. Small Anim. Clin., 76:1479, 1981.

Drudge, J.H., Lyons, E.T., Tolliver, S.C., and Kubis, J.E.: Clinical trials of oxibendazole for control of equine internal parasites. Mod. Vet. Pract., 62:679, 1981.

Drudge, J.H., Lyons, E.T., Tolliver, S.C., and Swerczek, T.W.: Use of oxibendazole for control of cambendazole resistant small strongyles in a bowel of ponies—a six year study. Am. J. Vet. Res., 46:2507, 1985.

Duncan, J.L.: Internal parasites of the horse and their control. Eq. Vet. J. *17*:79, 1985.

Duncan, J.L., McBeath, D.G., and Preston, N.K.: Studies on the efficacy of fenbendazole used in a divided dose regime against strongyle infections in ponies. Eq. Vet. J., *12*:78, 1980.

French, D., and Chapman, M.: Tapeworms of the equine gastrointestinal tract. Comp. Cont. Educ. Pract. Vet., *14*:655, 1992.

Gaughan, E.M.: Cecocolic intussusceptions in horses. Proc. Eq. Colic Res., *4*:14, 1991.

Hackett, G.E., and Buonafide, J.: A comparison of equine anthelmintics by route of administration. Prac. 33rd Ann. Mtg. Am. Vet. Parasitol., Abstract 54, 1988.

Herd, R.P.: Equine parasite control—problems associated with intensive anthelmintic therapy. Eq. Vet. Educ., 2:41, 1990.

Herd, R.P.: Epidemiology and control of equine parasites in northern temperate regions. Vet. Clin. North Am. (Equine Pract.), 2:337, 1986.

Herd, R.P.: Epidemiology and control of equine strongylosis at Newmarket. Eq. Vet. J., *18*:447, 1986.

Herd, R.P.: Parasite control in horses seasonal use of equine anthelmintics. Med. Vet. Pract., 67:895, 1986.

Herd, R.P., Miller, T.B., and Gabel, A.A.: A field evaluation of probenzimidazoles and nonbenzimidazole anthelmintics in horses. J. Am. Vet. Med. Assoc., *179*:686, 1981.

Jacobs, D.E., Pilkington, J.G., Fisher, M.A., and Fox, M.T.: Ivermectin therapy and degradation of cattle feces. Vet. Rec., *123*:400, 1988.

Love, S.: Parasite associated equine diarrhoea. Comp. Cont. Educ. Vet. Pract., *14*:642, 1992.

Lyons, E.T.: Prevalence of Anophocephala perfoliata and lesions of praschia megastoms in thoroughbreds in Kentucky at necropsy. Am. J. Vet. Res., *45*:996, 1984.

Lyons, E.T., Drudge, J.H., Tolliver, S.C., and Granstrom, D.E.: The role of intestinal nematodes in foal diarrhoea. Vet. Med., 320, 1991.

Lyons, E.T., Drudge, J.H., Tolliver, S.C., and Swerczek, T.W.: Pyrantel pamoate: Evaluating its activity against equine tapeworms. Vet. Med., 280, 1986.

Łyons, E.T., Drudge, J.H., Tolliver, S.C., and Swerczek, T.W.: Vet. Med. Small Anim. Clin., *81*:280, 1986.

Madigan, J.E.: Ivermectin use in the horse. Calif. Vet., *9*:29, 1984.

Mair, T.S., DeWesterlaken, L.V., Cripps, P.J., and Love, S.: Diarrhoea in adult horses: A survey of clinical cases and an assessment of some prognostic indices. Vet. Rec., 126:479, 1990.

McKellar, Q.A., and Scott, E.W.: The benzimidazole anthelmintic agents—a review. J. Vet. Pharmacol. Ther., 13:223, 1990.

Munsell, R.: A practical approach to verminous arteritis in horses. Vet. Med. Small Anim. Clin., 78:393, 1982.

Owen, R.H., Jagger, D.W., and Quan Taylor, R.: Caecal intususseptions in horses and the significance of A. perfoliata. Vet. Rec., 124:34, 1981.

Reinemeyer, C.R.: Small strongyles: Recent advances. Vet. Clin. North Am. (Equine Pract.), 2:281, 1986.

Reinemeyer, C.R., and Rohrbach, B.W.: A survey of equine parasite control programs in Tennessee. J. Am. Vet. Med. Assoc., 196:712, 1990.

Rew, R.S., and Felterer, R.H.: Mode of action of antinematodal drugs. In Chemotherapy of Diseases. Edited by R.D. Campbell and R.S. Rew. New York, Plenum Press, 1986.

Scott, P.: A review of some modern equine anthelmintics. N.Z. Vet. J., 25:373, 1977.

Slocombe, J.O.D., Cote, J.F., and McMillan, I.: Effectiveness of oxibendazole against benzimidazole resistant strongyles in Ontario. Proceeding Practice 31st Annual Meeting American Association Veterinary Parasitology, 1986.

Tritschler, J.P., Giordano, D.J., and Coles, G.C.: Resistance to benzimidazoles. J. Am. Vet. Med. Assoc., 191:391, 1987.

Waller, P.J.: Anthelmintic resistance and the future for roundworm control. Vet. Parasitol., 25:177, 1987.

CHAPTER 18

THERAPY OF EQUINE JOINT DISORDERS

18.1 Introduction
18.2 The Normal Joint
18.3 Pathogenesis of Degenerative Joint Disease
18.4 Drug Therapy
18.5 Septic Arthritis/Osteomyelitis Syndrome
18.6 Navicular Disease
18.7 Drug Therapy
18.8 Laminitis
18.9 Drug Therapy

18.1 INTRODUCTION

Degenerative joint disease (DJD) is considered to be one of the most frequently encountered debilitating diseases of performance horses because of the extreme stress placed on their joints. Excess stress on a joint causes injury to chondrocytes, the only living element in articular cartilage. Chondrocytes are responsible for the continued replacement of the proteoglycans of the articular cartilage.

DJD (osteoarthritis, osteoarthrosis) is an aseptic inflammatory disease that constitutes a relatively high percentage of all lameness diagnosed in performance horses or in older horses. Repeated trauma on the joint, owing to severe, frequent, and intensive stress, results in DJD being a common form of lameness diagnosed by the veterinarian. The disease usually affects the more highly mobile joints, such as the carpal and metacarpophalangeal joints in the young performing horse and the intertarsal and interphalangeal joints in the older animal. This results in damage to the articular cartilage and, with progressive deterioration, to bone damage, soft tissue damage, release of inflammatory enzymes, and changes in the synovial fluid. Periosteal proliferation, narrowing of the joint space, subchondral bone sclerosis, synovitis, and joint effusion usually accompany the condition. DJD is regarded as a "wear and tear" disease in which trauma, joint stress, joint loading, age, or joint instability may precipitate the condition. Primary causes may be "wear and tear," in which excessive stress on the joint cartilage damages the normal load bearing and shock-absorbing capacity of the joint. Secondary causes may be those arising from trauma, inflammation, osteochondritis, osteomalacia, or sometimes following an infectious process.

Treatment of DJD warrants specific therapeutic measures based on an understanding of joint structure, function, and pathogenesis of the condition. Trauma may damage not only the joint capsule or ligaments, but also the articular cartilage, synovial membrane, and underlying bone. The problem is particularly acute in highly competitive performance horses, in old horses, and in young horses subjected to continuous hard work and extensive fast training sessions on a regular basis.

18.2 THE NORMAL JOINT

The normal synovial joint is composed of the articular cartilage, synovial fluid, a lining synovial membrane, the joint capsule, and ligaments. The capsule itself is composed of a dense fibrous outer layer containing a rich vascular and nerve supply. The inner capsular layer is the synovial membrane.

The synovial membrane is also vascular and capable of a major inflammatory response. Its role includes maintenance of the internal environment of the joint and regulation of the matrix and synovial fluid regeneration. The layer is smooth, moist, and relatively inelastic.

Articular cartilage consists of hyaline cartilage. This covers the bony extremities and protects them from stress and pressure. The only living elements of the articular cartilage are the chondrocytes, which are responsible for cartilage metabolism and synthesis of the matrix. Chondrocytes are embedded in a complex meshwork of collagen fibers and the ground substance, which contains proteoglycans and glycoproteins. The articular cartilage functions as a shock absorber and facilitates movement. It receives its nutrition from the synovial fluid. This is as a result of its poor blood supply and poor capacity for autoregeneration.

Chondrocytes are specifically responsible for the continuous replacement of the proteoglycan ground substance of the articular cartilage. These proteoglycans are large, complex, spongelike molecules that are hydrophilic and thus trap water within their structure, conferring elasticity and resilience on the articular cartilage. Hyaluronic acid is synthesized by the synovial cells and has a molecular weight of approximately 2 million. Its metabolism is governed by the hyaluronidase enzyme system. This enzyme is present in lysosomes, which can be released during the inflammatory process. In synovial fluid, hyaluronic acid is organized in aggregates. For lubrication of the cartilaginous surface, hyaluronic acid must undergo binding with other specific lubricating glycoproteins. Hyaluronic acid constitutes more than 50% of the total glycosaminoglycan content of connective tissue, and acting as a viscous sponge, its hydrophilic nature enables it to trap large volumes of water. Because it is viscoelastic in nature, it is of critical importance in the functioning of the normal joint, acting as a shock absorber and load spreader. Apart from its role in the formation and functioning of the synovial fluid and matrix tissues, hyaluronic acid also prevents access of various inflammatory enzymes to the cartilage as well as regulating cell function and cell migration. The viscosity of the synovial fluid is proportional to both the concentration of hyaluronic acid in solution and to its molecular weight. Viscosity governs resistance to flow and distortions of physical form, whereas elasticity is the ability of the joint to retain its original conformation after being deformed. Solutions of hyaluronic acid are pseudoplastic and cushion the joint during compression and exercise.

Synovial fluid is a dialysate of plasma from the vascularized synovial membrane. The protein content is lower than that of the blood, but it also contains secretions from the synovium, especially hyaluronic acid. The function of hyaluronic acid is lubrication of the synovial membrane. It reduces and buffers the resistance of the joints to movement and mobility. Hyaluronic acid is an essential component of the viscosity and elasticity of the synovial fluid such that it is not displaced from its load bearing capacity between the bones during normal joint flexion and compression. The concentration and degree of polymerization of hyaluronic acid are critical factors in ensuring the normal functioning of hyaluronic acid as a component of the synovial fluid. This acid is a macromolecular mucopolysaccharide (glycosaminoglycan) and is a polymer of disaccharide and subunits of glucuronic acid with n-acetyl-glucosamine.

In addition, hyaluronic acid is an important component substance of the ground substance of connective tissue. Not only is it involved in determining the properties of synovial fluid, but also it links with the macromolecules and proteins to form the proteoglycans in cartilage connective tissue. The surface of the articular cartilage is covered by a slim layer of these proteoglycans, which function as a lubricant sliding layer.

PROTEOGLYCANS

These are specific glycoproteins that bind with hyaluronic acid and that are necessary for joint boundary lubrication. Proteoglycans are acid mucopolysaccharides and are composed of units of glycosaminoglycans, such as chondroitin sulfate and keratin sulfate, linked by a common protein core. On account of its hydrophilicity, a large polyionic complex structure is formed, which is able to resist compression and confer properties of resilience on the joint. Chondrocytes are responsible for continual regeneration and replacement of proteoglycans of the articular cartilage. Proteoglycans are also an integral part of the intercellular matrix. The molecular structure of the proteoglycans determines the biological properties of the articular cartilage. Similar to collagen, proteoglycans are synthesized by the chondrocytes and then secreted to the cell exterior.

18.3 PATHOGENESIS OF DEGENERATIVE JOINT DISEASE

Following intense, repeated stress on the joint, damage may be inflicted on the bone, cartilage, or associated soft tissues. The cycle of degeneration triggers off a cascade of sequential reactions, which ultimately constitute a vicious cycle.

Initial damage to chondrocytes precipitates release of lysosomal enzymes, hyaluronidase, prostaglandins, and superoxide radicals. Decreased chondrocyte metabolism impairs synthesis and release of the ground substance with ensuing loss of proteoglycan, softening of the cartilage, loss of resilience, inflammation, and perhaps synovitis. Although the role of the inflammatory process is unclear, deterioration of the articular cartilage and formation of the new bone in the subchondral areas occur. This is most noticeable in weight-bearing joints.

The synovial fluid undergoes marked changes both in consistency and in viscosity owing to the release of lysosomal enzymes, proteases, hyaluronidase, and prostaglandins. The increased vascularity and permeability of the synovial membranes contributes to the inflammatory process, with marked leukocytic invasion of the synovial fluid. Not all of the alterations in joint fluid, however, are derived from the inflamed synovial capillary supply.

Damage occurs also to the articular cartilage, which may be irreversible if left untreated, leading to an almost permanent loss of joint function. The chondrocytes, cartilaginous matrix, and collagen fibers undergo many changes. The surface collagen fibers became splintered and separated. Wear and tear on the joint causes loss of surface proteoglycans and a resulting deterioration in the elasticity of the articular surface. Damage to the cartilage leads to minute fractures and fissures and the liberation of cartilaginous detritus into the synovial fluid. Chondrocyte damage releases lysosomal proteases, which further attack the matrix and proteoglycan. Consequently, the synovial fluid becomes enriched with lysosomal enzymes, prostaglandins, and superoxide radicals, all of which are liberated from the injured tissues. Synovial fluid increases in protein content, and its viscosity decreases with the increased concentration of the enzyme hyaluronidase, which breaks down hyaluronic acid. A chain reaction is established whereby interaction of detritus with leukocytes releases further quantities of lysosomal enzymes and worsens the overall inflammatory response. Heat, swelling, and pain of the joint become clinically evident. Changes in the viscosity of the synovial fluid (the presence of breakdown products from cartilage, increased protein and enzymatic content, decreased concentration of hyaluronic acid) lead to changes in its elasticity and functioning. Both the degree of polymerization and the concentration of hyaluronic acid are decreased in DJD. When the joint space narrows, and with the reduced elasticity of the articular surface (from proteoglycan loss), ulceration, abrasion, and degeneration of the articular surface take place (Table 18–1).

Further trauma repeats and intensifies this cycle of events, with further proteoglycan loss and matrix degradation. As the matrix meshwork is broken down, enzymes, fragments, and debris are liberated into the synovial fluid. With progressive deterioration of the articular cartilage surface, the underlying bone becomes exposed, and osteophyte formation occurs. Sclerosis of bony tissue, with fragments of bone entering the joint cavity itself, may follow. Release of prostaglandins contributes to the overall pain, swelling, and inflammation, with increased permeability of the synovial vascular supply. Prostaglandins also suppress chondrocyte metabolism and proteoglycan synthesis.

18.4 DRUG THERAPY

DJD is essentially a catabolic process. Any therapeutic regimen must address itself to reversal of the cycle of degradative changes, i.e.:

- Promote synthesis of matrix components
- Reduce synovitis
- Relieve pain and swelling
- Retard degenerative metabolic processes
- Restore functioning of articular cartilage and synovial fluid to normal (Table 18–2)

In its purest form, DJD is an aseptic process. It may arise, however, secondarily from septic arthritis.

CORTICOSTEROIDS

These agents have been extensively used for treatment of DJD, especially when given by the intra-articular route. Such compounds are palliative only and act to suppress the inflammatory symptoms temporarily, without specifically addressing the fundamental underlying cause. Corticosteroids improve the stability and integrity of cellular membranes, including lysosomal membranes. This property can potentially reduce the quantity of lytic lysosomal enzymes present in joint fluid.

Two major classes of steroids have been used: water-soluble esters, such as succinates or phosphates, and insoluble suspensions of the acetate ester or free alcohol in polyethylene glycol. With the long-acting suspension types (Depo-Medrol), a major factor is the size of the particles in suspension, although corticosteroid-induced relief may persist for 3 to 4 weeks. With intra-articular injections, sterile aseptic precau-

TABLE 18–1
CYCLE OF DEGENERATIVE JOINT DISEASE

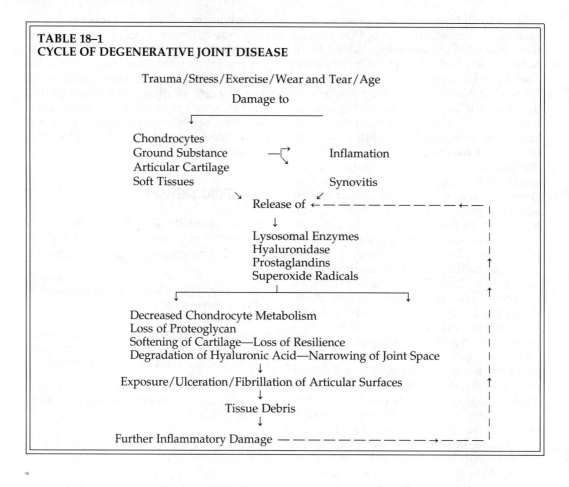

TABLE 18–2
DESIRABLE FEATURES FOR DRUG THERAPY OF DEGENERATIVE JOINT DISEASE

Retardation of catabolic processes
Reduction of inflammatory response
Promotion of synthesis of matrix
   components
Minimization of damage to articular
   cartilage
Restoration of viscosity, elasticity, and
   function of synovial fluid
Alleviation of pain
Restoration of joint function to normal
Avoidance of purely palliative effects

tions are most important. With a number of suspension-type formulations, joint flareups may occur after injection. Depression of growth and development of articular cartilage accompanies usage of these steroids, especially when used repeatedly. Corticosteroid-induced arthropathy may occur with resultant dry or locking joints.

With corticosteroids, clinical improvement is rapid and manifested by decreased joint distention, increased mobility, and decreased lameness, but many undesirable side effects occur that neutralize these effects. Chief among these are a transient postinjection flareup; osseous metaplasia of periarticular soft tissues; and arthropathy, on owing accelerated destruction of cartilage, with decreased cartilage elasticity, thinning, and fissuring. Ultimately the cartilage possesses decreased mechanical strength and elasticity.

Steroids can be useful in many horses affected with musculoskeletal problems and, by mitigating the inflammatory response, have enabled many horses to return to training. Long-acting steroids, such as methylprednisolone acetate, are successful in transient alleviation of pain and inflammation associated with degenerative and traumatic arthritis. They are totally ineffective, however, in treating the underlying cause. Most importantly, they possess catabolic activity, which is counterproductive in the therapy of this condition. Their catabolic effects suppress healing and regeneration of the cartilage and its ground substance. They adversely affect synthesis of proteoglycans and glycosaminoglycans.

Corticosteroids relieve the pain and inflammation but can suppress synthesis of components of the cartilage matrix and may result in steroid-induced degenerative arthropathy. The intra-articular use of methylprednisolone in horses has been shown to cause loss of proteoglycan with resultant DJD. In fact, corticosteroid-induced osteodegenerative lesions resemble those that occur in DJD. Such therapy may also predispose the animal to stress or chip fractures.

Corticosteroids should never be used as a substitute for correcting the underlying primary problem. They may be useful in cases of acute flareups.

Synthesis of hyaluronic acid is also suppressed by corticosteroids, which further impairs lubrication of the diseased joint. The catabolic osteodegenerative changes induced by corticosteroids can in fact resemble the DJD process itself.

Because they temporarily relieve pain, corticosteroids may obscure the true pathologic syndrome, allowing premature use of the limb and further injury and degeneration of the joint. Fracturing and chipping of bone may arise directly or indirectly from use of these catabolic steroids together with retardation of proteoglycan synthesis. Accelerated joint destruction and septic arthritis are associated risks of steroid therapy. Overall, corticosteroids are not indicated as primary agents in therapy of aseptic DJD.

NONSTEROIDAL ANTI-INFLAMMATORY DRUGS

Agents of this class, such as flunixin or phenylbutazone, although less liable to induce catabolic processes, simply provide palliative relief by virtue of their anti-inflammatory, antipyretic, and analgesic properties. Similar to the corticosteroids, they temporarily facilitate greater joint mobility during therapy but do not address the basic underlying pathologic process.

Phenylbutazone, which is a pyrazolone, is a nonsteroidal anti-inflammatory drug (NSAID) prescribed by veterinarians. After absorption, phenylbutazone is bound largely to albumin and may therefore influence the metabolism of other highly protein-bound drugs. Phenylbutazone is not a cyclooxygenase inhibitor; it is, specifically, an inhibitor of formation of prostaglandin E_2. As such, phenylbutazone may not be effective in patients whose clinical signs may relate to other vasoactive and neuroactive products of the inflammatory cascade at a given point in the disease process. Ketoprofen (a propionic acid derivative) has recently been approved for use in horses, although it has been used in humans in the United States since 1986. In horses, it apparently causes minimal gastrointestinal side effects and blocks both the cyclooxygenase and the lipoxygenase pathways. Thus one might reasonably expect that the efficacy of this drug might approach that of corticosteroids (which have a similar but not identical action), while avoiding the side effects of steroid use. NSAIDs have also been incriminated as contributory factors in the development of the gastric ulceration syndrome, especially in young horses, and so their protracted use should be avoided.

Aspirin (acetylsalicylic acid) is often selected because it is inexpensive and effective and because undesirable side effects (primarily gastric irritation) are few. The analgesic effects of aspirin are commonly attributed to its ability to block chemically induced (i.e., by bradykinin and other mediators) peripheral pain; in contrast to narcotics, aspirin has no central pain-relieving capability.

Recent experimental evidence suggests, however, that the use of aspirin and several other NSAIDs may decrease proteoglycan

<table>
<tr><td>

TABLE 18–3
EFFECTS OF POLYSULFATED GLYCOSAMINOGLYCAN

Binding to damaged cartilage
Enhancement of formation of new ground substance
Inhibition of catabolic processes
Inhibition of release of lysosomal enzymes, prostaglandins, hyaluronidase, and superoxide radicals
Protection of articular cartilage

</td></tr>
</table>

synthesis in joints affected by DJD, presumably by inhibiting early steps in the formation of chondroitin sulfate.

POLYSULFATED GLYCOSAMINOGLYCAN

This substance is now available for veterinary use in the treatment of degenerative and traumatic joint disease, although it has been available for osteoarthritic therapy in humans for many years. Polysulfated glycosaminoglycan (PSGAG) (Adequan, Luitpold) stimulates repair of cartilage and inhibits many of the processes that cause cartilaginous degeneration.

Proteoglycans are macromolecules that can trap water molecules within their structure. This trapping action gives normal cartilage its characteristic compression resiliency. PSGAG has a chondroprotective effect because it stimulates synthesis of new cartilage matrix. Joint stress also induces release of enzymes that can cause cartilage degeneration. PSGAG inhibits many of these enzymes, including prostaglandins (Table 18–3).

In DJD, degradation of collagens and proteoglycans reduces the elasticity of the cartilage and the overall ability of the joint to bear weight and stress. PSGAG inhibits prostaglandin synthesis and release and also inhibits other enzymes, such as hyaluronidase, which are responsible for catabolism of hyaluronic acid. This inhibitory activity against many lytic enzymes eventually stabilizes and reverses joint degradation and improves elasticity and joint fluid viscosity.

PSGAG is a complex, highly sulfated polysaccharide consisting of alternating units of galactosamine and glucuronic acid. After intra-articular administration, PSGAG binds selectively to the surface of the degraded or ulcerated articular cartilage, and high concentrations of PSGAG are found at the sites of the most severe degradation, where it binds with hyaluronic acid. It augments matrix formation, decreases the protein and enzyme content of the synovial fluid, and increases the level of viscosity.

Because cartilaginous degradation and debris formation are lessened, interaction of leukocytes with debris is reduced, and fewer lysosomal enzymes and prostaglandin-type autocoids are released. Hence inflammation is consequently suppressed.

In response to PSGAG, joint function is markedly improved; heat and swelling are reduced; and flexion, cushioning, load bearing, and mobility are restored to normal. Protein content of synovial fluid is lessened, and viscosity and elasticity are improved.

In 1984, the Food and Drug Administration (FDA) approved the use of exogenous PSGAG in horses for treatment of noninfectious degenerative arthropathy, traumatic joint dysfunction, and lameness, especially when associated with the carpal joint in the horse. Because of its strong electronegativity, PSGAG binds to the damaged cartilage. After intra-articular injection, therapeutic concentrations are detectable for up to 2 weeks. A parenteral (intramuscular) injectable formulation is now available, which shows equal efficiency to the yet intraarticular formulation minimizes the risk associated with joint injection. Exogenous PSGAG possesses a molecular weight of approximately 10,000. It is similar to the glycosaminoglycan of the cartilage ground substance.

When deposited intra-articularly, it selectively binds to damaged or degraded cartilage, augments formation of new ground substance, promotes healing, and prevents further articular damage. Because of the reduced cartilaginous degradation, the interaction between leukocytes and cartilaginous debris in the synovial fluid is also diminished. Thus release of lysosomal enzymes and prostaglandins is suppressed, contributing to an overall mitigation of the inflammatory response. Viscosity of the synovial fluid returns to normal, and healing of cartilage is enhanced.

In summary, the administration of PSGAG:

1. Promotes synthesis of matrix components
2. Possesses a chondrocyte protective effect
3. Retards the catabolic processes
4. Relieves pain and inflammation
5. Restores the functioning and consistency of synovial fluid to normal

Adequan (Luitpold) consists of a clear sterile aqueous solution of PSGAG—250 mg/ml in a 1-ml ampule.

The normal dosage is 250 mg (1 ml) injected into the affected joint once a week for 5 weeks. Aseptic precautions are the utmost importance for such technique. Occasionally blood coagulation time may be prolonged for a few hours after the injection. PSGAG therapy should be performed only after the initial infection (if any) has been treated successfully.

Intra-articular administration of 250 mg once weekly for 5 weeks is approximately the same in clinical efficacy to intramuscular administration of 500 mg every 4 days up to 28 days.

In contrast to steroids and NSAIDs, PSGAG inhibits proteolytic and lysosomal enzymes responsible for cartilage degeneration. It selectively binds to degraded cartilage and enhances the deposition of new matrix substance.

HYALURONIC ACID

The viscoelastic property of hyaluronic acid is of paramount importance to the horse undergoing severe joint stress. Exogenous injection of hyaluronic acid into the joint capsule promotes synthesis of the various matrix components, retards the catabolic processes, reduces synovial inflammation, restores synovial fluid to normal, and thereby relieves the pain. The molecular weight of the administered hyaluronic acid is of direct significance in terms of its duration of therapeutic effect. Because it is a polymeric macromolecule, its beneficial effects are attributable to its cushioning and shock-absorbing effect, impact on the inflammatory cells, migration and activity of phagocytes, and prostaglandin production. High-molecular-weight hyaluronic acid is more effective as a joint replacement fluid because of its particular viscosity and elasticity. The biological half-life of the high-molecular-weight compound is 16 hours in the horse, whereas that of the lower molecular weight acid is only 2 hours. The low-molecular-weight form is associated with a relatively higher incidence of postinjection flareup, whereas the higher molecular weight hyaluronic acid enables a horse to stay sound for longer periods of time.

Treatment of noninflammatory joint disease with intra-articular hyaluronic acid frequently produces beneficial results, with persistence of effect for 7 to 10 days after therapy. The acid forms a highly dispersed network with proteins and other mucopolysaccharides to form the ground substance. The molecule is a random, coiled-kinked configuration; is hydrophilic; and exerts its biological properties in proportion to the length of the chain. It possesses a significant difference from other anti-inflammatory agents and analgesics, which act only in a palliative fashion and which possess degradative and catabolic effects. Hyaluronic acid plays a key role in boundary lubrication of soft tissues and in the promotion of cartilage healing.

Usually 20 to 40 mg of hyaluronic acid is administered intra-articularly. It may be used repeatedly, with no detrimental effect on fracture healing, provided that it is injected aseptically. The molecular weight, the degree and extent of polymerization, and the concentration of hyaluronic acid are critical for its therapeutic effect. In synovial fluid, it exerts a molecular domain proportional to the length of the polymer chain.

Commercial formulations (Hylartin-V/Pharmacia) have a molecular weight of approximately 3.5 million and, when deposited into the joint, stimulate the local production of hyaluronate, while also lubricating the joint. In this way, hyaluronic acid promotes the long-term normalization of joint function.

High-molecular-weight sodium hyaluronate brings about normalization of the synovia, enabling it to resume its most important duties:

TABLE 18–4
EFFECTS OF HYALURONIC ACID

Improves soft tissue lubrication
Increases synthesis of high-molecular-
    weight hyaluronic acid
Has anti-inflammatory activity
Controls viscosity of synovial fluid
Is component of intercellular ground
    substance of connective tissue
Aids nutrition of articular cartilage

1. Lubrication of the soft tissues of the joint, thus reducing friction, alleviating pains, and improving joint mobility
2. Restoring the synovial barrier function and so inhibiting the invasion by leukocytes and enzymes
3. Contributing directly to a normalization of the nutrition of the articular cartilage in the treated joint (Table 18–4)

After treatment of 20 to 40 mg of high-molecular-weight hyaluronic acid intra-articularly, it is usually recommended that horses should receive 4 to 7 days' rest followed by a period of light work or training. Manufacturers usually state that approximately 20% of the hyaluronic acid remains in the joint after 22 hours.

The therapeutic benefits of intra-articular hyaluronic acid injection are attributable to the cushioning effect as well as to the compound's suppressant effect on cell migration, phagocytosis, and prostaglandin production. For successful treatment of DJD, it is necessary to have the drug present within the joint structures for as long as possible (Table 18–5). Treatment may be repeated at weekly intervals for a total of three treatments.

DIMETHYL SULFOXIDE

Dimethyl sulfoxide (DMSO) has many unique features. DMSO has the unique property of penetrating the unbroken skin rapidly and also aids the transcutaneous absorption of many other drugs. It enhances skin penetration without causing damage to the integrity of biological membranes. DMSO on its own possesses useful anti-inflammatory effects, local anesthetic effects, and antibacterial effects as well as diuretic and vasodilatory activity. High topical concentrations are usually necessary to bring about its pharmacologic effects when applied to the unbroken skin.

DMSO has a major anti-inflammatory action, second only to its activity as a skin penetrator. When inflammatory cells accumulate at the site of inflammation, various free radicals are released, which can be detrimental to the animal's own tissues. DMSO acts as a free radical scavenger, reduces tissue damage, and acts as an anti-inflammatory agent. Topical treatment with DMSO rapidly dissipates the inflammation and edema, and animals experience less discomfort and pain. Blood flow to the affected area is increased by DMSO through the enhanced formation of prostaglandin E, whereas the synthesis of other prostaglan-

TABLE 18–5
DRUGS FOR INTRA-ARTICULAR USE

Drug	Proprietary Name	Manufacturer	Concentration	Dosage
PSGAG*	Adequan	Luitpold-Pharmaceuticals	250 mg/ml	1 ml every 5 weeks
Hyaluronic acid	Hylartin V	Pharmacia	10 mg/ml	2 ml as required
Methylprednisolone acetate	Depo-Medrol	Upjohn	20 mg/ml 40 mg/ml	120–200 mg as required

*Now available for parenteral use also.

dins responsible for inflammation, PGG_2, PGH_2, PGE_2, and $PGF_{2\alpha}$ is inhibited. DMSO also stabilizes all organelle membranes and enhances similar stabilizing effects of glucocorticoids, blocks conduction of pain, increases blood flow, blocks polymerization of hyaluronic acid, inhibits fibroblast proliferation, and may modulate local immune responses.

When used topically, the toxicity of DMSO appears to be minimal. Although not more than 100 ml/day is recommended for topical use, larger amounts can be used intravenously in life-threatening situations. It has been suggested that DMSO can play a role in therapy of DJD because of its local analgesic properties rather than any specific anti-inflammatory effect.

ORGOTEIN

This is a nonsteroidal anti-inflammatory metalloprotein compound of bovine liver origin. It possesses superoxide dismutase activity. Superoxide radicals can cause degradation of hyaluronic acid, and the effect of orgotein is to stabilize neutrophilic lysosomes, thereby reducing the release of superoxide radicals. Orgotein also has a chemotactic effect on neutrophils, and usually the response to the drug is better in acute rather than chronic arthrosis. Orgotein accelerates the rate of conversion of superoxide radicals (chemically responsible for the edema, pain, and destruction of tissue cells) to water and oxygen. This breaks the cycle of chronic inflammation. Its anti-inflammatory action may be attributable to its ability to scavenge free radicals, stabilize cell membranes, and inhibit enzymes active in the inflammatory cascade. It is recommended in equine medicine for soft tissue inflammation associated with the musculoskeletal system. The dose for the horse is 5 mg by deep intramuscular injection on alternate days for 2 weeks, followed by twice-weekly injections for 2 to 3 more weeks. When given by the intra-articular route, a temporary marked increase in synovitis and severity of lameness sometimes appears. By inactivating the superoxide radical, it reduces the tendency toward depolymerization of the hyaluronic acid in synovial fluid and so maintains its viscosity

and lubricating properties. Its anti-inflammatory activity is somewhat limited compared with other anti-inflammatory agents, and it has little or no analgesic or antipyretic activity. Because of its large molecular size, superoxide dismutase does not easily penetrate normal membranes, so it probably does not readily penetrate target tissues in high concentrations after subcutaneous or intramuscular injection. The drug has been administered intra-articularly with equivocal results. In fact, in some studies, injecting it into joints actually increases inflammation and lameness. Clinical indications for orgotein have been limited to soft tissue inflammation in horses and spondylitic syndromes or vertebral disc disease in dogs. Side effects of the drug are uncommon.

Although osteoarthritic horses and humans have been believed to benefit from the use of this drug; the effects (if any) of orgotein on cartilage are unknown.

18.5 SEPTIC ARTHRITIS/OSTEOMYELITIS SYNDROME

Septic conditions in foals are frequently followed by the development of the septic arthritis/osteomyelitis syndrome. Although the primary site of sepsis may be elsewhere in the body, localization of bacterial infection in the synovial membrane or periarticular bone may occur in more than one joint. The condition is most common in, but not exclusive to, foals less than 2 months of age. Joint-ill, navel ill, or septic polyarthritis are alternative descriptions for this disease in bacteremic foals. Invading bacteria may reach the joint from the blood, from an external source, from a traumatic wound infection, or from an adjoining soft tissue cellulitis. Host factors that determine the likely severity of the condition include the anatomic properties of the tissue, bone, or joint; humoral or cellular immunity; and the repair capability of the damaged or traumatized tissue.

Sudden lameness and periarticular edema typical of this condition can flare up in young horses suddenly, and although there may be many predisposing causes, inadequate intake of colostral immunoglobulins is a major contributing factor. Joints such as the hock, stifle, carpus, or fetlock are most commonly involved.

Septic arthritis can develop from an infection through the blood stream, with or without corticosteroid injections. An infectious inflammatory reaction is established in the synovial fluids and synovial membrane. Release of leukocytes, proteolytic enzymes, hyaluronidase, and cartilaginous debris heightens the inflammatory response, leading to a further process of cartilage degeneration. Severe infectious or inflammatory erosion of the articular cartilage may ultimately elicit the development of the DJD syndrome. During the process of septic arthritis, fibrin clots form a large part of the inflammatory exudate. Fibrin can adhere to the articular cartilage, disrupting nutrition and the flow of nutrients from the cartilage. Collagenases and leukocytes can destroy cartilage and its ground substance. Therapy must be oriented toward removal of lysosomal enzymes, purulent exudate, and fibrin clots and treatment of the infection and inflammatory process.

Osteomyelitis is an inflammation of bone specifically involving the bone marrow, the cortex, or the periosteum. The age of the animal may influence the extent of periosteal and cortical involvement. Bacteria are not the only factors in the development of bone infection; disruption of bone supply or disruption of bone marrow is necessary before osteomyelitis can occur. Once bacteria are introduced into the bone and conditions are favorable for their growth, rapid destruction of bone can take place, especially in young animals. If a bacterial embolus is present, venous thrombosis may develop, with blockade of the nutrient capillaries resulting in transudation, local marrow necrosis, and development of an environment ideal for bacterial growth. Localization of circulatory bacteria may occur in the subchondral bone marrow in mature animals possessing closed growth plates.

Any damage to the periosteum, bone, and bone marrow enhances the bacterial infection. Necrotic tissue and clotted blood provide the ideal medium for bacterial growth. Ischemia is also an important aspect of osteomyelitis, and microorganisms thrive in avascular bone.

Among the bacteria commonly isolated from foals with septic arthritis/

osteomyelitis are *Escherichia coli, Salmonellae, Corynebacterium equi, Actinobacillus, Streptococcus, Staphylococcus aureus, Klebsiella, Pseudomonas,* and *Bacteroides.* Thus both aerobic and anaerobic bacteria may be involved. In general, infection caused by gram-negative rods carries a poor prognosis as compared with infection caused by gram-positive organisms.

Therapy of these conditions warrants the early and intensive use of systemic antimicrobial drugs, fluid and electrolyte supplementation, and the judicious use of anti-inflammatory drugs. Appropriate antibiotic therapy requires isolation of the causative pathogens from either the bone lesion or the blood. Therapy with antimicrobial agents must be intense and vigorous to take account of both the local and the systemic infectious involvement, the lack of satisfactory immunologic status of the foal, and the necessity to prevent rapid deterioration of the condition. Synovial aspiration, drainage with removal of debris, and distention or irrigation of the joint are important ancillary approaches that are often necessary to complement the systemic antimicrobial therapy. Saline or lactated Ringer's solution can be used for local joint irrigation. If abscessation or bone sequestration is evident, the abscess should be surgically decompressed and excised together with removal of dead bone and severely infected tissue. To obtain a joint aspirate, it may often be necessary to sedate the horse with xylazine and butorphanol. For extreme, nonresponsive cases of joint effusion, total anesthesia may be required to facilitate a thorough flushing of the joint with an electrolyte fluid containing gentamicin. Fluid aspirated from joints displaying septic arthritis usually has elevated protein levels and white cell counts containing many macrophages, neutrophils, synoviocytes, and lymphocytes.

Antimicrobial therapy must be based on culture and sensitivity testing whenever possible and must be regarded as adjuncts to other forms of therapy. With the exception perhaps of acute osteomyelitis, antibiotics alone are not the sole effective method of treatment. Many small-molecule antibiotics can cross synovial membranes, and so it is not automatically necessary to inject intra-articularly. Local injection of antibiotics is often contraindicated on account of giving rise to postinjection synovitis, which often accompanies such treatment. Antibiotics that attain useful therapeutic concentrations in joint fluid after parenteral (preferably intravenous) administration include penicillins, some semisynthetic beta-lactamase-resistant penicillins, cephalosporins, erythromycins, and aminoglycosides. In many refractory conditions, gentamicin, amikacin, carbenicillin, rifampin, and ticarcillin are especially useful. If the local pH is low and excess purulent material is present, the activity of aminoglycosides can be adversely affected, especially when gram-negative bacteria are involved.

Potassium penicillin and gentamicin sulfate, sodium ampicillin and gentamicin sulfate, or sodium ampicillin with potentiated sulfonamides are useful combinations with which to begin therapy while awaiting clinical or bacteriologic results. Care must always be exercised when using gentamicin because this nephrotoxic aminocyclitol antibiotic could cause severe kidney damage in a foal already suffering from decreased renal functioning and dehydration.

Regardless of the initial individual choice of antibiotic, vigorous therapy must be continued parenterally for 2 to 6 weeks to provide useful clinical results.

Depending on the extent of clinical response, bacteriologic culture results, and sensitivity testing, alternative antimicrobial drugs may have to be considered during the course of therapy. Quite often if response to gentamicin is clinically ineffective, a change to amikacin sulfate can be beneficial. Alternatively in the event of penicillin failure, the use of ticarcillin can give favorable results in many nonresponsive cases. Use of anti-inflammatory agents is frequently necessary to alleviate the swelling, pain, and inflammatory response associated with septic arthritis. Many of the liberated products of joint inflammation, such as lysosomal enzymes, prostaglandins, superoxide radicals, hyaluronidase, and proteases, can perpetuate the process of cartilage destruction, with the consequent exposure of underlying bone. A continual degradative process can thus be established.

Owing to their analgesic, antipyretic, anti-inflammatory, and antiprostaglandin properties, NSAIDs, such as flunixin meglumine, ketoprofen, and phenylbutazone, can be useful adjuncts for mitigation of the painful inflammatory response to the infection. They are specifically indicated when lameness is progressive. Because the NSAIDs have the capacity to contribute to the development of the gastric ulcer syndrome in foals, however, intravenous cimetidine, a histamine H_2 blocker, and ranitidine (these are gastric antisecretory agents) together with oral sucralfate, which coats ulcer sites and promotes healing, may be used to prevent the occurrence.

Once the infectious and inflammatory process has been brought under control, due cognizance must be taken of the damage and degeneration that has already occurred in the infected joint. Intra-articular administration with hyaluronic acid or PSGAGs can be beneficial by inhibiting many of the enzymes of inflammation responsible for cartilage degradation in addition to increasing the viscosity of synovial fluid and its lubricant properties. Such intra-articular medication protects articular cartilage, restores joint function to normal, and augments chondrocyte metabolism (Table 18–6).

18.6 NAVICULAR DISEASE

The cause and pathogenesis of navicular disease (distal sesamoiditis, podotrochlitis, podotrochlosis) still remain a much debated topic. Chronic podotrochlitis mainly affects working horses between 6 and 12 years of age, and it constitutes almost one third of all forelimb lameness diagnosed by the equine clinician. The condition affects the distal sesamoid (navicular bone) and its surrounding structures. It is a particularly painful condition characterized by periods of intermittent forelimb lameness. Only rarely is it diagnosed in the hind limbs.

There is still considerable controversy regarding the cause of navicular disease. Nonetheless, there are two popular theories: One is that the condition is mechanical, and the other is that it is vascular in origin. It appears that the condition may result from, or be caused by, a passive venous congestion in the foot and the navicular bone. In long-standing cases, the foot be-

TABLE 18–6
ANTIBIOTIC DOSAGES FOR SEPTIC ARTHRITIS IN FOALS

Drug	Trade Name	Manufacturer	Dosage
Aminoglycosides			
Amikacin	Amiglyde v	Bristol/Fort Dodge	6.6–11.0 mg/kg IV QID
Gentamicin	Gentocin	Schering	2.2 mg/kg IV TID
			50 mg locally
Kanamycin sulfate			5.0–8.0 mg/kg TID IM
Penicillins—Beta Lactam Antibiotics			
Potassium penicillin G			20,000–50,000 IU/kg IV QID
Sodium ampicillin	Amp-equine	SmithKline Beecham	10–50 mg/kg IV QID
Amoxicillin Trihydrate	Clamoxyl	SmithKline Beecham	10 mg/kg BID, IM
Ticarcillin disodium	Ticillin	SmithKline Beecham	110 mg/kg IV QID
Miscellaneous Antimicrobials			
Erythromycin	Erypar	Parke Davis	22–30 mg/kg PO
Trimethoprim-sulfadiazine	Tribrissen	Coopers/Pitman Moore	15–30 mg/kg IV BID
Rifampin	Rifadin	Merrill-Dow	10 mg/kg PO BID
Ancillary Therapy			
Flunixin meglumine	Banamine	Schering	1.1 mg/kg IM
Phenylbutazone	Butazolidin	Coopers/Pitman M	100 mg IV
Ketoprofen	Ketofen	Fort Dodge	2.2 mg/kg IV
Sodium hyaluronic acid	Hyalartin	Pharmacia	2 ml as required
PSGAG	Adequan	Luitpold	1 ml as required
Cimetidine	Tagamet	SmithKline Beecham	300 mg IV QID/480 mg PO
Sucralfate	Carafate	Marion	2 g PO QID
Aspirin			25.0–35.0 mg/kg TID

IV, Intravenous; IM, intramuscular; PO, oral; QID, four times a day; TID, three times a day; BID, two times a day.

comes abnormal in conformation with an upright narrow stance and a small frog.

Predisposing factors include defective shoeing, poor condition, poor hoof care, heredity and conformation, improper feeding, and excessive work on hard nonresilient surfaces. An immediate predisposing cause of the characteristic lameness is a diminished blood supply to the navicular bone, resulting in a chronic degenerative process. The condition is frequently observed in horses possessing a small foot relative to body size and especially if foot conformation is typified by a long toe and short heel.

The deep flexor tendon controls in part the overall articulation of the coffin joint, and during the process of normal locomotion, the deep flexor tendon glides smoothly over the posterior surface of the navicular bone. One of the longest held theories of the cause of this particular condition suggested that constant vibration and concussion led to damage to the tendon and cartilage, with this damage being restricted to the posterior surface of the navicular bone together with the tendon immediately overlying it. It is now established, however, that the interior of the navicular bone is profoundly affected in this condition.

Erosions of the cartilage, exposure of subchondral bone, and adhesions can develop between the navicular bone itself and the deep flexor tendon. The surrounding connective tissue may become highly vascularized consequent on the defects in the cortical bone structures.

The more widely held theory currently suggests that the major pathogenic changes are associated with ischemia of the navicular bone. Favorable results obtained with drugs that affect blood supply would tend to support this hypothesis. Ischemia within the navicular bone is caused by progressive arteriosclerosis and thrombosis within the major arteries supplying the bone. Sclerotic osteitis and bone necrosis are common sequelae of this reduction in cardiovascular nutritive supply. Angiography studies have indicated the occurrence of such vascular changes in the bone with thrombotic occlusion in the distal arteries. Such arterial occlusion can lead to the development of painful necrotic areas, reduced nutrition of bone, increased wear of the flexor tendon, and its consequent damage. Progressive lameness develops from this progressive ischemic state of the bony structures.

Mild local ischemia is associated with temporary lameness only, whereas ischemia involving the major primary arteries and arterioles through more widespread thrombosis formation can lead to severe vascular occlusion and bone necrosis and retards the revascularization process. Progressive lameness may develop from this severe ischemic state, although a secondary periosteal blood supply can develop to compensate for the diminished vascular nutrition of the ischemic navicular bone.

With the development of this local disease process, the hoof changes in shape, and the horse may adopt a characteristic pointing stance. In general, the prognosis of the condition is poor to variable owing to the chronic degenerative processes occurring.

Because navicular disease is attributable to ischemia caused by arterial thrombosis within the bone, tendon lesions are usually secondary to areas of ischemic necrosis immediately underlying the flexor cartilage. Frequently collapse of the fibrocartilage itself and lesion formation on the flexor surface of the bone follows (Table 18–8).

18.7 DRUG THERAPY

Because navicular disease is aggravated by arteriosclerosis and thrombotic developments, drug therapy is usually addressed toward rectifying the compromised circulation of the foot. This entails the encouragement of a periosteal blood supply and minimization of the vascular occlusion with the bony vascular supply.

Anticoagulants have been advocated to reduce the concentration of the clotting factors and thereby the clotting mechanism. Additionally, anticoagulants can be used to encourage the development of a secondary blood supply from the periosteum to counteract the vascular occlusion within the bone. Thrombosis of both the primary supply arteries and the secondary periosteal vessels contributes to the ischemic state and clinical manifestation of lameness.

WARFARIN

Warfarin (a dicumarol derivative) is the primary anticoagulant of choice owing to its oral availability, relative cheapness, and the fact that a specific antidote, vitamin K_1, is readily available. Warfarin not only acts to improve circulation through the foot but also possesses beneficial effects on erythrocyte flexibility and deformability as well as improving blood viscosity. The use of warfarin in the navicular case must be carefully monitored because of its widespread systemic effects on the blood clotting process. One of the problems inherent in warfarin therapy is the variation in dosages between individual horses because of individual susceptibilities, severity of the condition, and alterations in feeding and management. Treatment necessitates continual laboratory monitoring because the ultimate, clinically effective dose is near to the dose that causes severe general hemorrhage, sometimes with fatal results.

Monitoring of the one-stage prothrombin time (OSPT) must be performed at least twice over a 10-day period before starting treatment. This helps to establish the baseline OSPT. The objective of warfarin therapy is to increase the OSPT by 20% of the pretreatment level.

A normal starting dosage of warfarin is 1 mg/50 kg body weight daily, accompanied by monitoring of the OSPT twice weekly during the course of treatment. If no apparent clinical improvement is evident within the first 6 weeks of warfarin treatment, the starting dose may be increased by approx-

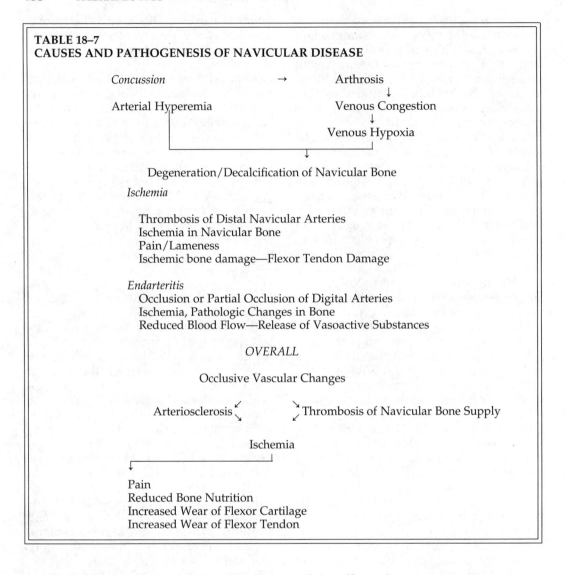

TABLE 18–7
CAUSES AND PATHOGENESIS OF NAVICULAR DISEASE

Concussion → Arthrosis
↓
Arterial Hyperemia Venous Congestion
↓
Venous Hypoxia

Degeneration/Decalcification of Navicular Bone

Ischemia

Thrombosis of Distal Navicular Arteries
Ischemia in Navicular Bone
Pain/Lameness
Ischemic bone damage—Flexor Tendon Damage

Endarteritis
Occlusion or Partial Occlusion of Digital Arteries
Ischemia, Pathologic Changes in Bone
Reduced Blood Flow—Release of Vasoactive Substances

OVERALL

Occlusive Vascular Changes

Arteriosclerosis Thrombosis of Navicular Bone Supply

Ischemia

Pain
Reduced Bone Nutrition
Increased Wear of Flexor Cartilage
Increased Wear of Flexor Tendon

imately 20%. Prolongation of the OSPT by 50% can be aimed for at this stage. Again twice-weekly monitoring of the OSPT is necessary. The ultimate daily dose of warfarin may vary between 1.0 and 8.5 mg/50 kg. When stabilization of the successive OSPTs has been established, monthly monitoring is adequate.

Duration of therapy with warfarin can be quite long term and extend for at least 6 to 9 months. After this therapy period, the drug may be gradually withdrawn, assuming that hoof care, corrective shoeing, regular exercise, and other ancillary measures are being attended to. Many horses remain sound after such a course of warfarin therapy.

Side effects that may accompany warfarin therapy include signs of hemorrhaging, painful joints, pale mucous membranes, hematomas, and general lassitude. Of particular significance is the fact that warfarin is extensively bound to plasma protein (>95%). Interaction with many other drugs and concurrent displacement from plasma albumin are hazards accompanying its usage. Highly bound drugs that compete for plasma albumin binding sites (e.g., phenylbutazone) may displace a significant amount of free active warfarin into the blood stream, thus causing a marked increase in OSPT. Because warfarin is so extensively bound to plasma protein, any displacement from this blood reservoir may

TABLE 18–8
SOME WARFARIN INTERACTIONS*

Drugs That May Cause Interaction	Drugs That Do Not Cause Interaction
Phenylbutazone	Acepromazine
Aspirin	Fenbendazole
Corticosteroids	Thiabendazole
Griseofulvin	Pyrantel pamoate
Barbiturates	Dipyrone
Antihistamines	Procaine pencillin with
Protein-bound antimicrobials	dihydrostreptomycin
Oxytetracycline	Orgotein
Sulfonamides	Bromhexine
	Clenbuterol
	Methindizate/dipyrone

*All drugs affecting liver function, highly protein, bound drugs, and analgesic anti-inflammatory drugs should be avoided.

increase the amount of free warfarin disproportionately. Accordingly, marked hemorrhaging is likely to occur in such instances, especially in the intestinal wall, abdominal cavity, ovary prepuce, joints, or retropharyngeal region. Any hemorrhage must be regarded as suspiciously significant. Hypovolemia, shock, gross anemia, and death can occur in severe cases. Highly protein bound drugs, analgesics, anti-inflammatories, and drugs affecting the liver (and thus the production of clotting factors) must not be used concurrently with warfarin. Some drugs are compatible with warfarin treatment (Table 18–8).

In the event of warfarin toxicity, either through overdosage or drug interaction, vitamin K_1 must be given immediately. Clinical response to this antidote is usually evident within 30 to 45 minutes. In severe life-threatening situations, whole blood transfusions, fluids, and plasma volume expanders may be necessary.

Reversal of warfarin-induced anticoagulation is required when clinical bleeding occurs or when the OSPT is too long. The subcutaneous route is more rapid and reliable than the intramuscular route for vitamin K_1. When given intramuscularly, vitamin K_1 may give rise to hematoma formation, and therapeutic response time can be erratic. A dosage of 300 to 500 mg every 4 to 6 hours is required for stabilization of the OSPT (or approximately 1 mg/kg).

With warfarin, improvement in lameness is seldom seen in less than 6 to 8 weeks. The drug is claimed to be effective in up to 60 to 70% of cases, and after cessation of treatment (which may run for up to 12 to 18 months), approximately 50% of cases remain sound. Warfarin must not be used in pregnant mares.

ISOXSUPRINE

Isoxsuprine hydrochloride was originally investigated because of its vasodilative properties. The original theory behind its use was that it would reduce ischemia in the navicular bone. It is now known that the navicular bone does not actually become ischemic in the navicular syndrome. Despite this, isoxsuprine hydrochloride has proved useful in treating navicular syndrome, although its mechanism of action is unknown.

This is a beta$_2$-adrenergic agonist, which, acting as a peripheral vasodilating agent, is used to treat ischemic disorders in humans. Assuming that arteriosclerosis and thrombosis are significant factors in the pathogenesis of navicular disease, it is logical that a vasodilatory agent may be of assistance in therapy. Isoxsuprine causes vasodilation by direct action on vascular smooth muscle. There have been no reports of abnormalities in the hematologic or serum biochemical values of horses undergoing treatment. Minor decreases in systemic blood pressure and vascular resistance, however, together with transient increases in heart rate and cardiac output may accompany its usage. Isoxsuprine can be considered superior to warfarin treatment in many ways because of fewer potential side effects and the lack of necessity to monitor patients during the course of treatment.

Acting as a beta$_2$ agonist, isoxsuprine increases blood flow to the foot. It also lowers the viscosity of the plasma and increases the elasticity of erythrocytes. Thus both plasma and erythrocytes can penetrate the dilated or constricted capillaries such that the original circulation is restored.

Therapy is performed over block periods of 3 weeks' duration. At each 3-week period, the dosage is adjusted in accordance with the observed clinical response. A loading dose is given at the outset, followed by one or more periods of either the loading dose again or a maintenance dose. Therapy is phased out over a period of weeks with a reducing dosage. Throughout each 3-week treatment course, the horse should be exercised to perform that amount of work which before therapy would have evinced lameness. In this way, adjustments of dosage may be deemed necessary. As with other forms of therapy, corrective shoeing and hoof care to restore the correct foot axis is a necessary ancillary supportive measure.

Treatment begins with the initial loading dose. This is usually followed by one or more 3-week periods during which the loading dose or an increased dose is administered. Therapy ends with a 3-week period of a withdrawal dosage.

Isoxsuprine is available for oral use in paste or capsular form. The capsules may be given in feed or in hay. Each capsule contains 40 mg isoxsuprine hydrochloride in a resin base. Slow release from this base ensures high, constant levels of this potent vasodilator in the blood. Paste formulations contain 40 mg isoxsuprine hydrochloride per milliliter in a palatable flavored base that is administered through an oral dosing syringe onto the back of the tongue.

The normal requirement for therapy is to begin dosage at 0.6 mg/kg twice a day. This dosage is given for a minimum of 21 days. If no improvement is noted after the first 3

weeks, the dosage can be increased by up to 100%. This dosage should be maintained until the horse can perform work for at least 14 days. If the horse becomes sound within the first 3 weeks, a further 3-week course should be given before beginning withdrawal therapy. Once clinical improvement and absence of lameness are maintained for at least 2 weeks, the scaled-down reducing dosage can be commenced. The withdrawal phase dosage is 0.3 to 0.4 mg/kg over a 3- to 6-week period. Dosage must always be adjusted in accordance with the clinical symptoms.

The dose of isoxsuprine hydrochloride may be safely doubled for the duration of treatment (1.2 mg/kg twice a day for 3 weeks, then 1.2 mg/kg s.i.d. for 2 weeks, and then 1.2 mg/kg once every other day for 1 week). Although this higher dose has not proved to be significantly more effective than the 0.6 mg/kg dose, responses of some severely affected horses may be better with the higher dose. No matter which dosage is used, the drug should be administered 30 minutes before feeding.

The normal course of therapy can vary from 6 to 14 weeks. Sudden discontinuation of therapy may result in a relapse to lameness within 10 to 20 days. Analgesic agents are best avoided during isoxsuprine therapy because they may mask accurate clinical evaluation of the symptoms presented.

Isoxsuprine is contraindicated during the last 3 months of pregnancy and also in mares within 1 month of foaling. A high percentage of treated horses become sound for prolonged periods after cessation of treatment (Table 18–9).

ORGOTEIN

This water-soluble metalloprotein has been used to alleviate the inflammatory components of navicular disease. Its anti-inflammatory action (inhibition of lysosomal enzyme release; enhanced phagocytosis of debris) may also assist in decreasing the extent of adhesion formation between the navicular bone and deep flexor tendon. Orgotein can be used systemically or preferably via juxtabursal injection as an adjunct to NSAID therapy and corrective shoeing. Juxtabursal injection is a relatively simple pro-

TABLE 18–9
GUIDE TO DRUG THERAPY FOR NAVICULAR DISEASE

ANTI-INFLAMMATORY DRUGS

Methylprednisolone	100 mg into navicular bursa or coffin joint
Phenylbutazone	1 gm BID orally

(Palliative only—longterm results not satisfactory)

Flunixin meglumine	1.1 mg/kg IV/IM
Ketoprofen	2.2 mg/kg IV/IM
Orgotein	5 mg local injection (better prognosis)

DRUGS AFFECTING CIRCULATION

Warfarin (anticoagulant, reduces plasma viscosity)

Starting dose,	1 mg/50 kg orally (monitor OSPT)
Eventual daily dose,	0.6–8.5 mg/50 kg (OSPT + 20%)

Isoxsuprine (peripheral vasodilator: beta$_2$ adrenergic agonist)

Initial dose,	0.6–0.9 mg/kg BID orally for 3 weeks
Maintenance dose,	0.6–0.9 mg/kg BID orally for 3 weeks
Reducing dosage,	0.3–0.4 mg/kg BID orally for 3 weeks;
	0.3–0.4 mg/kg BID orally on alternate days for 3 weeks

cedure, but it is extremely important that only a 1-inch, 20- to 22-gauge needle be used to avoid entering the bursa, scraping the articular surface, or traumatizing the digital cushion. A 5-mg injection of orgotein given in the area immediately palmar to the pastern is repeated at 1 and 2 weeks. Approximately 30 to 40% of horses given orgotein may remain sound for up to 14 months. This medication is no longer available in some countries, including the U.S.

OTHER ANTI-INFLAMMATORY DRUGS

Injections of corticosteroids into the navicular bursa or coffin joint have been popular treatment methods in the past. A dose of 100 mg of methylprednisolone temporarily alleviates the pain and inflammatory symptoms in a palliative fashion. Corticosteroids are not curative agents. NSAIDs, such as phenylbutazone, possess analgesic effects in addition to their anti-inflammatory activity. The usual dosage of phenylbutazone for navicular disease is 1 g/day orally twice a day. In conjunction with corrective shoeing and regular exercise, it may partially assist circulation in the foot and temporarily suppress local pain and inflammation. During therapy, it may extend the period of apparent soundness. Because navicular disease is not solely an inflammatory condition, anti-inflammatory drugs alone are devoid of longterm benefit, and frequently relapses occur. When using NSAIDs, if clinical improvement is not observed within 3 to 4 weeks, alternative drug therapy must be considered. Continual use of phenylbutazone can in fact hasten progression of the navicular syndrome and may have toxic effects, such as gastrointestinal ulceration and renal damage.

Prognosis of any therapy for navicular disease is influenced by conformation, such as small feet, contracted heels, and atrophied frogs. Accordingly, corrective shoeing must be oriented toward supporting the heels and increasing the overall weight-bearing surface with a view to establishing a straight hoof/pastern axis and normal foot conformation.

Treatment with isoxsuprine has been reported as successful, but many authors report a maximal success of 50%. This falls to about 20% of cases being sound in 12

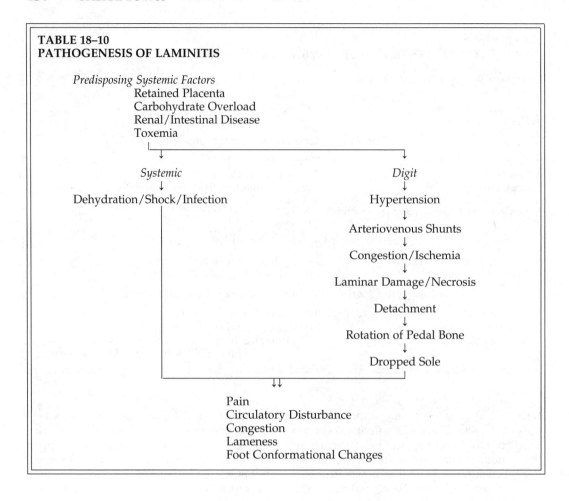

TABLE 18–10
PATHOGENESIS OF LAMINITIS

Predisposing Systemic Factors
    Retained Placenta
    Carbohydrate Overload
    Renal/Intestinal Disease
    Toxemia

Systemic → Dehydration/Shock/Infection

Digit → Hypertension
↓
Arteriovenous Shunts
↓
Congestion/Ischemia
↓
Laminar Damage/Necrosis
↓
Detachment
↓
Rotation of Pedal Bone
↓
Dropped Sole

⇓⇓

Pain
Circulatory Disturbance
Congestion
Lameness
Foot Conformational Changes

months after ceasing treatment. Treatment with warfarin is still quite popular, but the complications of monitoring and administering treatment with this drug have resulted in alternative treatments being used to a wide extent.

18.8 LAMINITIS

After colic, laminitis is the second most prevalent cause of death in horses. Most horses that recover are left with some degree of locomotor impairment that typically forces them into retirement. Laminitis in horses is frequently associated with concurrent systemic disease. Predisposing factors include overfeeding, rapid dietary changes, excessive intake of carbohydrates (grain overload), grazing of lush pastures, concus-sion accompanying exercise in unfit horses, renal disease, intestinal disease, colic, retained fetal membranes, exertional myopathy, toxemia, and liver disease (Table 18–10). When attempting to treat laminitis, the underlying cause must always be identified if further damage to the laminae is to be avoided.

Carbohydrate overload is the most common cause of laminitis, either through animals gaining access to a grain store or having overexposure to herbage. Cattle pasture that has received topping with nitrogen fertilizers seems particularly dangerous. In cases in which carbohydrate overload has been associated with the development of laminitis, degeneration of the intestinal epithelium has been demonstrated, with resultant transmural absorption of endotoxins. It is well established that most horses with laminitis have higher levels of detectable plasma endotoxin than nonlaminitic horses.

Carbohydrate overload appears to alter normal bacterial flora, resulting in increased cecal endotoxins and lactic acid concentrations. Absorption of lactic acid and endotoxins may cause the cecal lesions occurring in laminitis. In acute laminitis, digital laminar ischemia may progress to necrosis and coffin bone rotation.

In the event of grain overload, proliferation of lactobacilli can destroy large numbers of gram-negative bacteria, leading to liberation and absorption of endotoxins and increased production of lactic acid. Absorption of lactic acid and endotoxins may cause direct damage to the cecal epithelium in laminitis patients. Increased decarboxylation of histidine to histamine may elevate histamine levels. Hence antihistamines are sometimes used. Grain overload is usually associated with increased absorption of lactic acid, endotoxin, and histamine.

Laminitis is most frequently seen in small, overweight ponies, with usually the forelimbs being involved. The hindlimbs alone (rarely) or together with the forelimbs may also display characteristic symptoms. Affected animals in severe cases have pounding digital pulse; the distal limb and coronary band may become edematous. Before the onset of lameness, especially in cases of grain overload, diarrhea and coldness of the extremities may be evident. Insofar as laminitis is frequently associated with a systemic disease, many horses are systemically hypertensive. The increased blood flow to the foot gives rise to the bounding digital pulse.

Within the foot, many profound circulatory alterations occur. Central vasodilatation and peripheral vasoconstriction reduce the blood flow to the laminae. Arteriovenous shunts are established whereby blood is diverted to the venous return side. Ischemia and congestion of the capillary beds lead to laminar damage and necrosis. The hypertensive congestion is painful because the blood is being diverted away from the peripheral arteries. Separation of the hoof from the underlying tissues and rotation of the pedal bone by the traction of the deep flexor tendons may follow. To accommodate this new position, the sole alters shape, and sometimes penetration of the sole itself occurs.

In severe cases of laminitis, ischemia of the laminae leads to necrosis, swelling, detachment, abscessation, and perhaps drainage at the coronary band. Necrosis of the laminae arising from the decreased circulatory perfusion causes disruption of the attachment between the pedal bone and the hoof. Separation from the hoof wall and pulling of the deep flexor tendon rotates the pedal bone, which sinks within the foot, causing flattening of the sole.

18.9 DRUG THERAPY

Drug therapy of acute laminitis is aimed at alleviating pain and preventing sinking or rotation of the pedal bone. Damage to the laminae; circulatory changes, both local and systemic; hypertension; and foot conformational changes cause great pain, resulting in lameness. Obesity is one of the most common causes of laminitis in horses. Any systemic disease causing a toxic or septic focus, e.g., endometritis, pleurisy, or colic, can cause laminitis. The predisposing cause must always be treated before any improvement in laminitis can be anticipated.

The administration of corticosteroid drugs to susceptible or stressed animals can trigger an outbreak of laminitis. Hence their therapeutic use in laminitis is absolutely contraindicated.

Treatment must be started immediately after the earliest diagnosis of laminitis because of the risk of progressive damage to the internal structures of the foot. Therapy is aimed not only at relieving pain, but also toward normalizing laminar blood flow. Because the condition is reflective of changes in the general systemic state, any septicemia or shock must be vigorously treated.

In the presence of carbohydrate overload, fluids, purgatives, and antihistamines may be used. Antihistamines in many cases are clinically unreliable and of dubious benefit. In cases of carbohydrate overload, the animal should be removed from the pasture and its grain intake stopped until the gastrointestinal tract has recovered.

Symptomatic treatment with liquid paraffin by stomach tube aids excavation of the

---

TABLE 18–11
DRUGS AND LAMINITIS

Retained placenta/carbohydrate overload (possible causes)
    Fluids, purgatives, antihistamines
In addition:
    Analgesics, anti-inflammatories, and antibiotics (corticosteroids are contraindicated because
        of their deleterious effects on hypertension in laminitis)
    Pain in laminitis can be related to hypertension; consider the following therapeutic agents:
    Adrenergic agents:
        Isoxsuprine hydrochloride
        Phenoxybenzamine intravenously
    Analgesics:
        Phenylbutazone
        Ketoprofen
        Meclofenamic acid
    Antiprostaglandins for shock:
        Flunixin meglumine
        Ketoprofen

---

intestinal contents and may help to prevent further uptake of endotoxin (Table 18–11). Initial administration of NSAIDs is indicated for all cases of laminitis to relieve the pain and break the pain hypertension cycle. Low doses of acepromazine can be given three or four times daily for the first 48 hours to relieve anxiety and reduce hypertension.

Mares with retained fetal membranes should be given adequate systemic antibiotic treatment (penicillin/streptomycin or potentiated sulfonamide). Fetal membranes should be removed either manually or by oxytocin drip and the uterus lavaged. Uterine flushes are necessary if retention of the placenta is a predisposing factor. Antibiotics, anti-inflammatories, and analgesics are usually indicated.

Regardless of the therapeutic regimen instituted, however, prognosis is usually guarded. Many horses that recover from the clinical effects of laminitis experience some minor degree of impairment of locomotor function.

To treat systemic problems, 1 gallon of mineral oil acts as a laxative to expel toxins from the alimentary tract and minimize their absorption from the gut. In the event of endotoxic shock and dehydration, fluid therapy and NSAIDs are also beneficial for the local foot problem by virtue of their analgesic, anti-inflammatory, and antiprostaglandin properties.

Phenylbutazone therapy should be begun initially by the intravenous route and continued orally in doses not exceeding 4 g/day. (Ponies are particularly susceptible to gastric and oral ulceration following phenylbutazine therapy.) Flunixin meglumine may be used also at a dosage level of 50 mg/1000 lb, or ketoprofen may be used at 2.2 mg/kg intravenously. Aspirin is an underestimated NSAID. Aspirin can be used at a low dose of 5–20 mg/kg and displays potent antiplatelet activity at this level, thus counteracting the hypocoagulability of endotoxemia.

In the event of no response to the NSAIDs, DMSO can be considered. In gel form, DMSO may be applied topically two to three times per day at a total daily dosage not exceeding 100 g.

Although anti-inflammatory analgesics play a significant role by alleviating pain, a more rational approach is to attempt to control hypertension. Control of hypertension not only dramatically reduces pain, but also minimizes pedal rotation, which is a common complication of cases not diagnosed early enough or treated improperly at the outset.

The immediate treatment must aim to restore blood flow as rapidly as possible. The most effective vasodilator is acepromazine. As an aid to improve digital perfusion and to prevent thrombosis, alpha blockers can be considered. Phenoxybenzamine (beta-blocker) and heparin (anticoagulant) may thus be considered useful. The usefulness of low-dose aspirin has already been mentioned.

Acetylpromazine may be used not only as a tranquilizing agent, but also more importantly because of its peripheral alpha$_1$-adrenoceptor blocking activity. Acepromazine maleate given intramuscularly (10 to 30 mg/1000 lb body weight) every 6 hours reduces blood pressure.

Receptor-selective agents, such as phenoxybenzamine (an alpha$_1$ blocker) and isoxsuprine hydrochloride (a beta$_2$ agonist), reduce systemic and local blood pressure. The former inhibits adrenergic vasoconstriction; the latter directly causes vasodilation. During the first few days, oral isoxsuprine hydrochloride at a dosage of 0.9 mg/kg twice a day may be helpful to relieve peripheral vasoconstriction. Care must be exercised in using any such agent to reduce blood pressure because they may worsen any pre-existing shocklike systemic condition. Heparin given subcutaneously (40,000 U/1000 lb body weight) every 8 hours has also been advocated to prevent thrombus formation, disseminated intravascular coagulation (DIC) and consequent ischemia in the laminar supply blood vessels.

Corticosteroids are contraindicated in laminitis therapy. Their clinical use may in fact induce or worsen laminitis. Corticosteroids potentiate the vasoconstrictor effects of catecholamines and serotonin in the equine digital vessels. Occlusion of venous drainage from the digit by corticosteroids causes congestion and edema formation and can pharmacologically induce laminitis. Administration of corticosteroids to ponies often to treat sweet itch can lead to severe laminitis with pedal bone prolapse in all four feet within 48 hours.

Corticosteroids potentiate the catecholamines by a variety of mechanisms, including inhibition of catecholamine degradation, inhibition of extraneuronal catecholamine uptake, and an overall sensitization effect on the adrenoceptors. Histamine, serotonin, and adrenaline inhibit venous drainage from the vascular bed of the foot, leading to local congestion. Because the vascularity of the hoof is under sympathetic (adrenergic) vasomotor tone, corticosteroids create venous obstruction by enhancing the vasocontrictor potency of many endogenous biogenic amines. Corticosteroids also possess undesirable immunosuppressive and catabolic properties. Because gram-negative endotoxins can be predisposing factors in systemic conditions precipitating laminitis (especially in cases of carbohydrate overload), immunosuppressants are contraindicated. Glucose and insulin therapy may be indicated in obese horses, especially if prior use of corticosteroids may have worsened the condition.

Nerve blocks used in the early stages of the condition before pedal rotation can provide some symptomatic relief by lessening the pain, encouraging exercise, and thus increasing the local arterial blood flow. Nerve blocks can, however, increase the risk of rotation of the third phalanx if given at the inappropriate time, once the lamellar bed has lost its structural integrity.

Ancillary measures include administration of methionine because of its role in hoof keratinization (10 g/day for 7 days followed by 5 g/day for 21 days). Biotin (50 mg/500 kg body weight once daily) and zinc chelate (1 g/500 kg) are also recommended for optimal horn production (Table 18–12).

In long-established cases, cases treated with steroids, cases with a gradual onset, and cases occurring in the fall, the supplementation of the diet with sodium, potassium, and calcium salts is essential. Because an overlong toe may precipitate further separation of the laminae, foot care is necessary. Shortening the toe, lowering the heels, and protection of the sole and frog from pedal bone pressure by use of padded shoes are necessary.

In cases of chronic laminitis, hoof treatment and hoof care are required. In chronic cases, the element of pain may have lessened somewhat, and the degree of pedal bone rotation may have stabilized. The objective in such cases is to restore the normal alignment by lowering the heels, removing excess toe, and protecting the dropped sole. Necrotic areas of the laminae, corium, and

TABLE 18–12
LAMINITIS THERAPY GUIDELINES

Control
  Pain, inflammation
  Hypertension
  Infection
  Systemic involvement

Pain
  Flunixin meglumine,   1.1 mg/kg IM
  Phenylbutazone,   2 gm BID IV, PO
  Ketoprofen,   2.2 mg/kg IV
  Meclofenamic acid,   2.2 mg/kg PO
  Aspirin,   20 mg/kg
  DMSO,   50–100 g topically

Nerve Block
  Posterior digital block

Circulatory Changes/hypertension
  Isoxsuprine hydrochloride,   0.9 mg/kg BID PO
  Phenoxybenzamine,   600 mg in 500 ml saline IV
  Acetylpromaze maleate,   10–30 mg/500 kg every 6 hours IV
  Heparin   40,000 U/500 kg subcutaneously every 6 hours
  Aspirin   5–20 mg/kg IV

Systemic infection
  Procaine penicillin,   15,000–20,000 U/kg BID
  Trimethoprim/sulfadiazine,   15 mg/kg

Local infection
  Metronidazole
  Tincture of iodine

Dehydration/shock
  Fluids
  Plasma volume expanders
  Flunixin meglumine   0.25 mg/kg IV/IM
  Aspirin   5–20 mg/kg IV

Laxatives
  Mineral oil,   1 gallon

Dietary supplements
  Methionine,   10 g/day
  Potassium chloride,   15 mg/day
  Sodium chloride,   15 mg/day
  Biotin,   50 mg/day
  Zinc chelate,   1 g/day

IM, Intramuscular; IV, intravenous; PO, oral; BID, two times a day.

sole should be debrided to healthy tissue; the sole and frog should be protected and padded.

SELECTED REFERENCES

Byass, T.D.: Antidotal effect of vitamin K against warfarin induced anticoagulation in horses. Am. J. Vet. Res., 47:2309, 1986.

Carroll, C.L., Hazard, G., Coloe, P.J., and Hooper, P.T.: Laminitis and possible enterotoxemia associated with carbohydrate overload in mares. Eq. Vet. J., *191*: 344, 1987.

Coffman, J.R., Johnson, J.H., et al.: Orgotein in navicular disease: A double blind study. J. Am. Vet. Med. Assoc., *174*:261, 1979.

Colles, C.M.: A preliminary report on the use of warfarin in the treatment of navicular disease. Eq. Vet. J., *11*:187, 1979.

Colles, C.M.: Ischemic necrosis of the navicular bone and its treatment. Vet. Rec., *104*:133, 1979.

Eyre, D., Elmes, P.J., and Strickland, S.: Corticosteroid potentiated vascular response of the equine digit; possible pharmacologic basis of laminitis. Am. J. Vet. Res., *40*:135, 1979.

Golding, J., and Ghosh, P.: Drugs for osteoarthrosis. The effects of a glycosaminoglycan polysulfate ester on proteoglycan aggregation and loss from articular cartilage of immobilized rabbit knee joints. Curr. Ther. Res., *34*:67, 1983.

Hamm, D., Goldman, L., and Jones, E.W.: Polysulfated glycosaminoglycan: A new intra-articular treatment for equine lameness. Vet. Med. Small Anim. Clin., *79*:811, 1984.

Hood, D.M.: Studies on the pathogenesis of equine laminitis. PhD Thesis. Texas A & M University, 1984.

Jones, W.E.: Towards more rational joint therapy. Vet. Med. Small Anim. Clin., *79*:211, 1987.

Kruegar, A.S.: Ultrastructural study of the equine cecum during onset of laminitis. Am. J. Vet. Res., *47*:1804, 1986.

Martens, R.J.: Pathogenesis, diagnosis and therapy of septic arthritis in foals. J. Vet. Orthop., *2*:49, 1980.

Martens, R.J., Auer, J.A., and Carter, K.: Equine pediatrics: Septic arthritis and osteomyelitis. J. Am. Vet. Med. Assoc., *188*:582, 1986.

Matthews, N.S.: Cardiovascular and pharmacokinetics effects of isoxsuprine in the horse. Am. J. Vet. Res., *47*:2130, 1986.

McIlwraith, C.W.: Treatment of infectious arthritis. Vet. Clin. North Am. [Large Anim. Pract.], *5*:363, 1983.

McIlwraith, W.C.: Current concepts in equine degenerative joint disease. J. Am. Vet. Med. Assoc., *180*:239, 1982.

Nelson, J.D.: Antibiotic concentrations in septic joint effusions. N. Eng. J. Med., *284*:349, 1971.

Nizolek, D.J.H., and White, K.K.: Corticosteroid and hyaluronic acid treatments in equine degenerative joint disease. Cornell Vet., *71*:355, 1981.

Orsini, J.A.: Strategies for treatment of bone and joint infections in large animals. J. Am. Vet. Med. Assoc., *185*:1190, 1984.

Owen, R.: Intra-articular corticosteroid therapy in the horse. J. Am. Vet. Med. Assoc., *177*:710, 1980.

Rose, R.J.: The intra-articular use of sodium hyaluronate for the treatment of osteoarthrosis in the horse. N.Z. Vet. J., *27*:5, 1979.

Rose, R., Tennifer, R., and Hodgson, D.: Studies on isoxsuprine for the treatment of navicular disease. Eq. Vet. J., *15*:238, 1983.

Sprouse, R.F.: Plasma endotoxin levels in horses subjected to carbohydrate induced laminitis. Eq. Vet. J., *19*:25, 1987.

Stashak, T.S.: Navicular disease. *In* Adams' Lameness in Horses. Edited by T.S. Stashak. Philadelphia, Lea & Febiger, 1987.

Stick, J.A., Jann, H.W., Scott, E.A., and Robinson, N.E.: Pedal Boner rotation as a prognostic sign in laminitis of horses. J. Am. Vet. Med. Assoc., *180*:251, 1982.

Sweeney, C.R., and Markel, M.D.: Ticarcillin therapy in a foal with septic arthritis. Mod. Vet. Pract., *65*:841, 1984.

Turner, A.S., and Tucker, C.M.: The evaluation of isoxsuprine hydrochloride for the treatment of navicular disease: A double blind study. Eq. Vet. J., *21*:338, 1989.

Turner, T.A.: Management of navicular disease in horses—an update. Mod. Vet. Pract. *67*:24, 1986.

White, S.L.: Neonatal septicaemia. *In* Proceedings 3rd Annual Forum, and 13th Annual Science Program. XXX ADVIM, 1985.

Yelle, M.: Clinicians guide to equine laminitis. Eq. Vet. J., *18*:156, 1986.

REPRODUCTIVE THERAPY IN THE HORSE: BACTERIAL ENDOMETRITIS

19.1 Predisposing Causes and Infectious Agents
19.2 Principles of Therapy
19.3 Systemic Treatment
19.4 Local Therapy: Uterine Irrigation
19.5 Antimicrobial Drugs
19.6 Nonantibiotic Alternatives
19.7 Assisting Uterine Defense Mechanisms
19.8 Contagious Equine Metritis
19.9 Induction of Parturition
19.10 Induction of Abortion
19.11 Retained Placenta

19.1 PREDISPOSING CAUSES AND INFECTIOUS AGENTS

One of the main causes of infertility in mares is recurrent, persistent bacterial endometritis. Breeding, foaling, and routine examination procedures are all responsible for organisms gaining access to the mare's reproductive tract. Other complications, such as retained placenta, pneumovagina, and perineal laceration, greatly increase the risk of infection. In many mares, elimination of bacteria can be effected by the normal functioning of the local uterine defense mechanisms. Failure of these uterine defense mechanisms is a major factor in the establishment of bacterial endometritis. It has been established that endometritis in mares can cause premature luteolysis, with consequent elevations of prostaglandins E and F. Such an elevation of intrauterine prostaglandin levels can inhibit many of the humoral immune responses (e.g., antibody production and beta cell activation). This reduces further the resistance of the mare to uterine infection following a bacterial challenge.

The ability of the endometrium to resist and eliminate infections is highest during estrus. Phagocytosis and the rate of clearance of bacteria from the uterus are augmented by the influence of estrogens and diminished by progestogens. In mild infections, mares can recover from infection without undergoing antimicrobial treatment simply by going through one or two estrus cycles, which evacuate the infection and heighten local resistance. The indentification of a positive culture from a genital tract swab does not in itself indicate that an infectious reproductive problem exists.

Some mares have difficulty in resolving endometritis that is caused by bacterial contamination at mating. These mares can be highly susceptible to endometritis. In susceptible mares, impaired drainage of the uterus may partially contribute to the cause by leading to regular fluid accumulations. The breeding efficiency of mares can be adversely affected by bacterial invasion, but of prime significance is the change in the uterine defense mechanism, which can allow microorganisms of the normal flora of the genital tract to become invasive.

Management schemes oriented toward improvement in fertility in which susceptible mares are bred are based on reducing the bacterial contamination that accompanies breeding, killing the causative organisms with appropriate antimicrobial drugs, or assisting the natural local defense mechanisms of the body. Bacterial endometritis occurs frequently in mares, the most common isolates being beta-hemolytic streptococci and *Escherichia coli*. Natural host defense mechanisms are important in combating infection, but in the event of an ineffective response, antibiotic therapy can be useful.

A positive swab received from the genital tract may reveal the presence of a contaminant, a primary pathogen or a secondary invader. The widespread, frequently inappropriate use of antimicrobial drugs has not markedly reduced the incidence of metritis or infertility in mares but rather has caused a shift in the types and patterns of pathogens isolated, especially gram-negative organisms, such as *E. coli*, *Klebsiella*, and *Pseudomonas*. Complication with resistant strains or fungal overgrowth has also resulted from indiscriminate antibiotic usage.

Streptococcus, zooepidemicus, E. coli, and Staphylococcus aureus, are common opportunist-type pathogens isolated from cases of endometritis. When the infection is mixed, other environmental organisms, such as *Corynebacterium, Anthracoides, Streptococcus faecalis, Enterobacter*, and anaerobes such as *Clostridium* and *Bacteroides fragilis*, can enter the uterus. *Proteus, Pseudomonas aeruginosa*, and microaerophilic coccobacilli *Haemophilus equigenitalis* can be isolated from many refractory cases, the last mentioned being especially implicated in the venereally transmitted contagious equine metritis syndrome.

In routine cases of endometritis, beta-hemolytic streptococci tend to be the most commonly isolated bacteria, although in recent years there has been an increase in the proportion of gram-negative organisms isolated. These include *E. coli, Klebsiella, Enterobacter*, and *Pseudomonas*. *Klebsiella pneumoniae* (capsular types 1, 2, 5), *P. aeruginosa*, and *H. equigenitalis* are capable of acting as primary pathogens, whereas other organisms, such as *S. zooepidemicus, E. coli, Proteus*, and *Staphylococcus* species may act as secondary invaders once the devitalization process or defective local defense mechanisms are in existence.

Beta-hemolytic streptococci, *E. coli*, and staphylococci are opportunistic pathogens, and their isolation from the genital tract does not always indicate the presense of endometritis. Isolation of primary pathogens, *K. pneumoniae*, *H. equigenitalis*, and *Pseudomonas*, which are specific venereal pathogens, initiates the prompt instigation of appropriate control measures.

In previously untreated mares, the most commonly isolated pathogen is *S. zooepidemicus*. When mares have received previous, repeated treatment with antimicrobial drugs, *E. coli*, *K. pneumoniae*, and *P. aeruginosa* are commonly isolated.

During coitus or around the time of parturition, mares are at risk from infection by many of these organisms. The hormonal status of the animal at the time of infection can influence antibacterial efficacy, the capacity for leukocytic drainage, phagocytosis, and the extent of mechanical cervical drainage. Such endocrine status may modulate the neutrophilic chemotactic response and opsonization potential.

In recent years, the role of anaerobic bacteria in the mare's uterus has received more attention. For instance, *Fusobacterium necrophorum* and *Corynebacterium* pyogenes have a synergistic effect in terms of increasing the severity of postpartum infections in the cow. In the mare, anaerobic bacteria are believed to play a role in mares with endometritis that is accompanied by negative aerobic bacterial cultures.

Aerobic culture alone may not be sufficient to isolate all of the organisms that may be potential pathogens in cases of cervicoendometritis. Anaerobic culture is frequently recommended as an aid to diagnosis of endometritis in mares. It may prove to be particularly valuable when the results of aerobic cultures are not conclusive. Microaerophilic culture has become a routine procedure since the first recorded outbreak of contagious equine metritis, in which *Taylorella equigenitalis* was isolated as the causative organism. *Bacteroides*, *Fusobacteria*, and anaerobic cocci are regularly involved in the cause of many infectious infertility states in the mare. Isolation of anaerobic bacteria from the cervicoendometrium of

the mare will undoubtedly assume greater importance in the future. The widespread usage of a variety of antimicrobial agents in stud farm practice may suppress growth of aerobic bacteria and facilitate the growth of anaerobic bacteria, which may then become involved in the development of endometritis. Penicillins and metronidazole are drugs of choice for such anaerobic infections.

Bacillus cereus is a large gram-positive, spore-forming rod. It is a beta-lactamase producer and so is resistant to penicillins and cephalosporins. The organism is capable of causing outbreaks of human foodborne gastroenteritis as well as abortion in cattle and sheep. Recent attention has focused on the possible implication and involvement of this organism in cases of endometritis and abortion in mares also. Facultative anaerobes and strict obligate anaerobes have been isolated from mares with active postpartum metritis.

Diagnosis of endometritis rests on the history of reproductive failure, rectal palpation, vaginoscopy, ultrasonography, uterine culture, uterine biopsy, and uterine cytology. Bacterial cultures alone must be interpreted judiciously.

19.2 PRINCIPLES OF THERAPY

General therapy of endometritis in mares must be started after rectal and vaginal examination, bacteriologic culturing, and antibiotic sensitivity testing and possible histologic examination of uterine biopsy specimens. Successful treatment for bacterial endometritis must encompass the use of specific antimicrobial drugs, removal of predisposing causes as far as is possible, promotion of uterine drainage when there is a uterine discharge, and employment of techniques that assist compromised local uterine defense mechanisms. Overt clinical signs, a positive culture, and a history of infertility are clear indications for initiation of treatment.

Although intrauterine therapy is widely practiced, systemic treatment or preferably a combination of the two is the most efficacious clinical approach. The choice of antibiotic for acute bacterial endometritis must be made based on in vitro sensitivity testing. Specifically indicated antimicrobial drugs can be used systemically, locally, or by a combination of both routes. Although systemic therapy alone may not be sufficiently effective, it must be remembered that many locally used antibiotics can be irritant in themselves or may be associated with irritant vehicles. The regimen of treatment varies, in accordance with the severity of the infection, from single doses, daily administration extending over short or long periods, or administration before or after coitus. Local therapy may take the form of infusions or pessaries.

Despite various types of therapy over the years, no real impact has been made on the incidence of the disease. Proper, specific therapy is always indicated because improper treatment can lead to worsening of the condition. Many commonly used antiseptics and aminoglycoside antibiotics are highly irritating and can lead to damage of the endometrium. Indiscriminate use of antibacterials can lead to overgrowth of resistant organisms, pseudomonal infection, or suprainfection with yeasts or fungi. This illustrates the necessity for correct, specific use of appropriate antimicrobials in accordance with the culturing and sensitivity testing.

19.3 SYSTEMIC TREATMENT

Systemic administration usually results in uterine tissue and lumenal concentrations of antibiotic approximately equal to that of the plasma. Repeated treatments can be carried out without the risk of damage to the endometrium or the introduction of new infection locally. Also, because the drug is delivered parenterally, the presence of a purulent exudate or fetal membranes cannot adversely affect distribution. Many infectious processes are not always located or limited to the superficial layers of the endometrium, and hence systemic delivery ensures diffusion of the drug to the deeper layers of the uterus.

With regard to antibiotic therapy, generally following systemic administration, antibiotic concentrations are usually higher throughout the entire genital tract than after intrauterine therapy. Systemic therapy avoids having to invade the local tract and avoids the risk of introducing infection. Bet-

ter local distribution can be attained by using the intravenous route. Problems associated with this route, however, relate to dose size, cost, and the patient's ability to endure multiple injections.

Systemic administration results usually in concentrations of drugs in the genital tract similar to those of the plasma. Systemic therapy involves antibiotics, hormonal substances, prostaglandins, and antiinflammatory drugs (Table 19–1). Systemic hormonal preparations can stimulate cyclicity, promote ovulation, suppress estrus, prevent pregnancy, or synchronize estrus. Prostaglandins can shorten the diestrus interval, initiate myometrial contraction, and thus promote drainage of uterine fluids. To reduce the inflammatory response, anti-inflammatory drugs, such as corticosteroids, nonsteroidal anti-inflammatory drugs (NSAIDs) (phenylbutazone, flunixin), or dimethyl sulfoxide (DMSO) can be given.

19.4 LOCAL THERAPY: UTERINE IRRIGATION

Although many antimicrobial drugs are absorbed from the uterus after local infusion (e.g., sulfonamides, tetracyclines, penicillin, ampicillin, streptomycin, gentamicin), the presence of pathologic changes in endometritis can diminish the degree of local absorption. If absorption is hindered, high concentrations may be achieved in the uterine cavity itself and on the endometrium but not in the subendometrial tissues. The overall efficacy of intrauterine infusions is influenced by diverse factors, such as the prevailing local pH, oxygen, tension, and bacterial flora. The molecular size and structure of the antibiotic partially governs the degree of absorption; for instance, sodium benzylpenicillin is well absorbed from the mare's uterus, whereas some of the semisynthetic penicillins, such as ticarcillin, are not. Infusions are most commonly given during estrus, when the increased vascularity associated with estrogen assists local drug absorption.

An important factor regarding the success or failure of a local infusion is the type of antibiotic vehicle in the formulation. Many vehicles have a detrimental effect on the uterine tissue and retard the rates of ab-

TABLE 19–1
THERAPEUTIC APPROACH FOR BACTERIAL ENDOMETRITIS

Antimicrobial Drugs
Penicillins
    Penicillin G
    Ampicillin
    Ticarcillin
    Carbenicillin
Aminoglycosides
    Gentamicin
    Amikacin
Broad spectrum
    Tetracyclines
    Potentiated sulfonamides

Promotion of Uterine Drainage/Evacuation

Estrogens
Prostaglandins
Oxytocin
Washes/antiseptics/disinfectants (iodine, chlorhexidine, saline)

Augmentation of Uterine Defense Mechanisms

Homologous plasma, colostrum, hyperimmune serum
Induce estrus
Induce mild inflammation

sorption. Water-soluble vehicles are preferable. This is exemplified by gentamicin, with which the rate of disappearance from the uterine lumen is more rapid when given as a water infusion rather than in saline. In general, absorption from the uterine cavity is governed by the stage of the cycle and the volume and type of infusion. Prolonged, repeated, and unnecessary infusions with antibiotics can ultimately lead to infections with resistant organisms, *Pseudomonas*, or fungi, which in many cases can be difficult to treat.

The intrauterine route is useful because antibiotic concentrations in the uterine lumen and surface layers of the endometrium are usually higher and remain longer after intrauterine therapy than after systemic therapy. Daily infusion for 3 to 5 days during estrus is a commonly practiced routine or daily for 2 to 4 days after ovulation. Usually it is best to lavage the uterus on alternate days during estrus and to administer the antibiotic daily.

Intrauterine infusion must be made with sterile equipment and proper aseptic preparation of the mare. Total infusion volumes should not be excessive, and care should be taken to avoid excessive pressure.

When antimicrobial drugs are given locally, the endometrial concentration is higher than that of the blood. This is obviously desirable when the infection is restricted to the surface layer of the endometrium. Not all infections, however, are limited to the superficial lining of the uterus, and thus for deeper infections, systemic antibiotic therapy is warranted. A number of locally infused antibiotics can be degraded in the uterine lumen, preventing bactericidal levels of the drug reaching the site of infection.

Local therapy can also cause irritation and inflammation. Accordingly, local infusion of some drugs after breeding may be considered undesirable. The local infusion volume required varies—up to 200 ml has been advocated to distribute the antimicrobial agent adequately throughout the mare's uterus. Much larger volumes (up to 500 ml), however, are sometimes used to saturate the lumen and fill the uterus to overflowing. Local release of prostaglandin $F_{2\alpha}$ in response to local irritation by treatment with various chemicals does occur, and this can be beneficial as an aid to partial uterine evacuation.

Choice of delivery systems for local treatment include infusion pipettes, indwelling catheters, or volume infusion and recovery sets. Uterine irrigation solutions may contain a variety of substances: antimicrobial drugs, disinfectants, antifungal agents, anti-inflammatory drugs, mild irritants, or uterine resistance enhancers, such as plasma or colostrum.

Many physiologic infusions mildly stimulate the endometrium, resulting in the migration of inflammatory cells into the uterine lumen (e.g., tetracyclines, buffered gentamicin, dilute povidone-iodine solutions). Stronger irritants, (e.g., greater than 10% povidone-iodine, can give rise to a pronounced mucopurulent exudate, which may take some time to subside.

Infusions are commonly given during estrus to take advantage of estrogenic effects:

1. Increased blood flow
2. Increased excitability of the myometrium
3. Increased permeability of uterine blood vessels to leukocytes
4. Increased secretion of immunoglobulins to assist phagocytosis
5. Increased growth of the myometrium

Such infusions can be used to shorten diestrus and to treat endometritis at the time before the cycle in which the mare will be bred, thereby enhancing conception shortly after breeding. Intrauterine infusions possess more than just a simple antibacterial effect (e.g., with povidone-iodine or oxytetracycline). Interestrus periods are usually shortened in response to infusions given, especially between day 6 and day 10 of diestrus. Infusions can trigger a mild local inflammatory response, which may be overall relatively beneficial, but other adverse reactions can be provoked also, resulting in mycotic or pseudomonal overgrowth.

Lugol's iodine provokes a local inflammatory reaction with round cell infiltration and some degree of mucosal epithelial sloughing similar to that caused by povidone-iodine. Prior iodine treatment of the uterus, however, does result in a greater degree of absorption of poorly diffusible aminoglycosides, such as neomycin. Normally aminoglycoside concentrations are higher on the endometrial surface than in the plasma after local instillation. Anaerobic conditions and the presence of pus restrict the local efficacy of most aminoglycosides because their specific transportation mechanism into bacteria is oxygen dependent.

For local uterine infusion, antimicrobial drugs are not always necessary. Disinfectant/antiseptic solutions, such as chlorhexidine/iodine, may be preferred in many cases.

When infusing with 3 to 4 liters of saline, repeat flushings are necessary until the saline outflow from the uterus becomes visibly clear. Use of Lugol's iodine or 2% povidone-iodine is beneficial not only because of chemical activity, but also because of the mild inflammation, distention, and physical evacuation of the uterus that follows. If appreciable amounts of necrotic tissue or debris are present, a 2% solution of hydrogen peroxide can be instilled.

Occasionally the local infusion of DMSO can be used to reduce severe uterine inflammation and to increase the absorption of other locally applied drug substances. DMSO reduces inflammation by acting as a free radical scavenger. When inflammatory cells accumulate at the sites of inflammation, they release various free radicals that are toxic to the bacteria in inflamed areas as well as to the horse's own tissues. By scavenging these free radicals, DMSO reduces tissue damage and produces its anti-inflammatory response.

Other actions of DMSO that may contribute to its anti-inflammatory effect are its actions to stabilize lysosomal membranes because lysosomes contain some of the enzymes of the inflammatory response. DMSO penetrates rapidly, aids the transport of other drugs, decreases swelling, and promotes healing. Technically DMSO is called an apotic solvent, and some substances that are not soluble in either water or lipid solvents dissolve in DMSO.

DMSO has many good pharmacologic effects of its own. Among these are good anti-

TABLE 19–2
LOCAL UTERINE IRRIGATION

10% Lugol's iodine	5 ml in 250 ml saline
Strong Lugol's iodine	4 ml in 100 ml saline
Hydrogen peroxide 2%	As required
Chlorhexidine solution	As required
1% Povidone-iodine	500 ml
Sterile saline	1–4 liters
Homologous plasma	100 ml
DMSO	50–100 ml of 5% stock solution

inflammatory effects, local anesthetic effects, antibacterial effects, and diuretic and vasodilatory effects (Table 19–2).

19.5 ANTIMICROBIAL DRUGS

Mixed infections, aerobes, and anaerobes may all be involved in bacterial endometritis, and so a broad-spectrum approach is commonly taken. When particular pathogens are isolated, individual antimicrobial agents may be used based on in vitro sensitivity tests. Beta-hemolytic streptococci are still the most commonly isolated organisms, but there has been a noticeable increase in the number of gram-negative pathogens, including *E. coli*, *Klebsiella*, *Enterobacter*, *Pseudomonas*, and *Proteus*. Many of these pathogens are sensitive only to gentamicin, ticarcillin, amikacin, or other costly drugs.

When gram-positive cocci are isolated and pending results of culture and sensitivity testing, parenteral and local penicillin for 10 to 15 days or local 1% povidone-iodine, 500 ml, administered during estrus or with estrogen is a useful starting point. Gram-positive organisms are usually affected by penicillins (especially beta-hemolytic streptococci) or ampicillin. Sulfonamides are useful alternatives for treatment of gram-positive organisms, whereas many gram-negative organisms respond to gentamicin and amikacin. Neomycin can be considered for *Klebsiella* infection. The presence of *H. equigenitalis* in the reproductive tract is always of high significance. Ampicillin is one of the most effective antibiotics for *Haemophilus* infection. Overgrowth of *H. equigenitalis* by saprophytic organisms frequently presents problems in the recognition of infection.

Anaerobic bacteria can be present in significant numbers in many situations, including wounds, chronic skin lesions, and vaginal discharges.

Most anaerobes are sensitive to benzylpenicillin and most of the other beta lactam antibiotics. Other drugs include tetracyclines, potentiated sulfonamides, and the most potent drug of all, metronidazole. *B. fragilis*, which is commonly found in anaerobic infections, is a beta-lactamase producer, and so beta lactam antibiotics are useless against it.

Penicillin is well absorbed from the uterus of the mare. The duration of therapeutic blood levels is relatively short by this route, so treatment has to be repeated every 5 to 6 hours. Mechanical or chemical irritation of the uterus before infusion may increase the extent of absorption of the drug. When gram-positive cocci are found and pending results of the in vitro sensitivity evaluation, penicillin is a reasonable first choice. Local infusion of penicillin, however, may not be effective in cases of mixed infections because the drug may be neutralized by the enzyme beta-lactamase released by microorganisms other than the primary pathogen. Although ampicillin possesses a broader antimicrobial spectrum, it too is cleaved by beta-lactamase enzymes. The antimicrobial activity of gentamicin and amikacin is reduced under acidic and anaerobic conditions and also in the presence of organic debris.

Intramuscular injection of procaine penicillin (17,000 IU/kg) results in tissue concentrations in the endometrium approximately 50 to 70% that of the serum levels. Intravenous administration achieves high local levels also, although duration of action is shorter (<8 hours). Intravenous sodium ampicillin (7 mg/kg) provides tissue concentrations equal to or greater than serum for the first 4 hours. Both of these beta lactam antibiotics given parenterally are useful for attaining high bactericidal levels in the uterine tissues. Recommended doses are 20,000 to 50,000 IU/kg penicillin intramuscularly or 11 to 22 mg/kg sodium ampicillin intravenously. Such therapy is primarily indicated for beta-hemolytic streptococcal infection of the uterus.

The intrauterine infusion of 22000 IU/kg of sodium penicillin following prior infusion of 10% Lugol's iodine increases the absorption of penicillin from the uterus and is a reasonable first-choice drug when beta-hemolytic streptococci are involved. For broader spectrum activity, 2 g of intrauterine sodium ampicillin is useful. Useful first-choice local treatments include water-soluble mixtures of neomycin (1.0 g) or polymyxin B (40,000 IU). Five megaunits of crystalline sodium penicillin may be added to this combination and the infusate instilled into the uterus through a sterile catheter or pipette daily for 2 to 6 days depending on the severity of the infection and the clinical response.

One of the attendant hazards of prolonged uterine irrigation is the risk of mycotic infection locally. If mycotic infection of the mare's uterus is evident, 2.4 megaunits of nystatin or 100 mg of amphotericin B in 250 ml of normal saline can be considered.

Ticarcillin is a potent penicillin that is bactericidal against beta-hemolytic streptococci, *S. zooepidemicus, Pseudomonas, E. coli, Enterobacter, Haemophilus influenza,* and salmonellae but not *Klebsiella.* It is indicated primarily for beta-hemolytic streptococcal infection or especially for complications with *Pseudomonas.* Ticarcillin potentiated with calvulanic acid is available for anti-staphyloccocal activity.

Intramuscular injection of ticarcillin in mares yields therapeutic concentrations in the reproductive tract within 2 hours of injection. By local infusion, ticarcillin is non-irritant and produces high levels in the uterus and cervix. Systemic blood levels after local infusion with ticarcillin are quite low, indicating a high degree of localization and nonabsorption from the uterine tissue. For local infusion, 3 to 6 g of ticarcillin is infused in 250 ml of saline or sterile diluent.

When endometritis is complicated by pseudomonal infection, gentamicin may be considered. This may be used concurrently with ticarcillin to provide synergistic broad-spectrum cover. Carbenicillin has a similar spectrum of action as ampicillin but with the addition of certain strains of *P. aeruginosa, Proteus,* and *Enterobacter.* Carbenicillin may also be used simultaneously with gentamicin for antipseudomonal efficacy, but they must not be mixed in the same syringe.

Amikacin (2 g locally) is the aminoglycoside of choice when apparent resistance to gentamicin is present. Both gentamicin and amikacin are applied locally for endometritis caused by gram-positive organisms (especially staphylococci) and *Pseudomonas.*

For severe pseudomonal infection, a synergistic antimicrobial effect can be attained by combining an aminoglycoside, such as gentamicin or amikacin, with a beta lactam antibiotic, such as ticarcillin or carbenicillin. Polymyxins are cheaper alternatives for antipseudomonal activity, but they do not affect *Proteus* species.

Intrauterine gentamicin sulfate, 2.0 to 2.5 g/250 ml of normal saline, provides useful uterine antibacterial efficacy against many strains of *E. coli, Klebsiella,* and pseudomonal species involved in equine endometritis. When endometritis is associated with *Pseudomonas* infection, the use of three separate injections of prostaglandins (in addition to specific antipseudomonal antimicrobials) causes repeat ovulation (three times within 25 days) often with resolution of the infection.

Occasionally when bacteria cannot be isolated from cases of endometritis, dilute povidone-iodine solutions can be infused into the uterus and antibiotics given systemically. Only dilute solutions of povidone-iodine (1 to 2%) should be used. Intrauterine infusion of various disinfectants is a relatively common nonantibiotic alternative for treatment of uterine infections (Table 19–3).

TABLE 19–3
SOME ANTIMICROBIAL DRUGS FOR EQUINE ENDOMETRITIS

Drug	Parenteral dosage (mg/kg)	Intrauterine dosage
Amikacin	6.6	2.0 g
Amphotericin B		100.0 mg
Ampicillin	22.0	1.0–3.0 g
Carbenicillin	23.0–48.0	2.0–5.0 g
Gentamicin	2.2	2.0–2.5 g
Neomycin	10.0	1.0
Nystatin		2.4 megaunits
Penicillin	20,000–50,000	5.0–10.0 megaunits
Polymyxin B		40,000 IU
Spectinomycin		2–3 g
Sulfonamides		
Trimethoprim	15.0–30.0	6.0–12.0 g
Ticarcillin	44.0	3.0–6.0

19.6 NONANTIBIOTIC ALTERNATIVES

Although systemic and local antibiotics have prevailed as popular therapeutic approaches for uterine conditions, nonantibiotic alternatives must never be overlooked as useful ancillary agents. The importance of the resumption of normal cyclicity for spontaneous recovery from uterine infections is well established. Estrogens, oxytocin, and prostaglandins have an important supportive role to play in this respect. Estradiol benzoate, valerate, or cypionate (3 to 10 mg) are useful owing to their uterotonic effects. In the event of uterine atony, in which exudate has accumulated in the uterine lumen, small doses of oxytoxin (10 to 20 IU) can be of benefit if given within 4 to 6 hours of estrogen injection.

The administration of small amounts of estrogen during the postpartum period helps to protect the tract from infection and enhance uterine involution. In some cases of postpartum uterine atony, estrogen and oxytocin can be as effective as antimicrobial agents in the elimination of uterine exudate.

Endocrine status, especially ovarian hormonal activity, influences antibacterial mechanisms, polymorphonuclear cell response, phagocytosis, uterine motility, and cervical drainage. Ovarian hormones influence the resistance of the uterus to infection. High resistance is associated with the estrogen-dominated phase, whereas the progesterone-dominated phase tends to increase the susceptibility to infection.

Natural host defense mechanisms are of paramount importance in controlling local infection and should never be underestimated. Advantage must also be taken of the estrogen-related protective effects on the female genital tract. Hence treatment is preferable during estrus.

The use of prostaglandins may be beneficial to bring mares into estrus more frequently than is normal, thereby taking advantage of the favorable effects of estrogens. By artificially increasing the number of estrus periods within a short period, benefits may accrue from the protective effects of estrogens. Prostaglandins may be administered to bring about estrus within 2 to 4 days of injection by virtue of the luteolytic effect.

Alternatively, the estrus cycle can be shortened by intrauterine infusion of iodine. Mildly irritating solutions of iodine can induce estrus within 4 to 7 days, the normal strengths being either 5 ml Lugol's iodine in 250 ml saline or 4 ml strong Lugol's in 100 ml saline. These are given 3 to 4 days after the previous estrus. Such solutions infused during the early phase of the estrus cycle can precipitate release of prostaglandin F_α in similar manner to naturally occurring estrus (Table 19–4).

TABLE 19–4
NONANTIBIOTIC PARENTERAL THERAPY

Estradiol benzoate, valerate, cypionate	3–10 mg IM
Fluprostenol	250 µg IM
Oxytocin	10–20 IU IM

IM, Intramuscular.

19.7 ASSISTING UTERINE DEFENSE MECHANISMS

The local defense mechanisms of the mare's uterus play a key role in the determination of the severity of infection. Normal mares can efficiently eliminate the bacteria, and inflammation is a transient phenomenon: Such mares are usually resistant to bacterial endometritis. The normal equine uterus rapidly eliminates bacterial contamination that occurs during parturition or coitus. Uterine defense mechanisms commonly fail in mares with bacterial endometritis. Inadequate opsonization (the coating of bacteria with serum factors to enhance phagocytosis by neutrophils) may be involved. Although intense management, including repetitive antibiotic treatment, can enhance the fertility of some of these mares, it is unsuccessful in others.

The cellular response of the uterine defense mechanism in the mare is primarily neutrophilic phagocytosis of the invading organisms. This involves the migration of large numbers of cells to the site of infection and adherence of the bacterial cells to the membrane of the neutrophil (opsonization). Successful phagocytosis response on increased uterine muscular activity causes evacuation of the contents through the cervix.

In many cases of endometritis in which the uterine defense mechanisms have failed, this is reflected by depressed phagocytic activity of the polymorphonuclear cells. The primary defect appears to be at the level of bacterial opsonization and consequent failure of clearance of infectious material from the mare's uterus. Complement enhances (opsonizes) phagocytosis of bacteria. Opsonins coat bacteria, increasing their susceptibility to the inflammatory cells (neutrophils).

Susceptible mares may have an inefficient phagocytic response owing to incomplete opsonization. Infusion of homologous plasma as a source of complement has resulted in improved phagocytosis, and administration of intrauterine blood plasma has provided encouraging results. Such an infusion of plasma provides additional complement activity to compensate for the complement-deficient local immunity in the uterus of infected mares. This approach facilitates therapy and assists in the prevention of reinfection by promoting the natural defense mechanisms.

Mares with signs of active endometritis can be treated with intrauterine infusions of their own plasma (100 ml) for 5 consecutive days beginning on day 1 of estrus. The uterus is flushed with 3 liters of saline solution before the first infusion of plasma and on alternative days 3 and 5. Plasma may be collected from the mare at any time and used fresh or stored and frozen for later use.

Because estrogens enhance phagocytosis, it is preferable to treat the mare during estrus. Usually the uterus of the early estrual mare is irrigated with a large volume of sterile saline solution to remove excessive exudate, stimulate migration of neutrophils and opsonins to the lumen, and reduce bacterial numbers. Repeat flushings are made with sterile saline. Depending on the severity of the infection, two to four irrigations are performed and the saline aspirated to remove debris. The uterus is infused immediately afterward with 100 ml of the mare's own plasma. This plasma infusion can be repeated for 4 to 5 consecutive days. Saline solution flushing can be further repeated on alternative days if indicated by the presence of significant volumes of exudate. Hyperimmune serum, colostrum, or plasma with addition of antimicrobial drugs infused into the mare's uterus during estrus or diestrus has also been reported with beneficial results.

Activation of complement is necessary for phagocytosis of bacteria opsonized by serum factors. Heparin or citrate should be used as the anticoagulant for plasma. Ethylenediaminetetra-acetic acid (EDTA) should not be used because it blocks complement activation.

19.8 CONTAGIOUS EQUINE METRITIS

This venereally transmitted disease is a highly contagious disease of horses that is bacterial in origin and associated with poor fertility and breeding performance. The causative organism is a microaerophilic gram-negative coccobacillus designated *Haemophilus* (*Taylorella*) *equigentitalis*. The presence of this organism or of *Klebsiella pneumoniae* (type 5) is always of significance regardless of their numbers.

In infected stallions, *H. equigenitalis* in the smegma is transmitted at coitus. Mares develop endometritis 3 to 7 days after service, and this is characterized by a profuse sticky mucopurulent vulval discharge, with intense polymorphonuclear cell infiltration of the luminal epithelium sometimes accompanied by desquamation, vascular congestion, and hemorrhage. Stallions show no visible signs of infection. The pleomorphic coccobacillus *H. equigenitalis* is usually sensitive to a wide range of antimicrobials given topically, locally, or parenterally: benzylpenicillin, ampicillin, tetracyclines, erythromycin, neomycin, chloramphenicol, potentiated sulfonamides, and chlorhexidine. It is not always eliminated by a single course of treatment. Most strains are resistant to streptomycin. When *K. pneumoniae* and *P. aeruginosa* organisms are present, these can be quite difficult to treat with routine antibiotics. Polymyxin B and neomycin may be used as a first attempt, but gentamicin amikacin, ticarcillin, and carbenicillin are preferable.

Local infusions of the aforementioned antibiotics have been recommended. Infusion of the mare should be complemented by 5- to 7-day therapy with penicillin or ampicillin. Clitoral sinuses should be cleansed with 4% chlorhexidine and dressed with an antimicrobial ointment for several days.

For uterine infusion, water-soluble mixtures of neomycin sulfate, polymyxin B sulfate, and sodium benzylpenicillin are useful as broad-spectrum cover initially. For pseudomonal infection, gentamicin (2.5 g), ticarcillin (6 g), or amikacin should be used. Supportive systemic therapy in refractory cases is essential. (As already alluded to, a synergistic response is obtained when an antipseudomonal aminoglycoside, such as gentamicin or amikacin, is combined with an extended-spectrum penicillin, such as ticarcillin or carbenicillin).

Treatment of infected stallions includes the parenteral administration of gentamicin sulfate, 4.4 mg/kg twice a day intramuscularly or intravenously. This may be necessary for a 10- to 20-day course of therapy. Local treatment involves thorough cleansing of the penis with water and chlorhexidine and application of antimicrobial ointment for at least 6 to 7 days. The addition of polymyxin B sulfate (100 units/ml of extended semen) is also beneficial in the reduction of transmission of infection.

19.9 INDUCTION OF PARTURITION

The usual gestation length of the mare varies from 305 to 365 days, with a mean of approximately 340 days. The elective induction of foaling at a predetermined time ensures the presence of professional assistance and can minimize the occurrence of unsupervised delivery and its many associated problems. A number of mares foal at night, and so induced daytime foaling lends itself to convenience of management, economic considerations, and the presence of skilled labor and veterinary assistance at the crucial time of delivery. Apart from desirable economic and managemental considerations, induction of foaling may be desirable for other reasons; skilled supervision minimizes the risks associated with parturition to both the mare and the foal. If gestation is likely to be unduly prolonged (>365 days), parturition can be difficult with the delivery of a large foal and problems of dystocia. Complications for the mare and its offspring may arise in such cases. In arriving at a decision to induce foaling, medical and disease criteria must also be taken into account: preparturient colic, skeletal/arthritic problems, ventral rupture, uterine atony, loss of colostrum, or injuries to the mare. A history of premature placental separation can result in the delivery of weak, hypoxic, or dead foals. This risk is exacerbated when parturition is prolonged and difficult.

Whenever pharmacologic induction of parturition is initiated, it must be ensured that there is an adequate gestation length for the fetus to attain the maturity necessary for its adaptation to the extrauterine environment. Generally speaking, foals delivered before day 320 have little chance of survival. At this time, problems as a result of fetal immaturity are quite common. It is desirable that induction should not be attempted until at least 320 days. Before foaling is induced, adequate cervical dilatation must be present, and presentation and posture must be correct. Most experience of parturition induction in mares has been at full-term with single injections of oxytocin alone or in combination with estrogen. Other pharmacologic aids include corticosteroids, especially high dosages of dexamethasone; natural prostaglandin F_α; or fluprostenol, a synthetic prostaglandin analog in combination with flumethasone and estrogen.

Despite the obvious advantages of elective induction of foaling to schedule delivery at the most advantageous predetermined time, there are some hazards associated with the technique. Many commonly used inducing drugs are not quite as reliable, predictable, or safe in the mare as in other domestic species.

It is essential that induction be attempted only after an adequate gestation length to ensure viability of the offspring (day 320 to 330). Before this time, problems due to foal immaturity are quite common. The most successful results are obtained in mares showing impending signs of parturition.

CORTICOSTEROIDS

In mares, the widespread routine use of corticosteroids as induction agents is not as popular a technique as in other domestic species. This is because of the necessity of frequent daily injections, the variable waiting period until parturition is induced, and the inherent individual variability of response. The possibility of the birth of weak or hypoxic foals is another factor that has restricted the routine use of the technique.

Dexamethasone is a reliable inducing agent in many domestic species when administered in late gestation. In mares, however, the response to dexamethasone can be disappointing and unreliable. Doses used in mares must be appreciably higher than the dose used in other domestic species, and

when given to pregnant mares after 320 days of gestation, the response can be quite variable. Dexamethasone in quick-release formulation given at a dosage of 100 mg every day for 4 consecutive days beginning on day 321 of gestation results in parturition after 6 to 7 days. Usually foal survival and growth rate are satisfactory. Live, healthy foals can be expected by this technique, provided that treatment is not begun before day 320. Occasionally foals may be weak at birth but grow normally and improve considerably after 8 to 10 days. Milk letdown occurs at parturition, and retention of the fetal membranes does not usually occur. In pony mares, delivery takes place within a shorter period after the last injection—usually approximately 4 days. Dystocia has been noted in pony mares given 100 mg of dexamethasone. This is frequently associated with malpresentation.

Progesterone has been used in a similar fashion to corticosteroids as an inducing agent in mares, with the interval between injection at delivery being similar to dexamethasone. It is believed that progesterone acts through a process of biotransformation to corticosteroids in the adrenal gland or placenta.

PROSTAGLANDINS

Although prostaglandins produce both luteolytic and myometrial stimulant effects in mares, the precise parturition-inducing mechanism of their action has yet to be elucidated. At the moment of parturition, the concentration of endogenous prostaglandin F_α rises, and it is now well established that prostaglandin F_α is the uterine luteolysin that terminates the life of the corpus luteum in many species and that exogenous prostaglandin F_α can induce luteolysis in the mare. Side effects of exogenous natural prostaglandins in the mare include sweating, signs of abdominal discomfort, dyspnea, and transient drop in rectal temperature. Prostaglandins possess a tendency to worsen any pre-existing disorder of the alimentary tract or respiratory system owing to smooth muscle stimulant effects. Also on account of their potency, a relatively high incidence of dystocia due to malpresentation of the foal can arise. Although natural prostaglandins (F_α) have been used in mares, the general tendency is to use the synthetic analogs, such as fluprostenol, which are more potent and relatively freer of unwanted side effects.

The mechanism underpinning the induction process triggered by fluprostenol is not clearly understood. The absence of a high corpus luteum activity during late pregnancy in the mare would seem to preclude a luteolytic effect being the major mechanism. Also, fluprostenol is not a potent agent as regards myometrial smooth muscle contractile activity. Nonetheless, although the precise induction mechanism remains unclear, uterine contraction would appear to play a significant role in the initiation of parturition in the mare with prostaglandin analogs.

Fluprostenol is a potent inducing agent when used in mares between days 322 and 367 of gestation. It is more consistently effective than prostaglandin F_α, and when injected during the correct time frame, successful delivery can be anticipated within 4 hours. A single dose of 250 μg to ponies and 1000 μg to standard-bred mares usually suffices. (This is in contrast to natural prostaglandin F_α; in which single doses are not consistently effective. With prostaglandin F_α, it is often necessary to use repeat doses of 1.5 to 2.5 mg by injection every 12 hours.) Using analogs such as fluprostenol in late pregnancy, foaling can occur in 4 to 6 hours, with the fetal membranes being expelled 1.5 to 2 hours later.

The time from injection of fluprostenol to onset of second-stage labor ranges from 30 to 180 minutes. The appearance of the second stage of labor (sweating, uneasiness, abdominal discomfort, lengthening of the vulva) is normally apparent within half an hour of injection and persists for 10 to 30 minutes. After foaling, the membranes are expelled within 2 hours. Although success has been reported with fluprostenol usage in mares before cervical dilatation, malpresentation during parturition is an attendant hazard.

The general viability of foals after fluprostenol induction is good, but there have been some reports of hypogammaglobulinemia. This may be a result of reduction in volume of colostrum, because the immunoglobulin content of the colostrum itself is not necessarily diminished by the induction process. Hypogammaglobulinemia, however, can be a serious complication and may contribute to the overall weakness of the early foal during the vital first few hours of its extrauterine existence.

Although many mares foal within 3 to 4 hours of prostaglandin administration, alternative combination techniques can also be used with considerable success. One such technique involves an initial injection of estrogen with the synthetic corticoid flumethasone followed by another injection of flumethasone 12 hours later. Fluprostenol is then given at 24 hours, and foaling follows approximately 3 hours after the administration of this prostaglandin analog. Retention of the fetal membranes is a rare occurrence. The combination of estrogen and corticosteroid before prostaglandin administration is useful in stimulating milk production in addition to hastening the parturition process, especially in cases of advanced pregnancy in which signs of imminent parturition are not present. If induction is necessary before day 320 of gestation, two doses of fluprostenol, 500 μg every 2 hours, has been reportedly successful.

In instances in which induction is indicated but before an adequate gestation length, there is always the possibility of a premature foal. A combination of estrogen and flumethasone 24 hours before prostaglandin injection can be successful in stimulating milk production and inducing parturition in these cases.

The success or failure of prostaglandin techniques depends on the hormonal states of the mare at the time of the attempted induction. Overall, prostaglandins are more consistently successful when signs of impending parturition are present.

OXYTOCIN

Oxytocin is the most frequently used drug for induction of parturition in mares. Provided that the cervix is soft on palpation and facilitates the insertion of one or two figures into the external os and also that the foal is adjudged to be in normal presentation, oxytocin induces foaling usually within 15 to 60 minutes. In the absence of cervical ripening, an injection of estrogen may be necessary as a priming dose before administration of oxytocin.

The average parenteral dosage of oxytocin begins at 40 to 60 IU, and this facilitates a reasonably quiet foaling within 1 hour. Because the drug is such a potent tocolytic agent, it is always essential to attend to correct fetal presentation and positioning before administration, to ensure correct guidance of the forelimbs through the cervix during the phase of powerful uterine contraction. Oxytocin converts the normal weak, irregular, spontaneous contractions into more forceful, purposeful, and regular episodes. Thus correct fetal alignment is essential to avoid cervical damage or uterine rupture. Although estrogen can be given to relax the cervix before induction with oxytocin, some degree of cervical relaxation must be present if the decision-making process with regard to oxytocin usage is to be based on sound, safe principles. Oxytocin is given to best effect when foaling is imminent. When using oxytocin, it is important to be aware of the precise stage of gestation.

Oxytocin can be given intramuscularly, as a bolus intravenous injection, or intravenously in a saline drip. After intramuscular injection, foaling usually begins in 30 minutes with more pronounced sweating and discomfort than would be anticipated in a normal delivery. The most frequently employed route is the intramuscular route. Doses of 40 to 60 IU result in a delivery in less than 1 hour in nearly every case. (Higher doses are usually unnecessary and are likely to give rise to colic.) Ideally for best results with oxytocin induction, it is given at almost full-term when mares are showing signs of relaxation of the vulva and colostrum is present.

Assuming adequate veterinary supervision, there is a minimum of stress or trauma to the mare. Retention of fetal membranes is not usually a problem. The time for passage of the membranes can be influenced by the dosage of oxytocin employed. Doses of 20 units result in a slower foaling process with passage of the placenta after 3 hours. Higher dosages speed up delivery and cause a more rapid expulsion of the fetal membrane. A relationship between dose of oxytocin and placental expulsion may exist.

At the normal intramuscular dosage rate, preliminary activity marked by sweating and passage of excreta is evidenced within 10 minutes. At 20 minutes, anxiety and milk secretion is noticeable. After 30 minutes approximately, recumbency and straining are observed.

Doses in excess of 100 IU produce a more forceful contractile process with some degree of rolling in individual cases. If position, posture, and presentation are correct, however, together with adequate cervical dilatation, this should not necessarily result in a tumultuous contraction or violent parturition process.

Uterine atony responds to oxytocin injections, and retention of the placenta may be treated by administering 40 to 50 IU of oxytocin in saline by a slow intravenous drip over several hours. For a more controlled induction process, oxytocin can be given intravenously at a dosage of 5 IU three times at 15 minute intervals and then at a dosage of 10 IU at 15 minute intervals until parturition occurs. These smaller dosages allow for a more "physiologic" induction.

In general, dexamethasone poses the highest and fluprostenol the lowest risk to the fetus. Oxytocin is used clinically more routinely because it is more predictable and generally freer of side effects.

19.10 INDUCTION OF ABORTION

Elective abortion is indicated in mares when mismating has occurred or twin pregnancy exists. Intrauterine infusions containing saline, antibiotic, or dilute iodine solution can be used to good effect in these cases. Following instillation of 500 to 1000 ml of solution, abortion occurs within 48 hours.

Prostaglandins or analogs also terminate pregnancy, but consideration must be given to the stage of gestation if these agents are to be successful. In early pregnancy, when a functional corpus luteum is present but before the formation of the endometrial cups (35 days), a single injection of prostaglandin causes lysis of the corpus luteum, a sharp decline in progesterone production, termination of pregnancy, and a return to estrus.

Once the endometrial cups have formed, treatment must become more intense. Mares aborted after 40 days do not return to estrus until the endometrial cups cease functioning. Therapy with prostaglandin analogs around day 70 necessitates daily injection for 4 consecutive days. At 120 days, a double dose or repeat treatment at 48-hour intervals is necessary.

If fetal death and resorption occur after about the 42nd day of gestation, although prostaglandins induce luteolysis in the normal way, estrus and ovulation may not occur, and the ovaries gradually become smaller. This phenomenon is associated with the production and influence of pregnant mare's serum or equine chorionic gonadotropin (E.C.G.) secreted in large amounts between days 42 and 120 of gestation by the endometrial cups.

Thus administration of prostaglandin when a mare has been pregnant for fewer than 35 to 38 days causes onset of estrus in 3 to 5 days. If the prostaglandin is given after day 38 of gestation, the mare may abort but remain anestrus for a variable length of time. This anestrus is due to the functioning of endometrial cups present from day 42 to 150 of gestation. These cups start involuting about day 120 and have almost disappeared by 180 days.

This means that if rebreeding is intended in the same year, mares should be aborted before formation of the endometrial cup (days 35 to 40). Otherwise, return to estrus is delayed beyond 120 days.

19.11 RETAINED PLACENTA

Retention of the fetal membranes is a less common occurrence in the mare than in the cow. Normally the placenta falls away in the mare within 3 hours of foaling. Retention tends to be associated with uterine atony or the presence of an infectious process.

Oxytocin, 30 to 70 units subcutaneously, given every 2 to 3 hours beginning 4 hours after foaling hastens expulsion of the retained membranes. Occasionally signs of mild colic can be associated with this dosage regimen, and so a tranquilizer may be indicated. Large doses of oxytocin intravenously in the form of bolus injections (>60 units) can cause intense spasmodic contraction of the uterine muscle. If bolus injections are to be considered, doses of 30 to 40 units

only should be given intravenously every 15 to 20 minutes.

The preferable method is to give intravenous infusions of oxytocin, 80 to 100 units in 500 ml of saline, *to effect*. The mare must be constantly monitored for signs of abdominal discomfort when using this technique and the flow rate (and thereby the dosage) adjusted accordingly. Expulsion of the membranes can be expected in 30 to 45 minutes.

The contractility of the uterus can also be stimulated by the local infusion of a large volume of povidone-iodine solution. Approximately 10 to 12 liters of povidone-iodine diluted 1:10 are infused into the allantochorionic space by stomach tube. Elimination of the membranes using this technique takes about 30 minutes.

Antimicrobial therapy is warranted in many cases of retained placenta, especially when contamination is suspected. If the membranes have not been expelled within 8 hours of foaling, chemotherapy should be instituted. Parenteral therapy is preferred to local therapy not only because distribution of antibiotics to the uterine tissues is good, but also because it avoids the risk of introduction of infection locally. Intramuscular injections of sodium penicillin, 22,000 IU/kg twice a day, are useful first-choice approaches for systemic therapy. For local therapy, capsules of tetracycline (2 g) or gentamicin are useful agents. Intrauterine therapy must be practiced judiciously and selectively to avoid unnecessary introduction of local infection.

Antihistamines are indicated in protracted cases to prevent the occurrence of histamine-related disorders (e.g., laminitis). NSAIDs, especially phenylbutazone (2 g orally twice a day), are useful for prevention of the metritis-laminitis syndrome and also as analgesic agents to reduce pain caused by uterine involution.

SELECTED REFERENCES

Asbury, A.C.: Uterine defense mechanisms in the mare: The use of intrauterine plasma in the management of endometritis. Therio. *21*:387, 1984.

Baggott, J.D., and Prescott, J.F.: Antimicrobial selection and dosage in the treatment of equine bacterial infections. Eq. Vet. J., *19*:292, 1987.

Bennett, D.G.: Diagnosis and treatment of equine bacterial endometritis. Eq. Vet. Sci., 7:345, 1987.

Bennett, D.G.: Therapy of endometritis in mares. J. Am. Vet. Med. Assoc., 188:1390, 1986.

Boyd, E.H., and Allen, W.E.: Absorption of neomycin from the equine uterus: Effect of bacterial and chemical endometritis. Vet. Rec., 122: 37, 1988.

Brook, D.: The diagnosis of equine bacterial endometritis. Comp. Cont. Educ. Pract. Vet., 6:S300, 1984.

Buckley, T.C., and Leadon, D.P.: A survey of anaerobic bacteria isolated from cervicoendometrial swabs taken from mares present in Ireland during the 1986 thoroughbred breeding season. Irish Vet. J., 42:28, 1988.

Gustaffson, B.K.: Therapeutic strategies involving antimicrobial treatment of the uterus in large animal. J. Am. Vet. Med. Assoc., 185:1194, 1984.

Gustaffson, B.K., and Ott, R.S.: Current trends in the treatment of genital infections in large animals. Comp. Cont. Educ. Pract. Vet., 3:S147, 1981.

Haddad, N.S., Pederoli, W.M., and Ravis, W.R.: Pharmacokinetics of gentamicin at steady state in ponies: Serum, urine and endometrial concentrations. Am. J. Vet. Res., 46:1268, 1985.

Hinrichs, S.K., et al.: Clinical significance of aerobic bacterial flora of the uterus, vagina, vestibule and clitoral fossa of clinically normal mares. J. Am. Vet. Med. Assoc., 193:72, 1988.

Hirsch, D.C., and Jang, S.S.: Antimicrobic susceptibility of bacterial pathogens from horses. Vet. Clin. North Am. Equine Pract. 3:191, 1987.

LeBlanc, M.M., and Asbury, A.A.: Rationale for uterine lavage after breeding in mares. Proc. A.A.E.E.P. 33:623, 1987.

LeBlanc, M.M., Asbury, A.A., Lyle, S.K., et al.: Uterine clearance mechanisms during the early post-ovulatory period in mares. Am J. Vet. Res., 50:864, 1989.

Olso, J.D., Ball, L., and Mortimer, R.G.: Therapy of post-partum uterine infections. Proc. Ann. Meet. Soc. Therogenol., 1984.

Prescott, J.G., and Baggott, J.D.: Antimicrobial susceptibility testing and antimicrobial drug dosage. J. Am. Vet. Med. Assoc., 187:363, 1985.

Purswell, B., Ley, W.B., Spiranganathan, N., and Bowen, J.: Aerobic and anaerobic bacterial flora in the post-partum mare. Eq. Vet. Sci., 9:141, 1989.

Ricketts, S.: Vaginal discharge in the mare. In Practice (Vet. Rec.), 121:117, 1987.

Ricketts, W.W., and Mackintosh, M.E.: Role of anaerobic bacteria in equine endometritis. J. Reprod. Fertil., 35(Suppl):343, 1987.

Slusher, S.H.: Broodmare infertility. Medical therapy of reproductive disorders. Mod. Vet. Pract., 68:344, 1987.

Ward, A.: A new treatment for infertility in mares. Vet. Med., 65, 1985.

Washburn, M., Klesius, P., Ganjam, V., and Brown, R.G.: Effect of estrogen and progesterone on the phagocytic response of ovariectomized mares infected in utero with beta haemolytic streptococci. Am. J. Vet. Res., 43:1369, 1982.

Watson, E.D.: Uterine defense mechanisms in mares resistant and susceptible to persistent endometritis: A review. Eq. Vet. J., 20:297, 1988.

Watson, E.D., Stokes, C.R., David, J.S., et al.: Concentrations of uterine luminal prostaglandins in mares with acute and persistent endometritis. Eq. Vet. J., 19:31, 1987.

THERAPY OF MISCELLANEOUS EQUINE CONDITIONS

20.1 Foal Pneumonia—*Rhodococcus equi*
20.2 Strangles—*Streptococcus equi*
20.3 Chronic Obstructive Pulmonary Disease
20.4 Foal Septicemia
20.5 Gastrointestinal Disorders in Foals

20.1 FOAL PNEUMONIA—*RHODOCOCCUS EQUI*

Although foals are particularly susceptible to a primary bacterial pulmonary invasion, secondary bacterial pneumonia is common after an initial viral infection. Many causes predispose to foal pneumonia: management factors, overcrowding, stress, weaning nutrition, parasitism, individual susceptibility, congenital immunodeficiency, and inadequate intake of colostrum. Localization of infection in the respiratory tract can occur after inhalation or septicemia. Most infections are seen in foals over 1 month of age, with *Rhodococcus equi* infection being most common in the 4- to 8-week-old group. Foal pneumonia associated with *R. equi* is a severe disease process that presents many problems in treatment. The disease is insidious in onset and may present as a nonresponsive foal pneumonia, which can not only be an indication of possible antibiotic-resistant bacteria, but also evidence of consolidation and abscess formation in the lungs. A diagnosis of *R. equi* infection is frequently not made until initial broad-spectrum empirical therapy has failed. The condition may be chronic, with extensive bronchopneumonia, consolidation, and multiple abscess formation in the lungs and accompanying bacteremia. If appropriate treatment is not begun early enough, the mortality rate can be high (>70%). Variations in the antibiotic sensitivity patterns of *R. equi* isolates, multiple pyogranuloma formation, and irreversible lung damage renders antimicrobial therapy difficult.

R. equi pneumonia presents particular problems in terms of treatment because it is an intracellular organism, usually surrounded by purulent foci, and so antimicrobial penetration is difficult. Therapy with a combination of erythromycin, 25 mg/kg orally three times a day, and rifampin, 5 mg/kg orally twice a day, gives the best results.

Successful treatment of *R. equi* infections necessitates prompt administration of rationally indicated antibiotics together with supportive therapy and good nursing care. Ancillary therapy may include the use of bronchodilators, mucolytics, expectorants, antitussive agents, fluids, and antiprostaglandin drugs. Drugs used in treatment may be given parenterally, orally, or by nebulization and inhalation.

Treatment of *R. equi* pneumonia is generally most effective early in the disease. Antimicrobial therapy based on culture and sensitivity results usually consists of gentamicin, erythromycin, and rifampin. Bronchodilators, mucolytics, expectorants, and antitussives have also been used. Nebulization or bronchodilators, mucolytic, antimicrobials, and dimethyl sulfoxide (DMSO) has also been used. Fluid therapy can be used as needed, but corticosteroids are usually contraindicated.

ANTIMICROBIAL THERAPY

Antimicrobial therapy must be based on culture and sensitivity tests, and considerable variation occurs in the susceptibility of various isolates of *R. equi*. Most isolates are insensitive to penicillin, ampicillin, streptomycin, tetracyclines, and sulfonamides. The best response to treatment is seen in older foals or those with minimal abscess formation and lung involvement.

To treat *R. equi* infections successfully, an antibiotic must be well distributed in the lungs and possess the ability to penetrate abscesses and to kill organisms located inside macrophages and neutrophils.

Rifampin

Rifampin is a macrocyclic antibiotic that inhibits most gram-positive bacteria, including *Staphylococcus aureus*, *Corynebacterium*, and *Rhodococcus*. A distinct advantage of this bactericidal drug is its ability to penetrate cell membranes and to enter macrophages and polymorphonuclear leukocytes. Rifampin is soluble in both lipid and water at an acid pH, which makes it soluble in body fluids and capable of passing through lipid membranes. In the horse, peak serum levels occur about 4 hours after oral administration.

Undesirable side effects of rifampin include hepatotoxicity and an orange-red discoloration of the urine and saliva. Apart from *R. equi*, rifampin has been used to treat caseous lymphadenitis in sheep and goats; lung abscesses in calves; and umbilical infections, liver abscesses, and listeriosis in cattle, sheep, and goats. Rifampin is a potent inducer of hepatic enzymes, and with continued treatment, it may enhance its own excretion. Rifampin was originally intended as an antituberculosis drug and is currently used to treat *Neisseria meningitidis*. Rifampin should be used with another antibiotic because resistance to it develops rapidly. In veterinary medicine, rifampin has the potential for uses against a variety of organisms. A synergistic effect is seen when rifampin is given in combination with erythromycin for the treatment of pneumonia and cellulitis in foals caused by *R. equi*. It can be used to treat various staphylococcal infections in horses, including peritonitis and septic arthritis.

Rifampin, erythromycin, neomycin, kanamycin, potentiated sulfonamides, and chloramphenicol are effective against *R. equi* in vitro. Based on minimal inhibitory concentrations (MICs), rifampin is 90 times as potent as penicillin and five times as potent as gentamicin, whereas erythromycin is 30 times as potent as penicillin and twice as potent as gentamicin. Erythromycin and rifampin both penetrate cells and abscesses well, and when combined together a potent synergistic effect against *R. equi* is obtained.

Rifampin attains concentrations in the lung that exceed serum levels, and on account of its high lipophilicity, it is able to penetrate caseous material and suppurative tissues. Erythromycin and rifampin penetrate macrophages and neutrophils and thus can exert an intracellular antimicrobial effect. In combination, they are highly effective in infected foals even when severe, extensive abscessation has occurred.

The acid stable estolate or ethylsuccinate ester of erythromycin is given three times per day orally (25 mg/kg) in combination with oral rifampin. Both are well absorbed from the gastrointestinal tract. The absorption of the ethylsuccinate ester is enhanced with food. The intramuscular route of administration of erythromycin is associated with pain and inflammation. The intravenous use of the more expensive lactobionate salt offers no real advantage.

Oral erythromycin possesses the capability to alter the gastrointestinal flora, and so foals on erythromycin therapy must be observed for any side effects or signs of enteritis.

Erythromycin can be given as the estolate or ethylsuccinate salt at a dosage of 25 mg/kg orally three to four times a day. The dosage of rifampin is 5.0–7.5 mg/kg orally twice a day. This combination is clinically the most effective treatment of *R. equi* foal pneumonia.

The course of treatment is prolonged; therapy may have to be maintained over a period of months in severe cases. Using chest radiographs or plasma fibrinogen concentration as prognostic indicators, response to therapy with the combination can be monitored. The foal should be carefully observed for signs of enteritis because erythromycin can cause upset of the gastrointestinal tract flora. High doses of potentiated sulfonamides have proved effective in some early cases.

Alternative antimicrobial regimens used parenterally and with less predictable results include kanamycin sulfate, 5 to 8 mg/kg three times a day; gentamicin sulfate, 1 to 2 mg/kg three times a day; neomycin sulfate, 10 mg/kg twice a day; and formerly chloramphenicol, 50 mg/kg four times a day. Oral dosing with trimethoprim-sulfadiazine, 30 mg/kg three times a day, has proved effective in some early cases.

Gentamicin and neomycin are potentially nephrotoxic, especially in young foals subjected to longterm therapy. Hence renal functioning must be closely monitored in such patients. Chloramphenicol has a short half-life in the horse, and frequent administration is necessary to maintain effective concentrations in the tissues. Systemic antibiotic treatment must be maintained at high levels for at least 5 to 10 days after cessation of clinical signs. In horses, rifampin presents a number of advantages in the lengthy sojourn of the drug in the body and the ease of administration by the oral route. Cost and the potential for gastrointestinal tract side effects after oral administration to horses are negative factors meriting consideration.

Amikacin is a semisynthetic aminoglycoside antibiotic derived from kanamycin. The antibiotic resists degradation by most of the bacterial enzymes that inactivate other aminoglycosides. It exhibits broad-spectrum activity and has been shown to be effective against infections caused by *Pseu-*

domonas, Klebsiella, and *Escherichia coli.* Intramuscular injection of amikacin, 5 mg/lb three times a day for periods of 4 weeks or more, is useful for refractory respiratory infections in foals.

NEBULIZATION

Delivery of antimicrobials and other drugs by nebulization can be a useful way of treating foals with chronic bronchitis and bronchiolitis accompanied by a dry unproductive cough in the presence of a tenacious mucinous exudate. Nebulization treatment relieves bronchospasm, decreases mucosal edema, liquifies bronchial secretion, and kills bacteria in remote sites of the respiratory tree. Ultrasonic nebulizers can break up particles and disperse droplets less than 5 U in size into the terminal bronchioles and alveoli of the lung. Vaporizers produce a larger droplet size and deposit particles only in the upper respiratory tract and do not penetrate to the more distal sites.

Using a nebulization technique, the resultant aerosol is delivered through a loose-fitting face mask for inhalation periods of 10 to 30 minutes at 6- to 8-hour intervals. Nebulizer ingredients are usually a combination of a bland carrier substance, an antibiotic, bronchodilator, and mucolytic. For foals with *R. equi* infection, a useful nebulizing formula contains 180 ml half-strength saline (carrier), 5 to 10 ml of 20% acetylcysteine (mucolytic), 2 ml isoproterenol or 1 ml isoetharine hydrochloride (bronchodilator), and 150 mg gentamicin sulfate or 400 mg kanamycin sulfate (antibiotic).

A bronchodilator, such as isoetharine, relaxes the smooth muscle of the airways and alveolar system, producing dilation, diminishing secretions, and preventing airway spasm. Alleviation of spasm is particularly important if irritating mucolytics, such as acetylcysteine, are used.

An alternative ultrasonic nebulizer formula used with varied success for *R. equi* foal pneumonia contains 10 ml acetylcysteine, 10 ml isoetharine hydrochloride, 100 to 400 mg gentamicin sulfate or kanamycin sulfate, and 50 ml of saline. Nebulization is most successful in foals with diffuse bronchopneumonia and excessive mucopurulent exudate. The technique also assists the distribution of gentamicin and kanamycin, both of which are poorly absorbed from the respiratory system.

DMSO 90% can be added to a nebulization solution (10 ml/50 ml saline) to assist antibiotic penetration into the lung parenchyma. DMSO 40% has been used experimentally (1 g/kg IV) with intravenous antibiotics.

ANCILLARY TREATMENT

In cases in which large amounts of mucopurulent exudate are present in the airways, parenteral or oral administration of mucolytics, such as bromhexine hydrochloride or one of its phenolic benzylamine congeners (dexembrine), can be useful. Bronchodilatory agents can prove beneficial in relieving respiratory distress in severely affected foals, e.g., aminophylline, 5 to 10 mg/kg orally twice a day; terbutaline, 0.01 to 0.06 mg/kg orally twice a day; or clenbuterol, 0.8 μg/kg orally or intravenously twice a day.

Expectorants, such as iodides, guiacol, and volatile oils, loosen and mobilize respiratory secretions. Fluid therapy with balanced electrolytes is indicated in some cases to maintain hydration and promote mucociliary clearance and expectoration by reducing the viscosity of tenacious bronchial secretions. When fluids are used in severe cases, it must be remembered that iatrogenic pulmonary edema associated with fluid therapy can occur in pneumonic foals. Antiprostaglandin drugs, such as phenylbutazone, flunixin, or dipyrone (nonsteroidal anti-inflammatory drugs [NSAIDs]), ease discomfort and reduce fever in foals with pyrexia. Use of such antipyretic, analgesic drugs precludes the use of body temperature in the asssessment of success or failure of the therapeutic program.

Other useful agents include bronchodilators, such as glycopyrrolate.

20.2 STRANGLES—*STREPTOCOCCUS EQUI*

Strangles is an acute contagious suppurative disease caused by *Streptococcus equi.* Horses under 3 years of age are most commonly affected, but the condition can occur in older horses. The disease is characterized by mucopurulent inflammation of the upper respiratory tract accompanied by lymphadenitis and abscessation of adjacent draining lymph nodes.

Infection spreads by direct contact and environmental contamination from discharging infected horses. Although only one antigenic strain of *S. equi* is recognized, more than one strain may exist. The group is susceptible to penicillin and to a lesser extent to ampicillin and potentiated sulfonamide combinations. Antimicrobial therapy of strangles has always been a controversial issue. In the past, prompt therapy with penicillin G was advocated. It is now considered that the use of antibiotics before abscess drainage may suppress development of subsequent immunity. Therapy with penicillin G is indicated in nursing foals and in severe acute cases showing fever, anorexia, or obstruction of the upper airways. Stenosis of the airways owing to early abscessation is an indication for high-dose intravenous penicillin therapy (44,000 U/kg four times a day). Severe acute infection or a likelihood of pulmonary or joint involvement is another indication for antimicrobial use. Dosage of penicillin must be kept high and maintained over a period of 10 to 14 days in severe cases. Inadequate doses maintained for an inadequate period of time mask the symptoms, suppress the disease, delay abscess formation, and possibly increase the risk of development of encapsulated internal abscesses.

Although penicillin G is the drug of choice, potentiated sulfonamides have also been used for *S. equi* infection but with less clinical effectiveness. In general terms, the use of penicillin G or potentiated sulfonamides is best reserved for in contact animal to prevent disease outbreaks.

Antipyretic analgesics, such as phenylbutazone, can be beneficial in some cases to reduce pain and fever and to improve appetite. Fluid therapy may be indicated occasionally. When abscessation of lymph nodes has clearly occurred, they should be lanced, drained, and flushed with dilute 3 to 5% povidone-iodine solution for several days until discharge ceases.

20.3 CHRONIC OBSTRUCTIVE PULMONARY DISEASE

Similar to bronchial asthma in humans, chronic obstructive pulmonary disease (COPD) in the horse has a multifactorial etiology. This condition is a cause of chronic coughing in horses over 2 years old, and the incidence increases with age. Exposure to a moldy, dusty environment, especially poor-quality hay or straw, is associated with a high incidence of the disease (Table 20–1). The disease may be acute or chronic, the latter being more common. It may also be present in certain pastures. Genetic factors, diet, infectious agents, and inhaled allergens have all been implicated as causative factors. Infections of the air passages, allergic asthmatoid reactions involving the bronchi, and environmentally induced irritations of the bronchial tree can trigger off the reaction in a previously sensitized animal.

Once sensitized, a subsequent antigenic challenge can precipitate an outbreak of COPD depending on the individual susceptibility of the horse and the integrity of its pulmonary defense mechanisms. Defective clearance of foreign material may provide for continuous antigenic stimulation, leading to hypersensitization and exaggerated respiratory symptoms. This hypersensitive response leads to the accumulation of a viscous secretion in the airways and the development of bronchiolitis, bronchospasm, and emphysema. Although a primary infection may be involved, sensitization to environmental antigens, such as thermophilic actinomycetes, dust molds, fungal spores, and pollen, can initiate primary symptoms, such as dyspnea and coughing. Inhalation of small amounts of dust particles or environmental antigens to which a horse is hypertensive may subsequently cause clinical manifestation of COPD.

Initial viral infections followed by secondary bacterial colonization can also increase the viscosity of the tracheobronchial secretions, resulting in bronchial blockage with congestion and impairment of the expulsive mechanism of the respiratory tract. It may well be that viral agents will prove to be more important in the development of COPD in horses than previously thought. The syndrome tends to occur more fre-

---

TABLE 20–1
DEVELOPMENT OF CHRONIC OBSTRUCTIVE PULMONARY DISEASE

Antigen Challenge → Hypersensitivity
↓
Exudative Broncholitis
↓
Pulmonary Effusion
↓
Accumulation of Secretions
↓
Increased Viscosity of Secretions
↓
Decreased Mucociliary Clearance
↓
Reflex Bronchospasm/Respiratory Obstruction
↓
Impedance of Gaseous Exchange
↓
Respiratory Symptoms

---

quently in horses that have suffered a previous infection. Damage to the respiratory tract mucosa induced by viruses can predispose a sensitive animal, allowing airborne antigens in feed, bedding, or environment (e.g., pollen or fungal spores) to come into contact with immunoreactive tissue. Subsequent liberation of inflammatory mediators from mast cells results in a severe state of bronchospasm, leading to severe obstruction of respiratory function. Usually the disease is progressive, the horse displays reduced exercise tolerance, and a chronic cough with wheezing is usually present. Dyspnea becomes pronounced, with flaring of the nostrils during inspiration and a double expiratory effort ("heaving"). A mild nasal discharge and a hypersensitive response manifested by bronchiolitis, bronchospasm, bronchoconstriction, and emphysema become evident. COPD is most frequently seen in stabled horses, with respiratory distress being greatest during hot and dry weather.

ENVIRONMENTAL CONTROL

COPD is usually managed by strict environmental control to eliminate etiologic antigens, which may be present in hay, straw, or stable dust. Horses should be kept at

grass or in well-ventilated stables. Maintenance of a dust-free environment is essential, and mold or dusty hay and bedding should be avoided. The diet should be pelleted or cubed; vacuum-packed or dust-free hay only should be fed. Substitution of straw bedding by sawdust wood shavings or shredded paper is recommended. Removal of soiled material on a daily basis, avoidance of respiratory infections, and prompt treatment of bronchial disease must receive priority if the incidence is to be minimized. Although environmental control is essential, it may not always be possible, and in such instances, pharmacologic intervention may be necessary.

DRUG THERAPY

Therapy with pharmacologic agents is directed toward relief of the symptoms of respiratory embarrassment. The major problems necessitating medical management in horses with COPD are the result of functional and physical narrowing of the airways and excessive production of mucus. Short-term relief can be attained with the use of drugs, but in the absence of some environmental control measures, any improvement gained with drugs persists only for the duration of the treatment. Current

TABLE 20–2
DRUGS FOR CHRONIC OBSTRUCTIVE PULMONARY DISEASE

Therapy	
Bronchodilators	
Atropine	5–20 mg, IV, IM
Glycopyrrolate	3 mg, IV, IM, PO
Clenbuterol	0.8 μg/kg, IV, IM, PO
Theophylline	10–15 mg/kg, PO
	15 mg/kg, IV
Aminophylline	5 g, PO
Anti-inflammatories	
Corticosteroids	
Prednisolone	500 mg, IM, PO
Dexamethasone	20–40 mg, IM, IV
NSAIDs	
Flunixin	1.1 mg/kg, IV, PO
Meclofenamic acid	2.2 mg/kg, PO
Ketoprofen	2.2 mg/kg, IV
DMSO	—
Methylsulfonyl methane	15 mg, twice weekly
Expectorants/Mucolytics	
Bromhexine (Bisolvon)	48–90 mg, IM, PO
Dembrixine (Sputolysin) (Phenolic Benzylamine)	0.3 mg/kg, IV, PO
Iodides, Ammonium Chlorides	0.5 mg/kg, PO
Fluids:	
0.9% Isotonic saline	20–40 liters (10 liters/hour), IV
Hypertonic fluids	PO (expectorant effect)
Prophylaxis	
Sodium Cromoglycate	Single treatment (80 mg) by inhalation— protection for 3 to 4 days
	Four successive days treatment 80 mg/day—protection for 20 to 23 days

IV, Intravenous; IM, intramuscular; PO, oral.

medicinal treatments of choice include longterm therapy with bronchodilators, mucolytics, anti-inflammatories, and expectorants. Although these have all been used with varying degrees of success in affected animals, for the most part they counteract the respiratory symptoms for only short periods of time without addressing the fundamental underlying cause. Ancillary therapy must include some attempts to reduce inhalation of the aerosol particulate load on the mucociliary clearance system and measures to avoid viral infections of the respiratory system (Table 20–2).

Sodium Cromoglycate

Inhalation of sodium cromoglycate has long been used for prophylaxis of allergic respiratory disease in humans. It is a useful pro-phylactic measure for equine COPD, but it is not intended for therapy once the horse is showing clinical signs of the disease. Sodium cromoglycate has no direct bronchodilatory or anti-inflammatory effects, nor does it antagonize the cellular effects of histamine or leukotrienes. By causing blockage of calcium channels, it stabilizes mast cell membranes, preventing their degranulation after antigen challenge. This inhibits the release of many pharmacologically active mediators, such as histamine, 5-hydroxytryptamine, and slow-releasing substance of anaphylaxis. Given before anticipated antigen challenge to asymptomatic horses, the protection period increases linearly in accordance with the number of successive days of treatment. Usually a nebulizing dose of 80 mg/day is given by inhalation. This inhibits immediate and delayed hypersensitivity, preventing the outpouring of bronchoactive degranulation products from the respiratory tree. After a single inhalation of 80 mg, the period of protection is approximately 3 days, whereas inhalation over a period of 4 successive days can confer a period of protection of 24 days. As a routine prophylactic measure, sodium cromoglycate can be effective when given twice weekly. This is especially useful when horses are kept in an environment likely to precipitate COPD (i.e., on hay and straw).

Bronchodilators

Inhalational or parenteral administration of bronchodilators can bring about a temporary marked improvement clinically, indicating that airway spasm is directly involved in the pathogenesis of COPD. Partial effectiveness, short duration of action, and side effects limit the usefulness of many of these drugs. Bronchodilators include parasympatholytic anticholinergic agents, such as atropine, glycopyrrolate, and ipratropium; sympathomimetic drugs; and xanthine derivatives.

Atropine causes bronchodilation by decreasing the parasympathetic tone of the bronchial smooth muscle, thereby blocking reflex vasoconstriction. Although it is antisecretory, it can compromise mucociliary clearance by increasing the viscosity of the respiratory secretion. At doses of 5 to 10 mg intravenously, atropine can provide some immediate relief from bronchoconstriction. Because its duration of action in the horse is short (1 to 2 hours) and its use can be accompanied by many unwanted side effects, such as tachycardia, mydriasis, and ileus, it is not a primary drug for the symptomatic treatment of COPD.

Glycopyrrolate is a quatenary ammonium congener of atropine with similar pharmacologic activity but a longer duration of action than atropine (6 to 8 hours). In contrast to atropine, glycopyrrolate has a limited, restricted distribution in the body and so is less likely to give rise to undesirable side effects. Given intramuscularly at a dose of 3 mg, or subcutaneously at a dose of 1 mg, it can provide prompt relief. Effects are evident within 30 minutes of administration, and given two to three times per day, it can dramatically improve respiratory function, decreasing the respiratory rate by two thirds of the preadministration rate.

Sympathomimetic drugs include $beta_2$-adrenergic agonists such as clenbuterol, terbutaline, salbutamol, and fenoterol. These are prohibited in some countries. These adrenergic agents possess selectivity for the $beta_2$ receptors subserving bronchodilation and have fewer systemic and cardiac (than $beta_1$) side actions. In addition to their bronchodilatory actions, antiallergic activity and decreased mediator release from leukocytes may be present. Clenbuterol is a safe, effective bronchodilator and secretolytic agent in the horse. The duration of effect is in the range of 6 to 8 hours after single treatment, whether given orally or intravenously. It is commonly given twice daily by the oral route at a dose of 0.8 μg/kg. This is not permitted in the U.S. and is under review in Europe.

Xanthine derivatives, such as theophylline, aminophylline, or etamiphylline, have long been used in humans for relief of bronchospasm. In the horse, after intravenous administration, the effects are similar to those of clenbuterol but of shorter duration. With etamiphylline camsylate, intramuscular or subcutaneous injection repeated every 8 hours is necessary. Oral formulations are given twice daily. Cardiac stimulation and central nervous system activity may follow the use of xanthine derivatives. Theophylline is highly protein bound in the horse; the presence of other drugs can markedly affect its binding and clearance and can precipitate toxicity. Cimetidine and erythromycin are especially important in this respect. Theophylline is administered at a dosage of 10 mg/kg twice daily orally, etamiphylline camsylate is given three times per day at a dosage of 1 mg/kg body weight. Xanthine derivatives are indirect-acting sympathomimetics and also act as decongestants. Methylxanthines can increase mucociliary clearance by stimulating ciliary beat frequency, increasing water influx, and increasing secretion of mucus in the lower airways.

A number of bronchodilators are available for use in COPD. There are three types (pharmacologically) of bronchodilators:

1. Anticholinergics, such as atropine and glycopyrrolate

2. Beta agonists, such as clenbuterol and ephedrine
3. Methylxanthines, such as theophylline, which are phosphodiesterase inhibitors

Glycopyrrolate is less toxic than many other bronchodilators in horses. It is a quaternary ammonium compound that inhibits acetylcholine's action at receptors on postganglionic cholinergic neuron and smooth muscle. It is particularly water soluble and hence has a limited volume of distribution in the body and consequently fewer side effects. Glycopyrrolate used for COPD treatment results in reduced effort of breathing similar to atropine. Its advantage over atropine is its more specific respiratory action and less frequent effects on the heart and central nervous system owing to the charged nature of the molecule. When used intramuscularly, subcutaneously, or via nebulization, glycopyrrolate is a long-acting bronchodilator. A 1-mg subcutaneous dose is effective for up to 6 hours.

Mucolytics

Accumulation and hypersecretion of viscous mucoid material contribute to the overall impedance of respiratory exchange in COPD. Mucolytic agents, such as bromhexine hydrochloride (Bisolvon) and one of its congeners dembrexine (Sputolysin) (a phenolic benzylamine), reduce sputum viscosity and facilitate expectoration and expulsion of bronchial secretions. Bromhexine is given intramuscularly or orally at a dose of 48 to 90 mg/day.

Dembrixine is a phenolic benzylamine, trans-4[(3,5-dibromo-2-hydroxybenzyl amino)] cyclohexanol. The compound influences the secretory activity of serous glandular cells in the mucosa of the respiratory tract. The reduction in mucus viscosity, caused by the administration of dembrixine has both direct and indirect effects. Less viscous mucus is more easily removed by the mucociliary elevator and hence airway obstruction is reduced. At the same time, any reflex bronchospasm caused by the presence of abnormal mucus may be resolved.

As these events take place, a rapid return to normal respiratory function is observed. Often improvement is seen within 5 days.

Restoration of normal respiratory function leads to the return of fitness and performance in the horse.

Anti-inflammatories

Corticosteroids have had some success on a short-term basis in alleviating symptoms of COPD. Their actions include interference with antigen processing, inhibition of T lymphocyte responses to antigens, and suppression of tissue response to IgE-mediated releases of histamine from mast cells. Local synthesis of leukotrienes, prostaglandins, and thromboxanes is blocked, and inflammatory edema is decreased. In COPD, the initial dose of corticosteroid may be quite high: 500 to 800 mg of prednisolone given intravenously or intramuscularly or 30 mg of dexamethasone intramuscularly. Diminution of this dosage and alternate-day therapy may be possible as the symptoms regress. Laminitis, suppression of adrenocorticoid function, and increased susceptibility to infectious colonization of the respiratory tract can accompany longterm usage. Use of short-acting steroids, such as prednisolone, is therefore preferable. Corticosteroids produce only a temporary remission of signs and the rate and level of remission are not in general superior to many of the more selective bronchodilator drugs. NSAIDs, such as flunixin meglumine ketoprofen, or meclofenamil acid, decrease inflammation and pain by inhibiting synthesis of prostaglandins and kinins and to a lesser extent histamine and 6-hydroxytryptamine. NSAIDs can be considered in therapy for COPD, but response to them is variable owing to the multifactorial etiology of the condition and the complex role of chemical mediators of anaphylaxis in the pathogenesis of COPD.

Miscellaneous Agents

Antihistamines, formerly advocated to suppress coughing and to treat COPD, are clinically ineffective. Inhibition of the secretory activities of the bronchial tree results in a drying of secretions and reduction in mucociliary clearance. Because these drugs block only histamine, which is one of a large number of inflammatory mediators, antihistamines are unreliable and inconsistent when used as the sole means of therapy.

Diethylcarbamazine citrate, although primarily used as an anthelmintic, also inhibits the release of histamine, prostaglandins, and leukotrienes. It has been used in combination with corticosteroids in the theory of COPD at a dosage rate of 6 mg / kg. Whether leukotrienes are significant mediators of the condition is unclear, and definitive documented evidence of the clinical usefulness of diethylcarbamazine citrate in this condition is lacking. The use of various immunomodulators is currently being investigated.

Horses showing weak response to bronchodilatory agents may benefit from administration of large volumes of intravenous fluids. Infusion of 20 to 40 liters of saline (10 liters/hour) has been reportedly successful in some cases of COPD. Orally administered hypertonic electrolyte solutions are effective expectorants because they depolymerize complex proteins in sputum and attract water from the surrounding tissues into the mucus, rendering it less viscous and more easily eliminated. Ammonium carbonate, ammonium chloride, and iodide-containing compounds possess both an expectorant and a mucolytic effect by breaking down viscous mucoproteins and stimulating ciliary activity. Oxygen therapy may be warranted in severe cases of COPD.

Methylsulfonylmethane is an oxidation metabolite of DMSO and possesses many properties of DMSO. It acts as a free radical scavenger, inhibits inflammatory cell migration, and reduces inflammation. At a dosage of 15 g twice daily for a week, the compound can produce some relief in COPD.

The main problems requiring medical management in horses with chronic respiratory conditions are the result of functional and physical narrowing of the airways and excess mucus production. Management of these problems requires extended drug therapy with bronchodilators, agents that alter the viscosity and volume of mucus produced, and agents that help control the growth of a range of nonpathogenic and pathogenic microbial agents in the mucus. The corticosteroids are of comparatively little or no value in the management of these chronic problems.

20.4 FOAL SEPTICEMIA

Neonatal septicemia is a serious condition associated with high morbidity and mortality in foals less than 1 month of age. Many factors, especially relating to the dam, the foal, and the environment, may predispose to the development of sepsis in the newborn animal. Poor health and nutrition of the mare, uterine infection, uterine-placental derangement, dystocia, cesarean section, colic, endotoxemia, and premature lactation can result in fetal stress hypoxia and premature or weak foals. Even a normal healthy foal is immunologically less competent than the adult animal on account of the variation in complement levels, the less efficient phagocytic functioning, and the lack of anamnestic response to antigens owing to initial exposure. This increases its susceptibility to various pathogens. A common triggering cause of neonatal sepsis is failure of transfer of maternal colostral antibodies to the foal. Many organisms, either primary or secondary pathogens, can be involved in foal septicemia, which by hematogenous spread can localize in various body systems. Atlhough *Actinobacillus equuli, Escherichia coli, Klebsiella pneumoniae,* beta-hemolytic streptococci, *S. aureus, R. equi, Salmonella, Pseudomonas aeruginosa,* and anaerobic organisms may be isolated from clinical cases, in general gram-negative organisms are more commonly implicated. In utero infection is frequently caused by beta-hemolytic streptococci or *E. coli.*

Klebsiella, *E. coli,* and *Actinobacillus* are likely to cause problems in colostrum-deprived foals that have low serum globulin.

The main portal of entry of the infectious organisms from the environment or birth canal is through the umbilicus, gastrointestinal tract, or respiratory tract of the foal. The most important measure for preventing infection of newborn foals is ensuring adequate intake of colostrum (Table 20–3).

Symptoms of septicemia include diarrhea, respiratory distress, joint distention, seizures, colic, and uveitis. Treatment should include intravenous plasma (1 to 2 liters per foal), fluid therapy, and aminoglycosides or beta/actam antibiotics given systemically. (Oral antibiotics may lead to *Candida* overgrowths).

TABLE 20–3
BACTERIA COMMONLY ASSOCIATED WITH FOAL SEPTICEMIA

Organism	Likely Predilection Site
Actinobacillus equuli	Adrenal glands, kidneys, meninges
Escherichia coli	Joints, lungs, meninges, pleura
Klebsiella pneumoniae	Joints, meninges, lungs, peritoneum
Salmonella	Gastrointestinal tract, joints, bones, mininges, blood, kidneys, liver
Staphylococcus aureus	Joints, bones
Streptococcus	Blood, lungs, bones, joints, pleura, peritoneum, umbilicus, meninges

---

For the first 24 hours, the foal should receive nothing by mouth, but hydration, acidosis, and hypoglycemia must be corrected. Acetate and gluconate, being bicarbonate precursors, are preferable. Bismuth subsalicylate antagonizes prostaglandin and so possesses unique bowel activity.

Treatment of neonatal septicemia includes supportive care, use of antimicrobial agents, and immunologic assistance. Antimicrobial selections should be based on the results of culture and sensitivity tests; however, a combination of penicillin and an aminoglycoside (gentamicin or amikacin) can be used until test results indicate a change.

Therapeutic management of foal septicemia is based on:

1. Control of generalized infection
2. Treatment of the localized infection
3. Maintenance of homeostasis

Supportive care is critical in treatment of the condition (Table 20–4). The environ-

---

TABLE 20–4
SUGGESTED NORMAL ANTIMICROBIAL DOSAGES FOR FOALS

Drug	Dosage
Amikacin sulfate	7.5 mg/kg IV every 12 hours
Amoxicillin	
Sodium	22.0 mg/kg IM every 6 hours
Trihydrate	20.0–30.0 mg/kg PO every 12 hours
Ampicillin	
Sodium	20.0 mg/kg IV/IM every 12 hours
Trihydrate	11.0–22.0 mg/kg IM every 12 hours
Carbenicillin disodium	100.0 mg/kg IM every 6–8 hours
Cefazolin sodium	20.0 mg/kg IV every 8–12 hours
Cefotaxime sodium	20.0–30.0 mg/kg IV every 6 hours
Cephalothin sodium	20.0–30.0 mg/kg IV every 6 hours
Chloramphenicol succinate	50.0 mg/kg IV every 6–8 hours
Erythromycin estolate	25.0 mg/kg PO every 6 hours
Gentamicin sulfate	2.0–3.0 mg/kg IV every 12 hours
Kanamycin sulfate	7.5 mg/kg IV every 12 hours
Penicillin G	
Procaine	25,000–50,000 U/kg IM every 12 hours
Sodium or potassium	25,000–50,000 U/kg IV every 6–8 hours
Rifampin	5.0 mg/kg PO every 12 hours
Ticarcillin disodium	50.0 mg/kg IV every 6–8 hours
Sulfonamide-trimethoprim	15.0 mg/kg IV every 12 hours

IV, intravenous; IM, intramuscular; PO, oral.

ment is critical in the treatment of the condition. The environment should be warm, well ventilated, dust free, and clean. Provision of heat by lamps or blankets is necessary if the foal's rectal temperature drops below 99°F.

Infection is the most common cause of morbidity and mortality in neonatal foals. Most foals with bacterial septicemia have one or more predisposing factors present during fetal development, parturition, or early postnatal life. Poor health of the mare, prematurity of the foal, an improper umbilical disinfection favor infection of the foal.

Intrauterine infection is the most common cause of placental insufficiency during fetal development and can result in infection of the fetus. The most common predisposing factor of neonatal septicemia in foals is failure of passive transfer of maternal antibodies. Although foals are immunocompetent at birth, they are essentially immunologically naive to their environment. The principal portals of entry of infections are the umbilicus, gastrointestinal tract, and respiratory tract.

ANTIMICROBIAL THERAPY

Specific antimicrobial therapy must ideally be based on culture and sensitivity testing of the isolated microorganisms. Because both gram-positive and gram-negative bacteria can be associated with septicemia, broad-spectrum antibiotic therapy at high but safe doses must be started as soon as possible. Septicemia without localized signs should be treated for at least 10 days, and if localized signs are present, therapy should continue for 2 weeks after clinical signs disappear. Relatively few pharmacokinetic studies have been carried out in foals, and so drug dosages have largely been extrapolated from either adult equine or human infant dosage computations. A number of key considerations underline the safe, effective usage of antimicrobial agents in foals, and these must always be borne in mind before beginning therapy. Because septic foals are immunologically compromised, batericidal antimicrobial agents are preferable. Significant differences are present between the foal and the adult horse with respect to pharmacokinetic principles, and hence the ability of the young animal to cope with the drug, in terms of its efficacy or potential toxicity. Minor but significant pharmacokinetic differences also exist between premature and full-term foals.

Differences between neonatal and adult animals in their response to drugs can be attributed to altered disposition during the neonatal period. The major metabolic pathways for drugs, hepatic microsomal oxidative reactions, and glucuronide conjugation and the renal excretion mechanism, especially proximal tubular secretion, are deficient in neonatal animals. Development of the metabolic pathways, particularly the microsomal enzymes, proceeds at a variable rate among individuals and species after removal of the depressant effects of progesterone at the time of paturition. In foals, it is believed that functional maturity of the metabolic pathway occurs at approximately 2 weeks after birth.

Antibiotics are metabolized and excreted at entirely different rates in neonates than in adults. Increased absorption from the gastrointestinal tract, decreased plasma protein binding, increased volume of distribution, and altered routes of biotransformation and excretion account for some of the differences.

The extracellular fluid compartment of the foal is appreciably larger than the adult horse and this, coupled with a lesser degree of plasma protein drug binding, renders the volume of drug distribution greater in the foal with a consequent reduction in plasma concentration. Accordingly, higher doses are necessary in foals to attain the same blood levels as the adult horse. The foal is also deplete in hepatic drug metabolizing enzymes, and so the processes of drug biotransformation via the microsomal enzyme system is slower, thus prolonging the half-life of most drugs. Immature or compromised renal functioning retards elimination still further. Dosage intervals can therefore be longer with less frequent dosing than in the adult animal. The erythrocytes of the foal are particularly susceptible to oxidizing agents and thus to hemolysis and the development of hemoglobinuria. Potentiated sulfonamides can produce this effect in sensitive individuals. Other differences of significance in the neonatal foal include the increased permeability of the blood-brain barrier, allowing greater penetration of drugs into the central nervous system, and the erratic, unreliable absorption from the gastrointestinal tract.

Taking account of the foregoing consideration, certain generalizations can be made with regard to an antimicrobial drug intended for use in foal septicemia. The ideal drug should:

1. Be bactericidal with a broad spectrum of activity against gram-positive and gram-negative organisms
2. Be given by the parenteral route
3. Be eliminated without hepatic biotransformation
4. Be relatively nontoxic
5. Not be highly bound to plasma protein

The most common etiologic agents in foal septicemia include *A. equuli*, *Streptococcus*, *E. coli*, and *K. pneumoniae*. Of these, *Streptococcus* and *Actinobacillus* are almost always susceptible to penicillin. The enteric organisms (*E. coli*, *Klebsiella*) are the most unpredictable but are frequently susceptible to aminoglycosides. Anaerobes are usually sensitive to penicillin or potentiated sulfonamides. Metronidazole is the drug of choice for anaerobic infections.

Pending culture and sensitivity results, broad-spectrum bactericidal therapy should be started. Initial administration should preferably be by the intravenous route owing to the severity of the condition, the necessity for rapid response, and the possibility of a compromised peripheral circulation or inconsistent absorption. A good broad-spectrum choice is penicillin or ampicillin combined with gentamicin or amikacin. A trimethoprim-sulfadiazine combination or chloramphenicol, if permissible, is a useful second choice (Tables 20–4 and 20–5).

Penicillin G combined with an aminoglycoside (gentamicin sulfate, amikacin sulfate, kanamycin sulfate) is an excellent antibiotic for foal septicemia. Penicillin G is highly effective against streptococci and anaerobes, and most gram-negative rods and staphylococci are sensitive to aminoglycosides. Gentamicin and amikacin are more effective than kanamycin because fewer gram-negative organisms have gained resistance to them. Streptomycin is no longer

recommended because of the lack of sensitivity of most pathogens to this aminoglycoside.

Aqueous crystalline penicillin G may be given intravenously at 20,000 to 100,000 U/kg four times a day. Procaine penicillin is absorbed more slowly, and it may be given at a dosage of 20,000 U/kg twice a day. Sodium ampicillin should be given intravenously or intramuscularly at 11 to 22 mg/kg four times a day. Ampicillin is less effective than penicillin G against gram-positive organisms but is active against a number of species of gram-negative rods. *E. coli*, *Salmonella*, and *Actinobacillus* are resistant to sodium ampicillin. Ideally it should be used alone when aminoglycosides are contraindicated or a positive culture of a sensitive organ is obtained. Amoxicillin has a more marked, rapid bactericidal effect than ampicillin and can be given orally at a dose of 20 to 30 mg/kg. Amoxicillin intramuscularly at 22 mg/kg twice a day is usually effective against streptococci. More resistant organisms, such as *A. equuli*, require 22 mg/kg four times daily by the intramuscular route. Similar to penicillin G, ampicillin and amoxicillin are inactivated by beta-lactamase-producing organisms. Ticarcillin disodium has a broad bacterial spectrum (including *Pseudomonas*) and is given intravenously at 44 mg/kg every 5 hours or intramuscularly every 8 hours. Ticarcillin can be combined with clavulanic acid, as an amoxicillin, and in this form is effective against *E. coli*, *Klebsiella*, *A. equuli*, staphylococci, and *P. aeruginosa*.

Sodium oxacillin at 25 mg/kg intramuscularly every 8 to 12 hours treats beta lac-

---

TABLE 20–5
GENERAL THERAPY FOR GRAM-NEGATIVE SEPTICEMIA

Antimicrobials
Antiprostaglandins (flunixin, aspirin, indomethacin)
Corticosteroids
Intravenous polyionic fluids, electrolytes, buffers
Plasma, plasma volume expanders
Heparin

tamase-producing *S. aureus* infections. Third-generation cephalosporins, such as moxalactam and cefoxatime, display considerable activity against gram-negative organisms as well as posssessing useful tissue distribution properties. Moxalactam has been used in septicemic foals at 50 mg/kg every 6 to 12 hours. Because of its tendency to cause hemostatic abnormalities, its application in neonates is limited. Cefoxatime as the sodium salt is given at 10 to 40 mg/kg three times a day and is useful for coliform meningitis.

Of aminoglycoside antibiotics, gentamicin is the drug of choice for gram-negative sepsis. All of the aminoglycosides are eliminated by glomerular filtration, and they have potential to accumulate in renal tissues, causing nephrotoxicity especially in young animals subjected to decreased renal function subsequent to shock or dehydration. Gentamicin, given intramuscularly or intravenously at a dosage of 2 mg/kg two or three times a day, is one of the premier drugs for neonatal septicemia. Its excellent therapeutic properties are limited to some degree by its nephrotoxicity, signs of which include increased creatine and blood urea nitrogen, urinary tubular casts, and enzymuria. Efficacy tends to be more closely associated with high intermittent peak concentrations than continuous concentrations near or above the MIC. Gentamicin should be given only to foals with normal renal function. In such animals, clearance can still be variable. Aminoglycoside nephrotoxicity incidence increases 5 to 7 days after start of therapy, and if the duration of therapy exceeds 5 days, monitoring of serum drug concentration in addition to renal monitoring is advisable. Gram-negative organisms that are resistant to gentamicin frequently remain sensitive to amikacin, which may be given intravenously or intramuscularly at 10 mg/kg every 12 hours. Erythromycin estolate at 25 mg/kg orally four times a day should be used only if specifically indicated based on culture and sensitivity testing. Disturbances of gastrointestinal function are sometimes associated with erythromycin use in the horse. The drug is best reserved for treatment of *R. equi* pneumonia, in which in combination with oral rifampin (5 to 10 mg/kg twice a day) it exerts a potent synergistic effect.

Chloramphenicol is useful in foal septicemia and should be given intravenously as the succinate salt at 50 mg/kg every 4 hours or orally as the base or palmitate ester at 50 mg/kg every 6 hours. Chloramphenicol undergoes hepatic metabolism in most species and is then excreted in the urine. Much of the active drug as well as the metabolites circulate bound to plasma proteins. In foals, the half-life is short, and the drug must be administered every 4 to 6 hours to maintain effective blood levels. Chloramphenicol should not be used in foals that require sedatives or anticonvulsants because chloramphenicol can alter the microsomal enzyme activity in the liver, thus affecting the clearance of the latter drugs. The synergistic combination of trimethoprim and sulfadiazine provides broad-spectrum activity against many gram-positive and gram-negative organisms. Both drugs are well distributed throughout the tissues and are excreted primarily in urine. At a dosage of 15 mg/kg intravenously or orally twice a day, it is a good second choice for foal septicemia. High dosages of trimethroprim-sulfadiazine have been associated with transient neutropenia and acute toxic enteritis in horses.

Choice of antibiotics for foal sepsis must take account of a number of key considerations. Although a majority of neonatal septicemias are caused by gram-negative organisms, gram-positive and mixed infections also occur. This necessitates the use of broad-spectrum antibiotics. Bactericidal drugs should be used because the neonatal foal has an immature immunologic system, and stress and sepsis can depress immunocompetency. Intravenous administration is the preferred route of antibiotic delivery. The pharmacokinetic behavior of antimicrobial drugs in equine neonates differs significantly from that of the adult horse, especially in the first week after birth. Rational antibiotic choice would suggest either penicillin or ampicillin combined with an aminoglycoside, such as gentamicin sulfate, or if resistant strains are a problem, amikacin sulfate. Potentiated sulfonamides should be regarded as second-line antibiotics. Selection of a specific antimicrobial agent must be based on identification and susceptibility testing of the causative organism.

TABLE 20–6
FLUID THERAPY

Electrolyte	Gram Equivalents for Isotonicity Salt	g/liter for isotonic solution
Potassium	KCl	10.0
Bicarbonate	NaHCO₃	12.5
	Sodium lactate	16.0
	Sodium acetate	12.5
Sodium	NaCl	9.0
Calcium	CaCl₂	5.0
	Ca gluconate	30.0
Magnesium	MG SO₄	18.0

ADJUNCTIVE MEASURES

If failure of passive transfer is suspected, foals less than 15 hours old should receive oral equine colostrum. Commerical or donor plasma can be infused at 20 ml/kg. Hyperimmune and antiendotoxin serum gives promising results for the treatment of gram-negative septicemia.

Loss of fluid volume through sequestration in visceral and peripheral vascular beds is a common sequela of septicemia in young foals. Shock is not unusual, and because many foals suffer from gram-negative infections, they can also suffer from the deleterious effects of endotoxemia. Shock and endotoxemia can be treated with balanced polyionic fluids given intravenously. Lactated Ringer's solution given at 30 to 40 ml/kg/hour is the initial fluid of choice, given until adequate volume expansion is achieved. Because hypoglycemia is common, a continuous 5 to 10% dextrose intravenous infusion at 4 to 8 mg/kg/minute may improve blood flow, induce diuresis, and help to provide a metabolic substrate. Lactated Ringer's can be supplemented with 5% dextrose, or 2.5% dextrose in 0.45% saline can be given at 3 to 5 ml/kg/hour. Solutions of 50% dextrose are contraindicated because they are irritant and hypertonic and give rise to intracellular dehydration. Isotonic 5% dextrose solutions are suitable alternatives (Tables 20–6 and 20–7). Severe metabolic acidosis exists, intravenous infusion of isotonic 1.3% sodium bicarbonate should be given. Sodium bicarbonate can also be given in one-half strength saline or 2.5% dextrose. Such solutions should not be mixed with calcium-containing infusions, e.g., lactated Ringer's, because precipitation of calcium carbonate may form. In severe cases of hypovolemic shock, intravenous plasma (20 ml/kg) may assist in the restoration of blood volume.

If bradycardia is evident, positive chronotropic agents, such as atropine, epinephrine, dobutamine, isoproterenol, and

TABLE 20–7
MISCELLANEOUS DRUGS FOR GASTROINTESTINAL TRACT/SHOCK

Agent	Route of Administration	Dosage
Bismuth subsalicylate	Oral	1 oz/8 kg BW QID
Kaolin/pectin	Oral	1 oz/8 kg BW QID
Activated charcoal	Oral	0.25–0.5 kg BID
Flunixin meglumine	IM, IV	0.25 mg/kg TID

IM, intramuscular; IV, intravenous; BW, body weight; QID, four times a day; BID, two times a day; TID, three times a day.

calcium gluconate, can be considered. Atropine, however, can lead to stasis and gastrointestinal colic, whereas epinephrine and isoproterenol are potentially arrhythmogenic in hypoxia patients. Efforts to elevate arterial blood pressure with alpha-adrenergic agents can be counterproductive because the total peripheral resistance initiated by endotoxins is augmented still further to the detriment of tissue perfusion. For positive inotrophic activity, 1% dopamine intravenously at a dosage of 3 to 5 μg/kg/minute has been used with some success to counteract low cardiac output in foals. It is particularly beneficial when some degree of renal failure prevails on account of its vasodilatory effect in the splanchnic and renal vessels. To obviate states of hypercoagulability that can cause thrombosis in large veins, small doses of heparin, 40 U/kg subcutaneously three times a day, can be given with beneficial results. In the treatment of shock in the septicemic foal, the use of corticosteroids is controversial, and they are best avoided owing to their numerous unwanted side effects. Flunixin is more useful than corticosteroids owing to its lack of immunosuppressant effects and its potent antiprostaglandin, antiendotoxic activity. Flunixin must be used judiciously in hypovolemic foals because of its tendency to induce gastrointestinal ulceration and renal damage.

Shock, a common sequela of septicemia in young foals, is characterized by generalized inadequate perfusion and tissue hypoxia. Balanced polyionic fluids, such as lactated Ringer's solution, are often the initial fluid of choice. This can be administered at a rate of 30 to 40 ml/kg/hour until adequate volume expansion is achieved. Alternating lactated Ringer's with 5T dextrose or administering 2.5% dextrose in 0.45% saline solution at a rate of 3.4 ml/kg/hour has been done. A 50-kg foal that is 10% dehydrated requires 5 liters of replacement fluid. The maintenance intravenous fluid rate for a 50-kg foal is 200 ml/hour.

When metabolic acidosis is severe, intravenous infusion of isotonic 1.3% sodium bicarbonate solution may be given. Glucose solutions of 5% may be used to correct hypoglycemia and to supply a metabolic substrate. Sodium bicarbonate must never be mixed with solutions containing calcium (e.g., lactate Ringer's solution) because calcium carbonate precipitates may be formed. As an alternative, plasma at a dose of 20 ml/plasma kg body weight has been recommended. The plasma helps not only to restore circulating volume, but also to transfer immunoglobulins.

In the event of disseminated intravascular coagulation, heparin has been recommended at suggested treatment dosages of 80–100 units/kg at 4-hour intervals until clotting time doubles.

Corticosteroids have been used in the treatment of septic shock, but they can cause further immunosuppression in an already immunocompromised foal. NSAID, such as flunixin (Banamine), possess antiinflammatory and antiendotoxin effects, especially at a low dose of 0.25 mg/kg. Care must be taken, however, in their use because by inhibition of prostaglandin synthesis they may predispose foals to gastrointestinal ulceration and could be potentially nephrotoxic to hypovolemic foals.

When using NSAID, especially phenylbutazone, in foals, side effects are not uncommon. In some foals, therapeutic levels of phenylbutazone, 10 mg/kg/day, can produce signs of toxicity: oral and gastric ulceration, diarrhea, colonic edema, and marked protein loss from the gastrointestinal tract. They can also reduce renal blood flow through the kidney. The combination of dehydration and NSAIDs in neonatal foals markedly increases the incidence of these side effects.

When antimicrobials are employed for use in septicemic foals, it must be remembered that pharmacokinetics in neonates differs from that in adult horses, especially in the first 5 to 7 days after birth. Penicillin or ampicillin in combination with an aminoglycoside, such as gentamicin sulfate or amikacin sulfate, would be first choice. Potentiated sulfonamide is a reasonable second choice.

CENTRAL NERVOUS SYSTEM DISORDERS

Septicemic foals occasionally display seizures associated with hypoglycemia, electrolyte imbalances, or bacterial meningitis arising from a primary focus of infection in

TABLE 20–8
ANTICONVULSANTS FOR FOALS

Drug	Dosage
Diazepam	0.5–1.0 mg/kg IV
Pentobarbital	3.0–15.0 mg/kg IV
Phenytoin	5.0–10.0 mg/kg IV initially; then 1.0–5.0 mg/kg every 2–4 hours
Phenobarbital	1.0–10.0 mg/kg IV initially; then 0.5–1.0 mg/kg BID
Primidone	15–20.0 mg/kg oral, SID, or BID
Xylazine	0.44–1.0 mg/kg IV
Detomidine	40–80 μg/kg, IV/IM
DMSO	500–900 mg in 5% dextrose or 1 mg/kg in 5% dextrose IV.

IV, intravenous; BID, two times a day; SID, once a day

the lung, umbilicus, or gastrointestinal tract. In febrile infection, the blood-brain barrier permeability is increased, but despite this, considerable difficulty still exists with respect to penetration of antimicrobial agents into the central nervous system. Meningitis caused by Enterobacteriaceae poses many problems therapeutically because a number of antimicrobial agents that are rationally indicated fail to attain the critically effective levels in the central nervous system (e.g., gentamicin), whereas those that do penetrate centrally lack a potent bactericidal effect (e.g., chloramphenicol).

For treatment of coliform meningitis, intravenous trimethoprim-sulfadiazine, 24 mg/kg three times a day, is a reasonable first choice. Alternatively, third-generation cephalosporins, such as moxalactam and cefoxatime, should be considered because they display considerable activity against gram-negative organisms, easily penetrate the blood-brain barrier, and are effective in treatment of meningitis in human neonates and adults. The tendency of moxalactam to cause hemostatic abnormalities, however, has limited its use in the neonatal animal. Cefoxatime sodium, 10 to 40 mg/kg intravenously four times a day, is an effective drug for cases that have failed to respond to other broad-spectrum antimicrobials or in which organisms are isolated that are uniquely sensitive.

Anticonvulsants and sedatives may be indicated in foals with severe disorders of the central nervous system secondary to generalized septicemia. Diazepam is useful for seizures, but it possesses a noticeable lag period until its effects are noted. Because it does not abolish the focus of the seizures, other anticonvulsants may have to be considered if seizures are recurrent. Phenytoin limits development and spread from an active focus, but it can cause hyperactivity and nystagmus. Phenobarbital is a useful anticonvulsant agent that both elevates the seizure threshold and minimizes spread. It is not effective, however, in status epilepticus. Pentobarbital, another barbiturate, possesses a more rapid effect and has been used to stop seizure activity in foals. Its central respiratory depressant activity necessitates great care in its use, and hence it is not generally used unless diazepam is ineffective. Primidone is a congener of phenobarbital, possessing broadly similar actions to the latter.

Xylazine is a useful, readily obtainable sedative with predictable effects in horses that may be used for short periods. As an alpha$_2$ agonist, it can cause transient hypertension and so can exacerbate hemorrhage in the central nervous system. Detomidine is another useful and longer acting alpha$_2$ agonist. Phenothiazine derivatives are contraindicated in convulsing and septicemic foals because they decrease the seizure threshold and possess hypotensive actions. Intravenous DMSO at 500 to 900 mg diluted in 5% dextrose solution is reportedly beneficial for the treatment of cerebral edema (Table 20–8). Although foals with bacterial meningitis and cerebral edema may respond to DMSO, mannitol, or dexamethasone, corticosteroids can seriously compromise an already immunodeficient animal by facilitating the dissemination of bacterial infection throughout the body.

OCULAR INFECTIONS

Uveitis can be treated by topical cycloplegics, such as 1% atropine instilled every 4 to 6 hours, to relieve pain from ciliary spasm and prevent synechiae formation. Once effective cycloplegia is achieved, the frequency of administration can be reduced to once or twice daily for maintenance. For uveitis associated with septicemia, topical broad-spectrum antimicrobials, such as neomycin/polymyxin B, gentamicin, or chloramphenicol, are indicated. Topical corticosteroids (e.g., prednisolone acetate) reduce intraocular inflammation, whereas parenteral NSAIDs, such as flunixin meglumine or phenylbutazone, reduce intraocular inflammation and promote analgesia.

JOINT INFECTIONS

Septic arthritis or osteomyelitis is often a complicating feature of neonatal septicemia. Treatment of septic arthritis includes drainage and removal of debris from the joint and adjacent tissues as well as articular rest.

Septic arthritis may benefit from joint lavage using sterile polyionic solutions. Intra-articular antibiotics are not necessary because parenteral antibiotics (especially intravenous) provide therapeutic drug levels within the synovial fluid and in the synovial lining. Therapeutic concentrations of many antibiotics can be obtained in the synovial fluid after normal parenteral administration. Intra-articular injection can be used, but complications often ensue from this local method of administration.

Irrigation and lavage of the affected joints are beneficial because inflammatory debris and lysosomal enzymes, which are the major causes of cartilage destruction, can be removed. Septic arthritis is frequently associated with osteomyelitis. If osteomyelitis is identified early enough, specific systemic antimicrobial therapy is effective.

Ischemia, however, is an important aspect of osteomyelitis because microorganisms thrive in avascular bone. Gentamicin, cephalosporin, and ampicillin can be useful antibiotics by the intravenous route. Lincomycin, although good for bone penetration, must not be used in horses.

Systemic administration of NSAIDs is beneficial to relieve pain and diminish the effects of inflammation. Therapy with exogenous sodium hyaluronate (Hylartin V, Pharmacia) or polysulfated glycosaminoglycan (Adequan, Luitpold Pharmaceuticals) can be of benefit in decreasing synovitis; inhibiting enzymatic processes, which cause cartilage deterioration; and stimulating metabolic repair of cartilage.

Treatment of septic arthritis can benefit from intra-articular joint lavage with buffered sterile polyionic solutions. Irrigation and lavage of distended joints removes the inflammatory debris and exudate responsible for cartilage damage. Such a lavage can be performed after sedation of the foal with xylazine or detomidine. Intra-articular antibiotics are rarely warranted and may in fact induce local chemical synovitis, which is detrimental to the artricular cartilage.

Acute osteomyelitis requires intensive longterm antimicrobial therapy. If there is evidence of bone lysis, sequestration, or abscessation, surgical debridement and insertion of an indwelling drain are indicated.

UMBILICUS

To prevent infections of the umbilicus, the cord should be allowed to break spontaneously. The stump should be painted with a mild antiseptic, such as povidone-iodine solution or 2% tincture of iodine. Irritants must be avoided because they may directly induce necrosis of tissue, which then traps bacteria, causing a focus of infection for development of septicemia or a local umbilical abscess. Premature rupture of the cord can deprive the foal of appreciable quantities of blood, resulting in marked weakness and a disinclination to ingest adequate colostrum.

BACTERIAL PNEUMONIA IN FOALS

The respiratory tract is one of the main portals of entry for bacteria in foals, so it is not surprising that foal pneumonia constitutes one of the most frequently encountered infections in young foals. Infection of the lower respiratory tract may occur alone or in conjunction with more generalized infections. Bacterial pneumonia is one of the most common forms of lower respiratory infections encountered in the young foal. Bacteria most commonly involved are those associated with septicemia. Intrauterine infections of the dam and failure of passive transfer of maternal antibodies are among the most common predisposing causes.

Supportive care is of vital importance in the management of pneumonic foals, especially those with concurrent septicemia. Such care is usually necessary to maintain life until antibiotic therapy and the foal's immune system can control the infection. General measures include:

1. Provision of heat
2. Oxygen if the foal is hypoxic
3. Intravenous fluids to combat cardiovascular collapse. Balanced polyionic fluids, such as lactated Ringer's solution, are usually suitable administered at 30 to 40 ml/kg/hour. Dextrose saline (5%) can be used to counter any tendency to hypoglycemia.
4. If failure of passive transfer confirmed, plasma infusion indicated to boost circulating immunoglobulin levels. A dose of 20 ml plasma/kg should be administered slowly intravenously.

Streptococcus species are the most common bacteria involved in foal pneumonia, and in most cases they are susceptible to penicillins. A combination of a penicillin with an aminoglycoside (amikacin or gentamicin) or alternatively a potentiated sulfonamide is indicated for mixed infections. Ampicillin and especially amoxicillin reach high concentrations in the respiratory tract and secretions of foals. When gentamicin is used, regular monitoring of renal functioning is indicated.

The most commonly isolated organisms from the equine respiratory tract include *Streptococcus zooepidemicus*, gram-negative, nonenteric bacteria (*Actinobacillus* and *Pasteurella*), gram-negative, enteric bacteria (*Klebsiella, E. coli, Salmonella*), and miscellaneous organisms, such as *Bordetella, Pseudomonas,* and *Staphylococcus.* The most common anaerobe is usually *Fusobacterium necrophorum* followed by *Bacteroides.*

S. zooepidemicus is usually sensitive to penicillin, and this antibiotic should be the preferred drug for initial therapy of infectious equine respiratory tract disease. Procaine penicillin G, at a dosage of 25,000 U/kg body weight intramuscularly, is usually effective in these cases if the duration of therapy is suffcient and if the horse is rested in a reasonable environment.

Because streptococci are the most common bacteria involved in infections of the lower respiratory tract, penicillin is the logical choice for antimicrobial therapy. Penicillin is also effective against many isolates of gram-negative, nonenteric bacteria, such as *Pasteurella* and *Actinobacillus.* Aminoglycosides, such as gentamicin or kanamycin, can be combined with penicillins in the event of penicillin-resistant, gram-negative bacteria being involved. Used alone, aminoglycosides have poor activity against streptococci, although gentamicin is effective against staphylococci, *Pseudomonas, Klebsiella, Salmonella,* and *E. coli.* Additionally, aminoglycosides are expensive and potentially nephrotoxic, especially in young animals with reduced renal output secondary to dehydration. Amikacin is useful in many cases in which response to gentamicin or kanamycin is disappointing. When using penicillin, therapy should begin with high-dosage soluble sodium benzylpenicillin intravenously together with procaine penicillin intramuscularly, which provides lower but longer levels.

Other beta lactam antibiotics, such as ampicillin, amoxicillin, or cephalothin, provide useful levels in the respiratory tract and its secretions. Although broad spectrum in activity, the semisynthetic penicillins are less effective against gram-positive organisms than is penicillin G. The spectrum of ticarcillin is similar to that of ampicillin except that ticarcillin is highly effective against *Pseudomonas aeruginosa.* Amoxicillin and particularly gentamicin attain high levels in the bronchial secretions relative to their plasma levels. Potentiated sulfonamide preparations are good broad-spectrum agents on account of their wide range of antimicrobial efficacy and the high concentrations attained within the respiratory tract. Sulfadiazine attains high concentration in

TABLE 20–9
ANTIBIOTICS FOR FOALS WITH RESPIRATORY INFECTIONS

Drug	Dose	Route	Frequency
Procaine penicillin G	20,000–50,000 IU/kg	IM	BID
Potassium or sodium penicillin G	50,000 IU/kg	IV	QID
Sodium ampicillin	30–100 mg/kg	IV	QID
	20–50 mg/kg	IV, IM	TID
Gentamicin sulfate	2.2 mg/kg	IV, IM	TID
Amikacin sulfate	6.6 mg/kg	IV, IM	TID
Trimethoprim-sulfadiazine	30 mg/kg	PO, IV	BID
Erythromycin estolate	15–25 mg/kg	PO	QID

IM, intramuscular; IV, intravenous; PO, oral; BID, two times a day; QID, four times a day; TID, three times a day.

the respiratory secretions. Trimethoprim also attains relatively high, prolonged levels. Although penicillins are now the drugs of choice for most acute equine respiratory infections, which are usually caused by penicillin-sensitive streptococci, sulfadiazine-trimethoprim combinations may be more effective on account of significant beta lactamase production by gram-negative nonpathogens in the respiratory tract, which adversely affects penetration of the intact penicillin molecule. Potentiated sulfonamides also possess the advantage of being available in a suitable paste formulation for oral administration to young animals (Table 20–9).

Antibiotic therapy must be maintained for at least 5 to 7 days after cessation of clinical symptoms. If some improvement is not apparent within 3 to 5 days after initiation of therapy, the entire therapeutic regimen should be re-evaluated. Because pneumonia in neonatal foals can be complicated by atelectasis and respiratory failure, oxygen therapy may have to be considered. Intranasal humidified oxygen (4 to 10 liters/minute) may help to raise arterial P_{O_2}. A nonrebreathing resuscitation bag attached to a mask or endotracheal tube is a useful alternative means of oxygen supply. Nebulization of mucolytics, beta$_2$-adrenergic agonists (isoproterenol, salbutamol, terbutaline, clenbuterol), or aminophylline together with antimicrobials can be of benefit in acutely affected foals. In the event of severe respiratory distress and central respiratory depression, an analeptic agent, such as doxapram, may be considered. Bronchodilators are also indicated individually (Table 20–10).

Fluid therapy with balanced electrolyte solutions is indicated in some cases to main-

TABLE 20–10
BRONCHODILATORS FOR RESPIRATORY INFECTIONS IN FOALS

Drug	Mode of Action	Dose
Atropine	Parasympatholytic	0.01 mg/kg
Glycopyrrolate	Parasympatholytic	0.005 mg/kg
Theophylline	Phosphodiesterase inhibitor	12 mg/kg BID
Clenbuterol	Beta$_2$, adrenergic-agonist	0.8 μg/kg BID (Legal status?)
Terbutaline	Beta, adrenergic	0.06 mg/kg TID

BID, two times a day; TID, three times a day.

**TABLE 20–11
DRUG THERAPY FOR GASTRIC
ULCERATION**

Agent	Oral	IV
Cimetidine	8.8 mg/kg TID	6.6 mg/kg
Ranitidine	4.4 mg/kg BID	0.5 mg/kg
Sucralfate	2–4 gm QID	—

tain hydration and promote mucociliary clearance and expectoration by reducing the viscosity of tenacious bronchial secretions. Hyperhydration is practiced by some clinicians to assist further in mobilizing secretions, i.e., the use of intravenous hypertonic fluids.

20.5 GASTROINTESTINAL DISORDERS IN FOALS

During the first 6 months of life, diarrhea can affect up to 75% of foals, and if fluid and electrolyte balance is not monitored or imbalances treated early enough, mortality can be heavy. Foal diarrhea is attributable to many causes, including foal heat, parasitism, nutrition, bacteria, viruses, protozoa, and injudicious antibiotic therapy. Complications of foal diarrhea include impaction by meconium or foreign body, aerophagia, intestinal displacement and torsion, reflux aspiration pneumonia, and gastric ulceration in the glandular position of the stomach.

Klebsiella, *E. coli*, and *Actinobacillus* can cause diarrhea in foals with low serum globulin levels, especially when intake of colostrum has not been adequate. *R. equi*, although frequently associated with lung damage, can also cause primary diarrhea accompanied by fever.

Salmonellosis in foals less than 2 weeks old is characterized by an acute septicemia/bacteremia, which if severe enough can result in death before diarrhea develops. Symptoms of septicemia include seizures, colic, uveitis, joint distention, respiratory dysfunction and profuse watery diarrhea. Occasionally postoperative diarrhea may be due to invasion of *Salmonella* pathogens also. In very young foals, *Clostridium perfringens* types B and C and *Clostridium sordellii* can be responsible for severe hemorrhagic enteritis in the first few days of life. Other agents implicated from time to time include cryptosporidia and *Campylobacter*. Also, viruses (rota, corona, adeno, parvo) are now known to be of major significance.

Rotavirus infection primarily affects foals less than 2 months old and results in anorexia, depression, and a profuse watery diarrhea and severe dehydration. Coronavirus infection causes severe intestinal damage, and adenovirus can infect an already immunodeficient foal. Parvovirus infection results in villous atrophy and destruction of the crypt epithelial cells.

Some neonatal foals benefit from receiving an enema, *Lactobacillus* paste orally, tetanus antitoxin, and penicillin-dihydrostreptomycin soon after birth. At 4 days of age, more *Lactobacillus* paste can be given. Tetanus toxoid and vaccination against encephalitis influenza and pneumonitis should be given and the foal dewormed with a paste anthelmintic at 30, 60, and 90 days of age. The immunization and deworming are repeated at weaning, and deworming is done every month in first year of life. *Lactobacillus* pastes (probiotics) are useful in some foals in decreasing the risk of chronic diarrhea and unthriftiness.

Diarrhea, which is a clinical sign rather than a specific disease entity, can be secondary to systemic disease. The most important aspects of therapy for diarrhea are supportive care and maintenance of fluid electrolytes and acid-base levels. Antibiotics may be used when systemic involvement is evident. Flunixin meglumine, 1.1 mg/kg, may be helpful in suppressing diarrhea caused by enterotoxins and in decreasing inflammation of the bowel. Other agents, such as bismuth subsalicylate, intestinal lubricants, probiotics (*Lactobacillus* cultures), activated charcoal, and paregoric, can be considered also. Atropine, hyoscine, and methoscopolamine are best avoided because these drugs can easily decrease gut motility and induce ileus.

The ultimate cause of death in the diarrheic foal is attributable to dehydration, shock, and electrolyte imbalance. Thus fluid and electrolyte replacement therapy is the major factor in the management of the affected animal. Measures must be rapidly instigated toward replenishing the losses of sodium, chloride, bicarbonate, potassium, calcium, and water; counteracting any hypovolemia and decreased tissue perfusion; and preventing the occurrence of lactic acidosis and renal failure. Oral fluid and electrolyte therapy is satisfactory, especially with oral products containing glucose, glycine, and electrolytes.

The gastrointestinal mucosa can be protected by oral administration of bismuth subsalicylate. In the general treatment of gastrointestinal disease in the horse, there are three primary therapeutic considerations:

1. The elimination of the infectious agent(s)
2. The restoration of fluid, electrolyte, and caloric deficits
3. The prevention of any further metabolic deficits

Many cases of diarrhea can be controlled with supplementation of fluids and electrolytes alone. Care must be taken when using antimicrobial agents in horses for the control of diarrhea—in many cases, they may not only be clinically ineffective but may worsen the condition.

Simply to prevent secondary bacterial infection is not an adequate indication for antibiotic therapy, especially for salmonellosis in foals, because most broad-spectrum agents have potentially significant adverse side effects. Antibiotic-associated diarrhea is often associated with orally administered antibiotics.

FLUIDS AND ELECTROLYTES

Oral preparations for use in calves that contain glucose, amino acids, and electrolytes are beneficial in foals. For the first 24 hours of treatment, the foals should receive nothing by mouth. While milk is being withheld, however, a number of oral products may not meet the young animal's energy requirements, and so a risk of the development of hypoglycemia exists. Adequate energy supplementation must therefore always be ensured. A useful formula for oral use consists of sodium chloride, 30 g; po-

tassium chloride, 5 g; and sodium bicarbonate, 12 g per gallon of water to which 2% glucose can be added. Oral *Lactobacillus* cultures (probiotics) together with vitamin supplementation may be of use during the recovery period and also as prophylactic agents to in-contact or to high-risk foals.

Severely affected foals (weakness, dry mucous membrane, decreased skin elasticity) require intravenous fluid and electrolyte therapy. Intravenous fluids should preferably be isotonic, and Ringer's solution or lactate Ringer's solution are useful fluids for parenteral therapy. Although these readily available fluids are alkalinizing solutions, useful for the reversal of mild acidosis owing to bicarbonate loss, it may be necessary in cases of severe acidosis to administer parenteral sodium bicarbonate (1.3 g/liter) as an isotonic alkalinizing solution. Loss of potassium can be significant in diarrhea also, and supplementation at a rate of 20 meq/liter of potassium to all fluids may be beneficial initially. To prevent development of hypoglycemia, solutions of 5% dextrose are indicated.

Initially warmed polyionic electrolyte solutions should be infused at 40 m/kg. Intravenous 5% dextrose should be given to prevent hypoglycemia.

In the event of hypoproteinemia, when plasma protein content drops below 4.5 g/dl, plasma infusion may be required to augment plasma oncotic pressure to normal. Administration of 1 to 3 liters of plasma can produce a rapid effect in the reversal of hypoproteinemia in the clinically affected foal, especially when *Salmonella* species are implicated.

LOCALLY ACTING AGENTS

Drugs acting as gastrointestinal protectants are beneficial in foals affected with enteritis. Such agents, acting locally in the bowel, prevent further loss of fluid and electrolytes from the lumen of the gastrointestinal tract. Bismuth subsalicylate is one of the more useful agents locally because it also possesses some antibacterial activity, neutralizes bacterial toxins, and exerts an antisecretory effect through its local antiprostaglandin activity. The usual dosage is 4 oz every 6 hours. Preparations containing kaolin pectin and activated charcoal are also useful for protection of the inflamed enteric mucosa and adsorption of toxins.

Motility inhibitors, such as methscopolamine or atropine, are contraindicated in foals with diarrhea because of their innumerable side effects and local actions. These drugs can facilitate proximal migration of pathogens with the alimentary tract.

Although hypermotility may contribute to the diarrheic state, changes in motility patterns may be important in the pattern of resistance to the disease. Drugs such as opioids, which slow intestinal transit time, can increase bacterial proliferation, delay the disappearance of the organism for the feces, and prolong the febrile state. In horses with salmonellosis, such drugs may result in enhanced intestinal secretions and endotoxemia. In extreme cases, antisecretory agents (flunixin meglumine or aspirin) may be indicated, particulary when a severe dehydration or shocklike syndrome exists.

Prostaglandins stimulate intestinal secretions by increasing intracellular concentrations of cyclic adenosine monophosphate (cAMP) and by mediating the effects of calcium on secretion. Inhibitors of prostaglandin synthesis have a role to play as useful antidiarrheic agents in horses. Flunixin meglumine has a beneficial effect on hemodynamics in horses with acute diarrhea and endotoxemia; dosage is 0.25 mg/kg three times a day. NSAIDs have a number of side effects, however, which may contraindicate their use in foals, not the least of which is the associated risk of ulceration of the gastrointestinal epithelial lining by virtue of their antiprostaglandin activity.

ANTIMICROBIAL THERAPY

Foals should be given antimicrobials less frequently than adults because the immature hepatic microsomal system prolongs the drugs' half-life. Also, because the extracellular fluid volume of foals is proportionately nearly twice that of adults, the volume of drug distribution is greater, necessitating larger dosages.

Therapy with antibiotics must be restricted to those cases in which the considered view of the veterinary clinician indicates prudent, judicious use of chemotherapy on rational grounds. Many antimicrobial agents, especially broad-spectrum antibacterials, have potentially deleterious effects on the gut or its flora. Diarrhea in foals receiving antibiotic therapy can occur, especially in response to tetracyclines or potentiated sulfonamide combinations. After oral use of antibiotics, the normal intestinal flora can be altered, with the resultant overgrowth of pathogenic microorganisms or fungi, such as Candida. Diarrhea can be profuse, watery, and refractory to therapy, but it usually subsides in 24 to 48 hours after withdrawal of the implicated antibiotics. Aminoglycosides can be nephrotoxic in diarrheic dehydrated foals with compromised renal function.

The incidence of septicemia caused by gram-negative agents is extremely high. Therefore aminoglycoside antibiotics, gentamicin amikacin, and kanamycin, may need to be used therapeutically. Precautions to avoid aminoglycoside toxicity include pretreatment, measurement of blood urea nitrogen and creatinine, monitoring urine for casts and red blood cells, and monitoring of serum creatinine.

Although antimicrobial agents themselves do not dramatically alter the clinical course of enteritis, they can play an important role in minimizing the degree of systemic involvement and the likely risk of secondary foci of localized bacterial infections (e.g., septic arthritis, osteomyelitis), especially if severe septicemia exists (e.g., *Salmonella* infection).

In very young foals in which *C. perfringens* type B or C is a problem, treatment is by way of intravenous penicillin V combined with an aminoglycoside. *Actinobacillus* infection is best treated with intravenous ampicillin (22 mg/kg four times a day) combined with gentamicin or amikacin. Alternatively, trimethoprim-sulfadizine (30 mg/twice a day) may be considered.

Occasionally peritonitis results from the infection of the upper gastrointestinal tract, and this may be treated with either ampicillin or penicillin-aminoglycoside combination. It is not unusual to find anaerobic organisms involved in peritonitis. When anaerobes are implicated, penicillins should be used but not aminoglycosides. The most preferable drug for anaerobic infections is metronidazole, at a dosage of 15–20 mg/kg orally or by slow intravenous drip or injection. Potomac horse fever can be treated with oxytetracycline, 6.6 mg/kg SID for 5 days. Oxytetracycline usually relieves the fever but does not prevent the disease. Great care should be exercised when using this drug in horses because side effects in the gastrointestinal tract are not unusual.

SALMONELLOSIS

This disease is usually confined to large concentrations of horses in hospitals, farms, or studs, where stress and intimate contact is likely to occur. Transportation and intercurrent disease may be a precipitating factor. The most common mode of transmission is oral contact with the organism. Diarrheic cattle in contact with hospitalized horses can precipitate outbreaks of salmonellosis, especially in closely stocked or hospitalized horses. Recovered animals can continue to excrete *Salmonella* organisms in the feces for some time after clinical recovery.

Salmonella typhimurium, Salmonella enteritidis, Salmonella anatum, Salmonella heidelberg, and *Salmonella newport* are the most common serotypes associated with diarrhea in adult horses. Of the most commonly isolated salmonellae, only *S. typhimurium* is isolated with any degree or frequency from extraintestinal sites.

Of the 5 to 10% of horses believed to be infected at any one time, most are asymptomatic carriers or sporadic fecal shedders. Many clinical cases continue to excrete salmonellae during antimicrobial therapy even though in vitro culture tests may reveal sensitivity to the antimicrobial agents employed.

Clinically normal carriers of *S. typhimurium* can become symptomatic and initiate outbreaks following stress. Horses showing acute enteritis and diarrhea associated with *Salmonella* infection become markedly dehydrated and demonstrate a metabolic acidosis. Salmonellosis in young foals in usually manifested by an acute septicemia-bacteremia that often results in death before diarrhea even develops.

Isolation, avoidance of stress, and culture and bacterial sensitivity should be implemented in any suspected case of salmonellosis. Treatment must include primarily the correction of fluid and electrolyte imbalances, reduction of stress, and counteracting the effects of shock by the administration of NSAIDs or massive doses of corticosteroids. Antimicrobial drugs must not receive undue emphasis in treatment. Initial culturing is essential.

Antibiotics do not generally alter the clinical course of salmonellosis. Such therapy, if embarked on injudiciously, can prolong the fecal excretion of *Salmonella* organisms after the clinical disease has disappeared. Also, antimicrobial therapy may favor the development of antibiotic-resistant strains, which in turn can instigate generalized infections with resistant strains. Although antibiotics may reduce the number of susceptible organisms, transfer of resistance may be hastened by increasing the likelihood of contact between drug-resistant flora and *Salmonella* species. Thus indiscriminate therapy with antimicrobial drugs is counterproductive. Initial culture and sensitivity testing is essential, as is the specific initial treatment at the onset of the disease. Apart from the risk of increased carrier states, fecal shedding, and bacterial resistance, adverse effects, such as superinfection, mycotic colitis, and ulceration, have been observed in horses receiving antibiotic and corticosteroid medication. Oxytetracycline and lincomycin have been particularly implicated in many drug-induced disorders, culminating in colitis or diarrhea. They are contraindicated in salmonellosis therapy.

Antibiotic therapy frequently elicits highly variable results, particularly from infected horses or symptomless carriers. Therapy must be specific and directed toward isolates known to be susceptible to the antibiotic in question, especially in cases of bacteremia. Severe cases of salmonellosis with accompanying intestinal damage are unlikely to respond to antimicrobial drugs alone. Restoration of fluid and electrolyte balance, treatment of shock, and symptomatic control therapy for the severe diarrhea of salmonellosis is most important. Clinical recovery is more probable when vigorous supportive therapy and good nursing are employed.

When antimicrobial therapy is indicated, the parenteral route should be used. Oral antibiotic therapy with broad-spectrum drugs causes problems in the large intestine, where alterations of the bacterial flora may favor superinfections with microorganisms, such as clostridia or fungi.

Antimicrobial drugs are indicated in the early stages of acute salmonellosis. Depending on the sensitivity of the isolates, useful agents may include trimethoprim-sulfadiazine, ampicillin, gentamicin, amikacin, chloramphenicol, moxalactam, and polymyxin B.

Because salmonellosis is an intracellular infection, antibiotic sensitivity tests based on in vitro assays are not always useful. This is because of the difficulty of intracellular penetration in vivo. A reasonable first-choice antimicrobial agent is trimethoprim-sulfadiazine. Many foals with acute intestinal salmonellosis are also bacteremic, and ampicillin, gentamicin, and amikacin are useful antibiotics. Amikacin is usually more effective than gentamicin and is administered parenterally at a dosage of 6.6 mg/kg two or three times a day in foals more than 4 weeks of age. Moxalactam, a third-generation cephalosporin, given intravenously at 22 mg/kg four times a day, is beneficial in salmonellosis, but the cost of the drug limits its general use.

Overall, if the isolated salmonellae are sensitive to trimethoprim-sulfonamide, this combination is the initial drug of choice. Affected animals must be isolated and the environment disinfected. In the young septicemic animal, parenteral antibiotic therapy should be attempted, but in other animals, in which fluid therapy is the key to a successful outcome of the condition, such an approach is frequently futile.

GASTRIC ULCERATION IN FOALS

Gastric ulceration is a particular risk in young foals, especially those of the 1- to 6-month-old age group. Many factors predispose to this condition, and the use of NSAIDs has been implicated in its cause.

Gastric ulceration in foals has become a significant problem in recent years because of the increasing number of foals demonstrating clinical signs characteristic of duodenal ulceration and the higher incidence of sudden deaths from perforated gastric or duodenal ulcers. The advent of endoscopy has heightened awareness of the condition.

Several factors aid in protecting the lining of the stomach from digestion by hydrochloric acid. Principal among these are the mucous bicarbonate layer that covers the glandular mucosal surface, prostaglandin E_2, and mucosal blood flow. Prostaglandin E_2 enhances the secretion of bicarbonate-rich mucus, suppresses hydrochloric acid secretion, and promotes mucosal blood flow. Excessive use of NSAIDs results in ulceration of both glandular and squamous mucosal linings in foals and adult horses. Through inhibition of prostaglandin E_2, NSAIDs promote acid secretion, diminish mucosal blood flow, and compromise the mucus bicarbonate barrier.

Stress is another predisposing factor, as is infection. *Helicobacter* (formerly *Campylobacter*) *pyloris* is highly prevalent in humans with peptic ulcers and has been considered a primary pathogen in humans. Rotavirus, *Salmonella*, and *Candida* have also been associated with gastric lesions in foals.

Choice of drug option depends on location and severity of the lesions. Sucralfate (Carafate, Marion Merell Dow) is a mucosal protective agent. A sulfated polysaccharide, its mechanism of action is one of adhering to the ulcerated mucosa, stimulating mucus production, and enhancing prostaglandin E syntheses. It can be used as an adjunct to H_2 antagonists, although 2 hours should separate their application. H_2 antagonists suppress hydrochloric acid secretion through competitive inhibition of the parietal cell histamine receptor.

A dose of 4.4 mg/kg three times a day of ranitidine is usually given orally, although this can be increased to 6.6 mg/kg three times a day. The intravenous dose is 0.5 mg/kg. Cimetidine is somewhat less potent than ranitidine, and a recommended dosage is 8.8 mg/kg every 4 to 6 hours. H_2 antagonist therapy should be continued for 14 to 21 days. This may be sufficient to clear up the condition, although longer therapy may be warranted in more severe cases. Cimetidine intravenously is popularly used at 6.6 mg/kg every 4 to 6 hours or as a continuous infusion in intravenous fluids at 1.1 to 2.2 mg/kg/hour.

Antacids have not been widely used in horses. Approximately 180 ml of magnesium/aluminum hydroxide antacid given orally to horses results in an elevation of gastric fluid pH for 15 to 30 minutes. Administration of 250 ml magnesium/aluminum hydroxide is useful follow-up therapy for animals that have already responded to H_2 antagonists.

Antacids should be given after meals. Because of rapid gastric emptying, their effectiveness is slight on an empty stomach.

Specific H_2-receptor blocking agents, e.g., ranitidine and cimetidine, inhibit acid secretion, and cimetidine has been used on foals since 1982.

Sucralfate is a compound of aluminum hydroxide with a sucrose sulfate moiety. It is well tolerated by foals. It possesses weak antacid properties related to the slow release of aluminum hydroxide from the compound. When exposed to acid, sucralfate forms an adherent, viscous chemical complex at the site of ulceration. The compound's cytoprotective effects are related to its ability to inhibit the action of pepsin and the release of prostaglandin E into the luminal tract. The recommended dosage of sucralfate in foals varies from 2 to 4 g three to four times a day orally. Sucralfate might reduce the bioavailability of cimetidine when the drugs are not given 2 hours apart.

The incidence of gastroduodenal ulceration is highest in suckling foals younger than 4 months of age. The correlation between stress, NSAIDs, dietary factors, or infectious causes and ulceration is not completely understood. Successful therapy depends on early recognition and treatment with antacids and antisecretory or cytoprotective gastric agents.

PARASITIC INFECTION

Diarrhea associated with parasitic infection is common in young foals. *Strongyloides westeri* larvae are passed from the mare to the foal through the milk. Effective parasiticides include ivermectin, thiabendazole, cambendazole, and oxibendazole. Pain attributable to internal parasites can follow deworming of foals heavily infected with *Parascaris equorum* and subsequent impaction. This type of intestinal obstruction is more common when rapidly acting anthelmintics, such as piperazine or organophosphates, are used. The risk is less with more slowly acting drugs, such as benzimidazoles.

Acute abdominal pain, intestinal infarction, or enteritis can be seen with infection of *Strongylus vulgaris* larvae. Effective anthelmintics include ivermectin, fenbendazole, oxfendazole, and thiabendazole. (See Chapter 17.)

Strongyloides can be transmitted in the colostrum or possibly transplacentally and may cause moderate diarrhea. Treatment is with thiabendazole, 44 mg/kg; ivermectin, 200 µg/kg; or oxibendazole, at 10 mg/kg.

COLITIS

Colitis in horses often involves severe inflammation of the caecum and large colon and can give rise to diarrhea, fever, endotoxemia, and septic chock. Treatment of most cases of colitis must be intensive on account of the large volumes of fluid replacement necessary. Colitis in the horse has many causes: Infectious agents include *Salmonella enteritidis*, *Ehrlichia risticii* (Potomac horse fever). Certain of the clostridia viruses, antibiotics, NSAIDs, and grain impaction have also been implicated.

In colitis, regardless of the cause, tremendous losses of fluid, sodium, chloride, bicarbonate, and potassium can occur. Leakage of protein from the colonic epithelium can occur owing to the local toxins and inflammatory mediators. For this reason, hypoproteinemia, local inflammation, and extensive fluid and electrolyte loss typify the symptoms of equine colitis. Septicemia, bacteremia, and endotoxemia are common sequelae. Endotoxins are lipopolysaccharides found in the outer cell membranes of gram-negative bacteria. These are not normally absorbed from the bowel, but when the integrity of the colonic mucosa is damaged, these endotoxins are absorbed transmurally.

Metabolic acidosis frequently accompanies colitis because of the colon's failure to reabsorb bicarbonate. Hypertonic saline can be used to treat severe hypovolemic shock, acute hemorrhagic shock, and equine endotoxemia. Normal saline is 0.9% NaCl; hypertonic solutions are 2400 mOsmoL NaCl.

The mechanism of action appears to be vagally mediated and requires passage of the solution through the lungs for its effects to occur. The advantage is speed of administration and the small volume required.

Endotoxemia can be countered with 0.25 mg/kg dosage of flunixin meglumine. Early treatment with this NSAID can mitigate the systemic effects of absorbed endotoxin. DMSO possesses anti-inflammatory action and also scavenges free radicals produced by stimulated neutrophils. DMSO given intravenously as a 10% solution of 100 to 200 mg/kg/day can be effective for anti-inflammatory control in colitis.

Commercial equine endotoxin antisera are now available. These appear to be particularly useful in carbohydrate overload models with subsequent endotoxin absorption.

Antimicrobial drugs must be used judiciously in equine colitis if at all. The use of tetracyclines has always been controversial. For salmonellosis, specific sensitivities must be determined, and in many cases, antibiotics do not alter the course of the disease. When septicemia or bacteremia is threatened, careful use of broad-spectrum antibiotics is justified.

Control of secretions by means of bismuth subsalicylate, kaolin, or activated charcoal can be effective in limiting excessive colonic secretions. Other useful antisecretory drugs include NSAID, alpha$_2$-adrenergic agonists, and drugs that affect cellular calcium metabolism. See also Chapter 6.

SELECTED REFERENCES

Becht, J.L., and Semrad, S.D.: Gastrointestinal diseases of foals. Comp. Cont. Educ. Pract. Vet., 8:7S367, 1986.

Beech, J.: Chronic obstructive pulmonary disease. Vet. Clin. North Am. [Equine Pract.], 7:79, 1991.

Beech, J.: Drug therapy of respiratory disorders. Vet. Clin. North Am. [Equine Pract.], 3:59, 1987.

Beech, J.: Respiratory problems in foals. Comp. Cont. Educ. Pract. Vet., 8:S284, 1986.

Beech, J., and Merryman, G.S.: Immunotherapy for equine respiratory disease. Eq. Vet. Sci., 6:6, 1986.

Burrows, G.E., MacAllister, C.G., Beckstrom, D.A., et al.: Rifampin in the horse: Comparison of intravenous intramuscular and oral administration. Am. J. Vet. Res., 46:442, 1985.

Campbell-Thompson, M.L., and Merritt, A.M.: Effect of ranitidine on gastric acid secretion in young male horses. Am. J. Vet. Res., 48: 1511, 1987.

Caprile, K., and Short, C.: Pharmacologic considerations in drug therapy in foals. Vet. Clin. North Am. [Equine Pract.], 3: 1987.

Carter, G.K., and Brown, S.A.: Use of antibiotics in foals. Proc. Amer. Assoc. Eq. Pract. XX:209, 1986.

Carter, G.K., and Martens, R.J.: Septicemia in the neonatal foal. Comp. Cont. Educ. Pract. Vet., 8:S256, 1986.

Conboy, S.H.: Neonatal treatment techniques. Proc. Amer. Assoc. Eq. Pract. 28:369, 1982.

Divers, T.J., and Palmer, J.E.: Antimicrobial therapy in equine gastrointestinal disease. Proc. Amer. Assoc. Eq. Pract. XX:223, 1986.

Dixon, P.: Some observations on the penetration of antimicrobial drugs into the respiratory secretions of horses. In Lung Function and Respiratory Diseases in the Horse. Edited by E. Deegen and R.A. Beadle. International Symposium, Hannover, Germany, Hippiatrika, 1985.

Ellenberger, M.A., and Genetzky, R.M.: Rhodococcus equi infections. Literature review. Comp. Cont. Educ. Pract. Vet., 8:S414, 1986.

Feldman, M., and Burton, M.E.: Histamine 2 receptor antagonists. N. Engl. J. Med., 323:1672, 1990.

Firth, E. C.: Current concepts of infectious polyarthritis in foals. Eq. Vet. J., 15:5, 1983.

Furr, M.O., and Murray, M.J.: Treatment of gastric ulcers in horses with histamine type 2 receptor antagonists. Eq. Vet. J. 7(Suppl.):77, 1989.

Goetz, E.: Successful management of equine chronic obstructive pulmonary disease. Vet. Med., 79:1073, 1984.

Green, E.M., and Green, S.L.: Septicemia in neonatal foals. Part 2. Treatment. Mod. Vet. Pract., 68:90, 1987.

Hillidge, C.J.: Erythromycin and rifampin in combination for treatment of R. equi lung abscesses in foals. Proc. Ann. Med. Am./Assoc. Eq. Pract., 31:137, 1985.

Klein, J.D., Norton, C.R., Dashefsky, B., et al.: Selection of antimicrobial agents for treatment of neonatal sepsis. Rev. Infect. Dis. 5(Suppl.): S55, 1983.

Koterba, A.M.: Intensive care of the neonatal foal. Vet. Clin. North Am. [Equine Pract.], 1:3, 1985.

MacAllister, C.S., Sangiah, S., and Amouzedah, H.: The effects of cimetidine and ranitidine on gastric pH of fasted horses. Proc. 2nd Ann. Equine Colic Res. Symposium, 1987.

Madigan, J.E.: Caring for the newborn foal: The differences every practitioner should know about. Vet. Med., 63, 1986.

Morris, D., and Rutkowski, J.: Therapy in two cases of neonatal foal septicemia with cefoxatime sodium. Eq. Vet. J., 19: 151, 1987.

Morris, D.D., and Whitlock, R.H.: Therapy of suspected septicemia in neonatal foals, using plasma containing antibodies to core lipopolysaccharide. J. Vet. Intern. Med., 1:175, 1987.

Murray, M.: Diagnosing and treating gastric ulcers in foals and horses. Vet. Med., *86*:820, 1991.

Murray, M.J.: The progression of gastric lesions in young thoroughbred foals: An endoscopic study. J. Am. Vet. Med. Assoc., *196*:1623, 1990.

Murray, M.: Therapeutic procedures for horses with colitis. Vet. Med., *85*:510, 1990.

Nappert, G., Vrins, A., and Larybyere, M.: Gastroduodenal ulceration in foals. Comp. Cont. Educ. Pract. Vet., *11*:338, 1989.

Prescott, J.F., and Sweeney, C.R.: Treatment of Corynebacterium equi pneumonia of foals. J. Am. Vet. Med. Assoc., *187*:725, 1985.

Rifampin Physician's Desk Reference, 42nd ed. Oradell, NJ, Medical Economics Co., 1988.

Rouff, W.W., Read, W.K., and Cargihe, J.L.: An equine gastric ulcer model to test H_2 antagonists. Abstr. 68 Conf. Res. Workers An. Dis., *58*:10, 1987.

Sasse, W., and Deegen, E.: The efficacy of Sputolysin. Tierarzt. Umschau., *39*:941, 1984.

Sattler, F.R., and Remington, J.S.: Intravenous sulfamethoxozole and trimethoprim for serious gram negative bacillary infection. Arch. Intern. Med., *143*:1709, 1983.

Soma, L.R., Beech, J., and Gerber, N.H.: Effects of cromolyn in horses with chronic obstructive pulmonary disease. Vet. Res. Comm., *11*:339, 1987.

Wilson, J.H.: Gastric and duodenal ulcers in foals: A retrospective study. Proc. 2nd Eq. Colic Res. Symp. 1986.

21

NONSTEROIDAL AND STEROIDAL ANTI-INFLAMMATORY DRUGS IN HORSES

Nonsteroidal Anti-inflammatory Drugs
21.1 Introduction and History
21.2 Classification
21.3 Pharmacokinetics
21.4 Mechanism of Action
21.5 Toxicity and Side Effects
21.6 Pyrazolone Derivatives
Phenylbutazone
Dipyrone (Metamizole)
21.7 Oxicams
21.8 Salicylates
21.9 Propionic Acid Derivatives
Naproxen
Ketoprofen
21.10 Fenamates
21.11 Aminonicotinic Acid Derivatives
21.12 Clinical Uses
Steroids
21.13 Corticosteroids and their Formulations
21.14 Steroids and the Inflammatory Process
21.15 Shock
21.16 Other Effects of Steroids
21.17 Intra-Articular Therapy in Horses
21.18 Clinical Uses

21.1. INTRODUCTION AND HISTORY

The term "anti-inflammatory drug" refers to any pharmacologic compound that can inhibit one or several of the various stages of the inflammatory process. Many such compounds of diverse chemical structure recently have been introduced onto the market, and they tend to fall into two major groups—the steroid group (derived from the endogenous cortisone-type glucocorticoid of the body), which includes such potent members as prednisolone, dexamethasone, and betamethasone, and the nonsteroidal group typified by phenylbutazone, meclofenamic acid, naproxen, and flunixin. All these drugs can either suppress or reduce the inflammatory response and thus the cardinal clinical signs associated with the inflammatory process, such as heat, pain, swelling, hyperemia, and loss of function. They are often employed in equine practice as anti-inflammatory agents for the treatment of various acute or chronic conditions of the musculoskeletal system, and although the corticosteroids have been widely and successfully used in clinical conditions, the nonsteroidal group has attracted most interest in recent years. The constituent members of this group have become known collectively and logically as the nonsteroidal anti-inflammatory drugs (NSAIDs).

One of the major compounds of this group is undoubtedly phenylbutazone, which was introduced into human medicine in the 1940s and since has been widely used as an anti-inflammatory agent in humans.

The clinical application of phenylbutazone is accompanied by side effects, however, and because of these adverse reactions and toxicities, its application in humans has become more selective and judicious. Soon after its introduction into human medicine, phenylbutazone appeared on the veterinary pharmaceuticals market and quickly became the dominant NSAID used in the horse. During the last 20 years or so, phenylbutazone has been used with considerable success and clinical efficacy to treat various arthritic conditions of the horse. The spectacular success of phenylbutazone moved the pharmaceutical industry to devote considerable time and effort to researching new molecules with an efficacy comparable to or greater than that of phenylbutazone. Consequently, related compounds, such as meclofenamic acid, naproxen, ketoprofen, indomethacin, and flunixin also became available for equine use.

The origins of the nonsteroidal anti-inflammatory drugs are ancient. The Greek physician Hippocrates (460–377 BC), known as the "father of medicine," was aware of the analgesic properties of willow bark (*Salix alba*). Although the inherent therapeutic properties of the willow were forgotten by the medical profession for many centuries, the willow nonetheless continued to play a role in popular medicine.

Herb specialists administered boiled willow bark to their suffering patients. In 1763, Reverend Edward Stone gave the British Royal Society a report on experiments with salix (willow) bark on fevered patients. Because rheumatism was found primarily in damp geographic areas. Stone reasoned that the natural cure for such an illness also would be present in a wet vicinity. (Willow trees are most often seen at the water's edge.)

In 1829, Leroux extracted salicin, the glycoside responsible for the medicinal effects of the bark of the willow. Fifteen years later, Cahours prepared salicylic acid from oil of wintergreen (methyl salicylate). The synthetic production of salicylic acid from phenol was first accomplished in 1860. In 1876, proof of the antipyretic anti-inflammatory, and analgesic properties of salicylic acid were established in Berlin's Charite Hospital. Its major shortcomings, however, were an appalling taste and an irritant effect on the stomach.

In 1897, the chemist Felix Hoffman succeeded in refining salicylic acid by preparing it as the less irritant and soluble acetylsalicylic acid. In 1899, "aspirin" was introduced; "a" stands for acetyl and "spir" stands for "Spirsäure," the German word for "acid" (from Spirea.) Aspirin was introduced into medicine by Dreser in 1899.

The antiplatelet activity of aspirin has recently generated new indications for this old drug. In 1985, the U.S. Food and Drug Administration (FDA) indicated that a daily dose of acetylsalicylic acid could reduce the risk of a second heart attack by 20%, or by more than 50% in patients with unstable angina pectoris.

At present, chronic oral intake of low-dose aspirin is used to prevent arterial thrombosis. A dose of 75 mg daily is sufficient to decrease platelet stickiness and should also minimize side effects (gastric ulceration).

In 1990, low-dose aspirin (325 mg/day) was reported to alleviate the symptoms of migraine.

A recent development in human medicine has been the use of NSAIDs to inhibit the growth of colon tumors. In 1991, the use of regular aspirin in humans was reported to significantly reduce the risk of fatal colon cancer.

For decades aspirin has been the prototype NSAID against which all new introductions have been measured. In the last 30 years, NSAIDs and new formulations thereof have proliferated. They are all used in the symptomatic treatment of inflammation, e.g., in arthritis, tendinitis, and bursitis. Individual patient factors have an important effect on response to NSAIDs.

All NSAIDs possess a therapeutic threshold above which more medication does not provide greater analgesia. NSAIDs more effectively control somatic pain than visceral pain. They provide only symptomatic relief through their analgesic activity.

21.2. CLASSIFICATION

NSAIDs can be divided into two major groups—the enolic acids and the carboxylic acids. The enolic group can be subdivided further into (1) pyrazolone derivatives, such as phenylbutazone, oxyphenbutazone, and dipyrone, and (2) oxicam derivatives, such as piroxicam and meloxicam.

The carboxylic acids are comprised of (1) salicylic acid derivatives, such as aspirin and diflunisal, (2) propionic acid derivatives, such as ibuprofen, fenoprofen, flurbiprofen, ketoprofen, and naproxen, (3) acetic acid derivatives, such as indomethacin, sulindac, and tolmetin, (4) fenamates, such as meclofenamic acid, and (5) aminonicotinic acid derivatives, such as flunixin and clonixin (Table 21–1).

TABLE 21–1
CLASSIFICATION OF NSAIDs

Enolic Acids	*Pyrazolones*	Phenylbutazone
		Oxyphenbutazone
		Dipyrone
		Isopyrine
		Azapropazone
	Oxicams	Piroxicam
		Meloxicam
		Tenoxicam
Carboxylic Acids	*Salicylic Acids*	Aspirin
		Sodium salicylate
		Diflunisal
		Benorylate
	Propionic Acids	Ibuprofen
		Fenoprofen
		Flurbiprofen
		Naproxen
		Ketoprofen
	Fenamates	Meclofenamic acid
	Acetic Acid Derivatives	Indomethacin
		Sulindac (Prodrug)
		Tolmetin
	Aminonicotinic Acids	Flunixin
		Clonixin

TABLE 21–2
COMMON FEATURES OF NONSTEROIDAL ANTI-INFLAMMATORY DRUGS (NSAIDs)

- Highly acidic drugs.
- Highly protein bound in plasma.
- Act by inhibiting prostaglandin synthesis.
- Reduce pain in inflamed tissues by reducing tissue prostaglandin levels.
- Reduce fever.
- Accumulate in stomach, kidney, and small intestines and tend to produce lesions in these tissues.
- Difficult to detect in plasma.

In general, the mechanism of action and pharmacologic effects of all the NSAIDs are similar. All inhibit synthesis of central and peripheral prostaglandins.

Their pharmacokinetics vary, however, as does their enzyme affinity, and hence their clinical potency and side effects. Their primary actions are anti-inflammatory, analgesic, and antipyretic. These actions stem from their main mechanism of action—inhibition of prostaglandin synthesis. Many of their side effects, e.g., gastric ulceration, are also attributable to inhibition of prostaglandin synthesis.

All NSAIDs share several common features. As weak acids, they tend to penetrate the often more acidic environment of damaged or inflamed tissue. They are also well absorbed orally. When tissue is inflamed, the usual acidic pH ensures their local concentration at the site. They all have a pKa <4.5 (Table 21–2). Because of their low pKa values, these compounds have low water solubility. They are usually formulated as sodium salts to increase their water solubility. Such formulation also increases rate of absorption following oral administration.

Differences in pharmacokinetic patterns, affinity for cyclo-oxygenases (whether reversible or irreversible), bioavailability, and clearance times are responsible for the various potencies of the individual NSAIDs.

NSAIDs are effective primarily for the relief of minor musculoskeletal pain, but they are not effective in the treatment of severe visceral pain, such as that associated with visceral distention or torsion. Rates of renal clearance and half-lives vary for the different NSAIDs and also across species.

NSAIDs are used primarily for suppression of pain, inflammation, and pyrexia. They are also used for endotoxic shock and suppression of platelet aggregation.

21.3. PHARMACOKINETICS

The route by which the NSAIDs are administered has important consequences for their rate of absorption, metabolism, and elimination. The oral route is quite popular, and granules or powdered preparations in sachets are widely used. Numerous in-feed preparations of phenylbutazone have palatability problems, however, and as a result, several paste formulations administered by dosing syringe have been introduced.

As acidic drugs, NSAIDs are well absorbed from the gut. Irritancy is associated with the older salicylates; hence, buffered aspirin is used. Bioavailability differences following oral administration of various doses of NSAIDs among different breeds can be quite striking.

Aspirin is rapidly absorbed from the stomach and small intestine. Buffered aspirin is more soluble than is plain aspirin, but plain aspirin is less ionized in gastric juice. Following oral absorption, aspirin is hydrolyzed to acetate and salicylate in tissue and serum. Its pharmacologic effects are the result of plasma salicylate levels.

In the horse, phenylbutazone is absorbed mainly from the small intestine following oral administration, and peak plasma levels are reached after approximately 2–3 hours. (Oral doses of 4 g/1000 lb body weight usually give peak levels of about 20 µg/ml plasma). Several factors govern the rate and extent of absorption, and hence the overall bioavailability, of an oral dose of phenylbutazone and meclofenamic acid. Delayed absorption accompanied by lower peak plasma levels has been reported following oral administration on a full stomach compared to an empty stomach. Administration on an empty stomach results in higher peak plasma concentrations and a greater bioavailability of the oral dose.

Indeed, large variations in absorption rates and bioavailability may be observed in one animal. The pony displays a reduced capacity to absorb oral phenylbutazone and meclofenamic acid, and accordingly, the rate and extent of absorption of an oral dose are diminished in this species with a decrease in the overall bioavailability. This poorer absorption in the pony may lead to higher local concentrations in the large intestine. This feature may be related to the increased susceptibility of certain pony breeds to phenylbutazone toxicity.

Some drugs, notably phenylbutazone, dipyrone, isopyrin, flunixin, and ketoprofen, are available for parenteral intravenous administration. Flunixin is less irritant than phenylbutazone and therefore is recommended for intramuscular injection also.

Intravenous preparations of phenylbutazone are available for use in the horse, and these usually consist of phenylbutazone either alone or in combination with another pyrazole derivative, isopyrin. Isopyrin prolongs the half-life of phenylbutazone by competing for the phenylbutazone metabolizing enzymes.

Parenteral administration of NSAIDs can be painful upon injection. Consequently, several specific compounds may have to be rendered alkaline for injection. In horses, intramuscular administration of phenylbutazone can cause irritancy, local reactions, abscess formation, and sloughing. Local binding to protein at the muscle site may also delay its absorption (as long as 6 hours).

Most NSAIDs, including phenylbutazone, flunixin, ketoprofen, and dipyrone, are given to horses parenterally by the intravenous route.

The volume of distribution of NSAIDs is small because of the high degree of plasma albumin binding, which usually exceeds 96%.

Most NSAIDs have short half-lives. Also, these acidic compounds are rapidly excreted in the ionized form by the normally alkaline urine of the horse.

Despite their short half-lives, the clinical response to many NSAIDs is prolonged for several reasons. For most NSAIDs, no simple direct correlation exists between serum levels and concentrations attained at the inflammatory focus in the site of action. Even when plasma levels have declined or are no longer detectable, anti-inflammatory activity can still be present because of the binding and complexing with cyclo-oxygenases.

Some drugs, such as aspirin, bind irreversibly to platelet cyclo-oxygenase and hence display persistent activity. The analgesic and anti-inflammatory effects of aspirin are more short-lived because the binding to prostaglandin cyclo-oxygenase is reversible. In addition, some NSAIDs are converted into active metabolites, whereas most of the parent drugs accumulate more rapidly in inflammatory exudate, from which they are cleared more slowly than from plasma. Even drugs with a short half-life, such as flunixin (t1/2 = 1.6 hours) and meclofenamic acid (t1/2 = 0.9 hours), can achieve desirable clinical efficacy following once-daily administration in horses.

Despite the high plasma protein binding of these drugs, the level of drug in the inflammatory fluid often exceeds that in the plasma because some protein-bound drug can leak from the dilated permeable capillaries at the inflammatory focus.

Because of their high binding to plasma protein, they may displace or be displaced by other drugs from these binding sites. They can displace such anticoagulants (e.g. warfarin), hydantoins, sulfonamides, and some steroids.

These highly bound acidic drugs can compete with other highly bound drugs for the saturable binding sites on plasma albumin. Displacement of other highly bound acidic drugs, such as warfarin, can cause potentially serious results when such drugs are given simultaneously with phenylbutazone. For a highly bound drug such as warfarin (>96%), the displacement of only 2% from the albumin reservoir doubles the free unbound drug concentration with possibly serious results. A similar situation holds for phenylbutazone and sulfonamides.

NSAIDs must be used in strict accordance with dosage recommendations not only because of the "spillover" from saturation of plasma protein binding sites but also because of their innate toxicity.

Binding to muscle has been implicated in the slow rate of absorption of phenylbutazone from the intramuscular injection site.

Flunixin, meclofenamic acid, and phenylbutazone also can bind to dietary constituents and hay. Following oral administration, peak plasma concentrations may be delayed for as long as 18 hours. This delay may contribute to an increased local concentration in the large intestine and a consequent ulcerogenic effect.

With the notable exception of phenylbutazone, all the prostaglandin synthetase inhibitors are metabolized to pharmacologically inactive metabolites in the liver. Phenylbutazone is metabolized to oxyphenbutazone and hydroxyphenylbutazone, and together these derivatives comprise approximately 25% of the total drug administered. Oxyphenbutazone has clinical potency similar to that of the parent compound, and some of the anti-inflammatory properties of phenylbutazone probably result from oxyphenbutazone, which accumulates in the plasma following phenylbutazone administration and is then excreted. The metabolism is the primary and predominant factor responsible for reduction in plasma concentrations following drug administration. The dose-dependent kinetics of phenylbutazone in the horse, resulting in prolonged half-life and slower excretion at higher dosage rates, may reflect saturation of liver enzymes at high dosage levels and also inhibition of its metabolism by one of its metabolites.

An additive effect can be gained by combining two NSAIDs. For instance, phenylbutazone combined with isopyrin (enolic types) causes extension of half-lives and a longer-lasting effect because of competition for microsomal metabolizing enzymes.

Excretion in the bile in the form of glucuronides occurs for some NSAIDs. Cleavage to release the parent drug in the gut and enterohepatic cycling, however, have been demonstrated for several of these compounds.

Many NSAIDs, especially phenylbutazone, display zero order kinetics, i.e., half-life fluctuates in the body as levels are altered by changing dosages and by reduced elimination. This means that a constant amount, rather than a constant fraction, of the drug is continually excreted; thus, the half-life of the drug is dose dependent. This dose-dependent elimination occurs when processes other than simple diffusion play a major role. Drug metabolism, carrier-mediated transport, and plasma and tissue binding are saturable processes that exhibit a limited capacity for drug.

Oxyphenbutazone inhibits the rate of metabolism of phenylbutazone in the horse, and this inhibitory effect may be responsible for the dose-dependent effect on the plasma half-life of phenylbutazone. Hence, doses above the saturation levels can cause disproportionately high levels in plasma and tissues and varying half-lives. For instance, the half-life of phenylbutazone in the horse varies from 3.5–8 hours, depending on the dose administered.

Because phenylbutazone is a weak acid, the drug probably is preferentially excreted at a more rapid rate in an alkaline urine, whereas in an acidic urine, a slower, more prolonged excretion rate is probable. The rate of renal excretion of a pharmacologic compound is influenced by the extent of ionization in the uriniferous tubules, which in turn is regulated by the pH of the urine and the pKa of the individual compound. Because un-ionized drugs are preferentially lipid soluble, they tend to be reabsorbed by passive diffusion through the lipoid epithelium of the renal tubule, whereas ionized drugs, which are more readily water soluble, are more rapidly excreted. Because phenylbutazone is an organic acid, one would expect an acidic urine to result in less dissociation and consequently delayed excretion. Conversely, an alkaline urine should lead to increased ionization and thus more rapid secretion. Thoroughbreds during training excrete an acidic urine, whereas during rest a more alkaline urine is produced. Because of the usual alkalinity of equine urine, renal excretion of acidic NSAIDs is rapid.

Many of the NSAIDs possess short half-lives in the horse, e.g., naproxen, 4–5 hours; meclofenamic acid, 0.9 hours; and flunixin, 1.6 hours.

21.4. MECHANISM OF ACTION

Although the clinical use of phenylbutazone and especially of the salicylates has been extensive over the years, the primary mechanisms of action underpinning their anti-inflammatory, analgesic, and antipyretic activities have been identified only recently. Most evidence now indicates that the NSAIDs exert their action by inhibiting the local synthesis of prostaglandins that directly or indirectly mediate the inflammatory response. Because of their short half-life, the biological activity of prostaglandins resides in, or proximate to, their site of synthesis. Consequently, they are referred to as local hormones.

Mechanical, chemical, immunologic, or hormonal action initiates the release of phospholipase A_2 and C, which hydrolyze cell membrane phospholipids, thereby releasing fatty acids into the cell. The substrate arachidonic acid then enters a series of complex transformations, the so-called arachidonic acid cascade, leading to the production of an array of bioactive substances, the eicosanoids. This cascade involves four pathways:

1. The cyclo-oxygenase reaction leading to prostaglandins D_2, E_2, F_2, G_2, and H_2, the thromboxanes, and prostacyclin
2. The 5-lipoxygenase reaction leading to the leukotrienes
3. The cytochrome P-450 linked reaction leading to eicosatetraenoic acids
4. The 12-lipoxygenase reaction yielding a family of hydroxyeicosatetraenoic acids (12-HETE)

The prostaglandins arise from several sources, but the most likely initial source is injured tissue. All the possible sources have not been precisely isolated, however. Prostaglandins of the I and E series (PGIs and PGEs) have a prolonged vasodilatory effect and cause erythema. They also sensitize blood vessels to the permeability effects of other inflammatory mediators, such as histamine and bradykinin. The PGEs enhance the pain-producing effects of bradykinin. With respect to vasodilation, the prostaglandins have an action of equal potency but longer duration than that of histamine or the kinins. PGI_2 is the major product from the vascular endothelium of blood vessels, where it inhibits platelet aggregation. The prostaglandins also can counteract the vasoconstrictive effects of norepinephrine and angiotensin. They produce hyperalgesia at low concentrations, a cumulative effect that is related to the duration and concentration to which the tissues are exposed. In addition to these actions at the local level, the PGEs are thought to have a pyretic action, with high levels in the central nervous system associated with fever. Granuloma formation is enhanced by PGE, which causes proliferation of fibroblasts. In addition to prostaglandins originating from injured tissue, migrating leukocytes are also major sources of prostaglandins in rats.

Blood platelets exhibit a normal tendency to stick together ("clump") and to adhere to blood vessel walls. This tendency is controlled by another eicosanoid—thromboxane A_2. Thromboxane A_2 is a major cyclo-oxygenase product of platelets that causes aggregation of platelets and also acts as a vasoconstrictor. In this respect, thromboxane A_2 may also control hemorrhage at the site of injury. It is also produced by granuloma tissues. Its action on platelet adhesion is irreversible.

As arachidonic acid is released from phospholipids, it is also available to the lipoxygenase enzyme system. This system leads to the production of leukotrienes and 12-HETE. Leukotriene B_4 is produced in leukocytes and is a potent chemotactic compound. In addition, it is active with PGE_2 and PGI_2 in potentiating bradykinin, although it is not vasodilatory. Leukotriene B_4 appears to have a direct effect on vascular permeability.

Unstable intermediates can be formed via cyclo-oxygenase. This formation is accompanied by the generation of toxic free oxygen radicals, which are responsible for some of the tissue destruction present during the inflammatory process.

NSAIDs reduce inflammation by competitively inhibiting the enzyme (cyclo-oxygenase) prostaglandin synthetase. This suppresses synthesis of the unstable endoperoxides and PGE_2 and PGF_2. Prostaglandins, especially PGE_2 and PGI_2, produce vasodilation, increase vascular permeability, provoke pain (with bradykinin), and inhibit T-suppressor cells. All these roles of the NSAID contribute to anti-inflammatory actions. Prostaglandins are also released centrally from the hypothalamus during pyrexia.

The two classes of NSAIDs, i.e., carboxylic and enolic acids, may act on different enzymes. The carboxylic acids inhibit cyclo-oxygenase, and the enolic acids inhibit endoperoxide isomerase. This suggests that synthesis of PGE_2 would be blocked by phenylbutazone, which is an enolic acid, and PGI_2 synthetase would not be affected. A therapeutic dose of phenylbutazone blocks the synthesis of both compounds in the horse, however. Phenylbutazone undergoes peroxide-dependent co-oxygenation catalyzed by PGH_2 synthetase, thereby causing the inhibition of PGH_2 synthetase and prostacyclin (PGI_2) synthetase.

Phenylbutazone is now believed to be not simply a cyclo-oxygenase inhibitor, but specifically an inhibitor of formation of PGE_2. As such, phenylbutazone may not be effective in patients whose clinical signs may relate to other vasoactive and neuroactive products of the inflammatory cascade at a given point in the disease process.

The efficacy of the different NSAIDs in vivo correlates directly with their ability to inhibit cyclo-oxygenase in vitro, perhaps because some 17 NSAIDs inhibit cyclo-oxygenase irreversibly (meclofenamic acid, aspirin, and phenylbutazone), whereas the action of oxyphenbutazone (a biologically active breakdown product of phenylbutazone) is reversible. This pharmacodynamic hypothesis may explain the discrepancy between the short half-life and observed long duration of activity of most of the NSAIDs. Alternatively, some NSAIDs (flunixin and phenylbutazone) appear to be preferentially attracted to inflamed tissues. Another suggestion for the varying efficacy of the different NSAIDs is the occurrence of different cyclo-oxygenase isoenzymes that are inhibited to different degrees by the various NSAIDs. This may explain the disparity of efficacy with different inflamed tissues. Whatever the precise mechanism, however, NSAIDs unquestionably inhibit prostaglandin synthesis. Both phenylbutazone and flunixin inhibit the production of PGE_2 in inflammatory exudate at therapeutic doses.

The degree of inhibition of cyclo-oxygenase by a specific NSAID is correlated with the analgesic effect of the specific compound. This binding to cyclo-oxygenase may be reversible or irreversible. Aspirins, phenylbutazone, and meclofenamic acid are regarded as irreversible inhibitors, a characteristic that could explain their long-lasting analgesic effects despite their short half-lives.

Cyclo-oxygenase structure varies between species and between tissues, and NSAIDs differ in their ability to combine with them. These differences can explain differences in individual drug potency and species response. Whereas the horse requires phenylbutazone plasma levels of 10–25 $\mu g/ml$, humans require levels of 100–140 $\mu g/ml$ for a commensurate therapeutic effect.

Apart from cyclo-oxygenase, the arachidonic substrate is also acted on by another ubiquitous enzyme, lipoxygenase. This enzyme is found in the lungs, platelets, white blood cells, vascular endothelial cells, mast cells, and alveolar macrophages. Lipoxygenase action results in the formation of leukotrienes and hydroperoxy and hydroxyeicosa tetraenoic acids, which are other compounds important in inflammation.

Leukotrienes and prostaglandins affect chemotaxis, vascular dilation, and permeability. They potentiate the effects of other mediators, such as histamine and bradykinin. They are involved in fever, both from central release in the hypothalamus and by regulation of vascular smooth muscle.

Leukotriene B_4 is a potent endogenous chemotactic factor that enhances migration of leukocytes to the site of inflammation. Elevated concentrations of leukotriene B_4 have been found in the synovial fluids of humans affected with rheumatoid arthritis and also in inflamed joints in horses with soft tissue inflammation. Leukotriene B_4 potentiates bradykinin-induced vascular exudation and, with prostaglandin, mediates vascular exudation associated with inflammation. Leukotriene C_4 and leukotriene D_4 account for most of the slow-reacting substance of anaphylaxis.

Pyrogens precipitate the release of interleukin-1 by monocytes, macrophages, and Kupffer's cells. These pyrogens stimulate synthesis and release of prostaglandins in the hypothalamus, thus causing pyrexia. The antipyretic effect of NSAIDs occurs by inhibition of prostaglandin synthesis both centrally and locally.

The analgesic effect is accountable to the local suppression of prostaglandin synthesis (especially of PGE), which enhances the pain-producing effects of bradykinin.

Most NSAIDs do not affect lipoxygenase, and thus do not suppress leukotriene (chemotactic) synthesis. Indeed, blockade of cyclo-oxygenase by NSAIDs may allow redirection of arachidonate substrates toward the unaffected lipoxygenase pathway.

Because they possess little inhibiting effect on lipoxygenase, NSAIDs are not quite as potent as corticosteroids in reducing local inflammation.

Most of the NSAIDs currently used in equines do not reduce cell migration into inflamed tissue, thereby suggesting that they do not possess an antilipoxygenase activity. Consequently, leukotriene production is unaffected.

Research is currently directed toward finding a dual blocker—an NSAID that blocks both cyclo-oxygenase and lipoxygenase. Ketoprofen is the most recent addition to the equine medicines that inhibit both enzymes.

NSAIDs possess other characteristics that may be responsible to a lesser degree for their analgesic, anti-inflammatory, and antipyretic activity. Some act as antioxidants or scavengers for free radicals. Uncoupling of oxidative phosphorylation, inhibition of formation of kinins, depression of prostaglandin activity by competing for receptor sites, and inhibition of lysozyme activity may be other possible modes of action. They also facilitate cAMP-mediated membrane stabilization.

NSAIDs therefore reduce inflammation by preventing the release of prostaglandins which sensitize the blood vessels to the increased permeability caused by other mediators released locally, such as histamine and bradykinin. By preventing the release of local prostaglandins, the NSAIDs also prevent the sensitization of pain receptors. Because accumulation of phenylbutazone in the tissue is slow, and the drug only blocks synthesis of new prostaglandins, the anti-inflammatory and local analgesic effect of the drug is quite slow. Preformed prostaglandin concentrations must first decrease.

PGI_2 is a potent stimulator of cAMP accumulation, whereas thromboxane inhibits cAMP. Several NSAIDs, especially aspirin, not only inhibit cyclo-oxygenase, but, at lower dosage levels, block specific isomerases and synthetases, especially those involved in thromboxane formation.

The effect of NSAIDs on thromboxane synthesis results because platelets contain definite amounts of cyclo-oxygenase and cannot undergo de novo thromboxane synthesis. Therefore, NSAIDs that irreversibly inhibit cyclo-oxygenase prevent thromboxane A_2 production terminally. Their efficacy in this respect is therefore especially long lasting.

The balance between the cAMP-lowering activity of thromboxane in platelets and the cAMP-stimulating effects of prostacyclin in the vascular epithelium regulates platelet aggregation. Aspirin specifically inhibits thromboxane synthesis at doses far lower than the analgesic/anti-inflammatory dose. Aspirin also prevents release of bradykinin from damaged tissues. It increases bleeding times by decreasing platelet aggregation. Because aspirin inhibits platelet cyclo-oxygenase (thromboxane synthetase) formation, other types of antithrombotic drugs are currently being sought. These drugs include PGI_2 analogs, calcium antagonists, selective inhibitors of thromboxane synthesis, cAMP, and phosphodiesterase.

21.5 TOXICITY AND SIDE EFFECTS

Many of the toxic side effects of the NSAIDs are attributable to inhibition of prostaglandin formation. Commonly encountered side effects include gastric ulceration, fluid retention, renal papillary necrosis, blood dyscrasias, and skin rashes (Table 21–3).

Because NSAIDs affect cyclo-oxygenases, which are ubiquitous in all tissues (except red blood cells) the scatter of side effects can lead to diverse manifestations. The toxicity of phenylbutazone has been well documented in horses and especially in ponies. Ulceration of the gastrointestinal tract, including the oral cavity but predominantly the large bowel, is associated with protein-losing enteropathy and high-dosage oral use in some breeds of ponies.

Prolongation of bleeding time as a result of platelet aggregation by NSAIDs can be a

---

TABLE 21–3
ADVERSE REACTIONS WITH NSAIDs

1. Gastrointestinal upset: abdominal discomfort, nausea, ulceration, vomiting, dyspepsia, diarrhea, constipation
2. Major gastrointestinal bleeding, exacerbation or perforation of ulcer, protein-losing enteropathy
3. Toxic hepatitis
4. Skin rash: pruritis, urticaria, alopecia
5. Ocular: reversible blurring of vision
6. CNS toxicity: drowsiness, dizziness, lethargy, agitation, weakness, depression
7. Cardiovascular toxicity: arrhythmias
8. Sodium and fluid retention
9. Renal papillary necrosis

---

problem in patients susceptible to bleeding tendencies.

Ulceration of the stomach and alimentary tract is attributable to inhibition of the prostaglandins responsible for inhibiting the secretion of gastric (PGE_2) and hydrochloric acid (PGI_2) and of other prostaglandins responsible for stimulating the secretion of mucus and bicarbonate. Also, some NSAIDs (e.g., aspirin) may be a direct irritant of the alimentary tract mucosa.

PGI_2 is a vasodilator that regulates blood flow to the gut mucosa. Ischemia and hypoxia may be the underlying conditions that lead to erosion and ulceration. Bleeding into the gut and, in some cases, a protein-losing enteropathy result. Gastric and intestinal ulceration can be accompanied by secondary anemia and hypoproteinemia.

Prostaglandins locally are cytoprotective and decrease the volume acidity and pepsin content of gastric secretion.

Ulcerations associated with oral administration are most commonly seen in the large intestine (colon). Such ulceration is thought to result from the release of phenylbutazone from roughage during fermentation in the colon, which is the predominant site of fermentation in the horse. Biliary secretions may be important in this respect, especially following intravenous administration. Ulceration of the upper gastrointestinal tract is not as frequent as that of the colon, although buccal ulceration also has been seen. The dosage level used appears to be a particularly critical factor in the formation of these lesions.

Formulation of phenylbutazone has also been implicated as a factor in toxicity. Oral administration has been implicated as a causative factor in buccal ulceration. Care must be exercised with intravenous administration because extravascular injection can cause severe inflammation and sloughing with, in some cases, permanent occlusion of the jugular vein. Phenylbutazone can cause ulceration, hemoconcentration, and death from hypovolemic shock. Drug formulation, age, and breed play major roles in the incidence of such side effects.

Prolongation of bleeding time may occur with many of the NSAIDs. Aspirin at 20 mg/kg decreases platelet adhesion in the horse via inhibition of thromboxane synthesis. The gastrointestinal blood loss is potentiated by the antiplatelet effect on coagulation (i.e., impaired platelet adhesion).

Renal failure with papillary necrosis is another documented side effect of NSAIDs. It is more common in humans than in animals and may reflect not only a species difference but also the fact that humans are much older when they receive these drugs and consequently have impaired renal functioning. Renal papillary necrosis, however, can be a problem in horses receiving only the normal therapeutic dose of an NSAID.

The incidence of side effects in neonates is worsened in the presence of dehydration.

Prostaglandins are involved in renal physiologic processes, including regulation of renal blood flow, glomerular filtration, tubular ion transport, modulation of renin release, and water metabolism. NSAIDs can reduce renal blood flow through prostaglandin-mediated reactions and can increase blood urea nitrogen (BUN) concentrations.

Hepatotoxicity can also arise as a side effect leading to impaired drug metabolism. Blood dyscrasias are other relatively common side effects. Some NSAIDs (e.g., phenylbutazone) have a direct inhibiting effect on bone marrow hematopoiesis.

Experimental evidence suggests that the use of aspirin and several other NSAIDs may decrease proteoglycan synthesis in joints affected by degenerative joint disease, presumably by inhibiting early steps in the formation of chondroitin sulfate.

21.6 PYRAZOLONE DERIVATIVES

The pyrazolones are comprised of phenylbutazone, oxyphenbutazone, antipyrine, aminopyrine, dipyrone, and apazone.

PHENYLBUTAZONE

Phenylbutazone is the oldest and most widely used NSAID in equine practice. Its analgesic and antipyretic actions are similar to those of aspirin, and its anti-inflammatory actions resemble those of cortisone. Phenylbutazone is commonly used to control inflammation, especially laminitis and degenerative joint disease, and to treat postoperative disorders and postoperative pain.

Phenylbutazone is chemically related to aminopyrine (both are pyrazolone derivatives). Because of the ability of phenylbutazone to reduce inflammation and alleviate pain, horses otherwise unable to compete have been able to remain in training and race successfully. The anti-inflammatory action of the drug resembles that of the corticosteroids and has led to its widespread use in such conditions as arthritis, bursitis, chronic arthrosis, posterior paralysis, and chronic pain in muscle and soft tissue. It is not generally employed as an analgesic, although pain associated with inflammatory diseases can be relieved as a result of the anti-inflammatory activity of the drug.

Phenylbutazone is available for oral and parenteral usage. Oral formulations are administered as powders, tablets, pastes, and in one case a dosage-regulated bolus. Oral administration is often the preferred route because of the irritant action of the drug when injected intravenously. The presence of food in the stomach lowers the rate of passage and hence absorption. Though the NSAIDs are acidic, most of the absorption occurs in the duodenum. Variable absorption rates can occur in a single animal under constant conditions. Varying absorption rates have been reported in different breeds, with lower phenylbutazone absorption in ponies than in thoroughbreds. Different oral formulations of phenylbutazone appear to have higher bioavailabilities, e.g., paste has greater bioavailability than does powder.

After intramuscular administration, peak plasma levels are achieved in 6–10 hours. This slower rate occurs because phenylbutazone is fixed to muscle protein after intramuscular administration and consequently its absorption is delayed. Some local irritation occurs in both oral and intramuscular routes, and prolonged oral administration may lead to some gastric ulceration in the horse. This ulceration is a widely recognized side effect in humans.

Once phenylbutazone passes into the blood stream, it becomes highly bound to plasma proteins (approximately 96%). Despite this high affinity for plasma proteins, phenylbutazone has a short half-life in the horse. Indeed, the species variation in the half-life of this drug is marked (human = 72 hours; dog = 6 hours; horse = 3.5 hours). Because of the longer half-life of the drug in humans, and its slower rate of metabolism, the risk of cumulative toxicity is much greater in humans than in the dog or horse. (Remember that the half-life of a drug is the time required for the plasma concentration to fall by half.)

In the horse, the half-life of oxyphenbutazone is approximately the same as that of the parent drug, phenylbutazone, and it is bound to the extent of 87% to plasma proteins. Because it has lesser gastric toxicity (ulceration), it would appear to merit more serious consideration for oral therapy in animals. Oxyphenbutazone is available as a drug for use in human medicine.

Urinary pH influences the rate of excretion. The rate of excretion of any organic compound is influenced by the extent of ionization in the uriniferous tubule, which in turn is influenced by the pH of the urine and the pKa of the individual compound. Un-ionized particles tend to be reabsorbed by the kidney tubules, whereas ionized particles are readily excreted. The pKa of a drug refers to the pH at which half the drug is ionized and half is un-ionized. The pKa for phenylbutazone is 4.5. Accordingly, because phenylbutazone is an organic acid, one would anticipate that an acidic urine would result in less dissociation and consequently delayed excretion. Conversely, an alkaline urine should lead to increased ionization and thus more rapid excretion.

In the horse, phenylbutazone is a safe and effective agent. Its extensive use in equine practice without the problems experienced by its use in humans is a testimony to its safety and efficacy in the horse. The number of doses administered to horses over the years is exceedingly high, and yet the incidence of reported side effects is exceedingly small. This reduced incidence of toxicity in the horse is undoubtedly the result of several factors.

1. The lower dosage rate used in the horse (<4 mg/kg) as compared to that used in humans (<15 mg/kg).
2. The shorter half-life in the horse (3.5 hours) than in humans (72 hours), which accounts for its more rapid elimination from the equine systemic circulation.
3. The difference between the type of patient and type of condition being treated in equine and in human medicine. A high percentage of phenylbutazone treatment in humans occurs among elderly patients suffering from longstanding conditions with perhaps some degree of impairment in hepatic and renal function. The horse undergoing treatment is usually much younger and has relatively minor musculoskeletal damage.

The usual therapeutic dose of the drug in horses has resulted in no substantial evidence of blood dyscrasias, and although the horse is not particularly susceptible to gastric ulceration, one case of necrotizing phlebitis of the portal veins has been reported. Because phenylbutazone can increase the tubular reabsorption of sodium and chlorine by the kidney, the drug is contraindi-cated in patients with cardiac, hepatic, or renal dysfunction. Dehydration along with phenylbutazone use may cause renal papillary necrosis in the horse. Extensive use of the drug has been linked with chromosomal damage in humans, but this effect has not been documented in the horse. Some veterinarians have pointed out that a small percentage of horses may be slightly depressed or tranquilized after receiving a large dose and that rapid intravenous injection may occasionally precipitate excitement and incoordination. Although in general the NSAIDs do not alter the innate ability of the horse to compete, they enable the horse to perform nearer to its maximum capacity by relieving inflammation and its associated pain.

Certain pony breeds are particularly susceptible to phenylbutazone toxicity; oral phenylbutazone has been associated with protein-losing enteropathy syndromes resulting in shock and death. The underlying features are ulceration of the mucosa of the alimentary tract, loss of integrity of the epithelium, absorption of toxins, and shock. The overall toxicity syndrome may be partly attributable to poorer local absorption of phenylbutazone from the alimentary tract and resultant high local concentrations in the intestinal mucosa.

Because of its analgesic and anti-inflammatory actions, phenylbutazone has been used in dogs in the treatment of such painful conditions, as traumatic arthritis, osteoarthritis, ankylosing spondylitis, and muscle spasm associated with abnormalities of the vertebral discs.

Phenylbutazone is also used in horses as an anti-inflammatory analgesic agent and for various forms of lameness. One of the major indications for the therapeutic use of phenylbutazone is acute laminitis in horses, for which it is of great benefit in alleviating inflammation and pain. Also, in stud farms, a course of treatment with phenylbutazone can substantially extend the useful breeding life of aged stallions suffering from osteoarthritis or other painful conditions of the hind legs. In the racing thoroughbred, the potential value of phenylbutazone is undermined, to some extent, by the uncertain excretory times of the compound. This can pose a dilemma both for trainer and veterinarian presented with a lame horse shortly before racing. On the other hand, in horses other than racing thoroughbreds, e.g., working horses and hacks, in which phenylbutazone residues in the urine are of no importance, the drug can be an invaluable therapeutic agent in maintaining the usefulness of or in prolonging the active life of such an animal. Finally, the response to treatment and tolerance to the drug vary considerably. Withdrawal of the drug may be followed by the re-appearance of symptoms, thus indicating that the drug is not curative but is only palliative by virtue of its anti-inflammatory actions.

The usual dose of phenylbutazone is 4.4 mg/kg, which is effective for 24 hours despite its apparently short half-life.

DIPYRONE (METAMIZOLE)

Dipyrone (Metamizole) is related to phenylbutazone and is often combined with antispasmodic agents for use in colic in horses. Dipyrone is a pyrazolone derivative possessing antipyretic, analgesic, and anti-inflammatory properties. Its action is believed to be in part through the inhibition of kinin-induced muscle spasms. When given within the dosage recommendations of 10–11 mg/kg, the drug may be used repeatedly with little risk of masking the signs of cardiovascular deterioration frequently associated with the misuse of flunixin meglumine. The major advantages of dipyrone are that it has no major contraindications, it may be used repeatedly without markedly altering the apparent status of the animal, and it is a useful routine analgesic for controlling abdominal pain. Dipyrone has a short duration of action, and its effects are insufficiently pronounced to use alone with any degree of success in severe intestinal spasm or impaction. When used with antispasmodics, a synergistic effect is obtained, and the activity of both active ingredients is prolonged. (Dipyrone, phenylbutazone, and flunixin meglumine do not adversely affect cardiovascular status or gastrointestinal motility.) At the normal dosage rate, dipyrone alleviates mild pain and may be repeated more frequently than phenylbutazone or flunixin meglumine.

Clinical experience with dipyrone and flunixin meglumine in the treatment of colic indicates that both are effective in relieving pain associated with suspected intestinal smooth muscle spasm or mild colon impactions. Flunixin meglumine at 0.5–1.0 mg/kg is a potent analgesic that often provides 6 to 8 hours of relief. This effectiveness is not without untoward effects. If used injudiciously, without complete physical examination of the patient (including rectal examination and, in some cases, paracentesis), flunixin meglumine can mask the signs of intestinal ischemia-endotoxemia, thereby delaying lifesaving surgical intervention. Although other NSAIDs should perform similarly, the clinical problem of delayed surgery or referral is most evident with misuse of flunixin meglumine. This problem is not characteristic of dipyrone (Metamizole).

21.7 OXICAMS

Piroxicam is a relatively new NSAID used in human medicine. It displays potency similar to that of aspirin, indomethacin, and naproxen for the treatment of osteoarthritis or rheumatoid arthritis.

Another oxicam that has been introduced into veterinary medicine for small animals is meloxicam. This is used for musculoskeletal pain in dogs. It is also chondroprotective. It is given orally at a dose of 0.2 mg/kg.

21.8 SALICYLATES

The prototype member of this group is acetylsalicylic acid (or aspirin), which was introduced into human medicine many years ago and is still the most frequently used NSAID in humans. It is available in many "over-the-counter" remedies. Aspirin, however, still has not found widespread use in many of the animal species, although it can be an effective compound.

Although aspirin has a short half-life in the horse (similar to that of flunixin), the duration of clinical effect can last for up to 24 hours. At an acidic pH, aspirin is lipophilic, thus favoring rapid hydrolysis to salicylic acid and good absorption.

Salicylic acid is irritating and can only be used as a topical counterirritant, keratolytic, or linament. For oral use, salts or esters must be used to avoid tissue irritancy. Aspirin is the salicylic acid ester of acetic acid.

In comparative terms, the potency of acetylsalicylic acid in horses is quite low, and accordingly high doses must be employed: 75 mg/kg for loading dose and 25–35 mg/kg for maintenance.

Salicylate is a normal constituent of equine urine (from dietary sources) and is also detectable following topical application of methyl salicylate. Legumes, especially alfalfa, are high in salicylate. In the case of aspirin, rapid renal excretion is augmented by rapid tubular secretion also.

The use of salicylates in horses is superseded by use of the other NSAIDs for several reasons. (It is important to note that salicylic acid is rapidly excreted in the horse, especially in a horse with basic urine.) Salicylate is only 50% bound to plasma protein, whereas greater than 99% binding occurs for meclofenamic acid and naproxen. Nonetheless salicylates may be beneficial in preventing and treating milder forms of myoglobinuria or "tying up."

Low-dose aspirin (5–20 mg/kg) is particularly effective in preventing hypercoagulability of the blood in laminitis, colic and endotoxemia; the inhibition of thromboxane synthetose. This cyclo-oxygenase is very sensitive to low-dose aspirin, which irreversibly inhibits it.

21.9 PROPIONIC ACID DERIVATIVES

The propionic acid derivatives, naproxen, ketoprofen, and ibuprofen, share the analgesic, antipyretic, and anti-inflammatory activities of aspirin.

NAPROXEN

Naproxen is available in oral (granular) form only. It appears more palatable to horse than is phenylbutazone, for which palatability problems can arise. Bioavailability is reported at 50%, with peak plasma concentrations after 2–3 hours.

Naproxen is widely used in human medicine, but has a particularly high incidence of side effects (less so in horses).

In horses, the half-life of naproxen is 6 hours, and the drug is >99% bound to plasma protein. Naproxen seems particularly effective in cases of "tying up," i.e., in soft tissue inflammatory conditions. The clinical dose rate for naproxen of 2–4 g twice daily is effective for muscular inflammatory conditions.

Naproxen occurs at high levels in urine along with its major metabolite, 2-(5-hydroxynaphthyl) propionic acid.

KETOPROFEN

Ketoprofen is a highly potent and safe NSAID of the propionic acid group. (In general, the propionic acids are best tolerated.) Like the other NSAIDs, ketoprofen has a short half-life and does not tend to accumulate following repeat administration. The drug is rapidly absorbed, metabolized, and excreted. It is 99% bound in the blood stream to plasma albumin.

The metabolic pathway called glucuronidation leads to the formation of an unstable glucuronic ester that is excreted in urine. Conjugation and excretion can be relatively slower in older patients.

The effects of ketoprofen are longer lasting than its half-life (1 hour) would suggest. Delayed clearance from inflammatory fluid or a prolonged effect on mediators of inflammation may underlie these effects. Ketoprofen provides rapid yet long-lasting relief from pain and swelling. It is used in humans to treat osteoarthritis, rheumatoid arthritis, and ankylosing spondylitis. When compared to aspirin, ketoprofen displays much less gastrointestinal irritancy.

Ketoprofen is a "dual inhibitor," inhibiting both the cyclo-oxygenase and lipoxygenase branches of the arachidonic cascade. Potent analgesic and antipyretic activity is the result. Most other NSAIDs do not inhibit the lipoxygenase branch of the arachidonic acid cascade. Therefore, ketoprofen is much more effective in suppressing chemotaxis and inflammation, and in this regard approaches the corticosteroids in potency.

Related to ibuprofen, ketoprofen is indicated for the treatment of equine colic and musculoskeletal conditions. It is administered by the intravenous route at a dose of 2.2 mg/kg once daily for 3–5 days. Ketoprofen at up to five times the recommended dosage rate shows no evidence of gastrointestinal or other side effects. In comparative terms, ketoprofen is 50–100 times more potent than phenylbutazone as an analgesic. Although some NSAIDs can display destructive activity on cartilage in the medium term, research with ketoprofen has shown that chondrocyte damage and production of proteoglycans are not affected.

21.10 FENAMATES

Meclofenamic acid is formulated in oral and parenteral preparations. Absorption after oral administration is normally rapid; peak plasma concentrations occur between 30 minutes to 4 hours. Reports of its half-life vary from 2.6–8 hours. This discrepancy may occur because absorption can be delayed in horses with free access to hay.

Plasma clearance of meclofenamic acid appears to be quite rapid; total plasma clearance occurs in 24 hours following a single dose. Because meclofenamic acid does not accumulate in plasma, similar plasma clearance probably would occur after a course of treatment.

Metabolites of meclofenamic acid have not been reported, although conjugation with glucuronic acid has been suggested. From 10–14% of an oral dose is excreted in urine, and biliary secretion may also occur. Tissue residue levels have been established for meclofenamic acid. Highest levels occur in articular cartilage, omental fat, and hair.

A unique feature of meclofenamic acid is its slow onset of action, which takes 36–96 hours from the first dose. Its long duration of action and short half-life are similar to those of flunixin, although even more pronounced.

Although apparently more effective in the treatment of some conditions than others, meclofenamic acid is particularly useful in the treatment of acute and chronic laminitis and in skeletal conditions.

21.11 AMINONICOTINIC ACID DERIVATIVES

Flunixin is available in oral (granules), paste, and parenteral formulations. It is the only NSAID (except dipyrone) that is recommended for use intramuscularly. Flunixin meglumine is given parenterally for analgesic effect in equine spasmodic colic, but suppression of clinical signs may obscure the diagnosis. Such NSAIDs as flunixin meglumine suppress, but do not abolish, the acute inflammatory responses.

The analgesic effects of flunixin are superior to those of aspirin or phenylbutazone. In horses, clinically useful anti-inflammatory potency is present for as many as 30 hours despite a pharmacologic elimination time of only 1.6 hours. This is related to prolonged elimination from the inflammatory tissues and enzymes.

In horses, 1.1 mg/kg flunixin meglumine is given intravenously or intramuscularly once daily for as many as five days, according to clinical response. Although flunixin meglumine can be given intramuscularly, several different sites should be used. A slight swelling occasionally is observed at the injection site.

For oral or parenteral (intravenous and intramuscular) administration, similarly high bioavailabilities of 80% are reported. Free and conjugated flunixin occur in urine. Peak levels of urinary flunixin appear 2 hours after administration.

Clinical indications for flunixin in the horse include the alleviation of inflammation and pain associated with musculoskeletal disorders. It is also indicated for the alleviation of visceral pain associated with colic.

In horses, platelet aggregation is blocked by lower levels of flunixin than of phenylbutazone. (0.25 mg/kg)

The clinical application of NSAIDs in navicular disease may relate to their antithrombotic effects. Flunixin has been recommended for treatment of endotoxic shock. In this respect, it displays potency higher than that of either aspirin or phenylbutazone.

In shock, numerous early hemodynamic changes include portal hypertension, hepatosplanchnic pooling of blood, decreased cardiac output, and reduction in both central venous and systemic blood pressure. Arachidonic acid metabolites, such as thromboxane and prostacyclin, are elevated in animals with septic shock.

Reduced dosages of flunixin meglumine have been evaluated in experimentally induced endotoxemia. A low dose of 0.25

mg/kg flunixin meglumine reduces generation of arachidonate metabolites involved in shock. This lower-than-normal dose (the norm is 1.1 mg/kg) permits a more accurate assessment of the animals condition. Horses in hypovolemic shock are much more sensitive to the toxic effects of full doses of NSAIDs.

This dose of 0.25 mg/kg flunixin repeated at eight hourly intervals suppresses plasma thromboxane levels via cyclo-oxygenase inhibition, thus reducing the clinical effects of endotoxins. This low dose is less likely to mask clinical signs of colic.

Hypertonic saline can be used in conjunction with flunixin to counteract shock. Intravenous hypertonic saline with a tonicity eight times that of plasma (usually 7.5% NaCl) is used. Only a small volume of fluid given intravenously over 5–6 minutes is needed. This restores cardiac output and improves tissue perfusion.

21.12 CLINICAL USES

Various NSAIDs have proved more effective in the treatment of some conditions than have others. Meclofenamic acid, for instance, has useful efficacy against both acute and chronic laminitis. Naproxen, on the other hand, is more effective than phenylbutazone against experimentally induced myositis and clinically induced cases of "tying up." Flunixin meglumine is an especially useful compound in the treatment of colic endotoxemia and in the alleviation of symptoms associated with certain lamenesses. Flunixin meglumine can be given by the intramuscular or intravenous route at a dose of 1.1 mg/kg. Phenylbutazone, however, remains popular in the field because of its widespread, safe, and effective use over the last 20 years or so, and also because of its relatively lower cost (Table 21–4).

Clinically, phenylbutazone is an especially effective treatment for bone and joint inflammation and laminitis, as well as for soft tissue inflammation. In these conditions, its central analgesic effect, coupled with its local anti-inflammatory effect, renders it a potent and useful compound. Phenylbutazone blocks the synthesis of new prostaglandins locally, but its clinical effect does not become evident until the high concentrations of pre-existing prostaglandins have been reduced. Thus, phenylbutazone, as well as all the NSAIDs, require at least several hours for their clinical effect to become apparent, even after intravenous injection. Blockade of local prostaglandin synthesis returns the inflamed tissue to normality. When the critical blood level of the drug declines, the concentration of local prostaglandin in the inflamed tissue builds up again as a result of the effects of the various inflammatory stimuli, and consequently the pain, swelling, and attendant symptoms reappear. At this stage, another dose of the NSAID is required to maintain effective blood levels. In an adult horse of about 400 kg body weight, an oral dose of 4 g phenylbutazone produces optimal anti-inflammatory action, and subsequent doses

---

TABLE 21–4
NSAIDs—CLINICAL INDICATIONS FOR TREATMENT OF INFLAMMATORY CONDITIONS OF HARD AND SOFT TISSUES

- Arthritis and tendinitis
- Myositis
- Degenerative joint disease
- Laminitis
- Bursitis
- Colic
- Endotoxic shock (reduced-dosage flunixin)
- Navicular disease
- Enteritis
- Respiratory infections

TABLE 21–5
DOSES OF NSAIDs IN HORSES

Drug	*Dose*
Phenylbutazone	4.4 mg/kg orally, bid.
Naproxen	5 mg/kg intravenously; 10 mg/kg orally, bid
Meclofenamic acid	2.2 mg/kg orally, once daily
Flunixin meglumine	1.1 mg/kg intravenously, intramuscularly, orally, once daily
Ketoprofen	2.2 mg/kg intravenously, once daily

---

of about 2 g daily are then required to maintain the effect. Onset of action of the anti-inflammatory effects can be quite variable, depending on whether the horse has a full stomach. Because the effects persist for approximately 24 hours, once-daily administration is required. In addition, as the dosage of drug is increased, the blood levels also increase and the plasma half-life of the drug becomes more prolonged.

In the horse, approximately 10 µg/ml of plasma is the minimum effective blood concentration of phenylbutazone needed to provide a free unbound level of about 0.4 µg/ml. In the horse, an initial dose of as much as 4.4 mg/kg twice daily should be administered. Afterward, the dose is halved for an additional 4 days and then is reduced and administered daily depending on clinical effectiveness. Because of the increased susceptibility of ponies to the effects of phenylbutazone, a maximum dose of 2.2 mg/kg twice daily is recommended. Meclofenamic acid is administered at a dose of 2.2 mg/kg once daily, and the course of therapy is usually 5–7 days. Naproxen is administered twice daily at a dose of 5–10 mg/kg for as many as 14 days (Table 21–5).

Flunixin appears to be superior as an analgesic, especially in the treatment of flatulent and spastic colic. Growing evidence supports the potential use of NSAIDs in the treatment of endotoxic shock. Several studies have demonstrated improvements in endotoxin-induced changes in flunixin-treated ponies.

STEROIDS

21.13 CORTICOSTEROIDS AND THEIR FORMULATIONS

Corticosteroids are usually classified as either glucocorticoids or mineralocorticoids. This useful "classic" division is not accurate, however, because all the anti-inflammatory steroids tend to possess some mineralocorticoid activity to a greater or lesser extent. Although the NSAIDs are the most useful anti-inflammatory drugs in equine practice, the glucocorticoids (henceforth referred to as steroids or corticosteroids) are also used for a variety of conditions, such as pulmonary disease, arthritic conditions, and endotoxic shock.

Glucocorticoids are 21-carbon steroids derived from cholesterol. A wide range of potent synthetic corticosteroids is now available for veterinary use. The clinician must be familiar not only with the various mechanisms of action and formulations, but also with the possible side effects from steroid use to make a balanced judgment in a particular clinical situation. Steroids must always be used cautiously because side effects are common.

Although the natural and synthetic corticosteroids possess common qualitative features, they differ significantly in terms of their anti-inflammatory potency, biological half-life, propensity toward mineralocorticoid activity, side effects, and adrenal suppression (suppression of the hypothalamic-pituitary-adrenal [HPA] axis).

In the synthesis of newer more potent steroids, only minor molecular alterations are associated with disproportionately greater effects in pharmacologic activity. A high correlation exists between the desirable anti-inflammatory effects and the undesirable catabolic, mineralocorticoid, and adrenal suppressant effects. In addition, a close correlation exists between the anti-inflammatory potency of corticosteroids, their biological half-life, and their duration of action (Table 21–6).

In terms of inherent duration of activity, the corticosteroids can be regarded as (1)

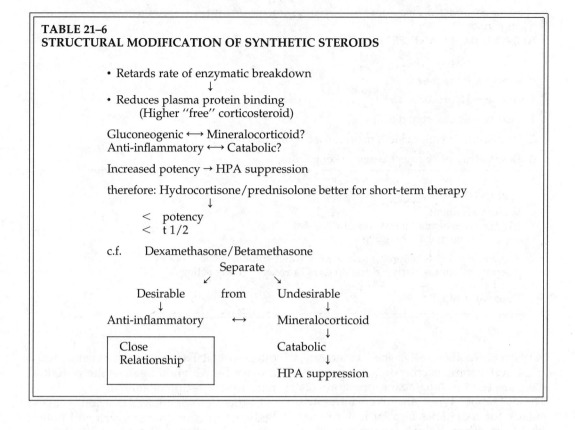

TABLE 21–6
STRUCTURAL MODIFICATION OF SYNTHETIC STEROIDS

- Retards rate of enzymatic breakdown
  ↓
- Reduces plasma protein binding
  (Higher "free" corticosteroid)

Gluconeogenic ⟷ Mineralocorticoid?
Anti-inflammatory ⟷ Catabolic?

Increased potency → HPA suppression

therefore: Hydrocortisone/prednisolone better for short-term therapy
  ↓
  <   potency
  <   t 1/2

c.f.   Dexamethasone/Betamethasone
                     Separate
              ↙   ↘
  Desirable   from   Undesirable
      ↓   ↓
Anti-inflammatory   ⟷   Mineralocorticoid
                                 ↓
  Close   Catabolic
  Relationship   ↓
                            HPA suppression

short acting, such as cortisone and hydrocortisone; (2) medium acting, such as prednisolone and triamcinolone; and (3) long acting, such as betamethasone, dexamethasone, and flumethasone (Table 21–7).

Despite this classification, however, the product form, the type and complexity of ester, and the overall ingredients of the formulation can affect the rate of release and the duration of therapeutic activity.

In reality, some of the steroids are prodrugs, e.g., prednisone is converted to the active prednisolone in the liver, as is cortisone to hydrocortisone. Steroid esters can also be regarded as types of pro-drugs because they must be hydrolyzed to release the free alcohol steroids in the body. These free alcohol steroid base forms can be pharmacologically classified into short acting, medium acting, or long acting.

Most of the free bases, cortisone, hydrocortisone, prednisone, prednisolone, methylprednisolone, dexamethasone, and betamethasone, can be used in the same way as

the water-soluble sodium phosphate or sodium succinate esters for intravenous injection. Because of rapid hydrolysis and solubility, the plasma half-life of the water-soluble esters is not significantly different from that of the steroid base.

Because only the free alcohol form of the corticosteroid is pharmacologically active, biotransformation of the water-soluble ester is needed to release the active form. A free alcohol form of betamethasone or dexamethasone is available for intravenous therapy.

Other short-acting preparations include alcoholic solutions or hydroalcoholic esters, such as succinate, hemisuccinate, sulfobenzoate, isonicotinate, phosphate, and phosphate disodium.

The water-soluble esters are often given rapidly intravenously to combat shock. Doses used in these situations are much higher than those required for anti-inflammatory use.

TABLE 21–7
STEROID BASES AND ESTERS

Steroid Bases (Free Alcohols)

Prednisone → Prednisolone ⎫
                    ⎬ Pro-drugs
Cortisone → Hydrocortisone ⎭

1. Hydrocortisone → Short acting

2. Prednisone/Prednisolone/Triamcinolone → Medium acting

3. Dexamethasone/Betamethasone → Long acting

Steroid Esters

1. Sodium succinate
                  → Short acting
   Sodium phosphate
   $t\,1/2 =$ Free alcohol intravenously
            (rate of ester hydrolysis)

2. Acetate/Acetonide/Dipropionate: Poorly water-soluble suspensions
   "Depot" intramuscularly—duration days to weeks → Long acting
           ↓
   Depression of HPA

Water-insoluble esters, such as acetate, trimethylacetate, acetonide, or dipropionate, are used in long-acting preparations. These "depot" types are given intramuscularly (or sometimes intra-articularly) for long-term effect. Release of the steroid is slow, and duration of biological action can range from days to weeks, depending on the specific type of depot preparation.

These long-acting preparations are more likely to cause adrenal insufficiency or increased susceptibility to infectious disease than are the short-acting steroids, especially when large doses are used or injections are repeated.

Dexamethasone trimethylacetate is a depot formulation for repository action frequently used for 2–3 weeks in horses. Other suspensions of insoluble steroid esters used in long-term therapy include methylprednisolone acetate, isoflupredone acetate, or triamcinolone acetonide.

Retarded absorption and hydrolysis ensure prolongation of plasma drug concentration varying from weeks to months. Use of depot preparations intra-articularly has been widely practiced for many years in equine therapy. Particle size is a crucial factor in the efficacy of some of these sterile suspensions. The use of this route of administration, which can provide dramatic and often spectacular short-term benefits, must always be weighed against the potential risks for the recipient animal.

Corticosteroids are well distributed in the body, and many dosage forms and potent formulations are available for topical, intra-articular, intramuscular, intravenous, and oral use.

Long-term therapy or use of depot preparations is closely associated with suppression of adrenocortical functioning in all species. This suppression is mediated via the extraneous supply of steroids acting via the servo mechanism to decrease production and release of adrenocorticotropic hormone at the hypothalamic-pituitary level.

The fluorinated steroids, dexamethasone, betamethasone, and flumethasone being the most potent and longest acting, tend to be the most closely linked with adverse side effects. Hence, accurate dosage and case assessment must always be carefully made when using these forms of steroids.

Steroids must be used with great care when infection is present, preferably using bactericidal cover if appropriate.

Because of their immunosuppressive activity, steroids must always be avoided when immunoincompetence is evident. Also, the triggering, predisposing cause of the individual condition must always be clearly evaluated, because steroids are simply palliative, not curative, in action.

21.14 STEROIDS AND THE INFLAMMATORY PROCESS

Steroids suppress the inflammatory response by inhibiting capillary dilatation, migration of leukocytes, and phagocytic activity. Accordingly, edema development, fibrin deposition, and collagen deposition are minimized.

Steroids also contribute to the maintenance of the normal circulation and cell membrane stability.

As anti-inflammatory drugs, corticosteroids act higher up proximate on the arachidonic cascade than do the NSAIDs. They thus block both the cyclo-oxygenase and lipoxygenase enzyme systems. In addition, they modify the activity of many other cells and tissues in the body.

When released, arachidonic acid is acted on by one of two enzymes, each producing a different and distinct class of product.

Drugs may inhibit prostaglandin synthesis at several levels.

1. Arachidonate release from a cell membrane can be inhibited by suppression of the activity of phospholipase A_2 via lipomodulin (e.g., steroids).
2. Inhibition of cyclo-oxygenase can inhibit the synthesis of prostaglandins (e.g., NSAIDs).
3. Inhibition of lipoxygenase can suppress formation of leukotrienes (e.g., some of the newer NSAIDs).

The steroids act by stimulating the formation of lipocortin (lipomodulin, macrocortin) in cells affected by various traumatic, mechanical, infectious, or toxigenic agents (Table 21–8).

Lipomodulin suppresses release of the enzyme phospholipase A_2, which would normally cleave the inaccessible phospholipids in cell membranes to release arachidonic acid and thus initiate the inflammatory process.

When arachidonic acid is released from damaged cell membranes, it acts as a substrate for the biosynthesis of various local hormones (eicosanoids). Cyclo-oxygenase activates production of prostaglandins from arachidonate; lipoxygenase catalyzes synthesis of the leukotrienes.

At the level of the arachidonic acid, suppression of the formation and release of the leukotrienes, PGE (vasodilation), PGF (vasoconstriction), PGI_2 (prostacyclin), and thromboxane is a major contributing factor toward the minimization and abolition of the local inflammatory process and chemotaxis. Blood platelets primarily produce thromboxane; prostacyclin is derived from vascular endothelial cells. Local injury results in release of arachidonic acid from platelets and the blood vessel wall. Platelets contain the enzyme thromboxane synthetase, which yields thromboxane. Thromboxane causes platelet aggregation and vasoconstriction. Another enzyme, prostacyclin synthetase, converts the arachidonate released from the injured cell wall into PGI_2 (prostacyclin), which in turn causes vasodilation and inhibition of platelet aggregation. The thromboxane-prostacyclin interaction is primarily a physiologic check-and-balance system operating in the body to maintain circulatory stability and homeostasis.

PGE is found in high concentrations in inflammatory exudates. It acts as a vasodilator, increases capillary permeability, and sensitizes local pain receptors. It may also act as a link between histamine and its receptors. The leukotrienes act as major chemotactic agents attracting polymorphs to the site of inflammation.

Leukotrienes also produce pain and cause hyperthermia. Biological roles of lipoxygenase products include increased leukocyte adhesion, chemotaxis, and degranulation, increased vascular permeability, bronchoconstriction, and vasoconstriction.

Steroids reduce the synthesis of all products of the arachidonic acid substrate, including products of lipoxygenase. (In shock, the formation of microthrombi, capillary bed shutdown, venodilation, and arteriolar constriction are critical elements traceable to the release of arachidonic acid.)

Corticosteroids are generally regarded as having a stabilizing effect on cell membranes (endothelial, lysosomal, and mitochondrial), thus preventing release of vasoactive amines, proteases, and hydrolases. Stabilization of endothelial phospholipid

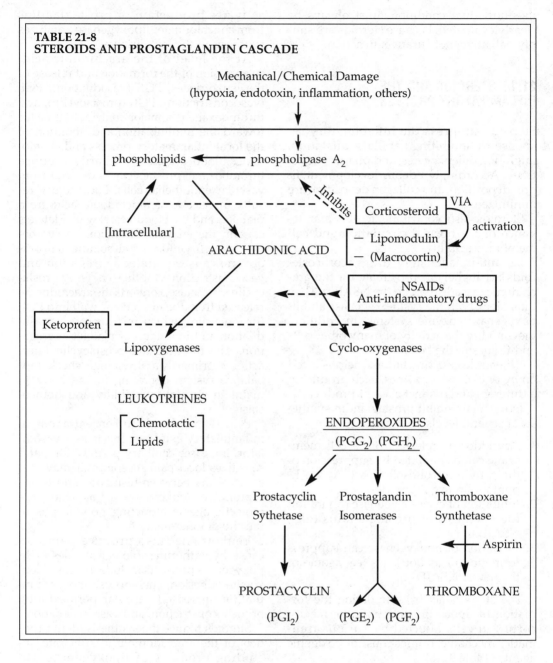

TABLE 21-8
STEROIDS AND PROSTAGLANDIN CASCADE

Mechanical/Chemical Damage
(hypoxia, endotoxin, inflammation, others)

phospholipids ◄——— phospholipase A_2

Inhibits

Corticosteroid VIA

[Intracellular]

— Lipomodulin
— (Macrocortin)

activation

ARACHIDONIC ACID

NSAIDs
Anti-inflammatory drugs

Ketoprofen

Lipoxygenases   Cyclo-oxygenases

LEUKOTRIENES

[Chemotactic
Lipids]

ENDOPEROXIDES
(PGG_2) (PGH_2)

Prostacyclin   Prostaglandin   Thromboxane
Sythetase   Isomerases   Synthetase

Aspirin

PROSTACYCLIN   THROMBOXANE

(PGI_2)   (PGE_2) (PGF_2)

via activation of lipomodulin is a major, but not the sole, mechanism of anti-inflammatory action. Some of the pharmacologic actions of steroids can persist in the absence of detectable drug concentrations. The half-lives can be appreciably shorter than the duration of effect. This characteristic is accounted for by the activation of lipomodulin, the results of which persist longer than do the levels of the steroids themselves.

Included in the defense systems of the body are interferon, complement lymphocytes, and substances of leukocytic action, such as lysozyme, lactoferrin, cationic proteins, and proteases. Interferon is particularly vital for combatting viral infections, and interferons also are depressed by corticosteroids.

Lymphocytes, neutrophils, eosinophils, and monocytes/macrophages are all affected by the steroids. Neutrophils lose their phagocytic potency, and a marked eosinopenia results.

Lymphocytes display a marked decrease in mitotic rate, thereby contributing to the overall immunosuppressive activity. Steroids can be a major cause of immunosuppression in domestic species and can easily exacerbate infectious disease by impairing host defense mechanisms. The increased rate of catabolism results in decreased antibody production. Corticosteroids reduce the number of lymphocytes, eosinophils, and basophils. Agranulocytosis often results from an increased rate of release of polymorphonuclear leukocytes from the bone marrow into the blood.

Lymphopenia results from the action of corticosteroids on lymphoid tissues. T cells (lymphocytes derived from thymus) tend to be more affected than B cells (lymphocytes derived from bone marrow). Redistribution of the T-lymphocytes accounts largely for the lymphopenia. The capacity of the lymphocytes to process antigens is diminished, and activation of lymphocytes previously sensitized to an antigen is inhibited.

Lymphokines are produced by lymphocytes following activation by antigen. A particular lymphokine macrophage migration inhibiting factor inhibits motility of macrophages, thereby allowing them to accumulate at the focus of inflammation. Because steroids suppress the effect of migration inhibiting factor on macrophages, local cellular accumulation does not build up.

Also, the release of interleukin-1 from macrophages is inhibited, which in turn inhibits production of T-lymphocytes. (The immediate stimulus for synthesis and release of T-lymphocytes is interleukin-2, but interleukin-1 is its immediate precursor.)

The neutrophilia produced by interleukin-1 appears to be caused by the direct action of the substance on bone marrow. Interleukin-1 also induces the production of acute-phase proteins, including haptoglobin, protease inhibitors, complement components, fibrinogen, amyloid A, and C-reactive protein.

Interleukin-1 causes fever by inducing an abrupt increase in PGE_2 in the anterior hypothalamus. This increase raises the thermostat set point.

Interleukin-2 is a protein secreted by the T-helper cells when they come in contact with macrophage-bound antigen. The overall function of the interleukin is to enhance the responses of the B cells to antigens. Corticosteroids act indirectly on cytotoxic T-lymphocytes by inhibiting interleukin-2 production.

Suppression of T-lymphocytes and macrophage activity, stabilization of cell membranes, especially lysosomal cell membranes, reduced phagocytosis, reduced antibody production, and inactivation of complement are important aspects of the anti-inflammatory effect. Because lipoxygenase activity is also blocked, leukotrienes are reduced, chemotaxis is minimized, and scar formation is weak and minimal (Table 21–9). (Another mechanism involved is prevention of the formation of plasmin (fibrinolysin), which assists leukocyte migration into the inflamed area.)

The net effects of steroids in the presence of acute inflammation are reduced edema, reduced fibrin deposition, and suppression of capillary dilatation, capillary permeability, leukocyte migration, and phagocytic activity.

21.15 SHOCK

A common indication for corticosteroid use is shock, especially that associated with endotoxemia, surgery, dehydration, or colic. Among the crucial factors that must be addressed when determining the potential efficacy of steroids in an animal in shock are:

1. The type of steroid to be used
2. The size of dose to be used
3. The timing, route, and rate of injection

Endotoxins alter membranes in many cell types and can trigger the alternate complement pathway. These effects may trigger disseminated intravascular coagulation. Microcirculatory disturbances include constriction of arterioles, dilation of venules, loss of erythrocyte plasticity, sticking and aggregation of granulocytes and thrombocytes to endothelium and each other, release of thromboxane A_2 from platelets, and increased permeability (loss of integrity) of capillary and venule walls.

TABLE 21–9
STEROID ACTIVITY

ENHANCEMENT OF ENDOTHELIAL INTEGRITY
↓
STABILIZES LYSOSOMAL MEMBRANES
↓
PREVENTS MITOCHONDRIAL DAMAGE
↓
PREVENTS DEGRANULATION OF POLYMORPHS

—HYDROLASES ↓
—PROTEASES ↓
—MYOCARDIAL DEPRESSANT FACTOR ↓

ALSO:
- INHIBITS MACROPHAGE RELEASE OF INTERLEUKIN-1
- INHIBITS LYMPHOCYTE ACTIVITY
- SUPPRESSES PHAGOCYTOSIS
- INHIBITS COMPLEMENT ACTIVATION
- INHIBITS VASOCONSTRICTION IN SHOCK

Early effects of endotoxin on the circulation are associated with abrupt generation of thromboxane. Afterward, the synthesis of prostacyclin is associated with vasodilation. Low blood pressure, splanchnic pooling, increased capillary permeability, and capillary shutdown can be attributed to release of arachidonate and generation of prostaglandins. Microthrombi may seal off blood flow in tissue beds.

High doses of steroids are necessary in shock therapy to stabilize cellular membranes adequately, inhibit the release of vasoactive compounds, stabilize the circulation, and prevent release of myocardial depressant factor.

Steroids act in various ways to counteract shock.

1. They enhance the stability and integrity of endothelial membranes, especially of the capillaries.
2. They interfere with the degranulation of polymorphonuclear leukocytes by stabilizing lysosomal membranes. This stabilization prevents release of acid hydrolase, which promotes formation of myocardial depressant factor.
3. They inhibit complement activation by endotoxin (Table 21–10).

The dosages used for shock therapy are much higher than those used for anti-inflammatory action. These high dosages may be given with safety only over a short period of time. High-dosage steroid therapy is not a substitute for aggressive fluid therapy and supportive care. Hypertonic fluids (7.5% NaCl) and plasma volume expanders may also be required intravenously. Both survival and reduction of cellular damage are influenced by early steroid administration. Effective therapy requires the administration of large doses given over a short but intensive period of time by the intravenous route.

A water-soluble ester—phosphate or succinate esters—therefore must be used for this purpose. The succinate ester is taken up rapidly into the cellular compartments. Methylprednisolone esterified with succinic acid enters tissue cells rapidly after intravenous injection. Significant differences in survival time have been observed between the same analog using different esters and between different analogs using different esters.

Because economic factors are a major concern at high-dosage rates in large animals, dexamethasone usually is preferred.

21.16 OTHER EFFECTS OF STEROIDS

Corticosteroids have numerous effects on the tissues and organs. They display a major catabolic effect on tissue, reflected by atro-

---

TABLE 21–10
USE OF ANTI-INFLAMMATORY/STEROIDS TO TREAT SHOCK

1. Enhance Endothelial Integrity $\rightarrow$

2. Prevent Degranulations of Polymorphs $\rightarrow$

Maximize
|
catecholamine
|
activity/tone

Degranulation
↓
enzymes-shock

3. Reduce Lymphocytes/Monocytes/T-lymphocytes
   • Block antigen-induced sensitization of lymphocytes
   • Suppress antibody formation
4. Depress Phagocytosis, Interferon Synthesis
5. Inhibit Ground Substance/Chondroitin Sulphate
   • Fibroblastic activity

---

phy of lymphatic tissues, reduced muscle mass, thinning of the integument, a negative nitrogen balance, osteoporosis, reduced calcium and phosphate absorption with their consequent enhanced renal excretion, and decreased fibroblast activity. Metabolically, steroids give rise to lipolysis and redistribution of fat, gluconeogenesis (formation of sugars from noncarbohydrate precursors, i.e., following lipolysis and proteolysis), muscular weakness (protein catabolism and potassium excretion), sodium and water retention, polyuria (inhibition of antidiuretic hormone), increased glomerular filtration rate, inhibition of the formation of the ground substance, and adrenal insufficiency (Table 21–11).

(One mechanism of the putative actions of anabolic steroids is the local displacement of corticosteroids from their catabolic binding sites on skeletal muscle.)

Other side effects of steroids include:

1. The possibility of gastrointestinal bleeding and ulceration (but not to the same extent as with the NSAIDs)
2. Diabetogenic effects, pancreatitis, and hepatic disorders

The effect of corticosteroids on early fetal development is still under debate, although in late pregnancy, the possibility of induced abortion must always be considered. In many species, administration of corticosteroids in late pregnancy can adversely effect the transfer of good-quality immunoglobulin to the suckling offspring. This problem would have obvious ramifications for the 1G status of the neonate.

Overall, the potent and visible signs of suppression of inflammation result in the absence of pain and inflammation and in a centrally enhanced feeling of well-being. This outcome can mask the presence of a serious disease state, however. Also, the tendency toward the spread of infection or reinfection must be borne in mind, as must the possibility of inducing a wide range of undesirable side effects.

LAMINITIS

In horses, corticosteroids tend to sometimes precipitate or worsen laminitis. This risk always must be assessed against the benefits of the steroid in a given clinical situation. Systemic use particularly of triamcinolone or dexamethasone to treat chronic respiratory problems in the horse can occasionally cause laminitis.

Steroids potentiate the effects of catecholamines on the vascular system of the equine digit. Hydrocortisone and betamethasone significantly potentiate the vasoconstrictor effects of catecholamines and serotonin on isolated muscle strips of the equine digital artery and vein. Because this vasoconstriction occurs more severely in

---

TABLE 21–11
OTHER EFFECTS OF STEROIDS

Metabolism

1. Carbohydrate—Protein—Fat → *Catabolism*
   Water and electrolytes → Retention/excretion
2. Endocrine system
3. Musculoskeletal system
4. Hematopoietic system
5. Anti-inflammatory

 I. Carbohydrate/Protein/Fat
    Gluconeogenic
    Fat mobilization   Protein catabolism
    Na^+ retention Ca^{++}, K^+, PO_4^+ excretion
 II. Suppression of ACTH release—Immunosuppression
III. Musculoskeletal
        Weakness → K^+, Ca^{++}, PO_4^+, N_2 ↓
        Protein catabolism
 IV. Hematopoietic:
        Lymphocytes, eosinophils ↓
        Thymus involution

---

the digital vein than in the artery in the same foot, poor drainage from the digit might cause congestion and edema formation, thus perhaps representing a pharmacologic basis for laminitis.

The venous system, which is more sensitive to the effects of steroids and catecholamines, tends to constrict, thus producing venous pooling of the feet and an ensuing laminitis. The mechanism of action of the steroid in the equine digit includes sensitization of adrenoreceptors, inhibition of catecholamine degradation by blocking the enzyme catecholomethyltransferase, and inhibition of extraneuronal catecholamine uptake. (Platelet dysfunction also may be involved in laminitis.)

By enhancing the venoconstrictor potency of several endogenous biogenic amines, steroids create venous obstruction in the digit. Adrenalin, serotonin, and histamine impede the venous drainage from the vascular bed of the hoof. This may represent a potential pharmacologic basis for the induced laminitis.

21.17 INTRA-ARTICULAR THERAPY IN HORSES

This area is undoubtedly highly controversial, although it has been practiced for more than 35 years by equine veterinarians.

Steroids tend to mask the signs of joint pain and should never be used as a substitute for correcting the underlying problem. Occasionally, however, the use of intra-articular corticosteroids might be considered to help to restore joint mobility and relieve pain quickly. Considerable care must be taken with this route, however.

Levels of corticosteroids achieved by the intra-articular route far exceed those that would be achieved by general systemic administration. Following intrasynovial administration, relief of pain is rapid, and duration of relief can last as long as 3–4 weeks, depending on the ester, steroid, and formulation. Although intra-articular therapy is widely practiced in the horse to avoid systemic side effects, some of the active drug may be absorbed into the circulation with usually minimal side effects.

When used in joint therapy, steroids improve stability and integrity of cell membranes, including lysosomal membranes. This tends to reduce the amount of lytic enzymes present in joint inflammation. Although the intra-articular route is relatively popular, problems from sepsis, mechanical damage, and catabolic effects have been attendant hazards. Catabolic effects mediated by chondrocyte suppression and diminution of synovial fluid synthesis have resulted in what is referred to as "dry, locking joints."

The use of depot preparations in particular has been widely practiced. Particle size, however, is a crucial factor in these local injections, which are intended to minimize absorption into the systemic circulation and hence to minimize the incidence of side effects.

Although inflammation and discomfort are greatly reduced when the steroid is injected directly into the joint, catabolism and destruction of articular cartilage are accelerated. The steroid also may encourage premature use of the affected limb, thereby worsening the condition.

In degenerative joint disease, corticosteroids can cause severe side effects. They may stimulate proteoglycan loss in normal or osteoarthritic cartilage after only a short period of administration.

Postinjection flareup, septic arthritis, accelerated rate of joint destruction, and worsening of degenerative joint disease are all problems of steroid use.

If the intra-articular route is to be used, the horse must be rested and stress put on the joint must be minimal. Steroids always are contraindicated when infection is in or near the joint, when fractures are present, or when osteoporosis exists.

Although intra-articular injection of long-acting corticosteroids reduces the immediate pain and inflammation associated with traumatic arthritis, these agents do not neutralize the agent causing the inflammatory response. In addition, the steroids slow the rate of proteoglycan synthesis and hyaluronic acid production.

Advantages of the intra-articular route include analgesia and reduction of joint swelling. Steroids suppress inflammation no matter what the cause. Intra-articular injection of long-lasting steroids, such as prednisolone, reduces pain and inflammation associated with degenerative and traumatic arthritis.

Steroids injected into joints, however, can mask the underlying condition and also encourage the following catabolic processes:

1. Inhibition of synthesis of matrix components
2. Inhibition of chondrocyte activity
3. Inhibition of synthesis of synovial fluid

Joint deterioration can occur because corticosteroids cause osteoporosis with suppression of normal osteoblast and chondrocyte activity, which leads to weakening of the articular surfaces.

Also, the analgesic effect of the steroids permits the horse to use the joint, perhaps resulting in the collapse of the articular cartilage.

On balance, corticosteroids should be used for arthritic conditions only in animals that fail to respond to other anti-inflammatory agents. These agents are useful in acute flareups in an animal that cannot be mobilized by more conservative means.

Intra-articular injection of corticosteroids is controversial, and must not be performed when fracture or sepsis is present, the articular cartilage is damaged, previous injections have been ineffective, or when premature use could further worsen the damage already present.

21.18 CLINICAL USES

Corticosteroids are indicated for many inflammatory conditions, such as those affecting the joints, gastrointestinal tract, skin, allergies, musculoskeletal conditions, myositis, polyarthritis, and some neoplastic disorders (Table 21–12).

The value of steroid therapy in veterinary medicine is unquestioned. When used to treat horses with musculoskeletal problems, steroids have enabled many horses to return to useful competition. Steroids suppress inflammation regardless of the cause. Steroids have also been employed for respiratory disease, for lymphosarcoma and tumors of the reticuloendothelial system, and occasionally for alimentary tract disturbances.

Specific equine disorders for which steroids have been used include traumatic arthritis and myositis, bursitis, tendinitis, eosinophilic myositis, and osteoarthritis. Natural repair processes are retarded and inhibited.

Nonetheless, the clinician must always consider whether the institution of steroid therapy

1. Will interfere with racing
2. Will cause hypoadrenocorticism
3. Will cause degenerative changes in articular surfaces

TABLE 21–12
APPLICATION OF STEROIDS

Inflammatory Conditions → Heat ↓ → Pain ↓
1. Allergic Dermatitis (sweet itch) ↘ Rubor ↓ ↘ Swelling ↓
    Myositis
    Tendinitis → Palliative only

2. *Arthritis*   ↗ Sepsis
     Contraindication ⇢ Fracture
               ↘ Damaged articular cartilage
               ↘ Degeneration
                   (Interfere with repair processes.)

3. *Shock*   High doses intravenously
4. *Respiratory*   Life-threatening situations
5. *Neoplasia of reticuloendothelial system* (lymphosarcoma)
6. *Induction of Parturition*

---

4. Will mask signs and pains from injury, thereby leading to premature use of a limb
5. Will spread infection
6. Will induce immunosuppression

Also, the potential risks of interfering with quality of colostrum and transfer of immunoglobulin from the mare to the foal or of precipitating labor must be considered when steroid therapy is used in mares in late pregnancy.

Side effects when using steroids in shock therapy include enhancement of bleeding, increased severity of acute pancreatitis, and steroid hepatopathy (Tables 21–13 and 21–14).

In the horse, as in other species, repeat administration can lead to suppression of the hypothalamic-pituitary-adrenal axis.

TABLE 21–13
ADVERSE REACTIONS/SIDE EFFECTS OF STEROIDS

- Mineralocorticoid effects:
   Severe potassium loss ⎫
                  ⎬ Long-term therapy
   Sodium/water retention ⎭
Also
- Protein breakdown → muscle weakness
- Fat mobilization
- Atrophy of skin
- Gastric bleeding
- Inhibition of bone growth → osteoporosis
- Decreased calcium absorption (vitamin D)
- Suppression of ACTH—Cortical suppression
- Susceptibility to infection
- Retarded wound healing — Fibroblast ⎫
                                  ⎬ Inhibited
               Collagen deposition ⎭
- Hyperglycemia ⎫ Polyuria
             ⎬
             ⎭ Polydypsia

TABLE 21–14
STEROID CONTRAINDICATIONS

- Diabetes mellitus
- Ocular problems—Glaucoma (fluid retention)
- Infection—sepsis
- Pregnancy
- Bone healing
- Immunosuppression } Relapses of viral infections
  Apparent improvement
- Osteoporosis
- Degenerative joint disease
- Fractures

TABLE 21–15
PRECAUTIONS TO REMEMBER WHEN CONSIDERING USE OF CORTICOSTEROIDS

1. Anti-inflammatory effects are potent and nonspecific.
2. Palliative only; therefore identify underlying cause of problem.
3. Risk of infection.
4. Use with antibiotics when necessary.
5. Immunosuppressive.
6. Spread of infection.
7. Premature use of affected area, e.g., foot.
8. Contraindication for laminitis in horses—especially triamcinolone dexamethasone.

TABLE 21–16
DOSES OF COMMONLY USED CORTICOSTEROIDS

Prednisone	100–300 mg intramuscularly, 50 mg intra-articularly
Triamcinolone	12–30 mg intramuscularly or subcutaneously, 6–25 mg intra-articularly
Betamethasone	10–50 mg intramuscularly
Isoflupredone	5–20 mg intramuscularly, 5–20 mg intra-articularly
Dexamethasone	2.5–5 mg intramuscularly
	5–10 mg by mouth daily
Dexamethasone sodium phosphate	1–2 mg/kg intravenously for shock
Flumethasone	1.25–5 mg intravenously, intramuscularly, or intra-articularly

---

Withdrawal signs following treatment may include diarrhea, electrolyte imbalance, hemoconcentration, depression, and myalgia.

The formulation of the drug product is one of the primary determinants of adrenal suppression. Soluble steroid forms can depress the adrenal gland for as long as 3–4 days, depending on the drug, dosage, and route of administration, whereas the insoluble esters (acetates) can depress the axis for as many as 7 weeks. Short-acting steroids should be used to minimize potential side effects (Tables 21–15 and 21–16).

SELECTED REFERENCES

NSAIDs

Abramson, S.B., and Weissmann, G.: The mechanisms of action of nonsteroidal anti-inflammatory drugs. Arthritis Rheum., *32*:1, 1989.

Alexander, F.: Effect of phenylbutazone on electrolyte metabolism in ponies. Vet. Rec., *110*:271, 1982.

Barrnett, H.J.M., Hirsh, J., and Mustard, J.F. (Eds.): Acetylsalicylic Acid: New Uses for an Old Drug. New York, Raven Press, 1982.

Betley, M., Sutherland, S.F., Gregoricka, M.J., et al.: The analgesic effect of ketoprofen for use in treating equine colic, as compared to flunixin meglumine. Equine Pract., *13*:6, 1991.

Boothe, D.M.: Controlling inflammation with non steroidal anti-inflammatory drugs. Vet. Med., Sept.:875, 1989.

Bottoms, G.D., Fessler, J.F., Roesel, O.F., et al.: Endotoxin-induced hemodynamic changes in ponies: effects of flunixin meglumine. Am. J. Vet. Res., *42*:1514, 1981.

Brune, K.: How aspirin might work: a pharmacokinetic approach. Agents Actions, *4*:230, 1974.

Buring, J.E., Peto, R., and Hennekens, C.M.: Low dose aspirin for migraine prophylaxis. JAMA, *264*:1711, 1990.

Burrows, G.E.: Therapeutic effect of phenylbutazone on experimental acute *Escherichia coli* endotoxemia in ponies. Am. J. Vet. Res., *42(1)*:94, 1981.

Chastain, C.B.: Aspirin: new indications for an old drug. Compend. Contin. Educ. Pract. Vet., *9(2)*:165, 1987.

Chay, S., Woods, W.E., Nugent, T., et al.: The pharmacology of nonsteroidal anti-inflammatory drugs in the horse: flunixin meglumine (Banamine). Equine Pract., *4*:16, 1982.

Clive, D.M., and Stoff, J.S.: Renal syndromes associated with nonsteroidal anti-inflammatory drugs. N. Engl. J. Med., *310*:563, 1984.

Collins, L.G., and Tyler, D.E.: Phenylbutazone toxicosis in the horse: a clinical study. J. Am. Vet. Med. Assoc., *184*:699, 1984.

Conlon, P.D.: Nonsteroidal drugs used in the treatment of inflammation. Vet. Clin. North Am. (Small Anim. Pract.), *18*:1115, 1988.

Davis, L.E.: Clinical pharmacology of salicylates. J. Am. Vet. Med. Assoc., *176*:65–66, 1980.

Ferreira, S.H., and Vane, J.R.: New aspects of the mode of action of nonsteroid anti-inflammatory drugs. Ann. Rev. Pharmacol., *14*:57, 1974.

Fessler, J.F., Bottoms, G.D., Roesel, O.F., et al.: Endotoxin-induced change in hemograms, plasma enzymes and blood chemical values in anaesthetized ponies: effects of flunixin meglumine. Am. J. Vet. Res., *43*:140, 1982.

Gandal, C.P., Dayton, P.G., Weiner, M., and Perel, J.M.: Studies with phenylbutazone, oxyphenbutazone and paraparadichlorophenylbutazone in horses. Cornell Vet., *59*:577, 1969.

Gerring, E.L., Lees, P., and Taylor, J.B.: Pharmacokinetics of phenylbutazone and its metabolites in the horse. Equine Vet. J., *13(3)*:152, 1981.

Goodwin, J.S.: Mechanism of action of nonsteroidal anti-inflammatory drugs. Am. J. Med. (Suppl. 1A), *77*:57, 1984.

Gunson, D.E., and Soma, L.: Renal papillary necrosis in horses. J. Am. Vet. Med. Assoc., *182*:263, 1983.

Gunson, D.E., and Soma, L.R.: Renal papillary necrosis in horses after phenylbutazone and water deprivation. Vet. Pathol., *20*:603, 1983.

Hall, R.C., Hodge, R.L., Irvine, R., et al.: The effect of aspirin on the response to endotoxin. Aust. J. Exp. Biol. Med. Sci., *50*:589, 1972.

Hamilton, H.B., and Withrow, S.J.: Antiplatelet therapy: A possible new therapeutic modality for controlling metastasis. Compend. Contin. Educ. Pract. Vet., *7(11)*:907, 1985.

Hardie, E.M., Kolata, R.J., and Rawlings, C.A.: Canine septic peritonitis: treatment with flunixin meglumine. Circ. Shock, *11*:159, 1983.

Harker, L.A., and Fuster, V.: Pharmacology of platelet inhibitors. J. Am. Coll. Cardiol., *8*:21B, 1986.

Henrich, W.L.: Analgesic nephropathy. Am. J. Med. Sci., *295*:561, 1988.

Henrich, W.L.: Nephrotoxicity of nonsteroidal anti-inflammatory agents. Am. J. Kidney Dis., *2*:478, 1983.

Higgins, A.J., and Lees, P.: The acute inflammatory process, arachidonic acid metabolism and mode of action of the anti-inflammatory drugs. Equine Vet. J., *16(3)*:163, 1984.

Higgins, A.J., and Lees, P.: Phenylbutazone inhibition of prostaglandin E2 production in equine acute inflammatory exudate. Vet. Rec., *113*:622, 1983.

Higgins, A.J., Lees, P., Sedgwick, A.D., et al.: Use of a novel nonsteroidal anti-inflammatory drug in the horse. Equine Vet. J., *19(1)*:60, 1987.

Higgins, A.J., Lees, P., and Taylor, J.B.: Influence of phenylbutazone on eicosanoid levels in equine acute inflammatory exudate. Cornell Vet., *74*:198, 1984.

Higgs, G.A., Eakins, K.E., Mugridge, K.G., et al.: The effects of nonsteroidal anti-inflammatory drugs on leukocyte migration in carrageenin-induced inflammation. Eur. J. Pharmacol., *66*:66, 1980.

Houdeshell, J.W., and Hennessey, P.W.: A new nonsteroidal, anti-inflammatory analgesic for horses. J. Equine Med. Surg., *1*:57, 1977.

Houston, T., Chay, S., Woods, W.E., et al.: Phenylbutazone and its metabolites in plasma and urine of thoroughbred horses: population distributions and the effects of urinary pH. J. Vet. Pharmacol. Ther., *8*:136, 1985.

Huskisson, E.C.: Osteoarthritis. *In* Drug Treatment of the Rheumatic Diseases. Edited by F.D. Hart. New York, ADIS, 1982.

Jackson, M.L.: Platelet physiology and platelet function: inhibition by aspirin. Compend. Contin. Educ. Pract. Vet., *9(6)*:627, 1987.

Jeffcott, L.B., and Colles, C.M.: Phenylbutazone and the horse—a review. Equine Vet. J., *9(3)*:105, 1977.

Johnstone, I.B.: Comparative effects of phenylbutazone, naproxen and flunixin meglumine on equine platelet aggregation and platelet factor 3 availability in vitro. Can. J. Comp. Med., *47*:172, 1983.

Jones, E.W., and Hamm, D.: Comparative efficacy of phenylbutazone and naproxen in induced equine myositis. J. Equine Med. Surg., *2*:341, 1978.

Judson, D.G., and Barton, M.: Effect of aspirin on haemostasis in the horse. Res. Vet. Sci., *30*:241, 1981.

Kantor, T.G.: Ketoprofen: a review of its pharmacological and clinical properties. Pharmacotherapy, *6*:93, 1986.

Kapravdh, M., Lumb, W.V., Wright, M., et al.: Effect of butorphanol, flunixin, levorphanol, morphine and xylazine in ponies. Am. J. Vet. Res., *45*:217, 1984.

Kauffman, G.: Aspirin-induced gastric mucosal injury: lesions learned from animal models. Gastroenterology, *96*:606, 1989.

Lang, E., and Steger, W.: A comparative study of efficacy and tolerability of ketoprofen and piroxicam. Br. J. Clin. Pract., *35*:167, 1981.

Lees, P., and Higgins, A.J.: Clinical pharmacology and therapeutic use of nonsteroidal anti-inflammatory drugs in the horse. Equine Vet. J., *17(2)*:83, 1985.

Lees, P., and Higgins, A.J.: Flunixin inhibits prostaglandin production in equine inflammation. Res. Vet. Sci., *37*:347, 1984.

Maitho, T.E., Lees, P., and Taylor, J.B.: Absorption and pharmacokinetics of phenylbutazone in Welsh Mountain ponies. J. Vet. Pharmacol. Ther., *9*:26, 1986.

Maylin, G.A.: Disposition of phenylbutazone in the horse. Proc. 20th Convention Assoc. Am. Equine Pract., pp. 243–249, 1974.

Meschter, C.L., Maylin, G.A., and Krook, L.: Vascular pathology in phenylbutazone intoxicated horses. Cornell Vet., *74*:282, 1984.

Paganini-Hill, A., Chao, A., Ross, R.K., and Henderson, B.E.: Aspirin use and chronic diseases: a cohort study of the elderly. Br. Med. J., *229*:1247, 1989.

Palmer, R.J., Stepney, R., Higgs, G.A., and Eakins, K.E.: Chemokinetic activity of arachidonic acid lipoxygenase products on leukocytes from different species. Prostaglandins, *20*:411, 1980.

Paulus, H.E.: U.S. clinical trials of ketoprofen: review of safety data. Sydney, Australia, Proc. Ketoprofen Symposium, 1985.

Piperno, E., Ellis, D.J., Getty, S.M., and Brody, T.M.: Plasma and urine levels of phenylbutazone in the horse. J. Am. Vet. Med. Assoc., *153*:195, 1968.

Read, W.K.: Renal medullary crest necrosis associated with phenylbutazone therapy in horses. Vet. Pathol., *20*:662, 1983.

Riley, R.G., Connor, G.H., and Beck, C.C.: Arquel as a treatment for equine laminitis. P.A.A.E.P. *21*:115, 1975.

Rosenberg, L., Palmer, J.R., Zauber, A.G., et al.: A hypothesis: nonsteroidal anti-inflammatory drugs reduce the incidence of large bowel cancer. J. Natl. Cancer Inst., *83*:355, 1991.

Ross, R.: The pathogenesis of atherosclerosis. An update. N. Engl. J. Med., *314*:488, 1986.

Simon, L.S., and Mills, J.A.: Nonsteroidal anti-inflammatory drugs. Part I. N. Engl. J. Med., *302*:1179, 1980.

Snow, D.M.: Non Steroidal Anti-inflammatory Agents in the Horse. In Practice. Sept. 1981. 23–30.

Snow, D., Baxter, P. and Whiting, B.: The pharmacokinetics of meclofenamic acid in the horse. J. Vet. Pharmacol. Ther., *4*:147, 1981.

Snow, D.M., Bogan, J.A., and Douglas, J.A.: Phenylbutazone toxicity in ponies. Vet. Rec., *105*:26, 1979.

Snow, D.M., Douglas, J.A., and Thompson, H.: Phenylbutazone toxicity in equidae: a biochemical and pathophysiologic study. Am. J. Vet. Res., *42*:1754, 1981.

Snow, D.M., Douglas, J.A., and Thompson, H.: Phenylbutazone toxicity in ponies. Vet. Rec., *105*:26, 1981.

Stafanger, G., Larsen, H.W., Hansen, H., and Sorensen, K.: Pharmacokinetics of ketoprofen in patients with chronic renal failure. Scand. J. Rheumatol., *10*:189, 1981.

Sullivan, M., and Snow, D.M.: Factors affecting absorption of nonsteroidal anti-inflammatory agents in the horse. Vet. Rec., *110*:554, 1981.

Templeton, C.B., Bottoms, G.D., and Fessler, J.F.: Effects of flunixin meglumine on hemodynamics, hematology, prostaglandins, and survival in ponies during chronic exposure to endotoxin. Fed. Proc., *42*:323, 1983.

Thun, M.J., Namboodiri, B.S., and Clark, W.: Aspirin use and reduced risk of fatal colon cancer. N. Engl. J. Med., *325(23)*:1593, 1991.

Tobin, T.: Pharmacology review—the nonsteroidal anti-inflammatory drugs. I. Phenylbutazone. J. Equine Med. Surg., *3*:253, 1979.

Tobin, T.: Pharmacology review—the nonsteroidal anti-inflammatory drugs. II. Equiproxen meclofenamic acid, flunixin and others. J. Equine Med. Surg., *6*:298, 1979b.

Tobin, T., Chay, S., Kamerling, S., et al.: Phenylbutazone in the horse—a review. J. Vet. Pharmacol. Ther., *9*:1, 1986.

Traub, J.L., Paulsen, L.M., and Reed, S.M.: The use of phenylbutazone in the horse. Compend. Contin. Educ. Pract., Vet., *5(6)*:S320, 1983.

Vernimb, G.D., and Hennessey, P.W.: Clinical studies on flunixin meglumine in the treatment of equine colic. J. Equine Med. Surg., *1*:111, 1977.

Williams, R.L., Upton, R.A., Buskin, J.N., and Jones, R.M.: Ketoprofen-aspirin interactions. Clin. Pharmacol. Ther., *30*:226, 1981.

Wolheim, F.A., Lindroth, Y., and Sjoblom, K.G.: A comparison of ketoprofen and naproxen in rheumatoid arthritis. Rheumatol. Rehabil., *17*(Suppl.):78, 1978.

STEROIDS

Anonymous: Are corticosteroids useful in shock therapy? J. Am. Vet. Med. Assoc., *177(5)*:453, 1980.

Barlow, J.E., and Rosenthal, A.S.: Glucocorticoid suppression of macrophage migration inhibitory factor. J. Exp. Med., *137*:1031, 1973.

Behrens, F., Shepard, N., and Mitchell, N.: Alteration of rabbit articular cartilage by intra-articular injections of glucocorticoids. J. Bone Joint Surg., *57(A)*:70, 1975.

Belling, T.H.: A better approach to intracarpal injections. Vet. Med., Feb.: 158, 1986.

Besse, J.C., and Bass, A.D.: Potentiation of hydrocortisone responses to catecholamines in vascular smooth muscle. J. Pharmacol. Exp. Ther., *154*:224, 1966.

Blackwell, G.J., et al.: Macrocortin: a polypeptide causing the anti-phospholipase effect of glucocorticoids. Nature, *287*:147, 1980.

Bottoms, G.D.: Endotoxin-induced physiologic changes in ponies: effect of flunixin meglumine, dexamethasone and naloxone. AAEP Newsletter, No. 2, pp. 39–42, 1982.

Casey, J.P., Short, B.L., and Rink, R.D.: The effect of methylprednisolone on hepatic oxygen supply and plasma lactate and glucose in endotoxemia. Circ. Shock, *6*:245, 1979.

Chunekamrai, S., Krook, L.P., Lust, G., and Maylin, G.A.: Changes in articular cartilage after intra-articular injections of methylprednisolone acetate in horses. Am. J. Vet. Res., *50(10)*:1733, 1989.

Claman, H.N.: Corticosteroids and lymphoid cells. N. Engl. J. Med., *287*:388, 1972.

Clermont, H.G., Williams, J.S., and Adams, J.T.: Steroid effect on the release of the lysosomal enzyme acid phosphatase in shock. Ann. Surg., *179(6)*:34, 1974.

Coppoc, G.L.: Relationship of dosage form of a corticosteroid to its therapeutic efficacy. J. Am. Vet. Med. Assoc., *186(10)*:1098, 1984.

Dinarello, C.A.: Interleukin-1 and the pathogenesis of the acute-phase response. N. Engl. J. Med., *311*:1413, 1984.

Dopson, L.C., et al.: Immunosuppression associated with lymphosarcoma in two horses. J. Am. Vet. Med. Assoc., *182(11)*:1239, 1983.

Eyre, P., and Elmes, P.J.: Corticosteroid-induced laminitis: further observations on the isolated perfused hoof. Vet. Res. Commun., *4*:139, 1980.

Eyre, P., Elmes, P.J., and Strickland, S.: Corticosteroid-potentiated vascular responses of the equine digit: possible pharmacologic basis of laminitis. Am. J. Vet. Res., *40*:135, 1979.

Fariss, B.L., Hane, S., Shinsako, J., et al.: Comparison of absorption of cortisone acetate and hydrocortisone hemisuccinate. J. Clin. Endocrinol. Metab., *47(1)*:137, 1978.

Ferguson, J.L., et al.: Dexamethasone treatment during hemorrhagic shock—effects independent of increased blood pressure. Am. J. Vet. Res., *39*:825, 1978.

Fox, A.C., Hoffstein, S., and Weissmann, G.: Lysosomal mechanisms in production of tissue damage during myocardial ischemia and the effects of treatment with steroids. Am. Heart J., *91(3)*:29, 1976.

Garcia-Leme, J.: Cellular Functions in Inflammation Hormones and Inflammation. Boca Raton, FL, CRC Press, 1989.

Gillis, S., et al.: Glucocorticoid-induced inhibition of T-cell growth factor. J. Immunol., *123*:1632, 1979.

Glade, M.J., Krook, L., and Schryver, H.F.: Morphologic and biochemical changes in cartilage in foals treated with dexamethasone. Cornell Vet., *73*:170, 1983.

Goetzl, E.J., and Goldstein, I.M.: Arachidonic acid metabolites. *In* Arthritis and Allied Conditions: A Textbook of Rheumatology. Edited by D.J. McCarty. Philadelphia, Lea & Febiger, 1989.

Grinstein-Nadler, E., and Bottoms, G.D.: Dexamethasone treatment during hemorrhagic shock—changes in extracellular fluid volume and cell membrane transport. Am. J. Vet. Res., *37*:1337, 1976.

Hirata, F., et al.: A phospholipase A2 inhibitory protein in rabbit neutrophils induced by glucocorticoids. Proc. Natl. Acad. Sci. USA, *77*:2533, 1980.

Imai, T., Sakuraya, N., and Fujita, T.: Comparative study of anti-endotoxic potency of dexamethasone based on its different ester types. Circ. Shock, *6*:311, 1979.

Jones, W.E.: Towards more rational joint therapy. Vet. Med., Feb.: 221, 1984.

Kemppainen, R.J., and Sartin, J.L.: Effects of single intravenous doses of dexamethasone on base-line plasma cortisol concentrations and responses to synthetic ACTH in healthy dogs. Am. J. Vet. Res., *45*:742, 1984.

Lewis, R.A., Austen, K.F., and Soberman, R.J.: Leukotrienes and other products of the 5-lipoxygenase pathway: biochemistry and relation to pathobiology in human diseases. N. Engl. J. Med., *323(10)*:645, 1990.

Meuleman, J., et al.: The Immunologic Effects, Kinetics and Use of Glucocorticoids. Med. Clin. North Am., *69*:805, 1985.

Moore, J.N., et al.: The effects of prednisolone sodium succinate in endotoxemia: comparison with flunixin meglumine. Proc. Equine Colic Res. Symp., Univ. of Georgia, Athens, 1982, pp. 176–178.

Nelson, A.W.: The unified concept of shock. Vet. Clin. North Am., *6*:173, 187, 227, 1976.

Nizolek, D.J.H., and White, K.K.: Corticosteroid and hyaluronic acid treatments in equine degenerative joint disease. Cornell Vet., *71*:355, 1981.

Parillo, J.E., and Fanci, A.S.: Mechanisms of glucocorticoid action on the immune processes. Ann. Rev. Pharmacol. Toxicol., *19*:179, 1979.

Pool, R.R., et al.: Corticosteroid therapy in common joint and tendon injuries of the horse. Part I. Effects on joints. Proc. 26th Ann. Meeting AAEP, Anaheim, CA, Dec. 1980, pp. 397–406.

Rhinhart, J.J., et al.: Effects of corticosteroid therapy on human monocyte function. N. Engl. J. Med., *292*:236, 1975.

Roth, J.A., and Kaeberle, M.L.: Effect of glucocorticoids on the bovine immune system. J. Am. Vet. Med. Assoc., *180(8)*:894, 1982.

Shatney, C.H., Lillehei, R.C., Dietzman, R.H., et al.: Influence of the salt moiety on the effectiveness of corticosteroid therapy in cardiogenic shock. Circ. Shock, 9:247, 1982.

Silberberg, M., Silberberg, R., and Hasler, M.: Fine structure of articular cartilage in mice receiving cortisone acetate. Arch. Pathol., 87:569, 1986.

Stevenson, R.D.: Hydrocortisone and migration of human leukocytes: an indirect effect mediated by mononuclear cells. Clin. Exp. Immunol., 15:417, 1973.

Toutain, P.L., Alvinerie, M., and Ruckebusch, Y.: Pharmacokinetics of dexamethasone and its effect on adrenal gland function in the dog. Am. J. Vet. Res., 44:212, 1983.

Toutain, P.L., Brandon, R.A., DePomyers, H., et al.: Dexamethasone and prednisolone in the horse. Pharmacokinetics and action in the adrenal gland. Am. J. Vet. Res., 45:1743, 1984.

Vane, J., and Botting, R.: Inflammation and the mechanism of action and anti-inflammatory drugs. Fed. Am. Soc. Exper. Biol. J., 1:89, 1987.

Vernimb, G.D., Van Hoose, L.M., and Hennessey, P.W.: Onset and duration of corticosteroid effect after injection of betasone for treating equine arthropathies. Vet. Med., 72:241, 1977.

Wilcke, J.R., and Davis, L.E.: Review of glucocorticoid pharmacology. Vet. Clin. North Am., 12(1):3, 1982.

DRUG CLEARANCE AND THE DOPING PROBLEM

22.1 Introduction
The Position in Europe
The Position in the United States
22.2 Types of Doping
22.3 Sampling for Drug Doping
22.4 Sample Analysis
22.5 Patterns and Problems of Doping
22.6 Problem Drugs

22.1 INTRODUCTION

The doping of horses is an undesirable practice for many reasons. First, it is an unfair, unjust, and dishonest practice. Second, the administration of the dope may cause permanent damage to the normal physiologic functioning of the animal. Third, it may interfere with the selection of animals for breeding and with the soundness of blood lines by conferring a false value on inferior animals. An animal must perform on its own inherent merits and according to its own natural ability without the assistance of chemical aids. In the United States, permissive medication is legally recognized in certain states for a variety of reasons.

In common with many other legal definitions, defining a dope is not easy. In European usage, animal doping is the administration of any substance, other than a normal nutrient, affecting an animal's speed, stamina, courage, or conduct in a race; performance in the show ring; or where it could confer a false value on an inferior animal.

Doping is frequently done to make a competitor's animal perform or show poorly. Tranquilizers, opiates, barbiturates, and other sedatives are used for this purpose. Doping to improve performance, such as using stimulants in racehorses, can cause serious side effects.

The best deterrent for the racehorse industry has been the detection of dope in the animal, with subsequent prosecution or suspension from racing activities of those individuals concerned.

With the advent of sensitive immunoassays, drugs or their metabolites are now detectable long after their pharmacologic effects have disappeared. This is useful in detecting low doses of potent drugs with no recognized therapeutic use in the horse. The number of cases in which residues of therapeutic or endogenous substances are found, however, will probably grow. The likely question is whether or not these substances could have been pharmacologically active at the detected level. This has, in part, prompted the call for thresholds.

THE POSITION IN EUROPE

In Europe, particularly Britain, Ireland, and France, doping is defined as earlier stated.

Rule 200 of the British Rules of Racing states that "any person who administers or allows or causes to be administered or connives at the administration to a horse of any amount of any substance (other than a normal nutrient), being a substance which by its nature could affect the racing performance of a horse shall be guilty of a breach of the Rules and may be declared a disqualified person or otherwise penalized by the Stewards of the Jockey Club in accordance with their powers under Rule 2 of these Rules."

The overall definition of a doping substance is loose and vague inasmuch as it is difficult to determine what constitutes a *normal* nutrient. In Britain, however, the position has been clarified somewhat by the publication of a list of categories of prohibited substances by the Stewards of the Jockey Club. The prohibited substances are listed under categories of drugs rather than as individual proprietary products. A prohibited substance is defined as "one originating externally, whether or not it is endogenous to the horse, which falls into any of the categories contained in the proscribed list published from time to time by the Stewards of the Jockey Club in the Racing Calendar."

In addition, the phrase, "nonnormal nutrient" has been replaced by "a substance, the origin of which cannot be traced to normal and ordinary feeding, and which by its nature could affect the racing performance." These changes in the Rules mean that if a prohibited substance is detected at the time of racing in the body fluids of a horse, regardless of concentration, grounds exist for an inquiry. The particular relevance of this to the veterinarian is that the therapeutic use of a prohibited substance at the time of racing is not allowed. Table 23–1 lists the categories of prohibited substances.

Doping may be divided into a number of categories: doping with intent to win or "stimulant" doping, when agents such as caffeine, amphetamine, or pentylenetetrazol are administered shortly before racing; doping with intent to lose when sedative agents such as the barbiturates xylazine, detomidine and choral hydrate, are administered. In addition to these major categories, the administration of a local anesthetic to mask lameness or of the various steroids for other purposes also constitutes doping. There are major distinctions between the United States and Europe with regard to legal racetrack medication.

TABLE 22–1
LIST OF CATEGORIES OF PROHIBITED SUBSTANCES, JOCKEY CLUB, 1977 (U.K.)

Drugs acting on the central nervous system
Drugs acting on the autonomic nervous system
Drugs acting on the cardiovascular system
Drugs affecting the gastrointestinal function
Antibiotics, synthetic antibacterials, and antiviral drugs
Antihistamines
Antimalarials
Antipyretics, analgesics, and anti-inflammatory drugs
Diuretics
Local anesthetics
Muscle relaxants
Respiratory stimulants
Sex hormones, anabolic steroids, and corticosteroids
Endocrine secretions and their synthetic counterparts
Substances affecting blood coagulation
Cytotoxic substances

THE POSITION IN THE UNITED STATES

CONTROLLED MEDICATION PROGRAMS

Many racing commissions in the 1960s and 1970s chose to allow a range of drugs to be used in performance horses under controlled conditions, e.g., phenylbutazone, furosemide, and the corticosteroids.

A controlled medication program is one under which certain drugs are approved for use in horses at times, most often including the last day before racing, and occasionally including medication on race day. California's controlled medication program served as the prototype for many of the controlled medication programs in the United States.

TABLE 22–2
SAMPLE ANALYSIS

Samples from winners
Samples from nonwinners
Samples from beaten favorites
Random samples
Horses seriously out of form
Quality control samples
Parallel testing
    (exchange negative samples comparing
    quality of analytical work)

This program called for detailed reporting of all medications administered, dispensed, or prescribed within the racing enclosure. The California Horse Racing Board approved phenylbutazone for use in horses up to the last day before racing in 1970 and approved furosemide for use in bleeders in 1975.

Currently, the major problems of racing in the United States are caused by too much racing. This has led to too few horses and small fields. Consequently many owners and trainers try to enter their horses too frequently and to race them when they are unfit to run.

This desire has led to constant pressure from horsemen through their organizations for so called "permissive medication". Started in the State of Colorado, this has grown until finally only a few states, continue to resist the pressure.

Proponents of the use of agents such as phenylbutazone suggest that if their use was restricted the number of horses fielded would be markedly reduced. On the other hand, opponents of the use of these drugs maintain that horses that need phenylbutazone to run should not be running under any circumstances, and to run horses on these drugs is inhumane.

Furosemide (Lasix®) used to help horses with bleeding in the respiratory tract, and with other respiratory or "wind" problems.

Usage control for both phenylbutazone and furosemide is relatively easy, since good analytic methods are available for these agents. Some states have endeavored to control phenylbutazone medication by quantitation, and while lower limits cause little difficulty, maximum allowable limits have caused problems.

A rule that is sometimes used when controlling medication is the "time rule". With this rule, the period before a race during which certain drugs cannot be administered is stipulated. As testing increases in sensitivity and the legitimate therapeutic use of relatively innocuous drugs such as phenylbutazone increases, more positives on drugs such as phenylbutazone are found through testing, although the trainers claimed the drugs had been given more than twenty-four hours before race time.

Once a horse is given the drug, it must continue to receive it through the season, regardless of whether it is therapeutically necessary or not. This is done to prevent any fluctuations in form. However, the belief is that because of the racing surfaces used plus the number of times the horses run each season, such permissive medication is essential.

The first introduction of permissive medication was by the State of Colorado permitting primarily the use of phenylbutazone (Butazolidin) for therapeutic purposes. A revision of Colorado rules issued information on allowable and prohibited drugs. Most important was that phenylbutazone, oxyphenbutazone and indomethacin also could be used up to approximately 24 hours before the race and when permitted would have to be used regularly until the horse was cured. This was controlled by the requirement that not more than 50 μg/ml of phenylbutazone and metabolites could be recovered from the urine sample.

Most states within the U.S. permit controlled use of phenylbutazone in racehorses within 24 hours of a race if the veterinarian declares the dosage rate and is prepared to certify the horse as raceably fit. However, levels of the drug above 50 μg/ml, are interpreted as evidence of administration of phenylbutazone within 24 hours of or on the day of the race.

Certain States in the United States of America allow the use of phenylbutazone provided this medication and the dosage rate is made known to the proper authority by the veterinary surgeon in charge of the case. The American Association of Equine Practitioners has suggested that 4.4 mg/kg administered intravenously is a "nonabusive" dose of phenylbutazone for a racehorse.

The State of California permits the controlled use of phenylbutazone and this means that a horse can be registered to race if the veterinarian states the dosage rate and is prepared to certify the horse as race fit. No drug is given within 24 hours of the race and the horse must be kept on the treatment until its name is removed from the register. These horses are expected to be positive to tests for phenylbutazone but amounts above 50 μg/ml of urine are taken as evidence of administration within 24 hours. The California horse racing board has also established that a test result of over 165 of phenylbutazone in μg/ml of urine is prima facie evidence of administration of race-day medication in violation of the rules.

The California controlled medication program clearly distinguishes between two classes of drugs, the Penal Code drugs, whose detection constitutes a "positive", and other medications, whose use *is* permitted within narrowly controlled conditions.

Many states have medication programs where phenylbutazone is prohibited within 48 hours of race time, pentazocine within 72 hours and procaine within 7 days. Kentucky allows the use of diuretics such as furosemide, anti-inflammatories such as phenylbutazone, the other nonsteroidal anti-inflammatory agents and salicylates, muscle relaxants such as methocarbamol, and the anti-inflammatory corticosteroids. Use of these drugs is carefully monitored by blood and urine analysis. In Ohio reports of "Controlled Medication" within 48 hours must be filed but the drugs can be administered up to 4 hours before post time. Other states within the USA do not permit use of phenylbutazone in the racehorse; presence of any level of the drug in urine is illegal.

22.2 TYPES OF DOPING

Various types of drugs are used to affect equine performance. First, there is doping to win, in which the horse is given a stimulant drug such as amphetamine, caffeine, apomorphine, or fentanyl to increase its speed. There is also doping to lose, or depressant doping, occurs when the horse is given a tranquilizer or depressant such as acepromazine or reserpine to make it run more slowly.

Drugs which stimulate the central nervous system (CNS) are thought to enhance performance by delaying the onset of fatigue. These drugs may decrease perception of the strenuousness of an event, increase alertness, decrease fatigue caused by sleep loss, and increase the amount of work an animal will perform for a reward. They may also mimic activation of the sympathetic nervous system and increase cardiorespiratory activity. Other classes of drugs may delay the onset of fatigue. Controversial aids such as bicarbonate, increased dietary fat, and erythropoietin are thought to buffer lactic acidosis, provide increased energy, and increase the oxygen carrying capacity of the blood, respectively. All of these may act to delay fatigue.

"Medications to win" are drugs that stimulate the central and or sympathetic nervous systems are included in this category. Sympathomimetic amines such as amphetamines increase locomotor activity, decrease fatigue and augment cardiorespiratory activity. Opiates, although depressant in man, have amphetamine-like effects in horses and raise pain thresholds. Anabolic steroids increase muscle mass and aggressiveness. Their ability to enhance performance, however, has been attributed more to their psychologic than musculoskeletal effects.

"Medications to lose" are those medications which generally decrease the functioning of the animal. Higher doses of putative sedatives (e.g., barbiturates, alpha-2 adrenoceptor agonists—detomidine xylazine), tranquilizers, (e.g., phenothiazines, butyrophenones, benzodiazepines) and hypnotics might decrease overall performance by depressing CNS activity.

A third form of doping occurs when a horse is given a drug to restore normal performance. Drugs such as phenylbutazone or furosemide come into this class, and while this is regarded as controlled medication in most of the United States, it is considered doping in most of western Europe. Thera-

peutic doping can compromise the veterinarian with trainers or animal owners.

The fourth form of doping is accidental or inadvertent causes of accidental "positives" include contamination of urine samples with nicotine and/or caffeine during sampling by the urine collector. Another cause of some inadvertent doping positives in England has been the inclusion of cocoa husk in horse rations by a feed manufacturer. Trainers who purchased and used this feed unwittingly fed their horses caffeine, which was metabolized to theobromine and turned up in the animal's urine. The methylxanthines, caffeine and theobromine, often occur as contaminants of manufactured feeds. They occur in potential components of compound feed such as cocoa and coffee products and from overenthusiastic administration of a popular tonic.

The occurrence of theobromine in postrace urine samples has been of concern in many countries. Because theobromine is a member of the xanthine alkaloid group of drugs and is closely related to the traditionally well-known stimulant caffeine, the significance of the detection of theobromine in a post-race urine sample is of major importance. The problems with the interpretation of the significance in these samples appear to have arisen from conflicting opinion regarding the classification of theobromine as a drug for the purposes of the Rules of Racing and the apparently innocuous sources of theobromine, e.g. chocolate or cocoabean meal based feedstuffs.

Plants containing substances closely related to cocaine, morphine, atropine, noradrenaline, and digitalis, are widely distributed naturally in the plant kingdom. Although they are not cultivated or used as horse food, they grow as weeds which can be ingested by racehorses who spend part of their day grazing. The widely-used pasture grasses of the phalaris species (canary grasses) contain bufotenine and other dimethyltryptamine compounds that are monoaminoxidase inhibitors and thus inhibit the degradation of serotonin and to a less extent the catecholamines, epinephrine, norepinephrine and dopamine. Under some growing conditions, the amounts of tryptamines are toxic but lower intakes raise catecholamine levels modestly and could have performance-enhancing effects. Tryptamine itself has an LSD-like action.

Results showing presence of some pasture plants that grow as weeds are likely to be classed as "prohibited", such as the opioid-containing wild poppy, the salicylate-containing willow which commonly grows in pastures and many others; however, a threshold for salicylate overcomes the possible problem caused by willow. The urine of horses and other herbivores normally contains small quantities of salicylate. This salicylate comes either from the grass and hay that the horse ingests or is a product of the horse's metabolism.

A very few cultivars of a yellow lupin contain sparteine, a cardiac stimulant in small doses which is available as a pure preparation and is used as an oxytocic and hypoglycemic substance in medicine. It is, therefore, a prohibited substance. It is occasionally detected in urine samples. Feed compounders, looking for sources of plant protein, might regard lupin seeds as a valuable source of protein for compound horse feeds.

In a urine test conducted in the U.K. by the Horse Racing Forensic Laboratory, traces of the banned substance 3-hydroxycamphor were found and the Jockey Club stripped the filly of its title. However, its owner, produced a number of independent experts who argued that the traces of the metabolite could have been the result of normal feeding.

It is well known that nikethamide (N,N-diethylnicotinamide) is metabolized very rapidly to nicotinamide. Hence, there is difficulty in proving that nikethamide has been used as a doping substance because nicotinamide is a normal physiologic metabolite in the organism as well as a vitamin preparation. However, an intermediate metabolite (N-ethylnicotinamide) is found in the urine of horses treated with Coramine. This is detected by gas chromatography/mass spectrometry, and synthesized and identified as being N-ethylnicotinamide.

Laboratories can find small quantities of prohibited substances that may have arisen endogenously within the horse (like anabolic steroids) or exogenously in the horse's normal diet (like salicylic acid) or also in processed feed (like theobromine). A threshold should be set for naturally occurring substances.

There are four substances involved, arsenic, salicyclic acid, 19-nortestosterone and theobromine. Traces of arsenic and salicyclic acid can be found in normal horse feed. Plants, such as lucerne especially, can be particularly high in the latter.

As with 19-nortestosterone the detection of administration of anabolic steroid preparations based upon testosterone to the colt presents major problems because of the endogenous nature of the parent steroid and its metabolites. Significant levels of testosterone and androstane-3, 17-diol have been detected in normal colt urine.

There is considerable debate about guidelines for defining and establishing drug thresholds. Differing perspectives have emerged from the United States and the international community. The need for establishing thresholds has arisen for several reasons. First, there are therapeutic drugs with legitimate uses in horses which could influence performance and be detected in trace amounts on race day. Second, there are dietary and endogenously occurring substances which could have been administered to produce a pharmacologic (performance altering) effect.

The international position is reflected in a set of guidelines proposed by the International Conference of Racing Authorities (ICRA) which considers endogenous substances and feed contaminants. In their guidelines "An endogenous or dietary prohibited substance (is) that (which) can be said to have arisen abnormally." Thresholds are levels above which these substances can be deemed to have arisen other than endogenous or through acceptable feeding.

REGULATIONS IN EUROPE

The Rules of Racing at present make it an offense to give a nonnutrient to alter performance at the time of racing. In other words, if a horse is lame and is restored to normality by the administration of phenylbutazone, its performance is affected at the time of racing by a substance other than a normal nutrient, and the animal is therefore by definition doped. This can pose a dilemma for the veterinarian in practice because on the one hand, he should give proper therapy to a sick animal, and on the other hand, he must not, however inadvertently, contravene the Rules of Racing. Threshold levels apply to five substances under Jockey Club (U.K.) Rules: arsenic, salicylic acid, theobromine, dimethyl sulfoxide and nandrolone conjugates.

The division between doping and legitimate veterinary therapy can, under some circumstances, be quite difficult to determine, and the criterion applied varies in different countries. In the United States for instance, many states now have "permissive medication" where certain drugs, such as phenylbutazone may be given, provided that the administration is openly declared. In addition, a horse once given the drug must continue to receive it throughout the season regardless of whether it is therapeutically necessary or not. This is done to prevent any fluctuations of form that might otherwise occur.

The Federation Equestre Internationale (FEI) has laid down a list of prohibited substances which must not be present in a horse's blood or urine during or after any official competition. This list, which appears below, is essentially similar to that prescribed by the British Jockey Club.

Prohibited substances are substances originating externally whether or not they are endogenous to the horse.

Substances acting on the nervous system

Substances acting on the cardiovascular system

Substances acting on the respiratory system

Substances acting on the alimentary system

Substances acting on the urinary system

Substances acting on the immune system

Antibiotics, antibacterial and antiviral substances

Antiparasitic substances

Antipyretics, analgesics and anti-inflammatory substances other than Phenylbutazone and Oxyphenbutazone

Endocrine secretions and their synthetic counterparts

Substances affecting blood coagulation

Cytotoxic substances

List of substances for which permissible concentrations have been established

Phenylbutazone = $2.0 \ \mu g/ml/plasma$

Oxyphenbutazone = $2.0 \ \mu g/ml/plasma$
Theobromine = $2.0 \ \mu g/ml/urine$
Salicylic Acid = $750.0 \ \mu g/ml/urine$
Arsenic = $0.2 \ \mu g/ml/urine$

It will be seen that the above list is very similar to that of the U.K. Jockey Club. There are however, a few significant differences:

Phenylbutazone and Oxyphenbutazone
A threshold level is permitted in order to allow treatment of horses in transit to a competition.

Theobromine
The permitted concentration is similar to that in the Jockey Club Rules, so it is important to emphasize that any feed for competition horses should be of a similar standard to that fed to racehorses.

22.3 SAMPLING FOR DRUG DOPING

In practical terms, four body fluids are available for sampling for dope testing: sweat, saliva, blood, and urine. Sweat is sometimes collected but can be unsatisfactory from a legal viewpoint in that it may be difficult to exclude contamination (e.g., nicotine from smoker's hands, theobromine from chocolate, or traces left from intramuscular injections many days earlier). For these reasons, sweat is not considered a satisfactory sample by most forensic authorities and is now rarely used in equine forensic chemistry.

Urine is generally accepted as being the best body fluid for analysis insofar as most drugs are excreted mainly or partly in the urine. Drug metabolites, in addition to unchanged parent drug, are frequently present in the urine, and in some cases (i.e., oxyphenbutazone from phenylbutazone), these metabolites are pharmacologically active. Urine testing has a number of advantages over blood testing for the detection of drugs or drug metabolites post-race.

A larger volume of urine is obtainable, and sufficient samples for split tests and confirmatory tests by other laboratories are often available. A further major advantage is that drugs and drug metabolites are often concentrated in urine.

Urine collection is normally made by acquiring a naturally voided sample from the

TABLE 22–3
METHODS OF ANALYSIS

Screening Methods
Used to detect the presence of an analyte or class of analytes at the level of interest. These
methods have a high sample throughput capacity and are used to sift large numbers of
samples for potential positives. They are aimed at avoiding false-negative results
Confirmatory Methods
Provide unequivocal identification of the analyte at the level of interest. These methods are
aimed at preventing false-positive results as well as having an acceptable low probability of
false-negative results
Sensitivity
Measure of the ability of a method to discriminate between small differences in analyte
content. Sensitivity is the slope of the calibration curve at the level of interest
Specificity
Ability of a method to distinguish between the analyte being measured and other substances.
This characteristic is predominantly a function of the measuring principle used but can vary
according to class of compound or matrix
Limit of Detection
Smallest measured content from which it is possible to deduce the presence of the analyte with
reasonable statistical certainty
Limit of Determination
Lowest analyte content for which the method has been validated with specified degrees of
accuracy and repeatability

animal into a suitable receptacle. It is important that a sufficient volume of sample is collected so the analyst will have sufficient material. It must always be ensured that any dope detected in a sample has been derived from that particular animal and not from any outside source or contamination; second, it must be ensured that a sufficient sample is taken to provide adequate material for the analyst to work on and, third, that the owner receives a sample for an independent analysis. This obviates any conflict or disagreement in the event of a positive result's being obtained from the analysis of one sample only. In addition, because it has to be clear to all concerned that all utensils and instruments used are free from dope substances, it would accordingly follow that the best way of sampling is by using a controlled technique. This involves using two containers—one for the actual sample and one for the washings from the empty containers. The contents of both containers, sample and control, are then analyzed, and a positive result is indicated only if the sample container alone is positive.

When a horse has won a race or has been picked for examination either by the veterinarian or the stewards, the animal is brought to the sampling area by one of the security men. A urine sample is collected or a blood sample taken if no urine is available. The urine sample is split, in the presence of a representative of the trainer, into two portions. The duplicate samples are placed in separate plastic bottles and the bottles sealed. All samples are coded so the laboratory knows only the number. The samples are delivered to the Unit under strict security. See Tables 22–3 to 22–6.

When blood is analyzed, it enables a quantitative interpretation of drug concentration to be given. In contrast, a urine sample may reveal only approximately how much was circulating when the sample was taken. Some drugs, however, can be detected in urine long after they have become undetectable in blood. Blood samples are not routinely taken because of the risk of injury to the horse and also the general reluctance of owners to permit them.

While blood can be very easily and rapidly obtained from horses, the volume available for use in a pre-race test is usually about 20 ml, less than a tenth of the usual urine volume. This small amount means

> **TABLE 22–4**
> **ANALYTICAL PROCEDURES**
>
> Initial screening/confirmatory tests
> Further examination for the presence of a prohibited substance
> Quantitation procedures

that the quantity of drug available to the analyst is correspondingly reduced. Further, some drugs or drug metabolites are found in lower concentrations in blood than in urine. A drug found in the bloodstream is usually found as the unchanged drug and not in the changed or metabolized form as found in urine. Virtually all drugs are more difficult to detect in blood than in urine. The principal exceptions are acidic drugs such as phenylbutazone and furosemide, which are highly bound to plasma proteins and are therefore present in high concentrations in blood.

Saliva was the principal body fluid used in the early days of dope detection, and in fact many positive results were reported. Today saliva is not commonly used, however, one of the principal disadvantages being that the volume obtainable is small. Also, experimental work suggests that many drugs do not pass readily into saliva from plasma. Factors affecting the salivary secretion of drugs have been reported in cows, horses, humans, and dogs.

The concentrations of drugs in saliva are low because that fraction of the drug which is protein bound in blood does not pass into the saliva. Thus, acidic drugs such as phenylbutazone, the other nonsteroidal anti-inflammatory drugs, and furosemide are found in saliva only in quite low concentrations.

Of interest to both the racing pharmacist and the veterinarian is the way a drug and its metabolites are distributed in the blood and urine, that is, the pharmacokinetics of the drug in the horse. Clearance times for drugs in racing horses is a central problem in equine medication control. Differences in urinary pH are well known to affect the urinary concentrations and rates of excretion of certain drugs.

The dose, formulation, route of injection, timing of injection, and halflife of the drug are other important factors. The sensitivity of the analysis test also affects the period when drugs may be detected in blood or urine.

22.4 SAMPLE ANALYSIS

In November, 1947, a group of chemists from the United States, Canada, France, and Mexico met in Chicago to form an organization of chemists serving racing authorities. This was the inception of the Association of Official Racing Chemists (AORC), which has since met yearly. In these meetings, problems arising in racing chemistry are discussed, and the discussions pub-

> **TABLE 22–5**
> **INITIAL SCREENING**
>
> Procedures are designed to examine a large number of samples quickly and to determine which are negative and those that require further examination
> Based on initial screening, further tests that are required are decided on. The selection of these further tests is most critical to prove conclusively whether or not prohibited substances are present in the sample and their concentration
> Interpretation of the screening data in this manner results in only a small number of samples being sent for further examination

TABLE 22–6
PROCEDURE

All samples are extracted
All samples are tested for salicylates using a color reaction
All samples are tested using thin-layer chromatography
Different thin-layer chromatography solvent systems are used to cover different groups of drugs, such as stimulant drugs and diuretics. Detection procedures include ultraviolet light and suitable spray reagents for the different drug categories
All samples are tested using gas chromatography
Samples are screened by ELISA to cover the following drugs or groups of drugs:
  Generic barbiturate, generic benzodiazepine, generic bronchodilator, generic corticosteroid, generic promazine, butorphanol, clenbuterol, detomidine, dexamethasone, etorphine, fentanyl, methylprednisolone, nandrolone, stanozolol, and furosemide. Samples are analyzed by mass spectrometry. A computer data bank search is applied to these samples

Confirmation
Owing to the serious consequences of confirming whether or not a sample is positive, the sample is further reanalyzed to prove beyond any doubt that a prohibited substance is present. Various chromatographic procedures are used, the most important of which is mass spectroscopy. Mass spectroscopy provides a molecular "fingerprint" of the particular drug and is now required as part of evidence in all legal proceedings

lished as proceedings. The primary purpose of the AORC is to increase the knowledge and professional skill of its individual members by sharing research and advances in techniques made by fellow members, and, as a result, perform a more effective service for racing. It seems unlikely, however, that doping will ever be eradicated completely because new compounds are being constantly brought onto the market, the metabolism of which must first be studied in the horse and for the detection of which new analytical methods must be worked out.

The published proceedings of these AORC meetings are confidential. The international symposia are attended by racing chemists and veterinarians who represent their racing authorities, and the proceedings are published for general circulation.

Each year the AORC circulates to members a list of drugs that have been detected in racing laboratories worldwide. Members of the AORC are required to notify the Association of drugs detected in their countries each year. The most complete statistics on drugs detected in horses are those of the Association of Official Racing Chemists.

Racing chemistry is a specialized branch of microtoxicology applied to the control of drug abuse as it pertains to horse racing. The racing chemist must be able to detect drugs and metabolites in biological samples taken from the horse at a race meeting and identify these substances positively beyond any legal doubt.

The modern laboratory undertaking routine analysis for the racing industry must be able to look for a range of drugs in a number of samples. The laboratory must analyze samples in a short time at reasonable cost. The equipment used should have sufficient sensitivity to detect the small amounts of drug and its metabolites excreted.

The first step in the analysis is to extract the drug and/or its metabolites from the biological fluid received from the race track (Tables 22–6 and 22–7).

In considering diffusion of drugs across biological membranes, it is necessary to bear in mind most drugs are either weak acids or weak bases that exist in solution as a mixture of ionized or non-ionized forms. These compounds are more lipid soluble than water soluble in the non-ionized form, and consequently the non-ionized form permeates readily across the lipid cell membranes, whereas the ionized form does not. The ratio of ionized to non-ionized drug in body tissue therefore is important and de-

---

TABLE 22–7
PERFORMANCE CHARACTERISTICS

Specificity—the ability of a method to respond only to the substance being measured
Accuracy—refers to the closeness with which the measurement approaches the true figure
Precision—refers to the repeatability of the measurement. It denotes the closeness with which the measurement approaches the average of a long series of measurements made under similar conditions
Reliability
Cost-effectiveness
Ruggedness—refers to a method's performance not being adversely affected by minor deviations from its well-described procedural steps
Portability—refers to the ability of a method to be transferred to other laboratories and analysts, while maintaining the same standards of method
Performance
Availability

---

pends largely on the dissociation content (pKa) of the drug and the pH of the medium. For drugs which ionize, it is possible to find at equilibrium unequal concentrations of the total drug (i.e., ionized plus unionized) on either side of the membrane. Only the non-ionized molecules readily cross this lipoid barrier and achieve the same equilibrium concentration on both sides of the membrane; the ionized molecules are virtually excluded from transmembrane diffusion ("ion-trapping"). If a pH difference exists across a biological membrane (e.g., plasma-saliva; plasma-renal ultrafiltrate; plasma-milk), the drug ionizes to a different extent on each side of the membrane; the result is unequal total concentration (ionized plus un-ionized) of drug on each side of the membrane.

Diffusion of drugs from plasma into the saliva depends on many factors: viz, the nature of the drug (whether acidic, basic, or neutral), its dissociation constant pKa, its fat solubility, its molecular size, and the extent of binding of the drug to plasma proteins. Other factors are the flow rate and pH of saliva. In general, the factors involved in the passive diffusion of drug molecules from plasma into saliva are similar to those for urine. Basic drugs concentrate into a saliva that is more acidic than the plasma, and acidic drugs concentrate into a more alkaline saliva.

The specific chemical procedures used by analytical chemists to identify drugs in samples of body fluids vary but in general, consist of solvent extraction followed by various screening procedures applied to these extracts. In early dope testing, the microcrystalline test was extensively used. This was based on the principle that many alkaloidal drugs could be precipitated from aqueous solutions as small crystals in the presence of heavy metal salts. The resulting characteristic shape and color of the precipitated crystals could be examined microscopically to identify the drugs. This test is still used in some dope testing laboratories. Other common, early tests were the various color tests, but in the last 30 years, the introduction of chromatography, spectrophotometry, mass spectrometry "molecular fingerprinting," and radioimmunoassay has improved the sensitivity and specificity of laboratory techniques in isolating and identifying drugs.

Mass spectrometry (MS) has become the standard instrumental method for the confirmation of the presence (and identity) of a drug in a sample. After a solvent extraction to partially isolate the drug from the sample, the material to be analyzed is further separated by gas chromatography (GC). The mass spectrum is characteristic of the particular drug. The pattern produced by the drug and its fragment ions may be visualized as a "molecular fingerprint" and thus the spectrum is routinely accepted as evidence of the drug's identity. The chromatographic characteristics of the drug also add to its confirmation. The mass spectrometer is sensitive down to the level of nanograms (one billionth of a gram) and rapid.

IMMUNOASSAY-BASED DRUG TESTING

Until recently, control of the use of illegal medication in horses in North America depended on thin-layer chromatography (TLC). Postrace urine samples taken from racehorses were shipped to postrace laboratories, extracted by liquid/liquid extraction, and subjected to thin-layer chromatography. Samples showing evidence for the presence of drugs were subjected to further testing, including gas chromatography/mass spectroscopy confirmation. Medication control in racing horses in North America mostly depended on this technology.

While TLC-based testing is relatively inexpensive, and sensitive enough to detect many medications, particularly in urine testing, there are medications which are difficult for it to detect. For these drugs the only test with requisite sensitivity and flexibility has generally been immunoassay, suggested to be the most practical approach to equine medication control.

More recently, however, a panel of ELISA-based tests have been developed for use in equine drug testing, and these ELISA tests can provide sensitive, and effective, screening for drug abuses.

These ELISA tests can be particularly effective in drug detection. They can be as sensitive as radioimmunoassays (RIA), and completed rapidly. A good ELISA is comparable to a RIA for accuracy.

The increased potency of drugs used to affect equine performance has required extremely sensitive tests. Simple one-step ELISA tests for drugs in racing horses are now available to detect drugs or drug metabolites at nanogram and subnanogram concentrations in blood or urine. These tests are effective in prerace testing and increase the effectiveness of postrace testing for many medications. Additionally, antibodies to commonly used therapeutic medications have been raised to permit development of rapid, sensitive, and economical quantitative assays for medications used in racing horses.

The ELISA test is capable of both improving the quality and reducing the cost of testing for acepromazine in racing and show horses. A competitive binding immunoassay, which is easily adaptable to other drugs, has been developed for the narcotic fentanyl. The ELISA test is very sensitive to furosemide (about 20 μ/ml). The test is rapid and can be read with an inexpensive spectrophotometer. The inability to detect basic drugs is a serious deficiency in an equine race testing system. The (ELISA) test antibody cross-reacts with hydromorphone, oxymorphone, nalorphine, levorphanol and codeine.

The ELISA tests operate as follows. The antidrug antibody is linked to flat bottom microtiter plates and drug-hemisuccinate is linked to horseradish peroxidase (HRP) to give rise to covalently linked drug-HRP complex. The assay is started by adding the standard, test, or control samples to each well, along with the drug-HRP solution. During this step, the presence of free drug or cross-reacting metabolites competitively prevents the antibody from binding the drug-HRP conjugate. The antibody/drug-HRP binding is therefore inversely proportional to the amount of drug. After incubation, the fluid is removed from the microtiter well, and the well washed. Substrate is added to all wells and their absorbance read in a microwell reader.

The urine or blood received must be examined for the presence of drugs or metabolites. Methods of routine analysis vary because there is always more than one way of performing a satisfactory analysis. Basically the laboratory is trying to separate the drugs present from the biological material received. Drugs can be broadly divided into three different types—acidic drugs, basic drugs, and a small number of neutral drugs—the basic is largest.

Usually if a drug is present in a body fluid, it may be present at too low a concentration for detection, and accordingly most screening procedures make extensive use of solvent extraction. The basis of this is simply that the drug is extracted into a solvent, the solvent is then evaporated so the drug can then be concentrated many times and is ultimately present at a detectable level. In the same way as it is largely the non-ionized drug that is lipid soluble and that can penetrate lipid cell membranes, so too in the laboratory it is mainly the non-ionized drug that diffuses into the solvent and is extracted.

Chemically there are three major categories of drugs:

TABLE 22–8
QUANTITATIVE ANALYSIS AFTER POSITIVE IDENTIFICATION

Extraction and preparation of sample
Extraction and preparation of blank urine sample
Extraction and preparation of reference sample
Extraction and preparation of spiked urine samples for setting up a standard curve.
Quantitative analysis by gas chromatography/mass spectrometry

To measure the amount of drug present in urine or blood, it is necessary to establish a standard curve for that drug. At least 3 spiked urine or blood samples are quantitatively analyzed at 5 different drug concentration levels. This information is used to establish a standard curve. Two aliquots of the sample are analyzed after the same procedure. The information from the sample is compared with that obtained for the standard curve, and the concentration of the drug present is measured

(1) Acidic compounds (barbiturates, salicylates, phenylbutazone)—ionized in alkaline solution and extractable from acid solution
(2) Neutral compounds (choral hydrate, trichlorethanol)—not ionized at any pH and extractable at any pH and
(3) Basic compounds (antihistamines, local anesthetics, caffeine, amphetamine)—ionized in acid solution and extractable from alkaline solution

Basic drugs include the narcotic analgesics, which have been used in racing horses for at least 100 years, and most stimulants, depressants, local anesthetics, and tranquilizers. Many of these drugs are active in low concentrations, with doses commonly about 10 mg/horse or less, which makes their detection in postrace urine challenging.

By adjusting the pH of the body fluid, the analytical chemist can influence the extent to which a drug can exist in the ionized form and thus facilitate its diffusion into the solvent for extraction. In this way, he can separate these three categories of drugs. Once the drug has been extracted, the specific techniques of detection and identification are used. The extracts may have to be further purified and concentrated before the sample is subjected to such procedures.

Once the solvent extraction has been made, the solvent is reduced to concentrate the extracts. A small portion of the acidic extract is spotted on a thin-layer plate and chromatographed. Other common maneuvers with acidic extracts include ultraviolet spectrometry (UV analysis) and, increasingly, high-performance liquid chromatography. If positive indications for the presence of a drug appear in any or all of these tests, the urine extract may be examined by gas chromatography/mass spectrometry.

From these initial examinations, either the sample is reported as negative, or it is indicated that further work is needed to determine whether a drug is present. When it becomes evident that a drug is present, a detailed study of the material is initiated (Tables 22–8 and 9). The final identification of the material present is achieved by as

TABLE 22–9
QUALITY CONTROL

Adding of drugs to blank urine samples
Samples processed through system (identity of selective samples not revealed)
Different drugs added to different samples

many different methods of analysis as possible, involving thin-layer, gas-liquid, and paper chromatography and mass spectrometry.

Gas chromatographs with mass spectrometers have been the most significant tool offered for the identification of detected drugs and the characterization of unknown substances occurring in sample extracts. Some drugs, such as anabolic steroids and corticosteroids, do not fit well into the existing routine analytical system and have to be tested for separately. Anabolic steroids and corticosteroids are screened for using either a radioimmunoassay technique or gas chromatography/mass spectrometry.

22.5 PATTERNS AND PROBLEMS OF DOPING

The pattern of horse doping has changed somewhat over the years. Narcotic-type drugs were perhaps the most commonly used doping substances years ago, but after the end of the World War II, this gave way to the use of agents such as amphetamine and other sympathomimetic compounds; followed by the use of local anesthetics, such as procaine; and then in recent years the use of anti-inflammatory drugs, such as phenylbutazone, anti-inflammatory steroids, and anabolic steroids. Although there has been little change in the proportion of positive cases internationally, the pattern has changed insofar as there has been a decrease in the incidence of criminal doping (e.g., by the use of central nervous system stimulants and depressants, such as caffeine, amphetamines, and barbiturates) and an increase in "therapeutic doping" mainly by the use of anti-inflammatory drugs.

It is this latter area that can pose numerous problems for the veterinarian in practice because any banned drug detected in the body fluids of horses at the time of racing may constitute a doping offense regardless of the reason for which the drug was initially administered. For instance, procaine is a commonly used drug in doping, in which it has been used either as a local anesthetic to mask lameness or as a stimulant in the horse. In fact, procaine has a pronounced stimulant effect in the horse being about 20 times more potent than in humans.

Procaine however, is also commonly employed therapeutically as procaine penicillin as which it functions as a simple organic base from which free antibiotic is released.

Doping is defined as the administration of any substance that can affect the performance of a horse at the time of racing. If a horse is lame and it is restored to normality for a race by giving it a drug, its performance is affected at the time of racing by a substance other than normal nutrient, and the animal is therefore by definition doped. In Europe, unless the Rules of Racing contain a clause permitting legitimate medication, the horse cannot be treated and raced. Although NSAIDs do not augment the performance of a healthy fit horse, they can restore normal performance at the time of a race. In recent years, the phrase "nonnutrient" has been replaced by the term "prohibited substance," and a list of categories of prohibited substances has been published by the stewards of the Jockey Club in the U.K. If a prohibited substance is detected at the time of racing in the body fluids of a horse, regardless of concentration, there are always grounds for an inquiry. The particular relevance of this to the veterinary surgeon is that the therapeutic use of a prohibited substance at the time of racing is not allowed. This can pose a problem for the veterinarian in practice because he must provide appropriate therapy for a sick animal, and must not inadvertently contravene the Rules of Racing, impugning either his own or the trainer's integrity.

In 1977, the Racing Authorities from many European countries drew up a list of prohibited substances (see Table 22–1), which defined a dope by its pharmacologic action rather than by its chemical name. The veterinarian now must walk a tightrope in a difficult situation because of

1. The shortage of pharmacologic information indicating consistently reliable drug clearance times in the horse
2. The progressive increase in the sensitivity of detection methods in the analytical laboratory, whereby smaller and smaller amounts of drug may now be detected at periods more and more remote from the time of administration
3. The tightening of international doping regulations.

Under Federation Equestre Internationale Rules at present, a list of prohibited substances similar to the Jockey Club Rules bans the use of certain drugs in competing horses. Following intensive discussion and debate, however, phenylbutazone has been permitted for use in equestrian events, provided that at the time of blood sampling the plasma level of phenylbutazone does not exceed a threshold level. Phenylbutazone is particularly effective in removing symptoms of lameness associated with osteoarthritic and osteoporotic conditions, which account for anything up to 75% of the clinically lame horse. In show-jumping season, the nature of the sport subjects the horse's feet to constant concussion. Many of these horses are older and some degree of pathologic change may have occurred in the feet. Phenylbutazone undoubtedly could assist the horse in such case. The question is frequently raised, however, concerning the ethics of keeping a horse in work that requires the constant administration of pain-relieving drugs. If a horse is suffering from an incurable condition, should such a horse be considered to have finished its useful working life? Because the NSAID acts only to restore a horse to its natural innate ability, some authorities believe that competing presents no moral problems. Against that must be stated that an animal must compete on its own inherent merits and according to its own natural ability without recourse to chemical aids or drugs. In other words, how can one horse be deemed better than another horse at a given time and place if it is necessary to use drugs to maintain its performance? Unsoundness surely should not be masked by drug administration.

Various arguments have been put forward suggesting that permissive medication, especially with phenylbutazone, could lead to abnormal requests on the horse's ability—that masking of pain, being contrary to the welfare of the horse, might encourage the progression of existing lesions and inhibit the resolution of the inflammatory process in the absence of appropriate rest, with consequent detrimental effects. It has been argued that banning of compounds such as phenylbutazone might conceivably lead to an increase in the undesirable practices of neurectomies, and that horses can be maintained successfully for

years on these compounds without any adverse effects and can compete successfully and consistently. Few animals competing under FEI rules are used for breeding, and therefore the same risks to bloodlines do not occur. Generally speaking, one sachet of phenylbutazone, or a maximum of 2.2 mg/kg body weight, should keep blood levels of the drug within the permitted level. On account of the great variation from horse to horse, however, the time of administration must allow a gap of at least 24 hours before the horse is likely to be sampled. The time for the clearance of drugs from the horse is important to the veterinarian who has been asked to treat a horse scheduled to race at some future date. It is increasingly difficult for the veterinary surgeon to give appropriate therapy to a sick animal, on the one hand, and, on the other hand, not to risk permitting his client to contravene unwittingly the rules of competition. As in so many other areas relating to the use of drugs in animals, the importance of emphasizing to clients the need to observe drug clearance times becomes greater as medicines become more potent, analytical detection methods more sensitive, and regulations stricter.

As already stated, in the United States, the concept of permissive medication has been accepted in most states. The stewards of the Turf Clubs of Ireland, Britain, and France view this as undesirable, and a joint statement to this effect was issued by these bodies in October, 1971, the point being that phenylbutazone could jeopardize the soundness of bloodlines.

Subsequently the Royal College of Veterinary Surgeons endorsed this statement and advised all veterinary surgeons to study the implications of the statement for the profession. It is also pointed out that the elimination of a drug such as phenylbutazone varies widely between individual animals and that this fact should be given due cognizance by the veterinarian before initiating treatment in the racing animal. Further, it drew attention to the fact that owing to improved laboratory techniques, small residues of the drug can be detected in an animal at a period remote from the time of administration. Accordingly, it was suggested the veterinary surgeon discontinue the use of phenylbutazone not less than 8 days before racing. This was hoped to be an adequate period to permit excretion of the drug from the body and thus avoid residue detection.

It is important therefore for the veterinarian to have some knowledge of the clearance times of the more commonly used, important drugs. By clearance time is meant the time that must elapse after the last administration of the drug for a dope test on the body fluid submitted for analysis to be negative. The clearance time for any particular drug depends on a number of factors, such as the dose used, the route of administration, the diet, the acidity or alkalinity of the urine, presence of other drugs, the sex and age of the animal, and its physiologic condition. Of importance to clearance time is the sensitivity of the analytical method employed, because a method that can detect a nanogram shows the presence of a given drug longer than one that can detect a microgram.

As analytical methods improve, more sensitive techniques evolve that can detect smaller and smaller residues at an interval more and more remote from the time of administration. This can be illustrated in the case of phenylbutazone, in which the difference in clearance times reported in the literature can be explained by several factors, not the least of which is the different methods of detection used by different laboratories. The earliest published methods relied on spectrophotometry for the estimation of the amount of drug present, a method that is considerably less sensitive than the more recent methods using radioactivity and gas-liquid chromatography. The overall concept of clearance times of drugs in racing animals is therefore complex and not confused because there are no agreed acceptable levels that do not interfere with form.

Current evidence suggests the urine pH of horses maintained on pasture is consistently alkaline and a substantial proportion of postrace urine samples of racing horses is acidic. Because urine pH can affect the urine concentration of some drugs, uncertainties are created when data generated in grazing horses are compared or extrapolated to racing horses.

CLEARANCE TIME OF THE NONSTEROIDAL ANTI-INFLAMMATORY DRUGS

Prerace Testing

Prerace testing is based entirely on blood sampling in North America, although at one time prerace testing in Hong Kong was done on urine. The blood sample is drawn two to four hours before the race and subjected to screening and, if possible, gas chromatography–mass spectrophotometry (GC/MS) analysis. In theory prerace testing allows the chemist to detect a medicated horse before it runs.

Obviously it is important for both the racehorse trainer and the veterinarian to be aware of the time limits involved between administration of the drug and the point at which a horse may race and be free of all traces or acceptable levels of that drug. In this respect, detection of a drug is directly related to the sensitivity of the method of detection. Clearance time of NSAIDs from horses may vary also with different circumstances. Precise withdrawal of treatment with NSAIDs is therefore precarious, and the general practice is to leave a wide margin of safety. In postrace testing, only a fraction of the horses running are selected for testing, the winners are usually selected, and the beaten favorites, and any other horses that have aroused the suspicions of the stewards or commission veterinarians.

The objectives of the forensic toxicologist are (1) to isolate and identify chemical agents using appropriate analytical procedures, (2) to measure quantitatively any identifiable chemical substances in the specimens, (3) to further confirm and interpret the results of the analyses as to cause and effect of the substance on the animal's health or well being, and (4) to express a conclusion based on the facts.

Phenylbutazone displays dose-dependent kinetics in the horse, with reported half-lives in plasma ranging from 3 to 8 hours. It is easily detected in urine, and high doses have been reported as detected in urine for 8 days. It is safe to assume, that plasma and urine are clear 48 to 60 hours after the last dose.

Naproxen is also an easy drug to detect in the horse because both it and its main metabolite absorb ultraviolet light and can be detected by spectrophotometry. Its half-life is about 6 hours in urine, and it has been suggested that 48 to 60 hours should be allowed for it to clear urine.

Flunixin has a short half-life of 1.6 hours in equine plasma. When administered at the recommended dosage of 1.1 mg/kg body weight, the drug was still detectable in urine 48 hours after the last dose.

Meclofenamic acid has a plasma half-life of six hours in the horse. Following the recommended dosages (2.2 mg/kg body weight), it has cleared plasma by 24 hours. After cessation of a course of treatment, the drug is reportedly detectable for 96 hours, although levels are low after 48 hours.

Clearance times for NSAIDs can be summarized as follows:

Phenylbutazone: 48–60 hours
Naproxen: 48–60 hours
Flunixin meglumine: 48 hours
Meclofenamic acid: 48–96 hours

22.6 PROBLEM DRUGS

Sedatives

Acepromazine and related phenothiazine tranquilizers have been used to illegally affect the performance of both racing and show horses. Treating nervous horses with a small amount of tranquilizer before a race or show event is done to allow them to settle down sufficiently to make a concentrated effort. The phenothiazine derivatives, particularly acepromazine and propriopromazine, are commonly used in this regard. They are readily available in veterinary circles and as extremely potent drugs, are given in small amounts, and so are difficult to detect with traditional detection methods.

Detomidine (Domosedan®) is a sedative/analgesic approved for use in horses. The sedative and analgesic properties of this group result primarily from their agonist activity on spinal and supraspinal α_2-adrenoceptors. Detomidine was created out of a need for a drug that produced long-acting sedative effects combined with an analgesia that is distributed uniformly throughout the body.

Anti-inflammatories

The anti-inflammatory drugs used in racehorses can be divided into the salicylates, dimethyl sulphoxide (DMSO), adrenocorticotrophic hormone, the corticosteroids and the NSAIDs.

The legal status of corticosteroids in racehorses differs among international racing jurisdictions. Corticosteroids are not permitted in England, Ireland, France, Australia, and in most states in the US, although it appears they are not expressly prohibited for training in the US. They were permitted in Florida in 1990.

Flunixin is commonly used at the California racetracks, not only as a colic treatment but as one of the four non-steroidal anti-inflammatory drugs permitted by the California Horse Racing Board. This approved and authorized drug may be administered after the horse is entered to race, but not later than 24 hours before post-time for the race in which the horse is entered.

Furosemide

Exercise-induced pulmonary hemorrhage (EIPH), which has been demonstrated to occur in 26–75% of racing horses, has potential for serious injury to horses and humans in a race when a horse abruptly stops as a result of EIPH. Several treatment regimens have been proposed to control EIPH, however, furosemide (Lasix) is the most commonly used drug for this purpose.

Occurrence of epistaxis bleeding during a race can cause the affected horse to slow or stop abruptly, posing a serious threat to horses and jockeys. In an effort to control this condition during races, many racing jurisdictions allow the prerace use of furosemide.

The improvement in the racing time of a "bleeder" after the administration of furosemide has been attributed to the effects of furosemide on modifying the severity of EIPH and this is the reason for the improvement in racing times. The possibility exists that furosemide, under racing conditions, has a direct effect on the performance of the horse.

Furosemide is the most controversial drug in racing. It is a potent diuretic, which causes up to a fiftyfold increase in the amount of urine voided in horses and man. Sometimes furosemide is administered to horses to facilitate the collection of a urine sample, but this can give rise to detection problems with other drugs. For example, if a horse is treated with phenylbutazone, the urinary concentration of the drug measured, and then furosemide administered, one finds that furosemide can reduce the urinary concentration of phenylbutazone up to fiftyfold. This is sufficient to interfere with routine screening for phenylbutazone. Blood sampling overcomes this problem.

There is a relationship between the changes in urine specific gravity (SG) and the concentration of drugs in urine. Racing jurisdictions which allow the use of furosemide require the administration of the medication between 3 and 5 hours before post-time, allowing the specific gravity of urine to return to near normal levels.

Beta-agonists

In humans, these agents are mainly used in the treatment of respiratory conditions, e.g., asthma where bronchoconstriction hinders normal breathing. As well as causing bronchodilation, other adrenergic responses may occur, especially following intravenous or oral administration. Sweating, muscle tremor and an increase in heart rate have been reported.

Sodium Bicarbonate

Standardbred racehorse trainers often dose their horses with sodium bicarbonate drenches prior to racing with the hope of improving their horse's performance by delaying the onset of fatigue. During high intensity exercise there is an accumulation of lactate and hydrogen ions within the muscle cells, resulting in a decrease in muscle cell pH. This decreased intracellular pH is thought to be a major factor in fatigue. Administering sodium bicarbonate causes blood pH to rise which then increases the efflux of hydrogen ions out of the muscle cell, thereby reducing the intracellular acidosis. This has posed a particular problem for authorities because of the normal biological variation in blood bicarbonate concentrations.

SELECTED REFERENCES

Alitalo, I., Vainio, O., Kaartinen, L., and Raekillio, M.: Cardiac effects of atropine premedication in horses sedated with detomidine. Acta Vet. Scand., 82(Suppl.):131, 1986.

Blake, J.W. and Tobin, T.: The gas liquid chromatograph and the election capture detector in equine drug testing. Br. J. Sports Med., 10:129, 1976.

Chay, S., Woods, W.E., Rowse, K., Nugent, T.E., Blake, J.W., and Tobin, T.: The pharmacology of furosemide in the horse. V. Pharmacokinetics and blood levels of furosemide after intravenous administration. Drug Metab. Disp. 11:226, 1983.

Clarke, A.F.: Exercise-induced pulmonary hemorrhage—the state and the status. Vet. Ann., 26:156, 1986.

Clarke, E.G.C., and Moss, M.S.: Veterinary aspects of doping. Eq. Vet. J., 9:27, 1977.

Clarke, K.W., and Taylor, P.M.: Detomidine: a new sedative for horses. Eq. Vet. J., 18:366, 1986.

Combie, J.D., Nugent, T. and Tobin, T.: The pharmacology of furosemide in the horse. IV. The duration of reduction of urinary concentration of drugs. J. Eq. Vet. Sci. 1:203, 1981.

Edwards, W.C.: Animal doping. Vet. Med. Small Animal Clin., 78:317, 1983.

Gabel, A.A., Tobin, T., Ray, R.S., and Maylin, G.A.: Furosemide in horses: a review. J. Eq. Med. Surg., 1:215, 1977.

Hopes, R., and Frank, C.: Medication tests in racehorses and competition horses. XXX Journal 2:96, 1990.

Kammerline, S., Wood, T., DeQuick, D. et al.: Narcotic analgesics, their detection and pain measurement in the horse: A review. Eq. Vet. J., 21:4, 1989.

Kelso, T.B., Hodgson, D.R., Witt, E.H., Bayly, W.M., Grant, B.D., and Gollnick, P.D.: Bicarbonate administration and muscle metabolism during high intensity exercise. In: Equine Exercise Physiology 2. Edited by Gillespie, J.R. and Robinson, N.E. Davis, CA, ICEEP Publication, 1987. Pp. 438–447.

Lawrence, D. and Livingston, A.: Opiate-like analgesic activity in general anaesthetics. Br. J. Pharmacol., 73:422, 1981.

Lawrence, L., Kline, P., Miller, J., Smith, J., Siegel, A., Kurcz, E., Fisher, M., and Bump, K.: Effect of sodium bicarbonate on racing standardbreds. J. Animal Sci., 68:673, 1990.

Lowe, J., and Hilfiger, J.: Analgesic and sedative effects of detomidine compared to xylaine in a colic model using I.V. and I.M. routes of administration. Acta Vet. Scand., 82(Suppl.):85, 1986.

Maybin, G.A.: Pre-race testing. Cornell Vet., 64:325, 1974.

McDonald, J., Gall, R., Wiedenbach, P., et al.: Immunoassay detection of drugs in racing horses. III. Detection of morphine in equine blood, by a one step ELISA assay. Res. Comm. Chem. Pathol. Pharmacol., 59:259, 1988.

Milne, D.W., Gabel, A.A., Muir, W.W., et al.: Effects of furosemide on cardiovascular function and performance when given prior to simulated races: A double-blind study. Am. J. Vet. Res., *41*:1183, 1980.

Moss, M.S., and Clarke, E.G.C.: A review of drug "clearance times" in racehorses. Eq. Vet. J., *9*:53, 1977.

Moss, M.: Modern techniques in dope detection. Vet. Rec. Suppl. *110*:87, 1982.

Nilsfors, L., and Kvart, C.: Preliminary report on the cardiorespiratory effects of the antagonist to detomidine, MPV-12. Acta Vet. Scand., *82(Suppl.)*:121, 1986.

Pascoe, J.R., McCabe, A.E., Franti, C.E., et al.: Efficacy of furosemide in the treatment of exercise-induced pulmonary hemorrhage in Thoroughbred racehorses. Am. J. Vet. Res., *46*:2000, 1985.

Pascoe, J.R., and Wheat, J.D.: Historical background, prevalence, clinical findings and diagnosis of exercise-induced pulmonary hemorrhage (EIPH) in the racing horse. Proc. AAEP 26th Annual Meeting, 1980. Pp. 413–420.

Roberts, B.L., Blake, J.W., and Tobin, T.: Drug interactions in the horse: effect of fursemide on plasma and urinary levels of phenylbutazone. Res. Commun. Chem. Pathol., *15(2)*:257, 1976.

Short, C.E., Matthews, N., Harvey, R., and Tyner, C.L.: Cardiovascular and pulmonary function studies of a new sedative/analgetic (Detomidine/Domosedan) for use alone in horses or as a preanesthetic. Acta Vet. Scand., *82(Suppl.)*:139, 1986.

Soma, L.R., Laster, L., Oppenlander, R., and Barr-Alderfer, V.: Effects of furosemide on the racing times of horses with exercise-induced pulmonary hemorrhage. Am. J. Vet. Res., *46*:763, 1985.

Stein, B., Laessig, R.H., and Indrikson, A.: An evaluation of drug testing procedures used by forensic laboratories and the qualification of their analysts. Wis. Law Rev., *3*:726, 1973.

Sweeney, C.R.: Effects of furosemide on performance and on exercise-induced pulmonary hemorrhage: A review in Proceedings, 36th Annual Conv. Am. Assoc. Equine Pract., 1990, p. 199.

Sweeney, C.R., Soma, L.R., Maxson, A.D., et al.: Effect of furosemide on racing times of Thoroughbreds. Am. J. Vet. Res., *51(5)*:770, 1990.

Tobin, T.: The effects of drugs on equine performance, and the use of ELISA tests in equine medication control. Eq. Vet. Sci., *9*:160, 1989.

Tobin, T., and Woods, W.E.: Aust. Eq. Vet., *7(Suppl. I.)*:1989.

Tobin, T.: Drugs and the Performance Horse. Springfield, IL, Charles C Thomas, 1981. Pp. 111–131.

Tobin, T.: Pharmacology review: a review of recent research on furosemide in the horse. J. Eq. Med. Surg., *2*:314, 1978.

Tobin, T., Roberts, B.L., Swerczek, T.W., et al.: The pharmacology of furosemide in the horse. III. Dose and time response relationships, effects of repeated dosing and performance effects. Equine J. Med. Surg., *2*:216, 1978.

Food Animal

23

C H A P T E R

MASS MEDICATION AND DISEASES OF SWINE

23.1 Introduction
23.2 Systems of Medication
23.3 Use of Antibiotics as Growth Promoters
23.4 Infectious Atrophic Rhinitis
23.5 Swine Pneumonia
23.6 Swine Pleuropneumonia
23.7 Colibacillosis
23.8 Swine Dysentery
23.9 Salmonellosis
23.10 Porcine Infectious Arthritis and Mycoplasmal Polyserositis
23.11 Residues in Swine Production
23.12 Sulfonamide Residues

23.1 INTRODUCTION

Enzootic pneumonia and atrophic rhinitis, both of which may be complicated by secondary bacterial pneumonia or pleuropneumonia, together with swine dysentery and bacterial enteritis are probably the most important diseases affecting the pig industry today. They result in severe financial loss, poor feed efficiency, and increased mortality.

With respiratory diseases, there is usually rapid spread of infection, high morbidity, debilitation, and depression of food conversion efficiency. In many fattening units, the most that can be hoped for is to keep the disease at a low level. There have been three main problems in the pig industry during the past 10 years: scours/enteritis, pneumonia/rhinitis, and insufficient growth rate coupled with poor feed conversion efficiency. The success of growth promoter antibiotics has been ensured in a sense by the continuing availability of broad-spectrum antibiotics. Despite the current legislation regarding the incorporation of antibiotics in feedstuffs, pig production still apparently continues to require the backup availability of these broad-spectrum products.

Therapeutic medication of feeding stuffs in pig production is perhaps the area of most significance from the viewpoint of drug residue formation owing to the wide variety of therapeutic agents that may ultimately make their way into the human food chain. Salmonellosis, swine dysentery, coliform infections, enzootic pneumonia, and atrophic rhinitis are all major problems that commonly necessitate antimicrobial medication in feed or water.

Respiratory infections of whole herds are generally associated with mycoplasmas and because of the chronic widespread nature of this condition in a herd, medication is generally provided as part of the concentrate diet. Oxytetracycline, tiamulin, and tylosin are frequently used for treatment of this condition. Bacterial pneumonias caused by *Haemophilus* or *Pasteurella* respond to in-water medication with substances such as tetracyclines, ampicillin, or phenoxymethyl-penicillin, which is especially useful for *Haemophilus* actinobacillus bronchopneumonia. The precise cause of atrophic rhinitis is still unclear, but strains of *Borde-*

tella and toxigenic strains of *Pasteurella* have been implicated. Sulfonamides, tylosin, and tetracyclines have been used with satisfactory results in this condition.

Control and avoidance of most swine problems revolve around managemental control measures, i.e., attendance to ventilation, stocking rates, temperature fluctuations, and so forth. Although this can appreciably reduce the incidence of disease in swine units, it also has added the bonus of decreasing the reliance on antimicrobial medication and hence the risk associated with the occurrence of antibiotic residues in swine carcasses. Antibiotic medication is no substitute whatsoever for good management practices. Generally, when infectious disease outbreaks do occur, it is necessary to attack the problem on four fronts:

1. Management of predisposing factors
2. Individual therapy of the severely affected clinical cases
3. Followup medication at therapeutic levels in feed or in water
4. Blanket medication programs at lower inclusion levels for in-contact animals on a prophylactic basis.

Pigs are subjected to numerous stresses at various times of their lives, stresses that can precipitate serious outbreaks of disease. These stresses generally occur at the following times:

Farrowing
Thrust into a hostile environment
Navel cord clipped and disinfected
Needle teeth clipped
Tail cut
Ears marked
Injected with iron
Weaning
Removed from dam into an unfamiliar environment
Change in feeding
Transportation
Mixing with other litters
Castration
Vaccination
Growing/fattening
Overcrowding of pens
Poor ventilation
Temperature fluctuations
Mixing of batches

Dusty environment
High ammonia levels

Antimicrobial drugs may be used as injectables, in feed medicants, in water medicants, or as growth promoters. The overuse of many such antibiotic formulations in the swine industry is a controversy that concerns both the veterinarian and the lay public.

The use of water-soluble drugs has been a traditionally popular method, especially for cases of subacute pneumonias or as supportive therapy in cases of viral pneumonia and for swine dysentery. Using nipple watering devices with pressurized water lines, drugs can be added at the rate of 1 to 4 oz/gallon into the daily water. Water medication is an advantage when pigs are anorexic and not eating. It is also quicker to administer, and this can be critical when in certain conditions speed of treatment is of essence. Disadvantages with water medication are that it can work out to be more expensive for certain drugs, the medicated water may be wasted more so than medicated feed, and water stability, or the fact that no suitable water-soluble drug may exist is a major determinant of this form of therapy.

Feed medication, although a cheaper form of treatment and less laborsome, does have the disadvantage that in many conditions the animal may eat little or no feed and consequently little or no drug. It may also lead to considerable drug wastage and residue problems because stockmen are loath to discard antibiotic-medicated feed from large feed hoppers.

Another class of in-feed antimicrobals are the feed additive growth-promoter antibiotics. These can be used only at approved levels, and these levels are far less than those necessary to achieve blood and tissue levels that would effectively treat respiratory disease conditions especially. Such low-level inclusion is really restricted to prophylactic medication and to supportive therapy in chronic enzootic pneumonia cases. As it happens, acutely ill animals fail to consume the normal amount of feed, and hence their drug intake is limited in any case.

Feed additives are strictly regulated by the Food, Drug, and Cosmetics Act. They are approved for only labeled dosage rates, and the amount of drug that can be added to feed is strictly controlled under the drug approvals convention of the Center for Veterinary Medicine (CVM) of the Food and Drug Administration (FDA). With regard to approved feed additives for swine, veterinarians hold no power of prescription (Rx drugs), but they can advise their clients with respect to usage and application in certain disease states. It must be emphasized that the extralabel usage of feed additives and antibiotics is not permitted by law and that such illicit use carries with it inherent liability and culpability for damages should violative levels of residues in excess of tolerances or maximum residue limits (MRLs) be detected.

Because feed-additive antimicrobial drugs are used at less than 50% of the therapeutic levels, their continued use is an issue of intense debate from the standpoint of induction of antibiotic resistance and also whether such practice is really in the long-term interest of the pig industry. The addition of certain medications in concentrate form to animal feeds may require that the user operate under the guidelines of the FDA forms No. 1800 and 1900. These guidelines permit concentrated drug premixes to be blended into feed and provide for periodic inspection of feed preparation facilities and of feed preparation and the analysis of samples of finished feed to determine drug concentration.

23.2 SYSTEMS OF MEDICATION

Modern intensive systems of pig husbandry can present major problems for antibiotic medication owing to the fact that most common housing and feeding systems do not allow in-feed or water medication of specific groups of pigs. In the past, the most traditional method was in-feed antibiotic medication because many drugs were not available in water-soluble form. Although drug residues should not be present in animal tissues at slaughter, if manufacturer's instructions on drug withholding times are followed, nonetheless a problem does exist in pig units insofar as current practices for selecting slaughter-weight pigs do not easily allow a definite withdrawal period to be observed, especially if a large column of medicated feed still remains in the bulk hopper.

FEED MEDICATION

The most popular method of administering therapeutic drugs to finishing pigs is in the feed. Residue problems may result from errors on the farm or at the feed mill or even contamination during transport, but if certain principles are applied, most problems should be avoided.

1. Use antibiotics early and at therapeutic levels. This is considered early strategic medication; e.g., a pig purchased through many sources should be treated during the period of maximum danger, i.e., from 90 to 120 lbs weight.
2. Withdraw all medicated feed at least 2 weeks and preferably 4 weeks before slaughter.
3. Organize a flow of pigs around the unit so pigs of one age are in one area.
4. Use veterinary advice to ensure informed, effective results, e.g., select as far as possible drugs that have no application in human medicine, and are of known quality in terms of mixing characteristics and effectiveness, and have stated withdrawal periods.

Some drugs, such as penicillin, are unstable in feed, and losses can reach up to 60% if moisture levels are high or acidic materials are used in the feed. The presentation of medicated feed in pig units depends on the type of feeding system in use on the farm. Hand mixing of drugs into feed may be useful when a single animal is being dosed and amounts of drug are carefully calculated and weighed out. When bulk feed is medicated by the manufacturer and automatic pipeline feeding systems connected to a bulk hopper are used, problems may arise by virtue of residual trace amounts of antibiotic-containing feed remaining in the pipeline. In-feed medication, although it may be relatively cheap, does possess many significant disadvantages. One of the principal disadvantages is that sick animals frequently become anorexic and therefore may not ingest adequate amounts of medicated feed. Conversely, the less affected animals may ingest too much of the antibiotic-containing feed and therefore may be more at risk in terms of their potential for presenting tissue residues. Improper mixing of the antibiotic may pose similar problems. A significant point is that many antibiotics once added to feeding stuffs soon deteriorate and lose their potency. This means that the batch of medicated feed has to be consumed fairly quickly.

One of the prime advantages of water medication is that sick animals usually drink even if they refuse food. Water medication is also, generally speaking, a more convenient way for the farmer to medicate animals at all levels of stocking density. If enough header tanks are available, only those specific animals requiring treatment may be medicated. There are fewer problems with water medication programs in terms of planning a treatment regimen and in using up the excess that may remain. Although many modern drugs are soluble in water, care must always be taken to ensure adequate mixing and dissolution because otherwise the undissolved drug simply sediments to the bottom of the tank, forming an insoluble gel, resulting in inadequate dosage, which could ultimately encourage the development of bacterial resistance. Water medication is flexible but usually prohibitively expensive for fatteners. It is most useful for weaners and must be considered as a viable alternative for all young pigs.

Water medication has proved successful in the treatment of systemic salmonellosis, in early cases of *Pasteurella* pneumonia in young weaner pigs, and in swine dysentery. In-feed medication has been used for a variety of conditions, including enteritis, enzootic pneumonia, atrophic rhinitis, and streptococcal meningitis. Antibiotics for use in feed include those that are insoluble in water, which includes those that have high gut activity, i.e., not appreciably absorbed from the gut. With water medication, care must always be taken to ensure that only sufficient water to last 1 day is medicated and that further medication is added for the next day. Cost is a major factor in deciding between in-feed and water medication. In-feed medication usually works out to be less expensive. The lack in many pig units of suitable equipment to dispense medicated water to individual groups of animals is another factor that has prevented water systems from becoming the primary medicating system. In regard to minimizing the occurrence of drug residues in pig meat, water systems would appear to have considerable advantage insofar as the water supply can be switched off after medication has taken place; also, only small quantities of drug need to be added to water on a daily basis. This is impossible to do with medicated feed and is probably one of the main reasons why the limitations of feed medication systems have been implicated in the drug residue problem in pigs.

23.3 USE OF ANTIBIOTICS AS GROWTH PROMOTERS

Antibiotics have long been associated with growth-promoting effects in animals. Since the original use of chlortetracycline as a growth promoter in chicks, the application of many other antibiotics at low levels in feeding stuffs has increased in line with the rapid developments in intensive animal production systems. For growth-promoting purposes, they are usually included in the feed at low levels, where they also improve the efficiency of feed use. For therapeutic purposes, they are incorporated at considerably higher levels in the feed for their antibacterial effects. In the 1960s, the incidence of antibiotic resistance in bacteria pathogenic for farm animals reached a point at which it was seen to be complicating the treatment of disease, and it was suggested that the feeding of low levels of antibiotics at subtherapeutic levels for growth-promoting purposes was a significant contributory factor.

Penicillin-resistant and tetracycline-resistant pathogens in pigs and poultry were becoming a real problem. The phenomenon of transferable drug resistance compounded the worsening situation. Transferable drug resistance was demonstrated to be a phenomenon that occurred mainly in the Enterobacteriaceae, whereby resistance to one or a number of antibiotics could be transferred from donor to recipient bacteria. In the event of resistance being transferred to potentially pathogenic organisms, this could ultimately complicate the antibiotic therapy of clinical disease outbreaks in humans and animals. Resistant bacteria of animals were seen to constitute a potential reservoir of resistance transmissible to humans. Thus the therapeutic antibiotics, penicillin, streptomycin, and tetracyclines, were banned as growth-promoter antibiotics in all member states of the European Community. This is not the case in the United States, where therapeutic use of penicillin and tetracyclines causes continued debate.

GROWTH-PROMOTER ANTIBIOTICS

In the United States, the permitted feed antibiotics for promoting growth and efficiency are: Arsanilic acid, bacitracin, chlortetracycline, bambermycin, lincomycin, carbadox, penicillin, sulfamethazine combinations, sulfathiazole, tiamulin, tylosin, and virginiamycin.

In Europe, the present permitted list of antibiotics that may be incorporated as growth promoters in animal feeding stuffs is as follows: avoparcin, zinc bacitracin, virginiamycin, spiramycin, tylosin, bambermycin, and salinomycin. There is a tendency toward using antibiotics for growth-promoting purposes that are poorly absorbed from the alimentary tract. The molecular size of antibiotics may be of significance in this respect, and many of these substances are of large molecular weight.

All of the growth-promoting antibiotics act to improve average daily gain and feed conversion efficiency. Apart from reducing the time for animals to reach market weight, thus lowering overhead costs on buildings and labor, the effects of saving of feed (60 to 70% of cost) can be significant. Most of these growth promoters act by a disease control effect, i.e., control of pathogenic organisms capable of producing specific disease or nonspecific detrimental effects resulting from toxin production. A gut-thinning effect often results after antibiotic usage, and this may allow for better nutrient absorption. Various metabolic and nutrient-sparing effects also are associated with low-level inclusion of antibiotic growth promoters in feed.

Avoparcin is used solely for growth-promoting purposes and is not used otherwise in human or veterinary medicine. It is primarily active against gram-positive bacteria and has a large molecular weight. It is virtually unabsorbed from the gastrointestinal tract and is rapidly eliminated as the unchanged antibiotic.

Zinc bacitracin is another gram-positive antibiotic of large molecular weight (1488) and is used exclusively for growth-promoting purposes.

Bambermycin is not used therapeutically in human or veterinary therapy and has pharmacologic properties similar to zinc bacitracin.

Tylosin is a macrolide antibiotic, and although used therapeutically in veterinary medicine, it is not used in human medicine. It is active principally against gram-positive microorganisms and mycoplasmas. Although it does undergo systemic absorption, no detectable levels of residue are found in the carcasses of pigs after the use of growth-promotional levels of tylosin.

Spiramycin, lincomycin, and virginiamycin are members of the same macrolide family of antibiotics, which present minimal residues when used in accordance with the manufacturer's instructions.

Feed-additive medications are to be used only at approved levels, which are generally far less than the levels necessary to achieve blood and tissue drug concentrations that would effectively treat acute respiratory disease conditions. Variation in administration from labeled directions constitutes extralabel use—a situation that requires extension of withdrawal times and is a privilege granted, at least in theory, only to the veterinarian under a veterinarian-patient-client relationship. Specific conditions justify such extralabel use, but the responsibility for that use falls on the veterinarian and producer.

23.4 INFECTIOUS ATROPHIC RHINITIS

Atrophic rhinitis is a multifactorial condition, which although common is incompletely understood. This disease is widespread and has a high incidence in many hog units. Environmental, nutritional, managemental, and infectious causes are known to be involved in the etiology of the condition. Although it was formerly held that a dietary calcium and phosphorus imbalance was the primary cause of atrophic rhinitis, this view is now not generally held, although poor nutrition or nutritional imbalance can lower the resistance of the animal to extraneous stressful factors. The degree of atrophic rhinitis is determined by several components, as follows: the primary infection and the pattern of secondary infectious agents, the genetic strain of pigs, nutritional influences, climatic factors, and, most important of all, management and housing. Varying temperatures and high concentration of dust and ammonia appear to contribute to the disease process.

The disease occurs in pigs 3 to 5 weeks of age. The first indications are sneezing, blockage of the lacrimal ducts, and facial discharge. Nasal hemorrhage, shortening of the nose, and deviation of the muzzle are common signs.

Bordetella bronchiseptica is the major causative pathogen, which devitalizes the nasal passages and turbinate bones, producing favorable local conditions for secondary infection by *Pasteurella multocida*. Toxigenic strains of *P. multocida* types A and D accentuate the bony changes, intensify local damage, and promote further atrophy of the turbinate bones. The *Pasteurella* toxins produce fibrous changes in nasal turbinates, ultimately progressing to atrophic lesions. The upper jaw then grows more slowly than the lower jaw, with a resultant wrinkled skin on the shortened snout. Sneezing, coughing, and exudation of the snout are then the cardinal clinical signs. When the atrophy is more developed on one side, the snout is deviated to that side. Recent work indicates the porcine cytomegalovirus (PCMV) may be the primary infecting agent that acts together with *B. bronchiseptica* and that infection usually occurs neonatally with the sow acting as the reservoir. Growth rate in affected young pigs is severely reduced, and in some cases, pigs never reach slaughter weight. Atrophic rhinitis commonly occurs in conjunction with enzootic pneumonia because the same adverse environmental conditions exist, and degeneration of the turbinate bones exposes the lower respiratory tract to a greater challenge from invading organisms. Toxigenic strains of *P. multocida* alone do not produce turbinate degeneration but do so in the presence of *B. bronchiseptica.*

Many outbreaks of atrophic rhinitis respond to husbandry measures, such as reducing stocking density, improving ventilation, and periodically depopulating farrowing houses and weaning houses. Only when these measures are impossible or fail should routine medication programs be introduced. Drug therapy, however, usually benefits from the addition of such husbandry improvements.

Ammonia interferes with respiratory tract function and predisposes the pig to infection. The young pig is confronted with the causal agents of rhinitis early in life, and it is at this time that the turbinates are most susceptible to damage. To ensure that the inflammatory process does not develop to any degree, antibacterial medication must be started as early as possible and continued in some cases until 10 to 12 weeks of age.

Atrophic rhinitis is caused by toxin-producing strains of *P. multocida, B. bronchiseptica,* or both. Antibiotics are of little value in arresting the course of disease but are useful in a prophylactic program. Sulfonamides, tylosin, and tetracyclines have been used in such medication schemes to arrest the early progress of rhinitis in affected herds. Potentiated sulfonamides or tylosin-sulfonamide combinations tend to give better results because of the increasing incidence of resistance by *Bordetella* to sulfonamides alone.

Tylosin is a macrolide antibiotic produced from the fermentation of a strain of *Streptocyces fradiae.* It has in vitro activity against many gram-positive, gram-negative organisms and mycoplasmas. It is of significant benefit as an injectable drug for the therapy of atrophic rhinitis or swine pneumonia caused by mycoplasmas, *P. multocida* and *Corynebacterium pyogenes.* It should normally be given intramuscularly, 4 to 10 mg/kg daily for 3 consecutive days.

Tylosin in combination with sulfamethazine displays a synergistic effect with exceptionally good activity against not only *B. bronchiseptica,* but also *Pasteurella.* Because of the electrostatic properties of powdered sulfamethazine alone in feed, the risk of carryover and residue formation in meat is increased. The granule formulation of tylosin-sulfamethazine reduces the dust associated with powdered formulates and minimizes sulfonamide carryover in the mill because less drug sticks to the mixer.

Even though tylosin and sulfadimidine are individually relatively active against *Pasteurella,* the combination is synergistic. Synergism, however, is likely to occur in the pig only if both tylosin and sulfadimidine are absorbed at the same rate; synchronized blood and tissue levels are required for synergism. Too-small crystal size presents an increased surface area for dissolution, leading to an early peaking in blood levels; with an overlarge crystal, the reverse effect is evident.

The use of granular premixes reduces the dust associated with powder formulations. A reduction in dust levels in the mill leads to an improved environment and maximizes the amount of active ingredients in the feed. There is a strong move to recommend granulation of sulfadimidine premixes for incorporation into feed. Granules also effectively eliminate the electrostatic charge that builds up on the sulfadimidine crystals in powder formulations. This minimizes sulfonamide carryover in the mill because less sticks to the mixer. Therefore less is available to be inadvertently incorporated into unmedicated rations that may follow.

THERAPY OF AFFECTED ANIMALS

Bordetella is susceptible to tetracyclines and oxytetracyclines. Oxytetracycline LA (long-acting) given to pigs at 1, 7, 14, and 21 days of age combined with a *Bordetella/Pasteurella* vaccination program frequently gives good results. Alternatively, inject piglets with potentiated sulfonamides, oxytetracycline (L.A.), tylosin, or spectinomycin on days 1, 7, and 14 (or at least three times at weekly intervals). In less severely affected outbreaks, the first injection can be given at 3 to 4 days of age.

It may be possible to medicate creep feed until after weaning, but a more positive program is to inject tylosin or potentiated sulfonamides on weeks 1, 2, and 3 after farrowing.

When outbreaks are more severe, the timing of the injection can be brought forward to day 1, 1 week, and 2 weeks. In particularly badly affected units, the sow's feed can be medicated for 3 weeks before parturition, or she may be injected 3 weeks, 2 weeks, and 1 week before farrowing. Additionally, the piglets may in such extreme cases warrant one of the three injection courses. If atrophic rhinitis is an endemic problem, as an alternative to medication of sow's feed, the sow can be injected 3 weeks, 2 weeks, and 1 week before farrowing to complement the course of injections given to the piglets.

FEED MEDICATION—CONTROL AND PROPHYLAXIS

Various feed medication programs have been recommended to control this disease, including the following chemotherapeutic strategies:

1. Medicate sows with tylosin-sulfamethazine premix, 200 g/ton, for a minimum of 3 weeks before expected farrowing and during lactation. This is to reduce or eliminate *Bordetella* and *Pasteurella* shedding by the sow.
2. Incorporate tylosin-sulfamethazine premix, 5 kg/ton, in all creep and grower rations for 15 to 30 days (200 ppm). Medicate with sulfamethazine, 100 to 450 g/ton, in feed continuously for 4 to 5 weeks, or chlortetracycline 300 g/ton.
3. Alternatively, lincomycin, 44 g/ton, and sulfamethazine, 110 g/ton.
4. Medication of feed up to weaning time is important, but feed medication should also be considered in severe outbreaks from weaning to day 135. Drugs used in this form include: Oxytetracycline, 350 g/ton; sulfamethazine, 340–450 g/ton; chlortetracycline, 300 g/ton.
5. Tylosin, 100 g/ton, is useful in grower finisher hogs in the presence of atrophic rhinitis and combined with sulfamethazine is effective additionally against *Pasteurella* and *C. pyogenes*.

Although sulfamethazine, 100 to 200 g/ton, has been used in sow rations before farrowing to reduce shedding of *Bordetella*, this practice has tended to encourage development of bacterial resistance. Potentiated sulfonamides or tylosin-sulfamethazine combinations have generally given better results.

Sulfonamides in feed, presented as the sole food source, can be given until after weaning. Increased resistance to sulfonamides fed in this way, however, has been noted, and there is a general problem with excessive sulfonamide usage in pig units resulting in violative residues in carcasses. This has become a matter of great public concern and one about which the CVM and United States Department of Agriculture (USDA) have become particularly concerned.

There are obviously various possible permutations on the timing of these treatment regimens depending on the severity and incidence of the disease. If water medication is desirable, tylosin-sulfathiazole daily for 3 days in the drinking water, 2.5 g/gallon, can be useful or, alternatively, sodium sulfathiazole, 500 mg/gallon, for 4 weeks.

It is not easy to clear herds of this infection, but a number of ancillary managemental steps can be taken, e.g., reduced stocking density, early weaning, total depopulation and restocking, and good ventilation. High levels of colostral antibodies in sow's milk can be achieved by vaccination of sows with *Bordetella* vaccines. Adherence to good management practices reduces the necessity for dependence on antibiotics. Gilts and sows can be vaccinated with *P. multocida/B. bronchiseptica* vaccines to ensure transference of high levels of colostral antibodies to the suckling piglets and thereby provide protection for the first 6 to 8 weeks of life. When outbreaks are severe and maternal protection is not sufficient, pigs may be vaccinated also but not when less than 5 weeks of age.

Antibiotics may be of little value in arresting the course of the disease but are useful in a prophylactic program. When low levels of sulfonamides are added to the diets of pigs in herds affected with atrophic rhinitis, they help maintain weight and minimize disease effects. Continuous in-feed medication from weaning to slaughter appears to convey little advantage in terms of live weight gain or feed conversion efficiency. Antibiotic protection of at-risk piglets before weaning may have a part to play in controlling the disease. Important management aspects are often overlooked and compensated for by increased use of parenteral and in-feed antibiotics.

23.5 SWINE PNEUMONIA

Mycoplasmal pneumonia, commonly referred to as enzootic pneumonia, is a highly contagious respiratory disease caused mainly by the organism *Mycoplasma hyopneumoniae*. It is an important cause of economic loss. Up to 50% of pigs are found to have lung lesions at slaughter, with up to 90% of pigs in some herds having lung lesions. Mycoplasmal pneumonia, considered to be the costliest of all swine diseases by some researchers, has the ability to cut growth rate and feed efficiency by as much as 25%. By far the most common secondary infection superimposed on the *M. hyopneumoniae* infection is *P. multocida*.

Mycoplasmal pneumonia may be present in a herd, but pigs show no symptoms because stress levels are at a minimum, and the animals have only a low-level infection. As stress escalates, however, mycoplasmal pneumonia may express itself.

Although no effective means have been developed to immunize hogs against mycoplasmal diseases, research indicates that some compounds are effective in the treatment and control of mycoplasmal diseases. Sulfonamides in combination with trimethoprim are used by several veterinarians even though a relatively high proportion of the strains are resistant to sulfonamides. To treat the basic mycoplasmal infection, lincomycin and tiamulin are used.

Although *M. hyopneumoniae* is regarded as the primary pathogen, if secondary bacteria (such as *Pasteurella, Bordetella, Haemophilus, Streptococcus*, and *Corynebacterium*) are involved, a high temperature, dyspnea, chronic coughing, and anorexia are present. Usually the apical and cardiac lobes of the lung are the most affected, with consolidation and hepatization. The disease has high morbidity but low mortality, with resultant suppression of growth rate and food conversion efficiency. Mycoplasmal infection of the respiratory tract increases the likelihood of secondary bacterial infection.

Strategic medication and modification of management practices underpin the successful approach to this disease problem. Swine pneumonia is usually a chronic syndrome caused by many infectious agents but strongly influenced by environmental factors. Clinical pneumonia results when pigs are exposed to a challenge of virulent microorganisms at a time when their resistance is low owing to environmental stress. *M. hyopneumoniae* is usually the primary pathogen, which can cause damage to the respiratory ciliary functioning and can also suppress the cell-mediated immune response.

Lungs damaged by mycoplasmal infection become a common site for secondary infection. Mycoplasmal pneumonia usually begins in 4- to 8-week-old pigs soon after they are weaned. Adding lincomycin (200 g/ton of feed) to nursery diets reduces the severity of mycoplasmal pneumonia lesions and improves growth rates and feed efficiencies. Tetracycline compounds also help reduce the incidence of mycoplasmal lesions and often are fed to limit the severity of developing lesions in young pigs.

P. multocida is a common secondary invader in swine pneumonia, and in the presence of other primary pathogens, a purulent bronchopneumonia with pericarditis and pleuritis sometimes results. Many other organisms may be isolated from porcine pneumonic lungs, including *Salmonella choleraesuis, Haemophilus parasuis, Streptococcus suis, B. bronchiseptica, actinobacillus*, and beta-hemolytic streptococci. Viruses such as swine influenza or adenovirus contribute to the overall disease process by suppressing immune mechanisms and facilitating the colonization and multiplication by bacteria and mycoplasmae. Pseudorabies virus, responsible for producing neurologic disease and reproductive failure, has often been implicated as a primary cause of pneumonia. Failure to attend to parasite control programs properly (especially *Ascaris suum*, which undergoes lung migration) can contribute to the incidence of the pneumonic lesions. Ascarid control programs must be part of a prophylactic package for swine pneumonia.

The design of the building's ventilation system is critical in minimizing pneumonia in confined pigs. Absolute temperature, when it is below that which is comfortable for the pig, adversely affects the pig's ability to remove bacteria from its respiratory tract.

Ammonia interferes with respiratory tract function and predisposes the pig to infection. *M. hyopneumoniae* causes a decrease in ciliary function and subsequent ciliary loss that may persist for up to 16 weeks. Treating individually symptomatic animals with antibiotic injections is a common practice on many swine farms. Although this is helpful, the most effective approach in treating acute herd outbreaks of respiratory disease is to inject the entire group initially with the appropriate antimicrobial and then to retreat individual pigs as necessary. The three major drug groups used most often in parenteral treatment of respiratory disease are the tetracyclines, the penicillins, and the macrolide antibiotics, tylosin and erythromycin.

The choice of antibiotic obviously depends on the antimicrobial sensitivity pattern of the isolate pathogens. Generally, parenteral administration is preferable initially in acute cases. Medication of feed and water is a popular practice, but because pigs with acute respiratory disease may have severely curtailed feed and water consumption, they may ingest subeffective levels of antibiotics.

Pigs become infected very soon after birth, and severity depends on the level and virulence of the challenge, the immune status of the pig, and the presence of various stress factors. The spreading of disease by *Mycoplasma* mainly takes place between younger age groups and not from older immune animals to younger ones.

Many antibiotics and vaccinations used for treatment and control of mycoplasmal pneumonia have been largely ineffective. The fluoroquinolones danofloxacin and enrofloxacin, however, have been successful and have been shown to reduce the prevalence of size of lung lesions. Spiramycin displays activity against *Haemophilus, Mycoplasma*, and *Pasteurella* also. It is used in a number of countries, with or without doxycycline combination, for enzootic pneumonia and pleuropneumonia. Similar to many other drugs, it does not possess approval from the regulatory authorities for such use. Tiamulin is one of the most potent antimycoplasmal agents against *M. hyopneumoniae* currently available.

The fastest acting treatment is with an injectable antibiotic. Injections of tiamulin at a dose of 12.3 mg base (equivalent to 15 mg tiamulin hydrogen fumarate)/kg body weight/day intramuscularly for up to 3 consecutive days are effective. Tiamulin premix, at a level to provide 30 to 40 ppm of the active ingredient, tiamulin hydrogen fumarate, can be given shortly before slaughter.

USEFUL ANTIMICROBIALS

Tiamulin is a potent antispirochetal drug indicated for swine pneumonia. In feed at a level of 200 ppm, it is a good choice of drug for early weaning feeds, possessing high mycoplasmal specificity and concentrating well in respiratory tissues. Supplementary medication may be required against various secondary pathogens in individual animals.

Tiamulin can be included at 20 to 30 g/ton in combination with sulfamethazine 100 g/ton from weaners and growers up to 16 weeks of age. All the remaining breeding animals are medicated daily with a suitable antibiotic, e.g., tiamulin (6 mg/kg body weight corresponding to 100 to 120 ppm in the drinking water). Alternative choices are oxytetracycline, 100 to 400 g/ton, or 100 g/ton sulfamethazine and 150 g/ton tylosin. Tylosin may act to potentiate the activity of sulfamethazine by way of increased absorption of the latter as well as complementing its antimicrobial spectrum.

In young pigs in which enzootic pneumonia is a consequence of recent exposure and largely independent of husbandry, a 5-day course of water medicated with tiamulin or tylosin can give good results. Tylosin is also available for medication combined with sulfathiazole. Individual parenteral treatment for 3 consecutive days can be repeated when pigs are weaned at 4 weeks of age.

Lincomycin displays a particularly low minimum inhibitory concentration (MIC) against *M. hyopneumoniae*. For mycoplasmal respiratory disease or following infectious mycoplasmal arthritis or polyserositis, lincomycin can be given to piglets daily for 3 consecutive days (10 mg/kg). Treatment must be given early because mycoplasmosis can be a triggering disease for a number of other infectious syndromes. Infectious arthritis and polyserositis can be complicating secondary problems in cases of respiratory mycoplasmosis.

The antibiotic lincomycin combats *M. hyopneumoniae*, the disease-causing organism, very effectively. Lincomycin also has the ability to reach the site of the disease-causing organism. In experiments, Lincomycin had the lowest in vitro MIC of 51 compounds that were tested. Its MIC was 0.09 μg/ml (range 0.06 to 0.11 μg/ml) against *M. hyopneumoniae*. This was 2.5 times more potent than the next most potent compound (sulfathiazole), which had a MIC of 0.25 μg/ml. Against *Mycoplasma hyorhinis*, lincomycin was 10 times more potent than the next most effective compound (0.03 μg/ml versus 0.30 μg/ml for sulfathiazole).

Lincomycin is an excellent choice for treating and controlling mycoplasmal diseases. This program involves treating with injectable lincomycin at the first indication of a problem to baby pigs each day for 3 consecutive days. In most infected herds, this is the first 3 days of life.

For mycoplasmal pneumonia in 4- to 8-week-old pigs shortly after they are weaned, adding lincomycin, 200 g/ton, to feed reduces the severity of mycoplasmal pneumonia and improves growth rate and feed efficiency. Tetracyclines can be used in the same way prophylactically.

The efficacy of enrofloxacin in bronchopneumonia and enzootic pneumonia was studied after artificial infections with *M. hyopneumoniae* and in naturally infected animals. When administered prophylactically in the feed, dosage rates from as low as 1.25 mg/kg were 100% mycoplasmacidal. In controlled studies in herds with enzootic pneumonia, dosage rates from approximately 2.5 mg/kg enrofloxacin proved to be more effective than conventional drugs, whether administered via the feed or parenterally. The efficacy of enrofloxacin in pigs was tested primarily in cases of piglet diarrhea, colidiarrhea, bronchopneumonia, enzootic pneumonia, and salmonellosis. It was found that dosage rates of 1 mg/kg or more were highly effective in artificial and natural infections. Enrofloxacin also produced a good response in colidiarrhea and colienterotoxemia of weaners and growers at dosage rates from 1 to 2 mg/kg.

Ascarid migration or high ammonia levels intensify the mycoplasmal pulmonary lesions. Whole-herd infections are generally associated primarily with virulent mycoplasmas. On account of the low-grade, chronic nature of the infection, medication is normally provided by the feed continuously—oxytetracycline, tylosin, or tiamulin being commonly used. Subtherapeutic levels fed continuously do not treat clinical disease but help to keep an outbreak in check. Tylosin fed at 40 g/ton reduces mycoplasmal infection and reduces the risk of secondary bacterial pneumonia. Secondary pneumonia caused by *Haemophilus* or *Pasteurella* may respond to water medication with tetracyclines, sulfonamides, or phenoxymethyl-penicillin.

SPECIFIC ANTIMICROBIAL STRATEGIES

Tetracyclines, sulfonamides, macrolides, tiamulin, penicillins, or lincosamides are commonly used to treat individual animals systemically in the event of acute outbreaks. Re-treatment with these intramuscular injections is often necessary. Such parenteral treatment is the only way of ensuring adequate levels of drug at the focus of infection. It may be desirable to complement parenteral treatment with in-feed or in-water medication for affected batches or as a preventative strategy for in control animals.

Inject tylosin on the second, third, and 21st days of life (5 to 10 mg/kg). Tylosin may also be injected at weaning and on entry to the fattening house. Individual pig treatment is followed up by medication in feed or in water.

The affected unit can be treated in blanket fashion with tylosin/sulfamethazine premix in feed for 2 weeks. When the disease is significantly under control tylosin in feed, 40 to 100 ppm, can be continued for a further 2 to 3 weeks.

The following antimicrobials can be considered for parenteral therapy:

Tiamulin, 15 mg/kg for 3 days
Tylosin, 5 to 10 mg/kg for 3 days
Lincomycin, 4 to 10 mg/kg for 3 days
Spectinomycin, 10 mg/kg for 3 days
Oxytetracycline, 10 mg/kg for 3 days

Oxytetracycline LA, 20 mg/kg at 4-day intervals

Erythromycin 5 mg/kg for 3 days

CONTROL

Control dosages are as follows:

Oxytetracycline, 50 to 100 g/ton continuously; therapeutic level, 200 to 400 g/ton for 7 to 10 days

Chlortetracycline, 50 to 100 g/ton continuously; treatment inclusion rate, 250 to 400 g/ton

Lincomycin, 200 g/ton

Tylosin/sulfamethazine, 100 g/tylosin 100 g/sulfamezathine per ton

Tylosin, 40 g/ton

Tiamulin, 30 g/ton (fed for up to 8 weeks)

Lincomycin/spectinomycin, 40 g/ton fed continuously

Reduction in stocking rate, reduction in the amount of dust in the unit, and improvements in the ventilation system must be attended to if the disease is not to become a recurring problem.

23.6 SWINE PLEUROPNEUMONIA

Pleuropneumonia is caused by *Actinobacillus pleuropneumoniae* (formerly *Haemophilus pleuropneumoniae*). This is a highly contagious disease, and in endemic herds, sows are carriers and provide colostral immunity for 3 to 4 weeks. Acute cases may occur as early as 6 weeks of age onward.

A. pleuropneumoniae infection often results in reduced body weight gain, increased feed intake, increased rate of mortality, increased number of pigs condemned at slaughter, and increased costs of medicine and veterinary treatment. Several investigations have shown that it is difficult to contain the disease within the herd area. One reason is probably air-borne infection from one section to another with ventilating air.

Prophylactic vaccination against *A. pleuropneumoniae* is not always effective. Another problem of vaccination is that it is impossible to protect against all serotypes at the same time. Each of the vaccines available today protects only against one to three serotypes.

More than 11 different serotypes of *Haemophilus* have been described. Severe *Haemophilus* infection can be associated with pleurisy and high mortality or a more chronic form with reduced growth rate and feed conversion efficiency. The condition is often seen in pigs in connection with stress, such as weaning, change of feed, change of environment, or mixing when colostral immunity is low.

The pleuropneumonia-causing organism is transmitted from pig to pig by inhalation and from farm to farm by the introduction of carriers or chronically infected pigs into a previously unexposed herd. *Haemophilus* pleuropneumonia can cause sudden death as well as chronic poor performance in pigs. The organism tends to be very virulent, and spread from hog to hog is by aerosol or nose-to-nose contact.

In clinical outbreaks of pleuropneumonia, the organisms locate deep in lung abscesses, which possess a poor blood supply. Usually pleuropneumonia affects older fattening pigs and follows an acute course with a high morbidity, pyrexia, respiratory distress, and death in 2 to 3 days. The mortality varies from 20 to 80%. At necropsy, there is a bloody nasal discharge and pleurisy with a layer of fibrin over dark red, hemorrhagic areas on the lung surfaces. Histologically the lungs show hemorrhagic necrosis of airways and alveolar walls.

In natural infection, there is a certain cross immunity (protection) between the different serotypes. Herds with good immunity against one serotype are to some extent resistant to infection with other serotypes. The resistance seems to be local by nature (mucosal immunity) with IgA antibodies in the mucus of the lungs. The cross immunity is, however, not complete, and herds housing several serotypes exist.

TREATMENT

The antibiotics most commonly in use (and with the fewest resistant strains) are:

Penicillin, 20,000 mg/kg

Ampicillin, 10 mg/kg

Oxytetracycline, 10 mg/kg

Oxytetracycline, 20 mg/kg
Tiamulin, 10 mg/kg

Bacterial pneumonias involving *Haemophilus* may respond to in-water medications with substances such as the tetracyclines, tiamulin, or ampicillin, although penicillin V (phenoxymethyl-penicillin) may be used with considerable success. Also, special attention must be paid to humidity, ventilation, and stocking density.

Treatment must be started early and repeated for 2 to 3 days, preferably the entire pen. Sensitivity patterns can vary considerably so laboratory detection of antimicrobial susceptibility must be carried out with the modified Kirby-Bauer method in many cases. Traditionally penicillin, ampicillin, and tetracyclines were the drugs of choice. With shifting sensitivity patterns, however, about 30% of strains are resistant to tetracycline, but many strains are still susceptible to gentamicin, spectinomycin, or sulfachloropyridazine. For treatment, gentamicin must be administered parenterally, which limits its mass application because it is not absorbed from the alimentary tract. For mass medication, macrolides (tylosin, erythromycin), ampicillin, cephalosporins, phenoxymethyl-penicillin, tiamulin, and potentiated sulfonamides are good choices.

Pleuropneumonia should be treated as soon as it is detected. If possible, separate sick pigs into a "hospital" pen and inject them intramuscularly with tiamulin at a dose of 12.3 mg base (equivalent to 15 mg tiamulin hydrogen fumarate)/kg body weight for at least 3 and up to 5 consecutive days. Tiamulin is also effective and of benefit in pigs concurrently infected with mycoplasmas. Given at 120 ppm in water for 5 to 10 days, tiamulin can effect a rapid clinical recovery, possessing activity not only against spirochetes, but also against *Haemophilus*.

The only reasonable choice for water or feed medication is tiamulin because of its high absorption from the gastrointestinal tract, even though quite a lot of tetracycline is used. The efficacy of tiamulin given in drinking water at 60 ppm for 5 and 10 days and at 120 ppm for 5 days was evaluated after pigs showed clinical signs of infection with *Haemophilus* pleuropneumoniae. Com-

pared with nonmedicated controls, pigs treated with tiamulin at 120 ppm had significantly fewer ($P < 0.05$) days with coughing and nasal discharge.

To reduce losses in acute outbreaks, good results have been obtained by water medication of all pigs for 5 days (tiamulin, 100 to 120 ppm) and injection of the sick pigs with penicillin for 1 to 2 days (the most affected twice a day). In this way, the level and spread of infection are suppressed to a minimum. Long-acting parenteral penicillin or oxytetracyclines have proved useful, although many strains of *Haemophilus* are resistant to sulfonamides.

Vaccination at 2- and 4-week intervals with *Haemophilus* bacterins can provide satisfactory cover, although a massive exposure challenge can overcome any vaccine. Parenteral erythromycin, 4 mg/kg intramuscularly, is indicated for *Haemophilus* infection, with additional antimicrobial potency directed against *P. multocida*, *Pasteurella haemolytica*, and *Mycoplasma*.

Peracute experimental infections with *A. pleuropneumoniae* were rapidly cured by three intramuscular injections of 2.5 mg/kg enrofloxacin at 24-hour intervals. Enrofloxacin can also affect the reversal of experimental *A. pleuropneumoniae* infection with three daily injections of 5 mg/kg each. Prophylactic and therapeutic efficacy against salmonellosis and the mastitis-metritis-agalactia syndrome (frequently caused be *Escherichia coli*) has also been reported.

For clinically affected animals, injections of tiamulin, sulfonamides, potentiated sulfonamides, or oxytetracyclines are indicated:

Sulfadimidine 33 1/3% (injection), 150 mg/kg
Sulfonamide/trimethoprim, 15 mg/kg
Oxytetracycline, 7 mg/kg
Ampicillin, penicillin V, 10 mg/kg
Lincomycin, 10 mg/kg
Streptomycin, 12 mg/kg
Gentamicin, 1.0 mg/kg
Tiamulin, 10 mg/kg
Enrofloxacin, 2.5 mg/kg
Erythromycin, 4 mg/kg

Doxycycline hydrochloride possesses activity against *A. pleuropneumoniae*. Given orally in feed over a period of 7 days, doxycycline at a level of 100 to 200 ppm improves weight gain and feed conversion and reduces pulmonary lesions.

CONTROL

Control dosages are as follows:

   Oxytetracycline, 50 to 100 g/ton prophy-
      lactically or 100 to 400 g/ton for 10
      to 14 days as treatment
   Tylosin and sulfamethazine, 100 g/ton of
      each fed continuously
   Sulfamethazine, 100 g/ton fed continu-
      ously
   Lincomycin/spectinomycin, 40 g/ton fed
      continuously
   Tiamulin, 120 ppm in water

ENTERIC INFECTIONS

For neonatal pig scours, a wide variety of agents have been used: tetracyclines, neomycin, gentamycin, and water-soluble apramycin and enrofloxacin. Response to therapy in salmonellosis can be disappointing, although apramycin, enrofloxacin, potentiated sulfonamides, and ampicillin have yielded excellent results.

Swine dysentery is a problematic disease, and the major cost factor involved is in prophylactic medication, which is often given from weaning to slaughter. Many drugs, such as the organic arsenicals tylosin and dimetridazole, which have been in use for some time, are now losing their effectiveness. Other drugs have appeared on the market that are effective, but these are generally more expensive, and there may be other drawbacks with their usage. Carbadox has a 75-day withdrawal period before slaughter, and so it cannot be used if the disease occurs in fattening houses. Tiamulin, a water-soluble preparation, is effective, but for many practical reasons, medication of drinking water cannot be carried out on most farms for long periods. Tiamulin shares some characteristics in common with the macrolide group of antibiotics. After administration by mouth to pigs, tiamulin is well absorbed, and peak plasma levels are achieved within 2 to 4 hours of administration. The compound is metabolized in the liver, and excretion takes place mainly through the feces via the bile. Other useful compounds include tylosin and lincomycin.

WITHDRAWAL PERIODS

One of the most controversial areas associated with antibiotic use in pigs is the compliance or otherwise with stated withdrawal periods. The imposition of mandatory withdrawal periods, inconvenient to the farmer who has to change from medicated to nonmedicated feeding as the animal nears optimum slaughter weight, must be shown to be absolutely necessary. In many ways, the choice of antibiotic can have a marked influence on whether residues are present at slaughter or not. The use of antibiotics that deposit in the kidney results in residues being present in this organ for a much longer period than if an antibiotic is selected that is rapidly excreted in the urine. Similarly, long-acting depot-type will present greater residue hazards than short-acting preparations of the same drug. Strict observance of stated withdrawal times is especially necessary during mass medication programs near to slaughter. Antibiotic tissue residues are also less likely with water than with in-feed medication because it is much simpler to cut off the water supply than to stop using feed, especially when there are still several tons of medicated feed left in the bulk hopper. Tissue residues may also be avoided if antimicrobial substances that are not absorbed from the intestinal tract are used. In many cases, however, this is not possible because antibiotics possessing systemic effects may be needed. Sulfonamides present frequent residue hazards in pigs.

23.7 COLIBACILLOSIS

Colibacillosis is probably the most common disease affecting pig herds. A variety of clinical syndromes have been described, including both neonatal and postweaning scours. For diarrhea to be caused, the K88 antigen must become established in the small intestine, produce an enterotoxin, and usually adhere to the microvilli.

Colibacillosis in neonatal piglets is primarily the result of infection with enterotoxigenic *E. coli* (ETEC). ETEC strains may be identified by "O" somatic antigens or by pilus antigens. These pilus antigens are referred to K88, K99, 987p, F41, and F165. Although there are other subtypes of the K88 pili (K88ab and K88ad), K88ac appears to be the common subtype in pigs in the United States.

In contrast to colibacillosis in calves, there does not appear to be an age at which piglets fail to become infected. ETEC attach to the small intestine by means of the pili and elaborate a toxin that interferes with the biochemistry of the cell; this leads to a net secretion of fluid into the small intestine. Heat-labile toxin leads to the activation of adenylate cyclase, which, in turn, increases levels of intracellular cyclic adenosine monophosphate (cAMP). The net result of elevated levels of cAMP is increased secretion of fluids and electrolytes from the cell into the lumen of the small intestine.

E. coli have a capsule that is composed of polysaccharide. Pathogenic *E. coli* have an A type capsule, which is heat stable. There are at least 70 antigenically different types of capsules in *E. coli*. On serotype the capsule is recorded as K (from the German word for capsule, "Kapsule").

The O or somatic (body) antigen is part of the cell wall and lies just beneath the capsule. The O antigen is a lipopolysaccharide portion, which gives different antigenic determinants for serotyping.

Many *E. coli* organisms have adhesion factors on their outer surface, which allow them to anchor to the enterocytes lining the small intestine. Once anchored to the intestinal villi, *E. coli* cause noninvasive diarrhea by production of toxins that affect the target epithelial cells, causing a gross imbalance in the water flux of the intestine, resulting in a net fluid loss. *E. coli* that cause diarrhea by way of this mechanism are ETEC. The mechanism by which the *E. coli* enterotoxin causes the hypersecretion is unknown; evidence points to the site of activity as being in the crypts of the mucosa. Secretion of fluid may occur across the intact mucosa, and cell damage, if it does occur, would appear to be a complicating factor. It is thought that the enterotoxin possesses enzymatic properties, which may be responsible for the accumulation of intracellular messengers, e.g., cAMP within the mucosal cells.

The ensuing diarrhea results in dehydration, metabolic acidosis, hyperkalemia, and decreased plasma bicarbonate. This may lead to hemoconcentration, hypovolemia, and prerenal uremia, with the animal becoming depressed and hypothermic. It has also been shown that piglets infected with enteropathogenic *E. coli* can show depressed glucose uptake, and it is well recognized that in rotavirus infections, flattening of mucosal villi reduces the surface area available for absorption, and even in *E. coli* infection, villous atrophy can occur.

E. coli enteritis can occur as follows:

1. Neonatal, 0 to 4 days
2. Milk or 3-week scours
3. Postweaning

Clinical signs include diarrhea, yellow pasty feces, wetness, normal or subnormal temperature, and dehydration.

TREATMENT

Oral therapy is preferably combined with parenteral antibiotic treatment:

Potentiated sulfonamides
Oxytetracycline
Neomycin, gentamicin
Furazolidone
Ampicillin
Amoxicillin
Apramycin
Enrofloxacin
Spectinomycin

Initial treatment using a drug likely to control the bacteria (gentamicin) is recommended until sensitivity test results are available. Fluid and electrolyte therapy is an important component of the therapeutic program in coliform scours in baby piglets. A variety of factors may be involved in the cause of porcine enteritis, and careful consideration must be given before a decision is made to administer antibiotics. It is imperative that should any young pigs start to scour, immediate action is taken to ensure that such piglets are given the best care possible and if necessary treated with antiscour preparations. Replacement fluid therapy can be vital. Quite often by placing a small dish of glucose saline, with or without specific water-soluble medication, near the scouring piglets and by providing a warm, dry creep area, all but the weakest of piglets can be saved. Glucose saline intraperitoneally is useful also.

Fluid replacement therapy is an important component in the treatment of colibacillosis. Fluid therapy, which can be given orally or rectally, should attempt to control the electrolyte imbalance and replace lost fluids. Oral fluid replacement as a treatment of dehydration in diarrhea has been widely and successfully practiced in human medicine as therapy in cholera and noncholera diarrheas. It has also been successful in treatment of calves with *E. coli* infection either naturally or experimentally acquired.

Oral fluid replacement with a glucose glycine electrolyte formulation is based on the observation that glucose and glycine are actively absorbed by the small intestine, with accompanied absorption of sodium and water. If the net absorption so produced exceeds the net secretion that is producing diarrhea, the process of dehydration is reversed. Solutions containing an actively absorbed amino acid, such as glycine, together with glucose have been shown to be more effective than solutions containing glucose and electrolyte without glycine (both in cholera). Intestinal absorptive capacity for glucose and glycine remains sufficient to benefit from the oral rehydrating effect of a glucose glycine electrolyte (e.g., Resorb/Lectade) solution. Often the only remedy that is required here is application of oral electrolytes (with or without kaolin or pectin absorbents) and glycine. For neonatal scours, a variety of agents have been used, including oral tetracyclines, and water-soluble apramycin. Neomycin, gentamicin, and other aminoglycosides are useful also. Glycine-containing electrolyte products are indicated in severe cases to remedy the dehydration and electrolyte imbalance. Parenteral therapy includes sulfonamides, potentiated sulfonamides, ampicillin, and amoxicillin. The problem with antibiotic therapy in large in-testing units is that resistance develops rapidly to many products, and so antibiotics should be regarded as second-line defense agents when nonantibiotic antidiarrheal electrolyte prep-arations have been unsuccessful. The use of vaccines, which are generally effective, is widespread.

In addition to vaccines, controlling the environment within the farrowing crate to keep it free of drafts and cold surfaces and at a constant temperature helps reduce the prevalence of scouring pigs. In some situations, using prostaglandins to induce and concentrate farrowing ensures that workers are nearby to monitor neonates to make sure they receive enough colostrum or to transfer piglets from large litters to sows with small litters. Other control methods being studied include oral administration of monoclonal antibodies (anti-K88) to neonatal pigs. Because of the K88 adhesion and local prostaglandin production, aspirinlike drugs have proved to be successful ancillary aids in therapy.

23.8 SWINE DYSENTERY

This highly infectious disease affects pigs mainly in the post weaning period between 10 and 16 weeks. It is prevalent in large units, which are continuously buying weaners from many sources. Overcrowding, poor hygiene, and common dung channels exacerbate the condition. The mortality rate is quite low, but loss of productivity is severe. Recovered animals are carriers and readily break down when stresses occur. Most pig owners feel compelled to medicate the food constantly. There are many drugs on the market that are effective in suppressing the symptoms, but they do not eliminate the causal agent. Producers should aim at eliminating the stresses already mentioned rather than relying on the drugs.

The exact cause of swine dysentery is not clear. The primary infective agent thought to be responsible for the disease is *Treponema hyodysenteriae*, but experiments have shown that this organism alone is unable to produce the disease when given to gnotobiotic pigs. Only when other agents normally resident in the colon of the pig are present can *T. hyodysenteriae* exert its pathogenic effect. The disease is transmitted by the ingestion of feces from affected or clinically normal pigs carrying *T. hyodysenteriae*.

Swine dysentery is an extremely troublesome form of enteritis caused by *T. hyodysenteriae* combined with bacteria such as *Campylobacter coli, Bacteroides vulgatus, Fusobacterium necrophorum,* and some *Clostridium* species. Although normally associated with fattening units, it can have a depressing effect on breeding units. *T. hyodysenteriae* has been isolated from vermin and flies, so increased vermin control and the treatment of the buildings with a long-lasting fly killer are of value.

Bacteroides, Fusobacterium, and other organisms as yet unidentified may be incriminated. The exact roles of *C. (Vibrio) coli* and *E. coli* have yet to be elucidated. These organisms may produce factors that aid the growth or the ability of *T. hyodysenteriae* to colonize the cells of the colonic mucosa and may, by their presence, increase the severity of the disease.

Signs include reduction in appetite, hollowing of the flank, pyrexia, diarrhea containing traces of blood, poor thriving, poor feed conversion efficiency, and failure to grow. Diarrhea, varying from blood-stained mucoid to frank dysentery, occurs with severe dehydration, loss of condition, and death in severe cases. It has also been suggested that infection with *Trichuris suis* may predispose pigs to an upgrowth of spirochetes and vibriolike organisms in the large intestine.

Swine dysentery is widespread in all pig populations. In the breeding unit, the disease seldom causes clinical disease, but many carrier animals act as a reservoir of infection. In the feeding herd, in which the disease has its major economic effect, control of the disease usually requires strategic or continuous medication. If clinical disease occurs, the costs in terms of reduced growth rate, decreased food conversion, and mortality can have an economically devastating result. With increasing awareness and legislation in relation to antibiotic residues in pig carcasses, the unit with endemic swine dysentery can have potential problems in complying with medication withdrawal periods before slaughter.

Because the disease is primarily initiated by a single spirochete, *T. hyodysenteriae* (although in gnotobiotic pigs *F. necrophorum* and *B. vulgatus* are also necessary for expression of the disease), it should be pos-sible to use antibiotic therapy to eradicate the organism. Practical experience with attempts at eradication of the disease has resulted in the evolution of a range of criteria considered essential in the eradication program. Eradication is based on medication of the whole herd for a period of 5 to 6 months, plus a stringent hygiene program to prevent any carryover of infection from pen to pen. Success cannot be guaranteed; however, the expense can be justified because the cost of the eradication program is commonly less than the annual cost of dysentery control on a unit.

Swine dysentery is widespread, although largely as a mild or inapparent infection suppressed by drugs. The major cost of the disease is therefore prophylactic medication, which is often given from weaning to slaughter.

TREATMENT

Treatment may be in feed or in water, but water medication is probably best for swine dysentery because infected animals commonly do not eat. Affected animals are initially anorexic, and so the first approach must be to medicate the drinking water. This may be combined with parenteral treatment of the worst affected animals. Owing to the highly contagious nature of the disease, all animals in contact should be medicated.

Water medication may be followed by infeed medication at therapeutic levels until all clinical signs have disappeared. Many drugs that have been used for some time now are losing their effectiveness, whereas other more recent additions onto the market are more effective but generally more expensive. When inappetence is a problem, as in many pig diseases, water-soluble preparations are more effective than in-feed antibiotics.

It is not uncommon to experience outbreaks of swine dysentery in gilts and sows. Having had a diagnosis confirmed, it is important to deal with this problem in a radical fashion. It may be necessary to institute a blanket medication routine for all affected and in-contact stock. It is most useful, following isolation of affected clinical cases and a subsidence of actual scour, that medication be continued for at least 2 weeks. Basically this is a situation in which once the condition broadly described as swine dysentery becomes established in an area of an intensive unit, control can be best maintained by paying attention to hygiene and isolation of clinical cases together with the judicious use of medication. The choice of drug used is to some extent governed by the feed and water system involved. In a situation like this, it is useful to be able to include the medication in solution in the drinking water as soon as clinical symptoms are noticed. An arrangement of the water system to include header tanks and drinking bowls, rather than nipple drinkers coming from a main pipeline supply, can facilitate the efficient, economic use of expensive soluble drugs. Also, as an emergency procedure, some type of small mixing arrangement in which some medicated premix can be dispersed through 1 or 2 days' supply of feed can prove useful.

Swine dysentery has been the scourge of bought-in weaners for decades, but a variety of substances are available for in-feed use, water medication, and injection. Dimetridazole can be used at 500 to 700 ppm in water for treatment and 200 to 300 ppm in feed for prophylaxis. This is permitted in Europe but not in the United States. Other products include tylosin, lincomycin, and tiamulin. With swine dysentery, it is essential to halt the progress of the disease as rapidly as possible; otherwise serious losses occur. When administering treatment, the best route for clinically sick pigs is via the drinking water, but this may be followed by in-feed medication once the acute clinical disease has abated and the pigs have regained their appetite.

Because affected pigs continue drinking, tylosin soluble, 100 g/190 liters for 3 to 5 days, is indicated. Severely affected animals may require individual treatment with Tylosin injection, 5 to 10 mg/kg. Water-soluble tiamulin is also a useful alternative and is considered by many to be the drug of choice for swine dysentery.

Drugs useful for swine dysentery include:

Tylosin
Tiamulin
Lincomycin
Spectinomycin
Erythromycin
Oxytetracycline
Dimetridazole, ronidazole (Not permitted for swine in the U.S.)
Organic arsenicals
Gentamicin
Furazolidone (now prohibited internationally)
Spiramycin
Carbadox
Virginiamycin

Work has been reported that suggests that selenium can increase the resistance of pigs to swine dysentery, but in general, the current practice on treatment is antibacterial mass medication of the affected stock.

DRUGS USED IN DYSENTERY CONTROL

Many drugs, such as organic arsenicals tylosin and quinoxalines and nitroimidazoles, that have been in use for some time are now either losing their effectiveness or possess other attendant problems. Carbadox is known to be mutagenic and potentially carcinogenic. It can pose health hazards also to those in contact with the drug at the mixing level. (In countries where carbadox is permitted, protective clothing must be worn to prevent inhalation or skin contact with the drug.) It has a withdrawal time of 70 days in the United States and at least 28 days in Europe. Dimetridazole (similar to a number of other nitroimidazoles) is banned in the United States for use in pigs. Ipronidazole has still been retained for blackhead in turkeys in the United States.

Ronidazole, ipronidazole, and dimetridazole are available as water and in-feed premixes in Europe. In eradication programs, they are generally used as the advance guard to damp down the amount of swine dysentery present in the entire herd. Resistance to these drugs, including dimetridazole and ronidazole, has been widely described.

Carbadox has been widely used for control of swine dysentery as a feed premix. Recommended levels have to be adhered to because higher doses can depress appetite and lead to signs of toxicity. When used in sow feed, it can cause constipation, so laxatives or roughage may be necessary, particularly around farrowing time. It has a long withdrawal period but has been used in successful eradication programs. Its use is controversial in some countries because of its mutagenicity.

Lincomycin is available as an injection, water-soluble agent, and in-feed premix. It has been used in eradication programs as a feed premix with success. Within the body, the drug has the ability to penetrate tissue and so effect repair of chronic swine dysentery lesions in the bowel. At treatment levels for swine dysentery, it has effective activity against mycoplasmal organisms, the primary infective agents in enzootic pneumonia and mycoplasmal arthritis. Individual pigs can be treated with lincomycin, 8 mg/kg, intramuscularly at 24-hour intervals. Followup treatment may be in the feed, 110 ppm, or 150 mg lincomycin in 4.5 liters of water until symptoms disappear. Medicated water should be discarded in 2 days if it has not been consumed and made up freshly again.

Lincomycin is highly effective in short-term and longterm disease management programs. It is effective against *T. hyodysenteriae*, the causative agent in swine dysentery. In complete pig feeds, lincomycin is approved at 110 g/metric ton for the treatment of swine dysentery. Swine dysentery is a persistent disease, and further outbreaks on a unit after the discontinuation of treatment may be due to a high incidence of infection or poor hygiene on the unit. Lincomycin premix treatment over a 3-week period should provide a prolonged period of freedom from the condition, provided that appropriate hygiene precautions are taken. When the pigs have completed the 3-week course of treatment, the level of cleanliness must be maintained.

Another particular advantage of lincomycin premix is its short withdrawal requirement. It must be remembered that feed containing lincomycin premix is toxic for cattle, sheep, and horses, and within the feed-mill, care is necessary to prevent cross contamination of feeds for those species. Resistance to *T. hyodysenteriae* has been reported in some instances.

Tiamulin is available as an injectable, water-soluble agent, and in-feed premix. In vitro it is the antibiotic with the greatest ac-tivity against swine dysentery. The injectable preparation has given excellent results in treating clinical cases.

Tiamulin is a semisynthetic diterpene antibiotic with pronounced in vitro activity against *T. hyodysenteriae*, various gram-positive organisms, and *Mycoplasma*. It is widely used clinically in the following formulations—injectable, water-soluble powder, solution, and feed premix to prevent and treat swine dysentery, to treat and mitigate the economic effects of enzootic pneumonia, and to treat mycoplasmal arthritis in pigs. Within the body, the drug has great ability to penetrate tissue and so effect repair of chronic swine dysentery lesions in the bowel. At treatment levels for swine dysentery, it has effective activity against mycoplasmal organisms, the primary infective agents in enzootic pneumonia and mycoplasmal arthritis.

CONTROL

Tiamulin premix is given at a level to provide 30 to 40 ppm in the finished feed of the active ingredient, tiamulin hydrogen fumarate, throughout the period that the affected pigs are on the farm. Salinomycin is a monovalent cationic ionophore antibiotic used as a coccidiostat in chickens and now as a growth-promoting feed additive in pigs. Interaction is possible between tiamulin and salinomycin. The compatibility of the two products seems not to be influenced by the actual mode of application (90% of tiamulin applied in feed is also absorbed) but rather by the dosage in milligrams per kilograms body weight per unit of time. Maximum tiamulin blood levels are reached 2 to 4 hours after application, whether the daily dose is consumed in feed or drinking water throughout the day or applied in a single injection.

The concurrent administration of salinomycin (80 ppm) in feed with tiamulin in feed at the prophylactic level (30 ppm) does not result in any adverse clinical effects. However, the concurrent administration of salinomycin (80 ppm) in feed with therapeutic levels of tiamulin administered in drinking water (0.006%), in feed (120 ppm), or as an injection (15 mg tiamulin/kg live weight) can result, within 24 hours, in se-

TABLE 23–1
SOME DRUGS FOR FEED MEDICATION

Agent	Recommended Dosage Rate for Therapy (and Control) (per ton feed)	
Therapy	Control	Prevention
Carbadox	50 g	
Dimetridazole	500 g	(200 g)
Virginiamycin	100 g	(25 g)
Lincomycin	110 g	—
Ronidazole (Not in U.S.)	120 g	(60 g)
Tiamulin	100 g	(30–40 g)
Tylosin	100 g	(40 g)

vere clinical signs consistent with ionophore toxicity, i.e., a primary myotoxicity leading to death in some cases.

Successful swine dysentery eradication programs have been based on the following claims for the reported efficacy of tiamulin: that tiamulin administered at 10 mg/kg body weight for 5 days eliminates *T. hyodysenteriae* from the individual pig and that tiamulin administered at 2 to 5 mg/kg body weight prevents reinfection during the course of an eradication program. A 5-day course of Tiamulin injection to all animals in the herd can form the medication phase of a successful swine dysentery eradication program. If used as a feed premix, attention must be given to ensure that correct dosage rates are administered.

Other drugs that have been used for treatment of swine dysentery include carbadox (Mecadox, Pfizer), bacitracin methylene disalicylate, lincomycin, sodium arsanilate, tylosin, and virginiamycin. Dimetridazole and ipronidazole have been shown to be effective against swine dysentery but are not cleared for this use in the United States.

There are several limitations to the use of the use of some of the aforementioned cleared drugs. Carbadox has a 75-day withdrawal time. *T. hyodysenteriae* has the ability to develop resistance to some of the cleared drugs in a fairly short time. Also, constant medication becomes quite expensive.

Some question exists about the use of drugs that have not been officially cleared for use in pigs with swine dysentery. Some veterinarians interpret the FDA's off-label use policy to mean that if cleared drugs are found ineffective, nonapproved drugs can be used off-label under the following guidelines: A licensed veterinarian must prescribe the off-label drug, the veterinarian is then equally responsible with the owner for illegal residues and reactions, and an exaggerated withdrawal time must be observed.

In certain facilities, such as those with all concrete floors, swine dysentery can be eradicated. It can be fairly easy to eradicate *Treponema* from the pig, but it is more difficult to eradicate it from the environment. In general, an eradication plan is designed to treat all the swine with an effective drug for 30 days or longer. At the end of the treatment period, the pigs are moved to cleaned and disinfected pens.

SUGGESTED MEDICATION PROGRAM

1. Anorexia usually occurs in the early stages of the disease, but pigs continue drinking; therefore water medication should be used to initiate treatment—tylosin/sulfathiazole soluble, 100 g/190 liters. Therapy may need to be continued for 3 to 5 days. Treat all pens sharing the same drainage or in direct contact with the affected pen.
2. Severely affected pigs should be treated with tylosin injection using a dosage rate of 5 to 10 mg/kg body weight.
3. Maintain therapy with tylosin/Sulfamethazine premix in the feed for up to

TABLE 23–2
TIAMULIN DYSENTERY CONTROL PROGRAM

Day	Medication	Sanitation
14–0	Feed: 35 g/US ton tiamulin for 2 weeks	Scrape pens daily
1–5	Water: 180 ppm tiamulin for 5 days (1 pkg/43 gal)	Wash all pens at least once daily
6–27	Feed: 25 g/US ton tiamulin for 3 weeks	Scrape pens daily
28–32	Water: 180 ppm tiamulin for 5 days	Pressure wash all pens at least twice

15 days. Blanket medication of the whole site may be necessary.

4. Consider prophylactic medication of all pigs entering the unit.

SUGGESTED CONTROL PROGRAM

1. Improve general hygiene on the unit; in particular, thoroughly clean all pens after water medication.
2. Keep cleaned, disinfected pens empty for at least 14 days to prevent carryover of infection.
3. Control rodents and flies.

Improved herd security and professional rodent control measures must be implemented before the medication period. A central drinking water reservoir may conveniently be established to medicate the entire unit from a single source. Herd veterinarians should be intimately involved in the planning, implementation, and monitoring of all activities. Following the medication/sanitation program, no further medication specifically against *T. hyodysenteriae* should be used on the farm. In addition, a sanitation program is essential during a medication period. The rodent population must be eliminated. *Treponema* can also survive in manure slurry.

Tiamulin is regarded currently as the medication of choice and is widely used, because problems of resistance in vivo are widespread with dimetridazole, lincomycin, and tylosin. Carbadox and olaquindox are also used, but carcinogenic and mutagenic hazards restrict their usage. Pneumonia problems also dramatically decrease after the elimination of swine dysentery with tiamulin.

Salinomycin (an ionophore) at 60 ppm in the feed has a prophylactic effect against swine dysentery. Similar to monensin, salinomycin is extremely toxic to horses and turkeys and is incompatible with tiamulin.

Lincomycin, 10 mg/piglet daily for 2 days, can be administered parenterally to individual animals, followed by water-soluble lincomycin, 150 mg/4.5 liters. Freshly medicated water must be made up every 2 days. Lincomycin is effective against not only *Treponema* but also *Bacteroides* and *Fusobacterium*. In complete pig feeds, linco-

TABLE 23–3
INJECTIONS

Agent	Dose
Tiamulin	10 mg/kg
Tylosin (Tylan 200)	2–10 mg/kg
Lincomycin	10 mg/kg
Oxytetracycline	10–20 mg/kg
Neomycin	10–12 mg/kg

TABLE 23–4
WATER MEDICATION

Agent	Dosage
Tylosin water soluble	25 g/100 liters (3–5 days)
Lincomycin/spectinomycin soluble powder	12.5 g active drug (lincospectin)/200 liters for 4–7 days (12.5 g activity per 100 g pack).
Dimetridazole	62 g/100 liters, continued for 5–7 days
Ronidazole	0.006% in drinking water for 5–7 days (60 ppm)
Ipronidazole	0.005% in drinking water for 7 days
Gentamicin	50 mg/5 liters for 3–5 days
Sodium arsanilate	1 gm/16 liters for 5–7 days
Tiamulin	60 mg/liter (0.006%)

mycin is used at an inclusion rate of 110 g/ton as the sole ration for 3 weeks. Alternatively, ronidazole, 60 ppm; ipronidazole for 6 to 10 weeks; carbadox, 50 ppm; and or sodium arsanilate can be considered. An alternative to lincomycin in water is water-soluble tiamulin, 60 mg/liter for 3 to 5 days, or dimetridazole, 120 mg/liter of medicated water.

Treatment for whipworms with a parasiticide, such as dichlorvos, is an important aspect of dysentery eradication programs.

Treatment of swine dysentery in acute outbreaks must be by individual injection (Table 23–4) or medication through the drinking water. Feed medication is of little use because pigs are anorexic when affected with the disease. Water medication (Table 23–4) is suitable for followup or mass treatment in affected houses.

After individual treatment by injection followed up by water medication, it is important to switch to in-feed medication (Table 23–5) as a preventive to future occurrence. Swine dysentery produces little immunity, and outbreaks can recur when medication is withdrawn. Resistance has occurred to a number of drugs currently used as in-feed medicants; hence it may be necessary to vary treatments from time to time.

23.9 SALMONELLOSIS

SALMONELLA CHOLERAESUIS, SALMONELLA TYPHIMURIUM

This disease is more common in pigs of 3 to 4 months of age. Clinical signs may vary from dullness, depression, and pyrexia to purplish discoloration of the ears and skin, enteritis, and blood in the feces.

Salmonellosis can be difficult to treat, and results in many cases can be disappointing: The continuous low-level usage of antibiotics over recent years has induced the development of strains of salmonellae resistant to many products normally used to control this disease. Treatment if possible should be based on laboratory isolation of salmonellae and their sensitivity pattern.

This disease is often associated with poor-quality meat meals and substandard rations. It can also be involved as a secondary infection following swine dysentery. The disease can occur at any age. It usually is more severe in younger pigs and aggravated by cold stress. It ranges from an acute septicemia through to chronic colitis. Mortality and morbidity can be high. Clinical signs include elevated temperatures; blotching of the skin; petechial and ecchymotic hemorrhages of the skin; and diarrhea, often flecked with blood or mucus. In the chronic form, watery diarrhea is common. Pigs lose weight and become dehydrated.

TREATMENT

The continuous low-level use of antibiotics has made the treatment and control of this disease difficult. As a result of continuous exposure, there are many resistant strains of *Salmonella* to many of the antibiotic products normally used to control this disease. When it is necessary to treat salmonellosis,

TABLE 23–5
IN-FEED MEDICATION

Agent	Dosage
Tylosin	100 g/ton of feed for 4 weeks, reducing to 40 g/ton of feed thereafter
Lincomycin/spectinomycin	40 g/ton of feed L
Virginiamycin	100 g/ton initially for 7–10 days, phasing out to 25 g/ton feed continuously
Dimetridazole	200–500 g/ton
Lincomycin	110 g/ton
Sodium arsanilate	90 g/ton of feed
Carbadox	50 g/ton; must be withdrawn 70 days before slaughter
Ronidazole 120	120 g/ton
Tiamulin	30–100 g/ton
Spiramycin	20 g/ton

the use of high levels of antibiotics over relatively short periods of from 7 to 14 days is recommended. Chemotherapeutic use includes:

Ampicillin
Apramycin
Enrofloxacin
Oxytetracycline
Potentiated sulfonamides
Spectinomycin/lincomycin
Carbadox
Virginiamycin
Tylosin/sulfadimidine

When antibiotic therapy is recommended, the subsequent response can be disappointing, but in general apramycin, potentiated sulfonamides and ampicillin have given good results. Antibiotic therapy can, however, result in carrier animals. Recommended dosages are as follows:

1. Furazolidone: 200 to 400 g/ton for 7 to 14 days. Despite the wide, continuous use of this product, over the years it was regarded as an effective treatment of *Salmonella* outbreaks. At 400 g/ton, it caused some palatability problems, resulting in a dropoff of feed consumption. It is now banned due to residue hazards.
2. Neomycin sulfate: 200 g/ton for 7 days.
3. Oxytetracycline: 200 to 500 g/ton for 7 days.
4. Chlortetracycline: 200 to 500 g/ton for 7 days. Tetracyclines should be used to treat *Salmonella* infections based on a bacterial isolation and sensitivity testing.
5. Apramcyin: 20 mg/kg treatment; 100 ppm in-feed control; 7 to 12.5 mg/kg in drinking water.
6. Enrofloxacin: 2.5–5.0 mg/kg.
7. Potentiated sulfonamides: 30 mg/kg.

Enrofloxacin has been shown to possess high therapeutic efficacy in enzootic pneumonia, *A. pleuropneumoniae*, *E. coli* scours, and *Salmonella* infections in pigs. In artificially infected pigs, *Salmonella* organisms were not isolated after a 10-day treatment via the feed with the lowest dose tested of 200 ppm.

CONTROL

1. Carbadox: 50 g/ton continuously. This product is useful in preventing the occurrence of salmonellosis. Withdraw 70 days before slaughter per United States regulation, and 28 days in Europe.
2. Lincomycin/spectinomycin (Lincospectin): 40 g/ton of feed continuously. This product may cause fungal overgrowth if fed over prolonged periods.
3. Virginiamycin: 50 g/ton of feed continuously.
4. Tylosin/Sulfadimidine: 100 g/ton tylosin and 100 g/ton sulfadimidine fed continuously.

5. Neomycin sulfate Neomix: 50 to 100 g/ ton fed continuously. This drug is not always effective owing to the high level of bacterial resistance to neomycin and problems associated with fungal overgrowth. Usage should be based on bacterial isolation and sensitivity testing.

Salmonella is often introduced into a herd through a carrier, such as rats, mice, visitors from other livestock operations, feed, and so forth. Visitors should not be allowed into the sheds unless they are provided with boots and overalls. Strict vermin control should be carried out, and if possible, pigs should be fed only pelleted feed. Cold stress and environmental stress should be avoided, and age groups should be separated as much as possible.

23.10 PORCINE INFECTIOUS ARTHRITIS AND MYCOPLASMAL POLYSEROSITIS

Lameness in piglets can be observed as early as 3 to 4 days after farrowing, with joint distention being apparent within 7 to 10 days postpartum. Infectious organisms may enter via the tonsils or small intestine or when omphalophlebitis is present. The immune status of the piglet and colostral intake are critical. Isolates from such cases include *Steptococcus, Staphylococcus, C. pyogenes, P. multocida, Moraxella,* erysipelas *A. pleuropneumoniae,* and *H. parasuis.*

Vaccination of sows or use of appropriate antimicrobials in sow feeds and injection of piglets shortly after birth are commonly practiced. Therapy is seldom effective when there is visual joint distention because by then the joint structures have been extensively damaged. Streptococci tend to be the most common pathogens in the polyarthritic pig, and penicillins, potentiated sulfonamides, oxytetracycline, and semisynthetic penicillins are the drugs of choice.

Mycoplasma hyorhinis and *Mycoplasma hyosynoviae* can give rise to polyserositis that occasionally affects the synovial membrane. These organisms are common inhabitants of the nasal cavity of growing animals. Stressful influences increase colonization. The invading mycoplasmas are usually sensitive to tylosin, lincomycin, spectinomycin, or tiamulin.

Haemophilus polyserositis, Gläser's disease, is caused by *H. parasuis,* and piglets are usually affected between 3 and 10 weeks. Therapy must be administered early and in-contact animals can be treated via water medications. *H. parasuis* is normally sensitive to penicillins, tiamulin, sulfonamides, ampicillin, lincomycin, and tetracyclines.

23.11 RESIDUES IN SWINE PRODUCTION

A product used in food-producing animals usually carries recommendations for its safe use on the label. These recommendations include the species for which it is intended, the maximum recommended dose, and the withdrawal period to be observed before slaughter. If the product is used correctly, it should not leave a significant residue in the tissues, but if highly sensitive methods are used, it is possible that a small trace can be detected. This may be an "acceptable" level of residue in some cases. The presence of unacceptable levels of residues in tissues causes concern for human health, and suspicion is particularly directed toward compounds that are known or suspected carcinogens or teratogens and toward those that at low concentrations have a toxic effect at the organ or cell level. The objective of monitoring programs is to detect unacceptable levels of residue that are potentially harmful to humans or that result in economic loss to the food or livestock industries.

USE OF ANTIBIOTICS IN PIG PRODUCTION

Antibiotics have long been associated with growth-promoting effects in animals. Since the original use of chlortetracycline as a growth promoter in chicks, the application of many other antibiotics at low levels in feeding stuffs has increased in line with the rapid developments in intensive animal production systems. For growth-promoting purposes, they are usually included in the feed at low levels, where they also improve the efficiency of feed use. For therapeutic purposes, they are incorporated at considerably higher levels in the feed for their antibacterial effects.

In the 1960s, the incidence of antibiotic resistance in bacteria pathogenic for farm animals reached a point at which it was seen to be complicating the treatment of disease, and it was suggested that the feeding of low levels of antibiotics at subtherapeutic levels for growth-promoting purposes was a significant contributory factor. Penicillin-resistant and tetracycline-resistant pathogens in pigs and poultry were becoming a real problem. The phenomenon of transferable drug resistance compounded the worsening situation. Transferable drug resistance was demonstrated to be a phenomenon that occurred mainly in the Enterobacteriaceae, whereby resistance to one or a number of antibiotics could be transferred from donor to recipient bacteria. In the event of resistance being transferred to potentially pathogenic organisms, this could ultimately complicate the antibiotic therapy of clinical disease outbreaks in humans and animals. Resistant bacteria of animals were seen to constitute a potential reservoir of resistance transmissible to humans.

Therapeutic medication of feeding stuffs in pig production is perhaps the area of most significance from the point of view of drug residue formation owing to the variety of therapeutic agents that may ultimately make their way into the human food chain. Salmonellosis, swine dysentery, coliform infections, enzootic pneumonia, and atrophic rhinitis are all major problems that commonly necessitate antimicrobial medication in feed or water.

WITHDRAWAL PERIODS

One of the most controversial areas associated with antibiotic use in pigs is the compliance or otherwise with stated withdrawal periods. The imposition of mandatory withdrawal periods, inconvenient to the farmer who has to change from medicated to nonmedicated feeding as the animal nears optimum slaughter weight, must be shown to be absolutely necessary. Controversy surrounds the determination of permissible levels of antibiotic residues and their detection. A simple, relatively clear standard test to detect antibiotic residues, which can be quickly performed at

the abattoir without disrupting the progression of meat distribution, does not result in a high incidence of false-positive results, and can deal with many samples readily, is also needed. It should also be decided whether any test adopted will identify specific antibiotics or more simply the presence of bacterial inhibitory substances. The former is costly and probably not justifiable; the latter is complicated by the presence of natural inhibitors in animal tissue as well as the release of inhibitors, such a lysozymes, when tissues that have been frozen are then thawed. This would necessitate the use of fresh meat in analytical tests.

In many ways, the choice of antibiotic can have a marked influence on whether residues are present at slaughter or not. The use of antibiotics that deposit in the kidney result in residues being present in this organ for a much longer period than if an antibiotic is selected that is rapidly excreted in the urine. Similarly, long-acting depot-type formulations present more residue hazards than short-acting preparations of the same drug. The effects of certain antibiotics on nontarget species must also be considered, for example, small traces of lincomycin in ruminant diets can severely affect milk production. Similarly, monensin contamination in horse feeds can have dire effects. Monensin and tiamulin are incompatible and have severe effects if there are carryover traces within a mill system.

Long-acting preparations should be avoided in the last 4 weeks of life because of their prolonged withdrawal periods. There is also the problem of residues, tissue staining, and damage at the site of the injection regardless of whether or not the product is long acting.

Antibiotic tissue residues are less likely with water-soluble drugs than with in-feed medication because it is much simpler to cut off the medicated water supply than it is to switch to a nonmedicated feed, especially when there are still several tons of medicated feed left in the bulk hopper. Tissue residues may also be avoided if antimicrobial substances that are not absorbed from intestinal tract are used. In many cases, however, this is not possible because antibiotics possessing systemic effects may be needed.

RESIDUES AND THEIR FORMATION

The use of antibiotics in pig production may result in minute quantities of drug residues in tissues that may subsequently become a part of the human diet. Two primary concerns in the development of new animal health products are the presence or absence of residues and the safety of such products if residues are present. Residues consist of trace levels of parent drug, its metabolites, or decomposition products in tissues of the treated animals after exposure to the drug.

Residues usually appear after unintentional exposure to the drug in question by way of failure to withdraw medicated feed at the appropriate time before slaughter and emergency slaughter of animals that have been treated with antibiotics as part of a therapeutic program. With certain drugs used in animal production, a tolerance level of residue may be permitted. This is a level that relates to the acceptable daily intake for the consumer. With other more potentially toxic compounds, a zero tolerance or zero residue is the defined level of tolerability.

The formation of a drug residue is the result of the interaction of many dynamic processes. Some of the more important of these are (1) the amount of drug administered; (2) the formulation used; (3) the duration of intake; (4) the absorption, distribution, metabolism, and excretion properties; and (5) the potential for tissue binding and sequestration in body compartments. The withdrawal period for a particular drug is based in accordance with its inherent pharmacokinetic properties (i.e., absorption, distribution, excretion) and toxicologic significance that Insofar as most drugs, especially the antibiotics, are excreted through the kidney, largely unchanged, this particular organ is exposed to extremely high concentrations of drugs as they are eliminated from the body. This is one of the major reasons why kidney tissue is frequently used as the sampling or reference tissue for antibiotic residues in pig meat.

For monitoring the safe usage of a drug, the assay procedure is applied on a finite or negligible-tolerance basis. Although this is a relatively convenient concept in determining the presence or absence of residue, it places a heavy burden on the analytical procedure, which is forced to operate at or near its limits of performance. Any assay procedure for drug residue detection must demonstrate sensitivity, specificity, reliability, and practicality and be subject to validation. One of the most difficult aspects of drug residue studies is to define exactly what a "residue" is. About a decade ago, the term "residue" was accepted to mean a parent compound or a metabolite, such as a conjugate, from which the parent compound could be regenerated. Later, as better techniques for metabolite studies were developed, "residue" became defined as the parent drug plus its related metabolites.

The definition has changed to include all drug-derived residue, and this has helped to identify one of the most potentially interesting areas—the nonextractable residue fraction. This is the proportion of the residue that has undergone a high degree of covalent-type binding in tissues and that is not amenable to the normal, routine residue assay procedures. Questions have frequently been raised about the significance of bound or nonextractable residue, as to whether the bound residue itself is especially toxic. Many hormonal substances and a number of antibiotics, such as chloramphenicol, are capable of forming bound residues in animal tissues.

The depletion of drugs from animal tissues usually follows a first-order decay curve. This means that if 50% of a drug disappears from an animal in a certain period of time, half of the amount remaining would disappear in an equal length of time. Therefore the concentration of the parent drug can never reach zero. In practice, however, there is a point below which the presence of a drug cannot be measured. Below the limit of detectability, tissue from the control animal responds to the assay in the same way as tissue from treated animals. Recent analytical methods, however, have had a dramatic effect on this limit.

Sulfamethazine is an antimicrobial drug commonly administered orally to pigs at a concentration of 100 g/ton of feed. At this concentration, the sulfonamide in combination with tylosin, tetracycline, or penicillin is effective for control of atrophic rhinitis and enteritis. The drug, however, may be retained in the tissues of animals for extended periods after administration, thus requiring a withdrawal period to allow the tissue concentration of the drug to become depleted to or to fall below the specified tolerance for that drug. Tetracyclines, especially oxytetracycline, are among the most widely used antibacterials together with the sulfonamides in pig practice. The advantage of their broad spectrum of action and their economy contributes largely to this fact. They are also the two most commonly used therapeutic agents both by way of feed medication and by way of individual injection to diseased animals. It is not surprising that these two classes of antibacterial agents are held to be the most common source of tissue residue formation in pig meat.

One of the common reasons for antibiotic residues is that the additive has not been correctly used. There are many reasons for this, e.g., difficulty in interpreting the manufacturer's instructions, difficulty of application on the farm, attempts at costs reduction, and expectancy of a quick response to a chronic condition. Obviously if there could be an agreed standard inclusion rate for all premixes for the normal basic use, life might be simpler for the compounder and his employee. There would also be a reduction in the possibility of error. As far as pig production is concerned, withdrawal periods are frequently difficult to observe in practice. Complete pens are seldom sold for slaughter on the same day, and so it can be difficult to achieve the ideal withdrawal time.

ANTIBIOTIC RESIDUES and HUMAN HEALTH CONSIDERATIONS

The major potential risks to the consumer after exposure to antibiotic residues relate to hypersensitivity reactions and the acquisition of resistance to certain antibacterial substances.

Antibiotic allergy in humans is a complex subject. In general, antibiotics have a low molecular weight and are incomplete immunogens or haptens. To stimulate an immune response, the antigenic determinants must combine with a carrier protein, and antibiotics that undergo spontaneous or metabolic degradation to release potential antigenic determinants are those that are most likely to sensitize. Exposure of individuals to antibiotics through food as well as through medical therapy proves a significant factor in the progressive rise in the frequency of hypersensitivity to the antibiotics concerned. It is generally estimated that the incidence of allergy to various antibacterial agents is as follows: Penicillin, 10%; cephalosporin, 5%; tetracycline, 5%; sulfonamides, 13%; and trimethoprim, 3%.

Induced bacterial resistance is another potential feature associated with residues in pig meat. Continual exposure to trace amounts of stable antibiotic residues could conceivably induce antibiotic resistance in the enteric flora of the consumer. During prolonged exposure to subeffective antibacterial levels, microorganisms can evolve a pattern of acquired resistance through the elaboration of enzyme systems detrimental to the structural integrity of the antibiotic. Structural changes in bacteria may also be induced. The presence of residues can also mask infections that may be present in the tissues at the time of slaughter, and this is most significant in the case of emergency slaughtered animals. Abundant evidence also exists that consumers can become infected with organisms (especially salmonellae) of porcine origin. Many microorganisms of porcine origin (including the coliform group) act as reservoirs of R-factors, and through the mechanism of transferable drug resistance, resistance patterns can be transferred to pathogens of humans. The overuse of feed antibiotics in pig production has resulted in the exposure of the porcine gut flora to antibiotic levels on a consistently longterm basis. The resultant acquisition by the enteric *E. coli* of resistance factors, which code for up to six antibiotics, has ensured that microorganisms of porcine origin can act as a resistance reservoir for humans.

EFFECT OF PROCESSING AND STORAGE ON ANTIBIOTIC RESIDUES

Because certain processing is required before food animal tissues enter the human food chain, it is necessary to know what happens to drug residues during the procedure. Usually a great deal of processing is required (e.g., scalding, washing, freezing, cooling) before the animal carcass is finally prepared for the consumer. Many drugs are heat labile, and should be eliminated during the cooking process. When drugs are broken down, however, there is always the question of whether they are simply inactivated and destroyed or whether they are converted to pharmacologically inactive metabolites, which may still be of some potential hazard to the consumer. Many penicillins are susceptible to various cooking temperatures, and at 100°C, activities are eliminated or degraded within a few minutes. Streptomycin and chloramphenicol are relatively heat stable, and there is virtually no loss of streptomycin activity when it is heated at 100°C for 2 hours. Owing to their inherent stability, chloramphenicol, streptomycin, and dihydrostreptomycin are not seriously affected by processing, storage, or cooking. Tetracyclines, especially oxytetracycline, are resistant to the effects of smoking and curing, and a number of the breakdown products of tetracyclines may themselves possess some toxic potential.

The penicillin nucleus (6-amino-penicillinic acid) is susceptible to beta-lactamase enzymatic cleavage and acid hydrolysis, and the resultant compound, penicilloic acid, is devoid of antibacterial activity. It carries an antigenic determinant, however, of the penicillins. To stimulate an immune response, the antigenic determinant must combine with a carrier host protein—thus the penicillin itself acts as an incomplete antigen or hapten. The most frequently sensitizing antibiotic is without doubt penicillin, and following degradation in the tissues, the penicilloic acid conjugates with protein, thereby producing sensitizing antigens, which are capable of producing undesirable effects even in small amounts. Such sensitizing components ingested as residues in foods of animal origin can cause a reaction in the consumer. Thus it is clear that many antibiotics in animal tissues may survive a variety of processes and that antibiotics that are metabolized or degraded are still potentially capable of inducing reactions in the consumer.

CONCLUSIONS

In the last 15 years, a variety of antibiotic and antibacterial feed additives have been presented to the swine industry, most of which have been promoted for the combined control of disease and improved growth or food conversion rate. In many cases, there has often been a lack of specific diagnosis, incorrect and excessive use of the antibiotic, and accompanying development of bacterial resistance. There has also been a tendency to regard antibiotics as panaceas, to the detriment of the adoption of other necessary husbandry measures. The popularity of additives has in no small way been contributed to by the manufacturing and advertising schemes of overpromotion. From the feed compounders' point of view, usage rates of antibiotics are sometimes difficult to interpret, nomenclature can be confusing, and inclusion rates can be variable and obscure at times. There is a continuing need to remind the farmers that correct husbandry rather than antibiotic medication is often the first step to improve the economic performance of pigs. What is needed in the future is the introduction of effective additives properly promoted for improved growth and feed conversion as well as specific agents for use against enteritis, pneumonitis, and rhinitis. These should have the necessary attributes of efficacy and safety. Clarification of inclusion rates, use of water-soluble antibiotics, and attention to basic husbandry procedures may well go some way toward minimizing what could become a serious problem. The producer should be taught to understand that failure to observe withdrawal times leads to violationary residues, which in the long term will be counterproductive to a viable pork industry.

23.12 SULFONAMIDE RESIDUES

A study by the FDA's National Center for Toxicological Research (NCTR) has shown that the veterinary drug sulfamethazine may be a carcinogen. Historically the swine industry has not effectively controlled sulfamethazine residues in pork carcasses.

During the past decade, various Food Safety and Inspection Service (FSIS) efforts have reduced violations, but they are still occurring: 3.6% of swine tissue samples tested in 1987 had violative sulfamethazine residues. The current safe residue level for swine is set at 0.1 ppm (100 ppb). This level includes a 1000-fold safety factor, so a consumer exposed to levels slightly over the 0.1 ppm level will not suffer ill effects.

Concerns about sulfamethazine residues in swine began in the mid-1970s, when up to 13% of swine liver and muscle samples tested by the USDA exceeded established tolerance levels. Sulfamethazine levels over 0.1 ppm, the tolerance level for sulfamethazine in swine and cattle tissues set by the FDA to provide a wide margin for human safety, can cause significant economic losses to pork producers and damage the image of pork as a wholesome food source.

The NCTR conducted a longterm bioassay study in mice with moderate to high levels of sulfamethazine. A draft NCTR report to the CVM concluded that the drug produced tumors in the thyroid gland of male and female mice at the dosage levels used.

In the carcinogenicity study in mice, thyroid follicular cell adenomas occurred in male and female mice at a dietary level of 4800 ppm. In the carcinogenicity study in rats, thyroid follicular cell adenomas and adenocarcinomas occurred in females at a dietary level of 2400 ppm and in males at a dietary level of 1200 or 2400 ppm.

In the carcinogenicity study in mice, the no observable effect level (NOEL) for thyroid hypertrophy was 86 mg/kg body weight/day for females and 68 mg/kg body weight/day for males. In the carcinogenicity study in rats, the NOEL for thyroid hyperplasia was 2.4 mg/kg body weight/day for females and 2.2 mg/kg body weight/day for males.

In the study on thyroid function in rats, the NOEL for increased thyroid weight was 30 mg/kg body weight/day for females and 25 mg/kg body weight/day for males at 12, 18, and 24 months. In this study, the serum concentrations of triiodothyronine and thyroid-stimulating hormone were highly variable and were not significantly different at any dose or at any time. The concentration of thyroxine in the serum was decreased in females at doses of 1200 or 2400 ppm in the diet for 18 months and in males at doses of 600, 1200, or 2400 ppm in the diet for 24 months. The decrease, however, did not show a consistent dose response trend. After receiving a draft from NCTR on January 13, 1988, the CVM took the following steps to reassess the safety of sulfamethazine:

- The CVM issued a letter to manufacturers of the drug used in food-producing animals informing them that the CVM would undertake a complete reassessment of the data contained in their animal drug files. Manufacturers were requested to submit any additional safety information.
- In anticipation of the final report from the NCTR, the CVM set up an internal review team. The team reviewed the data with a view to making a decision on what action should be taken with the drug. This resulted in prioritizing sulfonamides, and maintaining constant surveillance on the situation.
- The USDA and swine producers were notified of the draft report in an effort to ensure that residues of the drug in animals would be reduced to the lowest possible level. (USDA and FDA have had a chronic residue problem with this drug in hogs over the past 10 years. Until recently, swine had a violative residue rate of sulfamethazine at 4% at time of slaughter.)

In the meantime, the FDA and the USDA are cooperating to reduce levels of residues of sulfamethazine to the lowest possible level.

The USDA (whose subagencies are responsible for monitoring the use of animal drugs, whereas the FDA sets guidelines as to how they should be used) responded to the sulfamethazine affair with a four-part action plan designed to eliminate violative residues. The FSIS noted that although a decade of agency efforts to counter violative levels as high as 13% have significantly reduced the violative percentage, a percentage of swine tested still exceed the FDA-stipulated maximum tolerance of 0.1 ppm.

U.S.D.A. FOUR-STAGE PLAN

Stage one of the plan was to see rapid implementation of a comprehensive swine identification program devised jointly by the FSIS and its sister agency, the Animal and Plant Health Inspection Service (APHIS). The joint FSIS/APHIS scheme addressed what was described in the plan of action as a persistent problem in enforcement of safe residues: the inability to identify the source of hog carcasses during processing.

The second element in the FSIS plan consisted of a program designed to intensify the action taken by the agency to prevent violative residues. The action was to hinge on an in-plant rapid sulfamethazine test, called the "sulfa-on-site" (SOS test), which permits swift identification of animals with high residue levels.

Recognizing that the prevention of residues during the production process is "the best if not the only way to achieve residue control," the agency continued to encourage approved veterinarians, producers, and others to perform the SOS test on animals before marketing. As part of this effort, the FSIS proposed regulations for a "verified production control" (VPC) program, which permits producers to participate with the agency and to advertise this fact through product labeling.

Stage four of the FSIS policy, provided for rapid development and verification of new or improved effective test methods. A new enzyme-linked immunosorbent assay (ELISA) card test is available that has the ability to detect smaller amounts of sulfamethazine than the SOS system. Simple both to operate and to interpret, the new test is said to offer the potential for use in testing live animals by the producer. The E-Z Quik card test and the new Charm sulfonamide detection tests assist in this effort.

Commenting on the safety concerns raised by residues of sulfamethazine above the tolerance level of 0.1 ppm in edible tissues of swine, the CVM pointed out that "high levels can cause an effect on the thyroid and kidneys in laboratory animals and may result in allergic reactions in man." If illegal residues of the drug are not reduced to a satisfactory level, "we may have to ban the use of sulfamethazine in swine feeds," said the CVM.

The FDA and USDA/FSIS warned hog producers that a relatively small number of violators are posing a threat to human health and consumer confidence because of an unacceptable 6% level of sulfamethazine residues in marketed pork. The two agencies mailed a checklist to pork producers for posting near feed-mixing equipment to help eliminate the problem. The checklist is en-

titled "Avoid Sulfa Violations . . . It's Good Business." In addition, the FDA has initiated on-site investigations of those persons marketing hogs in which the FSIS has found a violative sulfonamide residue in edible tissues to determine the cause of residues. The agency will take regulatory action against those persons found causing sulfa residues in hogs slaughtered for human food. An educational program for residue avoidance by producers was seen as an integral part of the care strategy.

SOS TESTING

In February, 1988, the FSIS announced a plan to strengthen regulatory efforts. This plan included a system for mandatory swine regulation; stepped-up testing of individual hogs with an in-plant rapid test, the SOS test; a regulation for lot testing; voluntary preslaughter testing of live hogs; and development of improved analytical methods.

In March, 1988, the FSIS began an enhanced sample collection program to detect violative concentrations of sulfamethazine in pork. Part 1 of this program consisted of weekly submission of two muscle tissue samples for sulfamethazine laboratory analysis from each of the 100 largest swine slaughter plants. During part 1, 1618 samples were received for analysis, 1607 tests were performed, and 29 violations were found. Part 2 of the program consisted of training FSIS veterinarians in the use of the SOS test and placing it in each of the 100 largest swine slaughter plants, while simultaneously phasing out part 1. Urine samples from six animals were collected and tested each working day in each of the 100 plants.

The SOS test is the screening test being used by the FSIS to estimate sulfamethazine status of pigs rapidly at slaughter. Sulfamethazine concentrations in urine from slaughtered hogs are predictive of the sulfamethazine levels in the carcass. A confirmed violative muscle concentration (over 0.1 ppm) results in a market embargo for the producer.

The incidence of violative residues of sulfamethazine is below 1% in the United States. Contributing to this decline has been the action by the National Pork Producers

Council and farmer groups. Many producers have stopped using the drug, and the tighter controls on producers have exerted an effect. The agency's SOS testing program is also a contributing factor.

Although the level of illegal sulfamethazine residues could be considered reasonable compared with other drugs, no violative levels will ever be acceptable to the FSIS, whose goal is to reach zero residues. Sulfamethazine is currently under review at the FDA, and decisions relating to the future regulation of the drug could mean that it might eventually be withdrawn from the market if the tolerance level set is so low as to make it impractical.

Monitoring data show that the violative rate for market hogs has declined from 3.6% in 1987 to 1.4% in 1988 and to under 1.0% currently. It is likely that the FDA is going to request new data on the mechanism of action before reaching a conclusion on the future regulation of sulfamethazine.

SULFONAMIDES IN THE EUROPEAN COMMUNITY

Several member states of the European Community have already adopted tolerances of 0.1 mg/kg (100 ppb) based on old data, a value that had also previously been fixed by certain non-E.C. countries and that was considered to provide sufficient margins of safety. In this situation, the Committee for Veterinary Medicinal Products came to the following provisional conclusions:

Having regard to the available toxicological data and current practice within the Community and third countries, the Committee recommends that an analytical procedure for monitoring the observance of appropriate withdrawal times for sulfonamide compounds sensitive to at least 100 ppb of the original drug substance should be used.

Considering:

(i) the available toxicological data which suggest that the metabolites of the sulfonamides are within the same range of toxicity as the parent compounds,
(ii) the available pharmacokinetic studies which suggest that metabolites of the sulfonamides are unlikely to be present in residues in foodstuffs in significantly greater quantities than the parent substances, and
(iii) the need to provide for simple analytical detection methods whenever possible,

the committee does not consider it necessary to recommend the inclusion of any of the metabolites within this tolerance at present.

Residues of sulfonamides can be routinely monitored at and below the above-required limits using, for example, high-performance liquid chromatography. Reliable confirmatory or reference methods should be based on known procedures using gas chromatography/mass spectrometry. JECFA (Joint Expert Committee on Food Additives) has reviewed the sulfonamides and has recommended a tolerance MRL of 100 ppb in meat.

SELECTED REFERENCES

Backstrom, L., Brim, T., Collins, M., and Evans, R.: The effect of short term therapy with lincomcyin or linocmcyin/sulfamethazine on AR and nasal microflora in swine. Proceedings 9th International Pig Veterinary Society Congress, Barcelona, 1986.

Backstrom, L., Chung, W.B., and Ose, E.: Tilmicosin in prevention of AR in swine. Proceedings IPVS Congress, The Hague, 1992.

Backstrom, L., Hoefling, D., and Morkoc, A.: The effect of atrophic rhinitis on production economy in Illinois swine herds. J. Am. Vet. Med. Assoc., 187:712, 1985.

Backstrom, L., and Walkter, D.: Comparison between efficacy of CSP-250 on AR in swine induced by toxigenic bordetella bronchiseptica and Pasteurella multocida. Proceedings of the American Association of Swine Practitioners Conference, Denver, 1990.

Bakerville, A.: Pneumonia of pigs. A review. N.Z. Vet. J., 29:216, 1981.

Chronic toxicity and carcinogenesis study of sulfamethazine in B6C3F1 mice. Jefferson, AR, National Center for Toxicological Research, 1988.

Clark, L.K., Scheidt, A.B., Armstrong, C.H., et al.: The effect of all-in/all-out management on pigs from a herd with enzootic pneumonia. Vet. Med., 86:946, 1991.

Cordle, M.K.: J. Anim. Sci. 66:413, 1988. (USDA/Regulation of residues in meat and poultry products).

Daniel, G.M., Freese, W., Henry, S., et al.: An up to date review of atrophic rhinitis. Vet. Med., 735, 1986.

Desrosiers, R., and Moore, C.: A review of some aspects of porcine pleuropneumonia. Proc. AASP, Minneapolis, 1986.

Fairbrother, J.M., et al.: Prevalence of fimbrial antigens and enterotoxins in non classical serogroups of

Escherichia coli isolated from newborn pigs with diarrhea. Am. J. Vet. Res., *49*:1325, 1988.

Fitzgerald, G.R., et al.: Diarrhea in young pigs: Comparing the incidence of the five most common infectious agents. Vet. Med., *83*:80, 1988.

Gropp, J.M., Englisch, W.O.P., and Wagner, H.W.: Protein sparing effects of carbadox in pig diets. *In* Veterinary Pharmacology, Toxicology and Therapy in Food Producing Animals. Vol. 1. Abstracts of the 4th EAVPT Congress. Edited by F. Simon. Budapest, 1988.

Hall, W.: A review of colibacillosis in neonatal swine. Vet. Med., *84*:428, 1989.

Hays, V.W.: Benefits: Antibacterials. *In* Drugs in Livestock Feed. Vol. 1. Tech. Rep. Washington, D.C., Office of Technology Assessment, Congress of the United States, 1979.

Henry, S.C.: Evaluating the alternative therapies for swine respiratory disease. Vet. Med., *81*:763, 1986.

Johnson, M.W., Fitzgerald, G., Welter, M.W., and Welter, C.J.: The six most common pathogens responsible for diarrhea in new born pigs. Vet. Med., *87*:382, 1992.

Larsen, H.P., Hogedahl, P., Jorgensen, and Szancer, J.: Eradication of Actinobacillus pleuropneumoniae from a breeding herd. Proc. 11th International Pig Veterinary Society Congress, Laussanne, 1990.

Matsuoka, T., Ose, E.E., and Tonkinson, L.V.: Therapeutic effect of injectable tylosin against induced pneumonia in pigs. Vet. Med. Small Anim. Clin., *78*:951, 1983.

McKean, J.D., De Witt, D.L., and Honeyman, M.S.: Management factors affecting sulfamethazine depletion rate in swine. Agric. Pract., *10*:27, 1989.

Miller, C.R., Scheidy, S.F., Philip, J.R., and Free, S.M.: Prophylaxis and treatment of swine dysentery with virginiamycin. Proceedings 76th Annual Meeting US Animal Health Association, 1972.

Miller, D.J.S., O'Connor, J.J., and Roberts, N.L.: Tiamulin/salinumycin interactions in pigs. Vet. Rec., *118*:73, 1986.

Muller, R.D.: The use of apralan feed medication in the control of postweaning scours in swine. Agric. Pract., *7*:47, 1986.

Nicolet, J., and Schifferli, D.: In vitro susceptibility of Haemophilus pleuropneumoniae to antimicrobial substances. Proceeding VII IPVS Congress, Mexico City, 1982.

Nocross, M.A., and Brown, J.L.: Food Safety and Inspection Service initiatives for tissue residue reduction in meat and poultry. J. Am. Vet. Med. Assoc., *198*:819, 1991.

Olson, L.D.: Probable elimination of swine dysentery after feeding ronidazole, carbadox or lincomycin, and verification by feeding sodium arsanilate. Can. J. Vet. Res., *50*:365, 1986.

Olsen, L.D.: Tiamulin in drinking water for treatment and development of immunity to swine dysentery. J. Am. Vet. Med. Assoc., *188*:1165, 1986.

Pickles, R.W.: Tiamulin water medication in the treatment of swine dysentery under farm conditions. Vet. Rec., *110*:403, 1982.

Program Report—Sulfamethazine (SMZ) control program, part 1. Washington, D.C., USDA Food Safety and Inspection Service, Science and Technology Program, 1988.

Riviere, J.E.: Pharmacologic principles of residue avoidance for veterinary practitioners. J. Am. Vet. Med. Assoc., *198*:809, 1991.

Rutter, J.M., and Rojas, X.: Atrophic rhinitis in gnotobiotic piglets. Differences in the pathogenicity of Pasteurella multocida in combined infections with Bordetella bronchiseptica. Vet. Rec., *110*:531, 1982.

Schultz, R.A.: Swine pneumonia, assessing the problem in individual herds. Vet. Med., 757, 1986.

Schultz, R.A.: Haemophilus overview, diagnostic tests and potential treatment. Agric. Pract., *6*:25, 1985.

Schultz, R.A.: Therapeutic and/or prophylactic modalities against pneumonia in swine. Swine Consultant. Lawrenceville, N.J., Veterinary Learning Systems, 1985.

Schultz, R.A.: Treatment of pneumonia in swine. Proceedings AASP, Kansas City, Mo., 1984.

Schultz, R.A.: Haemophilus pleuropneumoniae. Proceedings George A. Young Conference and Nebraska SPF Conference, 1982.

Schultz, R.A., Cue, T., and Anderson, M.D.: Evaluation of tiamulin water medication in treatment for Hemophilus pleuropneumonia in swine. Vet. Med. Small Anim. Clin., 1625, 1983.

Stephano, A., Velasquez-Rojas, F., and Diaz, S.: Enrofloxacin treatment against experimental Haemophilus pleuropneumonia in weaned pigs. XX World Vet. Congress, World Vet. Assoc., Montreal, 1987.

Straw, B.: A look at the factors contributing to the development of swine pneumonia. Vet. Med., 747, 1986.

Straw, B., et al.: Pneumonia and atrophic rhinitis in pigs from a test station. J. Am. Vet. Med. Assoc., *182*:607, 1983.

"Swine Dysentery": Practitioner Planning Guide for Herd Elimination Programs. US Livestock Conservation Institute, Madison, WI, in cooperation with American Association of Swine Practitioners, Des Moines, IA, 1990.

Takeo, S., Hamakawa, M., Yoon, C.S., et al.: Therapeutic effects of doxycycline hydrochloride on Actinobacillus (Haemophilus) pleuropneumoniae infection in pigs. Agric. Pract., *13*:23, 1992.

Taylor, D.: Scours in pigs. In Pract., Vet. Rec. Vol. 118 (Suppl.) 40, 1986.

Van Dresser, W.R., and Wickle, J.R.: Drug residues in food animals. J. Am. Vet. Med. Assoc., *194*:1700, 1989.

Walton, J.R.: Selection of antibiotics for use in pig practice. Vet. Rec., *115*:520, 1984.

Walton, J.R.: In feed and in water medication for pigs. In Pract., *170* (Suppl.):29, 1980.

Zimmerman, D.: Role of subtherapeutic levels of antimicrobials in pig production. J. Anim. Sci., *62* (suppl. 3):6, 1986.

24

GROWTH-PROMOTING AGENTS

24.1 Introduction
24.2 Antimicrobial Growth Promoters
24.3 Ionophores
24.4 Hormonal Growth Promoters
24.5 Biotechnology and Growth Hormone
24.6 Beta Agonists
24.7 Pro-Biotics
24.8 Quinoxalines
24.9 Future Developments

24.1 INTRODUCTION

With rapid expansion of the world population, the demand for edible protein now exceeds the supply, and this gap is continuing to widen. A vast amount of solar energy fixed in plants is not nutritionally available to humans because cellulose constitutes 50% or more of all the carbon in the world's vegetation. The ruminant species are in a more favorable position than other farm animals because they can use cellulose and convert it to products capable of being assimilated by humans. This process enables humans to make indirect use of nutrients from roughages and other products that otherwise would not be available to them. The role of the farm animal, however, in converting feed protein into edible protein for the consumer is not a particularly efficient process. Various approaches to meet this need have been explored and developed, including disease control measures, breed improvements, and altered patterns of management and housing.

Growth is a complex biological phenomenon involving interactions of hormonal, nutritional, genetic, and metabolic factors. Hormones play an important role in coordination and integration of biochemical signals and physiological responses to maintain a homeostatic state in the body. Many hormones interact to control the growth of muscle and other body tissues of the animal. This area of endocrinology is becoming more important as more traditional methods of increasing growth come under increased scrutiny by consumers. The development of sophisticated radioimmunoassays to allow measurement of hormones in blood and tissue is leading to an increased appreciation of the endocrine regulation of growth. In addition, more emphasis is being placed on the affinity, specificity, and degree of binding of different hormones to specific high-affinity receptors in muscle, liver, and adipose tissue.

Growth is clearly the principal component that governs the efficiency of animal production, and an ability to manipulate animal growth is an important component in human control of domesticated animals. To be productive, all animals must grow; not all are required to reproduce or lactate. An understanding of the detailed physiologic mechanisms governing the rate and efficiency of growth of vertebrates is therefore an essential prerequisite to manipulate them effectively to meet food requirements fully.

In the last 30 years, researchers have been concerned with the physiologic aspects of growth in terms of size, the proportions of lean versus fat, and the efficiency of partitioning feed energy and nitrogen between lean and fat. There is now more interest in the balance of processes of protein degradation compared with protein synthesis and between lipolysis versus lipogenesis. Beneath this lies a continuing interest in the genetic control of the underlying pathways and our ability to identify the sources of genetic variation in animals and therefore identify ways in which the desirable traits can be maximized by modern programs of improvement. In this area, the possibilities of gene manipulation and gene insertion offer the greatest scope for increasing the rate of genetic improvement, which, once achieved, could be sustained without further manipulation.

Nevertheless, there have been many important developments in the last decade in the control of growth and definite progress in three areas: (1) the use of anabolic agents to increase protein deposition and therefore the yield of edible muscle, particularly in ruminants; (2) the use of antimicrobial agents as food additives for all four major farm species to increase growth rate, or at least to prevent a decreased growth rate in relation to disease incidence; (3) the use of immunologic methods to enhance the rate of growth, and (4) the use of growth hormone and beta-agonists.

In addition, there has been a surge of research interest in another area, an aspect of quantitative physiology related to growth, particularly that concerning the identification of the mechanisms of hypothalamic pituitary control of growth and the identification of the endocrine feedback process controlling the growth of the whole animal as well as the humoral control of cellular growth. The advent of recombinant DNA technology offers exciting prospects for the further manipulation of animal growth involving one or more of these mechanisms. The biochemical nature and biological activity of polypeptide growth factors controlling cellular growth are now under study. The future availability of exogenous sources of these materials offers exciting prospects of further methods of control.

Other important developments include the potential use of growth hormone (somatotropin) and related compounds; the potential use of immunologic methods to enhance the rate of growth; the potential use of beta-adrenergic agonists, particularly to modify carcass composition by decreasing fat and increasing the rate of protein deposition; and the direct genetic manipulation of animal embryos to enhance the expression of a desirable trait, e.g., increased growth hormone secretion or leanness. Because of the vast economic potential for growth promoters, there is major investment both by research institutes and pharmaceutical companies into these alternative methods of growth promotion, and many of the products are based on new biotechnologic methods. Consumer acceptance is of critical importance if such methods are to become commercially viable.

HISTORY OF GROWTH PROMOTANTS

Products that improve the rate and efficiency of growth in livestock have been used for 30 years. Termed "growth promotants," these products include compounds that can generally be classified as antibacterial agents (antibiotics) or anabolic compounds (estrogens and androgens). Growth promotants in the United States are under the regulatory control of the Food and Drug Administration (FDA). About twenty-four growth promotants are FDA approved for use in food-producing animals in the United States. Twelve of the 24 used in beef production (Table 24–1) are listed here.

Growth promotants are administered to the animal in either feed-additive form or implant form. Feed additives are mixed with the animal's daily feed ration, and implants are inserted under the skin of the ear. Implants, in contrast to feed additives, provide activity for an extended time period.

The ability of antibiotics and anabolic compounds to stimulate growth was first recognized in the late 1940s. In 1948, the synthetic estrogen diethylstilbestrol was reported to improve daily gain in heifers. A

TABLE 24–1
GROWTH PROMOTANTS APPROVED FOR BEEF

Feed Additives	Implants
Bacitracin	Compudose
Bacitracin zinc	Ralgro
Chlortetracycline	Synovex-H
Erythromycin	Synovex-S
Lasalocid	Finaplix
Melengestrol acetate	
Monensin	
Oxytetracycline	

year later, the antibiotic chlortetracycline was identified as producing increased growth response in poultry. Commercial development of antibiotics and estrogens proceeded rapidly, with FDA approval of both antibiotic and anabolic compounds in the early 1950s. The growth-promoting properties of antibiotics and anabolic compounds are well documented. The mode of action of these compounds, however, is not clearly understood.

In general, improvement in live weight gain after administration of feed additives to finishing beef cattle are about 5 to 15% and improvements in feed conversion efficiency in the order of 3 to 4%. The responses vary depending on the roughage content of the diet. When feeding high-roughage diets, administering feed additives results in greater increases in growth rate, and with high-concentrate diets, less effect on live weight gain is seen, but feed conversion efficiency is improved. Feed additives can be categorized as ionophores and non-ionophores. The ionophores modify the movement of ions across biological membranes of rumen microbes. Ionophores are considered to enhance production of propionate in the rumen microbes and reduce acetate and methane production. Protein-sparing effects and increased dry matter and protein digestibility have also been observed. Non-ionophore antibiotics act by inhibiting the action of certain gut microorganisms. The net effect of these feed-additive compounds is to increase the metabolizable energy available for growth. In contrast to the hormonal growth promoters, feed additives do not have adverse effects on sexual development of animals. In addition, they can be recommended for use in male and female animals that are to be used for breeding because they do not affect gonadotropic secretion from the anterior pituitary and the onset of puberty.

CLASSIFICATION OF SUBSTANCES USED

The main substances that have been used as growth promoters are grouped as follows:

1. Antimicrobials - e.g., non-ionophore antibiotics and synthetic antibacterials
2. Ionophore antibiotics
3. Quioxalines
4. Hormones
5. Growth hormones
6. Beta-agonists
7. Probiotics

ANTIMICROBIAL COMPOUNDS

Antimicrobial growth promoters have been used in pig and poultry production systems for many years. Ruminants can digest fibrous material by fermentation, but this process is inefficient owing to energy losses in the form of methane gas and heat and from the production of acetate rather than propionate. Chemical agents have been developed that can manipulate rumen fermentation by altering the microflora present and can improve conversion efficiency and in some cases growth rate. These compounds are broken into three categories based on their modes of action:

1. **Ionophore antibiotics**. The ionophore-type feed additives (e.g., monesin and lasalocid) modify the movement of ions across biological membranes and can have a protein-sparing effect and increase dry matter digestibility and protein digestibility in ruminants. Administration of monensin to cattle results in a 2 to 10% improvement in live weight gain, an increase of 3 to 7% in feed conversion efficiency, and up to a 6% decrease in food consumption. Initially this compound was used only as a feed additive, but following the introduction of a controlled-release intraruminal bolus, the use of monesin has been extended to animals at pasture.
2. **Non-ionophore antibiotics**. Narrow-spectrum glycoprotein antibiotics (e.g., avoparcin) and phosphoglycolipid antibiotics (e.g., flavophospholipol) (bambermycin) alter the rumen flora by inhibiting the action of some gram-positive gut microorganisms and peptoglycan formation, giving similar production responses to those production units using ionophores. In addition to yearling and finishing cattle, these compounds can also be administered to calves, either fed in milk replacer or in supplementary concentrates. The means by which these compounds exert their antimicrobial effect differs for various products.
3. **Gut active growth promoters**. This category of growth promoter includes enzymes and probiotics. Enzymes that are supplemented in the diet include amylase, lipase, and protease. The pro-biotic feed additives consist of selected strains of lactobacilli and streptococci, which alter the microbial species present in the digestive system of the animal, to the benefit of the treated animal.

24.2 ANTIMICROBIAL GROWTH PROMOTERS

Antimicrobial growth promoters are attracting renewed interest in the 1990s concerning residues in meat and the consequences to the consumer. This relates to the theory that antibiotic resistance will or has developed in the enteric flora of livestock and that this may lead to untreatable or difficult to treat disease problems in humans. This is an important aspect in the overall discussion of feed additives. Modern analytical techniques permit detection of substances in small amounts; no longer is one talking in terms of milligram/kilogram. Today science has advanced to detect and quantify residues in the nanogram/kilogram range if not the picogram/kilogram range. Hence the question of residues arises. Producers must be educated to ensure that antibiotics are properly managed to aid the production of cheaper and more wholesome meat.

The first materials to achieve recognition in the field of feed additives were antibiotics and antibacterial agents. Their use at low dietary concentrations to promote growth and at therapeutic levels to combat disease is well known and has been practiced in many livestock-producing countries for about two decades. Their effects at low levels are predominantly manifest in the lumen or at the surface of the intestine; resulting in increased growth rate, improved efficiency of feed use; and a sparing effect on nutrients, such as vitamins, proteins, and certain minerals. The small amounts required to elicit such a growth response made the incorporation of antibiotics and antibacterial agents into animal diets economically feasible. Following the publication of various reports, however. The number of substances now officially recognized as "feed antibiotics" has been severely reduced, although numerous other growth stimulants are available.

Zinc bacitracin can be added to feeds for growing pigs, poultry broilers and layers, calves, and lambs. It is a powerful antibacterial growth promoter, which at levels of 10 to 100 g/ton for poultry, 10 to 100 g/ton for pigs and 40 to 100 g/ton for calves and lambs can improve feed conversion by up to 12% and growth rate by as much as 28% in young animals.

Additives are also available that can influence carcass composition, producing an end product that has an increased percentage of muscle and decreased percentage of fat. Hormone-based additives have been marketed for this purpose and are widely used for finishing cattle, sheep, and pigs.

The discovery of selective antimicrobial agents (antibiotics) approximately 50 years ago was a major advance in the history of human and animal medicine. These antibiotics are chemical substances produced by microorganisms that have the capacity to inhibit the growth or to destroy other microorganisms. In subsequent decades, research in this aspect of medicine has mainly centered on the search for a wider range of antibiotics effective against disease-producing microbial species. As well as expanding the range of antibiotics available, this research has resulted in the identification of chemical substances (chemotherapeutics) with selective antimicrobial properties.

The improved performance with growth promoters is accompanied by reduced morbidity and mortality. Growth responses to antimicrobials were first reported in the late 1940s. In the intervening years, many antibiotics and chemical substances (possibly close to 1000) have been shown to have growth-promoting capabilities. The continuous use of low levels of antibiotics in animal feeds (growth promoters) is considered by some as posing a danger to human health by making a quantitative contribution to the pool of resistant bacteria that may in turn be transferred to the human population. To preserve the effectiveness of antibiotics that are important in the therapy of human diseases, governments of most countries have regulated the use of growth promoters in animal feeds.

A major feature of the increased intensification of animal production systems has been the extensive, continuous use of antimicrobial compounds as feed additives. A feed growth promoter may be defined as a substance that when added to feed in the subtherapeutic dosage for an extended period produces an economic improvement in one of the following indices of productivity:

- Growth rate and feed conversion efficiency
- Mortality
- Morbidity

Improvement occurs without adding fat to the carcass or causing "gut fill" or water retention.

Essentially the products used fulfill one of two (and in some cases both) roles: (1) The enhancement of performance by increased growth rate or improved feed conversion in clinically normal animals receiving nutritionally adequate diets and (2) the maintenance of animal health in the face of environmental stress and the challenge of increased microbial activity associated with modern systems of animal production, especially under conditions of intensive production.

Feed additives under group (1) can usually be defined as substances other than dietary nutrients, which achieve their effects in healthy animals fed a balanced diet containing adequate quantities of all known nutrients. Those substances in group (2) act prophylactically to suppress disease organisms and are not essentially growth promoters in their own right. The situation is confused in that some substances, for example, the antibiotic monensin, is in group (2) for a disease in one species (coccidiosis in poultry) but when given to ruminants come under group (1) (improved feed conversion ratio), with an additional effect in relation to coccidiosis in lambs.

The response to growth promoters is not generally accepted as being solely due to their action on the microbial flora. There is considerable experimental evidence showing a lack of response to growth promoters with germ-free animals or poor response in well-managed herds observing good hygiene standards. There is, however, less agreement on the exact mechanism of the response.

Attempts to establish quantitative changes in the microflora of animals during antibiotic feeding have not given consistent results. Neither has it been clearly established that subclinical disease is reduced in antibiotic-fed animals even though experience would suggest that it is in many situations. What has been established is that the response to growth promoters is greater in younger, unthrifty, or stressed animals and with unfavorable environmental conditions. Equally it has been established that when animals are well cared for in good conditions the response is small or may be absent. This is demonstrated by the results of many experiments.

In discussing the mechanism of growth, it becomes clear that the lower the microflora contamination, the lower the growth response to antimicrobials, and, conversely, as an animal develops clinical signs of disease, higher growth responses are obtained. Within these extremes, the mode of action of growth promoters is difficult to define. Many theories, including nutrient-sparing effect, metabolic effect, better absorption, and disease control, have been postulated. All are likely to be secondary to the effect of growth promoters on the microflora.

FEED ADDITIVES

Antibiotics are the most widely used group of feed additives and by definition are compounds produced by one microorganism that inhibit the growth of another organism. Those that have been used extensively in cattle include chlortetracycline, oxytetracycline, bacitracin, erythromycin, tylosin, monensin, and lasalocid.

The ideal antimicrobial growth promoters should:

1. Improve growth or production quantitatively and qualitatively
2. Improve feed conversion efficiency and promote better use of expensive nutrients, such as proteins
3. Have general, nonspecific action on metabolism in addition to preventing diseases associated with the early phases of life
4. Eliminate Enterobacteriaceae carrying R plasmids or at least not induce such plasmids
5. Have at most minute, or better nil, residues in edible tissues after 24 to 48 hours withdrawal of supplemented feed
6. Have no unfavorable environmental effects, e.g., when distributed as slurry, in particular against nitrifying and methane-producing bacteria in the soil
7. Not cause cross resistance with other antimicrobials
8. Not cross react with substances used as therapeutics, e.g., growth-promotional levels of salinomycin with therapeutic levels of tiamulin
9. Be nontoxic to the animal, to nontarget species, and to feed mill personnel
10. Be stable after pelleting with a long shelf life and with a readily reproducible method of assay.

Most feed additives are regulated by the FDA. Some other compounds not so strictly regulated are designated "Generally Regarded As Safe" (GRAS).

Low-level use of antibacterials in feed has attracted major opposition from certain sections of the medical profession on three main counts:

1. That the use of antimicrobial agents at subtherapeutic levels would select bacterial strains resistant to that agent
2. That the continuing high prevalence of bacterial resistance in farm animal populations was a direct result of using subtherapeutic levels in feed stuffs

3. That bacterial resistance to antibiotics, especially transmissible antibiotic resistance in salmonellae, would rapidly spread from farm animals to humans, again under the influence of using subtherapeutic levels of antibiotics for animal feeds

The primary modes of action of antimicrobial growth promoters have been ascribed to:

1. Nutrient-sparing activity
2. Metabolic effects
3. Antimicrobial effects

The growth-promoting effect of antimicrobials in the rat have been found to be proportional to the degree of protein deficiency. Nutrient-sparing effects may be mediated by changes in absorption or in the microflora of the alimentary tract.

Antibiotics may reduce the dietary requirement for certain nutrients by (1) stimulating growth of desirable organisms that synthesize vitamins or amino acids, (2) depressing the organisms that compete with the host animal for nutrients, (3) increasing availability of nutrients via chelation mechanisms, or (4) improving the absorptive capacity of the intestinal tract.

Growth promoters act primarily in the digestive tract and are eliminated with the feces. They exert a beneficial effect on the composition of the microorganisms inhabiting the gut. It has long been known that a well-balanced intestinal flora bars the way to pathogens trying to enter the body.

At the same time, growth promoters also act to slow down bacterial metabolism. This reduces the rate at which the intestinal flora break down feed proteins to substances, such as ammonia and biogenic amines, that are toxic to the animals and interfere with the absorption of nutrients through the intestinal wall. Growth promoters thus increase the availability of nutrients and improve intestinal absorption. They also help to conserve energy, particularly in beef cattle—which is the same as saying that they raise productivity. Growth promoters also exert a positive effect on metabolism, increasing the rate at which animals lay down protein, thus improving weight gain and feed efficiency.

Antibiotics also directly effect that rate or pattern of the metabolic process. Metabolic effects, e.g., increased nitrogen retention, have been reported after the use of the carbadox in pig grower diets. A clear relationship between the presence of a bacterium (*Streptococcus faecium*) in the gut of chickens hatched germ free and growth depression has been demonstrated.

DISEASE CONTROL

Antibiotics suppress organisms that cause clinical or subclinical disease. Suppression is completed by inhibiting the multiplication of organisms that produce toxins or by limiting their capacity to produce toxins that reduce performance but result in no obvious symptom of disease. Antimicrobial growth promoters affect the resident flora in six possible ways:

1. Bacterial cell wall damage
2. Reduction in gut wall thickness
3. Increase of intestinal alkaline phosphatase
4. Reduction in ammonia production and metabolism
5. Reduction in toxin production
6. Energy metabolism

Non-ionophore antibiotics and antibacterial additives are thought to have their main effects by inhibiting the action of gut microorganisms, but in pigs and poultry, it is possible that the presence of the gut-active antibacterials results in a thinning of the intestinal epithelium, with consequent changes in metabolic energy costs or in the efficiency of nutrient absorption. In the cases of ruminants, the beneficial effects of antimicrobial growth promoters lies more clearly in their ability to influence the balance of microbial species inhabiting the reticulorumen, such that a higher level of rumen propionate is produced in treated animals at the expense of acetate and sometimes of butyrate production, and there are significant reductions in energy losses due to the ruminal production of methane. The total effect is to increase the metabolizable energy content and also possibly to increase the net availability of the metabolizable energy available for protein and fat production. In ruminants, the extent or importance of changes in the small intestine similar to those observed in nonruminants has not, so far, been documented.

MECHANISM OF ACTION

At first, it was thought that growth stimulation was simply a manifestation of increased feed consumption. Theories on the mechanism of action of growth promotion by antibiotics since have been proposed and refuted, with little definite result. There still is much evidence for some close connection between antibiotics and vitamins in this respect.

There is to date no consensus on the mechanism of action, but it seems reasonable to assume that the growth-promoting effect and the vitaminlike activity both involve some action on the microbial flora of the animal. Antibiotics do not stimulate the growth of germ-free chicks, and the fact that bacitracin given by mouth is a potent growth agent indicates that the site of action of antibiotics is primarily restricted to gram-positive bacteria in the intestinal tract. In addition to interfering with gram-positive organisms, feed antibiotics also act by encouraging the proliferation of *Aerobacter*, an organism active in the degradation of uric acid. In ruminants, antibiotics effect a significant redistribution of the bacterial population of the rumen.

There are differences between various antibiotics in their mechanism of action on the microbial flora. Penicillin acts to reduce the intestinal dominance of *Streptococcus faecalis*; it tends to cause greater rises in coliform bacteria and greater decreases in the *Lactobacillus* level than do other antibiotics. These differences, however, are neither clear-cut nor fully reproducible. Sulfonamides and some arsenicals have effects similar to antibiotics, and there is some evidence that they suppress the output of an unidentified toxin produced by the intestinal flora.

Additional evidence for the role of changes in intestinal flora is provided by the fact that antibiotics consistently reduce the weight of the intestinal tract. The weight of the small intestine is reduced in conventionally raised chicks fed antibiotics, whereas no such response is found in animals raised in a bacteria-free environment. The small intestine decreases in weight before body weight starts to increase, and levels of antibiotic too low to increase body weight still cause decrease in intestinal weight. The decrease in intestinal weight is in turn correlated with an increase in metabolizable energy. This suggests that the growth stimulation produced by antibiotics may be linked to an increased efficiency in absorption of calorigenic nutrients.

There is reason to believe then that the immediate environment exerts a strong effect on the nature of growth response to antibiotics and that in part this is a social effect, with members of a flock providing each other with chemical or biological messengers regulating individual growth. Normal animals carry a population of microflora adherent to the wall of the intestines. These organisms, which are both symbionts and commensals, are not causing a pathogenic effect. The large numbers of organisms interfere or suppress the use or absorption of nutrients that are needed for optimal growth and feed conversion. Antibiotic growth promoters influence these organisms. Gnotobiotic animals on purified diets do not respond to antibacterial growth promoters. It is somewhat incredible, but true, that an antibiotic at a concentration as low as 1 to 2 ppm activity produces a significant response in growth and feed conversion. This is quite different from a response needed to treat or prevent a disease, such as enteritis or pneumonia, in which experience shows that, in most cases, concentrations of 100 ppm or more are needed during the treatment period.

Hence it is important to appreciate (1) that the response to a growth promoter is different from the response needed to control disease and (2) that the appraisal of an antibiotic, especially when this concerns resistance development, must be considered in relation to its use either as a growth promoter (at low level) or as a therapeutic agent (at high level) because the type of organisms responding and the degree of selection pressure are different. High levels of antibiotic mean a higher selection pressure, and although this may lead to resistance by disease-producing organisms (e.g., a gut pathogen), it is not necessarily or generally associated with the development of resistance in the normal flora because animals still continue to respond to low concentrations by improvements in feed conversion or body weight. When an antibacterial is used at low level in feed as a growth promoter, insufficient selection pressure is applied to cause resistance by pathogenic bacteria. It is not generally appreciated that the biggest resistance problem is caused by therapeutic levels, but growth-promoter levels are not necessarily a serious contributory factor to this. For example, studies on *Mycoplasma* and *Pasteurella* show that pathogenic strains of these organisms do not become resistant to continuous exposure to growth-promoting concentrations of antibiotics, but they do when the concentration is increased to therapeutic levels. After 40 years, usage evidence shows that antibiotics remain effective as growth promoters in all classes of livestock that continually receive them under practical farm conditions.

Antimicrobial growth promoters (feed additives) have been used extensively in pig and poultry production for many years. Avoparcin is the active ingredient of Avotan. It is a narrow-spectrum glycopeptide antibiotic and is recommended for beef cattle of all ages. The recommended dose for beef cattle is 50–100 mg avoparcin/head/day (15–40 ppm in feed). Improvements in live weight gain ranging from 5 to 15% have been reported, and an increase of 6 kg in carcass weight has been reported in a trial that extended over a period of 21 weeks in finishing steers. Avoparcin has a dual action. It acts in the rumen, enhancing fermentation, and in the intestine, improving the absorption of nutrients.

In the rumen, billions of microorganisms ferment the feed and convert carbohydrates into acetic, butyric, and propionic acids, which are absorbed and used for maintenance and growth. Some of these microorganisms are beneficial; others have a negative effect. Avoparcin reduces the level of those that are negative and encourages those that are beneficial, making fermentation more efficient. It particularly encourages the production of propionate, which aids lean meat production. Avoparcin also reduces methane as production, so less energy is wasted and more is absorbed. In the intestine, avoparcin inhibits wasteful bacteria, which damage the gut lining and affect the absorption of amino acids through the gut walls. In the presence of avoparcin, more amino acids are absorbed, and with the extra energy produced in the rumen, these are converted into extra lean meat.

Flavomycin (bambermycin) contains flavophospholipol and is a phosphoglycolipid antibiotic. It is recommended for use in calves fed on milk replacer or in supplementary feed to beef cattle of all ages. Increases in live weight gain and feed efficiency of 9% have been obtained in calves given 16 mg flavophospholipol/kg milk replacer or 20 mg flavophospholipol/kg supplementary concentrates. Similar responses have been obtained in finishing beef cattle.

The use of antibiotics in animal feeds is regulated by the FDA and by, or in cooperation, with state regulatory agencies. The FDA requires proof of safety and efficacy before approval of a drug for use singly or in combination. The FDA's authority to require evidence of efficacy was provided by the 1962 Kefauver-Harris amendment of the Food, Drug, and Cosmetic Act of 1938, which only provided the authority to require proof of safety. A number of drugs or combinations of drugs were approved before 1962. Soon the efficacy of all of the old drugs will have been re-evaluated, and any not proved efficacious will have been withdrawn from the market. The decision on some drug combinations has been implemented.

Approval for use by the FDA means that the drugs have been properly tested, that inclusion of the drug in question as a feed additive has been found to result in a performance superior to that of animals fed nonmedicated control diets, and that feeding the drug at the tested and approved level and duration does not result in harmful residues. Approval by the FDA should not imply that all approved drugs are equally effective for their intended use, such as promoting growth or improving feed efficiency. A clear distinction between relative efficacy and FDA approval for use seems to be frequently confused in discussions or decisions related to substitute or alternative drugs.

For drugs to be used as feed additives, the FDA requires assurance that the drugs are safe for target animals and that when the drugs are used at approved levels and properly withdrawn before marketing, residues in tissues are insignificant. Unless it can be proved that a feed antibiotic is not absorbed from the gastrointestinal tract, a practical method to measure tissue levels must be developed. The time required for tissue clearance must be determined also to enable the FDA to establish the minimum time required between the last feeding of the drug and the marketing of the animals for food purposes. After approval of a drug for use in food-producing animals, the Food Safety and Inspection Service (FSIS) of the United States Department of Agriculture (USDA) (Meat Inspection Service) monitors the tissue levels to ensure compliance. The FDA and state feed control officials monitor feeds to ensure proper feed-manufacturing practices, including the use of approved drug levels and drug combinations and proper labeling of the marketed feeds. Noncompliance may result in embargo of the feed or animals and appropriate citation and legal action, if a violation merits such action. The testing and retesting of drugs for efficacy provides a continuous evaluation of drug safety in target animals.

The antibiotics used in livestock and poultry as feed additives include bacitracin, bambermycins, chlortetracycline, erythromycin, lincomycin, neomycin sulfate, oleandomycin, oxytetracycline, procaine penicillin, streptomycin, tylosin, and virginiamycin. Bacitracin is used as is or in the form of zinc bacitracin or bacitracin methylene disalicylate. These antibiotics are used as feed additives for one or more of the following purposes: to improve growth rate, to improve feed efficiency, to decrease mortality, and to reduce morbidity. Three of these antibiotics, bambermycins lyncomycin, and virginiamycin have been approved for use in the United States since 1970.

Flavomycin (bambermycin) is a macromolecule, which, because of its heteropolar behavior, tends to form complexes. It is therefore one of the performance promoters that is extremely difficult for animals to absorb. Histologic studies of enteric absorption demonstrate this. Balance studies with flavomycin proved that the active ingredient is not absorbed but is excreted in the feces as the intact, biologically active molecule. Flavomycin affects the growth of bacteria that have colonized the intestinal tract. As a result, the metabolic activity of the modified intestinal flora is changed in favor of the animal. This results indirectly in an improvement in the digestibility of the nutrients and their subsequent use. This in turn gives rise to better growth performance in poultry, rabbits, and pigs and an improved laying performance in hens.

Digestion of enzymes is effected in the rumen by the rumen flora, which are composed of bacteria and protozoa. Flavomycin intervenes in the metabolic processes of the rumen by selectively influencing the growth of certain groups of rumen flora. Because it is not metabolized in the rumen, flavomycin exerts an antibacterial effect in the intestine. Flavomycin prompts the growth of amylolytic and cellulolytic microorganisms and of those that can ferment both starch and cellulose, such as *Bacteroides succinogenes, Butyrivibrio fibrisolvens,* and *Clostridium lochheadii.* Flavomycin therefore accelerates the breakdown of cellulose by about 15%.

Flavomycin reduces the formation of the microbial metabolic by-products, carbon dioxide and methane. Because the energy-rich methane in the animal's body cannot be used further and is excreted by eructation, flavomycin reduces energy losses. Flavomycin increases the formation of volatile fatty acids, especially that of propionic acid. The fatty acids are absorbed by the rumen wall and are oxidized by aerobic metabolism by the ruminant to produce energy. In addition to this, propionic acid plays a particular role in protein synthesis. The reduction in the formation of butyric acid lowers the risk of ketosis.

Even at the low dosage rates used for performance promotion, flavomycin has a marked antibacterial effect on the numerous gram-positive microorganisms that are found in the digestive tract. Flavomycin inhibits their reproduction by intervening in the biosynthesis of murein, the structural substance of bacteria cell wall. Damage to the murein layer results in cell bursting.

The structure of murein is a three-dimensional network in which chains of sugar molecules are linked by protein bridges. A number of enzymes are needed for the biosynthesis of murein. One of these, glycosyltransferase, forms sugar filaments from the already completed cornerstones, which then have to be linked together. Flavomycin inhibits this important stage in the biosynthesis of murein.

Comparison of the structure of the cell wall cornerstone with that of flavomycin reveals a marked similarity. Theoretically glycosyltransferase cannot distinguish between the two molecules and also uses flavomycin to form the chain. This prevents murein synthesis from taking place, by blocking completion of the normal structure. Flavomycin is one of the most active substances inhibiting murein biosynthesis and is therefore effective in low doses. Flavomycin is effective mainly against gram-positive bacteria. Some gram-negative microorganisms, such as *Pasteurella* and *Brucella*, also proved to be sensitive to flavomycin.

Antibiotics may be used singly; in combination with other antibiotics; or with other chemical compounds, such as sulfa drugs, cocciodiostats, or histostats. Approved levels, combination claims, and so forth are published in the Federal Register. The antimicrobial agent include antibiotics, which are of microbial origin, and chemotherapeutic agents, which are chemically synthesized compounds. This latter group includes arsenical compounds (arsanilic acid, 3-nitro-4-hydroxyphenylarsonic acid and sodium arsanilate), nitrofurans (furazolidone, nitrofurazone), and carbadox and sulfa compounds (sulfamethazine, sulfathiazole and sulfaquinoxaline). Other chemicals are used as antiprotozoal agents to prevent coccidiosis and histomoniasis in chickens and turkeys, and one agent, monensin, is used to improve feed efficiency in beef cattle.

Changes in use of antibacterials have occurred in the past decade. New uses for some of the old drugs or combinations of drugs have also been approved. The use of certain combination drugs has also been approved. The use of certain combination drugs has been discontinued because of lack of efficacy or because no individual company wished to provide the efficacy data. For the most part, these were drugs or combinations of drugs that were used sparingly. In addition to the concern for bacterial resistance, some antibacterial agents are being scrutinized because of other potential risks, such as carcinogenic properties. The decade of discussion on safety and efficacy has encouraged a more critical evaluation of all drug programs. There is certainly no universal agreement on the risks or benefits from certain drugs.

A National Academy of Sciences' committee (1980) concluded that it is not possible to conduct a feasible, comprehensive epidemiologic study of the effects on human health arising from the subtherapeutic use of antimicrobials in animal feeds. The committee did recommend further research on the mechanism by which subtherapeutic levels of antimicrobials promote growth of animals, which could possibly lead to the development of other substances or procedures to accomplish the same effect. They further recommended continued monitoring and occasional review of the possible effects on humans resulting from the subtherapeutic use of antimicrobials in animal feeds.

The Council for Agricultural Science and Technology Task Force (1981) essentially concluded, although it was not expressed in such terms, that it is also impossible to conduct a feasible, comprehensive economic impact study that will clearly define the impact of a partial or total ban on the subtherapeutic use of antibiotics in animal feeds. In the EC and Scandinavia, the continuance in use of antibiotics as feed-additive growth promoters is constantly under review because of consumer discontent.

24.3 IONOPHORES AND QUINOXALINES

Polyether antibiotics are fermentation products of *Streptomyces* species. Monensin, salinocycin, narasin, and lasalocid are the most commonly used substances within this group. They are organic acids with pKa values ranging from 6.4 to 6.6. The bulk of the existing knowledge of ionophores is based on monensin. Monensin does not differ materially from other polyether antibiotics in regard to chemical structure, physical and chemical properties, mode of action, clinical efficacy, pharmacokinetic properties, and toxicity. Maduramycin and semduracin are newer ionophores.

Ionophores form complexes with monovalent and divalent cations, some of which, K^+, Na^+, Ca^{2+} and Mg^{++}, are biologically significant. Salts of ionophores are only sparingly soluble in aqueous solutions, whereas they are soluble in organic solvents. A high rate of diffusion of these complexes across lipid membranes, coupled with a high degree of cation selectivity, partially explains their activity at the cell level. Thus polyether ionophores have been synthesized that have up to several hundred thousand times greater affinity to certain metal ions than to other ions.

CHEMICAL MANIPULATION

A wide range of chemicals have been studied for their capacity to manipulate rumen fermentations in the direction of increased propionic acid production and decreased methane levels. Ionophores (large molecules capable of binding cations) increase the production of propionic acid. Of these, the most widely used is monensin sodium (Rumensin, Elanco Division, Eli Lilly Co., Ltd.,) Monensin increases propionic acid production and decreases acetate and butyrate output, coupled with a decrease in the production of methane. It tends to alter all fermentations, both from roughage and from concentrate diets, and it is suggested that its effects arise because it selects against hydrogen-producing microbes and promotes the growth of succinic-acid-producing organisms (a metabolic precursor of propionic acid). Its mode of action appears to be due to its effects on the transport of ions across membranes.

METABOLISM IN THE RUMEN

Besides attempting to maximize output of animal product per unit of maintenance energy, there are two further approaches to improving the efficiencies with which dietary energy is used by ruminants: (1) increasing the efficiency with which energy in the diet is transformed into the end products of digestion in the gut, mainly volatile fatty acids (VFA), and (2) improving the efficiency with which end products of digestion are used for maintenance and for synthesis of animal products.

The key to improvements in the efficiency of VFA formation in the reticulorumen is by a minimization of the amounts of combustible gasses (mainly methane), which are formed by rumen microbes. Methane is a rich energy source that cannot be used and ultimately is lost in the gasses that are eructated. Low levels of methane usually occur when high proportions of total VFA are made up of propionic acid. The precursors of methane (CO_2) and propionic acid (hexose) compete for metabolic hydrogen, and the balance arising from this competition is an important determinant of the efficiency of energy transformations in the reticulorumen. Two main strategies can be used to reduce the energy losses as methane and other combustible gasses:

1. Modification of the diet, including the levels of food intake, composition, and methods of processing the food
2. Use of chemicals to promote the production of propionic acid and to inhibit methane formation

Ruminant animals are the most successful ecologic group of herbivorous animals, and economically they outweigh any other group. The secret of their success is their remarkable four-compartment stomach, which allows them to process large quantities of plant material by means of a mixed bacterial protozoal and fungal fermentation in the first two compartments. Some of the microorganisms are highly desirable in that they hydrolyze and ferment the major plant structural polysaccharides cellulose, xylan, and pectin to a mixture of VFAs, which the animal can use, and to methane, which it cannot. One aim of rumen manipulation is to reduce this gaseous energy loss. A second aim is to reduce ruminal degradation of dietary constituents, which the animal can itself digest, most importantly protein and starch. Most of the protein that is fermented is converted to VFAs and ammonia, only small proportions being incorporated into bacterial protein. This represents a big loss to the animal, and there are a number of ways of limiting ruminal protein degradation. Ruminal degradation of starch represents a partial loss of energy to the animal, especially in acetate-rich fermentations because acetic acid has only 64% of the energy content of the carbohydrate from which it was derived. A by-product is hydrogen, some of which is used by methanogens to reduce carbon dioxide to methane, whereas some is more usefully consumed in production of propionic acid, which has 106% of the energy content of the carbohydrate from which it was made. It is also glucogenic,

TABLE 24–2
IONOPHORES

Drug	Synthesized by	Company	Trade Name
Monensin	*Streptomyces cinnamonenesis*	Elanco/Eli Lilly	Rumensin
Lasalocid	*Streptomyces lasaliensis*	Hoffmann-LaRoche	Bovatec Avatec
Narasin	*Streptomyces aureofaciens*	Elanco	Monteban
Salinomycin	*Streptomyces albus*	A.H. Robbins	Salocin

which is particularly valuable in growing beef animals. Other possible ways of manipulating the rumen are stimulating the incorporation of ammonia into protein by bacteria and overall rate of digestion of fiber.

A major type of manipulator, the so-called propionate enhancer, is the commercially successful—monensin, an ionophoric antibiotic produced by *Streptomyces cinnamonenesis*. It inhibits certain ruminal bacteria, notably streptococci and ruminococci, and because some of the latter are cellulolytic, there is an immediate decrease in the degradation of fiber. In beef cattle, feed intake is significantly depressed, and the rumen takes about 3 weeks to reach a new steady state in which bacteria capable of producing hydrogen have been decreased and many that produce propionate have increased in number, with the result in one experiment that the measured ruminal output of metabolic energy had increased by 12% entirely owing to enhanced propionate. A consequence of the alteration in production and use of metabolic hydrogen is that methanogenesis is reduced—typically by 30%. Monensin also increases the percentage of starch and protein, which is not degraded in the rumen.

Under appropriate conditions, monensin has many beneficial effects on the rumen fermentation, and this has led to its widespread use, especially in the feedlot beef units in the United States, but it has the disadvantage of sometimes inducing anorexia in the first 3 weeks of feeding. The other ionophore—lasalocid—seems to be freer from this defect, although its mode of action and potency seem similar. Although mo-

nensin is sold based on improvements in food conversion efficiency, the later ionophoric antibiotics may well be sold based on increased growth rate. This will have economical advantages.

EFFECTS OF IONOPHORES

Ionophore antibiotics currently in use are "monovalent cationic" substances, e.g., monensin, narasin, and salinomycin, and "divalent cationic" substances, e.g., lasalocid (Table 24–2). This divalent binding (e.g., Ca^{++}, Mg^{++}) by lasalocid is due to its sandwich dimeric structure. An ionophore is a compound that makes cations (ions that carry a positive charge) lipid soluble. These have a polyether structure. Differences exist among them. Several ionophores have been used commercially as coccidiostats in poultry. Some of the effects that have been observed from use of monensin and some other ionophores in cattle and sheep include:

1. Decreased feed intake (grain and feedlot cattle and forage in cows, meaning more cow-carrying capacity)
2. Improved feed efficiency of feed or grain (in feedlot cattle, stockers, and cows)
3. Improved daily gain (in stocker cattle, approximately 2 lb/day; in feedlot cattle, approximately 2% to 7% for monensin and lasalocid, with salinomycin showing even greater increases in gain)
4. Slight improvement in carcass quality traits
5. Earlier puberty (approximately 1 month) in heifers at the same weight

6. Increased propionic acid and decreased acetic production in rumen
7. Possible protein sparing in the diet (lower requirement) or improved protein use or efficiency
8. Decreased methane production and improved efficiency of fermentation in the rumen
9. Decreased rate of passage and rumen turnover
10. Increase in digestibility of low-quality forages
11. Increase (small) in starch digestion on high-grain diets
12. Less protein degradation in rumen and increased bypass shift of more organic matter digestion to intestines
13. Increase in protein deposition or accretion in cattle on low or marginal protein diets
14. Control of or substantial decrease in level and frequency of coccidiosis in cattle and sheep, especially at the 30 g/ton level
15. Effective against gram-positive, but no gram-negative, microorganisms
16. Decrease in *Streptococcus bovis* and other lactate-producing rumen microorganisms (important in reduction of acidosis)
17. Partial intake regulator in self-feeding programs
18. Decrease in excess hydrogen ion levels (energy-sparing action)
19. Improved cell membrane permeability for certain ions

Because of the wide variety of effects in the rumen, monensin has been used to treat ketosis in dairy cows, and also to control bloat in pastured dairy cattle. In the latter indication, monensin has been designed as a controlled-release capsule releasing 300 mg of monensin/day for 100 days.

MONENSIN

Monensin (Rumensin) is a polyether antibiotic produced by the fermentation of *S. cinnamonenesis*. It was the first of this class of compounds to be identified as a promoter of zootechnical efficiency in ruminant animals. The discovery of this attribute of the polyethers arose from a systematic application of in vitro rumen fermentation techniques in a search for compounds capable of shifting the balance of VFAs produced in the rumen toward increased propionic acid production. Monensin is able to effect this change and to sustain it over extended periods of time, regardless of whether rations are forage-based or contain a high proportion of readily fermented carbohydrate.

It has a coccidiostatic effect in poultry and has been a popular constituent for their feed throughout the world. In beef cattle, it improves efficiency by 10 to 15% owing to an increase in the production of more propionic acid, which yields more energy than acetic or butyric acids after ruminal fermentation. Monensin has also proved to be efficacious in the control of coccidiosis in lambs and calves.

The mechanism of action is associated with its ability as an ionophore to complex with certain cations and transport them across cellular membranes. Monensin increases intracellular sodium. This is followed by an increase in intracellular calcium.

Although monensin is well absorbed from the gastrointestinal tract of most mammals, extensive hepatic metabolism coupled with the relatively low dose used for therapeutic purposes results in only trace amounts of the antibiotic being absorbed into the central circulation. Monensin apparently selects not only for certain propionate-producing bacteria, but also metabolically modulates them to produce more propionate. Because cattle generally eat to fulfill their energy needs, animals fed a high-energy diet containing monensin (e.g., feedlot ration) intake the same amount of energy and have the same daily weight gain, while reducing feed consumption. Cattle on pasture often eat below their maximum energy level, so monensin can help a producer increase daily gain and feed efficiency in the herd. In addition, monensin spares dietary protein. Similar results have been attained in lambs.

Ionophores, such as monensin and lasalocid, have received much interest and have been the subject of considerable research. Monensin was the first ionophore to be cleared by the FDA for use in feedlot cattle (in 1976) and in stockers (in 1978). In 1982, lasalocid was cleared for use in feedlot rations. Other experimental ionophores in use at present include narasin, salinomycin, and polyether A, maduramicin and semduracin.

GROWTH PERFORMANCE RESPONSES

The optimum inclusion rate for monensin appears to be 200 mg/day/animal or 10–40 ppm in finished feed. The effect of monensin on the growth performance of grain-fed cattle in the American feedlot system was studied in many experiments. Further experiments demonstrated the compound's effects in cattle fed rations composed almost entirely of freshly harvested or conserved forage and in pastured cattle. In grain-fed cattle, the rate of average daily live weight gain was not altered, whereas feed intake was reduced. The optimal dosage of monensin was 33 ppm in the ration on a 90% dry matter basis. This inclusion level resulted in an improvement of feed conversion efficiency (FCE) of 10.6%. In contrast, when cattle were fed high-roughage rations, feed intake was little altered when average daily weight gain was increased by 14.7%, and feed conversion efficiency improved by 15.3%. In pastured cattle, the addition of 200 mg of monensin to the daily pasture supplement increased average daily weight gain by 16.3%. This well-demonstrated effect of monensin on the growth performance of cattle has led to its inclusion in the rations of more than 95% of cattle being finished in large US feedlots.

Extensive research programs conducted in the United States and throughout Europe have clearly demonstrated the ability of monensin to improve the efficiency with which cattle convert feedstuffs to meat. At the effective levels of use, the inclusion of monensin in the feed produces no detectable residue in any edible tissue. The use of this compound and the benefits it offers to animal production present no known hazard to the consumer. Until recently, monensin was licensed for use only in feed or feed blocks. At pasture, especially if the grass is of sufficient quality, it is often unnecessary or indeed impractical to provide supplementary feed. Therefore under the predominant management systems, a carrier for

monensin premix was unavailable for a large part of the summer grazing season. The farmer was thus unable to derive any benefit from an effective growth promoter. Romensin has now been incorporated in a ruminal delivery device, containing 16.5 g of monensin sodium designed to deliver monensin sodium over a period of 150 days. With this bolus, it is now possible to administer monensin throughout the year in beef systems based on summer grazing.

The ruminal delivery device is administered orally using a balling gun; after swallowing, it lodges in the reticulorumen. The ruminal fluids enter the perforated ends of the device and begin to dissolve the copolymer at the two exposed faces of the cylindrical core. As the copolymer is dissolved, monensin sodium is released at a steady rate. Each device contains monensin sodium dispersed in a solid cylindrical core, which is inserted into a mild steel cylinder and the whole enclosed in a high-density polyethylene sheath. The bolus has round perforated ends, which allow access by the ruminal fluids to the face of the core. The bolus is administered to cattle using a special balling gun. Once in the reticulorumen, monensin is released at a steady rate over a period of 150 days. Monensin is available for use in some countries for control of bloat and also ketosis.

LASALOCID

Lasalocid sodium (Bovatec) (Avatec) is a polyether divalent ionophore antibiotic produced by the fermentation of *Streptomyces lasaliensis* and is similar to monensin and salinomycin. It is used for the prevention of coccidiosis in broiler chickens and is also an effective coccidiostat in ruminants. In ruminants, however, lasalocid has a positive influence on rumen fermentation and feed efficiency by altering the proportion of VFAs in rumen contents toward higher propionate and lower acetate, while methane production is reduced at the same time. The addition of lasalocid to feedlot diets improves feed efficiency by reducing feed intake without adversely affecting growth rate. In most of the investigations, the antibiotic has an additional positive influence on the performance of feedlot animals.

It has been shown the lasalocid, depending on the dosage, can alter the bacteria population quantitatively as well as qualitatively. These observations are in good agreement with other results, which showed that lasalocid or monensin selects resistant strains, such as *Bacteroides*, which produce succinate, and *Selenomonas*, which decarboxylize succinate to propionate. Lasalocid, similar to other ionophore antibiotics (monensin), has been shown to bring on increased propionic acid production and reduced methane formation in the rumen. These effects are due to a selection of bacteria that produce succinate and that ferment lactate as well as to an inhibition of bacteria that produce acetate, butyrate, and lactate as end products and hydrogen as intermediary precursors to methane.

SALINOMYCIN

Owing to its structure and mode of action, salinomycin (Salocin) belongs to the group of polyether antibiotics. It exerts its ionophorous properties on the action transport through the cell walls of animal tissues of bacteria and of protozoa. This effect within the gastrointestinal tract influences growth and feed efficiency as well as coccidial infections in ruminants and nonruminants (pigs).

As for other polyether antibiotics, salinomycin markedly increases the propionic acid concentration in the ruminal fluid, whereas proportions of butyric acid and acetic acid, methane gas production, and cellulose catabolism are reduced. Thus the feed energy is better used in terms of economics. Salinomycin reduces the catabolism of feed protein in the rumen, as indicated by lowered ammonia concentrations and retarded microbial protein synthesis. These observations have been made partially in vitro but most of them in vivo.

Based on the dose-response curve, calculated from many feeding experiments, salinomycin can be recommended for fattening cattle at a dose of 100 to 200 mg/head daily. At the optimum level, weight gain and feed conversion are improved by about 11%, compared with the unmedicated control groups. This level corresponds to approximately 0.6 mg/kg body weight daily.

For fattening lambs, the recommended dosage of 10 to 20 parts/10^6 in the total feed allows an improvement of about 12 to 13% in weight and feed efficiency. The negative effect after high concentrations of salinomycin in the feed looks similar in lambs as in cattle.

Salinomycin is the first licensed ionophore performance promoter in pigs, and its unique mode of action ensures disruption to the growth and reproduction of certain intestinal bacteria. This particular mechanism also helps counteract the buildup of bacterial resistance, so salinomycin continues to improve growth performance in the long term. Inclusion rates for pigs range from 50 ppm in starter rations to 25 ppm in finisher rations. Tests have shown that most appears in the feces in the form of inactive metabolites, subsequently being degraded with a half-life of less than 50 hours.

The normal bacterial cell is a chemical balance between the inside of the cell and the outside environment. The balance is maintained by a mechanism called an ion pump. Salinomycin joins with potassium, transporting it through the cell wall into the bacterium. The cell's ion-pump attempts to rebalance the situation, using up its energy until this becomes depleted. As a result of the shortage of energy, the ion pump fails to operate efficiently. There is a chemical imbalance, with a greater ionic concentration of potassium inside the cell than outside. Water enters the cell owing to osmotic pressure. The cell swells and becomes disrupted.

Salinomycin exerts its performance-promotion effect in pigs in two ways:

1. Throughout the whole intestine, salinomycin favorably adjusts the intestinal flora of the pig, thereby reducing those bacteria responsible for the production of potentially toxic by-products, which may damage the intestinal wall and limit absorption of nutrients.
2. In the large intestine, this favorable rebalancing of bacteria content results in better digestion of the foodstuffs during the time they undergo microbial digestion in this part of the intestine. In turn,

TABLE 24–3
DISTRIBUTION OF ADRENERGIC RECEPTOR SUBTYPES

Type	Tissue	Actions
Alpha 1	Most vascular smooth muscle	Contraction
	Pupillary smooth muscle	Contraction (dilates pupil)
	Pilomotor smooth muscle	Erects hair
	Rat Liver	Glycogenolysis
Alpha 2		Probable multiple effects: sedation, post-synaptic central nervous system (CNS) adrenergic reactors
		Platelet aggregation
		Inhibition of transmitter release
		Adrenergic and cholinergic nerve terminals
		Some vascular smooth muscle contraction
		Fat cells inhibition of lipolysis
Beta 1	Heart, fat cells, CNS	Activates adenylate cyclase
Beta 2	Respiratory, uterine and vascular smooth muscle	Activates adenylate cyclase

the nutrients released are more easily absorbed into the body, and fewer are lost in the voided feces.

Animals, including birds, must not be treated with products containing tiamulin while receiving salinomycin or for at least 7 days before or after receiving food containing tiamulin. Severe growth depression or death may result.

IONOPHORE TOXICITY

Ionophores can be directly toxic to sheep, cattle and horses, by incorrect feed inclusion rates. They also display serious drug interactions. Toxic interactions have been described between monensin and various therapeutic antibacterials used in turkeys, chickens, pigs, and calves; between narasin and tiamulin in chickens; and between salinomycin and tiamulin in chickens. Clinical cases of monensin poisoning have been reported after the accidental feeding of horses with a poultry premix, a cattle feed supplement, and a contaminated ration (Table 24–3).

Monensin is extremely toxic to some domestic animals, especially the equine species, if they ingest poultry or cattle rations containing the drug. Their toxicity to cattle, and especially to sheep and lambs, must not

be overlooked. Correct inclusion rates in feed are of critical importance. Monensin at recommended doses may also precipitate nitrite toxicity in cattle fed rations high in nitrate. Monensin intoxication can lead to a variety of clinicopathologic changes, depending on the species and the organs most severely affected. In cattle and horses, mild clinicopathologic changes and decreased exercise tolerance may be seen after a sublethal dose of monensin is ingested.

Typical signs of intoxication are as follows: anorexia, ataxia, depression, dyspnea, paralysis, and myoglobinuria. Ionophore antibiotic intoxication may result in a high rate of mortality. Postmortem investigations show necroses in the cardiac and skeletal muscles in all species. The clinicopathologic profile of horses suffering from monensin intoxication reflects cardiac, skeletal muscle, and kidney-related disturbances.

Monensin toxicosis should be suspected when recent changes in an animal's feed are followed by anorexia, ataxia, mild diarrhea, depression, dyspnea, stiffness, weakness, recumbency, and death—regardless of species. These signs are most pronounced in the horse, in which nonspecific colic, sweating, hypovolemic shock, and sudden death may also occur. The first deaths in cattle may occur more than 60 hours postingestion. Cattle often die with no signs of hyperexcitability or struggle. The prominent features of monensin toxicosis in sheep, swine, and dogs are muscle weakness and myoglobinuria.

The toxic effect of ionophores at the cell level is attributable to the formation of lipophilic complexes with monovalent and divalent cations, such as Na^+, K^+, and Ca^{2+}, whereby the transport of these ions across cell membranes is changed. Monensin transport of Na across cellular ion gradients leads to increased intracellular concentration of Na^+ ions. Increased intracellular sodium concentrations increase the influx of Ca^{2+} from the extracellular fluid, and the further increased intracellular Na^- concentrations accelerate the emanation of Ca^{2+} ions from the mitochondria with the following net result: intracellular toxic levels of Ca^{2+} ions. Accordingly, necroses in the skeletal muscles are caused by increased intracellular Ca^{2+} concentrations rather than disturbed Na^+-K^+ balance. Increased intracellular Ca^{2+} concentrations lead to strong activation of calcium/adenosine triphosphate and distribution of mitochondria. This mode of action also explains the anticoccidiostatic and antibacterial effect of ionophore polyether antibiotics.

Cardiomyopathy is reported in most species after monensin poisoning. The heart seems particularly vulnerable because its high energy demands are compromised by disturbances in the cellular physiology, which are attributed to ionophore activities. It is established that after skeletal muscle damage, creatine phosphokinase is released rapidly and cleared quickly, whereas aspartate aminotransferase (AST, formerly SGOT) is released less rapidly but persists longer in the circulation.

Alterations in equine serum enzyme concentrations generally reflect monensin-induced disruption of cell membranes. Skeletal muscle damage causes moderate (twofold to threefold) to massive (1000-fold) increases in the serum concentration of creatine phosphokinase. Because creatine phosphokinase is a cytosolic enzyme, concentrations increase early in the course of the poisoning as compared with the other enzyme alterations, such as concentrations of lactate dehydrogenase (LDH), which increase later.

The membrane-bound, red-blood-cell-related LDH isoenzyme is usually most prominent early in toxicosis. Later the cardiac-related isoenzyme becomes the major LDH component in serum. AST concentrations may be increased because of injury to muscle and hepatocytes; monensin is metabolized and stored in the liver.

In cattle, increases in serum, AST, and creatine phosphokinase concentrations are thought to be due primarily to muscle damage. Transient decreases in serum, potassium, sodium, and calcium concentrations have been seen 1 to 2 days after the onset of monensin toxicosis. These electrolyte changes probably occur secondary to diarrhea and rumenitis.

The range of clinical signs with salinomycin poisoning in horses—anorexia, depression, sweating, colic, dyspnea, weakness, recumbency, and ataxia—are similar to those recorded in horses with monensin poisoning. Similarly, the clinical pathology observed, although not extensive, indicates the same trend in the clinically overt cases that have been reported following poisoning, i.e., raised creatine phosphokinase, AST, and serum alkaline phosphatase activities. Although ionophore toxicity is rarely reported in horses, they appear to be particularly susceptible, and it should therefore be considered as a differential diagnosis of digestive upsets or locomotory disorders at establishments where ionophore-treated feeds are used therapeutically in other species.

Animals dying from lasalocid toxicity display froth in the trachea or bronchi, congested and edematous lungs, thoracic fluid, and a dilated heart at necropsy. Tissue sections reveal cardiac lesions, including myocyte necrosis, increased eosinophilia, and vascular degeneration, plus pulmonary edema. Lesions of monensin toxicity are similar to those of lasalocid, i.e., cardiomyopathy and pulmonary edema.

The diagnosis of ionophore poisoning is difficult because none of the clinical signs are pathognomonic and tissue samples do not betray toxic levels, although the presence and quantity of ionophores in feed or gut contents may be determined in the laboratory.

MANAGEMENT OF TOXICOSIS

As has been emphasized, ionophore antibiotics have a narrow safety margin (low therapeutic index), and by simultaneous use with other drugs, the metabolism and elimination of ionophores from the animal are inhibited. This leads to relatively higher concentrations of ionophores in the tissues and the risk of intoxication. Also, excessive inclusion rates in feed, especially for lambs, can give rise to problems. There is no antidote to polyether antibiotic intoxication. Vitamin E therapy may, however, alleviate symptoms. In the case of ionophore toxicity in pigs, it is important to differentiate the diagnosis from selenium and vitamin E deficiency and from the porcine stress syndrome.

Treatment is primarily supportive. Because ionophores are lipid soluble, mineral oil given early in toxic cases may sequester any remaining monensin within the gastrointestinal tract. Large volumes of intravenous isotonic fluids combat dehydration and hypovolemic shock and minimize renal damage. In all surviving cases, the recovery is protracted, requiring extended convalescence and an awareness of the possibility of a persistent cardiomyopathy. Experimental pigs that had been treated with vitamin E and selenium before dosing with monensin subsequently produced fewer adverse clinical signs, but the effectiveness of this treatment in other species is as yet undetermined and, once toxicity has begun, is extremely dubious.

For supportive therapy, pigs pretreated with 0.25 mg of selenium (as selenite) and 17 IU of alpha-tocopherol acetate per kilogram intramuscularly 1 day before dosing with monensin at 40 mg/kg orally suffered fewer adverse clinical signs than control pigs. This is thought to result because the cell membranes are protected from peroxidation.

Monensin is known to act by selective transport of sodium and potassium ions between extracellular and intracellular spaces. Movements of sodium ions across cell membranes are associated with changes in behavior of cellular calcium ions. Excess calcium ions have been suggested to be of potential importance in monensin toxicity. The involvement of calcium ion may further be evidenced by reported pathologic lesions in cardiac and skeletal muscles of affected animals. Calcium channel blockers selectively inhibit entry of extracellular calcium through the "slow" channels and its movement intracellularly within the sarcoplasmic reticulum.

From a treatment standpoint, no specific compounds are known to alleviate or interact with monensin. Effects of some cardiovascular drugs that antagonize calcium influx in cardioskeletal and smooth muscle were evaluated in mice receiving varying lethal doses (80, 100, 120, or 140 mg/kg ip). Calcium channel blockers (verapamil, diltiazem, and lidocaine), a calmodulin antagonist (chlorpromazine), adrenergic-receptor blockers (yohimbine, tolazoline, and propranolol), and a cardiac glycoside (digoxin) were evaluated for their effects on monensin toxicity after 30-minutes pretreatments in mice ip. All the calcium modulators evaluated, apart from chlorpromazine, propranolol, and digoxin, potentiated monensin toxicity significantly ($P<0.05$) by decreasing the calculated LD 50 of monensin (108 mg/kg); the latter three drugs had no effect on monensin toxicity. Studies suggest that excess calcium ion influx may not be the only factor responsible for monensin toxicosis in mice.

VIRGINIAMYCIN

Virginiamycin, an antibiotic comprising two distinct chemical entities, has been used as a growth-enhancing agent in nonruminating animals. Virginiamycin has primarily gram-positive activity, with a unique synergism occurring between the two chemical components of the antibiotic complex.

Virginiamycin is an inhibitor of bacteria in the small intestine of the pig. Such inhibition produces energy sparing through reduced lactic acid formation in the gastrointestinal tract. Virginiamycin is selectively active against small intestine organisms, with little activity against fiber-digesting organisms of the cecal and large intestinal regions of the digestive tract.

Virginiamycin's selective inhibition of lactate-producing bacteria prompted study of its effect on rumen fermentation. Growth trials have also been conducted, along with measures of virginiamycin's safety in cattle. Virginiamycin, monensin, and lasalocid were all shown to manipulate rumen fermentation in vitro toward increased propionic acid production. The ionophores monensin and lasalocid produce the greatest shift in VFA formation, whereas virginiamycin appears to produce initial manipulation at lower concentrations (0.15 to 0.5 parts/10^6) than the ionophores. VFA production is not inhibited by monensin, lasalocid, or virginiamycin. D- and L-lactic acid production is inhibited by virginiamycin at concentrations of 0.05 parts/10^6 or greater. Ionophores are less effective than virginiamycin in blocking lactic acid production.

Virginiamycin produces increased growth and feed use efficiency in steers. The major response to virginiamycin occurs early in the fattening period. During the growing phase, virginiamycin improves growth rate by 6.25% and feed use by 3.3%. Response to virginiamycin is smaller during the fattening phase, leaving an overall virginiamycin response of 2 to 3% for both growth and feed use efficiency.

An equally exciting challenge is to implant cultured cells fed to pigs at a rate of 15–50 ppm to 34 kg/4 months), the use of proprietary nondusting formulations, and the wearing of protective clothing when mixing carbadox in the ration.

The importance to pigs of quinoxalines started about many years ago, when quindoxin was marketed as an antibacterial growth promoter. Because of deleterious effects on humans handling this compound, it was rapidly withdrawn from use. A number of analogs were subsequently studied to fill the niche created by the withdrawal of quindoxin. Of these, carbadox was initially the main drug in use, but suspicion of its safety arose, and toxicologic data concerning human safety became paramount as prerequisites for the introduction of new quinoxalines. One aspect was the phototoxicity of quinoxalines. Quindoxin caused persistent photocontact dermatitis in several agricultural workers. According to the results of research and the clinical data on quindoxin, olaquindox, and carbadox should also be regarded as potential photoallergic agents.

The growing concern of consumer groups and of policy makers in drug regulatory agencies regarding the mutagenic and carcinogenic potency of the quinoxalines and their possible residues in food animal products has caused much debate.

24.4 HORMONAL GROWTH PROMOTERS

A significant, and controversial, pharmacologic development has been the introduction of the various anabolic-type hormonal growth promoters for use in beef cattle. That these substances are effective growth-promoting agents is beyond dispute, but some additional information may yet be required to underline their absolute potential uses, their precise pharmacologic and physiologic effects in treated animals, and their potential hazards to the food-producing animals and ultimately to the consumer.

The metabolic processes of animals, their growth rates, and therefore their speed of fattening are controlled and coordinated by hormones produced within the body. The various processes and accompanying behavioral effects can be modified by the simple surgical interference of castration in the male and spaying in the female. Bulls grow faster and lay down more lean meat in the carcass than steers; steers grow faster with a higher feed conversion efficiency than cows.

The differences in growth rates can be attributed to the hormonal status differences between the various animals. The hormones that have received most study and investigation in this context are the sex hormones produced by the gonads, which in untreated animals are responsible for the large differences in growth rate and rate of maturity (i.e., speed of fattening between intact males and females).

In ruminants, the sex hormones are responsible for the large differences in the rate of growth and fat deposition between males and females. The decreased level of androgens in castrated males results in the intermediate performance of the steer and is of course responsible for the desirable absence of secondary sexual characteristics. The possibility has arisen of modifying the effect of or supplementing the endogenous hormones by the administration of exogenous hormonal substances from outside the body. Anabolic agents possess physiologic properties similar to the natural sex steroids—testosterone is the parent androgen, and estradiol 17β is an estrogen. These hormones, or semisynthetic derivatives of them, can be implanted into cattle or sheep to supplement and complement the endogenous level of sex steroids, and this creates the hormonal status most favorable for growth.

To achieve maximum growth stimulation potential, androgens and estrogens must be present in concentrations that approximate to those circulating in entire bulls and cows. The objective has been the development of products that would restore the growth potential removed by castration and at the same time retain docile characteristics.

The use of appropriate anabolic agents creates a hormonal situation in castrates, females, and young stock that is similar to that found in intact males and pregnant females. Accordingly, the greatest benefits are seen in cows treated with androgens, bulls treated with estrogens, and castrates treated with combined preparations of androgens and estrogens.

PRINCIPLES IN USING GROWTH PROMOTERS

In general, the principle that dictates which type of hormone to be used is to supplement or replace the particular hormone type that is deficient in the animal to be treated:

- Females—produce estrogens normally, so better results obtained from the administration of androgens, e.g., trenbolone acetate. In some cases, however, anabolic responses are obtained by giving supplemental estrogens, e.g., culled cows.
- Steers—because the testes produce both androgens and estrogens, maximum anabolic responses obtained in steers from a combination of an estrogen and an androgen.
- Bulls—produce high quantities of androgens; therefore estrogens the hormones of choice to use in bull beef production. It must be remembered that estrogens suppress gonadotropic output (luteinizing hormone and follicle-stimulating hor-

mone secretion) from the pituitary, and this results in the suppression of testes growth. In beef production, this can be an advantage, but the corollary is that estrogens should not be used in males.

Age of the animal affects response, with variable responses being obtained in calves and consistent responses obtained from yearlings onward.

FORMULATION

Most anabolic-hormonal-type agents are presented in the form of implants, which are sterile preparations designed specifically so depots of drug can be stored at a site in the body tissues to release active drug slowly. They are usually pellets or small tablets, with or without excipients, compressed under aseptic conditions and implanted in the dorsal surface of the ear. As a practical means of medication, the pellet is limited to drugs of high potency, and to date only hormones have met this requirement. The implant is in essence a small sterile tablet manufactured by compression. It may be composed of essentially pure drug or contain other adjuvants, which act to modify the rate of absorption. Experimental data are usually required to produce a pellet, with a desired release characteristic giving a slow steady "pay out" of active principle over a period of time. Usually the first approach is one of compression of essentially pure drug into small pellets implanted in the target animal, and the plasma levels coupled with growth promotional effects are then determined over time. These preliminary data indicate whether the absorption rate of pellet must be increased or decreased.

A minimum concentration of anabolic agent in the blood and tissues is necessary to obtain the maximum growth response in animals. An ideal formulation supplies the agent at a constant rate. The release of drug from an implant should be of a zero order nature, i.e., the release of drug is independent of the amount of drug remaining in the pellet. This type of release may not always be attained because as the implant is absorbed, its geometric shape alters also, thus presenting a smaller surface area for absorption. What tends to occur is that the most rapid rate of absorption occurs initially, with an ever-decreasing amount being released as the pellet erodes. Thus after a few months, the concentrations in blood and tissues are too low to be effective. The initial level of drug in the plasma must therefore be substantially above the minimum effective level so an effective concentration is still obtained at the end of the desired release period. Although this necessitates the use of an agent of a high safety margin, it also necessitates much wastage of drug, a considerable portion of which may remain as a residue at the site of implantation in the ear. In combined implants, the rate of absorption of estradiol 17β, a natural estrogen, is reduced and persists for much longer than when estradiol is implanted alone or at a separate site. Further, estradiol 17β is released at a more constant rate from a pellet containing an intimate mixture of two steroids than from a pellet containing estradiol alone. A number of preparations are available containing estradiol 17β in combination with either testosterone or progesterone, and the efficacy of these products may be attributable in part to the slower release of the estradiol into the circulation. The effect of androgen and progesterone on estradiol absorption is probably a physical effect at the site of implantation, resulting from an intimate mixing with a higher amount of a second steroid. There may also be a pharmacokinetic dimension, however, insofar as the liver clearance and half-life of some steroids is influenced by the administration of others.

One particular polymeric material, silicone rubber, has been extensively studied as a matrix base for various hormonal implants. The permeability characteristics together with tissue compatibility of Silastic polymers provide the basis for their use as novel drug delivery systems. The rate of drug transport through or across the silicone rubber matrix depends largely on the lipophilicity of the drug, the concentration of the drug in the matrix, the surface area and thickness of the encapsulating polymer, and its diffusional characteristics. Estradiol 17β is now available in the form of an impregnated Silastic polymer, and this is claimed to give a more uniform release than a simple compression pellet of estradiol alone. Previous studies in sheep and cattle have shown that the rate of absorption of estradiol 17β from compressed pellets was delayed when the pellets contained an intimate mixture of estradiol 17β with trenbolone acetate. Further, the estradiol 17β was released at a more nearly constant rate from a pellet containing the mixture than from a pellet containing estradiol 17β alone.

Anabolic agents are available commercially in which estradiol 17β is combined with testosterone, progesterone, and in Synovex-H and Synovex-S (Syntex) preparations for heifers and steers, respectively. The efficacy of these formulations may be due in part to the possibility that the estradiol 17β is released into the circulation more slowly and steadily in the presence of the second steroid.

CLASSIFICATION OF COMPOUNDS USED

According to their biological activity, hormonal growth promoters can be classified into compounds with estrogenic, androgenic, and gestagenic activity and according to their chemical structure into endogenous steroids, extraneous steroids, and nonsteroidal extraneous compounds.

Stilbenes

These compounds, which were used in animal production, have now been banned in Europe and the United States because of their potential carcinogenic activity.

Natural Steroids

These three hormones, estradiol 17β, testosterone, and progesterone, are produced as part of the normal reproductive processes in mammals. They can now be produced synthetically in sufficient quantities and at a cost that allows their use as anabolic agents.

The major physiologically active estrogen, estradiol 17β is produced by the ovarian follicle in the female. Its production follows a cyclical pattern during the normal estrus cycle of farm animals and causes the behavioral changes associated with estrus. During pregnancy, estrogen concentrations rise and reach high levels before parturition.

Either estradiol 17β or derivatives of it, which are broken down to release the natural compound, are used as growth promoters in livestock production. Other compounds that have similar physiologic effects to estradiol are said to be estrogenic. Estradiol 17β can be produced synthetically.

Testosterone, the male sex hormone, is the major steroid produced by the Leydig cells of the testis. It is responsible for the development and maintenance of male sexual characteristics. Other compounds that have similar physiologic effects to testosterone are said to be androgenic.

Testosterone is produced by bacterial fermentation, using *Acetobacter pasteurianum*, from androstendiol. Further steps, involving precipitation with digitonin and formation of the semicarbazone, are required to produce pure testosterone.

Progesterone is the major hormone involved in the maintenance of pregnancy in farm animals. It is produced by the corpus luteum, which develops in the ovary after ovulation. High concentrations of progesterone are maintained throughout pregnancy or until just before the next ovulation in a nonpregnant cow. Compounds having similar physiologic effects to progesterone are said to be progestagenic. Progesterone is synthesized chemically.

Zeranol

Zeranol is a nonsteroidal compound with estrogenic activity, which is manufactured by International Mineral and Chemical Corporation under the trade name Ralgro. Zeranol is produced by reduction of the natural product zearalenone, which is produced by fermentation from the mold *Giberalla zeae*. This mycotoxin from *fusarium* species was originally identified by its estrogenic effects on sows fed moldy grain.

Trenbolone Acetate

Trenbolone acetate is a synthetic steroid with androgenic activity, some 10 to 50 times greater than that of testosterone.

COMMERCIALLY AVAILABLE ANABOLIC PREPARATIONS

Synovex-S

This implant contains 200 mg of progesterone and 20 mg of estradiol benzoate (which is metabolized by the animal to estradiol) in eight pellets. The progesterone principally helps offset side effects of the estrogen (such as "bulling"), although it also stimulates faster growth to a limited extent. Synovex-S is registered for use in steers, and its effects are claimed to last for 90 to 200 days. There is no withdrawal period for Synovex-S.

Synovex-H

This implant is registered for use in female cattle. It contains 200 mg testosterone propionate and 20 mg estradiol benzoate in eight pellets and has no statutory withdrawal period.

Synovex-C

This implant is designed for calves and contains 100 mg progesterone and 10 mg estradiol benzoate, and there is no withdrawal period.

Compudose 365 and 200

Compudose 365 is an implant containing 45 mg of estradiol 17β Compudose 200 is a similar implant but contains 24 mg of active ingredient. The unique feature of this product is that the steroid is impregnated into a silicone rubber cylinder, which forms the implant. This mode of delivery reduces the initial rate of drug release and prolongs the period for which the implant can be used. The amount of drug delivered depends on the surface area of the implant (size, 3 cm long and 4.8 mm diameter), and the thickness of the impregnated coating determines the duration of the implant's active life.

The implant is inserted subcutaneously into the ear and lasts for either 200 or 365 days. Controlled release of estradiol 17β is claimed to occur for 200 days (Compudose 200) or approximately 1 year (Compudose 365). It is easily seen and palpated in situ, in contrast to other implants. It is suitable for all ages of steers and has no withdrawal period. Compudose is currently registered for use in steers and cull cows, although there is also interest in its use in entire bulls and heifers destined for slaughter.

Ralgro

Zeranol (Ralgro) is licensed for use to improve weight gain and feed efficiency in cattle. The dose is 36 mg, contained in three small pellets. It is most widely used and is probably most advantageous in steers, although there is also evidence of some beneficial effects in heifers, cows, and bulls, and suckling calves. Its effects appear to last for approximately 100 days.

Finaplix

Trenbolone acetate (Finaplix, Hoechst) is licensed for use in steers, heifers, and cull cows being fattened for beef. The implant consists of 300 mg trenbolone acetate contained in 15 pellets. Ten implants are contained in each cartridge. Because it is androgenic in nature, trenbolone is used to greatest advantage in heifers and cows. It is used in steers preferentially as a finishing implant, i.e., during the last 3 months before slaughter. The maximum growth effect is obtained when combined with an estrogen.

MODE OF ACTION OF ANABOLIC AGENTS

Protein synthesis (anabolism) and protein breakdown (catabolism) are functions of all active cells and occur continuously. These are inherent properties of normal physiologic functioning, but they are capable of modification by many influences, especially by anabolic and catabolic hormones and their derivatives. The major anabolic hormones include androgens, estrogens, growth hormone, and insulin. The major catabolic hormones are corticosteroids, thyroxin, and adrenaline. Many other factors, such as the nutrient energy supply, oxygen tension, electrolyte, and acid-base balance, affect the anabolism-to-catabolism ratio. Anabolic or myotrophic effects are reflected by an increased nitrogen retention and the growth and development of bone. The main clinical applications of anabolic agents rest on their ability to promote a positive nitro-

gen balance by increasing the level of protein synthesis, without altering absorption or metabolism in the alimentary tract.

Most of the anabolic hormones and sex steroids act directly on the muscle cell by interacting with specific receptors. The steroid is released at its target cell, and it then enters the cell itself, where it binds to a specific cytoplasmic receptor (cytosolic receptor), which after undergoing a transformation enters the nucleus and binds to chromatin. This complex then activates RNA polymerase activity and the consequent synthesis of RNA, which then returns to the cytoplasm to initiate protein synthesis at an increased rate.

In androgenic compounds, these substances are believed to act locally on muscle cells through specific local receptors, acting to regulate protein synthesis and degradation, promoting protein accretion, and decreasing protein turnover rates. Testosterone, the parent androgen is usually reduced to the dihydrotestosterone form by 5 alpha reductase before it can bring about its androgenic effects, and it has been postulated that differences exist in the nature of the receptors responsible for androgenic as distinct from anabolic activity. This difference in selectivity has enabled synthetic anabolic derivatives to be prepared with high affinity for the anabolic-type muscle receptors and minimal affinity for the androgenic-type receptors. Another mechanism of action of androgenic-type compounds is one of reducing protein degradation by displacing the catabolic corticosteroids from their receptor sites. Thus the overall anabolic action at the local tissue level may be more of an anticatabolic effect resulting in a net increase in protein synthesis, with a consequent enhancement of feed conversion efficiency.

One of the secondary, indirect effects of treatment with trenbolone acetate in steers is a reduction in the plasma concentration of total thyroxine. This relative hypothyroid state may also result in improved growth and efficiency of feed use.

In contrast to the androgens, the estrogenic-type anabolic agents most likely act through the various hormones controlling energy metabolism. After estrogen treatment of ruminants, plasma concentrations of both insulin and growth hormones are increased, and elevated levels of these substances at the muscle cell result in increased protein accretion by increasing amino acid uptake. The major anabolic effects of estrogens occur via increased outpouring of growth hormone from the pituitary, and the raised plasma insulin concentrations are secondary to the changes in plasma glucose. The increase in secretion of growth hormone also results in a small increase in plasma glucose concentration. The combination of increased growth hormone and insulin in the muscle cell probably increases protein accretion.

Estrogens do not appear to have a direct effect on muscle cells but act on the hypothalamus or pituitary gland to increase the secretion of growth hormone. Most of these anabolic effects mediated by growth hormone are exemplified by nitrogen retention, increased protein deposition, and greater retention of calcium and phosphorus. Insulin secretion is also affected by estrogen compounds.

The net effect of all these steroids is to increase protein accretion (accumulation) inside the muscle cell. In trenbolone at least, this seems to be brought about by decreasing the natural rate of protein catabolism (breakdown) rather than increasing the rate of synthesis. The overall effect is to increase the rate of daily live weight gain, feed conversion efficiency, and proportion of lean meat in the carcass. Owing to the increase in feed intake, the percentage increase in efficiency is approximately half that of the increase in growth rate.

ADMINISTRATION

For all these hormonal substances to exert their desired effect, the method of administration to the animal is important. The best method is one in which the desired hormone level is sustained for as long as is necessary. Further, the preparation should leave only minimal, safe residues in the carcass. For this purpose, the anabolic agents are usually administered in pellet form as subcutaneous implants in the ear. This site is chosen because it is a relatively avascular area, thus retarding the rate of pickup of the drug into the blood stream. This allows for a controlled slow release of the active prin-

ciple, which is then gradually absorbed into the blood stream over a period of time, exposing the animal to a constant hormonal stimulating effect of the anabolic agent, which then modulates growth rate of the animal. At the end of the withdrawal period, up to 10% of the initial dose may still be found at the site of implantation in some cases. It is therefore important that all implanting is done on the dorsal surface of the ear beneath the loose skin overlying the conchal cartilage. This area is then discarded at slaughter. Care must always be taken to avoid the major blood vessels and to avoid crushing or wetting the pellets because this could result in rapid absorption, possible behavioral effects, and failure to obtain proper growth promotion and elevated blood and tissue levels. The overall rate of absorption of an agent from an implant can be influenced by a number of factors, including technique of administration; integrity of the pellets; total dosage given; presence of a second steroid in the pellet; implant size, shape, and hardness; and nature of the base materials used. These pellet-type implants have an effective duration of 90 to 100 days, and additive responses are obtained in beef systems when they are given every 100 days or so. In general, best results are obtained in animals from 1 year of age onward because the younger animal is growing close to maximum efficiency when well fed.

ANIMAL BEHAVIOR AFTER IMPLANTS

All implanted cattle succumb to stress more easily than nonimplanted cattle. The major problem arises from the use of estradiol as a growth promoter. Its use has been associated with increased mounting behavior and aggression. These effects generally last for 1 to 10 days after implantation and then subside. In some cases, size of rudimentary teats can be increased. In extreme circumstances, however, there have been a small number of reports of undesirable behavior in steers that has lasted for 1 to 10 weeks. To minimize these effects, it is important:

• Not to crush the implant when inserting it in the ear
• Not to implant cattle on wet days

- Not to have group sizes of implanted steers greater than about 40 in one area
- Not to mix steers with strange cattle and to avoid sudden changes in diet and environment

HAZARDS TO THE ANIMAL

If incorrectly implanted into breeding heifers, reproductive function may be severely impaired by androgenic anabolic steroids. The type and degree of impairment probably depends on the timing and duration of the implant, but the following hazards have been demonstrated with either trenbolone acetate or trenbolone acetate plus estradiol given to heifer calves at 4 months and again at 7 months of age:

1. A delay of 10 to 18 weeks in the age of puberty
2. Virilization of external genitalia
3. Impaired udder development with subsequent severe reduction in milk yield
4. A high incidence of dystocia

These changes persist for a considerable time after the anabolic steroids are no longer detectable in the plasma.

Some impairment of reproductive function also occurs with estrogenic anabolic agents. Although little information has been published, there is enough to indicate that no long-acting anabolic steroid should be implanted in breeding stock. Subsequent infertility may result caused by gonadotropin suppression.

Changes in behavior after implantation can also be a hazard. In a major survey in the United States, 3.7% of illness in feedlot steers was due to mounting and riding. The incidence has been rising with the increased use of anabolic agent implants.

RESPONSES TO GROWTH PROMOTANTS

In numerous trials carried out under many different husbandry and feeding systems, growth-promoting agents have increased the rate of live weight gain. It is still difficult to predict the magnitude of a growth response, although it is known to depend on a variety of factors. The main principles involved and known causes of variation in response are as follows:

- Growth responses are generally greatest in castrated animals with lower levels of circulating endogenous hormones and less in entire animals. Also, younger and lighter cattle respond less than older and heavier cattle.
- Estrogens are more effective in entire males, and androgenic agents are more effective in females, whereas in steers, most benefit derived is from a combination of the two. This may be a consequence of a higher level of specific enzymes for metabolism of the main natural circulating hormones for each sex, that is, less capacity for breaking down excess androgens in females and estrogens in males.
- Cattle that are growing at a fast rate (at least 1.0 kg/day, e.g., steers on good quality pasture or in a feedlot) respond better than those on a low plane of nutrition. Little response has been reported on feed supporting growth of less than 0.5 kg/day.
- The combined use of implanted anabolic agents and dietary ionophores (e.g., monensin, lasalocid), which modify rumenal fermentation, has an additive effect of feed conversion efficiency. The growth promotant increases both feed intake and growth rate; the ionophores usually reduce feed intake of concentrates, while either not affecting or increasing daily gain.

Since zeranol first became commercially available in the United States, numerous studies have demonstrated its effectiveness in improving weight gains in yearling steers, which are probably the most responsive class of cattle. Zeranol has been especially favored for use in intensive production systems, in which weight gains generally have been increased by 10 to 15% (8 to 20 kg) in 70 to 100 days, with feed conversion efficiency increased by 6 to 7%.

Estradiol benzoate-progesterone implants (Synovex-C) have been specifically registered for use in calves and are reported to have increased growth rate by between 4.3 and 10% in steer and heifer calves weighing about 70 kg at implantation. Experiments in the United States using estradiol 17β in lot-fed steers showed increases in average daily gain of 15.6% (12 kg extra over 124 days) compared with an increase of 8.1% (6 kg) by feeding monensin alone. Together the responses were additive and increased average gain by 27.4% (21 kg).

It appears that provided that steers have sufficient good quality pasture to support weight gains of at least 0.6 kg/day, the minimum extra gain that can be expected after treatment with zeranol is approximately 6 kg in 50 to 100 days. On better pastures, the increment in weight gain is more than 10 kg (>0.1 kg/day). Similar increases have been shown in Australia in steers treated with estradiol 17β. The best response reported in Australia is a weight advantage above controls of 42 to 50 kg in 203 days after repeated implantation with zeranol.

RESPONSE IN HEIFERS

Growth promotants cannot be recommended without qualification for use in heifers that may be used for breeding. Development and function of the reproductive organs can be impaired by longterm implantation with growth promotants. Zeranol (Ralgro), which is weakly estrogenic (between 1/300 and 1/800 times that of estradiol 17β) has been shown to interact directly with estrogen receptors and evoke many of the same biological and biochemical responses as the natural estrogen, estradiol. Longterm implantation can therefore stimulate negative feedback systems to the pituitary, disrupt cyclical activity, retard development, and compromise normal fertility. Responses to implantation of heifers in the United States also include about 10% higher rates of gain. Similarly, Australian experiments with trenbolone acetate (Finaplix) using heifers and culled cows have shown weight gain advantages of 10 to 26% (15 to 25 kg increase depending on the initial weight of the heifers or cows) above those of controls produced in 90 to 100 days.

SAFETY ASPECTS

It is important that the correct implantation technique is followed. The recommended location for implants other than zeranol is under the skin in the center one-third of the back of the ear. Zeranol should be implanted under the skin at the base of the ear. Errors that are commonly made include:

- Crushing the implant (pellet-forms), which releases the active ingredient too quickly, reduces its life span, and may increase the side effects. After insertion, the needle should be partially withdrawn before injecting the implant to allow space for the implant.
- Inserting the implant into the cartilage, where there is minimal blood supply, results in no absorption of the active agent. If implanted into the skin, the absorption rate is also reduced.
- Severing a blood vessel in the ear can occur. If the implant is deposited in the resultant hematoma, absorption is too rapid.

SIDE EFFECTS

In steers treated with estrogenic-type implants, one common side effect is an increased incidence of raised tail head settings; this may adversely affect market value. The phenomenon is caused by a relaxation of the sacrosciatic ligaments, which allows the tailbone to move slightly upward and over the rump. It usually develops within 1 month of implanting and often disappears by the time the cattle are marketed. There is no evidence to suggest that this effect adversely influences carcass yield or quality. Other side effects in steers include an increase in bulling behavior, attempted mounts and head-to-head contacts for the first few days after implantation, and some mammary development and enlargement of the testes.

In females, the main side effects of anabolics relate to their influence on the reproductive system already noted, although raised tailhead settings, increased bulling behavior, and mammary development have also been reported in heifers. The effect of estrogenic anabolics on reproduction in heifers appears to be mainly a delay in the age of attainment of puberty and lower conception rates of heifers implanted repeatedly or in those still containing.

POSSIBLE CONSUMER CONCERNS— ENDOGENOUS STEROIDS

Two naturally occurring female sex hormones, estradiol and progesterone, and one male sex hormone, testosterone, are used as growth promoters in beef cattle. The use of any kind of drug in food-producing animals requires a risk-benefit analysis. In discussing the safety of anabolic agents, a convenient distinction has been made between the natural and the synthetic hormones. One of the major concerns has been that perhaps these substances could enter the human food chain at unacceptably high levels and so put the consumer at risk. In animals and humans, there are specialized metabolizing pathways by which the naturally occurring endogenous compounds are broken down to inactive compounds in the liver and then rapidly excreted. They also possess a short half-life in the body, and for the most part they are not orally active. In addition, they are produced in large amounts in the human body depending on factors such as sex, age, and physiologic status. The sex hormones are secreted by the gonads, the adrenal gland, and placenta, the level of secretion being controlled by a complex but well-established feedback mechanism. They exert their hormonal effect at target tissues by binding to specific cytosolic receptors and initiate major physiologic effects in only trace amounts.

When steroids are administered orally, a considerable fraction of the total dose is inactivated in the liver and possibly also in the intestinal mucosa. The absorbed fraction of the dose is carried to the liver via the portal system, and the consequent rapid rate of metabolism in the liver results in the rapid excretion of inactive metabolites and a relatively short half-life for the drug. Attempts have been made to prolong the short half-life of many hormones by altering the chemical structure, especially at position 17 of the molecule (site of conjugation and metabolite formation). This considerably increases the resistance of the compound to inactivation by the liver and ensures that a major portion of an oral dose form reaches the general circulation in an active form. Ethinyl estradiol is one such form of estradiol that is used commonly in human medicine for oral administration. Although this modification of the molecule at C-17 increases the oral bioavailability of the hormone, it is still necessary for the oral dose to exceed considerably the parenteral form for comparable biological activity. Thus, although absorption of the natural parent steroids from the intestinal tract is relatively rapid, because of their susceptibility to rapid hepatic degradation and conjugation, they have relatively low oral bioavailability and are not regarded as orally active.

Most of the catabolism of endogenous steroids occurs in the liver, most likely during the first passage of the hormone, and enterohepatic circulation may then occur, with the metabolites exerting little if any biological activity. In cattle, most of the steroids are eliminated along the fecal route, where 60 to 90% of the metabolites are found in the free form, whereas the steroids excreted with the urine are predominantly conjugated.

Conjugated estradiol 17α is the major circulating estrogen after implantation of estradiol 17β. A large percentage of these metabolites is excreted directly in the bile after conjugation (glucuronides, sulfates), and metabolites, both free and conjugated, may be found in the tissues, particularly in the kidney and liver.

The development of well-validated radioimmunoassay methods to detect natural hormones in body tissues has allowed quantification of the normal physiologic levels of these substances and permits baseline comparisons with levels attained after the use of natural hormones as implants. Owing to the natural production of endogenous steroids in animals, the residues of these steroids are qualitatively indistinguishable from those derived from the use of these same steroids as anabolic agents. Using sensitive analytical techniques, levels of estradiol 17β have been measured in untreated animals and in animals treated with estrogenic implants. Comparisons have also been made between the production of endogenous estrogens by humans and animals as well as the estrogenic content of meat and milk. In other words, studies have been directed toward determining the residues in animal tissues resulting from implantation with natural hormones and comparing these levels with the normal physiologic levels of the body.

Results have indicated that the treatment of animals with exogenous natural steroids results in residues in edible tissues that are of orders of magnitude lower than those occurring in mature males, females, and pregnant females. In addition, the daily production rates of these same hormones by humans vastly exceeds those that could be ingested by consuming meat from implanted animals. The low oral bioavailability (10 to 15%) of these steroids and the existing pharmacologic barriers at the level of the liver and placenta effectively prevent any adverse effects from the ingestion of these trace residues.

SYNTHETIC STEROIDS—TRENBOLONE

Trenbolone acetate is a synthetic steroidal substance with hormonal-type activity that affects physiologic processes in the animal body. Although chemically related to testosterone, it possesses minimal androgenic activity but greater anabolic activity. It is also chemically less stable than testosterone because it possesses three conjugated double bonds. After insertion of trenbolone implants in the ear, the compound is released slowly, and at slaughter 65 days after implantation, levels of trenbolone are lower than those of testosterone in muscle, liver, and fat. Trenbolone acetate is rapidly hydrolyzed to trenbolone in the body, and its metabolites are rapidly excreted as the glucuronides and sulfates, mostly in the bile. The major metabolite of the trenbolone in cattle is 17-hydroxytrenbolone. Of the residue in cattle liver, it has been shown that approximately 10% is 17β hydroxytrenbolone, and 90% is 17α hydroxytrenbolone. The biological activity of 17α hydroxytrenbolone is estimated to be one twentieth of the 17β metabolite. Thus in this extraneous steroid trenbolone, a catabolism to biologically less active metabolites occurs in the liver, accounting for the low oral activity of this particular steroid.

As with other growth promoters, the metabolic and excretory tissues contain the highest residues of trenbolone acetate. After implantation with 300 mg radiolabeled trenbolone acetate, the liver shows the highest tissue concentration (33 ppb equivalents) (mean value) 60 days postimplantation. The bioavailability of this residue when fed to rats reportedly is 12%, so the effective residue level could be regarded as being 12% of 33 ppb, i.e., 4 ppb. Of this 4 ppb absorbable residue, 3.6 ppb constitutes the 17α metabolite and 0.4 ppb the 17β metabolite (metabolite studies). The biological activity of the 17α metabolite is estimated to be only one twentieth of the 17β metabolite, so in terms of biological activity, 0.2 ppb of the 3.6 ppb residue possesses biological activity. This gives a total residue in liver in terms of biologically active absorbable residue 60 days postimplantation of 0.4 plus 0.2 ppb. In other words, from a total liver residue in cattle of 33 ppb, approximately 0.6 ppb is biologically active and absorbable.

The residue values quoted are those of total radioactivity resulting from implantation with radiolabeled trenbolone. These residues are therefore a combination of parent compound plus metabolites. More specific methods of analysis, such as radioimmunoassay, would indicate far lower residues because the more specific the assay method, the more metabolites that are ignored. It is quite possible that in different species, different metabolic pathways and hence different metabolites occur after the administration of trenbolone. Using fairly standard longterm toxicologic procedures in the rat, it is possible that these metabolites may not be evaluated because the rat does not produce these types of metabolites. It could therefore happen that the human consumer could be exposed to these metabolites, which occur in beef tissue.

One way around this, however, is to use the relay toxicity technique, which simply involves feeding various tissues from the target species containing total residue (extractable and unextractable metabolites) to the rat. These tissues then contain metabolites to which humans may be exposed. To date, these relay toxicity studies indicate low oral bioavailability of the residues to the rat (10%) and little evidence of toxicity. Relay toxicity studies involving feeding tissues from treated veal calves to rats, involving a safety factor of 100, have given no indication of any adverse teratologic effect on reproductive performance nor any other toxicologic effect.

Because many hormonal-type substances have the potential to bind to protein, this area also has received considerable attention in evaluating the potential toxicity of many of the anabolic-type substances. In the cases of trenbolone, protein-bound residues seem to form a sizable fraction of the total residue formed. It has also been established that certain estrogens may covalently bind to proteins. The biological significance of this phenomenon is not clearly understood to date but such residues appear to have low oral bioavailability, based on subsequent refeeding experiments to rodents (relay toxicity tests).

Potential genotoxicity and carcinogenicity can be evaluated by mutagenicity tests and by the capacity for DNA binding. From the available evidence to date on the results of the Ames test, the mouse lymphoma forward mutation assay, the mouse bone marrow cytogenetic assay, and DNA binding studies, there is little evidence that either natural or synthetic agents are mutagenic. It has been pointed out that zeranol and trenbolone are not given to humans, and once covalently fixed to DNA, they can no longer be detached in the primitive state and fixed to another DNA, thus posing negligible risk to the consumer.

In short, trenbolone is metabolized in the animal body to a 17β compound with much lower biological activity. At slaughter, 65 days after implantation, levels of trenbolone are minimal and are lower than those of testosterone in muscle liver and fat. Meat from cattle implanted with high doses of trenbolone and fed to rats indicated toxicity in the rat and indicated also low oral bioavailability.

ZERANOL

This compound belongs to the chemical group known as the resorcyclic acid lactones. Zeranol is obtained by hydrogenation of zearalenone, which in turn is a mycotoxin produced by several of the *Fusarium* species of fungus, in particular *Gibberella zeae*. Zeranol is a nonsteroidal anabolic semisynthetic agent possessing some (minimal) estrogenic properties. The metabolism of zeranol has been studied in many species, including cattle and sheep, and the major metabolite is zearalenone. A minor metabolite, taleranol, has been identified in the rabbit. Most orally administered zeranol is absorbed and eliminated in the feces and urine as both free drug and conjugated metabolite.

After subcutaneous implantation of 36 mg of tritiated zeranol in cattle, the biological half-life is predominantly a function of the rate of drug release and absorption from the implant because the rate is slow compared with the rate of elimination of the drug. Based on the zeranol content of implants recovered from implanted cattle, 96.3% of the zeranol is absorbed from the implant in 65 days. Zeranol and its major metabolite zearalenone are excreted through the bile in all species except rabbits and humans: In the latter two species, urinary excretion is predominant. Most orally administered zeranol disappears from the tissues within 24 hours except for the liver and kidney. The compound may be regarded as an impeded or mimetic estrogen, and in terms of endocrine-related biological activity, it has some affinity for estrogenic receptors, with in vitro assays indicating that it possesses about 20% of the estrogenic activity of estradiol. Zeranol and its metabolites are of a low order of toxicity, and the acute oral LD 50 for the mouse and rat exceeds 40,000 mg/kg. This toxicity could be regarded as insignificant when compared with other drugs. Zeranol has undergone longterm toxicity testing in rats, dogs, and monkeys: No increase in the incidence of neoplasia was observed in any of these studies. A 10-year feeding study in female rhesus monkeys using doses of 75 mg/kg/day (approximately 27,000 times the dosage for steers) showed some hematologic changes at the highest dose level. Interim sacrifices performed during the course of this longterm study indicated no pathologic signs other than those that were attributed to excessive stimulation of the endocrine system. Several studies have been conducted to investigate the effects of zeranol on mammalian reproduction. In a 3-generation study on male and female rats, at levels up to 20 ppb in the diet, no drug-related changes were observed, and fertility, gestation, and viability indices were comparable for both control and drug-treated groups. Zeranol has also been evaluated for mutatoxicity, and using several concentrations in the Ames test (*Salmonella typhi*), zeranol was seen not to be mutagenic.

For estrogenic compounds, generally the oral no-effect level (nonhormonal level) is the highest dose (in mg/kg/day) that produces no estrogenic effect. One method used to study the no-effect level uses ovariectomized monkeys, in which therapy with exogenous estrogen restores the reproductive tract of the animal to the precastrate state. On this basis, the oral no-effect level for zeranol in primates has been established at 0.225 μg/kg/day.

RESIDUES OF ANABOLIC AGENTS

The distribution of residues of the anabolic agents in animal tissues depends on their mode of metabolism and excretion. Residues are found in muscle, fat, liver, and kidney as well as in urine, bile, and feces. In general, the concentrations tend to be higher in the excreta than in tissues.

IMPLANTATION SITES

Residues of anabolic agents are highest at the site of implantation; for this reason, implants are given in the ear, which is discarded at slaughter. In addition, the amounts of the endogenous steroids present in meat from treated animals are insignificant by comparison with the amounts in other foodstuffs as well as with the endogenous hormone synthesis in humans. The concentrations of estradiol 17β in muscle, liver, kidney, and fat of implanted steers averaged 5 to 20 pg/g, with the levels of progesterone and testosterone in muscle 120 pg/g. Safe levels of endogenous steroids were established by the FDA by limiting individual exposure to residues of 1% of the amount of steroid produced by de novo synthesis in prepubertal boys and girls, i.e., the lowest daily production.

EXTRANEOUS HORMONES

Establishment of safe levels of exposure to these substances is more complicated than for natural hormones. Because there is no daily de novo synthesis to serve as a convenient denominator to be used in the risk analysis of the agent, toxicologic testing must be conducted.

In Europe, the working group chaired by Lamming examined the data available on the xenobiotics, trenbolone and zeranol, up to 1982. They then requested additional data, which was provided by the companies concerned. The new evidence was reviewed by the group, which was about to prepare a draft document on the use of the xenobiotics in autumn 1985. The scientific committee, however, was suspended by the Agriculture Commissioner before it could present a report.

The conclusions of the working party were presented by Lamming. Similar to the three natural steroid hormones, trenbolone and zeranol were considered to have nongenotoxic tumorigenic effects in hormonally dependent target tissues. It was thought that sufficient data were available for zeranol to allow calculations of safe daily intakes of both the parent compounds and their major metabolites. Some anterior pituitary adenomas had been observed with high doses in male rats.

The no-hormonal-effect level was put at 1 μg/kg for 17-beta trenbolone and 10 μg/kg for the metabolite 17-alpha OH trenbolone. For zeranol, a no-hormonal-effect level of 25 μg/kg, with a level of 1 mg/kg for its metabolites talanerol and zeralanone, was proposed, subject to further detailed evaluation of the new data being made available on these compounds.

PROMOTIONAL ACTIVITY OF ENDOGENOUS SEX STEROIDS IN CARCINOGENESIS

Historically as early as 1932, it was shown that there was a casual association between the endogenous natural sex steroids and the neoplastic process. Since then, experimental data have accumulated indicating that estrogen administration is followed by routinely reproducible tumors in five species of animals and eight organ sites. These included tumors of the breast, cervix, endometrium, ovary, pituitary, testicles, kidney, and bone marrow, in mice, rats, or rabbits.

At present, the consensus of opinion the scientific experts, from the accumulated evidence from the literature, is that these hormonally active substances are not carcinogenic per se but act as promoters once the carcinogenic process has been initiated by chemical, physical, or viral agents. This promoting action appears to be reversible and thresholdable in nature.

This is in contrast to the situation with diethylstilbestrol. Diethylstilbestrol has been demonstrated to be genotoxic and would therefore be considered as capable of irreversibly initiating the carcinogenic process even at small concentrations. Because of this, the United States has banned the use of diethylstilbestrol in food-producing animals, on account of its direct toxicity.

The endogenous sex steroids have not been shown to be genotoxic agents; that is, they are negative when tested in mutagenicity assays. When experimental animals were treated with natural sex steroids alone, tumors were seen only in animals given extremely high doses for prolonged periods of time, doses that exceeded by many orders of magnitude the daily production rate of the species under study.

Evidence exists that tumors caused by sex steroids develop only in endocrine target tissues. Therefore it is reasonable to believe that natural sex steroids cause tumor formation through an epigenetic mechanism. The steroid-hormone receptor epigenetic interaction, which is central to endocrine activity, is a thresholdable, dose-related, reversible phenomenon.

Levels of estradiol in the implanted animals are extremely low compared with the human de novo synthesis rate of this hormone. Estradiol 17β levels in the muscle, liver, kidney, and fat of implanted steers averaged from 5 to 20 pg/g, with levels in fat being approximately three times higher than muscle.

A 500-g portion of estradiol-treated meat contains an amount of estradiol that is 15,000 times less than the average daily production rate in men and several million times less than the production rate in pregnant women. Even in the most sensitive human group, prepubertal boys, the added estradiol derived from ingestion of treated meat is a thousand times less than the daily production rate.

Based on these studies, the FDA has concluded that although regulatory analytical methods for monitoring the residues of animal drugs considered to be carcinogens are normally required, in the unique case of these endogenous hormones, a regulatory method is not needed for an assurance of safety because the maximum increased exposure to hormones, even considering misuse of the drug, is demonstrated to be far below those concentrations considered unsafe.

The FDA also recognizes that it would not be possible to enforce a ban on these compounds effectively because analytical methods cannot distinguish between the estrogen, testosterone, and progesterone that occur naturally in food-producing animals and that might remain from the use of these hormones for growth promotion.

SYNTHETIC SEX STEROIDS

In contrast to endogenous sex steroids, there is no daily de novo production rate for these synthetic compounds, which can serve as a common denominator to be used in the risk analysis of the agent. In addition, a complete package of information on the metabolic rate and persistence of the metabolites is not available. Therefore toxicologic testing is required, and it is necessary to demonstrate that the residue depletes below the concentration considered to be safe.

It is further mandatory to demonstrate that the synthetic hormonal agent is not genotoxic. This can be accomplished through the application of a battery of mutagenicity assays. The following mutagenicity assays are required:

Unscheduled DNA synthesis in mammals (UDS)
Two of the three following assays: (1) Ames test, (2) Drosophila-sex-linked recessive lethal assay, (3) in vitro mammalian cell gene mutation assay

The use of a hormonal no-observed-effect level affords a sensitive criterion for the establishment of the safety of potential steroid hormone tissue residues. It is based on the critical relationship, both in quantity and in time, between the various hormones that play a major role in the control of the reproductive process.

The FDA has determined that zeranol used under the approved conditions of use is safe for the consumer. No residues may be found in edible tissues of cattle and sheep as determined by a method with a limit of detection of 20 ppb.

For trenbolone acetate, radiotracer studies in cattle demonstrated that total residues of the drug are in the low parts per billion at 15 and 30 days after implantation.

CONCLUSIONS OF JOINT EXPERT COMMITTEE ON FOOD ADDITIVES, 1988

The Joint Expert Committee on Food Additives (JECFA), established under the World Health Organization/Food Additive Organization (WHO/FAO), issued its conclusions on the safety of hormonal growth promotors in 1988. The priority study list of the committee included the natural hormones, estradiol, progesterone, testosterone and the synthetic hormones trenbolone acetate, and zeranol.

Natural Hormones

''Estradiol 17β alone or in combination with other hormonally active substances, is administered to bovine animals by subcutaneous implant, usually in the ear, to improve the rate of weight gain and food efficiency. The release rate from one type of commercial implant is approximately 60 μg per animal daily.

''The committee considered an ADI unnecessary for a hormone that is produced endogenously in humans and shows great variation in levels according to age and sex. The committee concluded that residues arising from the use of estradiol 17β as a growth promoter in accordance with good animal husbandry practice are unlikely to pose a hazard to human health.

''Progesterone, in combination with estradiol 17β, is administered to steers and calves by subcutaneous implantation in the ear to improve the rate of weight gain and feed efficiency. The committee deemed it unnecessary to set an ADI for a hormone that is produced endogenously in humans and shows marked physiologic variation in levels according to age and sex. The committee concluded that residues arising from the use of progesterone as a growth promoter in accordance with good animal hus-

bandry practice are unlikely to pose a hazard to human health.

''Based on its safety assessment of residues of progesterone and in view of the difficulty of determining the levels of residues attributable to the use of this hormone as a growth promoter in cattle, the committee concluded that it was unnecessary to establish an acceptable residue level. A similar conclusion was drawn for testosterone. Hence a zero withdrawal time was adopted.

Trenbolone Acetate

After administration to cattle, trenbolone acetate is rapidly hydrolyzed to hydroxy-trenbolone acetate, the major metabolite being α TBOH, occurring in the excreta, bile, and liver. In muscle, most of the TBOH is present as β TBOH. Experiments with implantation of 200 mg of radiolabeled trenbolone acetate in calves and heifers showed that maximum levels of residues occurred about 30 days postimplantation. The highest mean concentration of residues as TBOH equivalents was 50 μg/kg in liver, and muscle contained 3 μg/kg.

The committee reaffirmed the opinion expressed at its 27th meeting regarding the results of longterm feeding studies with trenbolone acetate with rats and mice. It considered that the liver hyperplasia and tumors in mice fed high doses of trenbolone acetate (0.9 to 9 mg/kg of body weight/day) and the slight increase in the incidence of islet cell tumors of the pancreas of rats fed trenbolone acetate at 1.85 mg/kg of body weight/day (the highest dose in the study) arose as a consequence of the hormonal activity of TBOH. The committee therefore concluded that its safety assessment could be based on establishing the no-hormonal-effect level.

The major residue in liver and kidney is α-TBOH. Because this epimer has one tenth of the hormonal activity of β-TBOH, the committee established a temporary acceptable residue level of 14 μg/kg in liver and kidney. The committee recommended a temporary acceptable residue level of 1.4 μg/kg for β-TBOH in bovine meat based on daily intake of a 70-kg person of 500 g of meat. This was revised by JECFA in 1989 to an MRL of 2 μg/kg for β-TBOH in muscle, and 10 μg for α-TBOH in liver, based on a new ADI of 0.02 mg/kg.

Zeranol

"Zeranol is a nonsteroidal anabolic agent administered to cattle by subcutaneous implant in the ear to improve the rate of weight gain and feed efficiency. Studies with radiolabeled zeranol orally administered to rats and monkeys and implanted in cattle have shown that zeranol is metabolized to zearalenone and taleranol. In cattle the rate of depletion of the implant peaks at 5–15 days and slows with time. At 65 days, approximately 60% of the initial dose remains at the implant site.

"In a cattle study, when zeranol was administered according to good animal husbandry practice, the maximum mean residue levels calculated as zeranol equivalents did not exceed 0.2 μg/kg in muscle, 10 μg/kg in liver, 2 μg/kg in kidney, and 0.3 μg/kg in fat at any time after implantation. Zeranol was shown to be a weak estrogen in longterm studies in the mouse, rat, dog, and monkey. Most of the changes noted occurred in mammary glands and organs of the reproductive tract. Zeranol did not cause changes in other reproductive parameters in rats and was not teratogenic in mice or rats. Zeranol and its metabolites zearalenone and taleranol were not mutagenic in tests in bacterial and mammalian systems.

"An acceptable daily intake of 0 to 0.5 μg/kg of body weight was established for zeranol. An acceptable residue level was established for zeranol when used according to good animal husbandry practice: 10 μg/kg for bovine liver and 2 μg/kg for bovine muscle. (The latter is the lowest level consistent with the practical analytical methods available for routine residue analysis)."[*]

Codex (1991)

What should in theory have been an automatic acceptance of the maximum residue levels recommended by JECFA turned into an episode of politics superseding science at the Codex Alimentarius Commission meeting (1991). The Codex Committee on Residues of Veterinary Drugs in Foods (CC/RVDF) adopted the draft standards at its October 1989 meeting. Having cleared that hurdle, it was expected that they would

proceed to the final stage in the Codex procedure for final adoption by the Commission without event.

The European Community delegation to the 19th biennial meeting of the Codex Alimentarius Commission in Rome made history on July 4th, 1991, by successfully blocking the Commission's adoption of MRL standards for growth-promoting hormones.

The Codex Commission's failure to adopt the proposed MRLs for the three natural hormones (estradiol, progesterone, and testosterone) and one synthetic hormone (zeranol) as growth promoters in livestock was unexpected. It indicated a refusal to accept scientific evaluations on their own merit; overriding political deliberation seemed to obtain over science.

The failure to set international MRLs for the four hormones also has serious implications for the General Agreement on Trade and Tariffs (GATT). Many countries approve the use of these hormones, with the exception of the EC. Why undertake a scientific review if at the end of the day the views of the scientific experts are secondary to political considerations, albeit consumer driven?

The United States would like to see a change in the rules for acceptance of JECFA standards by the Codex Commission to the effect that, unless a delegation has prepared new scientific evidence, a vote at the final step of the procedure would not be permitted. This would eliminate the possibility of consumer preference overriding science.

Other Growth-Promoting Sex Hormones

Melengestrol acetate is a synthetic progestogen that is orally active. Given as a feed supplement either in liquid or dry form, it is recommended for use in feedlot heifers at a dosage rate varying from 0.25 to 0.5 mg/day. A withdrawal period of 48 hours must elapse before the treated animals are slaughtered for human consumption. The progestational activity of melengestrol acetate is approximately 125 times greater than that of progesterone when measured by estrus cycle inhibition in cattle. It possesses a little glucocorticoid activity but no estrogenic activity.

The drug is not effective in steers or spayed heifers. By suppressing heat in feed-

---

[*]From JECFA, *op.cit.*

lot heifers, melengestrol acetate is an effective agent in promoting growth and improving feed use. Weight gain is increased by 10 to 11.2% and feed efficiency by 7.6%. Large unovulated follicles develop, which release high quantities of estrogen, over the feeding period of 140–185 days.

A bolus of melengestrol acetate is presently being developed with an intention of obtaining a 120-day delivery of the drug. Residue studies using melengestrol acetate as the marker compound and fat as the marker tissue demonstrated that melengestrol acetate levels in fat remain well below the active level of 25 ppb, even when animals are still consuming the drug. Although widely used in the United States, MGA is not approved for use in the European Community.

24.6 BIOTECHNOLOGY AND GROWTH HORMONE

Because growth hormone is a known anabolic hormone and its release has been implicated as a possible mode of action of the anabolic steroids, there is great interest in the potential use of exogenous growth hormone for growth-promoting purposes. Growth hormone is a protein molecule. Bovine growth hormone is also called bovine somatotropin (BST), and until the advent of recombinant DNA technology, its only source was that extracted from animal pituitaries.

Somatotropins are essential substances found naturally in all animals. Being proteins, they are composed of a chain of amino acids; however, their precise structure depends on the species. Thus BST—the somatotropin found in the cow—has maximal biological activity in cattle and none in humans.

BST is produced by the pituitary, a gland at the base of the brain that is responsible for the production of a number of biological messengers. BST used to be called bovine growth hormone because in the early 1900s its only known role was that of stimulating growth. It is now understood, however, to have a profound influence on many bodily functions. For this reason, its original name has been replaced by the more accurate one of BST.

Although BST's actions are now known to be complex, its role can be summarized as that of channelling the energy derived from food into vital bodily functions. One of these is growth; another is the production of milk. BST's effect on lactation in the dairy cow is of particular interest here.

The development of natural growth hormones for livestock and poultry represents a major means for improving animal production, and genetic engineering techniques have made this development a reality both for logistical and for economic reasons. The synthesis of a variety of beneficial proteins is possible through this technology. Although the number of genetically engineered proteins in production is still limited, research is working toward the development of new tools to improve many aspects of life, including agriculture and medicine.

One vital therapeutic product, however, has been commercially available through biotechnology since 1982. This is human insulin (Humulin, Eli Lilly). The production process has been tried, tested, and proved safe over a number of years. It involves the fermentation of genetically engineered bacteria, programed to synthesize the insulin molecule. There is no direct release of either genetic material or the bacteria used. Another such product is human somatotropin (Somatonorm, KabiVitrum), developed for the treatment of hypopituitary dwarfism (growth failure) in children. This "biotech" product replaced the previously used pituitary-derived hormone owing to its greater safety. (Kreutzfeldt-Jakob syndrome transfer has been associated with natural growth hormone.)

A similar process is now being used to manufacture BST. Several groups have now cloned bovine growth hormone to expression in bacteria and yeast. The recombinant DNA procedures employed were similar to those used for cloning virus genes pertinent for subunit vaccination production. A mRNA species from pituitary gland enriched for bovine growth hormone nucleotide sequences is first reverse transcribed into DNA, and then this DNA copy is inserted into plasmids for expression in bacteria and yeast. Because this bovine growth hormone gene lacks the required regulatory features necessary for these microorganisms to express this gene, some additional restructuring of the gene is required. One of these maneuvers results in the addition of amino acid (methionine) at the beginning the bovine growth hormone gene so it differs slightly from naturally occurring growth hormones.

Nevertheless, despite the presence of this additional amino acid at the beginning of genetically engineered bovine growth hormone, preliminary clinical studies have indicated that it is as effective as naturally occurring bovine growth hormone in stimulation of milk production. For instance, although milk yields were increased 10.3% for natural bovine growth hormone over a 6-day period of treatment, milk yields were increased by 12.9% for recombinant bovine growth hormone. Milk fat, lactose, and protein percentages were not affected by the treatment. Feed efficiency (kg milk/kg feed) was improved by 9.5 and 15.2% for natural and recombinant bovine growth hormone, and no adverse effects were observed based on body temperature and somatic cell counts.

Thus recombinantly derived bovine growth hormone enhanced milk production and improved feed efficiency in a manner similar to the biological responses observed with natural bovine growth hormone. Genetically engineered approaches to improving animal production appear to be directly applicable to hormones and other growth promotants in which availability of the natural substance is limited and the costs to obtain the natural hormone exceed reasonable marketing considerations. Further studies are required to determine the safety of recombinant bovine growth hormone for both treated animals and consumers of their milk. An additional growth promotant presently under development is porcine growth hormone.

GROWTH HORMONES

The anterior pituitary gland receives both stimulatory and inhibitory signals from the hypothalamus in the form of growth-hormone-releasing factor and somatostatin. Growth hormone release causes the secretion of insulin from the pancreas and insulinlike growth factors or somatomedins from the liver. Insulinlike growth factors mediate many of the metabolic effects of growth hormone.

There are also feedback loops that regulate hypothalamic activity, in turn controlling growth hormone release. Growth hormone activity could theoretically be manipulated by modifying any of these peptides in the control pathway.

The effect of growth hormone on milk production (its galactopoietic effect) was discovered at least 40 years ago. Commercial exploitation, however, has had to await the technologic ability to synthesize large protein molecules by recombinant DNA techniques. The exact mode of action of BST is still not clear as to whether is acts via a direct effect on secretory cells, an indirect effect on secretory cells, an effect on mammary blood flow, a general repartitioning of body nutrients, or a combination of the four.

Although some of the direct effects of growth hormone on body metabolism are known, its indirect effects on the level of activity of the somatomedins are still largely unexplored. Polypeptide growth factors are known to be required for the proliferation of mammalian cells in culture and to act as regulators of the cellular development of bone, muscle, and fat; they therefore affect the productivity of the whole animal. Before these growth factors can be used in commercial animal production systems, however, further basic work is required concerning their structure, metabolism, and physiologic effects. Initially attention is focused on the insulinlike growth factors or somatomedins (IGF 1 and IGF 2) because the use of exogenous sources may fortunately not generate the feedback effects thought to control the circulating levels of endogenous growth hormone.

Somatomedins stimulate an increase in the number and size of a wide range of cell types, and specific receptors have been identified in many of these, e.g., cartilage, muscle, placenta, liver, and fibrous tissue. Of particular importance is their stimulatory effect on bone growth, which then allows the greater deposition of soft tissue. There is additional interest in fibroblast growth factor, platelet-derived growth factor, and epidermal growth factor and the interrelationship between these factors and insulinlike growth factors.

So far, IGF 1 and IGF 2 have been purified from human plasma and their structure determined, and it is known in humans that production of IGF 1 depends on growth hormone and that it appears to be the major factor regulating growth hormone effects on skeletal growth. The content of IGF 2 is highest in fetal plasma, and thus it has been proposed that it may be important in controlling fetal growth and development.

Classically somatomedins are thought to be produced by the liver under the influence of growth hormone. It is also clear, however, that other tissues, e.g., kidney, produce somatomedins and that other hormones also influence their production, e.g., prolactin, insulin, corticosteroids, and thyroid hormones. High rates of growth in farm animals have been correlated with high levels of somatomedins, and recent experiments have demonstrated an increase in the growth rate of laboratory animals after the administration of somatomedins.

Although its existence has long been suspected, the hypothalamic growth-hormone-releasing factor has only recently been isolated. Growth-hormone-releasing factor is a polypeptide consisting of 44 amino acids. Synthetic analogs of the factor have now been prepared and have been shown to stimulate the release of growth hormone in animals. There is some evidence that exogenous anabolic steroids act at least partially at the level of the brain by influencing the rate of growth-hormone-releasing factor release, although some steroids may also act at the level of the pituitary by influencing its responsiveness to growth-hormone-releasing factor.

One of the reasons for the long delay in the discovery of growth-hormone-releasing factor was subsequently found to be the concurrent existence of a growth-hormone-inhibiting factor also in the brain. This compound, known as somatostatin, is also a peptide but consists of only 14 amino acids. Somatostatin inhibits the release of growth hormone and insulin. There has been much recent interest in the practical exploitation of both growth-hormone-releasing factor and somatostatin in controlling the growth of farm animals by the development of analogs of growth-hormone-releasing factor and by immuno-neutralization in the case of somatostatin.

Growth-hormone-releasing factor is protein hormone that is episodically released from the hypothalamus. The effects of growth-hormone-releasing factor on animal production are increased milk production in cattle and increased nitrogen retention in sheep. These are mediated by way of increased growth hormone production. On account of the pulsatile intermittent release of natural growth-hormone-releasing factor, it is difficult to design a delivery system that mirrors the endogenous release pattern.

EFFECTS OF SOMATOTROPIN IN ANIMALS

Longterm administration of growth hormone to growing pigs, lambs, heifers, and steers has been shown to increase live weight gain. The increased gain is typically associated with increased protein accumulation, decreased fat content, and improved feed conversion efficiency. In cattle experiments, live weight gain responses to the administration of growth hormone have been lower than those normally observed with steroid implants. Much more work is required, however, to determine the optimum dose and mode of administration.

Perhaps of more immediate practical importance is the possible application of growth hormone in improving the efficiency of milk production in dairy cows. It has been known for many years that growth hormone is the major hormone limiting the rate of milk secretion during much of lactation in the cow and that daily injections of it resulted in increased in milk production.

Treatment might be expected to increase milk yield by 20 to 40%, although the short-term higher increases seen in some experiments may be difficult to achieve in practice. The minimum effective dose is between 5 and 10 mg/day. It should be emphasized that the effect of growth hormone is to increase the efficiency of milk production, not milk yield per se, by improving the efficiency of feed use. The physiologic mechanism of action is not clear, but it may involve improved blood flow through the udder and increased supply and extraction of substrates by the mammary gland from the blood.

At present, experimentally the treatment is given usually from 3 to 4 weeks after calving to about 40 weeks by a series of injections varying in frequency from daily to weekly. For the commercial product, a 2- to 4-week slow-release injection regimen is envisaged. There is considerable commercial rivalry in the development of hormone delivery systems and it is difficult to know which delivery system will be preferred, but it appears unlikely that an implant-type formulation will be developed in the near future, to obviate frequent injections. Because it is a protein, it cannot be given orally.

There appear to be several formulations of BST that may be marketed. These are daily dose, a 7-day prolonged-release, a 14-day prolonged-release, and a 28-day prolonged-release preparation. Some of these formulations are based on methionyl BST (14- and 28-day formulations), (Sometribove) and others (daily) are based on homology with natural BST. The less frequently given preparations contain larger doses of BST.

Once released into the circulation of an animal, the active life of Somatotropin is short. Consequently, injections have been given daily or much larger doses given in a slower release form over intervals of 2 to 4 weeks. These injections have rarely produced a local inflammation.

Indisputably somatotropin drives the metabolism of animals faster. What is in dispute is whether somatotropin might drive all or some animals too hard so as to create a welfare problem ("turbo cows," "bovine burnout"). Because metabolic stresses and production diseases in dairy cows are restricted almost entirely to the first 3 months of lactation, it might fairly be argued that BST administered after that time could increase milk yield in the declining phase of lactation and that this could be sustained without increasing the requirement for concentrate feed.

In this and a few other selected circumstances, BST might, in the light of existing knowledge, be administered to dairy cattle without significant insult to their welfare. If preparations containing BST were approved for use in lactating dairy cows, should the product be administered only by a veterinary surgeon at intervals of not less than 4 weeks and not until 90 days after

parturition or at such time as the cow has been diagnosed pregnant with her next calf? The first commercial BST likely to reach the market will possibly be formulated in 14- to 28-day prolonged-release systems. There has been no evidence in clinical trials of reduced health or longevity, and the milk from treated cows contains no more BST than that from untreated cows. (Optiflex, Somatech, Somidibove, and Sometribove are major BST products now in the regulatory phases.)

Bovine growth hormone appears to be relatively species specific and is inactive in humans. Perhaps more importantly from the point of view of human safety, because it is a protein, it is digested into its constituent amino acids after ingestion and is therefore inactivated in the gut. Thus there are not likely to be any significant toxicologic or residue difficulties.

Secretion of BST is pulsatile and may be influenced by adrenergic and cholinergic agonists, amino acid infusion, magnesium, cholecystokinin, vasoactive intestinal peptide, sleep, stress, glucagon, insulin, and free fatty acid levels. There is no evidence that BST per se has a direct galactopoietic effect on mammary tissue because no receptors for somatotropin have been identified in mammary tissue. In contrast, an indirect action apparently is exerted on the gland through the insulinlike growth factors.

In early lactation, there is an increased loss (compared with controls) of glucose from the body, increased plasma free fatty acids, and increased turnover of free fatty acids associated with BST use. BST has a diabetogenic action of decreasing the sensitivity of peripheral tissues to insulin and elevating blood glucose levels. Increased uptake of glucose oxidation and increased oxidation of long-chain fatty acids in the mammary gland occur. Elevations in plasma free fatty acid levels result from the use of BST. BST has not been demonstrated, however, to have a direct lipolytic action on adipose tissues. Elevation of blood ketone levels have also been reported.

EFFECTS OF BOVINE SOMATOTROPIN IN DAIRY COWS

Milk Yield

Short-term studies with BST (4 to 10 days) have shown increases of 1 to 15% in milk yield. Experiments of longer duration (70 and 84 days) have shown increases in milk yield of between 30 and 50% compared with control animals. A 20% increase in milk yield is the average figure recorded. Most of the results to date have been recorded in high-yielding Holstein cows on high planes of nutrition.

The increased milk yield resulting from the use of BST may lead to increased somatic cell count. Adequate monitoring of cell counts is required before and during treatment; if these exceed 400,000 ml, cows should not be treated with BST.

Feed Intake

It has been found that BST-treated cows have a higher feed intake than untreated cows. This is thought to occur because of a link between BST and appetite. The extra feed that is taken in is more efficiently used for milk production. This is to be expected because a greater proportion of this extra feed is used for production and not maintenance. In effect, the way in which BST acts appears to be similar to that mediating increased milk yield in genetically superior cows.

Milk Composition

Longterm administration of BST has no effect on milk composition. Short-term supplementation with BST has marginal effects on milk fat percentage and milk protein percentage. This is seen only in cows in early lactation or on short-term experiments in which feed intake does not increase quickly enough to meet the requirements of increased milk production. The overall yield of fat and protein, however, is higher because of the increased yields of treated cows. The present consensus is that BST-treated milk is nutritionally safe for human consumption.

POTENTIAL SIDE EFFECTS OF BOVINE SOMATOTROPIN

Animal Health

To date, extensive research with BST has shown no major adverse effects on cow health. One might expect ketosis to be a potential problem in these high-yielding cows, but to date this has not been documented. No significant increase in somatic cell counts has been found in BST-treated cows, and there has been no reported increase in the incidence of lameness. It is important to mention that all the research to date has been carried out on selected farms where the animals were maintained on a high plane of nutrition.

The possibility that BST treatment increases the risk of mastitis must be considered, and in particular, there is a need for multilactational trials to assess the effect of continued high milk yield on cows. Increasing importance is also being placed on the need to safeguard the "welfare" of the livestock kept on farms, with main concern directed at high-producing animals kept under intensive conditions of management. Many dairy cows are considered to be in this category; thus the use of BST to increase milk output by the dairy cow further is being questioned on welfare grounds. To date, there are no reports of increased metabolic disorders, such as ketosis, milk fever, or hypomagnesemia.

Reproductive Efficiency

Reports in the literature to date suggest that BST has no effect on reproductive parameters in dairy cows. Further research is needed to examine the longterm effects, if any, of BST on reproductive efficiency. This information is needed because any adverse effects on reproductive performance reduce the chances of the farmer achieving a target of one calf per cow per year. It is important to mention that reduced reproductive efficiency might negate some of the benefits of increased milk production. Lowered fertility in dairy cattle has been related to the magnitude of energy deficits in the immediate postpartum period.

OTHER CONSIDERATIONS

It is known that BST, even if there are significant residues in milk, is likely to be digested in the human gut into its constituent amino acids. However, is there any effect within the human gut before digestion? Similarly, insulinlike growth factor concentrations are increased in animals treated with somatotropin. What are insulinlike growth factor levels in milk? Do these affect the human gut?

Extensive clinical trials are in progress in many countries under government supervision. To date, it is unlikely, unless unforeseen problems emerge, that registration based on safety, quality, and efficacy will not be possible. Political and public acceptability, however, is another matter.

Few trials have been conducted with the examination of those physiologic and homeostatic mechanisms essential for good health as a first priority, yet it is just such trials that are needed to help decide whether somatotropin is acceptable. Some of the most important questions that need to be asked include:

1. Effects of immune status, in particular, cell-mediated immunity in the mammary gland of the dairy cow and in the mesenteric lymph nodes of growing animals
2. Effect on calcium and phosphorus status, bone metabolism, and pathology, particularly in young growing animals
3. Longterm effects of BST over a number of lactations on udder and hind leg conformation
4. Carryover effects of exogenous growth hormone on the ability of animals to produce endogenous growth hormone and thus on subsequent, unsupplemented performance.

Many companies have now reached agreement with the FDA, stating the "two lactation and three gestation periods would suffice to indicate safety for the time being."

Longterm assessment of the safety of BST is now addressed to the following factors:

1. Multiple lactation safety studies (designed to identify any tendency toward "burnout" or adverse cumulative effects of increased lactation of cows). As mentioned earlier, each cow supports her increased milk yield by adjusting her feed intake as necessary. This is a natural, self-regulatory process by which the cow reaches a new, more efficient equilibrium between feed energy and milk output. One hopes the notion of "burnout" is unfounded; test results show that cows treated with BST maintain body weight and body scores equivalent to those of untreated animals.

Key remaining issues include:

1. BST will not be commercially available in any country before it has been thoroughly tested and regulatory approval obtained. After this, consumer acceptance will have to be obtained.
2. Reproductive function (whether BST affects conception rates and the ability to produce a normal fetus).
3. Effect on offspring (e.g., growth rates).
4. Food consumption data and milk production.
5. Resistance to naturally occurring disease.
6. Mammary gland health (incidence of mastitis and recovery rate).

A wide-ranging, structured, postmarketing study of at least 2 years is needed to determine the effects of BST on the incidence of mastitis and associated metabolic disorders.

SAFETY OF BOVINE SOMATOTROPIN

BST occurs naturally in cow's milk at variable levels, generally less than 2 ppb but may occasionally range up to 10 ppb. No increase in BST levels in milk has been observed in cows supplemented with BST at expected use levels.

BST present in the milk cannot present a risk to the consumer. This is because BST is a protein, and similar to all proteins in our diet, it is broken down into its constituent amino acids by the digestive system. Once digested, BST can have no biological action in humans; it is active only in the cow after direct injection. Milk from cows treated with BST is in fact identical in all respects to milk from untreated animals. It is just as wholesome and of exactly the same high quality; it has the same levels of butterfat, protein, minerals, and lactose and has identical processing properties. Perhaps of more importance to the consumer, the milk is identical in terms of taste and smell.

BST's inactivity in humans has been demonstrated conclusively in the past; attempts in the 1950s to stimulate growth in children with hypopituitary dwarfism (i.e., who lacked somatotropin) by injecting BST were remarkably unsuccessful. Despite the high doses given, however, there were no ill effects, again proving BST's safety. Residues of Optiflex 640-treated animals do not present any risk to consumers of meat or milk from treated animals, according to EC regulatory agencies. Not will its use affect the quality of milk or meat or adversely affect the industrial processing of milk into yogurt or cheeses. No withdrawal period will be required.

The indications to date are that, provided that it is properly used, BST will be given a clean regulatory approval. These conditions might be that only sustained-release preparations could be used, and daily injections would be prohibited (this would be possible to monitor because sites of frequent injections can be detected). The revised site of administration of Optiflex (from the shoulder to the tailhead) is now deemed acceptable because local reactions observed are substantially reduced at the latter site.

Structurally BST products have differed by 0.5 to 5% in amino acid sequence from pituitary BST at the terminal end of the molecule. These differences arise from additions or deletions of amino acids.

In contrast to smaller steroid hormones (molecular weight, 275 to 350 daltons), which can be orally active, somatotropin is a large protein hormone (22,000 daltons) and is not absorbed from the digestive tract. When consumed, proteins undergo enzymatic digestion in the gastrointestinal tract. This destroys their ability to act on body functions and is why protein hormones, such as insulin and BST, must be injected rather than fed.

Milk from all cows contains minute levels of BST. Numerous studies have shown milk composition to be unaltered in BST-supplemented cows. The scientific community at the moment seems convinced that somatotropin concentrations in milk are not significantly elevated in BST-treated cows. There tends to be more prolonged debate, however, about the effects on insulinlike growth factor levels in milk. Insulinlike growth factors or somatomedins are produced mainly in the liver in response to somatotropin and are probably involved in mediating the action of somatotropin on milk production. Of the two insulinlike growth factors, IGF 1 concentrations in plasma and milk have been shown to be slightly elevated in BST-treated cows. Although IGF 1 is a peptide molecule and therefore digested in the gastrointestinal tract into its constituent amino acids, it is important to establish that these elevated concentrations do not affect the human gut epithelium before digestion. IGF 1 concentrations in milk are also elevated early postpartum in cows and in humans; therefore any adverse effect in humans is unlikely. A further consideration is the effect of residues of IGF 1 truncated form in the milk of treated animals. The truncated form may be more active than IGF 1 itself.

CODEX

The Codex Committee has included the two growth hormones, BST and porcine somatotropin, on its priority list of drugs to be reviewed. Their inclusion, at what is an early stage in their life cycle, is due to the experience of the problems with the anabolic growth promoters. It was thought that it would be better to have an assessment of the safety of BST and porcine somatotropin by an internationally recognized expert body before rather than after questions of their use arose. Indeed, the JECFA has reached the opinion that residues of BST in milk of treated animals were safe.

At their meeting in Geneva from June 9th to 18th, 1992, members of the JECFA put forward recommendations for ADIs and MRLs for 10 veterinary compounds, including BST. Because the committee considered that there is a large margin of safety for the consumption of residues of BST, it concluded that the presence of such residues does not represent a health concern. The JECFA group therefore recommended that there was no need to specify a numerical ADI or MRL.

The FDA has repeatedly stated that it has no safety concerns as regards human consumption of BST in milk. Residues of bovine growth hormone in milk, either naturally occurring or as the result of the administration of bovine growth hormone, are not considered to be biologically active in humans and thus are presumably of no concern from a food safety point of view. Consumer acceptance, safety aspects, and the collective views of the dairy industry are separate concerns about the commercial introduction of BST.

PORCINE SOMATOTROPIN

The proportion of muscle to fat in swine carcasses is naturally controlled by various hormones and metabolic factors. As pigs mature, these factors change, and fat deposition replaces lean as the major portion of carcass gain. To counteract this partitioning of dietary protein and energy from lean to fat, two types of commercial products are being evaluated. Known as porcine somatotropin and beta agonists, both of these products act through different metabolic mechanisms but are most beneficial in heavyweight pigs.

Porcine somatotropin, also referred to as growth hormone, is a hormone that is produced normally by pig pituitary glands. Recombinantly produced porcine somatotropin has been found to enhance performance dramatically.

By inserting the pig growth hormone gene into the genetically simple *Escherichia coli* bacteria, it is possible to manufacture recombinant porcine somatotropin. As the bacteria rapidly multiply, recombinant porcine somatotropin is produced along with other bacterial gene products.

Because it is a protein, porcine somatotropin must be injected. If given orally, it is digested to amino acids and inactivated. Current research is generally based on daily injections, although studies are underway with longer duration implants. Much attention is being focused on developing of a practical oral delivery system because swine producers probably cannot justify the time and labor required for daily injections of porcine somatotropin. Porcine somatotropin research has typically been done with a daily injection, but research is underway with implants lasting up to 30 days.

Research indicates that the use of porcine somatotropin dramatically improves carcass composition and production efficiency in growing-finishing swine. Additionally, when porcine somatotropin is administered to lactating sows, milk production rises.

Increases in protein deposition and decreases in fat deposition after injections of recombinant porcine somatotropin have been found across breeds, nutritional levels, sexes, and various management systems in different parts of the world. Treated animals have grown on average 10% faster, whereas feed conversion has improved by 17% and lean tissue growth by 8%.

A new oral delivery system for proteins has been tested in pigs. Such an oral delivery system, which overcomes the expense of administering hormones by injection, is a technical breakthrough of substantial commercial potential.

The system, which can be formulated as granules, capsules, or liquid, is designed to protect the protein from attack by digestive acid or enzymes, while still permitting its absorption through the intestinal wall intact. Growth hormone is normally broken down to an inactive form and digested like food when administered orally. The potential worldwide market for growth hormone in pigs has been estimated at over $300 million per annum.

The potential for an acceptable product largely depends on the availability of a practical delivery system. An ear implant that is capable of delivering porcine somatotropin for 4 to 6 weeks would seem to be another convenient product.

It is not completely understood how porcine somatotropin stimulates increases in feed efficiency, rate of gain, and muscling in hogs. After it is released from the pituitary gland into the blood stream, porcine somatotropin causes hepatic release of another small protein known as somatomedin-C. Somatomedin-C then binds to selected tissues, such as muscle, and causes cell multiplication and growth. Porcine somatotropin also alters the animal's intermediary metabolism, which decreases fat storage and increases protein (muscle) accumulation. Because of this, fatty acids are mobilized from fat depots to serve as preferred energy sources for body processes. The reliance of fatty acids spared carbohydrates and protein as energy sources, making them available for lean tissue development.

A negative effect of porcine somatotropin treatment is that treated pigs produce more heat as a result of higher maintenance energy requirements.

The liver, heart, and kidney of porcine-somatotropin-treated animals enlarges as the daily doses of porcine somatotropin increases. An immediate consequence of enlarged internal organs is a reduction in dressing percentage.

Many questions still need to be answered concerning porcine somatotropin before the substance can be given final approval, in particular with regard to the relevance of altered IGF 1 levels for consumer safety. Metabolism of IGF 1 might result in formation of active fragments. These questions did not prevent the FDA from authorizing the use of porcine somatotropin for efficacy studies without a withdrawal period.

If approved by the FDA, porcine somatotropin will be an important compound in economically and efficiently producing pork products with lower fat content. This approval, of course, hinges on a demonstration that porcine somatotropin is safe for swine and people consuming porcine-somatotropin-treated pork and confirmation that it is efficacious. However, currently BST is higher on the FDA's priority list than PST.

24.7 BETA AGONISTS

Interest has focused on a range of synthetic beta-adrenergic agonist drugs. An example of this type of compound is clenbuterol (benzyl alcohol, 4-amino-a-(t-butylamino) methyl-3.5-dichloro). This drug is used in veterinary medicine as a uterine muscle relaxant and as a bronchodilator, but it also achieves the desired end of producing a lean carcass in sheep and cattle.

Chemical control of fat deposition using implants, feed additives, or injectables have not consistently improved carcass fat-to-lean ratios while maintaining animal performance. Therefore, there appears to be considerable commercial potential for a product to improve meat animal composition. Beta-adrenergic agonists are a new class of feed additives that have been being investigated as a means of enhancing growth in meat-producing animals.

Recent advances in basic biomedical research have led to the development of clinically useful drugs known as second-generation adrenergic-receptor stimulants (agonists) and blockers (antagonists). Adrenergic receptors are now differentiated into four distinct subtypes: $alpha_1$, $alpha_2$, $beta_1$, $beta_2$. The new drugs are more receptor selective and tissue specific than older ones and hence have increased potential for

directed therapeutic action, with relatively fewer side effects on nontargeted organs. The $beta_2$-selective agonist clenbuterol causes bronchodilation with less $beta_1$ cardiac excitation than does the $beta_1$, $beta_2$ nonselective agonist isoproterenol. Compared with the latter, the $beta_1$-selective agonist dobutamine increases myocardial contractile force and cardiac output with less $beta_2$-mediated vasodilation and hypotension. The $beta_1$-selective antagonist metoprolol has advantage over the $beta_1$-$beta_2$ nonselective blocker propranolol for controlling $beta_1$ cardiac excitation in patients with compromised pulmonary function.

These new compounds have more restricted pharmacodynamic profiles and hence the potential for more selective therapeutic effects in particular situations. The basis for this selectivity resides with two interdependent discoveries: (1) the realization that alpha- and beta-adrenergic receptors actually comprised distinct functions in some tissues and (2) identification of drugs with relatively greater activity at one receptor subtype than at the others.

ADRENERGIC RECEPTOR CLASSIFICATION

The original differentiation of adrenergic receptors into the two main classes alpha and beta was based mainly on the relative potencies of the agonists norepinephrine, epinephrine, and isoproterenol in eliciting excitatory or inhibitory effects in a series of tissues e.g., heart, vasculature, lungs (Table 24–3). Excitatory responses were generally designated as alpha-receptor events, whereas, for the most part, inhibitory responses were designated as beta-receptor events. The excitatory beta receptors of the heart represented an important exception to this rule and pointed toward different types of beta receptors.

BETA$_1$- AND BETA$_2$-ADRENERGIC RECEPTOR SUBTYPES

Partly because of the potent beta-stimulatory properties of norepinephrine in some tissues (e.g., the heart) but not others (e.g., the lungs), it was suggested in 1967 that

TABLE 24–4
SOME TISSUE DISTRIBUTIONS OF BETA-ADRENERGIC RECEPTOR SUBTYPES

Effector organ	Receptor subtype	Effector response
Heart	Beta$_1$	Increased contractility, heart rate, conduction velocity, and arrhythmogenesis
Kidney	Beta$_1$	Renin release
Fat cells	Beta$_1$	Lipolysis
Skeletal muscle	Beta$_1$	Tremors
Eye	Beta$_1$	Increased aqueous humor
Noradrenergic neuron	Beta$_2$	Increased norepinephrine release
Lung	Beta$_2$	Bronchodilation
Vascular smooth muscle	Beta$_2$	Vasodilation
Intestine	Beta$_2$	Relaxation
Uterus	Beta$_2$	Relaxation
Pancreatic islets	Beta$_2$	Increased insulin secretion
Liver	Beta$_1$, beta$_2$	Gluconeogenesis

beta receptors actually comprised a heterogeneous population of two distinct subtypes: beta$_1$ and beta$_2$. Many tissues contain both beta$_1$ and beta$_2$ receptors in various ratios depending on species and other variables. One subtype usually dominates, however, and provides the tissue and organ with their functional classification as being under either beta$_1$ or beta$_2$ receptor control.

RECEPTOR LOCATION

The functionally prevalent beta receptor in the myocardium of most, if not all, mammalian species is the beta$_1$ subtype (Table 24–4). Activation of cardiac beta$_1$ receptors leads to the characteristic sympathomimetic response of the heart.

TABLE 24–5
BETA AGONISTS

Clenbuterol	
Salbutamol	"Designer" drugs
Cimaterol	
Carbuterol	Screening tests not necessarily specific
Terbutaline	→ Cross reactivity
Pirbuterol	
Ractopamine	
Fenoterol	

The beta-adrenergic receptors of the pulmonary airways and peripheral vascular beds are mainly the beta$_2$ subtype. The beta$_2$ pulmonary receptors subserve relaxation of bronchiolar smooth muscle and its accompanying bronchodilation, leading to an improvement in airway conductance. Vascular smooth muscle beta$_2$ receptors are present in various tissues, especially skeletal muscle, where they mediate vasodilation and reduced vascular resistance.

BETA$_2$-SELECTIVE BRONCHODILATORS

The beta$_2$-agonist effects of isoproterenol have been used successfully to improve airway diameter and conductance in obstructive pulmonary disorders, such as bronchitis, emphysema, and asthmaticlike syndromes. Because of equipotent beta$_1$ activity, however, cardiac excitation and tachydysrhythmias represent limiting side effects of isoproterenol when only beta$_2$-bronchodilator action is sought.

Metaproterenol, isoetharine, terbutaline, salbutamol, pirbuterol, and clenbuterol are new drugs that meet the requirements for high beta$_2$ and relatively less beta$_1$ agonist activity. Indeed these drugs are generally classified as selective beta$_2$ bronchodilators (Table 24–5).

MECHANISM OF ACTION

The mode of action of beta agonists is poorly understood, but their interaction with membrane-bound receptors increases lipolysis in adipose cells and stimulates hypertrophy in muscle fibers. Although beta-adrenergic agonists are known to stimulate the secretion of growth hormone and insulin, there is no direct evidence that these hormones mediate the tissue responses to the drug.

Activation of both $beta_1$ and $beta_2$ receptors results in activation of adenylate cyclase and increased conversion of ATP to cAMP. cAMP is the major "second messenger" of beta-receptor activation. For example, in the liver of many species, beta-receptor activation increases cAMP synthesis, which leads to a cascade of events culminating in the activation of glycogen phosphorylase.

In the heart, beta-receptor activation increases the influx of calcium across the cell membrane and its sequestration inside the cell. Beta-receptor activation also promotes the relaxation of smooth muscle. Although the mechanism is uncertain, it may involve the phosphorylation of myosin light chain kinase. Increased secretion of insulin, growth hormone, lipolysis, and glycogenolysis also underpin beta-agonist activity.

The beta agonists increase protein deposition, and this effect is a prolonged one in contrast to the relatively short-term effect of tachycardia (a $beta_1$ effect), which is also produced. The effects on protein deposition are mainly directed toward an increase in the levels of skeletal muscle deposition, and the effects on nonmuscle protein are by a decrease in the rate of protein degradation. In some experiments, evidence of an increased synthesis of protein was found, and this tended to occur in the initial period after the introduction of the compounds to the animal.

Clenbuterol and similar compounds act on the beta-adrenergic receptors and effect their response by the stimulation of cAMP production. Such compounds are called beta agonists, and because their effect on carcass composition is to increase the deposition of protein while reducing fat accretion, they are also referred to as repartitioning agents.

Beta agonists and catecholamines interact with specific cell membrane-bound receptors, leading to increased intracellular amounts of cAMP resulting in reduced lipogenesis and enhanced lipolysis. They also reduce protein degradation in muscle and stimulate the fractional protein synthesis rate, which results in hypertrophy of both fast and slow muscle fibers. The end result of these actions is that nutrient flow is directed toward muscle accretion and away from fat deposition, with consequential improvements in food efficiency and carcass composition. There are also indications that beta agonists can increase the basal metabolic rate, presumably by stimulation of beta receptors in brown adipose tissue. The evidence that some of the effects of these compounds may be exerted via the release of other hormones, such as growth hormone or insulin, is equivocal.

A therapeutic dose of clenbuterol for cattle is 0.3 mg/day for bronchial problems. For illicit use for growth effects, the dose is 10 to 15 times this scale. The beta agonist clenbuterol, however, has been licensed in some countries for use in cattle to relax the uterus at the time of parturition and for relaxation of the airways when bronchospasm occurs in cattle and horses. It is not licensed, however, for feeding at high doses as a repartitionary agent in cattle for growth. It is not approved by the FDA for any animal application in the U.S.

Clenbuterol appears to exert both $beta_1$ and $beta_2$ agonistic effects in that it produces cardiac stimulation ($beta_1$) and vasodilation ($beta_2$). Changes in metabolic rate and body temperature are typical responses to an adrenalinlike substance, but the reasons for the depression of appetite are less clear. The loss of appetite may be due to a feeling of malaise in the animal or possibly to the glycogenolytic and lipolytic actions of the drug having shut down the appetite centers; such a view is by no means universally accepted, but high doses of the beta agonist dl-isoproterenol injected into the cerebral ventricles caused hypophagia in sheep but not in cattle. A further point of interest, particularly in the sheep, was the differences in the time courses of the various responses to the drug. Heart rate and blood pressure were restored to normal levels within 24 hours and appetite within 5 days, but metabolic rate remained higher for 10 days, and in more recent experiments, it has remained higher for 3 weeks.

EFFECTS OF BETA AGONISTS

The net effect of a given drug in the intact organism depends on its relative receptor affinity (alpha or beta), intrinsic activity, and compensatory reflexes evoked by its direct actions. Adrenergic drugs or agonists act on the target cell via membrane-bound receptor molecules. The receptor responses were originally classified according to whether an adrenergic drug caused contraction (alpha) or relaxation (beta) of involuntary muscle. Alpha receptors are further subdivided according to whether they are postsynaptic (alpha$_1$) or presynaptic (alpha$_2$), and beta receptors are subdivided according to a tissue's response to beta agonists because some adrenergic drugs affect involuntary muscle in some tissues but not in others. Cardiac and intestinal smooth muscle are classified as beta$_1$, and bronchial, vascular, and uterine smooth muscle are classified as beta$_2$ receptors. Beta agonists that affect partitioning of body composition appear to act primarily on the beta$_2$ type of receptor.

CARDIOVASCULAR SYSTEM

Vascular smooth muscle tone is regulated by adrenergic receptors; consequently, catecholamines are important in controlling peripheral vascular resistance and venous capacitance. Alpha receptors increase arterial resistance, whereas beta$_2$ receptors promote smooth muscle relaxation. There are major differences in receptor types in the various vascular beds. The skin vessels have predominantly alpha receptors and constrict in the presence of catecholamines, as do the splanchnic vessels. Vessels in skeletal muscle may constrict or relax, depending on whether alpha or beta receptors are activated. Thus the overall effects of a sympathomimetic drug on blood vessels depend on the relative activities at alpha and beta receptors and the anatomic sites of the vessels affected.

Direct effects on the heart are determined largely by beta$_1$ receptors. Beta-receptor activation results in increased calcium influx in cardiac cells. Stimulation of beta receptors in the heart tends to increase cardiac output. A relatively pure beta agonist, such as isoproterenol, also decreases peripheral resistance.

RESPIRATORY TRACT

Bronchial smooth muscle contains beta$_2$ receptors that cause relaxation. Activation of these receptors thus results in bronchodilation.

METABOLIC EFFECTS

Sympathomimetic drugs have important effects on intermediary metabolism. Activation of beta$_1$-adrenergic receptors in fat cells leads to increased lipolysis. Human lipocytes also contain alpha$_2$ receptors that inhibit lipolysis by decreasing intracellular cAMP. Sympathomimetic drugs enhance glycogenolysis in the liver, which leads to increased glucose release into the circulation.

TOXICITY OF SYMPATHOMIMETIC DRUGS

The adverse effects of adrenergic agonists are primarily extensions of their receptor effects in the cardiovascular and central nervous systems. Adverse cardiovascular effects with pressor agents include marked elevations in blood pressure, which may cause cerebral hemorrhage. Increased cardiac work may precipitate severe angina or mycardial infarction. Beta-stimulant drugs frequently cause tachycardia and, more significantly, may provoke serious ventricular arrhythmias.

In human and veterinary medicine, clenbuterol and other beta agonists are used as bronchodilators for the control of bronchial asthma and also act as relaxors of smooth muscle contractions for control of parturition. Certain agents with beta-agonist activity have begun to be examined as human antiobesity agents because in obese rodents they produce a dramatic loss of adipose tissue with little apparent effect on lean body mass. This antiobesity activity could be produced by their known beta-adrenergic-mediated stimulation of lipolysis in fat cells and a parallel enhancement of the oxidation of the released fatty acids in brown adipose tissue.

In the early days of asthma treatment, nonselective $beta_1$ and $beta_2$ agonists were used in humans. They were effective for treating bronchoconstriction (via $beta_2$ stimulation) but also had heart action ($beta_1$), which was undesirable. Nowadays drugs are more selective, and drugs such as salbutamol ($beta_2$ agonist) are used for human asthma to dilate the bronchi, without affecting the $beta_1$ receptor in the heart. They target specific $beta_2$ receptors only. In veterinary medicine, the similar pharmacologic compound is a $beta_2$ agonist, clenbuterol, which finds in some centers wide therapeutic usage for respiratory conditions in horses and calves and which can be given by injection or by powder in feed for legitimate respiratory disease in large numbers of animals. All of these drugs are extraordinarily potent and are given in minute doses (micrograms). They also must be given several times per day because the body eliminates them rapidly. Asthmatics are well acquainted with this fact—they must inhale salbutamol three to four times a day. So, in short, these drugs are related to adrenaline, specifically target bronchial tissue receptors, and thus have minimal undesirable side effects at small doses.

At excessively high doses, however, with these drugs curious effects can be seen. We are all familiar with the adrenaline "flight or fight" reaction in stress. In stressful situations, adrenaline prepares us for evasive action—glucose levels are increased (our fuel for energy); glycogen (starch) in muscle is broken down; and blood vessels dilate, increasing blood supply and oxygenation to vital organs. The heart beats faster, and fat is broken down.

Similarly with excessively high doses of beta agonists in cattle, fat is broken down, blood supply and nutrition to muscle are increased, and an anabolic effect is induced. Growth hormone and insulin are released, muscle hypertrophies, and fat disappears. The net effect is not so much an overall weight gain but rather a conversion of fat

to lean. Hence the drugs are called repartitioning agents. For this reason, killing-out percentage is better, and financial incentives accrue to the producer.

Most published work has been carried out with clenbuterol and cimaterol, an earlier analog, and reports consistently show increases in muscle mass together with a reduction in fatness. Cimaterol increased daily live weight gain and feed conversion by 13 to 20% in ruminants but only by 1 to 3% in pigs and poultry. There may therefore be a difference between the magnitude of the responses of ruminants and nonruminants, but the relative dosage and duration of therapy may also exert some influence. Additionally, because protein is laid down at the expense of fat, this may negate any substantial increase in live weight gain. The effects of beta agonists on killing-out percentage have been consistent in improving this parameter. Females have tended to show greater improvements compared with males, and this apparently is related to the larger proportion of female tissue that is made up of fat.

The data with the related compound cimaterol show that fat content reduced by 16 to 25% in treated lambs (relative to controls), while growth rate was improved by about 20%, food conversion efficiency increased by 10 to 18%. Enhanced muscle growth is evidenced by an 18% increase in the cross-sectional area of the longissimus dorsi muscle. A study with cattle showed a similar pattern of response. Growth rate and food conversion efficiency were improved by 30%, carcass fat was reduced by 39%, and lean meat content and longissimus dorsi area increased by 17 and 41%.

The level of inclusion of beta agonists in the diet affects the response obtained. The optimum dose can vary for different production parameters. In cattle, administration of cimaterol increased growth rate (21%) during the first 5 weeks. Cimaterol had no effect on food intake but significantly increased food efficiency (18%) and killing-out percentage. Cimaterol administration reduced the proportion of bone and subcutaneous fat; there was a corresponding increase in meat content. The weight of the internal fat deposits was reduced significantly after treatment with cimaterol, and the area of the longissimus dorsi muscle was increased by 25%.

The effects of cimaterol on live animal performance and carcass traits in pigs and poultry were smaller than those observed in ruminants. The improvements in growth rate and food efficiency were between 1 and 3% in both species. In pigs, fat content was reduced by 18%, and there was a 13% increase in the area of the longissimus dorsi muscle. The effects of cimaterol on live animal performance traits are marginal. Its effects on a number of carcass traits, however, were more substantial. In general, the evidence shows that cimaterol causes a reduction in fat and an increase in lean in all species.

The results on the use of beta agonists in meat-producing animals have implications for livestock producers, the meat-processing industries, and consumers. For example, the reduction of carcass fat content by 10 to 20% would substantially reduce the amount of fat produced.

POTENTIAL HAZARDS ASSOCIATED WITH ILLEGAL USE OF HIGH DOSES OF BETA AGONISTS

On animal welfare grounds alone, excessive intake of beta agonists in feed can affect the heart of the animal. Although these are selective drugs for the blood vessel/bronchial $beta_2$ receptors, nonetheless at high doses they affect the heart ($beta_1$), causing hypertrophy and rapid heart rates with gross nausea and blood pressure changes in the affected animal. $Beta_2$ activation also drops the blood pressure so a compensatory rise in the heart rate takes place to normalize blood pressure. Muscle tremors and palpitations with possible anorexia are possible in animals receiving longterm high doses. At high doses, $beta_2$ receptor selectivity is not absolute, and so, some $beta_1$ effects can be seen.

Tachycardia, sweating, muscle tremors, colic, and lack of vitality accompany beta agonist use in farm animals. Those concerned with animal production and welfare should remember that many features of the circulation are controlled by the adrenergic nervous system and that these drugs may nevertheless have undesirable side effects; heart rates greater than 180/minute for periods of up to 2 hours represent a considerable physiologic insult. Compensatory deposition of fat often occurs after removal of beta agonists from the diet.

Meat from these animals is dark because of the increased blood supply to the muscle ($beta_2$ stimulation), poor in flavor (lack of glycogen), of poor keeping quality, tougher, and difficult to cut. The lack of fatty marbling takes away the traditional flavor. At factories, the hide is difficult to pull off the carcass because of the lack of subcutaneous fat.

For the unscrupulous operator using this material on cattle feeds, the hazards are significant. The drug is usually applied to the animal feed (usually skim milk powder), and the human inhalation intake in the cow shed can be colossal. Tachycardia, respiratory problems, fibrillation, muscle tremors, and deaths have been allegedly attributed to the human handling of this material. The adverse effects of adrenergic agonists are primarily extensions of their receptor effects in the cardiovascular and central nervous systems.

Adverse cardiovascular effects seen with pressor agents in man include marked elevations in blood pressure, which may cause cerebral hemorrhage. Increased cardiac work may precipitate severe angina or myocardial infarction. Beta-stimulant drugs frequently cause tachycardia and, more significantly, may provoke serious ventricular arrhythmias. Tachycardia, elevation of blood pressure, and fibrillation are associated known hazards from inhalation of high doses of clenbuterol.

There is currently a paucity of scientific information of the effects of these residues regarding consumer health. Clenbuterol and salbutamol are rapidly excreted from the animal body. Hence when used at normal low doses therapeutically and allowing the toxicologically established time for elimination, no major risk should exist. For illegal use in lean meat production, however, not only are high doses used, but also the drug is fed near to slaughter to obviate this elimination problem. Residues of beta agonists in carcasses could have the effect of nullifying beta blockers in the consumer, interfering with $beta_2$ tonicity in the pregnant uterus, elevating blood pressure, having adverse effects on diabetic patients and having adverse effects in patients suffering from angina.

Although to date it is believed that clenbuterol is not mutagenic, early experimental studies illustrated some incidences of leiomyomas in experimental animals. The glycogenolytic effect elevated blood glucose (diabetogenic effect) and reduced the keeping quality and palatability of meat.

A letter in the *Lancet* of 1990 drew attention to the possibility of alleged food poisoning in Spain illustrating that liver from treated Spanish cattle contained up to 150 ppb. This, however, was not a comprehensive scientific paper but rather correspondence on an observed syndrome. In March, 1991, a similar problem was reported from the Clermont-Ferrand region of France. Symptoms of palpitations, tachycardia, and muscle tremors were observed: typical signs of B_2 agonist intoxication. Clenbuterol was identified in the urine of affected patients. Owing to the problems detected in Italy, Germany, the Netherlands, Spain, France, and Belgium, the European Community, through its Committee for Veterinary Medicinal Products, has now put great emphasis on the elimination of this problem. Random residue tests have been developed for feed, tissues, urine, and liver. In 1989, Brussels suggested that member states should introduce specific laws into national statute books. The drug clenbuterol is expensive and is unlikely to be used at high levels for long periods in calves and beef animals. This would not necessarily hold true, however, for the cheap, illegal, black-market-imported products. European Community bodies are presently active in framing legislation on this problem. In 1992, further instances of clenbuterol food poisoning were reported from Spain.

In the United States, the concern is based on allegations of abuse of the drug, which is not approved for veterinary use, in exhibit animals at shows. Potential problems have come to the fore in show animals that appear to have significant muscle mass, giving them a competitive edge. Some urine samples from these show animals have tested positive. It has been suggested that the source of the clenbuterol may be from Canada, where the drug is approved as a bronchodilator in horses.

In the United States, show horses that proved positive for clenbuterol in urine samples have proved negative for liver samples according to the USDA. The FDA has sent letters out to State Departments of Agriculture and the USDA to enlist their assistance in preventing any illegal use of clenbuterol.

High-performance liquid chromatography, mass spectrometry, radioimmunoassay, enzyme-linked immunosorbent assay, and thin-layer chromatography tests have all been used in screening and confirming analysis. ELISA methods can now be used to examine plasma, urine, bile, and liver. Liver contains the highest level for the longest time, and a detection level of 1 ppb in this tissue has been established.

Clenbuterol is unlikely to be marketed as a repartitioning agent, but other synthetic beta-adrenergic agonists are being developed that, it is hoped, will produce comparable or enhanced repartitioning between fat and lean in the carcass with less significant side effects. Clenbuterol is a potent repartitioning agent in farm animals. The control of abuse of this substance relies on detection of small concentrations of the drug in animal tissues after its withdrawal from the diet.

POTENTIAL USE IN PIGS

Beta agonists produced naturally in animals include epinephrine and norepinephrine. Analogs of these compounds have been produced by several companies and fed to finishing pigs. They have increased gain in muscle mass and decreased fat deposition in finishing pigs. Several companies are now commercially developing synthetic beta agonists. Ractopamine (Eli Lilly and Company) is the most advanced in testing, having consistently improved daily gain, feed efficiency, and carcass quality when fed to finishing swine.

Although some parts of the world permit the use of beta agonists as repartitioning agents (especially in pigs for leaner carcasses), clenbuterol is highly likely to be banned even for therapeutic use in the European Community in the near future. Nonetheless beta agonists such as cimaterol have been used in many countries, and Ractopamine ("Paylean") is licensed in some countries in South America and the EC.

Ractopamine will be receiving special attention from the Codex Alimentarius Committee in Washington in the near future.

24.8 PRO-BIOTICS

Antibiotics are substances of microbiologic origin that depress the multiplication of bacteria and some other organisms. "Probiotic" means the opposite, a material of biological origin that promotes the multiplication of bacteria. The word also describes products containing live bacteria fed to livestock.

In recent years, interest has been generated in feeding selected microorganisms to animals to improve production. Strains of *Lactobacillus, Streptococcus, bacillus subtilis* or related microorganisms recovered from the intestinal tracts of birds and mammals have been used. Use of certain strains of these organisms has shown some degree of success in the control of enteric disease and has improved weight gains.

The benefits of lactic-acid-producing bacteria similar to *Streptococcus faecium* were first postulated by Metchnikoff. He believed that the growth of putrefactive organisms could result in gut adsorption of toxins detrimental to the host and suggested that lactic-acid-producing bacteria would prevent this phenomenon from occurring. *S. faecium* was once classified as a *Lactobacillus acidophilus* but has been separated by specific biochemical techniques. Other streptococci have been studied, including *Streptococcus faecalis* and *Streptococcus diacetylactis*.

LACTIC ACID BACTERIA

Lactic acid bacteria have been used in the treatment of gastrointestinal disorders since the beginning of the century. Metchnikoff was the founder of *Lactobacillus* therapy in 1908. He advocated the use of yogurt because of its high proportion of lactic acid bacteria and recommended it in gastrointestinal and other disorders. Because the bacteria in yogurt do not multiply in the intestinal tract, however, the therapy gradually moved toward *L. acidophilus* and organisms capable of multiplying within the intestine.

Many studies of the effects of *L. acidophilus* therapy were carried out over a period of years, with promising results. In the gut, lactobacilli are present, both floating free and attached to the gut wall. They are present normally in considerable numbers. Generally about one third of all the organisms in the gut are lactobacilli, and they function by increasing beneficial intestinal bacteria and interfering with attachment of enteric pathogens to the intestinal mucosa. They also cause a reduction in intestinal pH by the production of lactic acid and may reduce the intestinal oxidation reduction potential, thereby inhibiting aerobic intestinal pathogens. This may also reduce the production of undesirable metabolic by-products in the intestinal lumen.

Within the first few hours after birth, lactobacilli, picked up from the surroundings and particularly from the mother's teat, become established in the gut. An early intake of colostrum is also vital to ensure adequate antibody levels. Stress, such as disease, cold, hunger, or exhaustion, has the rapid effect of reducing the population of lactobacilli in the gut, probably through alterations in gut acidity. Born with a neutral gut environment, the neonate would, in its natural habitat, rapidly acquire protective microflora from its mother's teats. Intensive farming techniques deprive the animal of this opportunity, however, by separating mother and offspring almost immediately, leaving the latter highly vulnerable to pathogenic attack.

Rapid reductions in *Lactobacillus* populations have been found to follow animal stress in its various forms. Diminished competitive population pressure at these times probably plays a significant, although as yet unquantified, part in allowing potential pathogens, such as *E. coli*, to become dominant.

DEVELOPMENT OF MODERN PRO-BIOTICS

Although lactic-acid-producing microorganisms have been suggested from time to time, they have not proved successful until now. The reasons include:

- The use of inappropriate and therefore ineffective strains
- Low stability of the products (sharp decrease in the number of viable cells within a short time)
- No guarantee of a minimum content
- Prejudice against the whole group, owing to some products of low technical and qualitative standard

In veterinary medicine, the first tests in the prophylaxis of diarrhea in pigs were not carried out until 1965, which is relatively late.

In all the studies, the researchers repeatedly stressed the need for a stable product in which the cells retain their viability over a long period. Many strains are sensitive to temperature, humidity, and other environmental factors. Others are sensitive to acids, which lowers the chances of survival of the bacteria during their passage through the stomach.

The organisms most commonly involved are lactobacilli, which occur naturally in the small intestine of animals and humans. Lactobacilli are prolific producers of enzymes, notably the carbohydrases, which aid digestion. By assisting the breakdown of food in the small intestine, lactobacilli help to prevent the overflow of relatively undigested food material into the large intestine, where it would provide a rich environment for the nourishment of other, potentially pathogenic organisms, such as *E. coli*. In addition, a side effect of their enzyme action is the production of acids, toward which the coliforms are less tolerant. Based on this knowledge, products have arisen, largely for in-feed use, that contain lactobacilli in dried culture form, with the aim of enhancing growth and feed use.

New organisms, such as *S. faecium* and *Lactobacillus bulgaricus*, have a more specific antienterotoxic effect, which fulfills the requirements with regard to efficacy, stability, and environmental tolerance. One strain that appears promising is the probiotic *S. faecium*. It has been used successfully as a feed additive for many years. It is a potent lactic acid producer.

The lyophilized bacteria reach the intestinal tract undamaged (only slight losses occur in transit through the stomach—high acid tolerance). *S. faecium* has a generation time that is far shorter than that of other strains. It can therefore compete with the development of fast-growing pathogenic microorganisms. Multiplication means metabolism—in this case, production of large amounts of lactic acid. This produces a local gut environment in which pathogens cannot survive. *S. faecium* also "crowds out" other pathogenic bacteria and prevents their gut adhesion.

In the intestine, the microorganisms undergo activation and begin to multiply. Distribution in the whole intestinal tract is assured. This lactic-acid-producing organism appears to benefit the host by:

1. Aiding the host's digestive process
2. Colonizing the lower intestine and crowding out undesirable pathogens
3. Changing the oxidation/reduction potential
4. Producing antibacterial substances (bacteriocins)
5. Lowering the pH of the intestinal tract
6. Producing antitoxins

In other words, beneficial lactobacilli are stimulated, crowding out *E. coli*, and lactose is converted to lactic acid, thereby maintaining optimum gut conditions and improving digestion of milk.

Different modes of action of lactic-acid-secreting bacteria have been proposed, such as adhesion to the intestinal epithelium as a criterion for colonization. In that case, it must be speculated whether some competition for binding sites is taking place between *E. coli* and lactic-acid-secreting bacteria. The production of bacteriocins by *S. faecium* has been documented and has been proposed as an active component in diarrhea prevention. The lowering of pH in the small intestine by lactic acid has been investigated as a means of reducing the effects of intestinal pathogens. The reduction of *E. coli* numbers in the presence of lactic-acid-secreting bacteria appeared to promote a more favorable enteric flora balance. The neutralization of the effect of *E. coli* enterotoxin by *S. faecium* has been documented and proposed as a mode of action.

Strains of various *Lactobacillus* species are known to associate with the surface of stratified squamous epithelium in the stomachs of mice and rats, the pars eosophagia of swine, and the crops of chickens. In associating with the epithelial cells, the bacteria undoubtedly adhere to them. The adhesion may be mediated by acidic polysaccharides and lipoteichoic acid and involves some specificity from animal species to animal species.

Feeding *Lactobacillus* results in reduction of both coliform and *Clostridium* bacteria, particularly in stressed animals. Fed prophylactically, they minimize outbreaks of enteric disease, thereby effecting an optimization of growth potential. With the increasing emphasis on natural products, antibodies, and immunomodulators as well as consumer concerns over drug residues in edible products, it will be interesting to observe the comparative efficacies of pro-biotics and antibiotics as growth-promoting agents.

24.9 FUTURE DEVELOPMENTS

Biotechnology in the pharmaceutical industry is already well established. In the production of antibiotics and steroids by fermentation, increasing the yields of microbial strains and creating new ones by gene transfer and hybridization have been early goals of genetic engineering. The search is also on for the "new avermectin": Screening of new microbial isolates and the use of unusual precursors in culture broths to generate novel analogs of existing chemicals are now commonplace. Even the production of pharmaceuticals by more complex organisms, such as sheep, is now a possibility.

E. coli and *Bacillus* are in general use to produce materials of interest, but there is a move away from these prokaryotes, stimulated by their inability to secrete proteins in a form that is biologically active in animals and their all-too-efficient degradation of foreign materials before these can pass through the bacterial cell wall. Yeasts and vertebrate cells are now increasingly used to manufacture and release desired products in an active form.

In common with more traditional pharmaceuticals, the proportion that will be developed specifically for veterinary use is likely to be small, and most products will probably be "borrowed" from human use.

Nevertheless, there is a great deal of research activity in the extension of the use of these materials into animal health.

GROWTH AND PERFORMANCE

Somatotropins are undoubtedly the focus of the greatest biotechnologic effort by the pharmaceutical companies. BST itself is expected to obtain regulatory clearance in the near future, and fish somatotropins should follow soon after. An important factor in the acceptance of these aids to animal productivity will be the improvements in quality, not necessarily quantity alone, which are expected from their use. Other products of genetic engineering in the field could include growth-hormone-releasing factor, a much smaller molecule that is not species specific; prolactin, which is a performance enhancer in fish and poultry; and vaccines prepared from somatostatin, luteinizing-hormone-releasing hormone, or androstenone, which are still in development and require refinement before commercialization.

Active and passive immunization procedures have some potential for influencing the activity of the major endocrine pathways or to change the relative impacts of negative or positive feedback systems. Such immunization procedures encompass immunization against gonadotropin-releasing hormone, immunization against somatostatin, or immunization against adipocytes.

Immunologic neutralization of gonadotropin-releasing hormone is an alternative system to castration in cattle to control sexual behavior. Reduction in testosterone production and of the testicles and docile behavior result from this technique. Inhibition of production of gonadotropin-releasing hormone in male cattle reduced testicular growth and blood levels in testosterone. The effects of immunization last for 4 to 5 months, with an increased lean content of the carcass. Such active immunization against gonadotropin-releasing hormone, also termed immunocastration, results in faster growth rates in cattle and sheep and increased food conversion efficiency.

The rationale for immunization against somatostatin is to reduce the negative feedback effects against growth hormone and the somatomedins. Production of antibodies to somatostatin growth hormone inhibiting factor has been shown experimentally to enhance growth rate in sheep.

Reduction of fat levels can also be achieved by immunization against the fat cells or adipocytes. Elevation of adipocyte antibody levels by passive immunization in sheep has demonstrated a 40% reduction in body fat, with an accompanying increase in body protein and water.

Manipulation of the photoperiod by exposing animals to artificially long daylight has been reported to increase growth rate in sheep and cattle and milk yield in cows. The underlying mechanism currently remains unclear, but prolactin and especially melatonin appear to play a significant role. Melatonin is already a major research avenue for breeding control in sheep.

The development of transgenic animals offers exciting prospects for direct manipulation of the animal's growth and production. Experiments to date have concentrated on the transfer of cloned DNA sequences coding for growth hormone production into the mammalian embryo. The potential of gene transfer has been demonstrated in laboratory animals, and the most widely used method is the microinjection of DNA into one pronucleus of fertilized eggs. The use of gene transfer and recombinantly derived food animals offers interesting opportunities in biotechnologic procedures.

The production of large quantities of peptide hormones, particularly growth hormone by recombinant DNA technology, marks the beginning of a new era in the field of growth control in domestic animals. The first challenge is to develop methods for administering these peptides under practical conditions. At the moment, economically feasible slow-release vehicles for peptide hormones are not commercially available. Little is known of the longterm effects of administered growth hormone, somatostatin, growth-hormone-releasing factor, or somatomedins in domestic animals.

24.8 QUINOXALINES

Within the class of quinoxaline-1,4-dioxides, carcinogenicity has been reported for the parent substance of the group, quin-

doxin. Other substances in the group show positive responses in various tests for mutagenicity. This mutagenic activity seems to be connected with the mechanism of antibacterial action, thereby indicating that quinoxaline-1,4-dioxide with antibacterial and therefore growth-promoting efficacy will also inevitably show mutagenic activity to some extent. If mutagenicity is considered to indicate potential carcinogenicity, long-term tests would give the relevant information.

With regard to human safety, only minimal threat to the consumer's health is imposed by these compounds if they are used according to the licensing conditions (long withdrawal times) owing to the rapid excretion of these drugs and metabolites by the pig, render the metabolites less toxic than the parent drug. There are, however, major concerns for the health of the workers in the feed industry and on self-mixing farms. All quinoxalines are suspected of inducing photoallergy and phototoxicity. These effects, together with the genotoxic and mutagenic activity, involve risks for people handling these drugs as premixes or medicated feeds. The widest exposure could occur from residues of the parent drug in edible tissues of treated animals or from excretion and accumulation in the environment.

Humans can be exposed to an additive in several ways:

By skin contact with the additive, premix, or feed

By inhalation of dust generated during mixing and feeding

By skin contact with excrement or slurry from treated animals

By residues present in meat of slaughtered animals

Safety label recommendations were established to protect the health of workers and to avoid any exposure to the additives, especially by contact or inhalation.

In pigs, carbadox is metabolized rapidly to quinoxaline-2-carboxylic acid, a methylcarbazate, with the intermediary formation of desoxycarbadox. No residues of desoxycarbadox are found in edible tissues 72 hours after withdrawal of the carbadox-supplemented feedstuff (limit of determination, 5 μg/kg). Carbadox and its intermediary metabolite desoxycarbadox, however, are hepatotoxic, causing dose-related nodular hepatic hyperplasia in longterm studies in rats. They have also been shown to be mutagenic in in vitro and in vivo tests but no mutagenic effects have been observed with their metabolic products. Therefore it was concluded that the residues of carbadox have low toxicity because the parent compound and desoxycarbadox are not detectable 72 hours after administration of the product.

Nonetheless, human contact with carbadox must be kept to a minimum at the mixing stage, and protective clothing worn. In the United States a withdrawal time of 70 days applies to carbadox in pigs. In the United States, a zero tolerance has been set, with 30 ppb as the limit of detection.

SELECTED REFERENCES

Adams, H.R.: New perspectives in cardiopulmonary therapeutics: Receptoselective adrenergic drugs. J. Am. Vet. Med. Assoc., 185:966, 1984.

Ahlquist, R.P.: A study of adrenotropic receptors. Am. J. Physiol., 153:586, 1987.

Anderson, T.D., Wannalstine, W.G., Ficken, M.D., et al.: Acute monensin toxicosis in sheep, light and electron microscopic changes. Am. J. Vet. Res., 45:1142, 1984.

Aschbacher, P.W.: Diethylstilbestrol metabolism in food-producing animals. J. Toxicol. Environ. Health, (Suppl. 1):45, 1976.

Baker, P.K., Dalrymple, R.H., Ingle, D.L., and Ricks, C.A.: Use of a beta agonist to alter muscle and fat deposition in lambs. J. Anim. Sci., 59:1256, 1984.

Baldwin, R.L., and Middleton, S.C.: Biology of bovine somatotropin. National Invitational Workshop on Bovine Somatotropin, St. Louis, 1987.

Baldwin, R.S., Williams, R.D., and Terry, M.K.: Zeranol: A review of the metabolism toxicology and analytical methods for detection of tissue residues. Reg. Toxicol. Pharmacol., 3:9, 1983.

Barraud, B., Lungnier, A., and Dirheimer, G.: In vivo covalent binding to rat liver DNA of trenbolone as compared to 17-betaestradiol, testosterone and zeranol. In Proceedings Anabolics in Animal Production, Public Health Aspects, Analytic Methods and Regulation, Office International des Epizooties, Paris, 1983.

Bauman, D.E., Eppard, P.J., DeGeeter, M.J., et al.: Responses of high producing dairy cows to long term treatment with pituitary somatotropin and recombinant somatotropin. J. Dairy Sci., 68:1352, 1985.

Bauman, D.E., Peel, C.J., Steinhour, W.D., et al.: Effect of bovine somatotropin on metabolism of dairy cows; influence on rates of irreversible loss and oxidation of glucose and nonesterified fatty acids. J. Nutr., 118:1031, 1988.

Bechtel, P.J., Easter, R.A., Novakofski, M., et al.: Effect of porcine somatotropin on limit fed swine. J. Anim. Sci., 66 (Suppl. 1):282, 1988.

Beerman, D.H., Hogue, D.E., et al.: J. Anim. Sci., 62:370, 1986.

Bekaert, H., Casteels, M., and Baysse, F.X.: In Beta-Agonists and Their Effects on Animal Growth and Carcass Quality. Ed. J.P. Hanrahan. New York, Elsevier Applied Science, 1987.

Berger, L.L., and Ricke, S.C.: Comparison of lasalocid and monensin for feedlot cattle. J. Anim. Sci., 49 (Suppl. 1):357, 1980.

Berger, L.L., Ricke, S.C., and Fahey, G.C.: Comparison of two forms and two levels of lasalocid with monensin on feedlot cattle performance. J. Anim. Sci., 53:1440, 1981.

Boucque, C.V., Fiems, L.O., Sommer, M., et al.: In: Beta-Agonists and Their Effects on Animal Growth and Carcass Quality. Ed. by J.P. Hanrahan New York, Elsevier Applied Science, 1987.

Bouffault, J.C., and Willemart, J.P.: Anabolic activity of trenbolone acetate alone or in association with estrogens. In Anabolics in Animal Production. Proceedings of International Office of Epizootics Symposium, Paris, 1983.

Boyd, R.D., Bauman, D.E., Beerman, D.H., et al.: Titration of the porcine growth hormone dose which maximizes growth performance and lean deposition in swine. J. Anim. Sci., 65 (Suppl. 1):218, 1986.

Boyd, R.D., Beerman, D.H., Roneker, K.R., et al.: Biological activity of a recombinant variant (21 kd) of porcine somatotropin in growing swine. J. Anim. Sci., 66 (Suppl. 1):256, 1988.

Brockway, J.M., MacRae, J.C., and Williams, P.E.V.: Side effects of clenbuterol as a repartitioning agent. Vet. Rec., 120:381, 1987.

Bryan, K.A., Carbaugh, D.E., Clark, A.M., et al.: Effect of porcine growth hormone (pGH) on growth and carcass composition of gilts. J. Anim. Sci., 65 (Suppl. 1):244, 1987.

Burvenich, C., Vandeputte-Van Messom, G., Roets, E., et al.: Recombinant bovine somatotropin and intramammary Escherichia coli challenge in cows during early lactation. In Proceedings of the Seventh International Conference on Production Disease in Farm Animals, 1989.

Busby, W.D.: Effect of propionate enhancers on the performance of grazing steers and sexual development of beef bulls. M.S. Thesis, 1980.

Buttery, P.J.: Mode of action of zeranol and other anabolic agents. In Proceedings of Management for Growth, Orlando, FL, 1985.

Campbell, R.G., et al.: Effects of porcine pituitary growth hormone (pGH) administration and energy intake on growth performance of pigs from 25–55 kg body weight. J. Anim. Sci., *65* (Suppl. 1):244, 1987.

Chene, N., Martal, J., de la Llosa, P., et al.: Growth hormones. II. Structure-function relationships. Reprod. Nutr. Develop., *29*:1, 1989.

Cleays, M.C., et al.: Skeletal muscle protein synthesis and growth hormone secretion in young lambs treated with Clenbuterol. J. Anim. Sci., *67*:2245, 1989.

Confer, A.W., et al.: Light and electron microscopic changes in cardiac and skeletal muscle of sheep with experimental monensin toxicosis. Vet. Pathol., *20*:590, 1983.

Corah, L.R., and Riley, J.G.: Effect of feeding Rumensin during the growing phase of subsequent reproductive performance of yearling heifers. KS Agri. Expt. Sta Report of Prog., *494*:62, 1977.

Council for Agricultural Science and Technology: Antibiotics in Animal Feeds. Report No. 88. Ames, IA. 1981. P. 79.

Davis, S.R., Collier, R.J., McNamara, J.P., et al.: Effects of thyroxine and growth hormone treatment of dairy cows on milk yield, cardiac output and mammary blood flow. J. Anim. Sci., *66*:70, 1988.

Dixon, S.N., and Heitzman, R.J.: Measurement of synthetic anabolic agents in the tissues of farm animals. *In* Anabolics in Animal Production. Proceedings of International Office of Epizootics Symposium, Paris, 1983.

Dixon, S.N., and Mallinson, C.B.: Radioimmunoassay of the anabolic agents zeranol. III. Zeranol concentrations in the faeces of steers implanted with zeranol (Ralgo). J. Vet. Pharmacol. Therap., *9*:88, 1986.

Dixon, S.N., Russell, K.L., Heitzman, R.J., and Mallinson, C.B.: Radio-immunoassay of anabolic agent seranol. V. Residues of zeranol in the edible tissues, urine, faeces and bile of steers treated with Ralgro. J. Vet. Pharmacol. Therap., *9*:353, 1986.

Donoho, A.L.: Biochemical studies on the fate of monensin in animals and in the environment. J. Anim. Sci., *58*:1528, 1984.

Donoho, A., Manthey, J., Occolowitz, J., et al.: Metabolism of monensin in the steer and rat. Agric. Food Chem., *26*:1090, 1978.

Drennan, M.D., and Roche, J.F.: Effect of monensin sodium and Finaplix on performance on heifers at pasture. Anim. Prod. Res. Rep., An Foras Taluntais, Dublin, 1978.

Drennan, M.D., and Roche, J.F.: Influence of growth promoters on the efficiency of beef production. Anim. Prod. Res. Rep., An Foras Taluntais, Dublin, 1977.

Drennan, M.D., Roche, J.F., and L'Estrange, J.L.: Effect of monensin sodium, resorcyclic acid lactone and trenbolone acetate on performance and feed intake of finishing cattle. Anim. Prod., *28*:416, 1979.

Droumev, D., Pahov, D., Jourbinev, D., et al.: The effect of salinomycin (K-364) on calves for fattening. Vet. Sci. (Bulg.), *10*:34, 1981.

Elasser, T.H., Rumsey, T.S., and Hammond, A.C.: Influence of diet on basal and growth hormone-stimulated plasma concentrations of IGF-1 in beef cattle. J. Anim. Sci., *67*:128, 1989.

Emerging Developments in Veterinary Biotechnology. Office of Planning and Evaluation and the Center for Veterinary Medicine, Food and Drug Administration. Washington, D.C., 1986.

Eppard, P.J., Lanza, G.M., Hudson, S., et al.: Response of lactating dairy cows to multiple injections of sometribove, USAN (recombinant methionyl bovine somatotropin) in a prolonged release system. Part I. Production response. J. Dairy Sci., *71*:184, 1988.

Erherton, T.D., Wiggins, J.P., Evock, C.M., et al.: Stimulation of pig growth performance by porcine growth hormone. Determination of the dose-response relationship. J. Anim. Sci., *64*:433, 1987.

Evaluation of Certain Veterinary Drug Residues in Food. 32nd Report of Joing FAO/WHO Expert Committee of Food Additives. Geneva, WHO, 1988.

Farber, T.M., and Acros, M.: A regulatory approach to the use of anabolic agents. *In* Anabolics in Animal Production. Edited by E. Meissonnier and J. Mitchell-Vigneron. Paris, Office International des Epizooties, 1983.

Farber, T.M., Acros, M., and Crawford, L.: Safety evaluation standards in the United States. *In* Anabolics in Animal Production. Edited by E. Meissonnier and J. Mitchell-Vigneron. Paris, Office International des Epizooties, 1983.

Ferrando, R., and Vanbelle, M.: B-agonistas y produccion de carne: consideraciones y reflexiones. Rec. Med. Vet., *165*:91, 1989.

Food and Drug Administration (FDA): Fed. Regist. 46 (84/Friday, May 1), 24694–24696. Washington, D.C., 1984.

Food and Drug Administration (FDA): Fed. Regist. 49 (69/Monday, April 9), 13872–13873. Washington, D.C., 1981.

Foreyt, J., Parish, S.M., and Foreyt, K.M.: Lasalocid for improved weight gains and control of coccidia in lambs. Am. J. Vet. Res., *42*:57, 1981.

Future Trends in the Animal Health Care Market—A Survey of Industry Opinion. Report compiled by Stategic Technologies Inc., available from V & O Publications, 18–20 Hill Rise, Richmond, Surrey, TW10 6UA, UK. Undated.

Gallo, G.F., Lefebvre, D., and Block, E.: GnRH-induced LH response by dairy cows injected with recombinant bovine somatotropin (rbST) J. Anim. Sci., *67*/J. Dairy Sci., *72*:343, 1989.

Gaspar, P., Evrard, P., and Maghuin-Rogister, G.: Zeranol residue levels in edible tissues, bile and urine of cattle. 3rd Congress, European Association for Veterinary Pharmacology and Toxicology, Ghent, Belgium, 1985.

Goodrich, R.D., Garrett, J.E., et al.: The influence of monensin on the performance of cattle. J. Anim. Sci., 58:1484, 1984.

Grebner, G.L., et al.: Carcass characteristics of pigs injected with different levels of porcine somatotropin (PST) from 57 to 103 kg weight. J. Anim. Sci., 65 (Suppl. 1):245, 1987.

Green, H.B., Syndner, D.L., Miyat, J.A., et al.: The effect of "Somidobove" sustained release formulation on second lactation performance of dairy cattle. J. Anim. Sci., 67/J. Dairy Sci., 72:453, 1989.

Griffin, T., Parekh, C., Singh, A., and Coulston, F.: No hormonal effect level of zeranol in the cynomolgus monkey. In European Toxicology Forum, 1983.

Hanrahan, L.A., et al.: Monensin toxicosis in broiler chickens. Vet. Pathol., 18:665, 1981.

Hart, I.C., Blake, L.A., Chadwick, P.M.E., et al.: The heterogeneity of bovine growth hormone; extraction from the pituitary of components with different biological and immunological properties. Biochem. J., 218:573, 1984.

Heitzman, R.J.: The absorption, distribution and excretion of anabolic agents. J. Anim. Sci., 57:233, 1983.

Heitzman, R.J., and Harwood, D.J.: Residue levels of trenbolone and oestradiol-17β in plasma and tissue of steers implanted with anabolic steroid preparations. Br. Vet. J., 133:564, 1977.

Henricks, D.M., and Torrence, A.K.: Endogenous estradiol-17β in bovine tissues. J. Assoc. Off. Anal. Chem., 61:1280, 1978.

Hoffman, B.: Aspects on tolerance levels of anabolic agents with sex, hormone-like activities in edible animal tissues. In Manipulation of Growth in Farm Animals. Proceedings CEC Programme of Coordination of Research of Beef Production, Brussels, 1982. Edited by J.F. Roche and D. O'Callaghan. The Hague, Nijhoff, 1984.

Hoffman, B.: Use of radioimmunoassay (RIA) for monotoring hormonal residues in edible animal products. J. Assoc. Off. Anal. Chem., 612:1263, 1978.

Hoffman, B., and Blietz, C.: Application of radioimmunoassay (RIA) for the determination of residues of anabolic sex hormones. J. Anim. Sci., 57:239, 1983.

Hoffman, B., and Evers, P.: Drug residues in animals. In Veterinary Science and Comparative Medicine. Edited by A.G. Rico. London, Academic Press, 1986.

Holden, P.J.: Repartitioning agents for swine. Agric. Pract., 11:25, 1990.

Horton, G.M.J., and Stockdale, P.H.G.: Lasalocid and monensin in finishing diets for early weaned lambs with naturally occurring coccidiosis. Am. J. Vet. Res., 42:433, 1981.

Huber, J.T., Willman, S., Sullivan, S.L., et al.: Milk yield responses of sometribove, recombinant methionyl bovine somatotropin, during two consecutive lactations. J. Anim. Sci., 67/J. Dairy Sci., 72:4, 1989.

Hubbert, M., Branine, M., Galyean, M.H., et al.: Influence of alternate feeding of monensin and lasal-

ocid on performance of feedlot Heifers. Preliminary Data. Clayton Livestock Research Report No. 47, 1987.

Jansen, E.H.J.M., Van Den Berg, R.H., Somer, G., et al.: A chemiluminescent immunoassay for zeranol and its metabolites. J. Vet. Pharmacol. Therap., 9:101, 1986.

Janski, A.M.: Development of a sensitive method for extraction and assay of zeranol residues in animal tissues and the use of the method in a multiple implant study in cattle. In Anabolics in Animal Production. Proceedings of International Office of Epizootics Symposium, Paris, 1983.

JECFA/FAO/WHO report: Evaluation of Certain Food Residues. Geneva, WHO, 1988.

Johnsson, O.D., and Spencer, G.S.G.: The potential of somatotropin to increase lean meat production. AFRC News, 1986.

Karg, H.L., Meyer, H.H.D., Vogt, K., et al.: Residues and clearance of anabolic agents in veal calves. In Manipulation of Growth in Farm Animals. Proceedings CEC Programme of Coordination of Research on Beef Production, Brussels, 1982. Edited by J.F. Roche and D. O'Callaghan. The Hague, Nijhoff, 1984.

Knight, C.D., Azain, M.J., Kasser, T.R., et al.: Functionality of an implantable six week delivery system for porcine somatotropin (PST) in finishing hogs. J. Anim. Sci., 66 (Suppl. 1):257, 1988.

Koulikovskii, A.: Review of FAO/WHO activities in the field of anabolics used in animal production. In Anabolics in Animal Production. Proceedings of International Office of Epizootics Symposium, Paris, 1983.

Lamming, G.E.: A scientific approach to the licensing of veterinary drugs. Paper presented at the International Animal Meeting of the Animal Health Institute, Fort Lauderdale, FL, 1986.

Lamming, G.E.: Current progress in the manipulation of animal growth. In Animal Health and Productivity RASE Symposium Proceedings, 1985.

Lance, V.A., Murphy, W.A., Sveras-Diaz, J., and Coy, D.: Superactive analogues of growth hormone-releasing factor (1–29) amide. Biochem. Biophys. Res. Comm., 119:265, 1984.

Lanze, G.M., White, T.C., Dyer, S.E., et al.: Response of lactating cows to intramuscular or subcutaneous injection of sometribove. USAN (recombinant methionyl bovine BST) in a 14-day prolonged release system. Part II. Changed in circulating analytes. J. Dairy Sci., 71:195, 1988.

Lauderdale, J.W.: Use of MGA (melengestrol acetate) in animal production. In Anabolics in Animal Production. Proceedings of International Office of Epizootics Symposium, Paris, 1983.

Lean, I.J.: Studies on bovine ketosis and somatotropin. PhD Thesis, University of California, Davis, 1990.

Lean, I.J., Troutt, H.F., Goddger, W.J., et al.: Bovine somatotropin: Industry implications. Compend. Cont. Educ. Pract. Vet., 12:1150, 1990.

Lomas, L.W.: Lasalocid for ruminants—application. In Proceedings of 37th Annual Kansas Formula Feed Conference, 1982.

Martin, J.J., Gill, D.R., Strasia, C.A., et al.: Comparison of ionophores for feedlot steers. Oklahoma Agric. Exp. Sta. Res. Rep. MP, 116:166, 1984.

Migdalof, B.H., Dugger, H.A., Heider, J.G., et al.: Biotransformation of zeranol: Disposition and metabolism in the female rat, rabbit, dog, monkey and man. Xenobiotica, 13:209, 1983.

Miller, M.F., Cross, H.R., Wilson, J.J., and Smith S.B.: Acute and longterm lipogenic response to insulin and clenbuterol in bovine intramuscular and subcutaneous adipose tissues. J. Anim. Sci., 67:928, 1989.

Moseley, W.M., and McCartor, M.M.: Articles affecting monensin on growth and reproductive performance of beef Heifers. J. Anim. Sci., 45:961, 1977.

Nagaraja, T.G., Avery, T.B., Bartley, E.E., et al.: Effect of lasalocid, monensin or thiopeptin on lactic acidosis in cattle. J. Anim. Sci., 54:649, 1982.

Nation, P.N., Crowe, S.P., and Harries, W.N.: Clinical signs and pathology of accidental monensin poisoning in sheep. Can. Vet. J., 23:323, 1982.

Neff, A.W.: Analytical methods for MGA (melengestrol acetate). In Anabolics in Animal Production. Proceedings of International Office of Epizootics Symposium, Paris, 1983.

Neuendorff, D.A., and Rutter, L.M.: Effect of lasalocid on growth and pubertal development of Brahman bulls. J. Anim. Sci., 61:1049, 1985.

O'Keefe, M.: Tissue levels of the anabolic agents, trenbolone and zeranol, determined by radioimmunoassay. Proceedings of the Symposium on the Analysis of Steroids, Szeged, Hungary. Edited by S. Gorog. Budapest, Akademiac Kiado, 1984.

Palmiter, R.D., Brinster, R.L., Hammer, R.E., et al.: Dramatic growth of mice that develop from eggs microinjected with metallothionein-growth hormone fusion genes. Nature (Lond.), 300:611, 1982.

Peters, A.R.: Correct use of growth promoting implants. In Pract., 7:14, 1985.

Phipps, R.K.: The use of prolonged release bovine somatotropin in milk production. Bull. Int. Dairy Fed., 228:2, 1988.

Phipps, R.K., Weller, R.F., Austin, A.R., et al.: A preliminary report on a prolonged release formulation of bovine somatotropin with particular reference to animal health. Vet. Rec., 122:512, 1988.

Powell-Jones, W., Raefore, S., and Lucier, G.W.: Binding properties of zearalenone mycotoxins to hepatic estrogen receptors. Mol. Pharmacol., 20:35, 1981.

Raun, A.P.: Monensin. Effect of energy efficiency. Presented at European Congress for Improved Beef Productivity, Paris, 1978.

Raun, A.P., Cooley, C.O., Potter, E.L., et al.: Effect of monensin of feed efficiency of feedlot cattle. J. Anim. Sci., 43:670, 1976.

Richardson, K.E., Hagler, W.M., Jr., and Mirocha, C.J.: Production of zearalenone, α- and β-zeralenol,

and α- and β-zearalenol by Fusarium spp. in rice culture. J. Agric. Food Chem., 33:862, 1985.

Rico, A.G.: Metabolism of endogenous and exogenous anabolic agents in cattle. J. Anim. Sci., 57:226, 1983.

Roberts, N.L., and Cameron, D.M.: Roussel-UCLAF Trenbolone Acetate Documentation. Hormonal effects of orally administered trenbolone, findings from three studies in the domestic pig. Huntingdon Research Centre, RSL 357, 581, 663, 1985.

Roche, J.F., Davis, W.D., and Sherington, J.: Effect of trenbolone acetate or resorcylic acid lactone alone or combined on daily liveweight and carcass weight in steers. Ir. J. Agric. Res., 17:7, 1978.

Roche, J.F., Davis, W.D., and Sherington, J.: Effects of time of insertion of resorcylic acid lactone and trenbolone acetate and type of diet on growth rate in steers. Ir. J. Agric. Res., 17:249, 1978.

Ryan, J.J., and Hoffman, B.: Trenbolone acetate (TBA): Experiences with bound residues in cattle tissue. J. Assoc. Off. Anal. Chem., 61:1274, 1978.

Schams, D.: Somatotropin and related peptides in milk. In Use of Somatotropin in Livestock Production. Bovine Somatotropin Symposium, Brussels, Belgium, 1988. Edited by K. Serjrsen. New York, Elsevier Applied Sciences, 1989.

Schelling, G.T.: Monensin mode of action in the rumen. J. Anim. Sci., 58:1518, 1984.

Stallones, R.A., Alexander, E.R., Antle, C.E., et al.: The Effects on Human Health of Subtherapeutic Use of Antimicrobials in Animal Feeds. Washington, D.C., National Academy of Sciences, 1980. P. 379.

Stanton, T.L., Birkelo, C.P., and Grover, P.: Rumensin, Bovatec, ionophore rotation and Synovex/MGA effects on finishing Heifer performance. Fort Collins, Colorado State University Beef Program Report, 1989.

Timmerman, H.: In: Beta-Agonists and Their Effects on Animal Growth and Carcass Quality. Ed. by J.P. Hanrahan. New York, Elsevier Applied Science, 1987.

Topel, D.G.: Development and status of repartitioning agents for use in the swine industry. Proc. Univ. III, Pork Ind. Conf. Champaign, IL, 1987.

Truhaut, R.L., Shubik, P., and Tuchmann-Duplessis, H.: Seranol and estradiol 17-β: A critical review of the toxicological properties when used as anabolic agents. Reg. Toxicol. Pharmacol., 5:276, 1985.

United States Department of Agriculture, Food Safety and Inspection Service: Quantitation and Confirmatory Method for DES and Zeranol in Beef Tissue. Chemistry Division Laboratory Guidebook. Part 5, No. 5.051. Washington, D.C., 1986.

Van Der Wal, P., and Berende, P.L.M.: Effects of anabolic agents on food producing animals. In Anabolics of Animal Production. Proceedings of International Office of Epizootics Symposium, Paris, 1983.

Van Vleet, J.F., et al.: Clinical, clinicopathologic and pathologic alterations in acute monensin toxicosis in cattle. Am. J. Vet. Res., 44:2133, 1983.

Van Werden, E.J.: In: Beta-Agonists and Their Effects on Animal Growth and Carcass Quality. Ed. by J.P. Hanrahan, New York, Elsevier Applied Science, 1987.

WHO IPCS Report: Principles for Safety Assessment of Food Additives and Contaminants in Food. Geneva, WHO, 1987.

Windholz, M. et al.: The Merck Index, 10th Edition. Rahway, NJ, Merck and Co., 1983.

Zinn, R.A.: Influence of lasalocid and monensin plus tylosin on comparative feeding value of steam-flaked versus dry-rolled corn in diets for feedlot cattle. J. Anim. Sci., 65:256, 1987.

Zoa-Mhoe, A., Head, H.H., Bachman, K.C., et al.: Effects of bovine somatotropin on milk yield and composition, dry matter intake, and some physiological functions of holstein cows during heat stress. J. Dairy Sci., 72:907, 1989.

CHAPTER

25

BOVINE MASTITIS

25.1 Introduction
25.2 Intramammary Formulations
25.3 Intramammary Therapy
25.4 Treatment of Clinical Mastitis
25.5 Antibiotic Therapy During the Dry Period
25.6 Defense Mechanisms of the Mammary Gland
25.7 Staphylococcal Mastitis
25.8 Coliform Mastitis
25.9 Summer Mastitis—Dry-Cow Mastitis
25.10 Miscellaneous Mastitis
25.11 Vaccination and Intramammary Devices
25.12 Control Policy

25.1 INTRODUCTION

Bovine mastitis is a major cause of economic loss in all countries where dairying is practiced. The losses associated with the disease arise from reduced milk yields from infected quarters, loss of milk sales during antibiotic therapy, culling of chronically affected cows, and, occasionally, death in peracute cases.

This highly complex disease involves the interaction of bacteria, management, and the environment. Because it cannot be eradicated, it must be controlled. A successful control program must be economic, practical, and effective.

Although several different bacteria cause mastitis, *Streptococcus agalactiae, Staphylococcus aureus* and *Actinomyces pyogenes* are the most common causative agents. Only a small percentage of total mastitis infections is caused by coliforms, such as *Escherichia coli* or *Klebsiella*, and other mastitis organisms.

Streptococcus agalactiae survives in the mammary gland and lives only a short time outside the gland. Thus, it can be eradicated from dairy herds. When present, however, *S. agalactiae* can be found on the teats, udder, tonsils, vagina, and skin of the cow. The organism enters the gland through the teat opening and resides in the ducts and on the gland tissue surfaces. The infection damages gland tissue and reduces milk production.

Once present in the milk of infected cows, *S. agalactiae* may contaminate everything the milk contacts, including the hands of the milker, the equipment, and even bedding. When spread during the milking process, the organisms may be present at levels high enough to affect the bacterial and somatic cell counts of the entire milk production of a herd.

S. agalactiae was first identified as a causative pathogen in clinical bovine mastitis in 1884 and remained the prime etiologic agent until the introduction of penicillin into veterinary therapeutics in 1944.

Staphylococcus aureus assumed increased importance as a mastitis pathogen with the decline in significance of *Streptococcus agalactiae*. Initially, *Staphylococcus aureus* was sensitive to penicillin, but subsequently developed resistance as a result of selection for penicillinase activity (beta-lactamase).

Intensification in dairying has led to modified husbandry and management practices over the winter housing period. These modifications, in turn, have helped such opportunist organisms as *Escherichia coli* and *Streptococcus uberis* to precipitate an environmental type of mastitis. Coliforms can become pathogens in dairy herds. These disease organisms are derived from manure and inadequately cleaned milking machines and can be spread by improper milking procedures.

Good herd management, including a clean environment and the milking of only clean, dry teats, can reduce the incidence of coliform infections. If environmental contamination at and between milkings is limited, the problem should subside in 1 to 2 weeks. Newly reported pathogens include mycoplasmas, anaerobes, and fungal causes of mastitis. These appear to be increasing in incidence.

Bacteria, fungi, mycoplasmas, increasingly anaerobic bacteria, and even algae have been associated with the development of mastitis. On an overall basis, however, *Staphylococcus aureus* or *Streptococcus agalactiae* seem to be involved in 50% of all cases of bovine mastitis; just 10–12 species of bacteria account for most cases of bovine mastitis (Table 25–1).

The organisms abundant in the environment are rarely causes of intramammary infection unless their usual low new infection rates are for some reason exacerbated. At present, concern is focused on three environmental infectious agents that are relatively uninfluenced by current mastitis control programs: *Escherichia coli, Klebsiella pneumoniae*, and *Streptococcus uberis*. Less common are infections caused by *streptococcus* species other than *agalactiae, Pseudomonas*, other gram-negative bacteria, *Nocardia asteroides*, various yeasts, *Bacillus cereus*, and mycoplasmas.

B. cereus is an aerobic sporing anthracoid that is ubiquitous in soil and commonly found in the farmyard environment, where it usually behaves as a harmless saprophyte. *B. cereus* is well known to dairy bacteriologists as a cause of spoilation in milk and cream.

Herd problems may be caused by *Klebsiella* from dirty straw or contaminated wood

TABLE 25–1
BOVINE MASTITIS—CAUSATIVE AGENTS

Agent	Stain Characteristics
Streptococcus agalactiae	Gram + cocci
Streptococcus dysgalactiae	Gram + cocci
Streptococcus uberis	Gram + cocci
Streptococcus zooepidemicus	Gram + cocci
Staphylococcus aureus	Gram + cocci
Escherichia coli	Gram − rod
Enterobacter (Aerobacter)	Gram − encapsulated rod
Aerogens	
Klebsiella species	Gram − encapsulated rod
Proteus species	Gram − rod
Clostridium perfringens	Gram + rod
Actinomyces pyogenes	Gram + rod
Nocardia asteroides	Gram + acid fast
Pasteurella multocida	Gram − ovoid rod
Pseudomonas aeruginosa	Gram − rod
Mycoplasma species	Pleomorphic
Mycoplasma Agalcta var bovi	Pleomorphic

shavings, *Serratia* from contaminated teat dip cups or other sources, *Escherichia coli* or Group D streptococci from environmental contamination, or *Streptococcus agalactiae* and *Staphylococcus aureus* from contaminated milking equipment. Susceptibility testing is necessary to choose an appropriate antibiotic and to eliminate ineffective therapy.

Important sources of infection within a dairy herd are infected mammary glands, colonized teat ducts, or infected teat lesions. Transmission of the pathogens in question, primarily *Staphylococcus aureus* and *Streptococcus agalactiae*, occurs predominantly during milking. This mode of transmission is also characteristic of the less common agents, such as mycoplasmas.

Such pathogens as *Streptococcus uberis* and *Escherichia coli* are more commonly located on extramammary sites on the cow or in the environment. Control of these infections by milking time is poor, and therefore, transmission is considered to occur mainly between milkings.

Transmission of pathogens to, and subsequent infection of, nonlactating glands may account for more than 20% of all new infections, particularly with regard to *Streptococcus uberis*, whereas "summer mastitis"

is almost entirely limited to heifers and non-lactating cows.

Milk is a good medium for bacterial growth. Lactose is used as a source of carbon, and hydrolysis of casein provides an adequate supply of nitrogen. When inflammation develops, compositional changes in the secretion, partly the result of leakage of plasma into the udder, are likely to stimulate bacterial growth.

An important factor in susceptibility to infection is the resistance mechanism within the mammary gland itself. During the dry period when the gland is fully involuted, most of these resistance factors, including phagocytic cells, immunoglobulins, and lactoferrin, are present in high concentrations. At the beginning and end of the dry period, which are times of both functional transition of the mammary gland and high susceptibility to infection, these systems may be compromised.

Persistence of infection may result, in part, from suboptimal stimulation or suppression of the mammary immune system.

The main problem in antibiotic therapy of mastitis is the selection of an effective drug and the maintenance of adequate antibiotic concentrations of that drug at the site of infection. Problems also relate to distribution and binding of the antibiotic to serum and milk protein. High lipid solubility seems to assist tissue penetration.

Factors that control antibiotic concentration and the duration of contact with bacteria can be considered in the following categories:

1. The organism's location and susceptibility
2. Host-animal factors
3. Pharmacokinetics of the administered drug (distribution and elimination of the drug)

25.2 INTRAMAMMARY FORMULATIONS

Many different cerate formulations have been developed in recent years in response to the changing patterns of infection and the varying demands of the dairying industry. The dramatic increase in mastitis caused by gram-negative organisms has led to the introduction of more cerates possessing broad-spectrum antimicrobial activity. Arguments continue regarding whether the systematic reduction in gram-positive infections occasioned by mastitis control and dry-cow therapy has caused a subsequent reduction in protection against gram-negative mastitis organisms.

The development of antibiotics for mastitis therapy must take into account the results of in vitro studies regarding the appropriate spectrum of action of the antimicrobial agent against specific mastitis pathogens. In addition, effective antimicrobial levels must be attained in the presence of milk. The selected antibiotic must be stable both in milk and in the presence of degradative enzymes produced by bacteria, e.g., beta-lactamase. The drug must also be safe for use. This safety aspect is usually assessed by monitoring the white blood cell counts in milk, which serve as an index of the inherent irritancy of a particular cerate. Intramammary preparations for use in milking and dry cows must be thoroughly evaluated and tested to ensure that no significant rise in blood cell count occurs and that no blood or clots appear in the milk after infusion. Such characteristics indicate an irritant preparation.

Efficacy of a particular product depends not only on the antimicrobial levels attained in the gland after infusion, but also on the persistence of these levels. The persistence of an antibiotic in the udder depends primarily on the base in which the antibiotic is formulated and, to a lesser extent, on the nature of the actual antibiotic salt employed, i.e., whether a sparingly soluble salt is used. Bases for milking-cow cerates frequently contain oils and wetting agents to ensure that antibiotics diffuse rapidly in the udder. Dry-cow cerates, on the other hand, are usually formulated in specialized long-acting bases to promote antibiotic persistence. Once a potentially useful antibiotic has been selected, identified, formulated, and evaluated for safety and efficacy, in vivo studies relating to antibiotic elimination in milk must be carried out using microbiologic diffusion assays. Residual levels of antibiotics are measured using specific tests capable of detecting minute levels of antibiotic. Finally, clinical trials (animal trials) are carried out to assess the efficacy of the new formulation under field conditions. Both bacteriologic and clinical criteria are used as a basis for the assessment of the efficacy of the product under practical conditions of use.

COURSE OF INFUSED ANTIBIOTIC

The fate of an infused antibiotic in the udder may be broken down into three main phases:

1. Pharmaceutical phase
2. Pharmacokinetic phase
3. Pharmacodynamic phase

Pharmaceutical Phase

This phase covers the disintegration of the infused dosage form and the release of the active principle (antibiotic) from the ointment, base, vehicle, or depot formulation into the aqueous and lipid fractions of the milk. This type of pharmaceutical availability can be modified by physical or chemical manipulations of the formulation, e.g., by using sustained-release formulations, by adsorption to insoluble inert bases, by varying the degree of micronization of the active ingredients, or by incorporating insoluble salts of the antibiotic to retard the rate of release. Many bases have been developed, including vegetable and mineral oils and aqueous suspensions with or without wetting agents. Considerable care is required at the manufacturing level to obtain a uniform release rate of antibiotics, and the physical properties of such bases, including the viscosity, must be taken into account, especially when physically stable preparations are stored at different temperatures. Three different types of bases have evolved to allow long action (for dry cow), medium retention, or quick release. The major development of a mineral oil base with 3% aluminum monostearate has enabled the use of certain antibiotics in the dry period, thereby allowing a steady rate of release of antibiotics from the base over a period of weeks. An insoluble salt, such as cloxacillin benzathine or penicillin G benzathine, is often incorporated to retard the rate of release. Also, the persistence of drug in its base sometimes can be increased by increasing the total dosage. Many dry-cow products, for example, would contain perhaps 500 mg cloxacillin, whereas products designed for use in lactating cows would contain perhaps 200 mg. All products for use in the dry cow must be completely nonirritant to the udder.

Quick-release bases, on the other hand, frequently contain procaine penicillin G or other appropriate antibiotics in a vegetable oil base. These quick-release bases are commonly employed in the routine treatment of individual quarters when clinical recovery and early return to the sale of milk are important. The inclusion of other ancillary pharmacologic agents, such as corticosteroids, in a preparation has been justified on the grounds that these substances may remove any alleged chemical irritancy of the formulation itself or could help to suppress the inflammatory response in the udder. The U.S. Food and Drug Administration (FDA) has now released stringent guidelines regarding inclusion criteria for intramammary products, and combination products or polypharmacy are discouraged and indeed not generally approved for use. Aqueous solutions of antibiotics provide short-lived udder levels and are unsuitable for many penicillin-containing formulations.

Pharmacokinetic Phase

Several physiochemical properties influence the concentration of drug in the central udder compartment, e.g., binding of drug to milk, to udder secretions, or to plasma proteins, or the degree of lipid solubility, and the degree of ionization of the drug. Antibiotics administered via the teat canal diffuse rapidly to the top of the udder provided there is no blockage or obstruction by inflammatory debris. Some of the antibiotic is absorbed from the udder into the blood stream (and vice versa), depending on the degree of protein binding, pKa of the drug, and pH of the milk. Frequently in mastitis, the pH of the milk rises, thus tending to increase the udder concentration of parenterally administered acidic drugs, such as penicillin and sulphonamides, because of pKa partitioning and the "on-trapping" phenomenon. Excretion of drug from the udder is governed by the type of base, amount of milk production, characteristics of the antibiotic, and health status of the gland.

Pharmacodynamic Phase

This phase covers the interaction of the drug molecule with the pathogenic microorganisms inside the target compartment, i.e., the antibacterial actions within the inflamed udder tissue. Various factors attributable to the pharmacologic properties of the drug itself determine the intensity of the clinical effect, e.g., its action against the common pathogens of mastitis, the minimum inhibition concentration (MIC) required for different organisms, and the sensitivity or resistance of the various microorganisms to the released antibiotic. The necessary exposure time of each organism to the antibiotic levels in excess of the MIC also determines the success of treatment.

DESIRABLE PROPERTIES OF AN INTRAMAMMARY ANTIBIOTIC

1. Use in Lactating Cattle
   a. Minimal irritation to the udder
   b. Low MIC
   c. Low degree of binding to milk and udder proteins
   d. Low degree of ionization in the udder

e. Quick release rate from ointment or vehicle base

f. Adequate exposure time for antibacterial action

g. Short milk withholding times

2. Dry-Cow Therapy

a. Completely nonirritant to udder tissue

b. Bactericidal action (long exposure time)

c. High degree of binding to udder secretions

d. Stability of antimicrobial activity

e. Slow release rate from base

f. Large molecular weight

25.3 INTRAMAMMARY THERAPY

Intramammary treatment is the most common method of treating bovine mastitis. In streptococcal mastitis and in staphylococcal mastitis, such therapy usually results in clinical cure, but the bacteriologic cure rate is low. In acute mastitis, failures in intramammary therapy with antibiotics are the result of poor or uneven distribution of the drug throughout the intensely swollen udder parenchyma and of compression or blockage of the milk duct system by inflammatory products. Furthermore, staphylococci are tissue invaders, and intracisternally administered drugs may be unable to gain access to these organisms. Therefore, bacteriologic failures may occur even when the organisms are sensitive to the antibiotics used. Systemic treatment as an adjunct to intramammary treatment has been advocated as a means of overcoming these problems and, occasionally, as the only route of administration.

In the early days of mastitis therapy, penicillin resistance and development of resistance were the main explanations for unsatisfactory results from antibiotic therapy. Many strains of staphylococci became resistant to penicillin as they produced and secreted penicillin-destroying enzymes (penicillinases = beta-lactamase). Penicillin resistance within the genus *Staphylococcus* increased as a result of the use of antibiotics, but the resistance may have stabilized during the last few years. The resistance patterns vary greatly, however, from one geographic location to another and from herd to herd.

The bacterial mechanisms used to overcome the effects of host responses are becoming better understood. Mastitis-pathogenic strains of *Staphylococcus aureus* typically form a slimy polysaccharide capsule to protect them from host factors. Encapsulated strains present problems of effective opsonization. Mastitis-pathogenic staphylococci and streptococci also typically collect on their surface a shield composed of host proteins, including casein, fibrinogen, and immunoglobulin. Inhibition of inflammation and chemotaxis, resistance to intracellular killing by phagocytes, and immunosuppression are typical mechanisms interfering with host defenses.

The problem of staphylococcal resistance has been met by the production of beta-lactamase-resistant penicillins, such as cloxacillin. On a molar basis, however, these resistant penicillins are several times less effective than penicillin G. Penicillin G is still the most effective antibiotic for eliminating streptococci and most strains of staphylococci. Another approach toward penicillin-resistant staphylococci has been the use of other types of antibiotics, such as the macrolides erythromycin, tylosin, or spiramycin. Resistance may also become a problem for these antibiotics.

Some developments have been made toward dealing with beta-lactamase-producing staphylococci and gram-negative bacteria. Beta-lactamase-resistant penicillins, such as cloxacillin, are widely used in mastitis therapy, especially in dry-cow preparations. Wide-spectrum antibiotics are not used for this purpose because gram-negative organisms do not generally thrive nor survive within the dry udder. Another therapeutic approach for beta-lactamase-producing bacteria has been to combine a beta-lactamase antibiotic with a specific inhibitor of bacterial beta-lactamase. Such inhibitors include clavulanic acid or sulbactam. Although the inhibitors themselves have limited antibiotic activity, they inhibit microbial beta-lactamase irreversibly so that the coadministered antibiotic is not destroyed. The greatest benefit is obtained when the inhibitor is combined with a broad-spectrum penicillin, such as amoxicillin.

Antibiotics act in conjunction with endogenous inhibitors. Antibiotics are administered via the intramammary route for the treatment of chronic or mild mastitis, and are administered parenterally for acute clinical cases of mastitis, which require good systemic bioavailability.

For local use during lactation, penicillin, especially in a peanut oil base containing 3% aluminum monostearate, could give a success rate close to 100% for infection with *Streptococcus agalactiae* when administered at a dose of 100,000 I.U. at 48-hour intervals. Cloxacillin, which is not degraded by the staphylococcal beta-lactamases, is widely used (200 mg daily for three days) alone or combined with ampicillin (75 mg) against *Staphylococcus aureus*. Novobiocin (25 mg daily for three days) can cure clinically 96% of animals affected by *S. aureus* as compared to a 16% rate for penicillin-streptomycin. Other antibiotics, such as rifamycin, kanamycin-spiramycin, ampicillin, and tylosin, such as cure the majority of animals affected by *S. aureus* and mycobacteria.

Antibiotics for infusion in dry-cow therapy must be nonirritant to the udder. Benzathine cloxacillin eliminates 84% of *S. aureus* and 94% of *Streptococcus agalactiae* infections. Penicillin with novobiocin or with neomycin are other major active ingredients. Efficacy of erythromycin against staphylococci compares favorably with that of cloxacillin. Frequently, systemic injection produces the best results when combined with intramammary injection as an additional safety measure. Few reports are available on the bacteriologic efficacy of the procedure because the effect of intramammary treatment cannot be evaluated separately. Oxytocin and frequent milking at 1- or 2-hour intervals are recommended to remove toxic material from the udder and to maintain milk duct patency. Unless these steps are taken, intramammary treatment alone cannot be justified for acute cases.

Neomycin had been the chief ingredient in combination drugs for treating mastitis because of its wide antimicrobial spectrum. Erythromycin, polymyxin B, bacitracin, and penicillin G were added because of erythromycin's activity against *Staphylococcus aureus*, because of the synergistic and antifungal activity of polymyxin B, and because penicillin G and bacitracin possibly enforce the activity of neomycin. Although in practice these combinations were ostensibly better against streptococcal and staphylococcal infections than was penicillin G alone, such multiple combinations have a doubtful role in mastitis control.

Kanamycin possesses a broad spectrum of action, including E. coli, salmonella, Klebsiella, enterobacter proteus, and staphylococci and is often used in intramammary therapy.

In some countries intramammary treatments include many combination products that are of doubtful value and often not successful in eliminating infection. Moreover, the milk concentration achieved by any one antibiotic in such preparations is likely to be lower than the optimum required for treatment and thus could facilitate the development of resistance. Until relatively recently, broad-spectrum activity, including activity against beta-lactamase-producing staphylococci, could only be achieved by using antibiotic combinations. Although intramammary multiple antibiotic therapy continues to be of value in specific cases, the cephalosporins, which possess broad-spectrum activity, may provide a replacement for antibiotic combination.

Broad-spectrum activity is theoretically preferable to either gram-positive or gram-negative activity alone. Oxytetracycline provides this activity, but once again resistant organisms of both categories tend to develop relatively quickly. One reason that oxytetracycline is not used extensively is the instability of the formulation in plastic syringes. Penicillin G provides activity against streptococci and non-beta-lactamase-producing staphylococci. Most (50–60%) *S. aureus* isolated from mastitis infection produce beta-lactamase and are, therefore, penicillin G resistant. The introduction in 1962 of cloxacillin—an isoxazolyl penicillin stable in the presence of beta-lactamase—extended the spectrum of activity against gram-positive cocci. Erythromycin, a macrolide, has activity similar to that of cloxacillin. Erythromycin-resistant strains of organisms are comparatively rare, and resistance is short-lived.

A penicillin-novobiocin intramammary infusion product (Albacillan) and a solution of 1.2 million I.U. procaine penicillin G in 10 ml of sterile saline are both effective against *Streptococcus agalactiae* mastitis. Another popularly used intramammary antibiotic is novobiocin for staphylococcus aureus and streptococcal infections.

ERYTHROMYCIN INTRAMAMMARY

Erythromycin intramammary is a specially developed formulation of erythromycin for intramammary infusion that combines the known high degree of activity of erythromycin against *Staphylococcus aureus, Streptococcus agalactiae, S. dysgalactiae*, and *S. uberis* with the ability to penetrate alveolar tissue to an unusual degree.

The ability of the erythromycin to penetrate the alveolar tissue allows it to reach organisms residing in lesions and occluded milk ducts. In addition, the rapidity with which the antibiotic penetrates the tissue ensures that drug residues are eliminated from the udder much quicker than with other commonly used treatments.

The control of bovine mastitis with erythromycin administered parenterally is now widely accepted, and clinical studies confirm its efficacy.

Erythromycin exhibits a spectrum of activity covering most pathogens responsible for bovine mastitis, including penicillin-resistant staphylococci.

The cephalosporin group of antibiotics has been accepted for the treatment of a broad spectrum of gram-positive and gram-negative infections in humans. Cephacetrile is a semisynthetic cephalosporin antibiotic that was introduced into clinical use in human medicine several years ago. Its mode of action is bactericidal and similar to that of the beta lactam antibiotics. Other cephalosporins include cephalonium (for dry cows), cephalexin, and cefoperazone.

Cephacetrile is active against many gram-positive isolates. The drug is equally active against *Staphylococcus aureus* strains that are benzylpenicillin-sensitive and benzylpenicillin-resistant, and strains with multiple antibiotic resistance. Cephacetrile concentrations of 4 μg/ml inhibited growth of 10 of 15 strains of *Escherichia coli* tested. Cephacetrile is relatively stable to beta-lactamase degradation. Many useful cephalosporins are now on the market for mastitis therapy in the lactating and dry period. Cephalexin is effective against gram-positive organisms and E. coli.

In due course, undoubtedly, newer and more effective drugs, such as third-generation cephalosporins, florphenicol, and fluoroquinolones, will become available for mastitis treatment. The development of an optimal formulation of an antibiotic for the treatment of mastitis in lactating dairy cows involves several candidate formulations that are tested in many clinical experiments in cows. Criteria used for formulation selection are: milk levels in the udder, which should at best remain at effective levels for some time and then fall quickly; udder irritation, which should be as low as that experienced with competitor products; and efficacy, which should be maximized without making the product too expensive or leading to excessively long milk-withholding periods. Whatever intramammary treatment is used, frequent and thorough stripping of the infected quarter in acute clinical infections is recommended to remove both pus and endotoxins. Parenteral oxytocin injections can help to achieve more complete emptying of the gland prior to infusion.

Suggestions for intramammary treatment of lactating cows include using cephapirin, cloxacillin, kanamycin, novobiocin potentiated penicillins, and penicillin/dihydrostreptomycin.

Suggestions for combination treatments for lactating cows include:

- Ampicillin at 10 mg/kg, twice daily, intramuscularly for 3 to 5 days;
- Erythromycin at 5 mg/kg, twice daily, intramuscularly, or at 300 mg twice daily, intramammary, for 3 to 5 days; and
- Oxytetracycline at 20 mg/kg, daily, intravenously or intramuscularly for 3 to 5 days.

25.4 TREATMENT OF CLINICAL MASTITIS

PARENTERAL THERAPY

Successful systemic therapy depends on the effective passage of the drug from the blood into or near foci of infection in the udder. Passage of drugs across the blood-milk barrier takes place by passive diffusion. Similar to all biological membranes, this barrier is only penetrated by the nonionized, nonprotein-bound, lipid soluble fraction of the drug. The optimum properties of an antibiotic intended for mastitis therapy are:

1. High bioavailability from the injection site
2. Low protein binding
3. Low MIC against udder pathogens
4. High lipid solubility and nonionizable
5. Extended half-life in the udder

No single antibacterial drug meets all these requirements, but an examination of the pharmacokinetic properties of the commonly available drugs shows which are most likely to be useful in the systemic treatment of mastitis caused by gram-positive and gram-negative pathogens.

Occluded milk ducts might prevent the direct spread of an antibiotic administered intramammarily. Therefore, a combination of parenteral treatment with intramammary treatment seems to give better recovery rates than do intramammary treatments alone. Parenteral treatment, especially the intravenous route if possible, is recommended in the acute phase of mastitis when swelling of the tissue occludes the milk ducts.

The key to the successful treatment of acute clinical mastitis with antibacterial drugs is early detection and combined systemic and intramammary therapy with drugs possessing the lowest MIC against the most common pathogens involved and possessing the best penetration and distribution properties in the udder. When an accurate diagnosis is lacking, broad-spectrum antibiotics are preferred; however, the number from which to select is small. In acute coliform mastitis, intravenous oxytetracycline, intravenous sulfonamide and trimethoprim combinations, or intramuscular polymyxin B or gentamicin appear to be the preferred drugs. For the treatment of acute mastitis caused by gram-positive udder pathogens, combined parenteral and intramammary application of macrolide antibiotics appears to be the logical and rational choice on bacteriologic and pharmacokinetic grounds, but new drugs, such as the cephalosporins, should be as useful.

ABSORPTION AND DISTRIBUTION

Absorption from the administration site determines the rate of concentration decline and affects the systemic concentrations achieved. Several factors alter the rate of absorption from administration sites—notably the proximity and volume of blood supply and the nature of the antibiotic molecule and preparation. Intravenous administration is, in effect, injection into an area with an unlimited blood supply. It produces a transient, peak plasma concentration that provides the driving force to deliver drug molecules into the tissues. Intramuscular administration provides a high local concentration that diffuses into adjacent blood vessels but does not readily reach high concentration in the plasma and, therefore, may not be readily distributed to tissues in the rest of the body. Absorption from an intramuscular site can be variable because of the differences in blood flow to different muscle masses, the presence of connective tissue, and the volume of the drug injected.

For systemic mastitis therapy, effective passage of the drug from blood into and near the foci of infection must be achieved. The only known way to assess the accessibility of an infecting organism to the drug is by measuring drug concentration in the milk. The extent to which a drug gains access into milk from the circulation is largely governed by three properties of the drug molecule:

1. Lipid solubility
2. Degree of ionization
3. Extent of protein binding in plasma and in the udder

Logically, a drug molecule attached to a protein of large molecular weight is not as readily able to diffuse along its expected concentration gradient and does not achieve tissue distribution as rapidly. The equilibrium between bound and unbound drugs is based on the affinity of the protein for the molecule and the concentration of the drug. The binding proteins considered important in drug distribution are those in the circulatory system.

Milk has a normal pH of 6.5, which is more acidic than plasma. The greater availability of hydrogen ions in milk, as opposed to in serum, tends to favor the nonionized state of penicillin. Nonionized penicillin molecules that have scavenged hydrogen ions in serum then diffuse down a concentration gradient into milk, where they are likely to remain in their nonionized form. This favors diffusion back into serum.

In the case of mastitis, the pH of milk increases and can approach that of serum owing to increased tissue permeability. The possibility of the penicillin molecule getting into milk is the same, but it more readily becomes ionized again and, thus, becomes "trapped" in the milk.

When an erythromycin molecule achieves a nonionized state in the serum and then diffuses into the udder, it encounters a relative increase of hydrogen ions in normal milk compared to those in serum. Thus, the erythromycin molecule is more likely to become ionized and, therefore, be retained in the milk. In milk with an elevated pH caused by mastitis, this trapping of erythromycin is less likely.

The fact that the ionization state of a drug molecule can alter its ability to cross cell membranes raises the possibility of trapping molecules in different compartments as a result of the differences in pH between those compartments.

Conclusions that can be drawn from this consideration of drug distribution as a function of ionization include the following:

1. That weakly acidic antibiotics are present in milk at lower concentrations than in serum, but their distribution is shifted toward the udder in cases of mastitis
2. That, conversely, weakly basic drugs can achieve higher concentrations in milk, but this effect is reduced in mastitis

In general, ionized molecules do not cross membranes because of their lipophobic nature. As with protein binding, however, the equilibrium that exists between the ionized and nonionized forms of a drug is a function of the pKa of the molecule and the pH of the surrounding medium.

Cell membranes and tissues through which the drug molecules must pass to follow its concentration gradient serve as barriers because of their lipid matrix. Drug passage through such structures relates to the molecular size and polarity of the molecule and its degree of protein binding and ionization. Conditions that reduce the conti-nuity of a cell membrane tend to increase the ability of a drug to pass through. In general, a drug crosses lipid structures if it is of small size and polarity and is neither highly protein bound nor ionized.

For parenteral use, high availability to the infection site is desirable. A drug that is weakly basic or otherwise highly ionized in serum and sufficiently lipid soluble is indicated, e.g., a macrolide such as erythromycin. The bioavailability of erythromycin (pKa = 8.8), however, is influenced by "ion trapping" in the rumen, especially when the animal is fed on concentrates, i.e., at a pH close to 5.5. The mean tissue concentration in the udder, which is about eight times that of the plasma, decreases during mastitis because of pH changes (pH 7.5). By contrast, the pH changes in milk during mastitis may enhance the tissue concentration of such substances as sulphonamides and penicillins, which are usually poorly distributed to the udder.

Gram-Positive Pathogens

Antibiotics of the penicillin group that concentrate extracellularly because of poor tissue distribution work well in the milk phase. Sensitivity of the organism may be determined retrospectively by sensitivity testing or may be predicted from a knowledge of the likely infecting organism based on clinical signs and on herd history and its typical antimicrobial sensitivity. Sensitivities of organisms also vary between geographic regions.

The effect of formulation on drug persistence is well demonstrated by long-acting cloxacillin preparations, which have greatly extended persistence when the particle size is reduced.

The acidic penicillin G, ampicillin, cloxacillin, and cephalosporins can gain limited access to normal milk, and slightly higher concentrations can be attained and maintained in mastitic milk, but higher doses are required. The weak base ester of penicillin G, penethamate, can produce high concentrations of penicillin G in normal, more acidic milk, but lower concentrations are reached in the alkaline mastitic milk.

Only a fractionally small percentage of penicillin G molecules are nonionized in the serum; thus, the concentration in milk, owing to diffusion and retention, is slow relative to the concentration in serum. Penicillin molecules that get into milk in an animal with mastitis have a greater chance of staying there because they are retained in an ionized state by the higher pH of mastitic milk.

Until recently, broad-spectrum activity, including proven activity against beta-lactamase-producing staphylococci, could only be achieved by using antibiotic combinations. Although multiple intramammary therapy continues to be of value in specific cases, the cephalosporins, which possess broad-spectrum activity against many gram-negative udder pathogens and beta-lactamase-producing staphylococci, may provide replacement for antibiotic combinations. Intramammary cephalosporin therapy is often preferred in cases of acute staphylococcal mastitis.

In high doses, sodium benzylpenicillin can provide milk levels in excess of the MICs for many sensitive microorganisms for 12 hours or more, whereas most work with procaine penicillin indicates that, for bacteriostatic levels to be maintained for 24 hours, doses of approximately 16,500 I.U./ kg must be administered. Higher penicillin levels can be achieved in the udder by intramuscular injection of penethamate hydriodide, a basic hydrolyzable ester of benzylpenicillin. It achieves a concentration in milk five to seven times that in plasma. Once diffused into the udder, it is hydrolyzed to benzylpenicillin, which diffuses relatively poorly out of the gland again. Ampicillin penetrates the udder slightly better than does benzylpenicillin. A dose of 10 to 20 mg/kg is needed to maintain an MIC against highly sensitive organisms for 24 hours. Cloxacillin and cephalosporins also gain access to milk, but doses of 25 mg/ kg cloxacillin and 12.5 mg/kg cephalosporins are necessary to maintain an effective concentration for 4 to 8 hours.

Few antibiotics achieve effective intracellular concentrations to eliminate *Staphylococcus aureus* when the bacteria are sequestered within the phagocytes, especially in their acidic phagolysosomes. Rifampicin seems to be the most effective antibiotic when tested on phagocytozed *S. aureus* in vitro. Some of the high activity of rifampicin for intracellular *S. aureus* is caused by potentiation of its activity in the intracellular acidic compartment of the phagolysosome. Similar to rifampicin, paulomycin, and ciprofloxacin reduce viable intracellular *S. aureus* bacteria in the macrophage system. Enrofloxacin, now registered as a veterinary product, is a quinolone similar to ciprofloxacin with potential for treating intracellular infections.

The pH gradient between blood and normal milk favors the transfer of organic bases, such as erythromycin, tylosin, and spiramycin, from blood to milk. These macrolide antibiotics diffuse readily across the blood-milk barrier because of high lipid solubility, and they become trapped in the milk phase because of ionization. For instance, the blood-milk equilibrium of erythromycin stabilizes at 1:6.

Spiramycin levels in milk are maintained beyond what would be predicted from pharmacokinetic data on blood.

The macrolide antibiotics can be concentrated in the milk, and even though lower concentrations are reached in mastitic milk, these concentrations appear to be maintained at effective levels against *S. aureus* for at least 12 hours. Regardless of how high these concentrations are, they are below the MIC for even the most sensitive coliforms.

The macrolide antibiotics (erythromycin, spiramycin, tylosin, lincomycin, clindamycin) can be concentrated in the udder, and effective concentrations can persist in the milk for at least 12 hours after treatment. After systemic administration, erythromycin reaches levels in milk four to five times greater than those present in plasma. Similarly, tylosin achieves a concentration in milk 1.6 times higher than that in plasma. Both antibiotics at a dose of 12.5 mg/kg maintain for 24 hours milk levels in excess of the average MICs for staphylococci.

Whenever the pathogen is known to be sensitive to a drug that can be administered by both parenteral and intramammary routes, high bacteriologic cure rates can be expected with spiramycin, tylosin and erythromycin. The macrolide antibiotics are the ideal candidates for this approach when attempting to eliminate persistent gram-positive udder infections.

The macrolide antibiotics show a potential advantage over other antimicrobial drugs for parenteral treatment of acute mastitis caused by gram-positive bacteria. (Polymyxin B and the macrolides are narrow-spectrum antibiotics and should not be used without an accurate diagnosis.)

Sulfonamides and sulfonamide-trimethoprim combinations must be administered intravenously to reach effective milk concentrations and due to a partial loss of antibacterial activity in milk, concentrations attained are sufficient to inhibit only the most sensitive isolates. Oxytetracycline has only limited use against *S. aureus* because of its high MIC value against some strains.

The ability of several aminoglycoside antibiotics, which chemically are ionized bases and are poorly lipid soluble, to penetrate across the blood-milk barrier and to reach and maintain effective concentrations against *S. aureus* is limited. The lower MIC of especially kanamycin and gentamicin against *S. aureus* is the major determinant of the ability of these drugs to maintain effective milk concentrations for 8 to 12 hours.

Gram-Negative Pathogens

Dihydrostreptomycin is a base with low lipid solubility. High doses (10–20 mg/kg) must be injected every 6 to 12 hours for an effective concentration against highly sensitive isolates. Because of its low bioavailability, intramuscular injection of oxytetracycline does not give therapeutic levels in milk. Following intravenous injection, however, appreciable amounts enter milk and are effective against moderately sensitive isolates. Chloramphenicol is more highly bound to serum protein than is oxytetracycline, and the MIC of chloramphenicol against coliform bacteria is also higher than that of oxytetracycline. When administered intramuscularly at a dose of 50 mg/kg, chloramphenicol produces effective concentrations for 10 to 24 hours against moderately sensitive isolates. Chloramphenicol use is prohibited in food-producing animals, however.

Different sulfonamides appear in different concentrations in milk. The marked potentiation of effect between trimethoprim and sulfonamides may result in a tenfold increase in activity for each drug. Trimethoprim readily enters milk, but has a short half-life. Intravenous administration of a trimethoprim-sulfonamide combination at a dose of 40–50 mg/kg could provide effective concentrations against moderately sensitive organisms for 4 to 8 hours. Polymyxin B at 5 mg/kg and gentamicin at 3 mg/kg can produce effective concentrations against highly sensitive organisms for 10 to 12 hours. (Novobiocin, erythromycin, and beta lactam antibiotics are useful for gram-positive infections; oxytetracycline, sulfonamides, apramycin, kanamycin, gentamicin, broad-spectrum penicillins/cephalosporins, and spectinomycin are useful for gram-negative and mixed infections.)

25.5 ANTIBIOTIC THERAPY DURING THE DRY PERIOD

Antibiotic therapy during the dry period is one of the most effective mastitis control measures now available. Its advantages are cure rates higher than those obtained with lactational therapy without the need to discard milk from treated cows and with only minimal risk of antibiotic contamination of milk to be sold.

The manner by which antibiotics are administered at drying off may influence the number of new infections that develop during the dry period. The method of cannula insertions may affect treatment efficacy in quarters infected at drying off.

The first few days of the dry period is a crucial time for the milk cow in terms of mastitis because the cow undergoes the stress of no longer being milked and the teats are no longer cleaned and dipped on a daily basis. Thus, the cow becomes susceptible to new infections that can result in clinical mastitis during the dry period or at freshening. As many as 40% of new infections are established during the first 2 weeks of the dry period.

In addition, many cows already have a subclinical mastitis infection when they are dried off. Although not outwardly obvious to the dairyman, such an infection has the potential to develop into clinical mastitis.

Dry-cow therapy controls as many as 50 to 60% of existing infections. The organisms most commonly involved include *Staphylococcus aureus*, *Streptococcus agalactiae*, *S. dysgalactiae*, and *S. uberis*. Dry-cow therapy, along with proper udder preparation, helps to control the infections caused by these organisms. The number of somatic cells in the gland will subsequently be reduced, which is desirable from a milk quality standpoint.

Ideally, an antibiotic formulation for infusion at drying off should maintain its concentration in udder secretion for most of the dry period at a level sufficient to eliminate infections present at drying off and also to prevent new infection by the major pathogens in the dry period. It should not persist, however, after parturition to contaminate milk. In practice, most products are either semisynthetic penicillins or combinations of penicillin and streptomycin in slow-release bases. The udder is largely naturally resistant to gram-negative organisms because lactoferrins produced at this time inhibit their establishment.

Of infections present in quarters that are not treated at drying off, 90% persist into the following lactation. When infected quarters are treated with appropriate formulations after the last milking of lactation, about 40% of staphylococcal infections and fewer than 10% of those caused by *S. agalactiae, dysgalactiae,* and *uberis* persist. The elimination rates are higher than those achieved with therapy in lactation.

In cows untreated at drying off, particularly those infected in one or more quarters, the new infection rate is high for a short period after drying off. *S. uberis* is the most common pathogen. Dry-cow preparations have been designed with both carrier and molecular modification to reduce the rate of drug diffusion from the udder. The presence of aluminum monostearate—a large, inert molecule to which antibiotic can absorp—in the infusion product and the use of benzathine combined to cloxacillin inhibit the movement of active drug across membranes. These formulations create a prolonged local concentration of drug that is ideal for dry-cow preparations.

One shortcoming of conventional dry-cow therapy is that some cows treated at drying off have mastitis at calving. Frequently, these cases of mastitis are the result of new infections contracted during the dry period, and they indicate a failed prophylactic effect of the dry-period therapy. These failures may occur because dry-cow products are formulated for effect against gram-positive bacteria, but in some herds, gram-negative bacteria cause many of the new dry-period infections. Also, antibiotics infused at drying off provide protection in the early dry period but not in the prepartum period.

For instance, the administration of a lactating-cow product containing novobiocin and penicillin G procaine 1 to 3 days before calving appears to reduce effectively new *S. uberis* infections present at calving. A lactating-cow product containing a broad-spectrum antibiotic given shortly before calving might reduce new gram-negative infections. Unfortunately, predicting exactly when cows will calve poses some difficulties.

FACTORS IN SUSCEPTIBILITY AND RESISTANCE IN THE DRY PERIOD

The new infection rate is high in the early dry period, decreases as involution is complete, and then rises again as parturition approaches. The reasons for this changing susceptibility are only poorly understood. Factors influencing susceptibility might be broadly grouped as follows:

1. Changes in bacterial populations on the teat skin
2. Changes in the penetrability of the teat canal by bacteria
3. Changes in the effectiveness of defense mechanisms within the mammary gland itself

IMPORTANCE OF NEW INFECTIONS IN THE DRY PERIOD

Overall, the average new infection rate over the dry period is approximately 10% of quarters. This high rate of new infections means that, in the absence of effective control practices, the prevalence of infection is higher at calving than at drying off.

Another way to assess the importance of the dry period in the mastitis complex is to compare the number of infections established during the dry period with those originating during lactation. Approximately 45% of all infections occur while cows are dry.

Dry-period infections are also the cause of most of the clinical mastitis that affects many cows in early lactation.

Bacteria including most of the streptococci other than *Streptococcus agalactiae* and the coliform bacteria are most likely to reach the udder from the environment. Clearly, control measures effective against one of these categories of bacteria are not necessarily as effective against the other.

The numbers of *S. agalactiae* and *Staphylococcus aureus* infections occurring during lactation and during the dry period are usually similar. Infections caused by "green streptococci" (probably comprised largely of *Streptococcus uberis*) are more common in dry than in lactating cows, however. Studies have suggested that environmental bacteria cause most dry-period infections in some herds (*Streptococcus agalactiae*, *Staphylococcus aureus*, and other streptococcal and coliform infections).

25.6 DEFENSE MECHANISMS OF THE MAMMARY GLAND

The ability of the organisms to establish themselves in the sinus, ducts, or alveolar tissue depends on their ability to adhere to mucous membrane and to colonize the gland, despite the specific and nonspecific defense mechanisms of the cow.

The unmilked gland is more vulnerable to infection than is the gland milked at regular intervals. One obvious explanation is the absence of the flushing of the canal that occurs with regular milking. Another reason is that the increase in intramammary pressure that occurs for several days after drying off might shorten and dilate the teat canal, thus increasing its penetrability. Evidence does show that heightened susceptibility in the dry period is caused by enhanced penetrability of the teat canal.

Changes in the histology of the teat canal epithelium have also been noted. The thickness in the area of the stratum granulosum, which gives rise to the teat canal keratin, decreases throughout involution. This change is probably a result of continuing keratinization, which by day 16 of the dry period sometimes causes the formation of a plug of loose keratin completely occluding the teat canal. This greater mass of keratin may be a factor in reduced penetrability of the canal at later stages of involution.

Also of interest are changes in the teat cistern epithelium detected by scanning electron microscopy. The epithelium lining the teat cistern is arranged in numerous longitudinal folds. The surface of the epithelium is made of flattened hexagonal cells, usually with prominent microvilli on their surfaces. Some cells, however, do not have these microvilli. These nonmicrovilliated cells are thought to be mature cells in the early stages of degeneration. They are important in mastitis because some bacteria adhere preferentially to these nonvillous surfaces. The teat canal also contains antimicrobial proteins. These proteins, at physiologic pH, carry a positive charge and bind electrostatically to mastitis pathogens, which at the same pH carry a negative charge.

Many of the factors that inhibit bacterial growth within the teat canal remain to be identified. Nevertheless, proteins and lipids have been implicated. Esterified and nonesterified fatty acids, particularly myristic acid, palmitoleic acid, and linoleic acid, play an antimicrobial role. These fatty acids are present in the teat canal keratin, and the unsaturated fatty acids have been implicated as the most inhibitory factors.

Several nonspecific antibacterial components, including lactoferrin, the lactoperoxidase system, and lysozyme, operate in lactating or dry mammary glands. Increased concentration of lactoferrin in the dry period inhibits growth of *Escherichia coli*, because lactoferrin binds iron, thus making it unavailable to these iron-dependent bacteria. Lactoferrin does not influence organisms with a low iron requirement. The antibacterial properties of the lactoperoxidase system manifest themselves in the presence of other factors, which are normally absent in milk. The potential positive effect of the lactoperoxidase system within the gland is unclear. The concentration of lysozyme in cattle and its significance in relation to udder infection have been the subject of much discussion. An apparently genetic variation in lysozyme concentration between animals seems to exist.

Once microorganisms have penetrated the teat canal, they encounter the specific defense systems consisting of both humoral and cellular immune components. These systems eliminate most of the invading microorganisms. Immunoglobulins (IgG, IgM) in the mammary secretion opsonize bacteria, thereby facilitating phagocytosis by macrophages and polymorphonuclear leukocytes. The predominant immunoglobulin in the mammary gland is IgG1. IgG1, and to some extent IgG2, is selectively transported into milk, whereas IgA, and to some extent IgM, is synthesized in the gland, although the concentrations of IgA and IgM are low. In addition to the opsonizing effect, IgA and IgM may also prevent adhesion of gram-positive bacteria to the glandular mammary epithelium, thus contributing to their "flushing out" during milking. IgA and IgG1 may also enhance the bacteriostatic effect of lactoferrin.

Immunoglobulins alone, predominantly IgG2, can opsonize microorganisms by binding to specific antigenic sites on the bacterial surface. The antibody-antigen complexes (immune complexes) usually react with complement, another of the humoral defense components in the gland. Complement thus seems to act as an immune effector in the acute inflammatory phase. The bactericidal role of the bound antibody-complement complex is effective against only certain gram-negative bacteria and is less effective against gram-positive bacteria.

Polymorphonuclear leukocytes, lymphocytes, and macrophages produced in bone marrow migrate through capillaries and across alveolar and ductal epithelium into the milk. Polymorphonuclear leukocytes and macrophages possess Fc receptors for IgG and IgM, as well as for complement. The number of polymorphonuclear leukocytes increases with the severity of the mastitis. In chronic cases, the number of mononuclear cells may increase. Polymorphonuclear leukocytes and macrophages are motile phagocytic cells that find their target by chemotaxis.

INTRINSIC ANTIBACTERIAL FACTORS IN MILK

Specific antibacterial factors are:

1. Immunoglobulins produced by B-lymphocytes
2. T-lymphocytes
3. Phagocytes, polymorphonuclear leukocytes, and macrophages
4. Complement components

Nonspecific Antibacterial factors are:

1. Lactoferrin
2. Lactoperoxidase
3. Lysozyme

The lactoferrin-dependent iron-binding system does not effectively withhold iron from bacteria if the milk contains hemoglobin or other such compounds as occur in mastitic milk.

EFFECT OF DRUGS ON MAMMARY LEUKOCYTE ACTIVITY

Treatment of mastitis frequently involves drugs that adversely affect the ability of leukocytes to destroy bacteria. When mastitis-causing bacteria produce intramammary infection, polymorphonuclear leukocytes respond by phagocytosing bacteria and killing organisms intracellularly.

Tiamulin, Kanamycin and tetracycline are inhibitory to phagocytic activity only in high concentrations. Penicillin alone or combined with streptomycin or neomycin has no detrimental effect on PMNS, nor has cephalothin, ampicillin-cloxacillin, or sulfadiazine-trimethoprim. Tetracycline and gentamicin in vivo are more detrimental to phagocytic activity of polymorphonuclear leukocytes than is chloramphenicol. Overuse of antibiotics in intramammary infection may lead to drug resistance, yeast infections, and sensitization.

Anti-inflammatory agents have been used to ameliorate the clinical signs of intramammary infection. Methylprednisolone in vitro stabilizes polymorphonuclear leukocytes and does not affect phagocytic function, but flumethasone decreases their viability. Ibuprofen enhances phagocytosis and bacterial destruction. In endotoxin-infused quarters, anti-inflammatory agents are ineffective in lowering somatic cell counts, but ibuprofen-treated cows have less milk loss and recover more rapidly in milk production than do those given other anti-inflammatory agents.

25.7 STAPHYLOCOCCAL MASTITIS

Subclinical infections with staphylococcal infections are best treated when the cow is dried off. Hastening the drying off may be a wise decision.

S. aureus causes mild to severe mastitis, which may, in some cases, result in death. This organism grows well in wounds and is found on skin surfaces. It can be introduced into a herd by milkers or other people carrying the infection in a wound or scratch on their hand. Likewise, animals carry the organism and may spread it among the herd.

Serious *S. aureus* infections are often related to problems of mechanical milking. If a teat is damaged by improper milking procedures or malfunctioning equipment, there is a greater possibility the organisms will be transmitted to the udder.

Staphylococcal infections are usually difficult to treat in lactating cows. This is true regardless of the route of treatment and the drugs selected. Although clinical recovery can be expected, bacteriologic cure is not likely. Reports of treatment by intramammary infusion show about a 10% recovery. Reports of combined systemic and infusion treatment indicate a higher rate of recovery—up to about 30% over spontaneous cure. Dry-cow infusion with properly formulated and tested products however, improves bacteriologic cure to 75% to 85% of cases of staphylococcal infection.

The treatment effectiveness of *Staphylococcus aureus* intramammary infections by lactation therapy varies in experimental and field trials. Chronic infections are characterized by the inability of the gland to eliminate the micro-organisms, which results in continuous or intermittent shedding in the milk. This may be accompanied by intermittent clinical or subclinical infection. Intermittent *S. aureus* shedding is attributed to the presence of microabscesses or phagocytized intracellular organisms, in which the organisms survive and are released to re-establish active infections. The increase in *S. aureus* isolation following freezing and thawing of milk samples may support the proposed mechanism of disrupting milk leukocytes which have phagocytized but not killed all *S. aureus*. These intracellular micro-organisms are protected from most antibiotic activity. However, other research has reported the presence of an unstable L-form phase of *S. aureus* in milk samples that may also act as a mechanism for organisms survival. Cell wall defects in *S. aureus* and other gram positive organisms have been reported in bovine mastitis and other infec-tions as unstable L-forms, protoplast phase, spheroplast phase, transitional phase or stable L-forms.

Two features in the pathogenesis of mastitis contribute to the relative inaccessibility of the causal organisms to antibiotics and to variable cure rates:

1. Alveolar duct occlusion caused by epithelial hyperplasia, cellular desquamation, and periductal edema forms a physical barrier to antibiotic distribution. This has been illustrated by autoradiography.
2. Survival of intracellulary located *S. aureus* within epithelial and polymorphonuclear cells. A proportion of these organisms survives phagolytic enzyme assault. Because they are not actively dividing, they survive also the effect of such antibiotics as penicillins, which penetrate the leukocyte but rely on inhibition of cell synthesis for their activity.

An approach to deal with penicillin-resistant staphylococci has been the use of other types of antibiotics, such as the macrolides erythromycin, tylosin, or spiramycin, as well as novobiocin, kanamycin or potentiated sulphonamides. Resistance may also become a problem for some of these antibiotics, although of less frequent occurrence.

Another therapeutic approach for beta-lactamase-producing bacteria has been to combine a beta-lactam antibiotic with a specific inhibitor of bacterial betalactamase. Such inhibitors include clavulanic acid. Although the inhibitor has limited antibiotic activity in itself, it inhibits microbial betalactamase irreversibly so that the coadministered antibiotic is not destroyed. The greatest benefit is obtained when the inhibitor is combined with a broad-spectrum penicillin, such as amoxicillin.

Many new cephalosporins seem to have significant advantages in terms of beta-lactamase resistance, spectrum of activity, and lack of toxicity. Gram-negative infections have been treated with broad-spectrum antibiotics. Broad-spectrum penicillins, e.g., ampicillin, seem to be susceptible, however, to inactivation by beta-lactamases. Antibiotic resistance is also a problem with many other broad-spectrum agents, such as tetracyclines.

Cephalosporins, novobiocin, kanamycin, and erythromycin are also likely to have good activity against beta-lactamase-producing *S. aureus*, and the activity of cephalosporins against beta-lactamase-producing gram-negative bacteria increases with succeeding generations.

Antibiotics may penetrate these cells poorly. Even when they gain access to the cell, they may not distribute into phagolysosomes. Antibiotics of the fluoroquinolone group are effective against intracellular *S. aureus*.

As already mentioned, antibiotic concentration, as measured in the fluid phase of milk, may not be relevant for *S. aureus*, which is an invasive organism and may be present intracellularly, as well as extracellularly, in the milk phase.

25.8 COLIFORM MASTITIS

The clinical presentation of coliform mastitis is variable and ranges from local clinical symptoms of inflammation to severe systemic signs of disease accompanied by enormous losses in milk production. Adequate preventive measures for control of coliform mastitis are not available, and effective therapeutic regimens, especially for severe cases, are needed.

Coliform mastitis is recognized as a major cause of acute mastitis in many dairy herds. Cows with peracute and acute coliform mastitis frequently suffer from severe local quarter inflammation characterized by watery to serous secretions. Fever, depression, anorexia, ruminal stasis, and other systemic signs are also observed in severe cases and have been attributed to endotoxemia. Practitioners are familiar with these signs and must select appropriate therapy for the disease. Systemic and/or intramammary antibiotics are frequently administered to treat acute coliform mastitis. Removal of the secretions from affected quarters is considered to be an important aspect of therapy in acute coliform mastitis. In the management of peracute and toxic cases of coliform mastitis, reversal of the effects of endotoxin and administration of intravenous isotonic solutions are considered important.

The causative organisms are classified as environmental pathogens. Environmental sanitation and milking hygiene are important in their control. Coliforms are a group of bacteria that are lactose-fermenting gram-negative rods belonging to the family Enterobacteriaceae. This group includes the genera *Escherichia coli, Klebsiella, Enterobacter,* and *Citrobacter*. These genera are most commonly represented in mastitis caused by gram-negative bacteria. Coliforms are widely disseminated in nature. *Escherichia coli (E. coli)* is found in large numbers in manure of cows.

The incidence of acute coliform mastitis appears to be increasing. Control measures have reduced the level of contagious mastitis caused by *Staphylococcus aureus* and *Streptococcus agalactiae*. Mammary glands devoid of other infections and with low somatic cell counts are susceptible to new intramammary infections. Housing has an effect on incidence. Animals concentrated in confinement housing are exposed to more environmental bacteria, especially *Escherichia coli*. Stress caused by calving, ketosis, increased production, or concurrent disease has been associated with an increase in acute coliform mastitis.

Control measures for contagious mastitis have had little effect on controlling coliform mastitis. Gram-negative bacteria induce systemic reactions by the release of endotoxins. These endotoxins must enter the vascular system before systemic reactions occur. Endotoxins are part of the cell wall of gram-negative bacteria and are released upon death of the bacteria. Multiplication of bacteria in the gland induces local inflammatory response.

The influx of polymorphonuclear leukocytes into the milk is massive. These phagocytic cells ingest and degrade the coliform bacteria, and following degradation of the bacteria, the polymorphonuclear leukocytes release endotoxin. Endotoxin is generally considered a (the) major initiating factor in the production of damage to the mammary epithelium and increased vascular permeability. Additional factors may be involved, including other products of the coliform bacteria, polymorphonuclear leukocytes and their by-products (e.g., interleukins or endogenous pyrogen), and other tissue and serum factors (e.g., complement and coagulation factors.)

Clinical signs are referable to endotoxin release. If local inflammation prevents further multiplication of bacteria, complete recovery can occur. If endotoxin is released to the vascular system, toxemia and death can occur.

The formation of endogenous inflammatory mediators, such as interleukins, tumor-necrosis factor, and probably others, within the udder and their subsequent release into the circulation, rather than the absorption of endotoxin, are probably responsible for systemic disease symptoms during coliform mastitis. This hypothesis is supported by evidence that demonstrated high concentrations of endotoxin in milk in cows with acute coliform mastitis, whereas endotoxin was not detectable in plasma. In contrast, concentrations of endotoxin in plasma and milk were high in cows with gangrenous coliform mastitis.

CLINICAL PRESENTATION

In the early stages, changes in the udder may be minor, but later, the quarter is swollen and sensitive and the secretion becomes abnormal. Signs of endotoxic shock, including marked depression, dehydration, diarrhea, recumbency, and normal or subnormal temperatures, may appear within a few hours. Hypocalcemia may also be associated with severe endotoxic shock. Following release of endotoxin from the infecting *E. coli*, local and systemic signs are elicited. The problem is one of toxemia rather than bacteremia.

The classic presentation of acute and peracute toxic coliform mastitis includes moderate to severe local inflammation of the quarter and systemic signs. Early systemic signs include fever, anorexia, depression, shivering, and gastrointestinal atony. Signs generally attributed to endotoxemia include depression, dehydration, endotoxic shock.

The fatal cases of *E. coli* mastitis result from a complex interaction of the effect of endotoxins on the circulation and the impaired ability of the cow to excrete endotoxin. Because the blood tends to coagulate more easily and capillaries become more permeable, the circulating blood volume and blood pressure fall. Sequestration or "pooling" of large volumes of fluid in the hepatoportal system means that less blood flows through the liver and kidneys. As a result, the elimination of toxins from the body is reduced. Extensive fatty infiltration of the liver in two thirds of newly calved cows may impair endotoxin catabolism and contribute to glycogen depletion in liver cells. Fatalities may be caused by liver and circulatory failure. Gangrene of the quarter may occur.

Peracute coliform mastitis is often misdiagnosed in recumbent cows that have recently calved because of its clinical resemblance to parturient hypocalcemia and of the subtle or delayed changes that may occur in the gross appearance of the milk following *E. coli* infection. Parturient hypocalcemia may precede coliform mastitis during early lactation, presumably because of increased contamination of teat ends with feces during recumbency.

E. coli mastitis apparently does not occur in a subclinical form, and the dry udder is resistant to *E. coli* for 1 week after drying off until 2 to 3 days before calving because of the inhibitory action of naturally occurring "lactoferrin." For these reasons, dry-cow therapy is not a satisfactory method of control for *E. coli*, although it effectively controls other pathogens of the dry udder.

Coliform mastitis usually occurs close to the time of calving—from a few days before until 1 or 2 months after. It is usually a severe, acute condition that may endanger the life of the cow and usually requires veterinary attention with supportive therapy to combat the acute systemic reaction, e.g., systemic antibiotics, fluids, and ancillary therapy.

MEDIATORS OF INFLAMMATION

The mediation of inflammation observed in acute coliform mastitis is not well defined. Arachidonic acid metabolites (prostaglandins, thromboxanes, and leukotrienes), vasoactive amines (histamine and serotonin), kinins, complement by-products, toxic oxygen radicals, and other factors may all be involved.

Locally generated histamine, serotonin, leukotriene B_4, PGF_2, and other eicosanoids are involved in the pathogenesis of acute coliform mastitis. Arachidonic acid metabolites may participate in production or expression of most, if not all, of the classic signs of inflammation and are implicated in the pathogenesis of endotoxic shock.

The arachidonic acid cascade results in the production of prostaglandins, thromboxanes, and other potential mediators of inflammation. Inflammatory stimuli activate phospholipases, which result in the eventual release of arachidonic acid from phospholipids in cell membranes. In the cascade, arachidonic acid has three major fates.

1. The lipoxygenase pathway may produce leukotrienes and monohydroxy metabolites of arachidonic acid.
2. Chemotactic lipids may be produced via the action of activated oxygen species or ultraviolet light.
3. The prostaglandins and thromboxanes may be produced.

Steroidal agents reduce or inhibit the eventual release of arachidonic acid from cell membranes. Steroids may reduce the yield of all products of arachidonic acid. In contradistinction, the nonsteroidal agents act at the level of cyclo-oxygenase and reduce production of the thromboxanes and prostaglandins. Following therapy with nonsteroidal agents, lipoxygenase products and chemotactic lipids may be unaffected or increased. Current evidence suggests that leukotrienes, such as the slow-reacting substances of anaphylaxis, may be important in inflammation.

The arachidonic acid metabolites apparently play some role in the mediation of inflammation in acute coliform mastitis. The role of these metabolites in the onset of acute coliform mastitis, however, is not understood completely and evidently does not always represent a clear case of direct cause and effect, at least as measured by increased concentrations of arachidonic acid metabolites in blood and milk.

The role of these metabolites in the onset of acute bovine coliform mastitis was studied in experimental cases of coliform mastitis induced by intramammary introduction of viable *E. coli*. Small but statistically significant increases of PGF_2 and thromboxane B_2 were found in milk. An *E. coli* endotoxin model revealed significant increases of thromboxane B_2 in milk over time in endotoxin-treated quarters of lactating cows.

The inflammatory and systemic changes observed during the course of acute coliform mastitis are believed to result from the release of lipopolysaccharide endotoxin (LPSE) from the bacteria. Much of the release of this endotoxin occurs following bacterial phagocytosis and killing by neutrophils; however, some release may occur during rapid bacterial growth. Subsequent activation of the cyclo-oxygenase and lipoxygenase pathways results, thereby releasing arachidonic acid metabolites that are potent mediators of local and systemic inflammatory events.

Free radicals oxidatively attack cellular and subcellular membranes, as well as nucleic acids and enzymes.

The antioxidant nutrients selenium and vitamin E reduce the severity and incidence of coliform mastitis and thus lend indirect evidence of oxygen radical involvement in this disease process.

Thus, a reduction in severity of acute coliform mastitis requires either the inhibition of bacterial growth to reduce the exposure of the quarter and the cow to lipopolysaccharide endotoxin or the neutralization of the effects of the lipopolysaccharide endotoxin release.

E. coli isolates are usually sensitive to cephalosporins, to tetracyclines, to ampicillin, to erythromycin, to gentamycin/kanamycin, and 30% to sulfonamides. Because of the pathogenesis of acute coliform mastitis, one is more often confronted with endotoxin-induced shock rather than infection as the primary problem. A severely affected cow may require 40 to 60 liters of fluid intravenously in the first 24 hours.

Anti-inflammatory agents, particularly those that suppress the effects of mediators derived from arachidonic acid, may decrease some of the endotoxin-induced effects. Antimicrobial treatment should only be considered an adjunct to fluid replacement and other supportive care.

Toward the end of lactation, the start of antibiotic therapy should be delayed until the dry period. The dry period is an excellent opportunity for systematic treatment and control of mastitis. An estimated 45% of new infections are established during the first 2 weeks of the dry period. As intramammary pressure stops milk production, the teat canal expands and the udder is stressed. Also, when cows are not milked, teats are not cleaned or dipped to remove bacteria. These factors increase the susceptibility of a dry cow to mastitis infections.

CONTROL OF COLIFORM MASTITIS

Control measures that are usually effective against the more common forms of infection (staphylococcal/streptococcal) have had little impact when used against environmental mastitis caused by coliform bacteria. The problem is usually confined to housed animals and results from increased exposure to these pathogens in heavily contaminated environments. Overcrowding of yards, inadequate bedding, and poor cubicle construction are also contributing factors. Sand is the ideal bedding material from a bacteriologic standpoint. Numbers of coliform bacteria and the environmental streptococci found in sand or crushed limestone are nearly always lower than numbers found in organic bedding materials. In general, wood products, such as sawdust and shavings, are associated with coliform numbers in excess of 1,000,000/g of bedding. Wet or damp areas in the back one third of free stalls and tie stalls lead to increased exposure to environmental pathogens.

Passage of more fluid feces from high-yielding dairy cows on heavy concentrate rations may also increase contamination, especially when bedding is wet or cleaning of passageways is inadequate. Transfer of coliforms to the teats of cows usually results from contact with the environment. The udder secretions of cows during the dry period contain lactoferrin. This substance is an iron-binding protein that inhibits replication of *E. coli*. When levels of lactoferrin decline at calving, however, the udder becomes more susceptible to coliform infection. Also, the systematic reduction in gram-positive infections occasioned by mastitis control and dry-cow therapy may result in a reduction in overall milk leukocyte count and a subsequent reduction in protection against gram-negative mastitis organisms.

THERAPY

Because the clinical signs of peracute coliform mastitis are caused by endotoxin, elimination of the toxin and neutralization of its effects are of major importance (Table 25–2).

The major problem in peracute coliform mastitis results from a complex interaction of the effects of endotoxins on the circulation and on the impaired ability of the cow to excrete endotoxin. Pooling of fluid occurs in the body, thus leading to less blood flow through the liver and kidney and reduced toxin elimination from the body. Fatalities result from a combination of endotoxic shock and liver and circulatory failure.

ENDOTOXIC SHOCK

Endotoxic shock often occurs before an animal is presented for treatment, and specific additional therapy to counter the hypotensive shock then must be instituted. Ten liters of saline can be administered intravenously in about 20 minutes and usually produces a rapid, almost immediate clinical improvement. Although colloid solutions are ideal, the cost is prohibitive usually. Hypertonic saline (8%) can be rapidly infused intravenously to improve hemodynamics and tissue perfusion.

Fluids

For cows in endotoxic shock, intravenous administration of large volumes (10–15 liters) of fluid is necessary (glucose saline). From 10 to 15 liters should be administered immediately and subsequent infusion given over the next 8 to 12 hours. The shock resulting from sequestration of fluids systematically causes metabolic acidosis, for which sodium bicarbonate (150–200 g) can be administered at a concentration not greater than 5%. The improved tissue perfusion resulting from intravenous hypertonic saline reduces the risk of anaerobic glycolysis.

Such fluid therapy in the form of oral or intravenous electrolyte solutions is useful in reversing endotoxic shock. These solutions counteract the dehydration and metabolic acidosis usually present in *E. coli* mastitis. Electrolyte therapy creates a forced diuresis

TABLE 25–2
COLIFORM MASTITIS

Escherichia coli → Endotoxins
↓
Endotoxic Shock
↓
Sequestration of Fluids—Dehydration, Acidosis
Shock: Hypoglycemia, Hypocalcemia, Infection, Toxemia

THERAPY

Fluids
1. 10–15 liters saline initially (repeat 6–8 hours)
2. $NaHCO_3$ 150–250 g—5% solution
3. Dextrose saline 10–15 liters

Oxytocin
20–30 I.U. intravenously

Calcium Borogluconate
20% 400–600 ml intravenously

B Vitamins
20–30 ml intravenously

Antiinflammatories
1. Dexamethasone 1 mg/kg intravenously or intramuscularly
2. Aspirin 30–40 g orally
3. Flunixin 1.1 mg/kg intravenously

Cardiac/Respiratory Stimulant
Etamiphylline camsylate: 1400 mg intravenously or intramuscularly

Antibiotics
Parenteral (Intravenous): Potentiated sulfonamide, oxytetracycline, ampicillin, spectinomycin, streptomycin, neomycin, gentamicin, erythromycin, cephalosporin.
Intramammary: Neomycin, streptomycin, gentamicin, ampicillin, polynyxin β, potentiated sulfonamides, kanamycin, cephalosporin

that maintains renal function and enhances excretion of toxic metabolites. Intravenous administration is ideal in peracute cases because absorption of oral electrolytes is reduced in cows with gastrointestinal stasis. Oral fluids, however, are often substituted under field conditions because of the practical limitations of intravenous administration.

The severe hypoglycemia and glycogen depletion may be countered by giving several liters of 40% glucose solution intravenously. Selection and use of antibiotics for the treatment of coliform mastitis can present problems. In acute cases, initial parenteral administration is usually recommended. Selection of drug, route, and dosage depends on the bioavailability of the compound in the serum, its ability to penetrate the blood-milk barrier, and the expected MIC against the causative agent.

Oxytetracycline, ampicillin, potentiated sulfonamide, spectinomycin, and aminoglycosides are useful systemically (intravenously). For intramammary use, gentamicin (250 g per quarter) has been recommended. Alternatively, neomycin, kanamycin, polymyxin, ampicillin, cephalosporins, or potentiated sulfonamide intramammary preparation may be used. Bactericidal antibiotics, effective against gram-negative organisms, should be prescribed.

The role of antimicrobials in the elimination of *E. coli* organisms from the udder is probably overrated because many coliform infections are self-limiting and would resolve without them. Not all infections respond spontaneously, however, and antimicrobials are still a necessary component of the therapeutic regimen for coliform mastitis. The danger lies in relying on them too much and ignoring measures to combat endotoxic shock. The combination of sulfadiazine and trimethoprim at the rate of 24 mg/kg has been recommended as therapy in both salmonellosis and coliform mastitis. The combination at this dose and sulfachlorpyradizine at 90 mg/kg intravenously have been clinically effective. Cephapirin sodium is also effective. Ampicillin and trimethoprim combined with sulfonamides may also be used effectively for intravenous administration.

Antibiotics for E. Coli Mastitis

Useful antibiotics must:

1. Reach high concentration in the udder
2. Be effective against toxin-producing *E. coli*

The following may be considered (preferably intravenous).

Parenteral. Oxytetracycline, spectinomycin, erythromycin, potentiated sulfonamides, neomycin/framycetin, gentamicin, streptomycin, ampicillin, and cephalexin.

Intramammary. Potentiated sulfonamides, ampicillin, neomycin, polymyxin, streptomycin, cephalosporin, kanamycin, and amoxycillin.

Intensive studies have been made on the specific effect of large doses of polymyxin B used alone to treat mastitis by neutralizing gram-negative endotoxins in the udder.

Polymyxin B sulfate is often chosen in these cases because of its ability to inactivate endotoxin in mastitic milk in vitro as well as its antibiotic activity against *E. coli.* Some intramammary products marketed in Europe contain 100 to 200 mg of polymyxin B sulfate and apparently are effective in improving the clinical condition of cows with acute coliform mastitis if administered early in the course of the disease.

Polymyxins would be suitable for intramammary treatment, because resistance to polymyxins is not common and absorption of this drug from the udder into the blood stream is limited. At present, polymyxin is not approved by the FDA for use in cattle.

The aminopenicillins, cephalosporins (especially third generation), some aminoglycosides, and tetracyclines are usually effective against coliforms.

Anti-inflammatory Shock Therapy

Clinical observations indicate benefits from the anti-inflammatory effects of antiprostaglandins.

Because of the severe inflammation observed in acute coliform mastitis and the probable role of arachidonic acid metabolites in mediation and/or modulation of this inflammation, anti-inflammatory agents may be indicated as adjunctive therapy. These agents include the steroidal and the nonsteroidal anti-inflammatory drugs (NSAIDs). The use of anti-inflammatory steroids to treat acute coliform mastitis has been suggested and is followed by some clinicians. Steroidal agents may decrease fever and local inflammation and produce an improvement in general attitude. Some studies have indicated minimal benefit from use of steroids in experimental endotoxin-induced mastitis. Potential negative factors include deleterious effects on host defenses and the possibility of abortion in late gestation.

High doses of corticosteroids, e.g., 40 mg/100 kg dexamethasone, may be indicated and may be repeated after 8 to 12 hours.

Some of the mechanisms that may explain the effects of dexamethasone are stabilization of lysosomal membranes of neutrophils, which thus prevents proteolytic enzymes from damaging surrounding cells, and inhibition of production of endogenous mediators, such as prostaglandins, interleukins, and probably others.

Severe coliform mastitis results from impaired functioning of host defense mechanisms. The use of steroids seems contradictory for coliform mastitis because they have detrimental effects on the functioning of both cellular and humoral defense mechanisms.

Although high doses of steroids are useful in treating hypotensive shock, the use of antibiotics and steroids is futile in the absence of fluid therapy to restore normal circulation.

Nonsteroidal Anti-inflammatory Drugs. By virtue of their antiprostaglandin action, flunixin and aspirin can be useful in shock. Like steroids, however, the cost can be prohibitive in some cases.

Flunixin meglumine at 1.1 mg/kg has been advocated as a treatment of advanced endotoxemia because of its antiprostaglandin properties. The dose of 1.1 mg/kg has been empirically and experimentally effective in altering the clinical signs of coliform mastitis.

Aspirin has also been suggested as a part of the therapeutic regimen for coliform mastitis. Aspirin at 30 to 50 orally every 12 hours is appropriate to reduce pain, inflammation, and shock, and to restore appetite.

Periparturient cows occasionally have clinical hypocalcemia as a complicating factor. Calves have also been shown to have mild hypocalcemia in experimentally induced *E. coli* endotoxemia. The mechanisms for this mild, nonparetic, endotoxin-induced hypocalcemia are not well understood, but are proposed to involve endotoxin-related interference with intestinal absorption of calcium. Research is needed to establish the possible influences of high levels of *E. coli* endotoxin on calcium metabolism.

Calcium borogluconate can be administered by slow intravenous infusion. It should be given with caution to animals in endotoxic shock because they are vulnerable to calcium-induced tachycardia and cardiac failure. The slow intravenous or subcutaneous administration of 20% calcium borogluconate (400–500 ml) is appropriate.

Other Measures

Frequent milking out of the affected quarter aided by intravenous oxytocin (20–30 I.U.) helps to remove some bacteria and their toxins.

Stripping the affected quarter by hand physically removes both endotoxins and bacteria and should be done hourly. Intravenous oxytocin may facilitate this evacuation; however, affected quarters are minimally responsive to oxytocin. Antibiotics should be infused into the affected quarter after it has been stripped the last time of the day.

Etamiphylline camsylate (millophylline) at 1400 mg intravenously can be employed as a cardiac and respiratory stimulant in severe cases.

Vitamins

Multivitamins administered at 25–30 mg intravenously can assist depressed hepatic and metabolic functioning.

25.9 SUMMER MASTITIS—DRY-COW MASTITIS

The damaging effect of mastitis in dry cows and heifers during the summer months is known to farmers and veterinarians throughout the country and has been the subject of studies in many parts of the world. Many criteria have been used to describe the disease, which is commonly referred to as summer mastitis or *Corynebacterium pyogenes* mastitis, or *Actinomyces pyogenes* infection.

The disease is characterized by an acute suppurative mastitis with a large amount of foul-smelling pus. Occasionally abscesses may break through the skin, and extensive necrosis and sloughing of tissues may take place.

The isolation of *A. pyogenes* is not a prerequisite for classification as summer mastitis, because other bacteria are frequently isolated and may be as important in the pathogenesis. *Corynebacterium pyogenes*, reclassified *Actinomyces pyogenes*, is the pathogen most commonly associated with summer mastitis, however. The response to treatment is poor unless initiated early in the infection process.

Bacteriologic analysis of summer mastitis secretion shows a complex infection. Usually *Corynebacterium pyogenes* predominates, and the severity of infection is related to the presence of anaerobes. *Peptococcus indolicus* the most common anaerobe, but *Bacteroides melaninogenicus* and *Fusobacterium necrophorum* are often found.

Peptococcus indolicus has not been frequently isolated with *Corynebacterium pyogenes* from infected quarters of lactating cows. The organism may be present with *C. pyogenes* routinely; however, its significance cannot be ascertained.

The severity of infection varies with the bacteria involved, but extensive damage to the secretory tissue occurs.

Experimental work has shown that *Peptococcus indolicus* enhances the production and activity of *Corynebacterium pyogenes* hemolysin. Numerous virulence factors (hemolysin, coagulase, hyaluronidase) are produced by the bacteria involved in summer mastitis and synergism is expected.

The foul odor of organic acids and indole in the secretion, produced by *Peptococcus indolicus*, is probably the most reliable diagnostic feature.

The term "summer mastitis" is apparently a misnomer because cases can occur throughout the year in animals of all ages.

PATHOGENESIS

Summer mastitis is a necrotizing suppurative inflammation of mammary tissue in the nonlactating bovine. It is a galactophoritis with only slight primary involvement of the acinar tissue. Abscesses are grossly visible where the exudate remains stagnant in the ducts. The usual sequela is complete fibrosis of the affected gland with irreversible loss of function.

The possible predisposing factors and exact mode of transmission of summer mastitis remain uncertain. The disease has traditionally been regarded as an arthropod-borne exogenous infection, and many of the control methods in use are based on this precept.

Summer mastitis is an acute mastitis that is mainly seen during the summer months in pasture, nonlactating cattle, i.e., dry cows and heifers.

Therapy is rarely successful, and the infected quarter is usually lost for milk production. Infected animals are often systemically ill and exhibit stiffness caused by an arthritis/tendinitis.

Experimental work has shown that infection by *Corynebacterium pyogenes, Peptococcus indolicus*, and both together is more easily established and more severe in the dry gland.

SUSCEPTIBILITY

1. Infection is most common in late gestation and at calving.
2. Specialized dairy breeds are more susceptible.
3. Older cows are more susceptible.

CLINICAL PRESENTATION

The disease syndrome is marked by temperatures of as high as 107° F. Tachycardia and dullness are quite marked, and stiffness of the hind legs may be apparent with or without hock swelling. The joint swelling and tendinitis are thought to result from bacteremia from the site of suppuration. Abortion and premature calving may occur during the febrile stage.

Front quarters are more likely to be affected than are hind quarters because the fly *Hydortaea irritans* usually approaches the udder of the animal from the belly. The affected quarter is usually hard, warm, and painful to touch. Gross teat lesions are not always present, and incidence is not always related to the prevalence of fly bites. The exudate in advanced cases is usually thick, purulent, and yellow-green. If detected in the early stages, however, the exudate is more likely to be watery or flocculent. The characteristic foul smell of the exudate has been attributed to the presence of *Peptococcus indolicus*. Severely affected quarters may eventually slough. The mortality rate in untreated cases is approximately 50%.

DISEASE TRANSMISSION

Both exogenous and endogenous modes of infection have been suggested.

Exogenous Route

The fly Hydrotaea (*H. irritans*), which also causes "broken heads" in sheep and therefore is referred to as the "sheep head fly," is universally regarded as a vector of summer mastitis. This fly has one generation per year. A reduction in the incidence of summer mastitis has been achieved using fly control methods.

Both biting and sucking flies have been implicated in the pathogenesis. The biting flies, such as *Stomoxys calcitrans*, cause the initial tissue damage to the point of the teat. Once this damage has been done, the sucking fly H. irritans is attracted to the site and if contaminated with pathogens can set up the infection.

Summer mastitis has been successfully transmitted to dry cows using the sucking fly *Hydrotaea irritans* that has fed on the teats of a field case of the disease.

The histamine release associated with the biting flies may lower local defense mechanisms and thus increase the risk of infection.

Endogenous Route

Endogenous routes of infection have also been considered. *Corynebacterium pyogenes* is widely distributed in nature and can be isolated from normal animals. *C. pyogenes* infections frequently occur in housed animals during the winter months, when fly activity is negligible. "Summer mastitis" frequent occurs outside the fly season and in regions where neither *Hydrotaea irritans* nor a readily identifiable substitute occurs.

C. pyogenes and *Peptococcus indolicus* are ubiquitous and, on the bovine, are easily recoverable from mucous membranes and particularly from abscesses in cattle.

Hydrotaea irritans probably is involved in secondary transmission in the summer peak of disease, but other mechanisms also operate.

TREATMENT

Successful bacteriologic cure of summer mastitis is rare in the dry period. Treatment must be instituted early to have any chance of success. One of the earlier signs of summer mastitis is flies pestering a single teat orifice. Such quarters should be assumed to be infected even if clinical signs are absent. Animals should be treated systemically and intramammarily, and affected quarters should be stripped as frequently as possible. The best therapy is to treat the animal with antibiotics intramuscularly, or intravenously strip the quarter frequently, and administer intramammary antibiotics in the evening. Beta-lactam drugs are the intramammary drugs of choice, especially 250 mg cephalonium. Intramammary infusion, however, is often a worthless exercise.

Generally, treating the animals with antibiotics does little to halt the progress of *Corynebacterium pyogenes* mastitis or to prevent loss of quarters, even though the organism is markedly susceptible to antibiotics in vitro. A high percentage of nonlactating quarters infected with *C. pyogenes* during the summer months also fail to respond to therapy. Considerable success has been achieved in treating *C. pyogenes* mastitis with a combination of antibiotics and trypsin. Success might be increased if treatment were initiated at an early stage of the infection. The difficulty lies not in the sensitivity of the organism, but rather in the penetration of the antibiotic through purulent masses to the focus of infection.

By the time the animal is seen, the damage to the quarter usually is irreversible. Treatment in these cases should be aimed at saving the life of the animal. Local intramammary therapy may not be indicated at this stage. Regular and thorough stripping of the affected quarter for at least 4 or 5 days is however an important part of the treatment regimen.

The clinical response to penicillin is poor; systemic tetracycline is the drug of choice. Large intravenous doses are preferable (10–20 mg/kg intravenously every 12 hours). This dosage represents 50 ml of a 10 to 20% oxytetracycline hydrochloride solution. A treatment course length of 4 to 5 days is recommended. Intravenous fluid therapy may be indicated in severe cases.

Phenylbutazone is useful when stiffness and hock swelling are marked. The loading dose used in cattle is 10–20 mg/kg, and the maintenance dose is 2.5–5 mg/kg.

Flunixin meglumine 1.1 mg/kg intravenously or subcutaneously is a useful drug in toxic cows that display severe pyrexia and inflammation.

When regular stripping of the quarter is impractical, e.g., with a fractious animal, amputation of the teat or lancing of the quarter (or teat) may be necessary to allow drainage.

PREVENTION

Attempts at preventing infection have been directed toward different stages of the infection.

FLY CONTROL METHODS

The range of control methods attempted may be summarized as follows:

1. Insecticidal and repellant sprays
2. Insecticidal ear tags
3. Teat sealants
4. Barriers

Insecticidal and Repellant Sprays. Studies in several countries have found varying results from the use of short-acting or long-acting insecticides in controlling infection.

The insecticide is usually applied by spraying, which is laborious because the animals must be rounded up.

These insecticides include the organophosphorous compounds, or pyrethroids, which are safer. The synthetic pyrethroid sprays, e.g., cypermethrin 5% solution are more popular, however. Although these sprays reduce the level of fly pesting, results suggesting a reduction in the actual number of cases of summer mastitis have been somewhat equivocal.

Insecticidal Ear Tags. In the last decade, polyvinylchloride (PVC) ear tags that release insecticides slowly have been developed, especially in the United States. The active ingredient is deposited on the animal by rubbing or by shaking of the head. Ear tags are efficacious for 3 to 4 months.

PVC ear tags are usually impregnated with synthetic pyrethroids, such as cypermethrin, permethrin and flucythrinate. Toxic concentration on the hair is maintained by prolonged diffusion.

An examination of the effect of flucythrinate-impregnated tags found a significantly greater reduction in flies around the head compared to other areas of the body. The study suggests that because a proportionately greater number of flies may congregate around the udder, summer mastitis control might be better achieved by using impregnated tail straps or leg bands.

Other reports have suggested that flies are controlled well by the synthetic pyrethroid insecticides, but two medicated ear tags per animal are needed to control flies on the teats. Ear tags and pour-on formulations are more labor efficient, longer acting, and probably safer. Work performed in Belgium has shown that ear tags reduced incidence of disease in heifers by 75%. Ear tags are preferable to antibiotic infusion, especially when performed by the unskilled.

Teat Sealants. Both internal and external teat sealants have been used to control mastitis with varying results. External sealants are only of limited value in preventing summer mastitis infections because they require repeated application every 2 to 5 days. An internal teat sealant found effective in reducing infections in spring-calving dry cows during the winter housing period did not significantly reduce summer mastitis infections when compared with the results of long-acting (dry-cow) antibiotic.

Actual plastering of the teats is popular as a control method in some countries. The plasters are applied on July 1 and are changed every third or fourth week. The method is time consuming, however, and requires good holding facilities. Protective plastic films that are sprayed on the animal have also been tried; however, they tend to fall off when exposed to water. Latex plasticizers have also been tried.

Barriers. Barriers (e.g., Stockholm tar) are another long-established method of controlling summer mastitis. Controlled efficacy data are not available, however. Teat bandages have been used effectively in Denmark, emphasizing the likely role that the fly and teat damage have in the pathogenesis of the disease.

Stockholm tar can be heavily applied to the udder and teats. Scientific information concerning the efficacy of this control method is lacking, however, and frequent retarring is necessary.

Dry-Cow Antibiotics

Long-acting intramammary formulations should give prophylactic levels of antibiotic in the udder for at least 3 weeks after infusion. Longer periods of protection can be obtained by repeated infusions. Dry cows should have a prophylactic level of antibiotic in the udder during the peak challenge period. If a second infusion is necessary, one of the cheaper long-acting penicillin preparations might suffice.

Reports have shown that the efficacy of cloxacillin and ampicillin in a dry-cow base differed significantly among a single-infusion group and a group that received infusions at 3-week intervals. Infection still occurred in the repeated-interval group, however, and a 2-week interval would probably be preferable. Hence, repeated dry-cow infusions are necessary to provide protection.

Good results have been obtained with long-acting antibiotics for almost 40 years. They remain indispensable, reducing infection rates by as much as 80%. Frequently, one application is insufficient and infusion should be repeated well before the expected calving date.

The teat should be protected from damage and bacterial contamination.

Summary

The well-recognized means of reducing the incidence of summer mastitis follow.

1. Use dry-cow treatment on all cows and repeat after 2 to 3 weeks when a history of summer mastitis exists.
2. Control flies from July to September by persistent methods, such as pyrethroid ear tags or pour-on formulations.
3. Treat all teat lesions and trauma promptly to limit attack by flies.
4. Consider teat bandages or repellents applied to teats.
5. Avoid high-risk pastures.
6. Feed animals properly.
7. Perhaps change the calving pattern.
8. Monitor animals (a close inspection at least twice daily) and segregate any suspect animal immediately.

25.10 MISCELLANEOUS MASTITIS

MYCOPLASMAL MASTITIS

Mycoplasmal mastitis, caused by a variety of *Mycoplasma*, has been described by several authors. The disease is usually regarded as a low-morbidity condition. When the morbidity rate is high, the economic effects of this disease can be devastating for the farmer because of the dramatic drop in milk production and its effect on subsequent lactation yields, the rapid spread of infection, and the failure to respond well to antimicrobial therapy, which may result in the culling of affected animals.

Macrolide drugs are particularly effective for mycoplasmal mastitis. The disease is in-creasing and is undoubtedly related to stress factors in housing and management, especially with high-yielding cows.

NOCARDIAL MASTITIS

Nocardia asteroides infections are more frequently confined to a single quarter of individual cows; however, other *Nocardia* organisms have been identified in multiple quarters when transmitted by a common source.

Clinical features of nocardial mastitis have been characterized as acute infections progressing to chronic granulomatous lesions occurring in the first 2 weeks after parturition.

Removal of infected animals from the herd is the primary consideration. Control is based on early detection, diagnosis, and prevention of spread. Regular milk sampling is effective for early diagnosis, thereby allowing removal of infected cows before spread occurs. Intramammary therapy should be restricted to approved individually packaged commercial products used aseptically.

Nocardial mastitis, in general, is refractory to therapy by antimicrobial agents. Antibiotic sensitivity is greatest for erythromycin, with decreasing sensitivity to ampicillin, novobiocin, neomycin, tetracycline, and kanamycin.

Sulfonamides and penicillin, alone or in combination, are the drugs of choice for parenteral use and intramammary infusions. Potentiated sulfonamides have been used to control bovine pulmonary nocardiosis in a calf. Clindamycin is a major drug for nocardial infections in small animals.

Miconazole nitrate given intravenously at a dose of 50 to 400 mg has been suggested as treatment for nocardial mastitis and has also been used to treat intramammary yeast infection.

Nocardia asteroides infections are usually confined to a few animals, but herd outbreaks can occur if contaminated drugs, drug vials, or infusion equipment are used. Subclinical infections may be a reservoir of the organism. Clinical infection is acute, with a febrile response progressing to chronic granulomatous lesions (suppurative with draining tracts) within 2 weeks post partum. Clindamycin may be useful.

ANAEROBIC MASTITIS

Several reports have incriminated various nonsporulating anaerobic bacterial species in the cause of bovine mastitis.

Anaerobic bacteria generally do not show up in the routine bacteriologic diagnosis of mastitis. Recent developments in techniques for the isolation of even the most fastidious genera of obligate anaerobic bacteria have provided new perspectives on their significance as infectious agents.

Their significant presence in cases of clinical mastitis poses the question of their susceptibility to antimicrobial treatment. Although most gram-positive strains are susceptible to penicillin-based antibiotics, the more frequently isolated gram-negative rods are resistant. Anaerobic bacteria are also mostly refractive to aminoglycoside antibiotics and tetracyclines.

Lincomycin has been widely reported for its activity against a broad range of nonclostridial anaerobic bacteria, including gram-negative rods.

Isolation frequencies of these organisms in pure culture or in association with others from a wide range of purulent human infections often exceed 60%.

The role of obligate anaerobic bacteria in the etiology of mastitis in lactating dairy cows has been investigated. In one experiment, anaerobes were isolated from 12% of lactating mastitic cows, which were representative of 50% of the 10 dairy herds examined. *Bacteroides fragilis* was the most frequently isolated organism (50%), followed by *Peptococcus indolicus* (33%), *Eubacterium lentum* (33%), and *E. aerofaciens* (17%). These obligate anaerobes were always isolated with organisms classically involved in mastitis. Overt clinical mastitis was induced in healthy lactating udders within 24 hours by infection with single pure cultures of anaerobes via the teat canal. All *Bacteroides fragilis* strains were resistant to penicillin G and tetracycline. In addition, one strain was also resistant to ampicillin, cephalothin, and amoxicillin. Anaerobic gram-positive cocci and bacilli were sensitive to most antibiotics. These findings imply an important role for anaerobes in the etiology of mastitis.

Lincomycin has been shown to be an effective intramammary drug for anaerobic mastitis.

FUNGAL MASTITIS

Fungal mastitis has shown a relative increase in recent years. Poor hygiene, intensivism, stress, or indiscriminate use of antimicrobial drugs may be predisposing causes. Although antimycotic drugs, such as nystatin, miconazole, or ketoconazole have been useful, they are not cleared by regulatory authorities for use in mastitis by the intramammary route.

PSEUDOMONAS AERUGINOSA MASTITIS

Because *Pseudomonas aeruginosa* bacteria require few nutrients to grow and multiply, *Pseudomonas* organisms are widespread in the dairy environment. Although mastitis caused by *Pseudomonas* is relatively rare, it is important because the infections are so difficult to treat, and culling usually results. Polymyxin B, gentamicin, amikacin or carbenicillin, and ticarcillin are effective against *Pseudomonas*.

KLEBSIELLA MASTITIS

Many outbreaks of *Klebsiella* clinical cases have been traced to the use of green sawdust or sawdust that had become wet or damp during storage.

25.11 VACCINATION AND INTRAMAMMARY DEVICES

Two main obstacles are encountered when considering the use of vaccination to induce immunity against mammary infection and inflammation.

1. The diversity of bacterial species, strains, virulence factors, and consequently antigens
2. The difficulty of obtaining antibodies in sufficient quantities

The concentration of immunoglobulins in milk is low, but high levels are present in the dry udder and in colostrum. Most of the immunoglobulin is of humoral origin and consists mainly of IgG as a result of a selective transport process. The local immune response in the mammary gland of the ruminant is poorly developed, but direct antigenic stimulation increases antibodies of the IgA class. The main activity of antibodies in the mammary gland is to increase opsonization in preparation for phagocytosis.

Numerous studies have been carried out to determine the efficacy of vaccination in mastitis prevention. These studies have involved both local and systemic stimulation of antibody production. Results have often been contradictory; the most frequently reported advantage of vaccination is a reduction in the severity of clinical infection.

One of the major difficulties preventing successful vaccination is the absence of specific antigens. The wide variety of pathogens isolated from intramammary infections, together with the number of immunologically different strains of each pathogen, have hindered the development of a successful vaccine. In most vaccination experiments involving *Staphylococcus aureus*, some protection was afforded within the homologous system and to closely related strains, but not to different phage or serotypes of staphylococci.

In the bovine, both specific and nonspecific immunity play a role in the inflammatory response to mastitis. Immunoglobulin levels are low in normal milk. After inflammation has begun, IgG enters the gland. IgG has a role in the opsonization process. Immunoglobulins are part of the humoral immune system. They are designed to attack specific antigens. Exposure through natural infections or vaccination is required to stimulate the body to produce specific immunoglobulins.

Effective vaccines have been prepared for *S. aureus* mastitis. Use of a *S. aureus* bacterin reduces the severity of systemic reactions and increases the rate of spontaneous recovery. Bacterins do not reduce the incidence of new intramammary infections.

Immunization as a means of heightening resistance to mastitis has been investigated for several decades. Most reported data have yielded little solid evidence that would yet favor vaccination as a routine means of mastitis control. The more recent sensitive methods of measuring the immune response in the bovine mammary gland have been developed and the defensive mechanisms are now better understood. The enzyme-linked immunosorbent assay (ELISA) has been adapted to the measurement of specific antibody in lacteal fluids and can also reveal its immunoglobulin isotype. Phagocytosis and antiadhesive activity are two defensive phenomena of the mammary gland that are of established importance. Both of these phenomena are probably mediated by antibody specific for surface antigen(s), although not of the same immunoglobulin isotype. The neutralization of toxins is likely to lessen the clinical effects of infection.

In the past few years, vaccination against staphylococcal mastitis has emerged as a real future possibility. Research has shown that the cow can mount an immune response in the lactating gland. Previously utilized vaccines have employed considerably less than the optimum dosage of antigen. Furthermore, recent evidence indicates that *S. aureus* may produce virulent antigens in vivo that are generally not expressed in vitro. Antigen content and concentration in vaccines consequently have been modified accordingly. Routes of inoculation, timing of administration, and inclusion of adjuvant preparations have also been re-evaluated.

Numerous, more or less empirical attempts at vaccination mainly against staphylococcal infection have been made. No vaccine until recently has proved effective, although reduction in severity against homologous strains and increase in spontaneous recovery of vaccinated cows have been seen. The classic approach has been to enhance the polymorphonuclear leukocyte recruitment and opsonization for phagocytosis. Studies have revealed that live vaccines are superior to killed vaccines in promoting neutrophil response. Live vaccine stimulates the synthesis of IgG_2 antibodies, which are cytophilic and have opsonizing activity. Killed vaccine in oily adjuvants primarily stimulates production of IgG_1 antibodies, which do not mediate the same immunologic protection. Whether live staphylococcal vaccines can protect against homologous and heterologous strains remains to be seen.

Because mastitis pathogens exhibit considerable antigenic and pathogenic diversity, attempts to stimulate the nonspecific protective mechanisms in the udder of the cow have been carried out by means of the intramammary device. One such intramammary device consists of a polyethylene loop inserted into the gland cistern. It causes a neutrophilia and elevates immunoglobulin concentrations in the milk to levels that afford protection against invading pathogens without affecting milk quality. Initial results are promising, and much effort is now being directed toward developing this area. Combinations of a specific stimulus (vaccine) in association with a nonspecific stimulus (intramammary device) may prove to be the most efficacious means for stimulating immunity of the mammary gland.

Elucidation of pathogenic mechanisms employed by mastitis-causing organisms is providing a new understanding of the disease. Specific bacterial adherence to mammary gland epithelium is an important factor in mastitis pathogenesis. In general, the ability of a bacterial strain to adhere can be correlated to the prevalence of that strain in causing mastitis. These factors have major implications for the inclusion of relevant antigens in vaccine preparations.

The variability of oligosaccharide (0 or somatic) antigens among gram-negative bacteria is well recognized. Combinations of hexose molecule numbers, composition, and linkage produce a wide array of antigens.

The administration of the *Escherichia coli* J5 vaccine is protective against natural challenges to the bovine mammary gland by gram-negative bacteria, and it significantly reduces the incidence of clinical coliform mastitis. Considerable research is ongoing in this area.

25.12 CONTROL POLICY

The five points in mastitis control policy are:

1. A monitoring system
2. An effective milking routine
3. Routine parlor testing
4. Milking and dry-cow therapy
5. A culling policy

A monitoring system may be based on somatic cell count or clinical incidence. Targets should be set for a particular time period and must be attainable. When they cannot be achieved, the farmer feels that the program is ineffective and thus loses interest. When the target can be attained, however, the dairy farmer strives to set even higher goals. Constant motivation is essential.

Teat dipping aims to kill pathogens before they can enter the teat canal after milking. All teats should be dipped after every milking. Teat dipping every now and again is of no benefit. The best teat dip drips from the teats of the cow as she leaves the parlor.

The efficiency of the milkings can be monitored by observation in the pit and also by *E. coli* counts.

ANTIBIOTIC TREATMENT

Antibiotic selection should be based on the organisms involved and the stage of lactation.

Toward the end of lactation, the start of antibiotic therapy should be delayed until the dry period. The dry period is an excellent opportunity for systematic treatment and control of mastitis. If mastitis infections are controlled during the dry period, damaged tissue in the udder has a chance to regenerate.

As intramammary pressure stops milk production, the teat canal expands and the udder is stressed. Also, when cows are not milked, teats are not cleaned or dipped to remove bacteria. These factors increase the susceptibility of a dry cow to mastitis infections.

PERFORMANCE MONITORING

Good records are invaluable to the producer who desires to maximize production in the herd, because the data for milk production, somatic cell count (SCC), fertility, and feed cost per kilogram of milk can help to pinpoint problems.

If milk production drops significantly or SCCs increase, records can alert the producer to mastitis problems and the need to address them.

Dairy farmers must emphasize overall management. Production records allow the producer to track the herd and determine which animals are an asset to the herd and which should be culled and replaced with higher-producing animals.

Dairying is a complex business, no single individual can have all the knowledge necessary to implement the most cost-effective management plant. A producer can no longer be satisfied that everything seems to be progressing well; new ways to improve productivity and efficiency must be constantly sought.

SOMATIC CELL COUNTS

When high SCCs are detected in the bulk tank, the veterinarian should examine the producer's records.

The SCC is the primary monitoring tool for mastitis. The SCC is a quantitative tool that makes goal-setting, easier, helps to find the source of mastitis, and is helpful for culling cows.

All cows have somatic cells in their milk; a normal, uninfected udder may have as many as 200,000/ml. When the number increases because of an influx of leukocytes (white blood cells) from the blood, udder tissue damage is indicated.

In response to bacterial toxins and tissue damage, the body sends leukocytes to the site of the infection. The leukocytes engulf and try to destroy the bacteria and tissue debris by flooding the infection site until most of the infectious organisms are gone. A high SCC indicates that udder damage is occurring or has occurred and that these cells are trying to rectify the situation.

Many factors influence SCC as detected in the quarter, the cow, or herd. Infection status of the quarter, the age and stage of lactation of the cow, the season, stress, injuries, and management procedures all affect SCC.

Dairy Herd Improvement SCC reports help dairy farmers to monitor and evaluate individual cow performance. These reports can help to determine whether production reflects the true genetic potential of a cow or whether production declines are the result of subclinical mastitis.

SCC reports can also help dairy farmers to evaluate the effectiveness of their management program. By determining the rate at which new infections occur in the herd and the rate at which infections are re-moved, a producer can measure how subclinical infections affect production. The dairy farmer and the veterinarian then must run a bacterial culture on the milk of cows with a high SCC and identify the organisms causing the inflammation.

The chance of isolating a major pathogen, such as *Streptococcus agalactiae* or *Staphylococcus aureus*, increases dramatically with SCCs above 200,000.

ADVANTAGES OF SCC PROGRAMS

1. SCC information indicates the seriousness of the mastitis problem.
2. SCC monitoring programs develop awareness of subclinical mastitis.
3. SCCs enable monitoring of the effects of preventive measures and treatment programs.
4. SCC information provides evidence of chronic mastitis, which can be used in making culling decisions.
5. SCC information is readily available and inexpensive.

Dairy Herd Improvement programs provide SCC values in composite milk samples on a monthly basis. Bulk tank counts are also a useful measure of milk quality.

The SCC gives a good indication as to the level of infection in the herd, and is the best monitor of the overall success of mastitis control. Some guidelines for bulk tank SCC interpretation follow:

BULK TANK SCC

0–300,000—Minimal infection present.
300,000–500,000—Infection suspected.
500,000–800,000—Infection present.
Over 800,000—Mastitis problem herd.

Examination of the SCC for the previous 12 months gives a good guide to the level of infection in the herd.

The incidence of clinical mastitis should be less than 1% of the herd at any one time. This includes both cows under treatment and those from which milk is being withheld following intramammary treatment.

A dramatic increase in the prevalence of subclinical infections during the lactation suggests a problem with cow-to-cow transmission of infectious organisms. Milking procedures and equipment should be checked.

Seasonal variations do occur—counts are lowest during winter and highest in July and August—but the reasons are unknown. Researchers speculate that housing and temperature changes may be the cause.

CULTURING

Total bacterial count (TBC) and bacterial culturing are two other important aspects of mastitis control programs. Culturing is crucial for identifying mastitis pathogens in the herd and for discerning their prevalence. After treatment has been initiated, culturing can help to monitor its effectiveness.

For an accurate diagnosis, proper culturing techniques must be followed meticulously. Attention to proper procedure prevents contamination of the sample, which could lead to inaccurate interpretations of antimicrobial sensitivity.

Zone Sizes

Accurate measurements of zones of inhibition—based on the Kirby-Bauer tables—are crucial. A template laid over the agar helps to ensure accurate zone measurements.

SELECTED REFERENCES

Anderson, K.L.: Therapy for acute coliform mastitis. Compend. Contin. Educ. Vet. Pract., *11*:1125, 1989.

Anderson, K.L.: Mastitis therapy and pharmacology of drugs in the bovine mammary gland. Bovine Pract., *20*:64, 1988.

Anderson, K.L., Kindahl, H., Petroni, A., et al.: Arachidonic acid metabolites in milk of cows during acute coliform mastitis. Am. J. Vet. Res., *46*:1573, 1985.

Boisseau, J., and Moretain, J.P.: Drug excretion by the mammary gland. *In* Veterinary Pharmacology and Toxicology. Edited by Y. Ruckebusch, P.L. Toutain, and G.D. Koritz. Boston, MTP Press, 1983.

Borelli, C.L., et al.: Effect of *E. coli* J5 Vaccination on Incidence of Clinical Coliform Mastitis and Milk Production Loss in Dairy Cows. Abstract 12. 11th Annual Food Animal Disease Research Conference, University of Nevada, Reno, NV, 1990.

Bramley, A.J.: Environmental mastitis. Proc. N. M.C./AABP International Symposium on Bovine Mastitis. 1990.

Bywater, R.J., Dorwick, J.S., Osborne, S.J., and Follett, G.A.: International Conference on Mastitis: Physiology or Pathology. Univ. Ghent, Sept. 18–22, 1990.

Carlsson, A., et al.: Lactoferrin and lysozyme in milk during acute mastitis and their inhibitory effect in delvotest P. J. Dairy Sci., *72*:3166, 1989.

Conner, J.G., Eckersall, P.D., Doherty, M., et al.: Acute phase response and mastitis in the cow. Res. Vet. Sci., *41*:126, 1986.

Craigmill, A.L.: Antimicrobial therapy and milk and tissue residues. Proc. 30th Annual Meeting Natl. Mastitis Council, Reno, NV, 1991.

Craven, N., and Anderson, J.C.: Phagocytosis of *Staphylococcus aureus* by bovine mammary gland macrophages and intracellular protection from antibiotic action in vitro and in vivo. J. Dairy Res., *51*:513, 1984.

Craven, N., and Williams, M.K.: Defenses of the bovine mammary gland against infection and prospects for their enhancement. Vet. Immunol. Immunopathol., *10*:71, 1985.

Cullor, J.S.: Mastitis in dairy cows? Does it hinder reproductive performance? Vet. Med., *86(8)*:830, 1991.

Cullor, J.S.: Mastitis and its influence upon reproductive performance in dairy cattle. Proc. International Symposium Bovine Mastitis, Indianapolis, IN, 1990.

Cullor, J.S., and Chen, J.: Evaluating two new OTC milk screening ELISA's: Do they measure up? Vet. Med., *86*:845, 1991.

DeGraves, F.J., and Anderson, K.L.: Anti-inflammatory therapy for acute coliform mastitis. Proc. International Symposium Bovine Mastitis. Indianapolis, IN, 1990.

Du Preez, J.H.: Treatment of various forms of bovine mastitis with consideration of udder pathology and the pharmacokinetics of appropriate drugs. J. S. Afr. Vet. Assoc., *59*:161, 1988.

Du Preez, J.H., Greef, A.S., and Kraft, U.: The effect of lincomycin-neomycin treatment on experimental bacterial bovine mastitis. J. S. Afr. Vet. Assoc., *54(4)*:243, 1983.

Eberhart, R.J.: Coliform mastitis. Am. Vet. Med. Assoc., *170*:1160, 1977.

Erskine, R.J., Eberhart, R.J., Grasso, P.J., and Sclolz, R.W.: Influence of selenium supplementation on E. Coli mastitis. Am. J. Vet. Res., *50*:2093, 1989.

Erskine, R.J., Tyler, J.W., Riddell, M.G., et al.: Theory, use and realities of efficacy and food safety of antimicrobial treatment of acute coliform mastitis. J. Am. Vet. Med. Assoc., *198*:980, 1991.

Erskine, R.J., Wilson, R.C., and Riddell, M.G.: The pharmacokinetics and efficacy of intramammary gentamicin for the treatment of coliform mastitis. Proc. International Symposium Bovine Mastitis, Indianapolis, IN, 1990.

Francis, P.G.: Update on mastitis. III. Mastitis therapy. Br. Vet. J., *145*:302, 1989.

Franklin, A., Horn, A.F., Rantzien, M., et al.: Concentration of penicillin, streptomycin and spiramycin in bovine udder tissue liquids. Am. J. Vet. Res. *47*:804, 1986.

Gingerich, D.A., Baggott, J.D., and Yeary, R.A.: Pharmacokinetics and dosage of aspirin in cattle. Am. J. Vet. Res., *167(10)*:945, 1975.

Giri, S.N., Chen, A., Carroll, E.J., et al.: Role of prostaglandins in pathogenesis of mastitis induced by *Escherichia coli* endotoxin. Am. J. Vet. Res., *84*:586, 1984.

Giri, S.N., et al.: Effects of endotoxin infusion on circulating levels of eicosanoids, progesterone, cortisol, glucose and lactic acid, and abortion in pregnant cows. Vet. Microbiol., *21*:211, 1990.

Hardee, G.E., Smith, J.A., and Harris, S.J.: Pharmacokinetics of flunixin meglumine in the cow. Res. Vet. Sci., *39*:110, 1985.

Hillerton, J.E.: Summer mastitis—the current position. In Pract., Vet. Rec., *123*:131, 1988.

Hogan, J.S., and Smith, K.L.: A practical look at environmental mastitis. Compend. Contin. Educ. Vet. Pract., *9*:341, 1987.

Hogan, J.S., Smith, K.L., Hoblet, K.H., et al.: Bacterial counts in bedding materials used on nine commercial dairies. J. Dairy Sci., *72*:250, 1989.

Hogan, J.S., Smith, K.L., Todhunter, D.A., et al.: Efficacy of *Escherichia coli* J-5 vaccine for preventing coliform mastitis. Proc. International Symposium Bovine Mastitis, Indianapolis, IN, 1990.

Jenkins, W.L.: Concurrent use of corticosteroids and antimicrobial drugs in the treatment of infectious disease in large animals. J. Am. Vet. Med. Assoc., *185(10)*:1145, 1984.

Jones, G.F., and Ward, G.E.: Evaluation of systemic administration of gentamicin for treatment of coliform mastitis in cows. J. Am. Vet. Med. Assoc., *197*:731, 1990.

Kaartinen, L., Veijalainen, K., Kuosa, P.L., and Sandholm, M.: Endotoxin-induced mastitis. Inhibition of casein synthesis and activation of the caseinolytic system. J. Vet. Med., *35*:353, 1988.

Kirk, J.H.: Diagnosis and treatment of difficult mastitis cases. Part I. *Staphylococcus* and *Pseudomonas*. Agric. Practice, *12(1)*:5, 1991.

Larson, V.L., Farnsworth, R.J., and Baumann, L.: Therapy of acute toxic mastitis. Proc. Natl. Mastitis Council, 1981.

MacDiarmid, S.C.: Antibacterial drugs used against mastitis in cattle by the systemic route. NZ Vet. J., *26*:290, 1978.

Mackie, D.P., Logan, E.F., Pollock, D.A., and Rodgers, S.P.: Antibiotic sensitivity of bovine staphylococcal and coliform mastitis isolates over four years. Vet. Rec., *20*:515, 1988.

McKellar, Q.A.: Intramammary treatment of mastitis in cows. In Pract., Vet. Rec. *129*:244, 1991.

Mercer, H.D., Geleta, J.N., Baldwin, R.A., and Shimoda, W.: Viewpoint and Current Concepts Regarding Accepted and Tried Products for Control of Bovine Mastitis. J. Am. Vet. Med. Assoc., *169*:1104, 1976.

Mercer, H.D., Geleta, J.N., Schultz, E.J., and Wright, W.W.: Milk out rates for antibiotics in intramammary infusion products used in the treatment of bovine mastitis. Relationship of somatic cell counts, milk production level and drug vehicle. Am. J. Vet. Res., *31(9)*:1549, 1970.

Miller, R.E.: Proposed intramammary infusion product guidelines. J. Am. Vet. Med. Assoc., *170(10)*:1203, 1977.

Moore, G.A., and Heider, L.E.: Treatment of mastitis. Vet. Clin. Nth. Am. July 1984 Sympos. Bov. Mast., *6*:323.

Norcross, N.L., and Kenny, K.: Evaluation of a vaccine for mastitis caused by *Staphylococcus aureus*. Proc. XIV World Congress Diseases Cattle. Dublin, Ireland, Vol. 2, 1986.

Oetzel, G.R.: Coliform mastitis and hypoglycemia in two dairy cows in midlactation. Compend. Contin. Educ. Pract. Vet., *7(4)*:S237, 1985.

Opdebeeck, J.R., O'Boyle, D.A., and Frost, A.J.: Encapsulated *Staphylococcus aureus* from bovine mastitis. Aust. Vet. J., *65*:194, 1988.

Owens, W.E., Watts, J.L., Boddie, R.L., et al.: Antibiotic treatment of mastitis. Comparison of intramammary and intramammary plus intramuscular therapies. J. Am. Vet. Med. Assoc., *169*:1104, 1988.

Pyorala, S., and Kaartinen, L.: Diagnostic method for evaluating therapy response in clinical mastitis. Proc. International Symposium Bovine Mastitis, Indianapolis, IN, 1990.

Rasmussen, F.: In vitro antibacterial activity of trimethoprim and sulphonamide on bacteria causing bovine mastitis. Acta Vet. Scand., *12*:131, 1971.

Report of the panel of the colloquium on bovine mastitis. J. Am. Vet. Med. Assoc., *170*:1119, 1977.

Rothbauer, D.L., Bucknmer, E.C., and Wells, S.J.: Effect of vaccination with *E. coli* on the incidence of acute mastitis. Bovine Pract., *23*:112, 1988.

Sanchez, M.S., Ford, C.W., and Yancey, R.J.: Evaluation of antibiotic effectiveness against *Staphylococcus aureus* surviving within the bovine mammary gland macrophage. J. Antimicrob. Chemother., *21*:773, 1988.

Sandholm, M., Kaartinen, L., and Pyorala, S.: Bovine mastitis—why does antibiotic therapy not always work? An overview. J. Vet. Pharmacol. Ther., *13*:248, 1990.

Sears, P.M.: Nocardial mastitis in cattle: diagnosis, treatment and prevention. Compend. Contin. Educ. Pract. Vet., *8*:F41, 1986.

Sears, P.M., and Heider, L.E.: Identification of mastitis pathogens. Mod. Vet. Pract., *62*:531, 1981.

Sisodia, C.S., and Stowe, C.M.: The mechanism of drug secretion into bovine milk. NY Acad. Sci. Ann., *111*:650, 1964.

Smith, B.P.: Understanding the role of endotoxins in gram-negative disease. Vet. Med., *81(12)*:1148, 1986.

Smith, L.K., Todhumter, D.A., and Schoenberger, P.S.: Environmental mastitis: cause, prevalence, prevention. J. Dairy Sci., *68*:1531, 1985.

Soback, S.: Mastitis therapy: past, present and future. Proc. International Symposium Bovine Mastitis, Indianapolis, IN, 1990.

Sundlof, S.F., et al.: Food animal residue avoidance databank (FARAD): a pharmacokinetic-based information resource. J. Vet. Pharmacol. Ther., *9*:237, 1986.

U.S. Department of Agriculture: Compound Evaluation and Analytical Capability, National Residue Program Plan. Washington, DC, USDA, 1990.

Van Damme, D.M.: Techniques of rapid identification and susceptibility testing in mastitis culturing. Vet. Med., *78*:1097, 1983.

Van Damme, D.M.: Use of micronazole in treatment of bovine mastitis. Vet. Med., *78*:1425, 1983.

Van Dresser, W.R., and Wilcke, J.R.: Drug residues in food animals. J. Am. Vet. Med. Assoc., *194*:1700, 1989.

Watts, J.L.: Characterization and identification of streptococci isolated from bovine mammary glands. J. Dairy Sci., *71*:1616, 1988.

White, M.E., et al.: Discriminant analysis of the clinical indicants for bovine coliform mastitis. Cornell Vet., *76*:335, 1986.

Wilson, C.D., and Gilbert, G.A.: Pharmacokinetics of cefoperazone in the cow by the intramammary route and its effect on mastitis pathogens in vitro. Vet. Rec., *118*:607, 1986.

Ziv, G.: (1980) Drug selection in mastitis: systemic vs. local therapy. J. Am. Vet. Med. Assoc., *176(10)*:1109, 1980.

Ziv, G.: Pharmacokinetics of antimastitis products. *In* Proceedings of the Symposium on Animal Health Products: Design and Evaluation. Edited by D.C. Monkhouse. Acad. Pharm. Sci Am Pharm Assoc., 1978.

Ziv, G.: Pharmacokinetic concepts for systemic and intramammary antibiotic treatment in lactating and dry cows. Proceedings Seminar on Mastitis Control. Int. Dairy Fed. Bull., *85*:314, 1975.

Ziv, G., Paape, M.J., and Dulin, A.M.: Influence of antibiotics and intramammary antibiotic products on phagocytosis of *Staphylococcus aureus* by bovine leukocytes. Am. J. Vet. Res., *44*:385, 1983.

DRUGS AND THE BOVINE GENITAL TRACT

26.1   Corticosteroid-Induced Parturition
26.2   Indications for Induction of Calving
26.3   Types of Steroids
26.4   Prostaglandins
26.5   Tocolytic Drugs and Postponement of Parturition
26.6   Therapy of Bovine Metritis
26.7   Antibiotic Therapy
26.8   Nonantibiotic Alternatives
26.9   Bovine Pyometra
26.10   Therapy for Retained Fetal Membranes

26.1 CORTICOSTEROID-INDUCED PARTURITION

Much experimental work has supported the concept that the fetal pituitary-adrenal axis has a role in the initiation of parturition. Demonstration of this role was first shown by hypophysectomy and adrenalectomy, procedures that were proved to prolong the length of gestation.

The possible role of the adrenal gland was suggested when Holstein calves born 11 to 15 days after normal term were discovered to suffer from hypoadrenocorticism. Thus, although fetal hypophysectomy or adrenalectomy prolongs gestation, frequently either an aplasia or hypoplasia of the anterior pituitary and adrenal glands of the fetus occurs in naturally occurring cases of prolonged gestation.

Subsequently, the converse of this relationship was observed; the injection of cortisone or adrenocorticotropic hormone (ACTH) into the fetus brought about premature birth. Thus, the fetal pituitary-adrenal axis seemed to determine the moment of birth, and artificial stimulation of the mechanism allowed for the premature induction of parturition at a predetermined moment.

The ability to induce parturition at a prescribed time near the end of gestation by means of parenteral injection of a drug could prove to be a valuable aid in animal production.

The importance of a functional fetal pituitary gland in the maintenance of a normal pregnancy was observed when prolonged gestation in a Guernsey herd was associated with a high incidence of fetal adrenohyphophyseal aplasia. A hormonal imbalance between the fetus and dam explained the prolonged gestation in this case.

A celebrated report concerned an 11-year-old Holstein cow that showed no signs of impending parturition as the expected date approached. A caesarean section was undertaken and a live calf was born. The calf was deformed, and so euthanasia was performed. On postmortem examination, histologic examination of the hypophyseal area of the brain stem revealed a relatively normal pars nervosa. No pars distalis, pars tuberalis, or associated anterior pituitary cell types could be demonstrated, however.

External and internal stimuli induce or suppress the formation and secretion of the luteinizing hormone/follicle-stimulating hormone (LH/FSH) releasing hormone (variously referred to in the scientific literature as LH/FSH-RH or GnRH). This releasing hormone is produced by specific nerve cells in the hypothalamus. External stimuli include light, sound, smell, state of nutrition, temperature, stress, and mounting by other animals. Other factors, such as age, also influence secretion of LH/FSH releasing hormone.

The releasing hormone passes via the blood vessels of the hypophyseal portal system to the anterior lobe of the pituitary gland. LH/FSH releasing hormone stimulates the anterior pituitary to release the gonadotropic hormones, follicle-stimulating hormone (FSH), and luteinizing hormone (LH). These hormones pass via the blood stream to the ovary.

PITUITARY CONTROL

The pituitary gland exerts its influence on the reproductive cycle by secreting the gonadotropic hormones FSH and LH. These, in turn, influence the reproductive cycle as follows:

Functions of FSH

1. Causes the growth of the graafian follicles and the production of estrogen by the ovary.
2. Together with LH is responsible for maturation of the follicle.

Functions of LH

1. Initiation of ovulation caused by a preovulatory peak concentration in the blood.
2. Stimulates growth of the corpus luteum from the granulosa cells of the ruptured graafian follicle. Thus, LH is responsible for the process of luteinization.
3. In the cow, the continued secretion of LH is essential for the maintenance of the corpus luteum and for its secretion of progesterone. This continued secretion of LH at a lower level is essential both during the luteal phase of the estrous

cycle and throughout early pregnancy. Thus, LH in the cow has a luteotropic action.

OVARIAN HORMONE CONTROL

Estrogen

The estrogens are steroid hormones secreted by the granulosa cells of the graafian follicle. The most important naturally occurring estrogen in the cow is estradiol.

Estradiol has three main functions:

1. To prepare the reproductive tract for conception
2. To cause the characteristic estrous behavior by its action on the central nervous system
3. The estradiol peak produced by the increasing secretory activity of the graafian follicle is involved in the preovulatory LH surge because it sensitizes the pituitary to LH/FSH releasing hormone and may perhaps cause release of LH/FSH releasing hormone.

Progesterone

Progesterone is a steroid hormone secreted by the lutein cells of the corpus luteum. Following ovulation, the corpus luteum develops from the granulosa cells and the theca interna of the graafian follicle. Under the influence of LH, the lutein cells secrete progesterone.

Progesterone has four main functions:

1. Prepares the uterus for the embryo to implant.
2. Maintains pregnancy by providing a suitable environment for the developing embryo and inhibiting the motility of the uterus.
3. Prevents further estrous cycles by inhibiting the secretion of LH/FSH releasing hormone. The release of preovulatory levels of LH from the pituitary thus is prevented. Enough FSH is released, however, to allow follicles to develop during the luteal phase of the estrous cycle and even during early gestation. Consequently, some cows exhibit signs of estrous even during the early stages of pregnancy.

4. May exercise control of the reproductive cycle by means other than that of negative feedback on the hypothalamus. When GnRH is administered during the luteal phase of the estrous cycle, an increase in LH in the blood stream is observed. Despite this increase in LH, however, ovulation does not occur, thus suggesting that progesterone has another mode of action that prevents the return of the cycle.

UTERINE CONTROL

The hormones that have been used for induction are

1. ACTH
2. Corticosteroids, both short-acting preparations and slow-release preparations
3. Prostaglandins F_{2a}, E_1, and E_2 ($PGF_{2\alpha}$, PGE_1, and PGE_2) and various analogs.
4. Combinations of corticosteroids and prostaglandins and of corticosteroids and estrogens.

The requirements necessary for successful induction are:

1. A known, accurate date for service or artificial insemination
2. Induction at 270 days to ensure that the calf can be expelled vaginally and is capable of survival
3. Absence of infection, especially mastitis

Physiology

The parturition-inducing signals normally emanate from the fetus. These signals are reflected by a marked increase in the maternal blood corticosteroid levels resulting from the increased activity of the fetal adrenal glands. Plasma corticosteroid concentrations in the fetus increase markedly beginning several days before birth. The concentration in the dam's blood is only moderately elevated at this time. This situation is largely the result of increased glucocorticoid secretion by the fetal adrenal cortex.

In cattle, cortisol concentrations are greater in calves than in their dams immediately after parturition. This rise in fetal corticosteroids prior to parturition has also been demonstrated in sheep and goats. These findings tend to support the hypothesis that fetal, rather than maternal, glucocorticoids are principally involved in the initiation of parturition. High concentrations of glucocorticoids may lessen resistance against various infectious agents, and the susceptibility of newborn calves to bacterial infection may be enhanced by high plasma cortisol concentrations at birth. This rise may exert an influence on the levels of maternal hormones, with the result that progesterone is decreased and estrogen and $PGF_{2\alpha}$ are increased.

The endometrium of the nonpregnant cow produces a precursor of $PGF_{2\alpha}$. This substance is produced locally, adjacent to the ovary bearing the corpus luteum, and is carried in the blood stream to the ovary. There it is converted to $PGF_{2\alpha}$ and causes the corpus luteum to regress. Following luteolysis, progesterone levels fall rapidly, thereby allowing a new estrous cycle to commence. If the cow conceives, the uterine luteolytic mechanism is inhibited by the embryo or its membranes and regression of the corpus luteum is prevented.

The initiation of labor in sheep may result from $PGF_{2\alpha}$. The site of synthesis is believed to be the maternal cotyledon, from which the prostaglandin passes by an unknown route to the myometrium. $PGF_{2\alpha}$ causes lysis of the corpus luteum, and following infusion of the compound in primates, a sharp decrease in progesterone secretion has been demonstrated. The actual mode of action of $PGF_{2\alpha}$ is unclear, although many possible mechanisms have been suggested.

Prostaglandins themselves also have oxytocic-like effects on the uterine musculature. Sufficient levels of blood corticosteroid apparently suppress progesterone production and also induce the prostaglandin tissue levels essential for normal or premature parturition. The increased levels of corticosteroids may also initiate synthesis of pulmonary surfactant in the fetal lungs as a result of activation of specific enzymes. This surfactant allows the lungs to expand more readily at birth.

The original work on the premature induction of parturition was achieved by the administration of ACTH or corticosteroid to the ewe or the fetal lamb. Although corticosteroid treatment of the fetal lamb in-

duced parturition, initial reports suggested that corticosteroid treatment of the pregnant ewe did not have such an effect. Subsequent trials with large doses, however, showed that parturition could be induced by treating the ewe. Similarly in the cow, large doses of corticosteroids injected into the pregnant animal induced parturition. One can assume that, when the drug is injected into the cow, it also acts on the fetus.

When premature parturition is induced by the administration of synthetic corticosteroids, the signal from the fetal calf is being mimicked in a crude manner. Some synthetic steroids, such as dexamethasone, readily cross the placenta from the maternal circulation and presumably activate or induce the placental enzymes, which are normally the target of endogenous fetal cortisol.

INDICATIONS FOR USE OF CORTICOSTEROIDS

The use of corticosteroids for the induction of parturition can be advocated for various reasons. Sound medical reasons may dictate termination of pregnancy shortly before anticipated parturition, e.g., toxemia of pregnancy, hydrops allantois or amnii, renal disease, fractures, and cardiovascular disease of late pregnancy when the life of the dam or fetus might be saved by premature parturition. Any dystocia problems that might arise because of relative fetal oversize could be prevented or reduced by the induction of calving 2 to 3 weeks before term. Also, the application of corticosteroids to synchronized breeding programs might be beneficial. The corticosteroids have no ecbolic effect on a dead or mummified fetus, thus confirming that a viable fetal pituitary-adrenal axis is a prerequisite. One of the main disadvantages of using corticosteroids to induce parturition has been the high incidence of retained placenta. The results in this regard, however, are quite variable. The future fertility of animals in which retention of fetal membranes has occurred apparently is not affected.

Corticosteroid-induced parturition has been routinely adopted in several countries using various steroid preparations. The steroids can be broadly divided into two groups—the short-acting steroids in the free alcohol or soluble ester form, which cause parturition within 3 days of administration, and the long-acting steroids in the insoluble ester form, which induce parturition within 3 weeks.

Induction of Parturition in Cattle

The incidence of stillbirths is high in the animals treated before day 260 of pregnancy. The incidence of retained placenta, however, is less in these animals when treated with long-acting corticosteroids than when treated with the shorter-acting drugs. Animals treated after day 260 of pregnancy usually do not show any adverse effects, but the response to treatment may be too delayed to achieve any advance in the calving date.

Using a single injection of dexamethasone (20 mg) in soluble ester form, the average interval between administration and parturition in animals more than 260 days' pregnant is approximately 48–72 hours.

When induction is attempted prior to the last month of pregnancy, the results can be quite erratic. Retention of the placenta following treatment with corticosteroids has been described as a frequent occurrence. Some degree of prematurity is common in calves induced early.

Reports using long-acting corticosteroids in an extensive study of 3000 cows in New Zealand, showed that calf mortality was disturbingly high, and was mainly the result of stillbirth. Diarrhea and prematurity are often the main causes of calf death within 2 weeks of birth, following early induction.

26.2 INDICATIONS FOR INDUCTION OF CALVING

The indications for the induction of calving are:

1. To synchronize the calving period with the availability of labor, thus facilitating the observation and management of calving and overcoming the inconveniences caused by late-calving cows.
2. To avoid or minimize dystocia and to terminate unwanted pregnancies. If the dam is immature with a small pelvis or

if pregnancy is prolonged beyond 280 days, as occurs in some exotic breeds, the calf may be too large to traverse the birth canal. Premature induction thus can reduce the likelihood of dystocia caused by fetomaternal disproportion.

In diseased or injured cows in which termination of pregnancy will alleviate the condition, or when a live calf can be obtained before slaughter, premature induction may be used. Cows suffering from hydrallantois frequently respond.
3. For the therapeutic termination of pregnancy for various clinical reasons.

Premature induction of calving has some disadvantages, however. The birth weight of the calf is lower than it would have been at term, and thus, the subsequent growth rate is reduced. The incidence of placental retention is high, as much as 53% when short-acting preparations are used (Table 26–1). Colostrum quality can also be adversely affected by corticosteroid induced parturition (immunoglobulin content less than normal).

The stage at which calving is induced must be a compromise between the birth of a calf that is small enough to be born unaided and yet is large enough to be viable and subsequently to have an adequate growth rate.

Several different hormones have been used successfully to induce calving so that a live calf is born. Because induction before 260 days usually results in the birth of a small, weak calf with poor prospects for survival, the date of service or insemination must be accurately known.

ACTH exerts its effect by stimulating endogenous corticosteroid production. Thus, although ACTH has been used to induce calving, it is best replaced by the direct administration of corticosteroids. Numerous potent synthetic corticosteroids are available in two types. Those referred to as quick-release or short-acting preparations are aqueous solutions of the steroid; slow-release preparations are insoluble esters or suspensions. The short-acting preparations, such as betamethasone, dexamethasone, and flumethasone, when given at the normal therapeutic dose, usually induce calving after a latent period of 2 to 3 days after injection. The slow-release preparations

---

TABLE 26–1
INDICATIONS FOR AND DISADVANTAGES OF INDUCTION OF PARTURITION

Indications

1. Synchronization or advancing the time of calving to match the availability of pasture.
2. Predetermined calving related to the availability of skilled labor.
3. Prevention of dystocia resulting from relative fetal oversize.
4. Disease or injury of the cow.
5. Fetal abnormalities, i.e., mummification.

Disadvantages

1. Smaller birth weight/prematurity.
2. A high incidence of retained placenta.
3. Longer calving conception interval, although perhaps only a slight reduction in fertility.
4. Delay in reaching peak lactation.
5. Reduced level of antibodies in the colostrum.
6. Higher calf mortality/less immunoglobulin absorption.

---

have latent periods of 7 to 18 days, depending on the stage of gestation at which they are given. The time interval is much more variable.

EFFECTS OF INDUCTION ON THE CALF

Calf mortality can be high following induced calving. Losses as high as 35% have been reported. This loss is largely a function of prematurity and is dependent on the time of injection.

Except when calving is induced close to term, calves are frequently hypogammaglobulinemic. When calving is induced more than a few days early, the colostrum available to the calves may have a reduced content of immunoglobulins. The composition of the colostrum may be altered further by the precalving milking, which is often necessary to avoid udder damage.

Long-acting glucocorticoids administered to cows near the end of gestation result in an impaired ability to transfer immunoglobulin G1 (IgG1) from cow serum to cow colostrum. Such impairment is potentially significant to the passive immunity acquired by the calf because IgG1 is the predominant immunoglobulin in both the colostrum and the milk of ruminants. By suckling IgG1-deficient colostrum, the calf has decreased transfer to passive immunity and hence an increased chance of disease.

Calves born to cows treated with long-acting corticosteroids also have an impaired ability to absorb immunoglobulins. This impairment occurs because the steroid is available to act on the fetus for a time sufficient to promote premature "closure" of the immunoglobulin absorption processes of the gut.

Effects of Induction on the Cow

Induction of calving markedly increases the incidence of retained fetal membranes by as much as 40%. The high prevalence of retained fetal membranes is largely a function of prematurity.

Whether subsequent reproductive efficiency is impaired by retained fetal membranes is debatable. Some degree of metritis, however, is present in all cows with retained fetal membranes subsequent to induction. Metritis, in turn, can lead to reduced fertility, depending on the success or otherwise of immediate therapy.

26.3 TYPES OF STEROIDS

Synthetic corticosteroids, such as dexamethasone and betamethasone, are sometimes described as long-acting glucocorticoids (long-acting in comparison to naturally occurring steroids, such as cortisol). These synthetic steroids, however, may be prepared as short-acting or long-acting formulations.

Short-acting formulations are injected as solutions or as dilute aqueous suspensions of fine particles that dissolve relatively rapidly in body fluids. Such short-acting formulations are rapidly absorbed, thus producing peak blood concentrations within a few hours of injection and being eliminated from the body within 3 days. They can be used to mimic the rapid, sharp increase in fetal cortisol that normally occurs in the last day or so before natural parturition.

So-called long-acting, or depot, formulations of corticosteroids may also be used to induce calving. Such formulations may be prepared by various methods that result in a preparation that is absorbed only slowly following injection. Usually a slowly-released ester in a sparingly soluble base is used. Depot corticosteroids take 2 to 4 days to achieve relatively low peak blood concentrations, which may, however, take 2 to 3 weeks to decline to undetectable levels. Such long-acting formulations can be used to mimic the gradual increase in fetal cortisol that normally occurs in the last 3 weeks or so of gestation.

DEXAMETHASONE SODIUM PHOSPHATE SOLUTION

Dexamethasone, as a rapidly absorbed short-acting aqueous solution of the sodium phosphate ester, has been widely used to induce calving. Administered by intramuscular or subcutaneous injection during the last 2 or 3 weeks of gestation, doses in the order of 20 to 30 mg have produced average response times of between 36 and 72 hours. The shorter response times occur in cows closer to term at the time of treatment or when higher doses are used.

Dexamethasone is a reliable agent for induction of parturition, with 20 mg given as a single intramuscular injection. The mechanism by which dexamethasone works is well understood. The exogenous steroid mimics the fetal cortisol and acts on the placenta from the maternal side in the same fashion as does fetal cortisol.

Complications from dexamethasone induction are increased calf mortality when done too early and increased instance of retained fetal membrane.

Dexamethasone, in various formulations, is the most widely used glucocorticoid suitable for the induction of calving. Dexamethasone in polyethylene glycol was the corticosteroid formulation used in the first reported study of induced calving. When doses of 20 mg are administered by intramuscular injection to cows during the last 2 or 3 weeks of pregnancy, average response times of between 36 and 72 hours may be expected.

BETAMETHASONE ALCOHOL

Short-acting suspensions of betamethasone alcohol administered as a 20-mg dose during the last 2 to 3 weeks of pregnancy produce results similar to those seen following the use of dexamethasone in polyethylene glycol administered at a similar stage of pregnancy.

INTRAVENOUS INJECTION OF CORTICOSTEROIDS

The response time following the intravenous injection of corticosteroids is no shorter than that for aqueous solutions administered intramuscularly. The incidence of dystocia may be greater after intravenous administration, however.

DEXAMETHASONE TRIMETHYLACETATE

Of the long-acting corticosteroid formulations, dexamethasone trimethylacetate suspension has been the most widely used for the induction of calving. Following intramuscular injection into cattle, this ester, which has little aqueous solubility, takes 2 to 3 days to produce peak blood concentrations of dexamethasone.

The earlier in pregnancy a cow is treated, the longer the response time. The response to dexamethasone trimethylacetate is more variable than the response to short-acting steroids, but cows may be induced to calve considerably earlier in pregnancy, to take account of the lag phase for absorption.

TABLE 26-2
INDUCTION OF PARTURITION

Soluble Corticoids
Dexamethasone sodium phosphate
• 20 to 30 mg intramuscularly Day 260+
Betamethasone sodium phosphate
• 20 to 30 mg intramuscularly Day 260+

Long-Acting Corticoids
Dexamethasone trimethylacetate,
 20–25 mg Day 250+

Luteolytic Prostaglandins
Cloprostenol 500 μg intramuscularly
 Day 260+
Fenprostalene 1 mg subcutaneously
Dinoprost 25 mg intramuscularly

Note: When a combination of prostaglandin and cholesterol is used, calving time is more predictable.

Dexamethasone trimethylacetate is widely used as the first injection of a two-injection regimen to induce premature calving.

DEXAMETHASONE PHENYLPROPIONATE WITH DEXAMETHASONE SODIUM PHOSPHATE

Calving can be induced with a dual formulation consisting of dexamethasone as the long-acting phenylpropionate ester suspended in a solution of dexamethasone sodium phosphate.

Prior to the last month of pregnancy, this twin formulation produces results essentially similar to those expected following the administration of a long-acting dexamethasone formulation. Nearer to term, however, the short-acting dexamethasone sodium phosphate component of this formulation probably achieves the desired result. (Table 26–2)

26.4 PROSTAGLANDINS

The name prostaglandin $F_{2\alpha}$ is derived from the chemical properties of this substance: the "F" for its solubility in phosphate (spelled fosfat in Swedish), the "2" for the 2 double bonds in its side chains, and the "alpha" for its stereochemistry. Because of its relatively simple structure, prostaglandin has been commercially produced as potent synthetic analogs.

Control of the time of parturition in beef cows allows for closer supervision of calving during planned time periods when labor can be used more efficiently. The ideal agent for parturition induction must be effective without causing deleterious side effects, and parturition must occur within a predictable interval from injection to calving.

Agents used for parturition induction have included corticosteroids, prostaglandins, or a combination of both.

Prostaglandins are naturally occurring, unsaturated fatty acids with widely ranging biological activity. They are derived from linoleic acid and arachidonic acid, which are essential fatty acids. All prostaglandins have 20 carbon atoms, a cyclopentane ring, 2 aliphatic side chains, and a terminal carboxyl group of the hypothetical parent "prostanoic acid." A 15-hydroxyl function is necessary for biological activity.

Prostaglandins are stored within cells only to a limited extent, and normal requirements are met by de novo synthesis from arachidonic acid. This precursor normally is present within intracellular phospholipid stores.

Other important arachidonic metabolites include the thromboxanes, prostacyclins, and leukotrienes. These compounds, along with the prostaglandins, have various effects on the reproductive, circulatory, respiratory, and other systems of the body.

Probably, most, if not all, actions of prostaglandins in biological systems are mediated by changing levels of cyclic nucleotides (cyclic AMP [cAMP] [adenosine 3':5'-cyclic phosphate] and cyclic GMP [cGMP] [guanosine 3':5'-cyclic phosphate]). Prostaglandins may either promote or inhibit concentrations of endogenous cAMP, depending on the cell type concerned.

Rapid breakdown of prostaglandins takes place in several tissues, particularly lungs, liver, kidney, and placenta. The plasma half-life for most natural prostaglandins is about 90 seconds, except for PGA_1 and PGA_2, which are relatively resistant to deactivation and are thus able to function as circulating hormones.

The prostaglandins and related compounds play a complex part in the genesis of the inflammatory response, and most anti-inflammatory agents inhibit the prostaglandin-synthetase cyclo-oxygenase enzyme.

Actual or potential therapeutic applications of the prostaglandins include:

1. Induction of parturition or therapeutic abortion
2. Treatment of asthma (bronchodilation: PGE_1)
3. Treatment of gastric ulcers (inhibition of secretion: PGE_2, PGE_1)
4. Treatment of hypertension (PGA, PGC, PGE_2)
5. Treatment of thrombosis (improvement of platelet survival: PGE_1)
6. Treatment of male infertility (low concentrations of PGEs in humans associated with low sperm counts)

One of the problems of therapeutic use is the short biological half-lives of natural prostaglandins. Various analogs either have been introduced to overcome this problem (fluprostenol, fenprostalene and cloprostenol).

Fenprostalene (Bovilene) is an analog of $PG-F_{2\alpha}$ formulated for subcutaneous injection in a polyethylene glycol 400 vehicle that has a biological half-life that is longer than that of $PGF_{2\alpha}$ or of the prostaglandin analog cloprostenol. A difference in the chemical structure of fenprostalene appears to be responsible for the increased resistance to metabolism observed in this compound. This structural difference, combined with formulation in a more viscous vehicle and subcutaneous rather than intramuscular injection, apparently accounts for the increased half-life of fenprostalene.

These structural analogs (fluprostenol, cloprostenol and fenprostalene) do not undergo such rapid metabolism and accordingly have longer half lives than natural $PGF_{2\alpha}$.

THERAPEUTIC USES

The use of prostaglandins in cattle falls into two main categories—therapeutic use and breeding management. Therapeutic uses of prostaglandins include treatment of nondetected estrus (subestrus or anestrus), pyometra, mummified fetus, unwanted pregnancies, and luteal cysts.

Prostaglandins influence many biological systems because of their primary effect on smooth muscle activity, which causes contraction of the smooth muscles. Of most concern to the field of reproduction is $PGF_{2\alpha}$ and its primary actions, which are its ability to cause lysis of the corpus luteum and its oxytocic action, or ability to cause smooth muscle contractions.

$PGF_{2\alpha}$ and it analogs are luteolytic in many species. In the sow and bitch, however, $PGF_{2\alpha}$ is not totally successful in its ability to cause luteal regression. The luteolytic mechanism of prostaglandin action on the ovary is not unequivocally established. Theories for its mechanisms include contractile effect on the utero-ovarian vein, resulting in reduced blood flow through the ovary and increased steroid metabolites; decreased stores of cholesterol esters (progesterone precursors); decreased esterase activity; antagonism with luteinizing hormone or prolactin; or promotion of fragility in lysosomes (an initial sign of luteal regression in sheep). A corpus luteum receptor for $PGF_{2\alpha}$ has been identified in the bovine species. The prime moving factor is one of affecting intracellular levels of cystic nucleotides.

The side effects of administering exogenous prostaglandin $F_{2\alpha}$ analogs are mainly attributable to the ability to contract smooth muscles. The most common side effects (sweating and decreased rectal temperature) are most often seen in the mare. Other reactions have been increased heart rate, increased respiratory rate, abdominal discomfort, locomotor incoordination, and recumbency. Mild colicky signs are caused by the increased gastrointestinal motility resulting from the stimulation of the circular and longitudinal smooth muscles of the gastrointestinal tract. These effects, usually seen within 15 minutes after injection of the prostaglandins, disappear within 1 hour.

Prostaglandins can be absorbed through intact skin. Hence, some precautions should be taken by humans handling the drug. Because prostaglandins of the F series are potent bronchoconstrictors, caution must be observed when this drug is administered by asthmatic persons or persons with bronchial or other respiratory problems. In addition, because $PGF_{2\alpha}$ is an effective abortifacient in humans, pregnant women probably should not handle this drug. Federal law restricts the use of $PGF_{2\alpha}$, or the ordering thereof, to licensed veterinarians.

Prostaglandins have quite profound effects on the activity of smooth muscle, whether in blood vessels or bronchi. Of paramount importance is their effect on the smooth muscle of the reproductive tract. Seminal fluid is a rich source of prostaglandins. After coitus, sufficient quantities are absorbed from the vagina to have detectable effects on the motility of the reproductive tract. They may promote the transport of spermatozoa into the fallopian tubes or help to hold the ovum in position for fertilization. Uterine smooth muscle motility is also affected by the prostaglandins; the pregnant myometrial response invariably is stimulatory. In fact, prostaglandins may play a major role in onset of labor. In humans, prostaglandins of the E and F series exert a more powerful effect on the myometrium than do prostaglandins of the A and B series. Those of the F series stimulate the pregnant human uterus at threshold doses that are less than one tenth of the dose required to stimulate the nonpregnant myometrium.

Generally, most prostaglandins, including those of the E series, inhibit spontaneous movements of the isolated, nonpregnant myometrium, whereas those of the F series stimulate contractions. The hormonal status of the animal, however, alters the uterine response to prostaglandins; the gravid uterus responds differently from the nongravid uterus. In humans, PGE_2 stimulates the pregnant uterus and inhibits the nonpregnant uterus.

In human medicine, most clinical research has been concerned with the possible uses of prostaglandins in inducing labor and abortion. PGE_2 and $PGF_{2\alpha}$ infused in large doses have been used successfully to induce labor and abortion. They have also been administered locally as vaginal suppositories. Trials have shown that PGE_1, PGE_2, and $PGF_{2\alpha}$ given as intravenous infusions stimulate abortion in more than 90% of women with pregnancies between 9 and 28 weeks.

Diarrhea is a common side effect of $PGF_{2\alpha}$. Following intravenous administration, a local tissue reaction in the form of a phlebitis may be seen at the site of infusion, particularly with PGE_2.

Initiation of labor in sheep may result from the action of $PGF_{2\alpha}$. The site of synthesis is believed to be the maternal cotyledons, from which $PGF_{2\alpha}$ passes to the myometrium by an unknown route. An oxytocic-like action results.

A second major effect of prostaglandins in the reproductive system occurs on the corpus luteum. In many species, cells of the corpus luteum undergo lysis following injection of $PGF_{2\alpha}$. A sharp decrease in progesterone secretion by the corpus luteum has also been demonstrated in primates following infusion of $PGF_{2\alpha}$.

The functional corpus luteum acts as a time clock to control the length of the estrus cycle in domestic animals. The corpus luteum stimulates the uterus to produce a substance that in turn destroys the corpus. This lytic substance is believed to be formed under the influence of progesterone in the endometrium, rather than the myometrium. Growing evidence shows that in the ewe, at any rate, this substance is $PGF_{2\alpha}$. The luteolytic factor seems to have only a weak systemic effect. In fact, $PGF_{2\alpha}$ infused into the systemic circulation of sheep with transplanted ovaries does not induce luteal regression. The diluting effect of the blood, and also the rapid metabolism of $PGF_{2\alpha}$ in the lungs, is believed to be responsible. Prostaglandins are local hormones and display a very short biological half life.

Thus, although prostaglandins have wide and diverse actions in the body, they exhibit two major effects on the reproductive system—oxytocic-like effects and luteolytic effects, both of which are important in determining the role to be played by prostaglandins in veterinary medicine and therapeutics.

CLINICAL APPLICATIONS

Pyometra

Postpartum infection of the uterus may lead to a chronic pyometritis under the influence of a persistent corpus luteum. A single treatment with cloprostenol regresses the corpus luteum and estrus. Voiding of the uterine contents usually follows in 2 to 6 days. Insemination of the animal at this estrus is worthwhile. If estrus is not observed, the injection can be repeated in 11 days.

Luteal Cysts

Several reports in the literature have described the application of cloprostenol for luteal cysts. Of the animals treated with cloprostenol, most show estrus in 3 to 5 days. One can assume that an ovarian cyst has luteal tissue present if estrous behavior is absent.

Control of Estrus

The classic method of controlling (and if required synchronizing) the time of estrus is well documented. The principle is that if two injections of cloprostenol are given to randomly cycling animals at 11-day intervals, the second injection will fall in the midluteul (day 5 to 17) part of the cycle and synchronize estrus in the entire group. An average of 60% or more of the animals will be in heat following the first injection. Desirable animals can be inseminated at this heat, and only the remainder are re-injected for fixed-time insemination.

Fixed-time artificial insemination, when used without heat detection, should be used at both 3 and 4 days following the second injection to cover the normal scatter in ovulation times.

Prostaglandin Analogs

$PGF_{2\alpha}$ and its analogs cloprostenol and fenprostalene may be used to induce calving when administered in the last 2 weeks of gestation. Most cows calve within 48 hours after administration of either 25 to 30 mg of $PGF_{2\alpha}$ or 500 μg of cloprostenol. At this stage of pregnancy, however, the prostaglandins have little advantage over short-acting corticosteroids for induction. Combined, they provide more accurate timing of calving. Results with prostaglandin appear similar to those of corticosteroid-induced parturition, including the relatively high rate of retained fetal membrane (50%) in cows that are induced.

Prostaglandins alone, or in combination with long-acting corticosteroids, are effective abortifacients. Alone they are effective from about 30 days to 150 days of pregnancy. During the first trimester, a 40-mg dose of $PGF_{2\alpha}$ is reported to be 100% effective, and a 20-mg dose is 80% effective. In comparison, 20 mg of estradiol cypionate (ECP) is reported to be effective in 70% of cases.

Because corticosteroid treatment does not induce parturition if the calf is dead, the prostaglandins have the advantage because they can be used in cases of fetal mummification and maceration. Prostaglandins are more effective than estrogens in the treatment of fetal mummification.

When calving is to be induced in cows within the last 2 or 3 weeks of gestation, single injections of the rapidly absorbed short-acting corticosteroid formulations or prostaglandin analogs produce reliable and predictable results. In most cases, calving occurs within 3 days of corticosteroid treatment or within 2 days of prostaglandin treatment. Many practitioners believe that prostaglandins are more reliable than short-acting steroids.

The rapidly absorbed corticosteroids are less effective, earlier in pregnency, the slowly absorbed long-acting formulations are more reliable. The response time to such long-acting formulations, however, tends to be variable and unpredictable.

In an attempt to improve the precision of the technique, two-injection treatment regimens have been developed. An initial priming dose of a slowly absorbed steroid, followed some days later by an injection of a rapidly absorbed steroid formulation or prostaglandin, produces a reliable and predictable response.

The blood corticosteroid profile produced in the cow by the two-injection schedules may more closely mimic that of the fetal cortisol that initiates natural calving.

CLINICAL INDICATIONS

Misalliance

A single injection of 500 μg cloprostenol causes regression of the corpus luteum, which is the sole endocrinologic supporter of pregnancy from approximately day 6 to day 150.

The interval from treatment to response is usually 2 to 10 days, depending on the stage of gestation. When gestation is too far advanced, the fetus is carried to full term without incident.

Mummified Fetus

This condition is invariably sustained by a corpus luteum. Following cloprostenol treatment, the mummy is expelled, but may have to be removed from the vagina. Subsequent examination therefore is recommended during the week following injection.

A single dose of prostaglandin usually induces abortion within 5 days in cows that are not more than 5 months' pregnant. After 5 months of gestation, $PGF_{2\alpha}$ has been used to induce parturition in cattle. Results have been similar to those of induction schemes using short-acting corticosteroids.

OTHER HORMONES FOR ESTRUS CONTROL

Norgestomet-Containing Implants (A Synthetic Progestogen)

Norgestomet treatment consists of two components: an injection of estradiol valerate with norgestomet and an implantation containing only norgestomet. These have long been used for the synchronization of estrus in cattle. The removable ear implants contain 3 mg of active ingredient (norgestomet). A small plastic implant is inserted into the top of the ear between the cartilage and the skin. This implant contains a highly active progesterone compound called norgestomet, which is slowly released into the blood stream over the next 9 to 10 days. At the same time that the implant is inserted, an intramuscular injection of norgestomet and estradiol valerate is given.

The implants are removed 9 to 10 days after insertion, and the heifers either are inseminated (whether they are showing heat or not) or are mated 48 hours later.

Norgestomet is a potent synthetic progestin with a potency factor of 100 to 200 times that of progesterone. Norgestomet inhibits the secretion of FSH and LH by the pituitary.

The norgestomet in the injection ensures an immediate inhibitory effect of the pituitary, whereas the estradiol valerate causes regression of the corpus luteum in animals that have recently ovulated.

The use of the implant with PMSG (equine chorionic gonadotropin) can be used for heat induction in cows with true anestrus. Norgestomet can be combined with prostaglandin $F_{2\alpha}$ for heat synchronization.

Norgestomet implanted in both ears has also been used to synchronize parturition in cattle. Inserting on day 262 of pregnancy and removing on day 270 leads to expulsion of the calf within 36 hours. Removal of the implant mimics the withdrawal of progesterone, as is seen with the use of prostaglandin $F_{2\alpha}$, although this is not a major use.

PROGESTERONE RELEASING INTRAVAGINAL DEVICE (P.R.I.D.)

This device acts as an artificial corpus luteum inhibiting gonadotropin output in cattle and delaying onset of estrus. After 12 days in the vagina, the device is removed, progesterone levels decline and cattle ovulate within 2 to 4 days.

The progesterone releasing intravaginal device consists of a silastic elastomer which is left in situ in the cow's vagina for 12 days. The device contains the natural hormone, progesterone (1.55 g) which is uniformly distributed throughout the elastomer. The hormone is released at a predetermined rate and absorbed through the vaginal wall, the entire device acting as an artificial corpus luteum. Following insertion, 10 mg of estradiol benzoate is released rapidly from a gelatin capsule attached to the elastomer. Upon conversion in the body to estradiol 17 beta, this steroid assists in the premature regression or prevention of formation of the corpus luteum. The device is for synchronization of estrus, acts via the pituitary, and does not require the presence of a functional corpus luteum.

26.5 TOCOLYTIC DRUGS AND POSTPONEMENT OF PARTURITION

PHARMACOLOGIC BASIS OF TOCOLYSIS

At the time of a normal delivery, the uterus is estrogen dominated. The effect of a beta-adrenergic agent on a uterus that is contracting under the influence of estrogen and oxytocin is therefore important. Beta-adrenergic agents, given beforehand, antagonize oxytocin-induced spasm of the isolated uterine horn of the rat in estrus.

According to results obtained in human medicine, beta$_2$-adrenergic agents bring about dose-dependent partial or total inhibition of uterine contractions in women, even in labor or abortion induced by PGF$_2$. The tocolytic effect extends both to the basal tone and to the intensity and frequency of contractions of the myometrium.

Beta-adrenergic blocking agents are substances that prevent the effect of beta-sympathomimetics on beta-adrenergic receptors. The mechanism of action is based on competitive displacement.

Beta-adrenergic Agents

Delay of the onset of parturition has become possible by temporarily abolishing uterine contractions. This delay is achieved by using beta-adrenergic agents, which stimulate the beta$_2$-adrenergic receptors to uterine muscle cells. One such drug, clenbuterol, and other beta-agonists has been used successfully in cows, sows, and ewes.

Tocolytic drugs inhibit uterine contractions and postpone labor. The smooth muscle of the uterus contains beta$_2$-adrenergic receptors, which, when stimulated, cause relaxation of the myometrium and abolition of uterine contractions. Clenbuterol (Planipart) is a highly selective and long-acting stimulator of beta$_2$-adrenergic receptors.

When cattle are treated with 0.3 mg (10 ml) of clenbuterol by intravenous or intramuscular injection during the first stage of labor, tocolysis occurs within 15 minutes and lasts for approximately 6 to 8 hours. When treatment is given during second-stage labor, calving is postponed for a shorter period.

Once the tocolytic effect of clenbuterol wears off, normal labor resumes. No adverse effects are seen, and deliveries are shortened and easier than usual, especially in heifers. This ease in delivery occurs because dilation of the cervix and softening of the birth canal continue during the period of tocolysis. Viability of calves is unimpaired and subsequent fertility is normal.

The effect of clenbuterol and another tocolytic drug, isoxsuprine, may be helpful in the correction of dystocias resulting from abnormal presentations, especially breech presentations. Embryotomies are often easier after a tocolytic drug has been administered, as are caesarean operations and repositioning of a prolapsed uterus. Clenbuterol may be used to postpone a dystocia while the cow is moved or assistance is sought.

A beneficial effect of clenbuterol in cases of dystocia is an improvement in the supply of blood to the placenta and fetus during the period of myometrial relaxation, mediated by beta$_2$ vasodilation of blood vessels.

The tocolytic effect of clenbuterol frequently can be reversed by the administration of oxytocin. Clenbuterol should not be used with general anesthesia because of potential hypotensive effects. Prostaglandin F$_{2\alpha}$ and oxytocin, antagonize its effects.

26.6 THERAPY OF BOVINE METRITIS

Chronic endometritis, characterized by slight to moderate enlargement of the uterus, often results from postpartum infections. Affected animals usually cycle, but the cycle is often irregular. Increasing the number of estrous periods within a short time to help recovery is a viable alternative to antibiotic therapy.

Bovine metritis varies in severity from acute postparturient septic metritis to barely detectable clinical endometritis. Treatment may include the use of antibiotics, hormones, or intrauterine infusions (Table 26–3). Most treatments are based either on stimulation of the uterus or on overcoming suspected uterine infection. Antibiotics usually have been the first line of therapy, but automatic reliance on antimicrobials alone may be questionable. The use of non-antibiotic alternatives is often highly successful. The ability of the uterus to withstand contamination and overcome infection varies with the hormonal environment during the estrous cycle. Uterine hyperemia, increased flow of mucus, and increased permeability and motility are actions of estrogens that aid uterine defense mechanisms. The use of prostaglandins in

---

**TABLE 26–3
ENDOMETRITIS TREATMENT**

Nonantibiotics

Estrogen
Oxytocin
Prostaglandin
Ergonovine
GNRH

Antibiotics

Penicillin
Ampicillin
Oxytetracycline
Streptomycin
Gentamicin
Sulfonamides
Neomycin
Polymyxin

---

cycling animals with nonspecific endometritis depends on the resistance of the uterus to the introduction of infection during the estrogenic stage of the cycle compared to the relative ease with which infection could establish itself during the luteal phase.

Nonantibiotic Drugs

For early postpartum problems, nonantibiotic drugs of interest are those capable of stimulating uterine contractility, e.g., oxytocin, estrogen, prostaglandin, and ergonovine, or of stimulating uterine defense mechanisms, e.g., estrogens and gonadotropin-releasing hormone (GnRH). Uterine atony caused by the blockade of the release oxytocin may be of greater significance as a cause of retained placenta than is generally thought. (Blockage of oxytocin release can be brought about by pain and stress via natural endorphins.)

Evidence suggests that attempts to increase the rate of uterine involution and to stimulate the return of estrous cycles are likely to accelerate the clearance of infections causing endometritis. The available drugs that could achieve this result are GnRH, prostaglandins, and estrogens.

Spontaneous recovery from uterine infections is associated with resumption of normal cyclicity. Estrogens increase the tonicity of the uterus and increase local resistance to infection by increasing local vascularization and motility. After calving, when estrogen levels have dropped, exogenous estrogen can assist involution and offer protection from uterine infection. Intramuscular estradiol benzoate, 3 to 10 mg, given twice at 3-day intervals, can often be as effective as antibiotic medication. In severe cases, 10–20 I.U. oxytocin, given within 4 to 5 hours of estrogen, may help to cause expulsion of uterine exudate.

When given immediately after calving, oxytocin itself can exert a preventative effect. Intramuscular oxytocin (10 I.U. repeated) can prevent development of retained placenta after difficult calvings and reduce the incidence of postpartum infections. The effects of oxytocin are heightened in a uterus sensitized by estrogen, thus perhaps explaining its efficacy immediately after calving, when estrogen levels are still elevated. Clinical postpartum metritis itself can respond to oxytocin therapy insofar as oxytocin has uterotonic effects. Treatment may be required over a period of 2 to 3 days and, when necessary, augmented by estradiol administration.

Postpartum infection in the cow often results in chronic endometritis characterized by a slightly to moderately enlarged uterus. Analogs of PGF_2 are indicated in special cases of chronic endometritis and pyometra, especially when associated with a persistent corpus luteum. Use of prostaglandin is based on the luteolytic effect, which brings the cow into estrus within 2 to 4 days of injection. Early therapy can enhance uterine involution because delayed involution may be associated with dysfunction of the postpartum prostaglandin release system. Apart from the luteolytic effects, prostaglandins also have contractile effects on the bovine myometrium. Intrauterine infusions with disinfectants are fairly common nonantibiotic alternatives to the treatment of postpartum infections. Irritating solutions, such as Lugol's iodine solution, can induce estrus caused by prostaglandin release in a pattern similar to that of a spontaneous estrus.

When postpartum infections occur in cycling animals, an artificial increase in estrous periods within a contracted space of time is valuable because of the beneficial effect of endogenous estrogen. Intrauterine infusion of irritating solutions of iodine during the early part of the estrous cycle can induce estrus in 4 to 7 days. Midcycle infusion does not tend to alter the cycle, whereas late-cycle infusions prolong the cycle by 4 to 5 days.

Infectious Origin

The prevalence of postpartum uterine infection differs with the management of the individual herd. Excessive contamination of the environment with pathogenic microorganisms can result in infection of the reproductive tracts of cows during the postpartum period. Isolation of cows with purulent discharges is necessary to prevent spread of infections because ordinary hygienic practices may not be sufficient.

Endometritis and metritis may progress to pyometra when gram-negative anaerobic bacteria act synergistically with *Corynebacterium pyogenes* in the progesterone-dominated uterus.

C. pyogenes is the bacterium commonly associated with endometritis in the cow. Most of the other aerobic isolates are probably commensals.

C. pyogenes is still considered the most significant pathogen found in the uterus. But several other fastidious anaerobic bacteria have been found, including *Bacteroides* and *Fusobacterium*.

Investigations into the role of anaerobic bacteria in some human infections have shown that such bacteria can depress phagocytosis. The effect is greatest with strains of *Bacteroides melaninogenicus* and *B. fragilis*, both of which have been isolated from the bovine uterus affected with endometritis. A possible synergistic effect of *Fusobacterium necrophorum* and *Corynebacterium pyogenes* occurs in bovine endometritis.

If both organisms are present together, the clinical signs and the associated infertility may be more severe than when only one of these organisms is isolated. *Corynebacteria* flourish because of the reduction in phagocytosis and, they may also produce a growth factor necessary for the proliferation of the anaerobes.

Clostridial species also have been implicated in endometritis. Toxic conditions can occur from mixed or pure gram-negative infection. Regardless of the causative organism, if the accumulation of fluid and necrotic debris is large, antibiotic therapy is rendered much more effective when the fluid and its toxic by-products are irrigated from the uterus.

As the postpartum period progresses in cows with metritis, however, the bacterial population of the uterus often changes from a mixed population to a population composed predominantly of *Corynebacterium pyogenes*, *Fusobacterium necrophorum*, and *Bacteroides*. All three of these bacteria are generally susceptible to penicillin. Penicillin is not a good choice for local intrauterine therapy in the early postpartum uterus because the population of bacteria is mixed and may produce beta lactamase. Systemic penicillin therapy, however, is a reasonable choice at this time because the bacteria likely to invade the endometrium from the uterine lumen are usually susceptible to penicillin.

26.7 ANTIBIOTIC THERAPY

In moderate to severe uterine infections, the infection is seldom localized and restricted to only the superficial layers of the endometrium. Accordingly, parenteral treatment must be considered. A single intrauterine treatment is justified in only mild cases of endometritis. Several antimicrobial agents are absorbed from the uterus—sulfonamides, tetracyclines, penicillin, ampicillin, streptomycin, and gentamicin. The absorption in the immediate postpartum period is considerably less than that following complete uterine involution. Endometritis itself further diminishes absorption because of exudates and membranes. Poor local absorption results in high concentration within the uterine cavity and on the endometrium, but adequate concentrations may not be attained in the subendometrial tissues, vagina, cervix, ovaries, or oviducts. The vehicle of the antibiotic also affects the degree of absorption; a water vehicle achieves deeper penetration.

INTRAUTERINE ADMINISTRATION

Many antibacterial drugs have been used and recommended for intrauterine treatment. Products that cause a severe inflammatory reaction should be avoided. If the uterus is filled with a large amount of exudate, this fluid should be siphoned off gently before the local administration of antibacterial drugs ensues.

The limitations of three antimicrobial groups should be mentioned at the outset. Penicillins are highly susceptible to cleavage by beta lactamase producers. Aminoglycosides are ineffective in an anaerobic environment. Sulfonamides lose activity in the presence of pus. They also possess residue hazards.

Drugs administered into the uterus may be absorbed into the circulation and may even pass into the milk in detectable amounts. Absorption of some drugs from the uterus may be enhanced by inflammation. Acidic drugs apparently are better absorbed than are basic drugs because the pH of the infected uterus tends to be acidic. Hence, more drug is present in the nonionized lipid soluble form.

The absorption of drugs from the uterus is influenced by the stage of involution. In the immediate postpartum period, the absorption of some drugs, such as penicillin, dihydrostreptomycin, and oxytetracycline, is relatively poor compared to absorption from the involuted uterus. The absorption of sulfamethazine and chloramphenicol is quicker and is less affected by involution.

Estrogens are often used as an adjunct to antibiotic treatment of uterine infections. The intramuscular or intrauterine administration of 10 mg estradiol benzoate significantly increases the absorption of penicillin from the uterus.

For antimicrobial treatment to be effective, concentration of drug must be achieved and maintained at the site of infection for an adequate period. Two main routes of administration are used to treat the uterus: local (intrauterine) and systemic (intramuscular, intravenous). Several antimicrobial agents are absorbed from the uterus (sulfonamides, tetracyclines, streptomycin, penicillin, ampicillin, gentamicin, and chloramphenicol). The presence of uterine pathologic changes (endometritis) can result in further decrease of absorption. Poor absorption results in a high concentration of the drug in the uterine cavity and on the endometrium. But adequate concentrations frequently are not achieved in suben-

dometrial tissues, vagina, cervix, or ovaries and oviducts. Absorption of antibiotics is enhanced by estrogen. The molecular structure and size of the antibiotic may influence its absorption from the uterus.

If intrauterine therapy is chosen, several factors should be considered before selecting the infusion product. Because the uterus of the cow becomes contaminated during calving, the microbiologic environment of the uterus should play an important role in determining intrauterine therapy. For example, antimicrobials that are ineffective in an anaerobic environment (e.g., aminoglycosides) should not be used in postpartum intrauterine therapy.

Several factors determine the efficacy of antimicrobial therapy of uterine infection. These include the following:

1. The antibiotic sensitivity of the organisms
2. The ability to attain therapeutic concentrations of the active antimicrobial agent in the uterine wall and lumen
3. The immune response of the host

Intrauterine administration during the early postpartum period (before day 30) is not recommended because mixed bacterial infections may render penicillin ineffective as a result of beta lactamase production by bacteria. Parenteral administration, however, provides adequate serum levels to treat puerperal metritis (22,000 to 45,000 I.U./kg procaine penicillin intramuscularly twice daily for 3 to 5 days).

Mixed bacterial infections in metritis occur more commonly than do infections involving single pathogens. The problem of beta lactamase-induced resistance does not occur with oxytetracycline therapy in mixed bacterial infections; thus, oxytetracycline is more effective than penicillin in treating these infections. Sulfonamides are relatively ineffective on account of diminished activity in the presence of pus and the formation of inactive metabolites locally.

Intrauterine infusion of natural penicillin (10 million I.U. of sodium penicillin in a midcycle uterus) gives satisfactory concentration in the lumen and in the endometrium for as many as 24 hours.

Gentamicin does not affect anaerobic bacteria and has less bactericidal activity in an acidic or anaerobic environment.

The intrauterine route, although providing high initial concentrations in the uterine lumen, has several disadvantages:

1. Repeated infusions for the continuation of treatment may not be convenient.
2. Infusion may damage the endometrium through trauma or cytotoxicity.
3. The infusate may be diluted by, bound to, or expelled with the exudates.
4. Transfer of infection or exudates up the uterine tubes may be encouraged.
5. Further infection may be introduced to the uterus.
6. The choice of dosage form may affect the efficacy of treatment.

In endometritis with copious production of pus, however, uterine infusion of solutions may be useful for lavage of the uterine and contents.

As already stated, systemic administration of antibiotics results in tissue concentrations in the genital tract that are comparable to blood levels. Such administration usually results in antibiotic concentrations in uterine tissue and lumen that are equal to blood plasma concentrations. The concentrations are generally the same in the normal and the infected uterus. The systemic administration gives a better distribution in the tubular genital tract and to the ovaries. Furthermore, fetal membranes and abnormal exudate cannot mechanically influence the distribution. Also, systemic administration eliminates the risk of damage to the endometrium. Repeated treatment can be carried out relatively simply and without introduction of new infections.

Several factors should be considered if antibiotic therapy is instituted. An anaerobic environment precludes the effective use of aminoglycosides because their antibacterial activity is markedly reduced under anaerobic conditions. The effectiveness of sulfonamides, nitrofurans, and aminoglycosides is reduced markedly by the presence of blood, pus, and tissue debris. In any case, some of these drugs cannot be used in food animals in the United States. Intrauterine infusions of penicillin might be contraindicated because penicillin might change the bacterial population to predominantly gram-negative species. Systemic penicillin is acceptable, however, because most of the bacteria actually involved in in-

vading the endometrium are gram positive and subsequently susceptible to penicillin.

Systemic administration of penicillins results in genital tract tissue and lumen concentrations similar to blood plasma concentrations in the cow and mare. A dose of 22,000 to 45,000 I.U./kg of sodium penicillin G is thus sufficient to combat most pathogens that are sensitive to penicillin.

Parenteral treatment can attain high uterine levels of antibiotic and better overall penetration and distribution, especially if given by the intravenous route. Although intravenous administration of ampicillin or penicillin G in particular results in high local levels, duration is short and treatment must be repeated after 6 to 8 hours. Membranes, placental debris, and exudates cannot adversely affect the distribution of a parenterally administered drug. The parenteral drug also can be given more frequently than the intravenous drug without the attendant risks of local damage or introduction of more infection locally. For moderate to severe uterine infections, systemic treatment must always be considered. Oxytetracycline, locally as well as twice a day parenterally, usually provides adequate levels in the uterus, as does parenteral penicillin/streptomycin. If penicillins are considered for intrauterine therapy, the semisynthetic type (ampicillin) is preferred because it is not absorbed as rapidly as is penicillin G. Gentamicin has a good effect on uterine pathogens also and provides effective antibiotic cover parenterally (twice a day/three times a day) or locally. Most uterine pathogens are sensitive to sulfonamides, which are absorbed better by the postpartum uterus than are other antibacterials. Parenteral treatment with sulfonamide-trimethoprim is a useful approach because of the good distribution and sensitivity of *Escherichia coli* to the combination.

The penicillins are nonirritant when infused into the uterus. Following intrauterine administration, high concentrations in the uterine lumen and endometrium may be attained.

Intramuscular injection of penicillin equal to or greater than 22,000 I.U./kg results in tissue concentrations in the endometrium that reach 50% of the serum levels. Intravenous injection shows the same trend, although tissue concentrations vary more and the duration of measurable amounts is not longer than 8 hours. Intravenous administration of ampicillin, 7 mg/kg or more, affords tissue concentrations that are equal to or greater than blood serum levels for the first 4 hours. Both ampicillin and penicillin, if given in appropriate doses, result in endometrium tissue concentrations that are high compared to blood serum levels. The doses recommended are 22,000 to 45,000 I.U./kg sodium penicillin G intramuscularly or 10 to 15 mg/kg ampicillin intravenously. Tetracyclines are another useful choice for intrauterine therapy because the bacteria involved usually are susceptible and because the activity of tetracyclines is reduced only slightly within the lumen.

Oxytetracycline is completely ionized at physiologic pH, has a low lipid solubility, and has a relatively large volume of distribution. For the treatment of uterine infections, the intravenous administration of oxytetracycline may be necessary because of the bioavailability variations of most intramuscular formulations.

After intrauterine administration of 5.5 mg/kg oxytetracycline, high levels in the endometrium can be maintained for 24 hours. Absorption of oxytetracycline from the uterus is poor, however, and low concentrations may be attained only in the uterine wall, ovaries, and blood plasma.

Tylosin and erythromycin are both highly lipid-soluble basic antibiotics with fairly low MICs. Intravenous doses of 10 mg/kg (erythromycin) and 20 mg/kg (tylosin) every 12 hours may maintain useful levels in the tissues. Fluoroquinolones are recent introductions which display a large volume of distribution, useful spectra, and unique mechanism of action. These can be usefully considered for parenteral treatment of metritis.

26.8 NONANTIBIOTIC ALTERNATIVES

Nonantibiotic drugs of interest in the early postpartum period are those that can stimulate uterine contractility (e.g., oxytocin, prostaglandin, ergonovine, estrogens) and/or the uterine defense mechanisms (e.g., estrogens, GnRH).

OXYTOCIN

Results of oxytocin for prevention of retained placenta and postpartum infections are mixed. Oxytocin (20 I.U.) intramuscularly immediately after calving, and preferably repeated 2 to 4 hours later, reduces retained placenta in cows, especially after difficult calvings. Uterine atony caused by blockage of oxytocin release, therefore, may be of greater importance as a cause of retained placenta than previously was thought. The blockage of oxytocin release may be provoked by an increased synthesis of endorphins caused by stress and pain. The effect of oxytocin on an evident postpartum metritis is not well established, but some evidence shows that oxytocin is uterotonic in the postpartum cow. The effect is better on a uterus sensitized by estrogens, thus perhaps explaining the beneficial effects of oxytocin immediately after calving.

Route of Administration

Probably the best way to administer oxytocin is by intravenous drip infusion (60 to 100 I.U. over 6 to 10 hours). Because frequently this route is not feasible, the second best approach is the administration of relatively small doses (20 I.U. to cow), intramuscularly 3 to 4 times a day as necessary, 2 to 3 days. In mild-to-moderate cases of acute postpartum metritis, this approach could be the sole treatment, especially if estrogens have been used to sensitize the uterus. Use of high doses of oxytocin are not advised because of the risk of uterine spasm.

Because oxytocin is quickly inactivated in the body, veterinarians should administer the drug only by a slow intravenous drip infusion. This technique extends the therapeutic effectiveness and offers the advantage of easily controlling the dosage during treatment.

The intramuscular route should be reserved only for animals too difficult to work with. This route requires a higher frequency of administration of oxytocin, because part of the dosage is destroyed following parenteral injection in the body.

Dosage

Because of its powerful uterine stimulating actions, oxytocin must be used with care. Sometimes, practitioners, hoping for a better response, overdose with oxytocin. This approach can cause problems. Rather than using a single large dose, oxytocin should be given in small quantities continuously during a certain period of time. An overdose of oxytocin can cause a prolonged myometrial contraction (tetanus uteri) and damage the uterus.

ESTROGENS

The importance of resumption of normal cyclicity for the spontaneous recovery from uterine infections is well established. The actions of endogenous estrogens on the uterus are well documented and include:

1. An increase in blood flow
2. An increase in the excitability of the myometrium
3. An increase in the permeability of uterine blood vessels to leukocytes
4. An increase in the secretion of immunoglobulins

Beneficial effects of estrogen are associated with its uterotonic effect. Administration of small amounts of estrogen during the postpartum period, with its low endogenous estrogen production, would seem to help to protect the cow from uterine infections and enhance the uterine involution. Estrogens are frequently used as the only treatment for mild-to-moderate postpartum infections with or without retained placenta, but they have been equally effective in combination with antibiotics. The doses recommended are 3 to 10 mg of estradiol benzoate, estradiol valerate, or estradiol cypionate intramuscularly. The treatment can be repeated twice at 3-day intervals. Uterine atony with accumulation of exudate in the uterus may benefit from low doses (10 to 20 I.U.) of oxytocin within 4 to 6 hours of estrogen injection.

Estrogens alone can be as effective as antibiotics for a mild postpartum infection. Intramuscular injections; repeated twice at 3-day intervals, are given. When atony of the uterus is accompanied by accumulation of exudate, the estrogen injection can be followed by small doses of oxytocin 4 to 6 hours afterward.

Infusion

Under certain circumstances, intrauterine infusions can cause the same effects on the estrous cycle as do exogenously administered prostaglandins. Since the late 1960s, practitioners have known that irritating solutions infused during the early part of the estrous cycle (day 4 or 5 of the cycle), induce estrus within 4 to 7 days of the treatment. Necrotizing endometritis occurs as early as 24 hours after the intrauterine infusion of a solution containing 5 ml of a strong Lugol's iodine solution in 250 ml of saline. By the time of estrus (day 10, when infusion is given on day 5 and the day of previous estrus is day 1), the endometrium regenerates. This premature estrus is induced by endogenous release of PGF_2 during endometrial repair, which commences 3 to 4 days after infusion.

Intrauterine infusion with various disinfectants is a relatively common antibiotic alternative to treatment of postpartum infections. Although positive results occasionally have been reported, results are equivocal.

When a weak Lugol's iodine solution is infused during the first part of the estrous cycle (3 to 4 days after the previous estrus), estrus is usually induced within 4 to 7 days.

Although little data are available from controlled experiments, empiric results suggest that intrauterine infusion with iodine might be an alternative to prostaglandin use for treatment of endometritis, especially in cases of repeat breeding with no or only mild clinical signs of endometritis. Various concentrations and volumes of infused Lugol's iodine solution have been used, e.g., 5 ml strong Lugol's iodine solution in 250 ml saline (100 to 200 ml infused) and 4 ml strong Lugol's iodine solution in 100 ml saline (100 ml infused). The infusions are given 3 to 4 days after previous estrus.

Studies have shown that infusion of iodine is followed by release of prostaglandins in a pattern similar to that of spontaneous estrus. The cycle is unaffected by infusions during estrus or midcycle. Infusions in late cycle (day 16 onward), however, prolong the cycle by 4 or 5 days. Infusion of Lugol's iodine solution appears to be a viable alternative to prostaglandins, especially in cases of repeat breeding with mild overt clinical signs.

The regimen that has been used consists of an intrauterine infusion of 1 to 2% Lugol's iodine solution (1 to 2 ml of a strong Lugol's iodine solution per 100 ml of saline) on day 4 or 5 of the cycle (day 1 is the day of previous estrus). The volume of the infused solution is not critical, because volumes as low as 5 ml of Lugol's iodine solution have proved effective in inducing estrus.

The intrauterine infusion of various disinfectants to treat postpartum infection is quite common. Little controlled evidence shows that this treatment works, however. In fact, infusion could suppress uterine defense mechanism, and therefore, the procedure is not recommended, until clear scientific data validate such procedures.

PROSTAGLANDINS

Prostaglandins and their analogs, fenprostalene and cloprostenol, have been used for their luteolytic effects to evacuate the pathologic content of the uterus. Dinoprost is the name of a synthetic $PGF_{2\alpha}$ compound. Fenprostalene is an analog of prostaglandin $F_{2\alpha}$ formulated for subcutaneous injection. This has a biological half life that is longer than the natural prostaglandin $F_{2\alpha}$ (Dinoprost) or the other synthetic analog, clostprostenol. The structural variation of fenprostalene coupled with its formulation in a viscous vehicle ensures retardation of biological cleavage and thus a longer half life. Bovine pyometra is the pathologic postpartum condition for which prostaglandins are most often used. Studies have demonstrated that intramuscular doses of 12.5 to 25 mg $PGF_{2\alpha}$ or of 0.5 mg cloprostenol, its synthetic analog, are effective in emptying in the uterus. Uterine evacuation starts as early as 24 hours after injection, and cows frequently come in heat 3 to 4 days after treatment. Usually, one treatment is enough to establish normal cyclicity. Cows can be inseminated at the first or the second estrus following the induced estrus. Pregnancy re-

sults obtained so far seem to be good (more than 60% of animals pregnant).

Chronic endometritis in cycling animals without an apparent accumulation of fluid in the uterus is another condition for which prostaglandins have been successfully used. This condition, often a result of postpartum infections, is characterized by an enlarged uterus caused by a thickening of the uterine wall. Cows with chronic endometritis are usually cycling, although the cycle length may be irregular. Endogenous estrogens produced near the time of estrus enhance recovery. An increase in the number of estrous periods brought about within a short period of time by prostaglandin treatments therefore could be useful.

The effect of PGF_2 and its analogs (cloprostenol, fenprostalene, dinoprost) on chronic endometritis in the presence of a corpus luteum, especially pyometra, is well established. A positive effect even in the absence of a corpus luteum cannot be ruled out. Also in pyometra, pus can interfere with the normal release of prostaglandin from the uterus. Hence, exogenous prostaglandin is one of the best treatments for pyometra and endometritis. Some evidence shows that retained placenta and delayed involution in postpartum cows is related to low amounts of prostaglandin or to inadequate duration of the postpartum release of prostaglandin. Field results indicate that twice-daily treatments with 25 mg of $PGF_{2\alpha}$ or its analogs intramuscularly during the first 10 days after parturition may enhance uterine involution. Successful single treatment of the early postpartum cow with no functional corpus luteum has been reported. The effect might be produced by increased uterine contractions or factors involved in the uterine natural defense. Prostaglandins possess oxytocic-like activity on the myometrium.

Prostaglandins are used to induce estrus via their luteolytic effect. Estrus occurs within 2 to 3 days of administration. The number of treatments necessary depends on the severity of the endometritis. One or two treatments 10 to 14 days apart are usually adequate in mild to moderate cases.

Prostaglandins administered twice daily for several days decrease the average time for the completion of uterine involution, but such an approach is not practical under field conditions. A synergistic effect occurs between estradiol benzoate and prostaglandins. When heifers in diestrus are treated with 200 μg of estradiol twice daily for 3 days and dinaprost (7 mg) is given concurrently with the last dose of estradiol luteolysis occurs in several cases (the recommended therapeutic dose is 25 mg). The same dose of dinaprost given alone to similar heifers can produce luteolysis. Prostaglandins available for food animals are as follows:

PROSTAGLANDIN	TRADE NAME	USUAL DOSAGE
Fenprostalene	Bovilene	1 mg Subcutaneous
Cloprostenol	Estrumate	500 μg Intramuscular
Dinoprost tromethamine	Lutalyse	25 mg Intramuscular

GONADOTROPIN-RELEASING HORMONE (GnRH)

GnRH, because of its demonstrated capacity to stimulate release of LH from the pituitary, has been recognized as a major aid for improving reproductive efficiency in postparturient dairy cows. The primary areas of GnRH application (other than cystic ovary treatment) have been the initiation of early ovarian activity in the early postpartum period (10 to 20 days post partum) or the improvement of conception rates when given at insemination.

Physiologically, the pituitary hormones are in low concentrations in the peripheral blood following parturition. These hormones, FSH and LH, are not present in sufficient concentrations during the first 10 days post partum to stimulate ovulation.

From field, and experimental work to date, it is clear that attempts to increase FSH and LH concentrations in the blood indicate that the pituitary gland requires at least 8–10 days after calving before GnRH treatment can trigger an increase FSH and LH concentrations in the peripheral blood.

If GnRH is administered at 10–14 or more days post partum, (a single 100- to 250-μg intramuscular injection) stimulates the pituitary gland to release LH. This LH surge mimics the normal preovulatory LH increase and causes the mature follicle to ovulate.

In cows treated with GnRH 10 to 20 days after calving, increased progesterone levels are found 5 to 7 days after treatment, thus indicating that ovulation has occurred. Physiologically, GnRH is synthesized in hypothalamic neurons, is then transported to the anterior pituitary gland by the specialized portal system in the hypothalamic-hypophyseal portal system. Specific receptors on the gonadotropic cells of the anterior pituitary respond by increasing LH and FSH in blood within 30 minutes that lasts for 4 to 6 hours. The intensity of the LH and FSH release depends on the dose administered and the endogenous hormonal status of the animal being injected. In cows with follicular cysts, GnRH or one of its potent analogs results in their rapid luteinization, and most cows show estrus 17 to 24 days after GnRH injection.

For follicular cysts, delayed ovulation, follicle atresia or improvement in conception rates, small synthetic analogs usually decapeptides, are available to promote release of LH after 1 1/2 hours and FSH 2 hours following I.M. injection. This release induces maturation of ovarian follicles and ovulation after a 24 hour time lag.

GnRH administered in the early postpartum period has resulted in a decrease in the calving-to-conception interval. This treatment stimulates the return of ovarian activity and increases the secretion of endogenous estrogens. GnRH is no longer effective after the signs of chronic endometritis have been established 3 or more weeks after calving; prostaglandins and/or estrogens should then be employed.

After parenteral administration, the synthesis and release of the gonadotropins LH and FSH are induced to develop their effect on the reproductive glands. Other endocrine processes are not disturbed by the course of these physiologic functions.

GnRH is used to reduce the interval between calving and the first ovulation. It also increases the number of ovulations during the 3 months after calving. Trials in the field have shown that, when the hormone is given on the 10th and 14th days post partum, conception is improved with or without a retained placenta.

Early Postpartum Use

The basis for giving GnRH 10 to 20 days postpartum is based on the observation that bovine fertility during the normal breeding period is directly proportional to the number of estrous cycles before breeding. The administration of GnRH should therefore enhance the chances of early resumption of cyclic activity.

Studies and field experience have shown that cows with periparturient disorders (reproductive, metabolic, or others) are likely to benefit from GnRH given 10 to 20 days postpartum. This benefit is probably associated with the observation that peripartient metritis problems frequently delay onset of cycling by somehow affecting the hypothalamic-hypophyseal-gonadal axis.

The administration of GnRH reduces the interval from calving to first ovulation and increases the number of ovulations during the first 3 months after calving. It is established that the administration of GnRH intramuscularly on days 10 and 14 after parturition increases the conception rate in cows with retained placenta and for all postpartum cows. Natural GnRH or analogs therefore may become useful, clinical alternatives to antibiotics to improve the fertility in cows with retained placenta.

Because GnRH acts centrally through its effects on LH release, late-ovulating repeat-breeding cows may also benefit from GnRH treatment that hastens ovulation and improves conception rates. Secretion of LH also may improve potential development of the corpus luteum and increase progesterone secretion, which could result in improved embryo survival. Higher progesterone levels occur in GnRH-treated repeat breeders than in untreated repeat breeders. Sometimes GnRH can cause an increase in uterine infections through phase. The development of luteal tissue and progesterone production in the early post partum.

Other application for GnRH include the following:

1. Follicular cysts
2. Delayed ovulation
3. Follicle atresia

Nutrition-Related Influences

Selenium is one of the most important trace elements as regards reproductive efficiency in dairy cows. Research with vitamin E-selenium has demonstrated its role in normal uterine function. Selenium is a component of glutathione peroxidase, and a direct correlation exists between the level of this enzyme and selenium. Glutathione peroxidase has a central role in cellular oxidation-reduction reactions. The enzyme catalyzes reactions that aid in the destruction of hydrogen peroxide and fatty acid hydroperoxides. Glutathione peroxidase and vitamin E (alpha-tocopherol) are believed to be important in protecting mammalian cells against oxidant damage. Increased incidences of metritis and mastitis can be attributable to selenium deficiency.

Vitamin E is believed to act as a scavenger of peroxides; with selenium, it thus protects cells from peroxides and allows them to continue functioning normally. Various disease conditions are related to vitamin E-selenium deficiency. Its implications in retained placenta and its effects on the immune system are important to toxic metritis. Selenium deficiency in muscle tissue, as occurs in white muscle disease, is a well-recognized syndrome; its effect on smooth muscle contraction apparently is the same. This lack of smooth muscle contraction in the uterus that causes abnormal involution, combined with the possible compromise of the immune system, might be a predisposing factor in toxic metritis.

The incidence of retained placenta in cattle can be reduced with selenium treatment where known deficiency exists. Perhaps no other single factor can influence toxic metritis more than another trace element, calcium has an important role in muscle contraction and also has a relatively volatile nature in lactating dairy cows. Nutritional intake, internal mobilization, and excretory drain is dependent on calcium. The major reason for post partum uterine inertia during parturition is hypocalcemia. The role of prostaglandins in myometrial contraction involves calcium ion transport. Progesterone blocks this effect. Postparturient hypocalcemia has long been recognized as an important disease in dairy cattle. Low calcium levels impair smooth muscle contraction and predispose the uterus to depressed involution, thereby preventing expulsion of uterine contents and subjecting the uterus to infection and toxic metritis. Copper is also well established as a key trace element for optimal performance of the body's defense mechanisms.

26.9 BOVINE PYOMETRA

Bovine pyometra is an infectious uterine disorder, usually a sequel to peripartum disturbances, such as dystocia, retained fetal membranes, and acute endometritis. Pyometra may also be associated with early embryonic death and may also follow as a sequel to artificial insemination. The condition is characterized by anestrus and a swollen, soft, doughy uterus containing varying amounts of pus. The ability of the uterus to form the uterine luteolysin $PGF_{2\alpha}$ is impaired, and thus diestrus is prolonged by the presence of a persistent corpus luteum. The most common infectious agent associated with pyometra is *Corynebacterium pyogenes* (C. pyogenes).

Pyometra is a pseudopregnancy type of condition. Mucopurulent exudate accumulates in the uterus, thereby causing persistence of the corpus luteum and the absence of estrus. Both cloprostenol and $PGF_{2\alpha}$ have been reported effective in inducing luteolysis and a positive response in greater than 90% of cows with pyometra. Luteolysis is relatively complete 24 hours after treatment, when uterine evacuation begins. The mummified fetus is expelled from the uterus about 96 to 120 hours after treatment.

True pyometra seldom shows spontaneous resolution. True pyometra in cattle is characterized by accumulation of purulent material, the persistence of a corpus luteum, and a physical state of anestrus. The retained corpus luteum is probably secondary to the pathologic change in endometrial tissue. Sometimes, abnormal hormonal influences, such as with corticosteroid-induced parturition, can cause retention of the placenta by not allowing softening of the connective tissue, and leading to a thick, leathery placenta. This is retained and then provides a suitable medium for growth of purulent organism.

Treatment

Drainage of accumulated pus followed by infusion of the uterus with antibacterial drugs is relatively ineffective. Only 20 to 30% of animals make a clinical recovery with such treatment, and a smaller percentage breed successfully.

Endometritis or metritis with fluid and pus accumulation in the uterus (e.g., pyometra) requires evacuation of the pathologic content so that the cow can cycle again regularly. A luteolytic agent, such as $PGF_{2\alpha}$, or analog is ideal, provided that the cow has a functional corpus luteum.

Abnormal contents within the uterus prevent the release of endogenous prostaglandins from the endometrium, thereby resulting in a persistent corpus luteum. A luteolytic dose of PGF is an effective treatment for pyometra. If an antibacterial drug is to be infused into the uterine lumen after treatment with PGF, penicillin is the drug of choice. Other antibacterials, such as tetracyclines or ampicillin, are likely to be more useful.

Parenteral estrogens produce good results also. For example, 5 to 15 mg estradiol benzoate may produce luteolysis with resultant estrus and uterine evacuation. This effect is not always consistent. The uterine contraction produced by estrogens may also permit the spread of infection to the oviducts, ovaries, and ovarian bursa, with resulting sterility. The use of estrogens, however, could also cause cystic ovaries. Repeated injections of estrogens give the best results but increase the risk of side effects. The infusion of antibiotics or Lugol's iodine solution about 1 week after estrogen treatment is believed to speed recovery. Clinical recovery can be expected in about 50% of animals, with about half of these regaining fertility. Because intrauterine use of disinfectants may suppress the uterine defense mechanisms, e.g., phagocytosis, the use of intrauterine infusions in the postpartum cow cannot be routinely recommended.

$PGF_{2\alpha}$ (dinoprost), cloprostenol, and fenprostalene are superior to estrogens for treating pyometra. $PGF_{2\alpha}$ and its analogs is the best treatment for pyometra and endometritis in cows with corpora lutea. Uterine pus interferes with the natural release of prostaglandin from the endometrium. After prostaglandin injection, which results in luteolysis and follicular development, the level of progesterone decreases and the level of estrogen increases.

Systemic administration of 25 mg $PGF_{2\alpha}$ (Dinoprost) intramuscularly fenprostalene 1 mg, or 500 μg of cloprostenol intramuscularly results in regression of the corpus luteum and evacuation of the uterus. Mucopurulent vaginal discharge is obvious by the third day after injection, and uterine evacuation is completed by 5 to 7 days. Evacuation of the uterus is associated with signs of estrus. The success of the treatment is indicated by the return of the uterus to normal condition, as assessed by palpation, within 7 to 10 days. The small percentage of animals that fail to show completely clear vaginal mucus after the initial treatment may be given a second prostaglandin injection 8 to 12 days after the first.

Prostaglandin given to animals with pyometra causes luteolysis and effects evacuation of the uterus. The cow with pyometra seems more sensitive to $PGF_{2\alpha}$, responding to as little as 5 mg. A normal luteal dose should be given, however. Because luteal tissue of a cow with pyometra may not behave as that in a cow with a normal cycle, 100 μg GnRH can be given 48 hours before $PGF_{2\alpha}$ is given. The release of luteinizing hormone stimulated by GnRH makes the luteal tissue more susceptible to the luteolytic agent. Conception rates following prostaglandin treatment of bovine pyometra are reported to range from 40 to 70%. Better results are generally seen when breeding is delayed for at least one cycle after treatment.

$PGF_{2\alpha}$ can be used as an effective abortifacient agent in the bovine species. Single doses of 30 to 45 mg $PGF_{2\alpha}$ have been used to induce abortion in cows during the first 30 days of gestation, in cows in gestation 40 to 120 days, and in feedlot heifers in the first trimester of pregnancy. Abortion is induced within 7 days after treatment or in the first trimester of pregnancy. Estrus begins at or near the time of abortion, and plasma progesterone levels decline to less than 1 mg/ml before abortion. These events indicate that the corpus luteum has regressed. Additionally, abortion earlier in gestation tends to enhance cyclicity in beef cattle. A single dose of prostaglandin will induce abortion in 5 to 7 days in cows that are not more than 5 months pregnant. After 5 months, the predictability of the prostaglandin wears off.

Prostaglandins can be used successfully for termination of pregnancies complicated by a mummified or a macerated fetus. After a 25- to 50-mg dose of $PGF_{2\alpha}$, the cervix becomes dilated and the fetus becomes lodged in the cervical canal. By day 4, cows show estrus and the fetus can be easily removed from the vagina. By day 8, the uterus is reasonably involuted and a corpus luteum can be palpated. The fetus is not totally expelled but is only delivered into the vagina. The fetus must be removed manually from the anterior vagina. Prostaglandins seem less effective for treating cases of macerated fetus than for mummified fetus. The mummified fetus may remain in the vagina unless manually removed.

Prostaglandins effectively terminate pregnancy to approximately 150 days of gestation.

26.10 THERAPY FOR RETAINED FETAL MEMBRANES

Although retention of the fetal membranes is the major side effect associated with induced calving, it may also be a problem following natural parturition. The fetal membranes normally are passed within 2 to 4 hours of calving.

Following delivery and separation of the cord, the fetal membranes lose their blood supply, and continuing contractions express some retained blood. The marked reduction in the blood supply to the uterus allows dilatation of the crypts of the maternal caruncles, which are all devoid of muscle.

Thus, the loosened membranes are shed normally during the third stage of labor by contraction and involution of the uterus between 2 to 4 hours after the birth of the calf. When the membranes are retained beyond 12 hours, a clinical condition exists.

Common sequelae to retained fetal membranes are endometritis, metritis, pyometra, salpingitis, perimetritis, and oophoritis, with subsequent reduced fertility. Less commonly, acute septic metritis, peritonitis, or septicemia may occur.

The causes of retained fetal membranes may be listed under four main headings: the first three are direct and the fourth is indirect:

1. Prematurity
2. Placentitis and cotyledonitis
3. Uterine inertia
4. Management and nutrition

The basic goals of therapy for retained fetal membranes are to prevent secondary complications and to return the cow to reproductive usefulness as soon as possible. Although unified opinion about the best treatment for retained fetal membranes is lacking, most practitioners agree that manual removal leads to an increase in the previously listed complications.

Retention of fetal membranes occurs more often after corticosteroid or prostaglandin-induced parturition than after normal parturition. The incidence of retained placenta is less if parturition is induced after the 276th day of gestation. The occurrence of retained membranes as related to day of calving is similar to that observed with glucocorticoid-induced calvings.

TREATMENT

Various measures either singly or in combination have been undertaken to treat this condition. They can be conveniently described under the following headings:

1. Manual removal
2. Antiseptics
3. Antibiotics
4. Ecobolics
5. Uterine evacuation

Clinically ill animals naturally require more intensive attention.

Manual Removal

Most reports state that, unless the fetal membranes come away easily or uterine inertia or obstruction follow, manual removal should not be carried out. Damage to the genital tract must be avoided because such damage increases the risk of septicemia and perimetritis. When performed, manual removal is usually first attempted 3 to 4 days post partum.

Antiseptics

Various antiseptics have been used in the past, including Lugol's iodine solution (500 ml of a 2 to 4% solution), which is an effective antimicrobial agent. Many antiseptics, however, are inactivated by the high levels of organic material present.

Antibiotics

Several sources report the use of tetracyclines at a rate of 1 to 2 g on alternate days, either in 500 ml of saline or as a powder. This treatment eliminates local infections and, if used promptly after calving or after clinical illness has developed, results in marked improvement. Subsequent conception rates are excellent.

Milk should not be used for human consumption for at least the required period after the last treatment. Absorption of antibiotics from the uterus in the immediate postpartum period is less effective than at other stages of the reproductive cycle, and blood therapeutic levels are maintained for a shorter period than after intramuscular injection.

Many antibacterial drugs have been advocated for both systemic and intrauterine administration to treat retained fetal membranes. Several workers report that the severity of the effects of retained fetal membranes associated with induced parturition may be reduced by routinely administering oral, parenteral, or local antibiotics. Systemic administration of sulfonamides, however, results in better subsequent fertility than does manual removal of retained fetal membranes followed by local antibacterial treatment. Lugol's iodine solution, 500 ml of a 2 to 5% solution, administered by intrauterine infusion every 2 to 3 days until the placenta is expelled, is an effective therapy. The systemic administration of penicillin is frequently used to treat retained fetal membranes.

Studies have shown that treatment of retained fetal membranes with one of the tetracyclines reduces the incidence of metritis and improves fertility. If fetal membranes are still present 24 hours after calving, 2 to 3 g (i.e., 4 to 6 pessaries) of one of the tetracyclines should be placed into the uterus every other day until the membranes have been expelled. Then, one additional dose should be administered after expulsion. Cows treated by this regimen have a subsequent fertility similar to that of healthy herdmates. When retained fetal membranes are left untreated, cows require more services per conception and have a longer calving-to-conception interval.

Ecobolics and Other Hormones

Oxytocin has been administered subcutaneously at the rate of 30 to 50 I.U. at 2 to 4 hours for as many as 4 treatments. It has little effect, however, when more than 24 hours have elapsed after calving.

Ergonovine at the rate of 1 to 5 mg has a more prolonged effect than does oxytocin and appears to be more effective.

Prednisolone administered on alternate days, combined with antibiotics, reportedly reduces considerably the amount of inflammation present.

When retained fetal membranes are associated with uterine atony caused by hypocalcemia, oxytocin and calcium borogluconate are likely to give good results. In this instance, oxytocin is given intramuscularly or subcutaneously, 30 to 50 I.U. every 2 hours for as many as 4 doses. Selenium/vitamin E should also be considered because of its role in normal reproductive physiology.

Estrogens A logical step in the treatment of retained fetal membranes is the administration of estrogens. These hormones increase uterine tone, myometrial activity, and the blood supply to the uterus, thereby making the uterus more resistant to infection. Estradiol, 1 to 4 mg, may be administered up to 4 times with no ill effects.

Uterine Evacuation

Evacuation of the genital tract by siphonage is another relevant technique when foul-smelling fluid is present in excessive amounts. Retained fetal membranes are also associated with deficiencies in selenium, vitamin E, iodine, and vitamin A. The incidence of retained fetal membrane can be significantly reduced by injecting the cows with selenium and vitamin E 4 weeks prior to calving. Iodine is another

trace element which in some geographic areas if deficient can lead to retained fetal membranes.

PROPHYLAXIS

Prophylactic measures include the diagnosis and prevention of abortion, prophylactic therapy with vitamin A, vitamin E, and, when appropriate, selenium or iodine, and observance of strict peri- and postpartum hygiene procedure.

Although doses of corticosteroids used for induction are too small to significantly affect the cow's resistance to infection, studies have demonstrated that doses as low as 40 mg/cow may impair the phagocytic and bactericidal activities of bovine leukocytes. Other adverse effects relate to the high incidence of retained fetal membranes, lower quality of colostrum, and less ability by the calf to ingest immunoglobulins.

The effect of retained placenta on future fertility differs with duration of retention and presence of other diseases. Retained placenta may predispose the cow to more severe forms of uterine disease. Whether the placenta is retained after induced parturition does not necessarily affect the time from calving to conception. Routine treatment (with systemic and intrauterine antibiotics) in cows requiring assistance at delivery or suffering with retained placenta does not necessarily help to prevent metritis. Treatment with oxytocin does not reduce retained placenta in cows that calve normally nor in cows that require assistance at calving. A single intrauterine administration of antibiotics or iodine given 15 days after parturition does not shorten the time required for recovery.

Retained placenta can frequently be a predisposing factor to uterine prolapse. When dealing with a prolapse, epidural anesthetic can be useful by postponing straining and reducing defecation. For large prolapses, oxytocin is useful at 50 I.U. intramuscularly, 10 I.U. intravenously, or 50 I.U. locally. Local application of hypertonic saline or sugar can cause appreciable shrinking of prolapsed uterus.

Clenbuterol (Planipart), 10 ml by intramuscular or slow intravenous injection, can facilitate replacement by causing relaxation,

TABLE 26–4
TREATMENT OF UTERINE PROLAPSE

Epidural anesthesia
Oxytocin
Hypertonic saline
Beta$_2$ agonists.

but it must not be used in conjunction with corticosteroids or epidurals. Legal controls on the availability of this beta-agonist are in place in some countries (Table 26–4). Clenbuterol and isoxsuprine, another beta$_2$ agonist, activate the uterine beta$_2$ receptors causing myometrial relaxation. Oxytocin, and prostaglandin F$_{2\alpha}$ antagonize their effects.

SELECTED REFERENCES

Aderibigbe, A.A.: Prompt treatment for uterovaginal prolapse is critical. Vet. Med., 79:1091, 1984.

Ayliffe, T.R., and Noakes, D.E.: Some preliminary studies on the uptake of sodium benzylpenicillin by the endometrium of the cow. Vet. Rec., 102:215, 1978.

Bosc, M.J., et al.: A comparison of induction of parturition with dexamethasone or with an analogue of prostaglandin 2 (A-PGF) in cattle. Theriogenology, 3:187, 1975.

Brand, A., DeBois, C.H.W., and Kommerij, R.: Induction of abortion in cattle with prostaglandin F$_{2\alpha}$ and oestradiol in cattle with prostaglandin F$_{2\alpha}$ and oestradiol valerate. Tijdschr. Diergeneesk., 100:432, 1975.

Braun, W.F.: A review of prostaglandin therapeutics in reproduction. VM/SAC, 75(4):649, 1980.

Bretzlaff, K.N.: Rationale for treatment of endometritis in the dairy cow. Vet. Clin. North Am., 3:593, 1987.

Bretzlaff, K.N., Ott, R.S., Koritz, G.D., et al.: Distribution of oxytetracycline in the healthy and diseased postpartum genital tract of cows. Am. J. Vet. Res., 44:760, 1983.

Cavestany, D., and Foote, R.H.: Prostaglandin F2 alpha-induced estrus in open cows and presumed abortion in pregnant cows with unobserved estrus in a herd monitored by milk progesterone assay. Cornell Vet., 75:393, 1985.

Cavestany, D., and Foote, R.H.: Reproductive performance of Holstein cows administered GnRH analog hoe 766 (Buseretin) 26 to 34 days postpartum. J. Anim. Sci., 61:244, 1985.

Dailey, R.A., Inskeep, E.K., Washburn, S.P., et al.: Use of prostaglandin F2 alpha or gonadotropin releasing hormone in treating problem breeding cows. J. Dairy Sci., 66:1721, 1983.

Day, A.M.: Cloprostenol for termination of pregnancy in cattle. A. The induction of parturition. NZ Vet. J., 25:136, 1977.

Elmore, R.G.: Putting prostaglandin F2a to work in your bovine practice. Vet. Med., 84:1093, 1989.

Elmore, R.G., et al.: Induction of Beef Cows Using Prostaglandin or Dexamethasone (Abst). Chicago IL, Proc. Conference Research Workers Animal Disease, 1987.

Garcia-Villar, R.: Fenprostalene in cattle: Evaluation of oxytocic effects in ovariectomized cows and abortion potential in a 100 day pregnant cow. Theriogenology, 28:467, 1987.

Greene, H.J.: Clinical study of the use of clenbuterol for postponing parturition in cows. Vet. Rec., 109:283, 1981.

Guedawy, S.A., Neff-Davis, C.A., Davis, L.E., et al.: Disposition of gentamicin in the genital tract of cows. J. Vet. Pharmacol. Ther., 6:85, 1983.

Gustaffson, B.K.: Use of drugs other than antibiotics in treatment of uterine disease in large animals. Mod. Vet. Pract., 66:389, 1985.

Gustaffson, B.K.: Therapeutic strategies involving antimicrobial treatment of the uterus in large animals. J. Am. Vet. Med. Assoc., 185(10):1194, 1984.

Gustaffson, B.K., and Ott, R.S.: Current trends in the treatment of genital infections in large animals. Compend. Contin. Educ. Pract. Vet., 5:147, 1981.

Gustaffson, B.K., Backstrom, G., and Equvist, L-E.: Treatment of bovine pyometra with prostaglandin F$_{2\alpha}$. An evaluation of a field study. Theriogenology, 6:45, 1976.

Herrler, A., et al.: Purified FSH supplemented with defined amounts of LH for superovulation dairy cattle. Theriogenology, 29(1):260, 1988.

Herschler, R.C., and Lawrence, J.R.: Inducing Parturition with a Bovine Prostaglandin. Vet. Med., 81(6):580, 1986.

Herschler, R.C., and Lawrence, J.R.: Studying the safety of prostaglandin induced parturition in dairy cows. Vet. Med., 81:674, 1986.

Herschler, R.C., and Lawrence, J.R.: A prostaglandin analogue for therapy of retained placentae. VM/SAC, 79(6):822, 1984.

Jackson, P.S.: Treatment of chronic postpartum endometritis in cattle with cloprostenol. Vet. Rec., 101:441, 1977.

Jackson, P.S., and Cooper, M.J.: The use of cloprostenol for the termination of pregnancy and the expulsion of mummified fetus in cattle. Vet. Rec., 100:361, 1977.

Jackson, P.S., and Cooper, M.J.: The use of cloprostenol (ICI 80996) in the treatment of infertility in cattle. Proc. World Assoc. Biuatrics, 1976.

Jayappa, G.H., and Liken, K.I.: Effect of antimicrobial agents and corticosteroids on bovine polymorphonuclear leukocyte chemotaxis. Am. J. Vet. Res., 44:2155, 1983.

Johnson, C.T.: Time on onset of oestrus after the injection of heifers with cloprostenol. Vet. Rec., *103*:204, 1978.

Johnson, C.T., and Jackson, P.S.: Induction of parturition in cattle with cloprostenol. Br. Vet. J., *138*:212, 1982.

Kindahl, H., Edqvist, L-E. Grandstrom, E., et al.: The release of prostaglandin $F_{2\alpha}$ as reflected by 15-keto-13, 14-dihydro-prostaglandin $F_{2\alpha}$ in the peripheral circulation during normal luteolysis in heifers. Prostaglandins, *11*:871, 1976.

Lindsell, C.E., et al.: Variability in FSH:LH ratios among batches of commercially available gonadotrophins. Theriogenology, *25(1)*:167, 1986.

Masera, J., Gustaffson, B., Afiefy, M.M., et al.: Disposition of oxytetracycline in the bovine genital tract: systemic vs intrauterine administration. J. Am. Vet. Med. Assoc., *176*:1099, 1980.

Mass, J.P.: Prevention of retained placenta in dairy cattle. Compend. Contin. Educ. Pract. Vet., *4(12)*:S519, 1982.

McCracken, J.A., Carlson, J.C., Glew, M.E., et al.: Prostaglandin $F_{2\alpha}$ identified as a luteolytic hormone in sheep. Nature, *238*:129, 1972.

Miller, H.V., Kimsey, P.B., Kendrick, J.W., et al.: Endometritis of dairy cattle. Diagnosis, treatment and fertility. Bovine Pract., *15*:13023, 1980.

Misra, S.S.: Observation on the therapeutic management of uterovaginal prolapse in bovine. U.P. Vet. J., *4*:55, 1976.

Olson, J.D., Ball, L., and Mortimer, R.G.: Therapy of postpartum uterine infections. Bovine Proc., *17*:85, 1985.

Ott, R.S., and Mansfield, M.E.: Fenprostulene vs fenprostalene in combination with dexanethisive for induction of parturition in beef cows. Agri—Practice 19, 1985.

Panongala, V.S., and Barnum, D.A.: Antibiotic resistance patterns of organisms isolated from cervicovaginal mucus of cows. Can. Vet. J., *19*:113, 1978.

Pharris, B.B., and Wyngarden, L.F.: The effect of $PGF_{2\alpha}$ on the progestin content of ovaries from pseudopregnant rats. Proc. Soc. Exp. Biol. Med., *130*:93, 1969.

Plenderleith, R.W.J.: Treatment of uterine prolapse. Proc. Br. Cattle Vet. Assoc., 55, 1981.

Plenderleith, R.W.J.: Induction of parturition in dairy heifers using prostaglandin $F_{2\alpha}$. Vet. Rec., *193*:502, 1978.

Putriam, M.R.: Parturition: A mechanism review. Induction intervention and calf viability. Bovine Proc., *15*:122, 1983.

Roth, J.A., and Kaeberle, M.L.: Effect of glucocorticoids on the bovine immune system. J. Am. Vet. Med. Assoc., *180(8)*:894, 1982.

27

DISEASES OF SHEEP

27.1 Classification of Diseases Causing Enteritis/Diarrhea
27.2 Causes of Scours in Lambs
27.3 *Escherichia Coli* Infection
27.4 Treatment of Coccidiosis in Lambs
27.5 Toxoplasmosis
27.6 Foot Rot

27.1 CLASSIFICATION OF DISEASES CAUSING ENTERITIS/DIARRHEA

1. **Bacterial**
   Colibacillosis
   Lamb dysentery
   Hemorrhagic enterotoxemia
   Salmonellosis
   Bacterial enteritis (*Campylobacter*)
2. **Viral**
   Rotavirus
   Coronavirus
3. **Parasitic**
   Most gastrointestinal parasites except *Haemonchus*
   Cryptosporidiosis (cryptosporidium)
   Coccidiosis (*Eimeria*)
4. **Nutritional/Managerial**
   Sudden feed changes
   Lush feed
   Overfeeding
   Poor-quality milk replacers
   Lactic acidosis
   Copper deficiency in association with molybdenum excess

PERINATAL MORTALITY IN SHEEP

The incidence of mortality among newborn lambs is a major limiting factor to income in the sheep industry. Many studies have shown that up to 20% of all lambs die prior to weaning. Nutrition, management, maternal instinct of ewes, colostrum intake, climate, and diseases influence lamb mortality. Birth weight is also important, with small lambs (less than 3 kg) and very large lambs (more than 4.5 kg) at increased risk of dying in the first 3 days of life. Predator activity in flocks, primarily by dogs, may also significantly affect mortality. Failure to nurse for any reason is a major cause of death from starvation and is characterized by an empty abomasum or an abomasum filled with dirt, hair, and feed.

Causes of perinatal mortality may vary between flocks and between geographic areas; however, the four dominant categories of lamb loss that consistently surface are:

1. Abortions
2. Hypothermia, starvation, and exposure
3. Pneumonia
2. Stillbirth and dystocia

Generally the greatest losses occur in the first few days of life, usually from *Escherichia coli* infection, but rotavirus/coronavirus may also be involved.

Diseases involving neonatal lambs usually occur suddenly. The consequences to the newborn are severe, and treatment is commonly unrewarding. Prevention of neonatal losses is a more feasible alternative to traditional treatment programs. The long-term economic benefit of prevention programs to both the producer and the veterinarian should be obvious. Veterinarians and producers, however, must recognize where, when, and how lamb losses occur before any preventive programs can be developed. Veterinarians and producers also must acknowledge the impact of management decisions on perinatal mortality and on the economic survival of the producer.

27.2 CAUSES OF SCOURS IN LAMBS

INTERNAL PARASITES

Nematodes

Despite the increased knowledge and awareness of nematodes by sheep producers, nematodiasis is still a major cause of scours and ill-thrift in sheep.

The main species that cause scours in sheep are *Ostertagia* and *Trichostrongylus*. *Haemonchus contortus* (barber's pole worm), which is a major parasite in summer rainfall areas, does not usually cause scours in sheep. The main signs of *Haemonchus* infestation are anemia, poor exercise tolerance, and death.

Nematodirus have eggs that are resistant to desiccation. Outbreaks of scours caused by *Nematodirus* infestation are usually seen in weaner sheep in spring or summer, especially if the same weaning paddock is used each year, and soon after drought or prolonged dry conditions. *Nematodirus* infestation causes severe scours and death in young sheep. Eggs can overwinter and it can thus be a lamb-to-lamb and year-to-year disease.

Trichostrongylus axei can cause scours in sheep, but outbreaks of nematodiasis caused by *T. axei* alone are not common. *T. axei* is significant because it infects both sheep and cattle. Grazing systems that employ sheep-cattle crossovers to control the major nematode genera, can break down because of *Trichostrongylus axei*. In normal circumstances, the benefits obtained from using a sheep-cattle crossover far outweigh the risk of a *T. axei* problem emerging.

Nematodirus, Ostertagia, and *Trichostrongylus* are the most important nematodes that cause ill-thrift and scours in sheep. The adult *Ostertagia* and *Trichostrongylus* nematodes reside in the abomasum and small intestine, respectively. These parasites cause scours in animals. Sheep with low adult worm burdens and low fecal egg counts and that display a high resistance to infection may still develop scours and ill-thrift when challenged by many larvae. This susceptibility is apparently the result of a hypersensitivity reaction to the ingested larvae at the gut level.

Methods to control the prevalence of gastrointestinal nematodes must be based on a combination of sound grazing management and use of strategic anthelmintic treatments. See Chapter 29 "Therapy of Endoparasites in Cattle and Sheep".

COLIBACILLOSIS

Outbreaks of colibacillosis are rare in paddock conditions, but can occur when lambing ewes are under severe stress. These outbreaks are usually associated with lambs receiving inadequate colostrum and with cold wet weather. The affected lambs develop acute diarrhea and death is common. Bacterial enteritis is most commonly seen in spring, in winter from cold stress, and in both seasons from nutritional stress. At these times, the sheep also must adjust to significant changes in the composition of the pasture.

Management factors are often involved in the cause of bacterial enteritis. Stresses associated with weaning, shearing, and dipping appear to predispose young sheep to bacterial enteritis. The disease is common in weaners stocked at high rates, irrespective of the pasture availability.

Another significant factor in the expression of the disease is intercurrent diseases, such as nematode infections and *Eimeria ovis* infection (coccidiosis). The significance of deficiencies in the trace elements, especially selenium and copper, must be investigated further. The role, if any, of viruses, e.g., coronavirus, in initiating or predisposing sheep to bacterial enteritis can not be ruled out.

Colibacillosis is more common in lambs that are born and reared indoors. It is also common in bottle-reared lambs.

Diagnosis is usually made at post mortem, and correction of the problem generally depends on improvement in ewe nutrition, hygiene, and husbandry.

COCCIDIA

Coccidiosis is seen under two similar circumstances, both of which involve young lambs under stress. These lambs are in feedlots and in heavily stocked lambing paddocks.

The disease is caused by a mixed protozoan infection by several *Eimeria* species. Diagnosis by fecal examination is difficult because most young sheep are infected and oocyst counts are not strongly correlated with clinical disease. Lambs can have high oocyst counts without clinical disease and vice versa. Affected lambs should be submitted for postmortem examination to confirm the field diagnosis.

In outbreaks, coccidiosis quickly affects a large percentage of lambs. Affected lambs exhibit diarrhea, occasional dysentery, depression, and anorexia.

Viruses/cryptosporidia cannot be overlooked as a cause of lamb scours either. Their incidence and significance appear to be rising.

TRACE ELEMENTS

Copper Deficiency

Clinical signs of copper deficiency include enzootic ataxia in lambs, bone fragility in weaner sheep, steely wool, and loss of pigmentation in black-wooled sheep. In chronic cases, signs may include anemia, ill-thrift, and scours.

Diagnosis of copper deficiency can be confirmed by blood tests and, if possible, liver tests for copper levels in a group of affected sheep.

The best treatment depends on the individual situation. Short-term deficiency can be overcome by using copper treatments, such as injection, on individual animals. Injection is best for secondary hypocuprosis, if molybdenum-induced. Long-term treatment is best attained with oral copper capsules containing copper oxide needles. Oral copper therapy is not indicated if oral intake of high amounts of molybdenum is the triggering factor. See also Chapter 28, Trace Elements.

Cobalt Deficiency

Cobalt deficiency is generally seen in lambs between 12 and 24 weeks of age that graze sandy coast soils in the flush of spring.

Clinical signs are ill-thrift, severe wasting, weeping eyes, and scaly ears. Diarrhea is often seen in later stages of the deficiency.

Diagnosis can be confirmed by response to treatment with an injection of vitamin B_{12}. Blood tests may also be used, but delays in reporting results are common.

Treatment of affected animals is achieved using injectable vitamin B_{12}. Longer-term remedies include top dressing with cobalt or use of foliar sprays. Adult sheep can be given cobalt bullets, boluses, or drenches, but bullets do not protect the lamb.

27.3 *ESCHERICHIA COLI* INFECTION

Escherichia coli infection in newborn lambs is appearing more and more frequently on farms. The infected lamb refuses to suck and begins to dribble at the mouth. The abdomen becomes swollen. Scours may or may not be obvious at first. The disease is often fatal within a few hours.

The epizootics of colibacillosis are often associated with:

1. Adverse environmental factors—cold windy weather with significant temperature fluctuations, and also
2. dirty lambing conditions leading to buildup of infection in the environment.

The *E. coli* organism is classified according to certain serologic characteristics, i.e., somatic "O" antigen, the envelope "K" antigen, and the flagellar "H" antigen, plus certain biochemical reactions.

In lambs, two different forms of the condition have been recognized, namely, the systemic and enteric, and different strains of *E. coli* have been associated with the disease.

E. coli infections in lambs can result in diarrhea, septicemia and/or meningitis, and polyarthritis. The diarrheic form (colibacillosis) is relatively common under intensive lambing and raising conditions.

The enteric form is most commonly seen in lambs from 12 hours to 8 days of age and often appears in the later stages of the lambing program, when continuous use of lambing sheds or paddocks has occurred and a buildup of infection has taken place. Entry of enterotoxigenic strains of *E. coli* is believed to be primarily through the umbilicus or nasopharyngeal route in heavily contaminated environments.

Although the exposure of the newborn to a heavily infected environment is obviously a contributory factor, other precipitating factors, such as failure to obtain and/or maintain adequate colostrum and devitalization resulting from chilling, are also involved. Coma and death occur in 12 to 72 hours from onset of symptoms.

The lamb in this instance is dull, inappetent, constipated, and fails to pass meconium. These lambs are often colostrum deprived.

The systemic or septicemia form is usually associated with the older lamb, i.e., 2 to 6 weeks of age, although it can occur in neonatal lambs 2 to 3 days old.

The septicemic and meningitis/polyarthritis manifestations also are commonly encountered and are assuming significance now as a cause of neonatal mortality. Enterotoxigenic *E. coli* cause a secretory diarrhea in newborn lambs. Enterotoxigenic strains should be distinguished from strains of *E. coli* that cause septicemia or chronic arthritis. Enteric infection in lambs and kids younger than 10 days of age causes acute, profuse, watery diarrhea. The diarrhea results from the secretion of electrolytes and enterotoxin produced by the *E. coli* colonizing the gut. The loss of sodium, chloride, potassium, bicarbonate, and water into the bowel lumen causes electrolyte imbalances that may be fatal. Diagnosis is based on age of onset, clinical signs, and isolation of the organisms in culture of the feces. The main differential diagnosis for diarrhea caused by *E. coli* is diarrhea caused by rotavirus. These two pathogens may also combine to cause outbreaks of diarrhea in neonatal lambs.

CLINICAL SIGNS

As stated, colibacillosis of lambs is characterized by profuse scours, dehydration, and depression. It may involve lambs only hours old, but lambs may show initial signs even when several weeks of age. Most cases are seen in lambs 2 to 8 days of age.

E. coli septicemia is a cause of "sudden death." The lamb usually is found dead with minimal signs of struggle. The affected animals are usually 4 to 8 weeks of age and among the best in the flocks. Losses are usually in the order of 1 to 5%, but may reach 20%.

Lambs with the meningitic form are usually found recumbent and paddling. They may have opisthothonus and/or nystagmus. Animals with arthritis, but little meningeal involvement, are still-gaited and depressed.

Thus, traditionally in lambs, two different forms of colibacillosis have been recognised:

(1) The enteric form, and
(2) The systemic form.

The enteric form seen in the first week or so of life usually peaks late in the lambing program where continuous use of lambing sheds has occurred and a severe build-up of infection takes place.

Adverse weather conditions, cold windy weather with temperature fluctuations, dirty lambing conditions, stressful delivery, and failure to acquire early colostrum precipitate the acute classic outbreak of *E. coli* scours. The affected lamb is dull, debilitated, anorexic, and ceases following the ewe. Diarrhea/dehydration follow rapidly. Death can occur within 24 to 72 hours from first onset of symptoms.

TREATMENT

Treatment for colibacillosis in lambs is similar to that used for white scours in calves, i.e., reduction of milk intake, fluid and electrolyte replacement, and general nursing (e.g., Lectade, Resorb, ionaid).

Oral fluid therapy and lamb warming, in conjunction with both oral and parenteral antibiotics, appear to be the most effective treatment. Glucose given only orally or by intraperitoneal injection may rectify any hypoglycemia, and treatment with anti-inflammatory agents, such as flunixin or dexamethasone, is probably indicated to help to combat the endotoxic shock.

An oral antibiotic not readily absorbed from the intestinal tract, administered as soon after birth as possible in conjunction with an oral laxative, e.g., 30 ml of a mixture of 60 g magnesium sulfate, 60 ml treacle, and 0.5 liter water, is an effective prophylactic treatment.

Specific antibiotics available in handy oral-dose form for sheep have proved quite effective, e.g., apramycin, spectinomycin, and gentamicin.

Prevention of *E. coli* infection is a better approach than cure, and provided that lambing pens are kept clean to minimize *E. coli* challenge, vaccination of the ewes with *E. coli* bacterins is a sensible way to prevent the problem in sheep flocks. Adequate intake of colostrum containing high titers of antibiotics then is suckled by the lamb in the early postnatal period. Prevention of *E. coli* diarrhea is based on good husbandry procedures, which include the provision of clean, dry lambing pens and sufficient colostral intake (50 ml of colostrum per kg body weight within 6 hours of birth). Fortunately, the disease does not appear in lambs as frequently as in calves. In problem flocks, vaccination of ewes with an *E. coli* bacterin prior to lambing should provide specific passive immunity to the lambs via the ewes' milk for the prevention of *E. coli* diarrhea. The most effective method of prevention is to ensure early and adequate consumption of colostrum for newborn lambs.

Enteric colibacillosis usually develops in the absence of the protective effect of colostrum.

Treatment of colibacillosis is rarely successful because the disease strikes rapidly, spreads widely, builds up environmental infectivity, and can devastate flocks.

CONTROL AND PREVENTION

Control of enteric colibacillosis is based on hygiene and management.

The greatest source of infective organisms is other lambs, particularly those with scours. Therefore, isolation of individuals or age groups assists in the containment of infection. Also, hygienic precautions, such as cleaning of feeding equipment and pens, are valuable.

Other forms of *E. coli* infection control are, at best, based on theoretic considerations rather than on practical results. Avoiding the use of permanent sheep paddocks is one suggestion. Mixing of different age groups to provide a wide range of colostral antibodies is another.

Colostrum

Good management procedures demand attention to colostrum intake, which is vital to the early health and vigor of the newborn lamb. The amount of colostrum a lamb drinks depends on the quantities available and on the success of suckling. Availability of colostrum is affected by breed, nutrition of the ewe during late pregnancy, and the number of lambs born.

When multiple births occur, the immunoglobulin transfer is reduced in proportion to the number of offspring.

Immunoglobulin deficiency in lambs is usually the result of poor colostrum production in the dam (low immunoglobulin) rather than of failure to suckle.

The colostrum may be used during the same or a subsequent lambing period, because when it is deep frozen ($-20°$ C), ewe colostrum does not deteriorate for at least a year. Whether thawing colostrum in a microwave oven damages the immunoglobulins is not known. Studies have given equivocal results, although overheating may denature the proteins.

Vaccination of Ewes

Vaccines are now commercially available for the active immunization of ewes against the strains of *E. coli* commonly associated with disease in young lambs.

In problem flocks, vaccination of ewes with an *E. coli* bacterin prior to lambing should provide specific passive immunity to the lambs via the ewes' milk for the prevention of diarrhea.

Lambs from vaccinated ewes must receive 1 liter of colostrum within the first 18 hours of birth; 50 ml/kg should be given within the first 6 hours.

Neonatal Protection

Several diseases that surround the newborn lamb in the first few days of life can be adequately controlled by strategic use of vaccination of the dam to pass on passive protection.

Because hyperimmune serum either is not available for economic reasons or is unacceptable for use, prompt active immunization of the ewe is necessary to gain this protection.

Colostral transfer of antibody in the sheep is efficient. The level of transfer is directly proportional to the titer of the ewe at lambing.

Active immunization of the ewe with *E. coli* bacterin significantly raises antibody titers in lambs. Dam vaccination given to ewes 3 to 4 weeks before lambing ensures high maternal titers of antibody in the dam. These antibody titers are transferred via colostrum to the lamb.

For adequate flock protection, all ewes should be vaccinated to prevent disease outbreaks in neonatal lambs that would otherwise act as reservoirs of infection.

E. coli vaccines also have the advantage of preventing the onset of a rapid and fulminating disease in weak or premature offspring for which diagnosis and treatment usually occur too late.

Probiotics may also play a useful role in accelerating recovery and shortening the convalescent period following colibacillosis.

Antimicrobial therapy of neonatal calf and lamb scour can be fraught with controversy and often ends in failure because of the numerous microbial agents implicated and the accompanying complexity of predisposing causes, mainly of a management and nutritional nature. The acuteness of the disease process, the serotypes and virulence of the microorganisms, and the varied pattern of antibiotic resistance render antimicrobial treatment difficult for the veterinarian. The inadequate immunocompetence of many calves also adds a significant dimension to the pathogenesis.

Despite the recent justifiable interest in the role of viruses and non-bacterial agents, evidence shows that enterotoxigenic *E. coli* is still the major cause of diarrhea in calves and lambs younger than 1 week of age. Viruses are more commonly implicated in calves and lambs aged from 1 to several weeks.

Importance of Colostrum

Colostrum is perhaps the most potent natural agent with which to combat neonatal scour. Ensuring the transfer of passive immunity to neonatal lambs is one of the primary determinants of survival rate. Numerous studies have compared passive immunoglobulin levels during the first few days of life with subsequent mortality. These studies show that lambs with low immunoglobulin levels are at increased risk. Additionally, not all ewes under natural conditions possess high antibody titers against *E. coli*.

Absorption of Maternal Antibody

Lambs are born deficient in circulating immunoglobulin antibodies and depend exclusively on acquired colostral antibodies for protection against environmental *E. coli* pathogens in the immediate postpartum periods. Newborn animals can absorb maternal colostral antibodies only for a period of hours. Closure of the intestinal absorptive gate by pinocytosis is progressive for approximately 24 hours. After this time, the maternal antibodies are restricted to the gut lumen.

Absorbed immunoglobulin protects against systemic disease, but unabsorbed immunoglobulin also plays an important role in protection against local gut colonization by *E. coli*. Overall protection of the highly susceptible neonatal calf or lamb depends on a combination of systemic (absorbed immunoglobulin) and local (unabsorbed immunoglobulin) immune mechanisms. Thus, the presence of antibody in the intestine after 24 hours also plays a significant role in scour protection.

Boosting Colostral *E. coli* Antibodies

E. coli produces watery diarrhea that is often fatal during the first 3 days of life. Exposure to pathogens and susceptibility to environmental stress are highest during this time when the calf cannot produce its own antibodies.

Prepartum immunization of the dam with *E. coli* bacterins can dramatically reduce mortality and morbidity by stimulating high levels of colostral *E. coli* antibody.

Flock history and the ability to ensure colostral intake are vital in determining whether dam vaccination will be economically justifiable. Dam vaccination has the added advantage of alerting the client to the importance of colostral intake and facilitates close collaboration between the veterinarian and the client in embarking on flock health and lamb protection programs.

Dam vaccines containing the K99 antigen are available. K99 is the gut adhesion virulence factor for *E. coli* that causes adhesion, seepage, and toxin production in the gut. Given to the lamb at least 2 weeks before lambing, these vaccines ensure high levels of *E. coli* immunoglobulin antibodies in the colostrum.

Absorption of antibodies protects against septicemic colibacillosis, whereas the antibodies remaining in the gut after 24 hours protect against *E. coli* scour.

Feeding of Colostrum to Lambs

Maximum colostral antibody transfer is achieved by feeding 200 ml/kg of colostrum within 18 hours of birth. Colostral immunoglobulin levels begin to decline rapidly soon after lambing; the third milking has only 20 to 30% of the immunoglobulin concentration of that taken immediately after lambing. Feeding lambs less or delaying the time of colostral intake causes a linear decline in the amount of immunoglobulin transferred.

Although colostral immunoglobulin can vary from ewe to ewe, the total amount ingested by the lamb is more important than the actual immunoglobulin level of colostrum. Thus, high levels of immunoglobulin in the lamb can be obtained from ewes low in immunoglobulin provided large volumes of colostrum are fed early. Early feeding is essential because of:

1. The rapid decline in maternal immunoglobulin levels
2. The decreasing ability of the lamb to absorb immunoglobulin systemically

In short, the critical factors are:

1. The availability of the colostrum
2. The speed with which it is ingested by the lamb
3. The amount ingested by the lamb

Thus, if the provision of colostrum is substantially delayed, a marked decrease in the level of immunoglobulin transfer can be expected, together with a correspondingly high rate of hypogammaglobulinemia as compared to the rate obtained when colostrum is given as the first feeding.

Colostrum can be stored and fed to lambs even after the intestinal absorption barrier has closed (24 to 27 hours). This unabsorbed immunoglobulin provides high protection against intestinal colonization.

When lambs suckle early and vigorously (with good "mothering behavior"), they tend to achieve higher immunoglobulin levels than do lambs left with their dam for 12 to 24 hours and allowed to suckle at will. Failure to suckle for whatever reason can be satisfactorily overcome by bottle feeding of early colostrum. Poor mothering may require this approach.

27.4 TREATMENT OF COCCIDIOSIS IN LAMBS

Coccidiosis is becoming recognized as an important obstacle to the production of fat lambs, and as the intensification of fat lamb production increases so do the risks of *Eimeria* infection.

Coccidia can be found in sheep of all ages, but they are most prevalent in young growing animals, in which manifestations of infection generally are observed. Older animals are the usual source of infection for the young by acting as parasite reservoirs.

Coccidiosis in sheep is caused by obligatory protozoan parasites of the genus *Eimeria* and is one of the most economically important diseases in the sheep industries. It is especially pathogenic in preweaned and recently weaned lambs. Coccidia are relatively common parasites in growing animals. Serious economic losses result from reduced rate and efficiency of gain in growing affected animals. Effects of subclinical or economic coccidiosis are not well documented, but they are important in terms of efficient production and herd health. Older animals are the usual source of infection for the young, and they often shed low numbers of oocysts in feces for months at a time.

Clinical disease is observed most frequently in 2- to 8-week-old lambs housed with their dams in lamb-rearing units; and in lambs 2 to 3 weeks after weaning; or intercurrent disease. The disease also occurs in ewes and lambs that are maintained for long periods of time on contaminated wet areas or heavily stocked pastures.

The most conspicuous sign of coccidiosis is diarrhea. The coccidia destroy many intestinal cells over a short period of time, thus resulting in watery diarrhea, dehydration, weight loss, tenesmus, and rectal prolapse.

The main sign of the disease is profuse scour, which can be rapidly fatal if left untreated. The young lamb has little or no resistance to coccidiosis. Consequently, once infection occurs in the surroundings, such as damp bedding, the disease spreads like wildfire to the young stock. Deaths from scour or severe stunting of growth can follow.

If the disease is not too severe, i.e., subclinical, scour will not be seen, but instead, loss of weight occurs from which the young lambs may never fully recover.

Another insidious effect of coccidiosis is the suppression of the immune system, thereby lowering the lamb's defenses and increasing its susceptibility to such disease as *Nematodirus* or *Escherichia coli*.

Although coccidia infections are self-limiting, small numbers of oocysts can be shed over long periods, and re-exposure to sporulated oocysts is probable.

The most obvious initial reservoir source of infection is the ewe. Coccidial oocysts shed by the ewe cycle through the lambs, thereby leading to a rapid buildup in environmental contamination. Each oocyst ingested by a lamb may lead to the shedding of many thousands in the feces. In the lamb's gut, the oocysts multiply and consequently destroy the gut lining, thereby causing severe diarrhea and dehydration. Some oocysts may overwinter on pastures and others may survive in the lambing accommodation if between-season cleaning is not adequate. The major source of infection for the lamb is, however, the ewe.

Damage to the host is primarily that of cell disruption caused by stages of the parasite invading and destroying cells. Because asexual reproduction occurs, one ingested oocyst can result in the destruction of thousands of cells during the oocyst formation process. Epithelial cells that transport nutrients and fluids into the body are usually damaged. Damaged cells allow the leakage of blood and plasma into the lumen of the gut and bacterial invasion from the gut into tissues.

CLINICAL ASPECTS

The disease is most common in young lambs kept under feedlot conditions, but is seen also in lambs and yearlings on pasture. The main signs are diarrhea, depression, and anorexia. Severely affected animals show weakness, weight loss, and dehydration, and in some instances, death supervenes.

Destruction of many intestinal cells within a short time often results in watery diarrhea (usually without visible blood), dehydration, weight loss, tenesmus, rectal prolapse, anaemia, and death. Immune complex glomerulonephritis has also been attributed to coccidiosis. Diarrhea often occurs about 2 weeks after ingestion of oocysts and coincides with massive destruction of intestinal or cecal epithelium by massive amounts of schizonts and gametocytes. Destruction of crypt cells often results in sloughing of intestinal mucosa and sometimes hemorrhagic enteritis.

Coccidiosis can be diagnosed in a live animal by observation of clinical signs and demonstration of many oocysts in feces. Watery diarrhea may be observed, but sheep as a species do not usually have the bloody diarrhea that is a characteristic of coccidiosis in cattle. Affected animals grow poorly, are depressed and anorexic, and often die.

The presence of several thousand oocysts per gram of feces is usually indicative of coccidiosis. Most sheep, however, pass moderate amounts of oocysts on a routine basis without experiencing clinical disease. Numbers of oocysts per gram of feces vary tremendously between individuals and change dramatically over a few days.

In uncomplicated coccidiosis, many oocysts (5,000 to 10,000/gm feces) are found in the feces. Remember, however, that lambs may have high oocyst counts without disease or low oocyst counts with disease.

On necropsy, the classic picture of ovine coccidiosis is marked enteritis with numerous white foci present in the small intestine. These are visible from both the mucosal and serosal surfaces and are filled with gametocytes and oocysts. On occasion, small papillomatous growths full of oocysts are found in the small intestine.

Occasionally, a low-grade enteritis associated with a granulomatous reaction to the coccidial parasites leads to significant villous atrophy and may be accompanied by a granulomatous lymphadenitis.

CONTROL

Several husbandry measures can be taken to reduce the risk of coccidiosis. Stress increases susceptibility to disease and consequently should be avoided whenever possible.

Crowding is another important factor, and areas where lambs congregate, i.e., around feeders and drinkers, should be kept clean. This degree of cleanliness can be achieved by moving feed and water troughs regularly and by using troughs designed to avoid spillage to ensure that lambs do not eat feed from coccidial-infected ground. Troughs should also be raised to reduce contamination with infected dung.

Because oocysts can survive on the pasture for at least a year, use of the same field for successive crops of lambs can lead to a buildup of infection. This buildup can be prevented by rotational grazing.

Coccidiosis in sheep is usually related to overcrowded conditions and fecal contamination. Proper sanitation greatly reduces the infection rate and the incidence of clinical disease. Affected sheep should be isolated, and special care must be taken to ensure that their feces do not contaminate the feed and water of unaffected sheep. Coccidian oocysts are generally resistant to disinfectants that can be used safely in animal-raising facilities.

HUSBANDRY AND MEDICATION

Any medication program aims to reduce or eliminate oocyst shedding in the ewe and to prevent the coccidia from cycling through the lambs.

Control can be based either on preventing heavy challenge and/or on chemotherapy.

High intake of infective oocysts is often associated with crowding of lambs in a moist warm environment. The prepatent period under ideal conditions is about 3 weeks; thus, buildup can occur rapidly. Prevention of infection under feedlot conditions is difficult unless the sheep are kept on slats. Lambs or weaners at pasture can be stocked at lower rates and/or placed in drier paddocks to reduce the magnitude of challenge.

All lambing accommodations should be cleaned out between seasons and, indeed if lambing pens are used, between lambing. If lambing is outdoors in straw yards, the site should be changed yearly. Pastures should be rotated so that lambs do not graze on fields used by sheep the previous year.

The overall philosophy of coccidiosis control is to prevent the clinical disease through use of proper sanitation and to administer a coccidiostat before anticipated outbreaks of disease. An effective coccidiostat should be given (1) when sheep are overstocked or are in wet, muddy areas; (2) before and when lambs are stressed by weaning, transport, or severe weather; (3) when lambs enter feedlots; and (4) when, based on record keeping, the disease is likely. Preventive treatment should be administered for 28 consecutive days or longer, depending on the severity of the situation, and should begin before the disease is predicted. A coccidiostat should be used at a level that causes shedding of a few oocysts, to allow the host to develop resistance to later challenge, but will prevent clinical or economic disease. In addition to preventing clinical disease and mortality, use of a coccidiostat usually results in significant increases in rate and efficiency of gain, as well as in a reduction in intercurrent disease, such as myiasis and bacterial diarrheas or nematodiasis.

Coccidiosis is difficult to treat entirely satisfactorily. Severely affected lambs are anorexic and do not ingest in-water medication. For them, individual treatment with amprolium, sulfadimidine, sulfadimethoxine, or sulfamethoxypyridazine and electrolytes is necessary. For less acute cases, in-water and in-feed medication (where possible) is usually sufficient. The advent of toltrazuril may well improve prophylaxis and treatment. Toltrazuril is used as a short, in-water dose during in-feed use of ionophores. Diclazuril is also being evaluated for coccidiosis.

DRUG TREATMENT

Several drugs have been used successfully for both treatment and control of ovine coccidiosis (Table 27–1). These include:

1. Decoquinate (Deccox)
2. Amprolium (Amprol)
3. Ionophores (monensin and lasalocid)
4. Sulfonamides

Most of these are used as coccidiostats in other species, and for several of them, the level of inclusion is critical to avoid untoward side effects (e.g., amprolium is a thiamine antagonist and excessive levels of ionophores may suppress appetite).

Of the modern coccidiostats used in the United States, the Food and Drug Administration (FDA) has approved lasalocid at 20 to 30 g/ton of feed for use in sheep. Decoquinate at 0.5 mg/kg of body weight for lambs, and monensin at 20 g/ton have also been used.

The recommended treatment schedule for preventing coccidiosis in sheep is to feed lasalocid in feed at approximately 0.5 to 1 mg/kg body weight per day.

Lasalocid is a polyether antibiotic isolated from fermentation products of *Strep-*

TABLE 27–1
DRUGS FOR OVINE COCCIDIOSIS

	TREATMENT	*CONTROL*
Decoquinate	100 ppm in feed (lambs) (0.5–1.0 mg/kg, body weight) 50 ppm (ewes)	100 ppm (lambs) (28 days) 50 ppm (ewes)
Amprolium	50 mg/kg orally (4–5 days)	50 mg/kg body weight for 21 days, in feed
Monensin	1–2 mg/kg orally (20 days) (Do not exceed 20 mg per head)	20 ppm in feed
Lasalocid	20–30 ppm in feed 0.5–1.0 mg/kg body weight	—
Sulfamethazine	140 mg/kg orally (3 days)	25 mg/kg (7 days)
Sulfamethoxypyridazine	22 mg/kg body weight by intramuscular injection	—
Totrazuril	20 mg/kg (in water)	

tomyces lasaliensis. The recommended schedule for preventing coccidiosis in sheep is to provide lasalocid in feed at approximately 0.5 to 1 mg/kg body weight per day. In a complete feed, this level would be achieved with 30 g of lasalocid per ton of feed.

Decoquinate at 0.5–1.0 mg/kg body weight is highly effective in preventing coccidiosis in experimentally infected lambs. Monensin fed prophylactically in feed at 10 to 30 g/ton effectively controls shedding of oocysts and increased feed conversion rates and weight gains.

Levels of monensin of more than 40 g/ton of feed may suppress production gains, and at 36 g/ton, sheep can reduce feed intake for several days. Monensin at these higher levels is quite unpalatable, and even higher levels can be toxic. Monensin is highly toxic for horses and should be used with extreme caution when horses are on the premises.

Amprolium prevented coccidiosis in feedlot lambs at 50 mg/kg per day when fed for 21 days. It is also available in water for treatment over 4 to 5 days, usually combined with ethopabate. Amprolium at 50 mg/kg body weight is quite effective, but because this drug is a thiamine inhibitor, care must be taken in circumstances in which polioencephalomalacia may occur.

Amprolium can cause laminar cortical necrosis (polioencephalomalacia) and death if used at high levels of 280 mg/kg body weight for 3 to 4 weeks.

Because the ewe is the primary source of infection for the lamb, medication ideally should adopt a three-pronged approach.

1. Medicate ewe compound rations for 3 weeks before lambing.
2. Medicate ewes post partum until weaning.
3. Medicate lamb creep rations with coccidiostat.

Proper administration of anticoccidial drugs can significantly reduce or eliminate clinical coccidiosis in sheep. The modern anticoccidials are termed "coccidiostats" because they inhibit the development of various stages of coccidia in the intestine and thereby prevent disease without affecting development of immunity.

Decoquinate (a 3-hydroxyquinoline) (Deccox) is indicated for use in sheep. At a dose of 0.5–1.0 mg/kg body weight, decoquinate effectively controls shedding of oocysts and thereby increases weight gains. Decoquinate acts at the early schizogony stage and is recommended for feeding to lambs or ewes for 28 days when coccidiosis is anticipated or is a hazard. The normal inclusion rate using the premix in lambs is 100 ppm active ingredient and in ewes is 50 ppm. Like many other coccidiostatic drugs (e.g., monensin), decoquinate is also effective against toxoplasma. Decoquinate at elevated dosages is extremely safe in ruminants, and toxicity has not been reported.

Use of ionophores, such as lasalocid or monensin, in growing sheep and goats may also increase feed utilization in addition to preventing coccidiosis through selective alteration of rumen microflora. Proper use of coccidiostats results in more economic production and greater profits for the producer.

Sulfa drugs, as sulfamethazine and sulfadimethoxine, are also used to treat coccidiosis. Sulfamethoxypyridazine ("Midicel") at a dose of 22 mg/kg is particularly effective for individual treatment of coccidiosis.

27.5 TOXOPLASMOSIS

Toxoplasmosis has long been recognized as one of the main causes of ovine abortion. Perinatal deaths caused by *Toxoplasma gondii* probably are more common than reported because diagnosis of abortion in sheep is difficult and expensive. (Other causes are important also, such as salmonellosis, iodine deficiency, selenium deficiency, and viruses.)

Abortion "storms" due to toxoplasma generally occur during the last 3 to 6 weeks of gestation, when most ewes are at a similar stage of pregnancy.

Toxoplasmosis abortions in the ewe flock have become an increasing problem for lamb producers and usually entail the expulsion of mummified fetuses. Abortion of sets of twins and triplets often involves combinations of mummified fetuses and more normal-appearing lambs.

Toxoplasmosis is usually transmitted by oral ingestion of a feed or bedding source contaminated with infected cat feces.

When abortions or stillbirths occur, toxoplasmosis is frequently diagnosed as an important cause of otherwise unexplained outbreaks of perinatal mortality in sheep. This problem creates major economic losses to the industry.

Toxoplasma oocysts shed in cat feces are easily dispersed by wind, rain, rodent movements, birds, humans, and farm machinery. These oocysts are the primary source of toxoplasmic infection in sheep. Cats, therefore, should not be allowed to contaminate foodstuffs or bedding destined for use by pregnant sheep.

From a management point of view, sheep that have aborted once because of *T. gondii* infection should be saved for future breeding because this parasite rarely causes subsequent abortion. Unfortunately, many sheep producers tend to sell ewes that have aborted and thus lose their valuable immune stock. *T. gondii* infections in sheep are sporadic, and the parasite is not transmitted from sheep to sheep. Infected sheep cannot be distinguished from noninfected sheep without a serologic test. Furthermore, the causes of abortion and neonatal mortality in sheep are numerous.

The economic impact of *T. gondii* infection to the sheep industry can be determined only by investigating and reporting the specific diagnosis of abortion. Simple, efficient, and inexpensive tests are needed for each infectious agent. The detection of *T. gondii* antibodies in fetal sera or fluids in the modified agglutination test meets some of the criteria for the diagnosis of toxoplasmic abortion.

Toxoplasmosis is a true zoonosis occurring naturally in humans, in domesticated and wild animals, and in birds. Survey data based on serologic findings indicate for the United States a high incidence in dogs, in cats, in cattle, in pigs, and also in goats, as well. Cats are an important reservoir for humans, as well as sheep.

Toxoplasmic infection of the pregnant woman has special epidemiologic significance because accumulated data support the concept that transplacental transmission occurs to the fetus. Congenital infection occurs in approximately one third of infants born to mothers who acquire infection during pregnancy.

Toxoplasmic infection has been estimated to be the cause of approximately 35% of cases of chorioretinitis in children and adults. Chorioretinitis occurs most often as a consequence of congenital toxoplasmic infection.

TOXOPLASMA ABORTION

Toxoplasmosis is one of the most commonly diagnosed causes of abortion in sheep. As already stated, high rates of infection with *T. gondii* occur in sheep, and cats are common carriers. Toxoplasmosis is one of the common causes of late abortion in sheep and deaths in neonatal lambs. When many abortions occur late in pregnancy, this parasite should be considered as a possible cause. Sporadic abortions in late pregnancy may reflect the susceptibility of individual ewes on a farm in which the disease is endemic.

Cats can amplify and spread the infection through their feces in the form of resistant oocysts, often by contaminating concentrated feed, hay, and bedding.

Abortions occur late in pregnancy, usually during the last 3 to 6 weeks. As much as 50% of the flock may abort, and a high neonatal death rate may accompany outbreaks. The parasite invades the placenta, thus producing a severe placentitis, and subsequently infects the fetus. The placental lesions consist of white flecks containing actively multiplying organisms.

Full-term lambs may be born dead or alive and weak, in which case they die in a few days. Few gross abnormalities are evident when lambs are aborted at full term or at an earlier stage.

Clinical effects of infection include neonatal death, abortion, stillbirth, and fetal death, mummification, and resorption. The severity of the disease is directly correlated with the ewe's stage of pregnancy when infected. Infection of ewes during early pregnancy (fewer than 50 days) commonly results in fetal death and resorption. Infection at midpregnancy (70 to 90 days) results in fetal death, stillborn lambs, or weak lambs that die soon after birth. Infection during late gestation (more than 100 days) results in congenitally infected lambs that will usually live. Clinical disease is rare in adult sheep.

Once animals have been infected with *Toxoplasma*, they are generally immune to the disease for the rest of their lives.

A single dose of a recently introduced toxoplasma vaccine gives a minimum of 2 years of protection from the disease. Vaccination does not prevent the animal from contracting natural *Toxoplasma*, but does protect against its harmful effects, i.e., abortion and infertility. Therefore, natural antibody should develop normally.

Regarding chemotherapy, treatment of toxoplasmosis has proved generally unrewarding. However, the incidence of fetal deaths following infection with *T. gondii* can be significantly reduced and the birth weights of the live lambs significantly increased if pregnant sheep are fed prophylactically with the coccidiostat.

To be effective against both abortion and barrenness, a medication must be fed during the whole gestation period. To date, monensin sodium, fed at 15 mg/head/day, is the most commonly used medication. Monensin at this dose has its major effect in the gut lumen, where it suppresses the subsequent orally acquired infection. Results have shown that it significantly increases both the weight and the number of live lambs born.

For monensin to be effective it is necessary to deliver the daily oral dose from before the time susceptible pregnant sheep are exposed to oocyst-contaminated feed.

Monensin is not ideal, however, because it is not licensed for use in sheep; the margin for error between the prophylactic and toxic doses is slight; and cross-contamination of feed at the mill can create a toxicity hazard for other animal species. Lasalocid and salinomycin are other ionophores that can be relatively effective.

Although the feeding of ionophores to prevent toxoplasma abortions in ewes is experimental, results suggest that in the absence of more specific medication, they may be worth using. With regard to ionophores, recent trials have shown that in-feed medication with 2 mg decoquinate/kg body weight/day for 8 weeks prior to lambing reduced abortions and perinatal losses from toxoplasmosis by 80% compared to abortions and losses in unmedicated ewe lambs. Earlier commencement of medication might provide more complete protection.

Experiments in nonpregnant sheep, decoquinate fed at 2 mg/kg body weight/day had the same effect as monensin in suppressing the early febrile response to challenge infection with *Toxoplasma*.

The 2-mg/kg body weight/day of decoquinate resulted in a statistically significant reduction in the severity of *Toxoplasma* infection in pregnant ewes, when compared to unmedicated controls. In addition, the high safety and good palatability of decoquinate may allow economical use at high concentrations in small quantities of feed.

Coccidiostatic agents therefore apparently can play a significant therapeutic/prophylactic role against these virulent unicellular toxoplasmic protozoa.

27.6 FOOT ROT

Foot rot is probably one of the oldest recorded diseases in sheep. It is a highly contagious infectious disease of mixed bacteria that can occur as a spectacular outbreak of lameness affecting practically all the sheep in the flock at the same time. It can cause severe lameness by affecting all four feet simultaneously. Extensive lameness in a flock of sheep can cause considerable economic loss from sheep of all ages. The main types of losses resulting from lameness are:

1. Poor performance in grazing sheep of all ages resulting from reduced feed intake
2. Reduced performance resulting from pain
3. Reduced fertility in rams
4. Premature culling
5. Cost of treatment in terms of time and medications
6. Death in severe cases

The effects of foot rot on production are:

1. Lower growth rates in infected lot-fed lambs
2. Decreased wool production in diseased animals
3. Additional losses resulting from emergency slaughter and poorly developed lambs born to diseased ewes

Losses from decreased wool production are caused by the infected animal's loss of condition and difficulty in breeding. The hind legs of both the ram and the ewe must be in good shape for the proper servicing to take place.

Under pen conditions, decreased weight gains and lower wool growth rates have occurred in sheep experimentally infected with foot rot. Weight losses attributable to foot rot, and also the magnitude of the loss, were related to the virulence of the infecting organism.

Foot rot is prevalent in sheep because a predisposing causative agent, the gram-negative anaerobe *Fusobacterium necrophorum*, (Sphaerophorus necrophorus) is nearly always present in a normal sheep environment.

Transmission of foot rot occurs in warm, moist conditions in animals already made susceptible by previous episodes of water maceration, frostbite, or mechanical trauma. *Bacteroides nodosus* and *Fusobacterium necrophorum*, pathogenic synergists, cause contagious foot rot. Other organisms, such as *Corynebacterium pyogenes*, often enter lesions and play an unknown role in the pathogenesis. Although *Fusobacterium necrophorum* plays a major initial role in the pathogenesis, the severity of the lesion depends on the virulence of *Bacteroides nodosus*. *Bacteroides nodosus* lives for just a few days in soil or pasture; therefore, infected animals must be present if the disease is to be spread. The disease, however, can persist for years in some sheep, thus making these animals subclinical carriers.

As stated, the invasion of the foot by these bacteria is assisted by climatic conditions. Adequate moisture and temperature are necessary for the bacteria to penetrate the skin. Consequently, this disease is quite common in lowland flocks grazing lush pastures.

Because one of the main etiologic agents is *Bacteroides nodosus*, elimination of *B. nodosus* from a flock, by either chemotherapy or culling of affected animals, can result in permanent eradication of the disease because *B. nodosus* does not persist in the environment.

The primary invasion site for foot rot is the skin between the claws. The resulting strain of the infection—benign or virulent—depends on the strain of *B. nodosus* involved. Virulent foot rot starts as an interdigital dermatitis and progresses to involve large areas of hoof matrix.

The pili of *B. nodosus* are the antigens used for the serologic classification of strains and also are the major antigens eliciting protection against foot rot in homologous, but not heterologous, serogroup challenge. Fimbrial antigens stimulate a serotype-specific immunity that has resulted in the development of multivalent vaccines. In the United States, at least 14 serotypes (I to XIV) have been described, although some of these are closely related by sharing major pilus antigens. (Nine major serotypes have been described in the United Kingdom, and 22 have been described elsewhere.)

Traditionally, chemotherapy of *B. nodosus* infections has been based on topical treatment using antibacterial compounds, such as formalin or zinc sulfate. The combination of the antibiotics procaine penicillin and dihydrostreptomycin sulfate administered at high dose rates, however, also effectively cures a high proportion of affected animals, providing that dry conditions prevail at the time of treatment.

This treatment, along with good management practices to maintain top sanitation and to keep animals as uncrowded and stress free as possible, can help sheep farmers to avoid the economic losses this highly contagious disease can cause.

Treatment of foot rot in sheep requires aggressive foot paring which is necessary to get good results from topical therapy of foot rot characterized by progressive necrotizing inflammation of the soft horn. The lame sheep should be treated individually by paring back the diseased horn and applying 10% formalin or antibiotics to the diseased tissue.

Normal sheep should have their feet trimmed and should pass through a clean footbath containing 10% formalin, stand on a clean area for a few hours, and then move to a fresh pasture.

Brought-in sheep should be footbathed on arrival and preferably kept in isolation for 3 weeks.

B. nodosus is susceptible to penicillin via parenteral injections or can be killed by direct contact with zinc sulfate, copper sulfate, or formalin. The more than 22 serotypes of *B. nodosus* have different invasive, virulent, and immunogenic properties.

Copper sulfate and formalin have been the standard materials used in footbaths. More recently, a 10 to 20% zinc sulfate solution with 2% sodium lauryl sulfate has proved as effective as formalin or copper sulfate.

The use of formalin must be preceded by foot paring and must be followed by a period of draining and drying on a hard surface to exert therapeutic effect.

Of the three topical chemical products currently used for footbath solutions (zinc sulfate, copper sulfate, and formalin), only zinc sulfate has no irritating fumes. It also is nontoxic to both shepherd and sheep, does not stain the wool, and is nonirritating to the skin. The penetration of zinc sulfate may be enhanced by increasing the footbathing time or using a penetrating agent, such as the anionic detergent sodium lauryl sulfate. Because moderately good results have been achieved with zinc sulfate, the agent is undergoing a renewal of interest.

Parenteral antibiotics have a fairly high cure rate and have the added advantage of reaching the undetected sequestered lesion.

Penicillin is still an effective antibiotic, even when compared with a wide range of antimicrobials tested, including the newer antibiotics cephalosporin and clindamycin. In field evaluation tests of penicillin, streptomycin, neomycin, oxytetracycline, erythromycin, and sulfonamides, only high doses of erythromycin, or penicillin with streptomycin, were effective in treating foot rot.

A lincomycin-spectinomycin combination has been increasingly promoted as an excellent fastworking treatment for foot rot. Because this combination has proved at least as efficacious as penicillin with streptomycin for the therapy of foot rot in sheep, it may be considered as a valuable alternative therapeutic treatment.

Two of the notable aspects of lincomycin-spectinomycin treatment for foot rot are its effectiveness against gram-negative anaerobic bacteria, such as *Fusobacterium necrophorum*, and its effective antibiotic penetration even into dense bony tissues.

The Lincomycin-spectinomycin combination alone and the lincomycin-spectinomycin combination plus formalin footbaths have proved to be highly effective against foot rot under fixed conditions.

SELECTED REFERENCES

Baker, N.F., Walters, G.T., and Fisk, R.A.: Amprolium for control of coccidiosis in feedlot lambs. Am. J. Vet. Res., 33:83, 1972.

Beattie, C.P.: The ecology of toxoplasmosis. Ecology Dis., 1(1):13, 1982.

Bergstrom, R.C., and Maki, L.R.: Coccidiostatic action of monensin fed to lambs: Body weight gains and feed conversion efficacy. Am. J. Vet. Res., 37:79, 1976.

Bergstrom, R.C., and Maki, L.R.: Effect of monensin in young crossbred lambs with naturally occurring coccidiosis. J. Am. Vet. Med. Assoc., 165:288, 1974.

Beverly, J.K.A., and Watson, W.A.: Prevention of experimental and naturally occurring ovine abortion due to toxoplasmosis. Vet. Rec., 88:39, 1971.

Boray, J.C., Crowfoot, P.D., Strong, M.B., et al.: Treatment of immature and mature Fasciola hepatica infections in sheep with triclabendazole. Vet. Rec., 113:315, 1983.

Bulgin, M.S., Lincoln, S.D., Lane, V.M., et al.: Comparison of treatment methods for the control of contagious ovine foot rot. J. Am. Vet. Med. Assoc., 189:194, 1986.

Bulgin, M., Lincoln, S.D., Lane, V.M., et al.: Evaluating an ovine foot-rot vaccine. Vet. Med., 80:105, 1985.

Buxton, D., Donald, K.M., and Finlayson, J.: Monensin and the control of experimental ovine toxoplasmosis: A systemic effect. Vet. Rec., 120:618, 1987.

Chetwin, D.H., Liardet, D.M., Kingsley, D.F., and Hindmarsh, F.H.: Foot rot in Ruminants: Proceedings of a Workshop, Melbourne, 1985. Edited by D.J. Stewart, et al. CSIRO, Div. of Animal Health/Australian Wool Corp., Glebe, New South Wales, 1986.

Craig, T.M.: Epidemiology and control of coccidia in goats. Vet. Clin. North Am. (Food Anim. Pract.), 2:389, 1986.

Day, S.E.J., Thorley, C.M., and Beelsey, J.E.: Foot rot in Ruminants: Proceedings of a Workshop, Melbourne, 1985. Edited by D.J. Stewart, et al. CSIRO, Div. of Animal Health/Australian Wool Corp., Glebe, New South Wales, 1986.

Demertzis, P.N., Spais, A.G., and Papasteriadis, A.A.: Zinc therapy in the control of foot rot in sheep. Vet. Med. Rev., 1:101, 1978.

Dennis, S.M.: Perinatal Lamb Mortality in Western Australia. Aust. Vet. J., 50(10):443, 1974.

Dubey, J.P.: Status of toxoplasmosis in sheep and goats in the United States. J. Am. Vet. Med. Assoc., 196:259, 1990.

Dubey, J.P., and Beattie, C.P.: Toxoplasmosis of Animals and Man. Boca Raton, FL, CRC Press, 1988.

Dubey, J.P., and Kirkbride, C.A.: Epizootics of ovine abortion due to Toxoplasma gondii in northcentral United States. J. Am. Vet. Med. Assoc., 184:657, 1984.

Dubey, J.P., Miller, S., Powell, E.C., et al.: Epizootiologic investigations on a sheep farm with Toxoplasma gondii-induced abortions. J. Am. Vet. Med. Assoc., 188:155, 1986.

Dubey, J.P., and Towle, A.: Toxoplasmosis in sheep: a review and annotated bibliography. Miscellaneous publication No. 10. London, Commonwealth Institute of Parasitology, 1986.

Dwyer, P.J.: Ovine perinatal mortality. In Sheep: Production, Disease and Marketing. Edited by P.J. Dwyer, J.F. Quinlan, and W.O. McMickan. Dublin, Dept. of Agriculture, Government Publications Office, 1984.

Eales, A.: Update: watery mouth. In Practice, 9:12, 1987.

Egerton, J.R., et al.: Protection of sheep against foot rot with a recombinant DNA-based fimbrial vaccine. Vet. Microbiol., 14:393, 1987.

Egerton, J.R., Parsonson, I.M., and Graham, N.P.H.: Parenteral chemotherapy of ovine foot rot. Aust. Vet. J., 44:284, 1968.

Foreyt, W.J.: Epidemiology and control of coccidia in sheep. Vet. Clin. North Am. (Food Anim. Pract.), 2:383, 1986.

Foreyt, W.J., and Hunter, R.L.: Clinical Fascioloides magna infection in sheep on Oregon pasture shared by Columbian white-tailed deer. Am. J. Vet. Res., 41:1531, 1980.

Foreyt, W.J., Gates, N.L., and Rich, J.E.: Evaluation of lasalocid in salt against ovine coccidia. Am. J. Vet. Res., 42:54, 1981.

Foreyt, W.J., Parish, S.M., and Foreyt, K.M.: Lasalocid for improved weight gains and control of coccidia in lambs. Am. J. Vet. Res., 42:57, 1981.

Gregory, E., Foreyt, W.J., and Breeze, R.: Efficacy of ivermectin and fenbendazole against lungworms. Vet. Med., 80:114, 1985.

Herd, R.P.: A practical approach to parasite control in sheep in northern United States. Compend. Contin. Educ. Pract. Vet., 6:S67, 1984.

Herd, R.P., Streitel, R.H., McClure, K.E., et al.: Control of hypobiotic and benzimidazole-resistant nematodes of sheep. J. Am. Vet. Med. Assoc., 184:726, 1984.

Herd, R.P., Streitel, R.H., McClure, K.E., et al.: Control of periparturient rise in worm egg counts of lambing ewes. J. Am. Vet. Med. Assoc., 182:375, 1983.

Hindmarsh, F., and Fraser, J.: Serogroups of Bacteroides nodosus isolated from ovine foot rot in Britain. Vet. Rec., 116:187, 1985.

Horton, G.M.J., and Stockdale, P.H.G.: Effects of amprolium and monensin on oocyst discharge, feed utilization, and rumen metabolism of lambs with coccidiosis. Am. J. Vet. Res., 40:966, 1979.

Houston, D.C., and Maddox, J.G.: Causes of mortality among young Scottish blackface lambs. Vet. Rec., 95:575, 1974.

Huffman, E.M., Kirk, J.H., and Pappaioanou, M.: Factors associated with neonatal lamb mortality. Theriogenology, 24:163, 1985.

Linklater, K.A.: Abortion in sheep. In Practice 1(1):30, 1979.

Masur, H., Jones, T.C., Lewipert, J.A., and Cherubins, T.A.: Outbreak of toxoplasmosis in family and documentation of acquired retinochorioditis. Am. J. Med., 64:396, 1978.

Pout, D.D.: Coccidiosis of sheep: A review. Vet. Rec., 98:340, 1976.

Quinn, P.J.: Toxoplasmosis in Irish sheep: Epidemiological and public health aspects of this zoonosis.

Proc. Eighth Int. Symposium of the World Assoc. Veterinary Food Hygienists, 1981.

Rook, J., Bartlett, P., Trapp, A., et al.: Lamb mortality—a reflection of flock health. In Proc., 65th Annual Postgraduate Conference, Michigan State Univ., College of Veterinary Medicine, East Lansing, January 25, 1988.

Salman, M.D., Dargatz, D.A., Kimberling, C.V., et al.: An economic evaluation of various treatments for contagious foot rot in sheep using decision analysis. J. Am. Vet. Med. Assoc., 193:195, 1988.

Samizadeh-Yazd, A., Rhodes, C.N., and Tott, A.C.: Ovine coccidiosis: Comparison of the effects of monensin and aureomycin on lambs infected with coccodia. Am. J. Vet. Res., 40:1107, 1979.

Smeal, M.G., and Hall, C.A.: The activity of triclabendazole against immature and adult *Fasciola hepatica* infections in sheep. Aust. Vet. J., 60:329, 1983.

Stewart, D.J., Peterson, J.E., Vaughan, J.A., et al.: The pathogenicity and cultural characteristics of virulent, intermediate, and benign strains of *Bacteroides nodosus* causing ovine foot rot. Aust. Vet. J., 63:317, 1986.

Stott, K.J.: Foot rot in Ruminants. Proceedings of a Workshop, Melbourne, 1985. Edited by D.J. Stewart, et al. CSIRO, Div. of Animal Health/Australian Wool Corp., Glebe, New South Wales, 1986.

Throley, C.M., and Day, S.E.J.: Foot rot in Ruminants. Proceedings of a Workshop, Melbourne, 1985. Edited by D.J. Stewart, et al. CSIRO, Div. of Animal Health/Australian Wool Corp., Glebe, New South Wales, 1986.

Tritschler, J.P., Giordano, D.J., and Coles, G.C.: Anthelmintic usage by New England sheep farmers. In Proc. Am. Assoc. Vet. Parasitologists, Las Vegas, NV, 1985.

Turner, K., Armour, J., and Richards, R.J.: Anthelmintic efficacy of triclabendazole against *Fasciola hepatica* in sheep. Vet. Rec., 114:41, 1984.

Uggla, A., Sjoland, L., and Dubey, J.P.: Immunohistochemical diagnosis of toxoplasmosis in fetuses and fetal membranes of sheep. Am. J. Vet. Res., 48:348, 1987.

Waller, P.J., and Thomas, R.J.: The natural regulation of *Trichostrongylus* spp. populations in young grazing sheep. Vet. Parasitol., 9:47, 1981.

Wescott, R.B., and LeaMaster, B.R.: Efficacy of ivermectin against naturally acquired and experimentally induced nematode infections in sheep. Am. J. Vet. Res., 43:531, 1982.

Whitelaw, A.: Survey of perinatal losses associated with intensive hill sheep farming. Vet. Annu., 16:60, 1976.

Whitelaw, A., and Fawcett, A.R.: Further studies in the control of bovine fascioliasis by strategic dosing. Vet. Rec., 109:188, 1981.

Winklen, C.E.: Lamb survival. Vet. Rec., 108:15, 1981.

Wolff, K., Eckert, J., Schneiter, G., et al.: Efficacy of triclabendazole against *Fasciola hepatica* in sheep and goats. Vet. Parasitol., 13:145, 1983.

Zimmerman, G.L., Jen, L.W., Cerro, J.E., et al.: Diagnosis of *Fasciola hepatica* infections in sheep by an enzyme-linked immunosorbent assay. Am. J. Vet. Res., 43:2097, 1982.

CHAPTER

28

TRACE ELEMENT DEFICIENCIES

28.1 Copper
28.2 Cobalt
28.3 Selenium and Vitamin E
28.4 Iodine

28.1 COPPER

Copper is one of the most complex trace elements involved in animal metabolism especially in cattle and sheep. It is required in the structure and function of many enzymes and is involved in most oxidative reactions, and metabolic pathways.

Surplus copper in the body is retained and accumulates in the liver where it is available for later use if required. Therefore, clinical signs of a copper-deficiency may not appear for many months, e.g., 4 to 5 months for scours or changes in coat color. When the period of copper deficiency is short, the liver stores may be adequate to make up the deficiency, by releasing stored copper into the circulation.

The classic signs of copper deficiency in cattle are scours and the typical change in coat color. Because copper is required in the formation of bone, a deficiency often results in increased bone fragility, the formation of shorter, broader long bones, and a lack of elasticity, e.g., in the pelvis. This latter effect may result in increased dystocia especially in heifers. Because of this, copper is essential for reproductive function. Responses to copper therapy in deficient animals result in increases in milk production and usually an increase in the conception rate.

Dietary copper requirements of cattle are higher than that of sheep. The amount of copper required depends on the presence of several other inhibitory dietary constituents that can affect copper absorption.

Copper is required for the metabolic function of a dozen or more enzymes involved in numerous specific oxidase-type reactions in animals. Grazing animals are usually affected by copper deficiency before plant growth is affected. In cattle, copper is required for mitochondrial function and energy transfer, for tissue and bone growth, for pigmentation of hair, and for leukocyte function. Copper is intimately associated with phagocytic function and the immune status of ruminants.

The lesions and signs caused by copper deficiency are the result of a reduced activity of specific copper-dependent enzymes. The fundamental biochemical basis for such lesions, however, has not been established, and various other aspects of cytology, development, and metabolism may be involved.

Although widespread supplementation of pastures and animals with copper, has been practiced clinical disorders caused by deficiencies of copper continue to be major problems in grazing cattle. Many problems in grazing animals are attributable to new methods of pasture management, introduction of different grasses by variations in seasonal pasture growth, by soil ingestion, by the use of modern fertilizers, and by the strong influence of other dietary components, such as molybdenum, sulfur, and iron, on copper absorption and storage. These inhibitory dietary sources are routinely present in many pastures.

Copper as a nutritional element is found in adequate amounts in pastures in most areas. Deficient areas have been reported in Florida and in the coastal plains region of the Southeast. Copper can be provided conveniently in deficient areas by adding copper sulfate to the salt at a rate of about 0.5%. Stores of copper in the liver serve as a reserve for as long as 4 to 6 months when animals are grazing copper-deficient forage.

AVAILABILITY AND REQUIREMENTS

Copper can form insoluble, or non-absorbable, complexes with many other elements. Copper interacts metabolically with many other substances, including zinc, iron, cadmium, molybdenum, sulfur, and ascorbic acid. The interaction between copper, zinc, and cadmium is probably the result of a decrease in the efficiency of absorption and partly of changes in the distribution among body tissues. This interaction appears to be directly related to competition for binding with the carrier protein metallothionein, a cysteine-rich protein that is found in hepatic, renal, and intestinal mucosal cells. The interaction between copper, molybdenum, and is of paramount importance in ruminants, and the formation of thiomolybdates have been suggested as the active components in this interaction. These compounds, which are synthesized in the rumen by microorganisms acting on dietary molybdenum and sulfur, reduce the absorption of copper from the gut and therefore lower the amount and availability of copper at metabolic sites of action. The copper, molybdenum, and sulfur content of pastures and forages varies with the species of plant, soil conditions, and fertilizers used. Grasses tend to be higher in molybdenum and lower in copper than are legumes grown in the same conditions.

Although the application of copper-containing fertilizers to soils low in copper-containing plants generally increases the copper content of the herbage, the amount and frequency of application required varies with the soil and climatic conditions. In particular, on alkaline soils, molybdenum levels can be very high and granite soils, heavy application of lime can significantly raise molybdenum levels.

ABSORPTION

Of critical significance is the syndrome of secondary copper deficiency, where the actual copper level of the herbage is considered adequate, but some other factor exerts an inhibitory influence on the availability of the ingested copper in the gut. Iron, molybdenum and sulfur all adversely affect the biological availability of copper, even where pasture copper levels are adequate. It is accepted that iron does not disturb copper metabolism in preruminant calves, but does disturb such after weaning. High dietary iron reduces copper in the liver and plasma of calves, but as a rule does not induce clinical signs of copper deficiency. High intakes of iron and reduced copper levels in calves, however, create susceptibility to the adverse effects of molybdenum on growth rate. Iron oxide also inhibits copper absorption from the ovine gut.

Molybdenum and sulfur are the most important ingested factors that suppress the extent of copper absorption. The antagonistic effect of molybdenum results from its combination with sulfur in the rumen to form thiomolybdates. The formation of these compounds is effected by the rumen microorganisms and the synthesis of sulfide from dietary sources of sulfate or sulfur amino acids. The resultant Thiomolybdates inhibit both the absorption of copper and its incorporation into the copper-dependent enzymes, such as caeruloplasmin, superoxide dismutase, and cytochrome oxidase.

The best known inhibitory factor is molybdenum. When the copper-molybdenum level ratio is less than 5:1, ingested copper and molybdenum can form insoluble copper molybdate complexes that are not available for absorption from the gut. Molybdenum is the primary cause of induced (or secondary) copper deficiency (hypocuprosis).

High molybdenum levels in pasture may occur under a number of circumstances:

1. Soil naturally high in molybdenum i.e., molybdeniferous marine shales; clover swards
2. Improved pastures. No top dressings have been used to increase the rate of production of nitrogen-fixing bacteria
3. Wet pastures. Molybdenum is absorbed from the soil to leaf more abundantly when soil is wet, and drainage is poor
4. Lime pastures. Again, liming can cause plants to take up high molybdenum levels from the soil
5. High soil pH, and clover dominated pastures tend to be high in Mo

High levels of sulfur in the herbage or diet lead to the formation of cupric sulfide in the rumen. Cupric sulfide is relatively insoluble and, as such, renders dietary copper unavailable to the animal.

Herbage Copper Concentration

Grasses generally contain lower copper concentrations than do clovers. Providing the cattle have enough pasture to eat and the diet does not contain excessive amounts of factors (molybdenum, sulfur, iron), that reduce the availability of the copper, deficiency should not be a problem.

High dietary intakes of molybdenum, sulfur, iron, zinc, cadmium, and calcium decrease the availability of dietary copper to animals. Liming of pastures can result in an overall decrease in the copper available to plants and animals.

The levels of inhibitory factors and the degree to which these various interactions may be present, and the intensity of their effects on different tissues, may lead to various copper-responsive conditions in cattle.

CLINICAL SIGNS OF DEFICIENCY

Because copper is involved in so many and varied metabolic processes, the clinical signs of deficiency may vary according to age, breed, nutritional status, and geographic location. Usually, all animals in a group do not show the same degree of clinical signs of copper deficiency at the same time.

Generally, copper deficiency is associated with decreased weight gain, scours, depigmentation of hair and wool, impaired keratinization, anemia, cardiovascular disorders, bone disorders, infertility, immune status dysfunction and the development of enzootic ataxia. In sheep, loss of wool crimp with the production of "steely wool," lack of pigment from wool, and the development of enzootic ataxia or "swayback" in lambs are the most common signs of copper deficiency. Lambs that are born with enzootic ataxia, the congenital form of the disease, may have cavities within their cerebral white matter.

Copper is also intrinsically connected with the immune competence, and phagocytosing, ability of the host animal. Increased disease susceptibility follows copper deficiency.

Hair Coat Abnormalities

The fading of coat color (a "burnt" color in black cattle) and the development of thin, sparse, dry hair are some of the earliest signs associated with copper deficiency in young cattle, e.g., brownish colored Herefords and golden-tinged black cattle. These signs of copper deficiency are usually seen before growth becomes stunted. The hair, particularly around the ear margins and eyes, usually shows the first changes, of discoloration.

Changes in color and texture of hair coat are not necessarily specific for diagnosis of copper deficiency because similar changes also occur with cobalt deficiency and also with retention of the winter coat caused by debilitation from severe internal nematode infection (e.g., Hemonchus).

Retarded Growth

This problem can be one of the earliest signs of copper deficiency. Copper or caeruloplasmin levels in plasma usually must indicate deficiency for at least 4–6 weeks before weight gains from copper supplementation occur.

Diarrhea

Diarrhea is a common but not consistent clinical sign of copper deficiency in cattle. It is nonspecific, and an association with copper deficiency can usually be suspected when cattle with diarrhea have not responded to anthelmintic treatments.

Scours may arise from primary or secondary copper deficiency. Low dietary intake of copper (the so called "primary" or "classical" copper deficiency) lowers cytochrome oxidase levels in intestinal epithelium, and partial atrophy of the villi occurs. This villus atrophy leads to malabsorption, loss of weight, ill thrift and variable diarrhea.

High molybdenum concentrations in lush herbage are commonly associated with diarrhea. This responds rapidly to copper given by injection. On pastures high in molybdenum, cattle may develop diarrhea before liver reserves have depleted and blood copper stores have decreased.

Miscellaneous Signs

Anemia can be a sign of copper deficiency that develops late in the disorder.

Skeletal defects in calves with copper deficiency may be seen as thickened epiphyses around the fetlock and as swelling and stiffness of the joints.

Infertility has also been associated with severe copper deficiency, Molybdenum excess has been regarded as important in reducing fertility in cattle.

DIAGNOSIS

Many factors should be taken into account when making a diagnosis of copper deficiency. The presence of certain aspects of a clinical syndrome may help in diagnosis, e.g., enzootic ataxia in lambs indicating copper deficiency. Determinations of copper in the diet, pasture, or tissue must be made, but the results are of limited value unless the concentrations of other interacting elements are also determined. Copper values in the liver (liver biopsy) may give a good indication of body stores, but as with copper levels in the blood, the normal range is variable, and levels can show rapid reductions during depletion while the animal remains clinically normal. Copper content of the blood changes during pregnancy and after birth, and the serum contains less copper than does plasma because caeruloplasmin is lost during clotting. Serial samples from a few individuals are much more likely to give useful information regarding copper status of a group than are single samples taken from many individuals. Copper values in hair and fleece have also been used to assess the copper status of animals.

Changes in the activities of several copper metalloenzymes, such as caeruloplasmin, cytochrome oxidase, and amine oxidase, in the blood and tissues have been used to diagnose copper deficiency. More recently, copper superoxide dismutase has been used also as a diagnostic tool and usually a useful indicator of copper status in ruminants.

Assessment of Copper Status

A good indication of the copper status of grazing cattle can be obtained from analysis of copper or copper-containing enzymes in plasma or erythrocytes or in liver samples. Individual samples from suspect herds or flocks are not very useful.

For diagnostic purposes, whole blood samples, collected in heparinized containers from a representative number of animals, or preferably from 10% of those at risk, should be sent to the laboratory. Follow-up, or serial, samples should be taken.

Erythrocytes usually contain less than one half of the blood copper. In erythrocytes, more than one half of the copper occurs as superoxide dismutase, an enzyme which also contains zinc. The remaining copper in the erythrocyte is more loosely bound to protein and in a more labile form. Then, the plasma caeruloplasmin and copper concentration decrease.

Copper Concentration in Plasma

Blood levels, although commonly used, are not reliable indicators of copper status. The caeruloplasmin contains approximately 80 to 90% of the copper in plasma. Low levels of copper or caeruloplasmin in plasma reflect depletion of copper reserves in the liver, but do not necessarily reflect the depletion of copper-dependent enzymes in tissues. Differences in these tissue enzyme changes appear to be necessary for development of the pathologic changes or reductions in production. These enzymes take about a month to become important after the copper level in plasma has decreased to low levels.

Copper Concentration in Erythrocytes

In the erythrocytes, up to 75% of the copper is present in the enzyme copper superoxide dismutase. Because the lifespan of erythrocytes is about 120 days, and copper superoxide dismutase is synthesized at the stage of erythropoiesis, copper concentration in erythrocytes therefore depends on the copper intake of the animal during the previous several months.

Overall, copper concentration in liver is the best indicator of copper sufficiency, or copper stores, whereas blood is a more convenient sample to obtain for estimation of inadequate intake. Also, plasma concentrations (free copper) reflect short-term copper nutrition, whereas enzyme-fixed erythrocyte concentrations reflect long-term copper nutrition. Simultaneous measurements of both of these indicators can determine whether the cattle are in an ascending, descending, or steady state of copper nutrition.

TREATMENT AND PREVENTION

Prevention of copper deficiency can be achieved by:

1. Oral administration of copper in sustained release formulations
2. Injection of copper salts
3. Inclusion of copper salts in concentrate feed or water
4. Ad libitum provision of mineral supplements
5. Top dressing pasture with copper salts
6. Altering pasture management

The two basic methods of prophylaxis against copper deficiency in ewes and

---

TABLE 28–1
COPPER TREATMENTS

Injectable Preparations	Oral Preparations
1. Copper glycinate	1. Copper sulfate
2. Diethylamine cupro-oxyquinolone sulfonate available copper 6 mg/ml	2. Copper oxide needles
3. Copper heptonate	3. Cosecure: 13.3% w/w Cu as CuO, 0.3% w/w Se as Na_2SeO_4, w/we Co as Co_3O_4.
4. Copper methionate	Controlled-release glass formulations
5. Copper calcium EDTA	

Injectable Therapy for CATTLE

1. 100 mg copper to pregnant animals at 6 to 7 months gestation (to supply fetus with adequate reserves)
2. 100 mg copper to cows post calving to restore blood levels before service
3. 50 mg copper to calves just prior to first grazing period at 2 to 3 months of age
4. 100 mg copper at 6 to 9 months of age to maintain levels
5. 100 mg copper repeated as required every 3 to 6 months.

Injectable Therapy for SHEEP

1. 40 mg copper at 4 to 6 weeks before lambing to supply fetus and avoid swayback
2. 90 mg copper methionine may be given to the ewe at lambing to maintain copper levels until weaning via milk

---

swayback in lambs that are currently available are:

1. Slow-release capsules introduced into the abomasum by mouth
2. Long-acting injectable organic copper compounds (Tables 28–1 and 28–2).

All forms of copper therapy are potentially dangerous to sheep.

The manufacturer's recommendations as to dose rate for each compound should be strictly observed and care must be taken to ensure that no other copper compounds are available to sheep. The susceptibility of some breeds to copper toxicity should be considered, and in all cases, a low concentration of copper in the blood must be ensured before administration.

Oral Administration of Copper

Typical oral doses of copper sulfate (usually the pentahydrate form containing 25% by weight of copper) for sheep are 10 to 15 mg/kg body weight.

In cattle older than about 4 months of age, oral doses of 4 g copper sulfate (1 g copper) have been used to correct copper deficiency.

Dietary manipulation or oral treatments are effective for chronic primary deficiency. In severe and acute deficiencies, particularly if alimentary absorption is impaired, parenteral treatments are best for restoring normal copper concentration in the animal. Because no significant transfer of copper occurs from cow to calf through milk, cows and calves require separate treatment.

Oral drenching with an aqueous solution containing copper sulfate is useful for primary copper deficiency only. Because as much as 95% of a single dose may be excreted, the treatment must be repeated frequently to be effective. Such treatment is not particularly useful if the diet contains high levels of molybdenum and sulfate.

As a rule, oral forms of copper therapy are not effective when molybdenum or other inhibitory factors in the diet induce secondary hypocupremia.

In sheep, especially, because of the risk of toxicity, whole-flock medication in feed or water is generally impractical. Individual treatment, therefore, is necessary. The main criteria for an ideal product follow.

1. One dose should provide sufficient copper to cover the risk period.
2. The duration of effect should allow administration at a convenient stage in the flock management routine, e.g., at tupping.
3. The copper given should enter the animal's system slowly to minimize the risk of toxicity.
4. Copper treatment can be combined with other management tasks without the risk of precipitating copper toxicity.
5. Risk of side effects associated with administration of the particular product should be minimal.
6. Sustained release of copper should be ensured to reduce substantially the chances of copper toxicity.

Administration is usually best in early pregnancy for control of swayback.

SUSTAINED RELEASE ORAL COPPER DOSAGE FORMS

Copper oxide needles

The use of fine needles of copper oxide has been developed and widely used in the last few years. These needles are given in gelatin capsules that lodge in the rumen, from which they are absorbed over a period of 6 to 8 weeks.

Doses of 5 g copper oxide needles for calves, 10 g for yearlings, and 20–25 g for adult cattle, approximately equivalent to dose rates of 2.5 to 5 g/100 kg live weight, should give protection for up to 6–8 months approximately.

The oral administration of copper oxide particles or wire was developed as a preventative agent and is proving to be a most useful method of protection. A single administration of 20 to 25 g oxidized copper wire per cow is sufficient to sustain elevated plasma copper levels for as many as 32 weeks post treatment. The administration of 4 g copper oxide needles to ewes in midpregnancy prevents the occurrence of swayback in their offspring.

Copper oxide needles are brittle rods (1-cm long) made by oxidizing fine copper wire. They are nontoxic when given by mouth, and they can be given in doses sufficient to establish long-lasting reserves of copper in the liver. Their properties were discovered when researchers found that the combination of small particle size and high specific gravity caused the needles to become trapped in the folds of the abomasum. Subsequent experiments showed that the needles are retained there for 30 to 60 days in sheep and cattle and slowly release copper in absorbable forms.

Copper oxide needles dissolve slowly, and some of the released copper is absorbed by the normal physiologic processes. They can be recovered from the sites of retention for several weeks after administration, and during this period, the reserves of copper in the liver, the principal storage organ, increase. The copper stored in the liver then acts as a depot from which copper can be slowly released to maintain normal concentrations in the blood during periods when the animal may be receiving an inadequate copper intake. They have been used most frequently in sheep, but they are also effective in cattle. Administration of 4 g of copper oxide needles to ewes during the first half of pregnancy protects their lambs from swayback. Administration of 2 g of copper oxide needles to lambs provides sufficient copper to prevent the development of hypocupremia until lambs are weaned.

The increased copper level in the liver extends protection from 6 to 10 months, depending on the level of antagonistic challenge on the farm. Dose rates vary from 20 g for a cow to 2 g for a lamb. More frequent (i.e., 6 monthly) use of smaller doses is preferable to a single annual large dose.

Oxidized copper wire particles given per os to cattle are an alternative to subcutaneous copper glycinate injections. Oxidized copper wire particles have been recovered from the stomachs of cattle slaughtered months after treatment. Treatment with oxidized copper wire particles (50 g) results in sustained higher copper concentrations in plasma than do subcutaneous injections of copper glycinate.

Most forms of copper are potentially toxic to ruminants, and therefore, one must know the safe and effective dose of copper oxide needles. Manufacturers dosage instructions should therefore be carefully adhered to at all times.

Controlled-Release Glass

Ruminal glass bullets have been developed for sheep and cattle and, from some initial experimental trials, show promise as a vehicle for supplying trace minerals to animals. The bullets apparently are retained in the reticulum, and perhaps copper ions are washed directly into the omasum, thereby resulting in a short residence in the rumen.

Physical constraint has been tried by using soluble "controlled-release glass." The rate at which the tissues of the recipient animal are exposed to the active element is governed by the rate of solution of the glass.

A unique technology used during the manufacturing process incorporates into the structure of the glass the three major trace elements—cobalt, selenium, and copper. Normally, glass contains 60 to 70% silica, but the glass bolus is made almost entirely of constituents that occur naturally in the ruminant diet—sodium, phosphorus, calcium, and magnesium oxides and the three trace elements.

Once administered to the animal, the bolus dissolves slowly and completely in the reticulorumen, from which a gradual and sustained release of trace elements ensures that continuously adequate supplementation levels are available to control and protect against deficiency.

Two different sizes of bolus are currently available, one for cattle and one for sheep. In cattle, a dose of two boluses per animal, and in sheep a dose of one bolus per animal, normally provides effective supplementation of all three trace elements for a year.

The slow-release action of the glass ("Cosecure") bolus as it dissolves gradually in the reticulorumen ensures a sustained, controlled supply of copper, cobalt, and selenium ions in a form and in amounts that can be readily absorbed and metabolized by the animal. This measured supply provides continuous adequate levels of supplementation rather than large peaks and troughs, thereby avoiding excessive demands on the metabolism of the animal and precluding the possibility of overdosing when the animal naturally is sufficient in one or another element. Overdosing is prevented because of the slow and specific rate of release from the bolus. Any excess in trace element absorption over metabolic requirements is un-likely to reach a significant level, even over a long period.

Use of soluble glass boluses produces normocupremia that lasts 3 months, but by 7 months up to two thirds of treated cows may have normocupremia. Copper oxide needles, on the other hand, produce normocupremia that lasts at least 7 months. This treatment possibly contributes to the higher copper values seen in calves from the calving subsequent to administration.

In summary, copper oxide needles administered in gelatin capsules or slow-release phosphate glass boluses containing copper both possess a long-lasting action and avoid carcass blemishes. The disadvantages are that capsules may rupture during administration and glass boluses can break unless care is taken.

A high level of oral dietary inhibition factors may interfere with copper absorption in the intestine. Regardless of the oral dose form of copper.

Copper Injection

Numerous copper compounds are available for subcutaneous or intramuscular injection, including copper sulfate, acetate, citrate oxychloride, heptonate, borogluconate, naphthenate, oleate, asparaginate, caseinate, methionate, ammonium sulfate, oxine (8-hydroxyquinoline), versenate (sodium ethylenediaminetetra-acetic acid [EDTA]), and glycinate. The criteria by which the suitability of the compounds should be judged are:

1. Minimal damage at the site of injection
2. Satisfactory liver storage (90 to 100% of the administered dose)
3. A safe margin between therapeutic and toxic doses

The various problems that have been encountered with different marketed copper chelates include large local reactions at the site of injection (methionates, glycinate), poor absorption, too rapid absorption, short-lived protection, and toxicity (oxyquinoline-copper complex).

Injectable copper is the preferred form of delivery when high dietary molybdenum can interfere with oral absorption of copper supplements (i.e., for secondary copper deficiency).

The three organic injectable copper preparations for clinical use in sheep are heptonate, diethyl copper oxyquinoline sulfonate (DCOS), and methionate.

Heptonate and DCOS cause little or no local tissue damage. Methionate is potentially more irritant, but if given subcutaneously, any reaction can be trimmed locally at slaughter without affecting the meat. The therapeutic index of heptonate and DCOS is in the region of 3:5, whereas the therapeutic index of methionate is 1:20 or higher. For this reason, copper methionate may be used safely in neonatal lambs for the prevention of delayed swayback.

Dosage of copper products may vary depending on the severity of the deficiency. Sheep are especially prone to copper toxicity, however.

Copper calcium edetate, copper glycinate, copper methionate, and copper heptonate and DCOS compounds are available for treating deficiencies. Some are restricted in use to either cattle or sheep.

Copper calcium edetate by subcutaneous injection produces a rapid rise of copper values in blood and liver, thereby relieving immediate symptoms of copper deficiency, and confers a longer-term effect in cattle.

After intramuscular injection of copper glycinate or the copper salt of methionine, the copper is largely removed from the site of injection and deposited in the liver.

The various disadvantages of injectable copper are that some provoke reactions at the site of injection, some translocate rapidly to the liver, and others translocate rather slowly. Their duration of action is inferior to that of the new oral compounds.

COPPER INJECTABLES

Amongst the advantages and disadvantages of copper injections are:

1. May cause local irritation
2. May cause symptoms of copper toxicity
3. Are not affected by dietary inhibitory factors
4. May be used for therapy of deficient animals
5. Can provide up to 5 months of supplementation
6. Are perhaps a more certain way of copper supplementation than are oral sustained-release presentations for secondary copper deficiency.

Injections can only give short-lived protection, however, usually because the copper that can be given safely in a single dose is limited. Therefore, repeat injections are commonly needed to maintain adequate protection.

Timing is also critical, especially in ewes. When injected too early, protection may wear off and thus increase the risk of swayback lambs. When injected too late, swayback is again the possible result.

Copper glycinate is the most frequently available compound, and is suitable for both primary and conditional (e.g., molybdenum-induced) forms of copper deficiency. A single subcutaneous injection of 400 mg copper glycinate containing 120 mg copper provides adequate copper for adult cattle more than 150 kg for 2 to 3 months; 60 mg copper is recommended for animals less than 150 kg.

A copper complex suitable for parenteral administration would have to possess the best attributes of DCOS and copper methionate, but their separate properties of rapid transport from the injection site and slow arrival at the storage sites would be difficult to combine.

The frequency of injection of the organic copper complexes depends on the product and on the severity of the copper deficiency. For instance, on soils high in molybdenum content, copper may have to be injected every 2 to 3 months to prevent copper deficiency, whereas in marginal situations, a single injection at the appropriate time may cover the period of greatest risk.

Cattle are not as susceptible to copper toxicity as are sheep, but deaths in calves 1 to 2 months old have occurred after they were given 12- to 24-ml injections of EDTA-hydroxyquinoline complex containing 6 mg/ml copper.

Chronic copper poisoning has occurred in dairy cows by oversupplementing prepared feed with as much as 22 g of copper sulfate per day.

Cattle require approximately 120 mg copper at 3-month intervals, depending on the rate of copper release from the formulated slow-release commercial product. Cattle grazing high molybdenum pasture usually require larger doses of copper to reverse clinical signs of molybdenosis. Injectable copper products bypass the oral inhibition of molybdenum.

The organic copper preparations apparently differ in their rate of translocation to the liver, in their toxicity, and in local reaction. DCOS is rapidly translocated, copper methionate and copper glycinate are slowly translocated, and copper calcium EDTA is intermediate with regard to translocation. The rapid translocation of copper from the site of injection when given as DCOS limits the dose that can be administered without the risk of acute toxicity.

Copper methionate and copper glycinate are slowly mobilized and hence have a low toxicity; however, they can cause local tissue reaction that may result in encapsulation of variable amounts of the dose at the site of injection. The copper methionate complex can be administered in doses up to 6 mg copper/kg body weight without deleterious effect. Copper calcium EDTA is a most effective treatment for cattle. They can tolerate the administration of up to 1 mg copper/kg body weight in the form of edetate as a single injection. Adverse reactions to injections of commercial preparations of copper-calcium EDTA have been observed in livestock. For treatment of copper poisoning, see Chapter 8.

28.2 COBALT (Co)

Cobalt is used by ruminal organisms to synthesize into vitamin B_{12}, which is absorbed in the small intestine and stored in the liver. Vitamin B_{12} is an essential coenzyme in the metabolism of propionic acid (a major energy source in ruminants) Gluconeogenesis and energy generation.

Growing animals are more susceptible to cobalt deficiency than are older animals, and sheep are more susceptible than are cattle. To deficiency symptoms.

Cobalt deficiency in ruminants is a manifestation of vitamin B_{12} deficiency brought about by the inability of the rumen microorganisms to synthesize sufficient vitamin B_{12} to meet metabolic needs when dietary cobalt is inadequate. Nonruminants cannot incorporate cobalt into its physiologically active form and must obtain their vitamin

B_{12} preformed in their food. Volatile fatty acids, especially acetic and propionic acids, are the primary sources of energy in ruminants. In cobalt-deficient sheep, the metabolism of propionate is adversely affected because of a malfunctioning key enzyme, methylmalonyl-CoA isomerase, which requires vitamin B_{12} to function properly. The impaired propionate metabolism leads to a marked increase in the urinary excretion of methylmalonic acid. In general, most soils are richer in cobalt than are the plants growing on them, and soil ingestion can provide a significant source of cobalt. Ruminants convert a high proportion of ingested cobalt into vitamin B_{12}-like compounds, however, and appear to have a limited ability to absorb the vitamin B_{12} that is produced.

The trace element cobalt is required for synthesis of vitamin B_{12} by rumen microbes. This vitamin B_{12} co-enzyme is required by methylmalonyl-CoA mutase, a mitochondrial enzyme involved in the major pathway through which propionate and several amino acids are metabolized. Propionate, derived from fermentation of dietary cellulose in the rumen, is the major precursor of glucose in the ruminant, and hence of prime significance for energy generation and utilization of nutrients.

Although cobalt intake is the major determinant of synthesis of vitamin B_{12} in the rumen, many other factors can be involved. In addition to vitamin B_{12} (cyanocobalamin), several natural analogs of the vitamin are also synthesized. In sheep, these are not absorbed and hence cannot be detected in the serum. In cattle these analogs can be absorbed, however, and they may constitute a variable proportion of the total serum vitamin B_{12} level as measured by many laboratory assays. High concentrate diets have a marked depressant effect on vitamin B_{12} synthesis in the rumen and can lead to production of more of the analogs.

VITAMIN B_{12} RESERVES IN THE LIVER

Cobalt deficiency syndrome is influenced largely by the reserves of vitamin B_{12} in the liver. In calves these reserves depend on transfer of the vitamin from the dam to the calf during gestation and on the consumption by the cow of a cobalt-adequate diet during pregnancy. Milk is a poor source of vitamin B_{12} for calves, and cobalt given to cows has little effect on levels of the vitamin in milk.

When the vitamin B_{12} concentration in the liver decreases, the ability of cattle to utilize propionate can be seriously impaired, and then severe signs of cobalt deficiency are seen.

FACTORS THAT AFFECT COBALT AVAILABILITY

Not all the low cobalt areas have been clearly defined. Soil type, cobalt concentrations in the soil, and availability of cobalt in the soil to plants are poorly correlated. Management and seasonal factors are important determinants affecting the cobalt levels in plants and animals in low cobalt areas. Application of lime has been associated with reduced cobalt uptake in pastures. This is true of other trace element deficiencies, as well.

Regarding soil deficiency, soil from acidic igneous rock, such as granite, generally lacks cobalt, whereas that of basaltic origin has adequate cobalt. Sedimentary and volcanic soils often reflect the cobalt content of the parent rock. Cattle usually do not become deficient on moderately deficient or marginally deficient soils. Cobalt content in the soil can be decreased by prolonged adverse weather conditions. Plants growing on waterlogged soils have cobalt levels many times higher than those of plants grown on the same soil types with good drainage. Other minerals can also affect plant uptake. Manganese and iron reduce cobalt uptake. Nickel is also a competitive element. Plants appear to take up nickel in preference to cobalt.

Low cobalt levels in pastures are suggestive of the possibility of deficiency in the animal but must not be used to diagnose unequivocally an animal deficiency. The pasture cobalt content can vary with the season and from year to year. On severely deficient soils, however, pasture cobalt tends generally to remain low all year.

In addition, certain plant species differ in their ability to take up cobalt from soil; legumes tend to have greater uptake than grasses. When cobalt in soil is low, differences in cobalt concentrations between grasses and clovers become negligible. Reduced soil acidity (e.g. by liming) reduces uptake of cobalt by plants.

DEFICIENCY AND CLINICAL SIGNS

Cobalt deficiency can be seen in ruminants grazing pastures upon which horses and other nonruminants remain healthy and grow normally. In situations of severe deficiency, wasting and mortality are pronounced in animals of all ages. Loss of appetite, failure of growth, loss of weight, changes in coat, depletion of body fat stores, and muscle wasting may occur rapidly and anemia develops. If the dietary deficiency is less severe, the signs may be much less pronounced; young animals may show a vague ill-thrift and mature animals may show reduced milk production and give birth to weak young.

Cobalt deficiency in cattle is characterized by poor growth, anorexia, depressed appetite, occasional diarrhea, anemia, and harsh coat. A predisposition to parasitism may also occur.

Calves with adequate vitamin B_{12} reserves in the liver must graze cobalt-deficient pastures for up to 9 months before vitamin B_{12} levels in the liver become depleted.

The signs of severe cobalt deficiency are nonspecific and may resemble those of starvation. Signs include retarded growth, rough hair coats, and diarrhea. In low cobalt areas, lambs are most sensitive to vitamin B_{12} deficiency followed by ewes, calves, and cows in that order. Severe signs in adult cattle are only seen in herds kept on wet pastures or where soils are sandy and low in cobalt.

Subclinical Cobalt Deficiency

Cattle with marginal cobalt deficiency usually display no specific clinical signs. Some cattle may have pale rough coats, but the deficiency can only be demonstrated conclusively by a growth rate response after oral cobalt supplementation or after vitamin B_{12} injections.

Very many areas deficient in copper also tend to be marginally deficient in cobalt. In temperate climates the important periods for both cobalt and copper deficiencies occur in the spring and winter periods.

Cobalt deficiency can predispose to the intensity of effects of parasitism. The ingestion of nematode larvae is high during the late winter and spring periods. This coincides with peak times of cobalt deficiency, for maximum growth rates of young cattle, anthelmintic treatments and strategic parasite control programs, in addition to treatment with both copper and cobalt, may be required. Many oral parasiticide drenches are supplemented with cobalt, although the levels are usually inadequate to combat deficiency.

DIAGNOSIS

The growth rate and body condition of cattle provides an indication of the likelihood of a cobalt deficiency problem. Herds grazing quality pastures, showing poor growth and wasting indicates that they may be deficient in cobalt. A marginal deficiency can be confirmed only by comparative growth rate measurements of treated and untreated groups grazing on the same pasture.

In cattle, the complex relationship between cobalt nutrition and vitamin B_{12} concentration in plasma is less correlated than in sheep. Plasma levels generally are of little help in assessing marginal deficiencies in cattle, because of the absorption of inactive analogs of Vitamin B_{12}. Many methods (including microbiologic assays) used to measure vitamin B_{12} in the laboratory do not distinguish between true vitamin B_{12} and its analogs. Folic acid measurement may provide a useful index of vitamin B_{12} status.

Laboratories frequently measure plasma vitamin B_{12} and folic acid together in one batch. Folate, being closely related metabolically to vitamin B_{12} is a useful but frequently underutilized indicator.

Vitamin B_{12} concentration in the liver provides an indication of the vitamin B_{12} reserves in the tissue. Vitamin B_{12} concentration in plasma indicates dietary cobalt intake and rumen vitamin B_{12} synthesis, and has a much shorter half-life than does vitamin B_{12} in the liver.

The liver is the storage organ for vitamin B_{12} and is the recommended sample site for diagnosing cobalt deficiency in cattle.

Serum vitamin B_{12} is a useful diagnostic test in growing sheep but to date has not been as thoroughly evaluated in cattle.

Some workers consider the minimum requirement for cattle to be similar to that for sheep. Cobalt levels in pasture may act as a guide to deficiency but should not be used to diagnose animal deficiency, because of the many variables affecting absorption.

The most conclusive diagnostic test is a weight gain or production response trial in which performance of cobalt-supplemented animals is compared with that of untreated animals.

TREATMENT AND PREVENTION

Cobalt deficiency in sheep and cattle can be treated and prevented by a range of cobalt supplements, such as drenches, licks, foliar sprays, and fertilizer top dressings, as well as intraruminal bullets, boluses, and vitamin B_{12} injections.

Cobalt Drenches

Sheep and cattle require regular and very frequent oral administration of cobalt to satisfy their vitamin B_{12} requirements. Doses of cobalt as cobalt sulfate must be given at weekly intervals. In areas of cobalt deficiency, vitamin B_{12} injections are recommended for deficient calves showing clinical signs of ill thrift. An injection of 4 mg cobalamin (intramuscular, subcutaneous) should provide adequate vitamin B_{12} levels for 3 months.

Vitamin B_{12} injections are effective when a rapid response is required. In sheep, appetite is restored rapidly with injection, whereas with oral administration of cobalt sulfate, appetite may not be fully restored for a week.

Forms of vitamin B_{12} available commercially are hydroxocobalamin and cyanocobalamin. Cyanocobalamin is chemically more stable. In general, parenteral injections of hydroxocobalamin are more effective than injections of cyanocobalamin in raising the vitamin B_{12} status of animals.

Cobalt pellets (20 g containing 90% cobalt oxide) may be used for immediate treatment of deficient calves and cattle, but calves younger than 2 months of age may not retain the pellets satisfactorily.

Cobalt Bullet Therapy

A cobalt bullet placed in the rumen continuously releases sufficient amounts of cobalt for conversion to vitamin B_{12} to meet the animals' needs. Bullets now available commercially contain about 30% by weight of cobalt oxide. The bullets are effective for as long as 5 years in sheep, but appear less satisfactory in cattle.

The choice between using pellets or vitamin B_{12} injections depends on cost effectiveness and on the time period for which animals require supplementation. Vitamin B_{12} preparations have become relatively less expensive in recent years.

TOXICITY

Both acute and chronic cobalt toxicity can occur. Cattle appear more sensitive to cobalt salts than do sheep. Doses equivalent to 7 mg/kg body weight may on occasion be lethal to cattle.

Feeding of cobalt in excess of 0.8 mg/kg body weight daily to dairy cows has been reported to be harmful, e.g., loss of appetite and incoordination.

Overzealous supplementation (1 mg/kg body weight) of calves may result in toxicity. The signs are not specific and include anorexia, listlessness, loss of weight, mild diarrhea, rough hair coat, and ataxia. Cobalt levels in the liver of cattle with cobalt toxicity have ranged from 4 to 70 mg/kg DM, in comparison to the normal range of cobalt levels in the liver of 0.08 to 0.22 mg/kg DM.

28.3 SELENIUM AND VITAMIN E

Both selenium and vitamin E have roles in the prevention of muscle damage by oxidants produced during metabolism. Selenium is an essential component of the enzyme glutathione peroxidase, which catalyzes the removal of metabolites of oxygen, such as hydrogen peroxide, which are potentially toxic to cells. Vitamin E is thought to protect cell membranes from the damaging effects of these oxidants. Cattle and sheep obtain plentiful vitamin E from green pasture. A selenoprotein resembling cytochrome C has been isolated from hair and muscles of normal lambs, but is absent in selenium-deficient lambs. Its function is not known.

Selenium has been recognized as an essential trace element for animals. In the United States, as elsewhere, forages from several regions have inadequate selenium concentrations to meet normal requirements.

Selenium has been added to total rations of confined cattle either as sodium selenite or in linseed meal to increase plasma selenium concentrations. Subcutaneous injections of sodium selenate at 0.5 mg selenium/kg of body weight increases serum selenium significantly ($p < 0.001$) in Hereford/Holstein and Charolais/Holstein steers.

The duodenum apparently is the main site for selenium absorption, and monogastric animals apparently absorb more of the ingested selenium than do ruminants. Absorbed selenium is carried in the plasma, and selenium undergoes a chemical transformation within erythrocytes. The expulsion from erythrocytes depends on adequate glutathione levels in these cells. Once expelled, selenium is largely taken up by beta-lipoproteins. Selenium enters all tissues, appears to be highly labile, and can be transmitted through the placenta to the fetus. It is excreted in feces, urine, and expired air. The main selenoprotein is glutathione peroxidase, which is present in many body tissues and fluids, with the highest activity in the liver.

Selenium interacts with arsenic, mercury, silver, copper, cadmium, sulfur, methionine, vitamin E, and dietary protein. The minimum selenium requirements vary according to the level of production used as criteria for assessment and the composition of the diet. The commonly accepted requirement for lambs and calves is approximately 0.1 ppm.

The selenium concentrations occurring in feeds vary widely depending on the plant species and on the selenium status of the soil in which the plant is growing. In areas where selenium-responsive diseases occur, the forages usually contain below 0.05 ppm, but in selenium-sufficient areas, the level is at least 0.1 ppm selenium on a dry matter basis.

The primary factor controlling the level of selenium in plants is the total selenium level in the soil. Although if soil concentration is adequate, selenium concentration in plants can be altered by other inhibitory factors.

1. In poorly drained soils anaerobic conditions are produced that reduce selenium to forms unavailable to plants.
2. Many pasture species have various abilities to concentrate selenium; legumes often have lower levels than grasses. When pasture selenium concentrations fall to low levels, however, differences between species tend to become negligible.
3. The presence of sulfur can depress pasture selenium.

Methionine, copper, vitamin E and polyunsaturated fatty acids interact with selenium. Soils in the low selenium areas are usually acidic and receive a high annual rainfall.

Applications of superphosphate fertilizers decrease the concentration of selenium in pastures and may also decrease the uptake of selenium by grazing livestock, thereby predisposing lambs to white muscle disease.

DEFICIENCY AND CLINICAL SIGNS

Both selenium and vitamin E are integral to the proper functioning of the immune system. Because of their immunomodulating function, deficiency states lead to a variety of signs. Selenium is necessary for growth and fertility in animals and is required to prevent liver necrosis and mulberry heart disease in pigs, exudative diathesis and pancreatic fibrosis in poultry, and white muscle disease in lambs, calves, and foals. Selenium-responsive ill-thrift occurs in young sheep and cattle. The condition varies in severity, and specific lesions do not appear in any organ system. Selenium is of critical importance for reproductive efficiency in cattle. Selenium deficiency has also been linked to some cases of bovine mastitis.

Selenium deficiency can result in nutritional muscular dystrophy in calves. Adequate selenium is necessary also for optimum performance of certain host defense mechanisms. This is true of the reproductive tract and mammary gland. When dams are supplemented with a sufficient level of selenium, calves are not deficient at birth.

Lamb losses can be prevented by a selenium/vitamin E (Selenium/Vite) dose given 1 month before lambing. Numerous studies have shown that injections of selenium and vitamin E mixtures may also reduce mortality in neonatal calves and the incidence of retained placenta in cows. Selenium is of major significance for normal reproductive function. The incidence of normal cycling metritis, and retained placenta is clearly linked to selenium status.

Clinical Signs

1. White muscle disease is a noninflammatory myonecrosis that occurs in skeletal and heart muscle of calves usually between 1 and 4 months of age. The heart lesions are generally most severe in the left ventricle. Stiffness, often with an arched back, and sudden death are presenting signs.

   Calves may have elevated heart rates (up to 200 beats/minute). Calves appear listless and have difficulty standing. Those than can stand often walk stiffly on the tips of their hooves, with their backs arched and tails raised. Calves suck the cow if assisted, and temperature remains normal.

   Calves with myopathy of skeletal muscles may have a stiff gait and show trembling of the limbs and weakness. Usually the muscles of the limbs are affected on both sides and may be swollen and firmer than normal.

   Myopathy of heart and skeletal muscles, known as white muscle disease, is the most serious clinical form of selenium deficiency in calves.

   Clinical diagnosis of white muscle disease in calves can be difficult. The respiratory signs may resemble those of pneumonia associated with septicemia and toxemia. The muscular disorder must be differentiated from traumatic injuries, polyarthritis, spinal cord depression, organophosphate poisoning, and blackleg. Elevated plasma creatine kinase activity (>1000 U/liter) indicates muscle damage. The levels return to normal within a few days following injections of selenium (0.1 mg/kg live weight) or of combined solutions of selenium and vitamin E.

2. A selenium-responsive ill-thrift can occur in all ages of dairy and beef cattle, particularly in the autumn and winter. It runs from subclinical growth defects to mortality. Much research is being undertaken to elucidate other functions of selenium in animals and to uncover factors that provoke the appearance of biochemical and clinical defects in animals deficient in selenium and vitamin E.

3. A selenium-responsive infertility characterized by early embryonic death is well recognized in sheep. In addition, deficiencies of vitamin E and selenium can cause depression of the immune response system, particularly cell-mediated mechanisms. Such a response can be manifested by increased genital tract infections and retention of fetal membranes.

   Data indicate that selenium readily crosses the placenta in beef cattle and that, when dams are deficient in selenium, fetal calves can partially compensate by apparently concentrating selenium. The selenium concentration in colostrum is significantly increased by supplementing selenium in pregnancy.

4. Birth of premature, weak, or dead calves has been associated with selenium deficiency.

5. Many reports describe a reduction in incidence of retained fetal membranes following treatment with selenium-vitamin E. Selenium deficiency is commonly overlooked as a predisposing cause of retained fetal membranes.

6. Milk production responses to selenium treatment are widely believed to occur. Results reveal that a milk production response is only likely when selenium levels in the blood are below 100 nmol/liter (8 μg/liter).

7. Selenium status can play a role in the ability to combat infection. Neutrophils isolated from the blood of selenium-deficient (blood selenium below 10 μg/liter) and selenium-adequate Holstein steers had similar abilities to phagocytize *Candida albicans*. Neutrophils from selenium-deficient animals, however, were less able to kill the ingested yeast.

Selenium and vitamin E mutually combat infection in three areas: phagocytosis, humoral responses, and the metabolism of arachidonic acid into prostaglandins, which influence smooth muscle function. Selenium augments immunity by enhancing antibody synthesis. Selenium also appears to have a role in the resistance of animals to disease.

DIAGNOSIS

The selenium content of tissues, feed, and soils also is valuable in diagnosis. Selenium is deposited in all tissues of the body. The hair of cattle from seleniferrous areas contains 10 to 30 ppm selenium compared to 1 to 4 ppm selenium in hair of cattle grazing in normal areas. Animals with selenium-responsive conditions usually have low selenium and glutathione peroxidase (a selenoprotein) values in their tissues. Glutathione peroxidase values are now being widely used as an aid in the assessment of the selenium status of animals.

Selenium status of cattle can be determined by measuring blood or liver selenium levels or blood glutathione peroxidase concentration.

The selenium levels in liver and, especially, blood are slow to respond to changes in nutritional selenium levels. In cattle, these changes occur in 3 to 4 months in liver and 6 months in blood. In contrast, the more rapid selenium intake from proprietary oral and subcutaneous selenium formulations results in a rapid increase in selenium concentration in tissues. Glutathione peroxidase levels in blood are slower to respond, however, because the glutathione peroxidase enzyme is incorporated into the erythrocyte during erythropoiesis and the concentration depends on the selenium status of the animal at this time. The life span of bovine erythrocytes is approximately 120 days; thus, changes in glutathione peroxidase levels in blood are not immediate.

Accordingly, when tests are being used to determine selenium status on a farm, one must know whether animals were previously treated with selenium and if so, at what dose, what type of formulation, and when dosing occurred.

TREATMENT AND PREVENTION

Application of selenium compounds to soil or herbage is not widely practiced because the selenium is poorly absorbed by the plants and surface contamination immediately following application may create a toxic hazard. The environmental impact of selenium is now attracting considerable attention from the FDA and environmental groups. Oral dosing successfully combats selenium deficiency in the short-term but is labor intensive. Selenium-containing mineral supplements, salt licks, ruminal bullets, and new boluses that release selenium for 120 days have been used successfully. Some intraruminal selenium pellets are claimed to provide sheep with selenium for at least 4 years, but some studies with commercially available pellets indicate that they provide selenium for only a much shorter time. Selenium oxide has been incorporated into phosphate-based glass that has been given to provide a controlled, slow release of selenium, following release from the rumen/reticulum.

Selenium preparations are marketed in the form of sodium selenate or selenite for use as a drench or as an injection (intramuscular or subcutaneous). Selenium pellets (30 g) containing 5 or 10% elemental selenium for oral use have been used on a trial basis in cattle.

Selenium Injection

Selenium, in the form of either sodium selenite or potassium selenate, is often given parenterally (by injection). Both of these forms rapidly raise the levels of selenium in the animal. Any excess amount not needed by the animal's immediate requirements is excreted. The selenium level then drops within a few weeks, thus leaving the animal once again deficient and in need of a repeat treatment. A depot preparation of barium selenate in paste form, for subcutaneous injection provides extended selenium levels. Depot selenium injections ("Deposel") allow the safe injection of a high level of selenium over a period of time, thereby continuously maintaining an adequate level in the animal.

Results suggest that an oil base is superior to a water base for selenium preparations containing sodium selenite, sodium selenate, or barium selenate and that the parenteral route is better than the oral route. The release of selenium from the injection site is delayed when given in an oil base as the barium rather than the sodium salt. A barium selenate preparation released on the market in some countries is suitable for parenteral administration to livestock.

One disadvantage of parenterally administered selenium salts (especially the intramuscular route) is occasional swelling at the site of injection. Furthermore, about 3 months must elapse before slaughter to allow time for the selenium to disperse. (This depends on the precise formulation used.)

In general, parenteral or oral doses of selenium of 1 mg to lambs, 5 mg to adult sheep, 5 to 10 mg to calves, and 25 to 30 mg to adult cattle every 3 to 4 months should be adequate to ensure selenium sufficiency without risk of toxicity in livestock on a selenium-deficient pasture.

Most commercial selenium preparations are recommended for use at a rate that provides only 0.05 mg selenium/kg body weight, and because this dose is so low, parenteral treatment may be necessary at weekly intervals (Table 28–2 and 28–3).

With the depot preparation of barium selenate, at a dose rate of 1 mg selenium/kg body weight, effective protection against deficiency should last for several months. One disadvantage is associated with the use of this insoluble preparation, however; large percentages of the original selenium remain at the site of injection (Table 28–4).

Injection of selenium and vitamin E is effective for specific times of risk, such as when cows approach calving. Administration of selenium to pregnant cows 2 months prior to calving provides good protection against white muscle disease in calves. Injections of selenium, with and without vitamin E, may decrease the incidence of retained placenta in the dairy cow. They also ensure optimum reproductive performance

---

TABLE 28–2
PARENTERAL PREPARATIONS OF COPPER

Copper methionate (20 mg/ml)	Cattle: 40–120 mg Sheep: 40 mg Lambs: 10 mg.

Copper calcium edetate (50 mg/ml)	Cattle: <100 kg, 50 mg
	      >100 kg, 100 mg
	      (up to 200 mg)

Copper glycinate (60 mg cu. ml)	Cattle: <150 kg 1 ml every 3–6 months
Diethylamine (DOS) (6 mg cu. ml)	Cattle: <250 kg, 12 mg/50 kg >250 kg, 120 mg Ewes: 12 mg
Copper heptonate (12.5 mg/ml)	Sheep: 25 mg

---

and assist the body defenses against mastitic organisms.

Injectable preparations of selenium and vitamin E have been used routinely in sheep and goats as a means of supplementation when concentrates and complete feeds are not available. Because selenium crosses the placenta readily, injections are most frequent and useful during the last trimester of pregnancy.

When using selenium veterinarians should remember its narrow margin of safety. Toxicity syndromes in animals, "alkali disease", or "blind staggers", are well known. Content of selenium in hair or urine may confirm toxicity, blood levels in animals with "alkali disease" are 1–2 ppm, in "blind staggers", they are 2–4 ppm. Deformed hooves occur in cattle. Selenium is also toxic to humans, and workers should always be cautioned when handling selenium preparations. The F.D.A., and the feed mill industry are becoming increasingly concerned about this issue.

Subcutaneous injections of either selenate or selenite are more effective than oral

---

TABLE 28–3
SELENIUM TREATMENTS FOR ANIMALS

Injectable formulations

1. Selenium injection (Sodium Selenite)
   Dose: 0.05 mg/kg
2. Dystosel (1.5 mg/ml Se as potassium selenate + 68 I.U. of DL-alpha-tocopherol acetate/ml)
Rapid release, suitable to treat clinical disorders. May require repeated treatments at 2–4 week intervals for calves.
Dose: 0.02–0.04 ml/kg (calves)
3. Barium selenate (Deposel or Zoselen La) (50 mg/ml)
Provides several months of protection in adult cattle and sheep. Slow release results from low solubility. Reduced risk of toxicity. Local deposition at site.
Dose: Cattle/sheep: up to 1.0 mg/kg

Oral Formulations

1. Selenium drenches
Dose: 0.1 mg/Se/kg body weight
2. Selenium pellets (18 month activity)
3. Selenium bolus (Dura S.E.) (4–8 months)

TABLE 28–4

IODINE   Soil/Plants
↓
THYROID GLAND   (Iodine Trapping)

↓ Formation of Hormones

THROXINE (T$_4$)
TRI-IODOTYRONINE (T$_3$)
↓

REGULATE —Metabolism in Entire body

—Growth

—Reproduction

—Resistance to Infection

—Milk Production

—Normal Functioning

drenching in elevating selenium levels in whole blood. Parenteral treatment bypasses rumen breakdown of soluble salts to elemental selenium and avoids any potential toxic interaction with other orally administered drugs. Risk of selenium toxicity in cattle is higher if parenteral treatment is used. The slow-release parenteral selenium product consisting of barium selenate suspended in an oil-beeswax mixture is available in some countries. This product produces a rapid (3 to 4 weeks) and prolonged rise in selenium concentrations and is relatively nontoxic.

Oral Selenium

Solutions of sodium selenate (usually the decahydrate form with 21.4% by weight of selenium) or sodium selenite (45.7% by weight of selenium) are often prepared at a selenium concentration of 1 mg/ml.

Currently available products for oral administration include specific nutritional supplements containing selenium, and also selenium-supplemented worm drenches.

The amount of selenium given orally is low and compensates a minor deficiency for, at the most, 2 to 3 weeks only. This route thus has the disadvantage of requiring subsequent repeat treatments, which is expensive in terms of product and labor and may also mean an extra gathering of animals at an inconvenient time.

In the case of moderate to severe deficiencies, however, such oral treatments do not provide animals with levels of selenium adequate to regain their correct status.

Selenium Bolus Therapy

A new selenium bolus (Dura SE) safely and effectively supplies selenium to pregnant cows. Evidence for the efficacy of the selenium bolus has been shown in several recent studies. This selenium bolus is an osmotic pump designed to release 3 mg selenium/day into the reticulorumen. The selenium bolus is designed to provide selenium supplementation for 120 days.

'Dura-SE-120' bolus elevates blood selenium levels for 4 to 8 months. The bolus is surrounded by a semipermeable membrane that absorbs ruminal fluid. Absorption activates an osmotically driven pump, which releases sodium selenite at a consistent rate of 3 mg/day. The pump achieves a steady state in 3 to 4 weeks and exhausts itself in approximately 120 days. The device contains a densifier of sintered iron to ensure that it remains in the rumen or reticulum. Oral selenium pellets are also available

---

TABLE 28–5

DEFICIENCY OF IODINE
1) Low Soil Levels
2) Low Plant Levels
↓
Lowered Production of Thyroid Hormones
↓
Clinical Signs of Iodine Deficiency

---

which elevate blood selenium for up to 18 months.

Selenium supplementation is a high-priority need for heifers and dry cows in selenium-deficient areas. In these areas, dairy workers usually add selenium supplements to the feed ration for all the cows in the milking herd; however, heifers and dry cows are often neglected.

Recently published research indicates the selenium bolus Dura SE (its generic equivalent) resulted in increased blood selenium concentrations for up to 7 months with a single treatment. University studies and field trials demonstrate prolonged elevation of selenium levels in whole blood in animals supplemented with Dura Se vs. unsupplemented controls.

Selenium Toxicity

Toxic single doses for cattle are 9 mg/kg body weight. Lethal doses of sodium selenite by injection are 1.2 mg selenium/kg body weight. The toxicity of oral doses of selenium is influenced by many factors, including the form of the selenium.

Concern has surfaced regarding the environmental impact of selenium used in animal feeds. Although at present little evidence links selenium in animal feeds to environmental toxicity, higher levels of the element in the future could create a problem.

The U.S. Food and Drug Administration (FDA) is currently appraising the environmental impact of selenium. Selenium is one of the most hazardous nutrients used in the feed industry. Feed mill operators can be at risk from the dust if adequate measures are not taken.

28.4 IODINE

Iodine is an important element for animals because of its role in the synthesis of the thyroid hormones thyroxine (T_4) and triiodothyronine (T_3). These hormones affect rate of metabolism; growth; reproduction; health and survival of offspring; lactation; and development of brain, lung, and heart. In ruminants the major site of absorption of iodine is the rumen, although absorption also occurs in the small and large intestines. The abomasum is the major site of endogenous secretion. They are also involved in the maintenance of reproductive efficiency and lactation. See Tables 28–4 and 28–5.

The iodine content of water and feeds depends on the availability of iodine in the soil and the amount of iodine content of fertilizer applied to the soil. Soils low in iodine produce plants low in iodine. In geographic areas where people and animals feed on plant and animal material from soils low in iodine, goiter is endemic. Iodine deficiency, simple goiter, has been recognized in both humans and animals for hundreds of years as an important metabolic disorder.

Iodine is not required as an essential nutrient by plants. The variation in iodine content of various pasture species is marked, however. Levels are high in perennial ryegrass and white clover, but low in some grasses: cockfoot and Yorkshire fog. A seasonal trend is apparent also, with highest

TABLE 28–6
ANTI-THYROID SUBSTANCES IN PLANTS—GOITROGENS
THESE BLOCK SYNTHESIS OF THYROXIN EVEN IF THERE IS NO DIETARY
IODINE DEFICIENCY

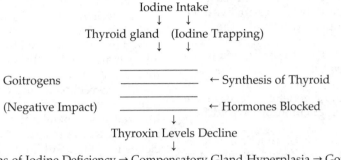

Naturally occurring *GOITROGENS* from Rape/Kale act as follows:

Iodine Intake
↓   ↓
Thyroid gland   (Iodine Trapping)
↓   ↓

Goitrogens ———————————— ← Synthesis of Thyroid

(Negative Impact) ———————————— ← Hormones Blocked
↓
Thyroxin Levels Decline
↓
← Clinical Signs of Iodine Deficiency → Compensatory Gland Hyperplasia → Goiter

Thus Sheep/Cattle in *Iodine Sufficient* Areas *May Need High Doses of Iodine* by Injection to Overcome Goitrogen Block.

New Faster Growing Grass Species)
High Usage of Fertilizers) Iodine Deficiency in Grasses
Higher Dependency on Grasses/Silage)

iodine levels occurring in pastures in winter. Some plants may contain goitrogens, which can induce clinical signs of iodine deficiency in animals with diets containing adequate iodine. The two main types of goitrogens follow.

1. The thiocyanate type, which inhibits the uptake of iodine by the thyroid gland, thereby resulting in a compensatory goiter. This condition can be treated by injection with iodine preparations.
2. Thiouracil type, which interferes with the oxidation of iodine in the thyroid gland.

White clover and *Brassica* species contain thiocyanate. The adverse effects of dietary goitrogens upon requirements for iodine mean that higher levels of iodine are necessary if crops high in goitrogen content (e.g., rape, turnips, kale) are used as winter fodder to pregnant animals. (Table 28–6)

Low soil iodine levels are associated with distance from the sea and annual rainfall. Iodine deficiency is most likely to occur when rainfall is heavy and iodine in the soil is continually depleted by leaching. The ability of the soil to retain iodine under conditions of high rainfall is directly related to its type and geological formation. Goiter does not occur regularly from year to year in animals, perhaps because of climatic or management factors.

Interest in iodine deficiency has been renewed in recent years. In many geographic areas, this interest is based on the increasing incidence of still-born calves or neonatal deaths in calves and lambs that show an enlarged and hyperplastic thyroid gland. This has led to these assumptions:

1. That the enlarged thyroid is related to cause of death
2. That the enlarged thyroid results from too little iodine in the diet

DEFICIENCY

Iodine deficiency in cattle is first observed as an enlargement of the thyroid glands in slaughtered cattle or newborn calves. Birth of goitrous calves is a sign of borderline or definite dietary iodine deficiency even though the cows may appear in normal condition. More than a year on low-iodine diets may be required before deficiency signs are noticed. Long-term deficiencies may result in decreased milk yields, low conception rates, and increased incidence of metritis.

Obscure iodine deficiencies in livestock can pass unrecognized because the deficiency may cause only stillbirths or weak hairless offspring. The origin of goiter when detected in calves must be determined. Goiter can result from iodine deficiency, goitrogens in the feed, or genetic defects in the production and regulation of thyroid hormones.

Goitrogens may be of practical importance because they are found as goitrin in most members of the *Brassica* family. These substances interfere with synthesis of thyroid hormone by limiting the capacity of the thyroid to "trap" iodine or to incorporate it into thyroactive substances. Other thioglycosides with antithyroid activity have been found in cruciferous plants, and cyanogenetic glycosides, which convert hydrocyanic acid into thiocyanate, have been found in tissues.

Application of lime to pasture can also reduce iodine content. By contrast with the common inorganic fertilizers, farmyard manure can exercise a powerful influence on iodine content of plants. It can decrease iodine levels of perennial ryegrass tenfold. The effect is probably attributable to the strong affinity of iodine for organic matter.

The signs of iodine deficiency can be produced by the presence of goitrogenic substances. Brassicas, such as kale, contain goitrogens of the thiouracil type that inhibit hormone synthesis in the thyroid, and their effects cannot be completely overcome by additional dietary iodine. Iodine supplementation by injection may be preferable in such cases. Cyanogenetic goitrogens are present in some clovers, and they inhibit the uptake of iodine by the thyroid. Their effects can be overcome by increasing the intake of iodine.

Goitrogen may interfere with the uptake of iodine by the thyroid gland or with the synthesis of thyroxin. Thiocyanate produced from cyanide in white clover may interfere with iodine uptake by the thyroid and exacerbate an iodine deficiency.

Because goitrogens occur in the *Cruciferae* family of plants, especially the *Brassica* species (kale, rape, turnips), pregnant ewes grazing these crops have produced goitrous lambs. The feeding of brassicas or fodder containing inadequate iodine results in calves with goiter. This outcome is caused by a goitrogen or by an insufficient intake of iodine. Differences in thyroid activity and improved iodine status have been observed in cattle switched from hay to silage. Silage may have less thyroactive substances than does the hay.

With respect to iodine deficiency symptoms commonly observed in ruminants, a lowered basal metabolic rate is seen in all animals. In the pregnant animal, a deficiency is apt to result in the birth of hairless (or woolless), weak, or dead young. Goiter results from changes in thyroid tissue cells, which undergo compensatory enlargement as a result of the deficiency of iodine. Goiter may be a symptom of a less severe deficiency than that characterized by the lack of hair or wool.

Clinical Signs

Failure to Reproduce. Iodine deficiency can cause the arrest of fetal development at any stage, thus leading to early embryonic death, resorption, or absorption. Substestrus in cows and loss of libido in bulls has also been reported.

Perinatal Mortality. Perinatal mortality is characterized by birth of weak or dead calves. This outcome can be associated with prolonged gestation and parturition and retention of fetal membranes. A catarrhal endometritis following normal expulsion of the placenta often appears to be associated with suboptimal iodine intake. Affected calves may show varying degrees of hairlessness and enlarged thyroid glands.

Other Clinical Signs. Lowered milk production is reported to be a frequent symptom of clinical iodine deficiency. Metabolic disorders of ketosis and hypomagnesemia have been suggested to be predisposed by hypothyroidism.

TABLE 28–7
IODINE DEFICIENCY—CALVES/LAMBS

— Unthriftiness
— Slow growth rate (interferes with growth hormone)
— Hairlessness
— Poor wool growth
— Low quality fleece
— Susceptibility to ectoparasites/endoparasites
— Lowered milk production
— Reproductive failure—difficult calvings—repeat breeders
— Fetal mortality—dead calves/lambs
— Enlarged thyroid gland—goiter—Compensatory Hyperplasia
— Anemia
— Retained placentas
— Susceptibility to infections—scours

Management

High protein intake or underfeeding has been suggested to interfere with the utilization of iodine by reducing serum globulins that bind thyroid hormones.

Such management practices, as ploughing up permanent paddocks can induce iodine deficiency, probably from increased leaching of iodine.

IODINE STATUS

Iodine deficiency can be detected by analysis of blood serum or milk for iodine. Total iodine concentrations of less than 40 μg/liter of serum or of 25 μg/liter of milk indicate iodine deficiency. When iodine in bulk herd milk is below 20 μg/liter, iodine in the diet may be too low. Iodine deficiency may appear in cattle on iodine sufficient diets if as much as a quarter of the feed is from strongly goitrogenic crops, especially *Brassica* forages.

Iodine status is commonly determined in the laboratory by measuring the plasma protein-bound iodine concentration, but this measurement does not correlate well with the secretion of thyroid hormones. The most reliable method is the measurement of the thyroxin (T_4) concentration in the plasma. A simple and useful technique for lactating cows is to measure the iodine content of the milk, which usually correlates well with iodine intake.

The iodine content of milk may be a useful indicator of iodine deficiency in a herd. Iodine values in milk of less than 25 μg/liter indicate a suboptimal intake in cows, and iodine concentrations in milk of less than 80 μg/liter indicate an iodine deficiency state in ewes. A sensitive diagnostic test of thyroid insufficiency arising from inadequate iodine nutrition in ewes may be to measure the change in thyroxin concentrations after iodine supplementation.

Protein-bound iodine (PBI) values of 3 to 4 μg/dl are currrently regarded as "normal" for adult sheep and cattle. Serum PBI values consistently below 3 to 4 μg/dl may therefore be regarded as suggestive of thyroid insufficiency in farm animals. Usually T_4 levels are measured in laboratory blood tests by radioimmunoassay. These are better indices for deficiency analysis.

The overall diagnosis of the cause of goiter involves assessment of the iodine nutrition of the herd, thyroid function tests, and chemical analyses of the feed for goitrogens. Iodine concentration in milk of less than 25 μg/liter indicates that cattle have a low iodine intake. Provision of salt licks containing stabilized iodine may overcome the deficiency.

IODINE IN PREGNANCY

The primary physiologic requirement for iodine is synthesis by the thyroid gland of hormones that regulate rate of energy metabolism. This is affected by the efficiency of dietary iodine content, thyroid collection of iodine fed, the presence or absence of goitrogens, the extent of iodine recycling within the body, and the rate of secretion of iodine from the thyroid.

Lactating cows require more iodine than do nonlactating cattle because a significant fraction of the iodine intake is normally excreted in milk. This amount may increase with the level of milk production. Although iodine needs of high-producing lactating cows are met under normal feed conditions nonetheless, cows in the last 2 months of gestation should be supplemented with iodine because of the possible harmful effect on the fetus if iodine is deficient.

DIAGNOSIS

Perinatal mortality is best diagnosed using weight of thyroid gland and histologic findings. Stillbirths, hairlessness and increased incidence of metritis are other indications.

Reproductive failure and lower milk production are more difficult to diagnose. They are general signs not necessarily solely attributable to iodine deficiency. However, low conception rates, and reproductive inefficiency are clearly linked to iodine deficiency. Currently, these conditions are best assessed by a response trial comparing iodine-supplemented and unsupplemented groups of animals.

Laboratory analytical tests that have been or can be used are as follows.

1. Milk iodine using a bulk herd milk sample. Iodoform disinfectants applied to the teats can affect this test, however.
2. About 90% of iodine bound to plasma protein is T_4; the remainder is T_3 and other iodine derivatives. Total serum iodine. This test more closely reflects dietary iodine intake than does plasma-bound iodine. Serum T_4 and T_3 levels, determined by radioimmunoassay (RIA), are used in humans to assess thyroid function. These RIA tests are now used routinely in animals to measure blood iodine status and thyroid function. Of the preceding analytical tests, T_4 and T_3 RIA are considered the most useful, because of their accuracy in reflecting iodine in-

take, thyroid trapping, and hormone formation.
3. Finally, pasture or dietary iodine levels can act as a guide to possible deficiency but should not be used to diagnose deficiency in the animal, because levels could be normal, but goitrogens might be interfering with their utilization.

TREATMENT AND PREVENTION

The daily requirement of iodine for a lactating cow is approximately 10 mg. This amount may need to be increased to 15 mg if large amounts of reversible goitrogens (thiocyanate type) are fed.

Iodine should be supplemented 3 months before parturition to prevent abortion, stillbirth and placental retention. When treatment is first initiated, abortions and perinatal deaths may not always stop at once. A few sporadic cases may occur for up to 2 months after commencing treatment. Supplementation may be performed orally by potassium iodide, potassium iodate, or by a depot oily injection.

An iodized oil preparation (475 mg iodine/ml Lipiodol) given by intramuscular injection (4 ml) is considered to be effective for 2 years in dairy cattle. Administration should be performed before mating.

Iodine and Lipiodol

Lipiodol is a slow-release depot iodine injection in poppy seed oil given by intramuscular injection. This method of administering iodine is most suitable because of the slow release and slow absorption of iodine over a prolonged period of time. This characteristic is particularly important in ruminant animals, in grazing animals, and in pregnant stock, in which the need for iodine intake is continuous and the demands for the developing fetus in pregnancy are increased. It has also been used in horses to augment reproductive efficiency.

1. To prevent abortion, stillbirth, and placental retention, the injection should be administered at least 1 month before calving or lambing, or 1 month before mating.
2. When flocks are feeding off *Brassicas* species, the injection should be administered

2 months before commencement of such feeding.

3. In known iodine-deficient areas, the depot injection should be routinely administered.

4. For optimum growth and reproductive performance in all stock, Lipiodol should be administered at least once, preferably at weaning. (Lipiodol is claimed to increase fleece weight by 20%.)

Cattle and horses should receive 4 ml intramuscularly every 2 years. Sheep, goats, and deer should receive 1 ml intramuscularly once in a lifetime.

This depot injection given to ewes before breeding can result in:

1. An increase in the number of live lambs born
2. A reduction in the number of deaths among young lambs
3. A better wool clip from the ewes
4. Better growth rates in lambs
5. Better reproductive efficiency in cows

SELECTED REFERENCES

Allen, W.M., Moore, P.R., and Sansom, B.F.: Controlled release glasses for selenium supplementation. *In* Trace Element Metabolism in Man and Animals. New York, Springer Verlag, 1982.

Ammerman, C.B.: Recent developments in cobalt and copper in ruminant nutrition: A review. J. Dairy Sci., *53*:1097, 1970.

Andrewartha, K.A., and Caple, I.W.: Effects of changes in nutritional copper in erythrocyte superoxide dismutase activities in sheep. Res. Vet. Sci., *28*:101, 1980.

Boila, R.J.: Cupric oxide needles for grazing cattle—growth and metabolic interrelationships. Can. J. Anim. Sci., *67*:577, 1987.

Boyne, R., and Arthur, J.R.: Effects of molybdenum or iron induced copper deficiency on the viability and function of neutrophils from cattle. Res. Vet. Sci., *41*:417, 1986.

Boyne, R., and Arthur, J.R.: Effects of selenium and copper deficiency on neutrophil function in cattle. J. Comp. Pathol., *91*:271, 1981.

Bray, A.C., Suttle, N.F., and Field, A.C.: The formation of tri and tetrathiomolybdates in continuous cultures of rumen microorganisms and their adsorption onto fibra. Proc. Nutr. Soc., *41*:67A, 1982.

Bremner, I., Mills, C.F., and Young, B.W.: Copper metabolism in rats given di or trithiomolybdate. J. Inorg. Biochem., *16*:109, 1982.

Caple, I.W.: Trace elements: deficiencies, nutrition and disease. *In* Proc. No. 68. Beef Cattle Production.

Post-Graduate Committee in Veterinary Science, The University of Sydney, 1984.

Caple, I.W., and McDonald, J.W.: Trace Mineral Nutrition. *In* Sheep Production and Preventive Medicine. Post-Graduate Committee in Veterinary Science, The University of Sydney, 1983.

Caple, I.W., Andrewartha, K.A., and Nugent, G.F.: Iodine deficiency in livestock in Victoria. Vic. Vet. Proc., *38*:43, 1980.

Cline, J.H.: Trace minerals, copper, zinc, and cobalt in health and disease. Proc. MSU Vet. Conf., 322, 1981.

Conrad, H.R., and Moxon, A.L.: Transfer of dietary selenium to milk. J. Dairy Sci., *62*:404, 1979.

Deland, M.P.B., Cunningham, P., Milne, M.L., and Dewey, D.W.: Copper administration to young calves: oral dosing with copper oxide compared with subcutaneous copper glycinate injection. Aust. Vet. J., *55*:493, 1979.

Deland, M.P.B., Lewis, D., Cunningham, P.R., et al.: Use of orally administered oxidized copper wire particles for copper therapy in cattle. Aust. Vet. J., *63*:1, 1986.

Dick, A.J., Dewey, D.W., and Gawthorne, J.M.: Thiomolybdates and the copper-molybdenum-sulphur interaction in ruminant nutrition. J. Agricultural Sci., *85*:567, 1975.

Eckenhoff, J.B.: Veterinary dosage forms using principles of osnosis. *In* Proc. Intl. Symp. Control Rel. Bioact. Mater., *15*:227, 1988.

Gay, C.C., Pritchett, L.C., and Madson, W.: Copper deficiency in ruminants. *In* Proc. 20th Annual Meeting, Am. Assoc. Bovine Pract., 1988.

Gleed, P.T., Allen, W.M., Mallinson, C.B., et al.: Effects of selenium and copper supplementation on the growth of beef steers. Vet. Rec., *113*:388, 1983.

Gooneratne, S.R., Buckley, W.T., and Christensen, D.A.: Review of copper deficiency and metabolism in ruminants. Can. J. Anim. Sci., *69*:819, 1989.

Gyang, E.O., Stevens, J.B., Olson, W.G., et al.: Effects of selenium vitamin E injection on bovine polymorphonucleated leukocytes, phagocytosis and killing of *Staphylococcus aureus*. Am. J. Vet. Res., *45*:175, 1984.

Halpin, C.G.: Plasma cobalamin (vitamin B_{12}) analogues in cattle. Proc. Nutr. Soc. (Aust.), *7*:184, 1982.

Judson, G.J., Brown, T.H., Gray, D., et al.: Oxidized copper wire particles for copper therapy in sheep. Aust. J. Agric. Res., *33*:1073, 1982.

Judson, G.J., Dewey, D.W., McFarlane, J.D., et al.: Oxidized copper wire for oral copper therapy in cattle. Edited by J.M. Gawthorne, J. McC. Howell, and C.L. White. *In* Trace Element Metabolism in Man and Animals. New York, Springer Verlag, 1982.

Judson, G.J., Mattschoss, K.H., and Clare, R.J.: Selenium pellets for cattle. Aust. Vet. J., *56*:304, 1980.

Julien, W.E., Contrad, H.R., Jones, J.E., et al.: Selenium and vitamin E and incidence of retained placenta in parturient dairy cows. J. Dairy Sci., *59*:1954, 1976.

Kuchel, R.E., and Buckley, R.A.: The provision of selenium to sheep by means of a heavy pellet. Aust. J. Agric. Res., 20:1099, 1969.

MacPherson, A.: Copper oxide wire for the bovine. In Trace Elements in Animal Production and Veterinary Practice. Edinburgh, Publication No. 7 of the British Society of Animal Production, 1983.

MacPherson, A., Moon, F.E., and Voss, R.C.: Biochemical aspects of cobalt deficiency in sheep with special reference to vitamin status and a possible involvement in the aetiology of cerebrocortical necrosis. Br. Vet. J., 132:294, 1976.

Mason, J.: Molybdenum-copper antagonism in ruminants: A review of the biochemical basis. Irish Vet. J., 35:221, 1981.

McClure, T.J., Eamens, G.J., and Healy, P.J.: Improved fertility in dairy cows after treatment with selenium pellets. Aust. Vet. J., 63:144, 1986.

NRC: Nutrient Requirements of Dairy Cattle. 6th Ed. Washington, D.C., National Academy Press, 1989.

National Academy of Sciences: Nutrient Requirements of Dairy Cattle. 5th Ed. Washington, D.C., National Academy of Sciences, 1978.

Naylor, J.M., Kasari, T.R., Blakely, B.R., et al.: Diagnosis of copper deficiency and effects of supplementation in beef cows. Can. J. Vet. Res., 53:343, 1989.

Paynter, D.I., Hucker, D.A., and McOwan, D.H.: Changes in erythrocyte Cu-An superoxide dismutase activity following thiomolybdate administration to sheep. Proc. Nutr. Soc. (Aust.), 7:185, 1982.

Phillipo, M., Humphries, W.R., Bremner, I., and Young, B.W.: Possible effect of molybdenum on fertility in the cow. Proc. Nutr. Soc., 41:80A, 1982.

Richards, D.H., Hewett, G.R., Parry, J.M., et al.: Bovine copper deficiency: Use of copper oxide needles. Vet. Rec., 116:618, 1985.

Sanders, D.E.: Cobalt in bovine nutrition. Compend. Contin. Educ. Pract. Vet., 11:757, 1989.

Stogdale, L.: Chronic copper poisoning in dairy cows. Aust. Vet. J., 54:139, 1978.

Sumner, G.J.: Safety and efficacy of a bovine sustained-release selenium device. In Proc. Am. Acad. Vet. Consultants. Trenton, NJ, Veterinary Learning Systems, 1988.

Suttle, N.F.: The interactions between copper, molybdenum, and sulphur in ruminant nutrition. Annu. Rev. Nutr., 11:121, 1991.

Suttle, N.F.: Bovine hypocuprosis. Vet. Ann., 23:96, 1983.

Suttle, N.F.: Dietary molybdenum reduces the effectiveness of oral and parenteral treatments for hypocuprosis. In Trace Elements in Animal Production and Veterinary Practice. Edinburgh, Publication No. 7 of the British Society of Animal Production, 1983.

Suttle, N.F., and Jones, D.G.: Recent developments in trace element metabolism and function: trace elements, disease resistance and immune responsiveness in ruminants. J. Nutr., 119:1055, 1989.

Trinder, N., Woodhouse, C.D., and Rentan, C.P.: The effect of vitamin E and selenium on the incidence of retained placentae in dairy cows. Vet. Rec., 85:550, 1969.

Underwood, E.J.: The Mineral Nutrition of Livestock. New York, Food and Agricultural Association of the United Nations and Commonwealth Agricultural Bureaus, 1981.

Underwood, E.J.: Trace Elements in Human and Animal Nutrition. 4th Ed. New York, Academic Press, 1977.

Whitelaw, A., Armstrong, R.H., Evans, C.C., et al.: Effects of oral administration of copper oxide needles to hypocupraemia sheep. Vet. Rec., 107:87, 1980.

Wikse, S.E., Herd, D., Feild, R., and Holland, P.: Diagnosis of copper deficiency in cattle. J. Am. Vet. Med. Assoc., 10(11):1625, 1992.

THERAPY OF ENDOPARASITES IN CATTLE AND SHEEP

29.1 Bovine Ostertagiasis

29.2 Lungworm Infestation in Calves (Parasitic Bronchitis)

29.3 Liver Fluke (Fascioliasis) in Cattle

29.4 Parasitic Gastroenteritis in Sheep

29.5 Fascioliasis in Sheep

29.6 Bovine Coccidiosis

29.7 Cryptosporidiosis

29.1 BOVINE OSTERTAGIASIS

The internal parasites of cattle can be divided into three main groups: roundworms (nematodes), which parasitize the abomasum, intestines, and lungs; tapeworms (cestodes), which parasitize the intestines; and flukes (trematodes), which parasitize the liver.

Nematodes that parasitize the stomach and intestines are collectively referred to as gastrointestinal nematodes, and the disease for which they are responsible is termed parasitic gastroenteritis. Although some 18 species of gastrointestinal nematodes are known to parasitize cattle, the stomach worm *Ostertagia ostertagi* is the most pathogenic and economically the most important. Parasitic gastroenteritis caused by *O. ostertagi* is referred to as ostertagiasis.

The important gastrointestinal parasites are *Ostertagia* (ostertagi), *Haemonchus*, and *Trichostrongylus axei* in the abomasum; *Cooperia oncophora, Nematodirus helvetianus, Bunostomum phlebotomum,* and *Stronglyloides papillosus* (in young calves) in the small intestine; and *Oesophagostomum radiatum* in the large intestine.

Nematodes that parasitize the lungs are called lungworms, and only one species, *Dictyocaulus viviparus*, occurs in cattle. It is responsible for the condition known as parasitic bronchitis, commonly referred to as husk or hoose.

The importance of the tapeworm *Moniezia* as a cause of poor production in cattle is open to question. At present, little evidence shows its importance in this respect.

Fascioliasis is another important parasitic condition of cattle. It is caused by the liver fluke, *Fasciola hepatica*.

The abomasal nematode parasite of cattle, *Ostertagia ostertagi*, has drawn a considerable amount of attention over the last 2 or 3 decades. It has been described as the singlemost pathogenic and economically important parasite of cattle in temperate areas of the world.

Ostertagiasis is widely known as a common disease entity in cattle throughout the country and is probably a cause of major production deficiency in subclinical parasitism. Ostertagiasis can be classified into two basic types. Type I ostertagiasis is commonly seen in young calves during their first season at grass. It can occur at any time from July to the end of the grazing season. In this type of disease, many larvae ingested with the herbage cause severe damage to the gastric glands during the course of their development into adult worms (usually completed in 3 weeks). Type II ostertagiasis or "winter scours" is commonly seen in yearling cattle in the late winter and spring of the year following their first season at grass. The disease is caused by the sudden resumed development of many arrested fourth-stage larvae that originally were acquired when the animals were at grass in the autumn of the previous year. Ostertagiasis can occur in both housed animals and those at grass.

LIFE CYCLE OF *OSTERTAGIA OSTERTAGI*

All gastrointestinal nematodes have life cycles similar to that of *O. ostertagi*. Adult female worms in the stomach lay eggs that pass out in the feces. In the fecal pat, the eggs develop and hatch, consequently releasing first-stage larvae. Development then proceeds through two larval stages until a third stage, infective larva, is produced. Under suitable conditions of moisture, infective larvae migrate from the fecal pat onto the herbage. When ingested by the grazing animal, the larvae pass to the abomasum, enter the glands that line the wall of this organ, and become fourth-stage larvae. Following a period of development and growth in the gastric glands, these larvae mature into adult worms, emerge from the glands, and lie on the surface of the stomach lining. Under normal conditions, approximately 21 days elapse between the ingestion of infective larvae and the appearance of adult, egg-laying worms in the stomach. The damage caused to the gastric glands by developing fourth-stage larvae results in digestive disturbances that are reflected in the common symptoms of loss of appetite, poor growth, and diarrhea characteristic of the disease.

Under certain conditions, the development and growth of early fourth-stage larvae in the gastric glands can be interrupted. The larvae then remain in a state of arrested development for as long as 6 months. The reasons for arrested development are complex, but larvae acquired from herbage during the autumn and early winter apparently tend to become arrested and can remain in this state until the following spring. At such time, development is resumed, and the life cycle is completed in the normal way.

EPIDEMIOLOGY

When weaned calves are turned out in spring onto pastures that have been grazed by cattle in the previous year, the calves immediately become infected with worms and, as a result, pass eggs in their feces for several weeks. These eggs undergo a period of development in the fecal pat and eventually form infective larvae. These larvae then migrate onto the herbage. The rate at which the eggs develop into infective larvae is governed by temperature. Eggs passed during the early part of the grazing season require 2 to 3 months to develop, whereas those passed in the midseason require only 1 or 2 weeks. All the eggs passed during spring and early summer thus tend to complete their development at about the same time. Consequently, many infective larvae suddenly appear on the pasture in midseason and persist at these high levels throughout the remainder of the year. The ingestion of many infective larvae during the second half of the grazing season and their subsequent development in the animal cause type I ostertagiasis.

Infective larvae that are not ingested persist on the herbage throughout the autumn and winter and into the spring of the following year. At this time, they begin to die off, and by early June, the larvae remaining on the herbage usually fall to insignificant levels. Although the numbers of infective larvae on pasture in spring are usually not high enough to cause disease, sufficient larvae remain to initiate new infections in calves turned out at this time. In this way, infections are maintained on pasture from year to year.

Depending on regional conditions, age, class of animals, management systems, and other factors, development of the parasite in the host after ingestion may proceed normally or may undergo a period of dormancy.

Type I ostertagiasis is the clinical entity during which many rapidly acquired larvae complete their development to the adult stage in 3 to 4 weeks. Cases in beef cattle may occur from the time of weaning until 18 months of age during winter and spring in southern temperate environments. In northern temperate environments, such infections are observed from mid-July to the end of autumn grazing in October. Most animals in a herd can be affected, but mortality is low if treatment is administered within a few days from the onset of clinical signs. Nearly any broad-spectrum anthelmintic is effective at this time.

A major feature of type I disease found at necropsy is many worms, most of which are adults. Type I represents the condition resulting from the strain with a cycle of 21 to 28 days. The fourth-stage larvae spend only a few days in the gastric glands and then emerge and rapidly mature to the egg-laying adult stage. After ingestion by cattle, *O. ostertagi* third-stage larvae enter gastric glands and molt to the fourth larval stage. This process requires about 4 days. In the course of normal development, the parasite grows and molts to the early or fifth stage at 10 to 12 days after infection. At this point, they emerge from the tissue, mature to adults on the mucosal surface, and mate. Total time required for development from third-stage larvae to sexually mature adults is about 3 weeks. Major pathologic changes in the abomasum and clinical signs occur when the young adults emerge from the tissue to the lumen.

Type II represents the condition caused by a strain of *Ostertagia* with a prolonged cycle. This long cycle is caused by the fourth-stage larvae, which persist in the gastric glands for 14 to 18 weeks. This strain overwinters in cattle in northern temperate areas and oversummers in southern zones. Most larvae ingested on pasture undergo the first parasitic molt to the early fourth stage in the gastric glands, but develop no further for a variable and often protracted period of time. The larvae at this stage are slightly longer than 1 mm and are largely undifferentiated. Histologically, they can be seen deep in the abomasal mucosa at the base of glands. Some practitioners have theorized that larval metabolism is depressed during the inhibited state. Host response to the larvae is little or none, and they are not susceptible to the effects of such drugs as thiabendazole, oxibendazole, levamisole, or morantel tartrate.

The terms larval hypobiosis and inhibited, arrested, or retarded development are used by various authors to describe the same phenomenon. Inhibition of this nematode has been likened to the state of dormancy, in which insect populations survive through periods of adverse climate. The diarrhea, weight loss, poor appetite, and other clinical signs observed in the host animal coincide with the damage caused to the mucosa as young adult worms emerge from the tissue. The adult worms, once free on the mucosal surface, are not the major factor involved in pathogenesis.

THERAPY

The control of ostertagiasis in young cattle should always be based on a prophylactic strategy that uses strategic dosing to limit the number of eggs and therefore the number of developing larvae on the pasture. Clinical outbreaks of type I ostertagiasis can be avoided by administering medication to cattle in the middle of the grazing season and then moving cattle to a clean pasture (i.e., not grazed that year). If this move is not feasible, 3 doses of anthelmintic should be administered 3, 6, and 9 weeks after turning out.

At the recommended dose rates in cattle, thiabendazole, oxibendazole, and thiophanate are effective only against adult and developing larval stages of the common gastrointestinal nematodes. (At an increased dose rate, however, thiophanate is effective against lungworms.) Albendazole, fenbendazole, and oxfendazole have broader spectra of activity that include nematode larvae arrested in their development. Albendazole and oxfendazole are also effective against tapeworms. The spectra for netobimin and albendazole are extended further to include adult *Fasciola hepatica*, although the doses must be increased to 20 mg/kg and 10 mg/kg, respectively, for efficacy against this parasite species. The higher dosage is recommended for netobimin used in the treatment of arrested nematode larvae (Tables 29–1 and 29–2).

The most appropriate anthelmintics for use against ostertagiasis type I are drugs that possess activity against lumen-dwelling adults and developing larvae. (Activity against the hypobiotic stage in the abomasal glands is not necessary for anthelmintics used in prevention or treatment of type I ostertagiasis). Thus levamisole, thiabendazole, or oxibendazole can be employed exclusively for type I ostertagiasis therapy. Organophosphates such as coumaphos at a dosage of 2 mg/kg for 6 days can also be used.

A recent development has been the introduction of a sustained-release bolus containing morantel tartrate. Following oral administration at turn out using a special balling gun the bolus settles in the reticulum rumen and then releases morantel over a 90-day period, during which establishment of ingested larvae is prevented. By the end of this period, i.e., toward the end of July, the amount of infective larvae on pasture is small and unlikely to be significant. (The oxfendazole pulsed-release bolus is another novel system which provides protection.)

Anthelmintics effective not only against adult and developing larvae but also against arrested larvae can be used at any time of year. The following classes of anthelmintics may be considered also for control of ostertagiasis type I:

1. Ivermectin
2. The insoluble benzimidazoles—albendazole, fenbendazole, and oxfendazole
3. The probenzimidazoles—febantel, netobimin, and thiophanate. These anthelmintics may also be used at housing in the late autumn to kill any hypobiotic larvae, thus pre-empting the possibility of ostertagiasis type II outbreaks from January onward. (The use of ivermectin, given at winter housing, for type II ostertagiasis, possesses the added advantage of ectoparasite control: lice, mites and hypoderma grubs.)

In routine use in dairy or beef calves, in situations other than the control of type II ostertagiasis, little difference in efficacy exists between any of the benzimidazoles, levamisole, or morantel, unless resistance is a particular problem. The ease of administration of injectable levamisole preparations, pour-

TABLE 29–1
GENERAL SPECTRUM OF ACTIVITY OF SOME COMMONLY USED ANTHELMINTICS IN RUMINANTS

Group	Chemical Name	Gastro-intestinal Nematodes	Inhibited Larvae	Lungworm	Fluke
Benzimidazoles	Luxabendazole	+	+	+	—
	Thiabendazole	+	—	—	—
	Parbendazole	+	+	—	—
	Fenbendazole	+	+	+	—
	Oxfendazole	+	+	+	—
	Albendazole	+	+	+	+
	Triclabendazole	—	—	—	+
	Oxibendazole	+	—	—	—
Probenzimidazoles	Febantel	+	+	+	—
	Thiophanate	+	+	+	—
Imidothiazoles	Levamisole	+	—	+	—
Pyrimidines	Morantel (Bolus)	+	—	Prevents Establishment	—
Avermectins	Ivermectin	+	+	+	—
Organophosphates	Haloxon/Coumaphos	+	—	—	—
Piperazine	Diethylcarbamazine	—	—	+	—
Salicylanilides	Rafoxanide	—	—	—	+
	Oxyclozanide	—	—	—	+
Substituted phenols	Nitroxynil	—	—	—	+
	Niclofolan	—	—	—	+
	Bithionol Sulfoxide	—	—	—	+
	Hexachlorophene	—	—	—	+
Aromatic amide	Diamphenethide	—	—	—	+
Sulfonamide	Clorsulon	—	—	—	+

on levamisole or ivermectin products, or intrarumenal oxfendazole injections gives them a significant marketing advantage.

Ivermectin, which is given by injection, or by pour-on technique has the advantage of ease of administration combined with a spectrum of activity that includes all the major nematodes, plus the sucking lice, mange mites, and some ticks and warble fly larvae. Its residual effectiveness confers a distinct clinical advantage related compounds moxidectin and doramectin are available in some countries. Ostertagiasis type II can be avoided by not moving calves back to original summer pastures before being housed in late autumn/early winter. A dose at housing should be administered. When the treatment is given in the autumn or winter, a large percentage of the larvae present probably are in the arrested or hypobiotic form. Thus, an anthelmintic that possesses a high efficacy against these inhibited larvae must be used.

Reliance formerly was placed on management techniques, particularly treatment in the grazing season combined with a shift to safe pastures. This procedure was difficult to implement on many properties, but the advent of ivermectin, fenbendazole, albendazole, oxfendazole, and febantel, which kill a high proportion of the dormant larvae, was a major breakthrough. The use of these compounds in the summer removes the hypobiotic larvae before they emerge and cause injury to the stomach.

Treatment of ostertagiasis type II is best accomplished using drugs that are effective against the arrested larval stages of the parasite, as well as against adult worms. Currently available anthelmintics with this activity are ivermectin, fenbendazole, oxfendazole and albendazole. Ivermectin

TABLE 29–2
SOME ANTHELMINTICS FOR CATTLE

Drug	Proprietary Name	Dosage	Route	Safety Index	Comments
Albendazole	Valbazen	7.5–10.0 mg/kg	Oral	20	Nematodes/Moniezia. Effective against mature fluke at increased dosage. Can be teratogenic.
Clorsulon	Curatrem	7 mg/kg	Oral	5	Fluke only—8 wks and upwards.
Fenbendazole	Panacur Safeguard	5–10 mg/kg	Oral	20	Nematodes/Moniezia. Ostertagiasis Type I, Type II Higher dosage for hypobiotic larvae and Moniezia.
Ivermectin	Ivomec	0.2 mg/kg	Subcutaneously	30	Nematodes/Ectoparasites. Osterlagiasis Type I and Type II Hypobiotic larvae. No effect on flukes or cestodes.
Ivermectin (bolus)	Ivomec	—	Oral	—	
Ivermectin/ clorsulon	Ivomec-F	1 mL/110 lbs	Subcutaneous	—	Nematodes/ectoparasites/Adult flukes
Levamisole	Levasole	7.5 mg/kg	Subcutaneous	5	Nematodes. No effect on hypobiotic *Ostertagia*.
Morantel	Paratect	22.7 g Bolus	Oral	30	Slow release of drug from bolus over 60–90 days. Prevention of *Ostertagiasis*.
Coumaphos	Baynix	2 mg/kg for 6 days	Oral feed additive	4–5	Nematodes in beef cattle.
Thiabendazole	Omnizole	66–88 mg/kg	Oral	15	Not effective against lungworm. Effective against Nematodes of gastrointestinal tract. Does not affect hypobiotic *Ostertagia*.
Triclabendazole	Fasinex	12 mg/kg	Oral	20	All stages of fluke from 2 weeks upward.

appears to have efficacy that approaches 100% and should eliminate most worms with a single treatment. Fenbendazole and albendazole and oxfendazole are slightly less effective, and removal of arrested stages may sometimes require twice the dosage recommended for adult parasites (Table 29–3).

The time of year may dictate the product used. With the older anthelmintics (thiabendazole and levamisole), treatment prior to placing cattle on pastures in spring should give best results. Ivermectin, (or moxidectin/doramectin) on the other hand, may be used to advantage in the fall for hypoderma grubs control and to eliminate immature *Ostertagia* that would be carried through the winter in infected cattle. In either case, one treatment per year should be sufficient. Although generally showing good to excellent activity against inhibited larvae at the approved dose of 5 mg/kg, fenbendazole may have some variability of efficacy against the inhibited forms. The variability has been demonstrated with all benzimidazole compounds, and its cause is largely unknown. The variability is essentially an incomplete removal of inhibited larvae from individual

TABLE 29–3
SOME ANTINEMATODAL DRUGS FOR CATTLE

Chemical	Drug	Route	>90% efficacy at recommended rate*				
			Gut	Worms		Dictyocaulus	
			A	DL	AL	A	DL
Benzimidazoles	Fenbendazole	Oral	+	+	+	+	+
	Oxfendazole	Oral	+	+	+	+	+
	Oxibendazole	Oral	+	+	—	—	—
	Albendazole	Oral	+	+	+	+	+
	Thiabendazole	Oral	+	+	–	–	–
Probenzimid-	Febantel	Oral	+	+	+	+	+
azoles	Thiophanate	Oral	+	+	+	+	+
	Netobimin	Oral	+	+	+	+	+
Imidazothiazoles	Levamisole	SC					
		Oral/SC	+	+	–	+	+
		Intramuscular					
		Pour-on					
Pyrimidines	Morantel	Bolus	+	+	–	(prevents establishments)	
Avermectins	Ivermectin/ Doramectin/ Moxidectin	Bolus/pour-on injection	+	+	+	+	+

*A = adults; DL = developing larvae; AL = arrested larvae (mainly *Ostertagia*)

treated cattle within a group. Fenbendazole, oxfendazole, albendazole, and ivermectin should be highly efficient in removing inhibited larvae during the pre-type II phase and in minimizing losses during actual type II disease outbreaks, particularly if the condition can be detected at its onset in a herd. In experimental trials, ivermectin has demonstrated a consistently high level of efficacy against inhibited larvae. Use of anthelmintics alone relies on frequent administration to totally suppress infection and pasture contamination, whereas integration with pasture management (safe pasture) can extend the effectiveness and reduce the frequency of treatment.

29.2 LUNGWORM INFESTATION IN CALVES (PARASITIC BRONCHITIS)

The epidemiology of this disease is complex and still not fully understood. Calves turned out in spring onto pasture grazed by cattle in the previous year may acquire low levels of infection from infective larvae that have overwintered on the herbage. First-stage larvae passed by these animals de-

velop into third-stage infective larvae. Many of these third-stage larvae can suddenly appear on pasture and cause disease at any time from midseason onward. Older animals that have acquired an immunity, but still harbor small numbers of lungworms, may contribute to the pasture contamination and, therefore, act as a source of infection for calves. The calf swallows worm larvae with the forage and thus infects itself with the lungworms. The susceptible calf (3 to 9 months of age) can become heavily infected.

Infection with adult lungworms produces a pneumonia with the clinical symptoms of coughing, some elevation of temperature, and, ultimately, varying degrees of lung consolidation. When a calf has consolidation of the lungs, a part of the lung tissue is replaced with scar tissue that remains for the rest of the animal's life. This type of lung damage stunts the calf as it grows older, and its lung capacity does not increase normally. Bronchitis and pneumonia may be caused by the migration of developing fourth-stage larvae through the lungs and by the presence of adult worms in the bronchi and trachea. The severity of the disease depends on the level of infection; it can vary from slight coughing when the level of infection is low, through bronchitis and pneumonia of varying degrees of severity, to sudden death when massive infection has taken place. Generally only calves in their first grazing season are affected; older animals usually have developed a strong immunity to reinfection.

Eggs laid by female worms hatch and release first-stage larvae while still in the lungs. These larvae are then coughed up, swallowed, and passed out in the feces. Here, the first-stage larvae develop into third-stage infective larvae, which migrate onto the herbage. When ingested by the grazing animal, the infective larvae pass to the intestine, burrow through its wall, develop into fourth-stage larvae, and pass by way of the blood stream to the lungs. Here they leave the blood vessels and enter the small air sacs and airways that make up most of the substance of the lung. They develop into adult worms that migrate through the airways until they arrive at the bronchi and trachea. Infective larvae develop into adult worms in 3 to 4 weeks.

THERAPY

As with ostertagiasis, the anthelmintic employed for the treatment of lungworm should be effective against the developing larvae and the adult parasite *Dictyocaulus viviparus*.

Successful removal of both prepatent and patent infections can be achieved by the use of the insoluble benzimidazoles, fenbendazole, oxfendazole, albendazole, febantel, and netobimin/thiophanate and also the use of ivermectin or levamisole.

Diethylcarbamazine citrate is available for use solely against the larval stages responsible for prepatent hoose. This drug, a derivative of piperazine, must be administered daily for 3 days by the intramuscular route.

Levamisole and febendazole remove arrested lungworm larvae, but the role of these hypobiotic stages is less well defined in parasitic bronchitis than in ostertagiasis. Fenbendazole is particularly effective against *D. viviparus*.

In cases of severe parasitic bronchitis with profound respiratory embarrassment, injectable products may be more advantageous than oral products because of their speedier onset of activity, higher bioavailability, and avoidance of inhalational respiratory problems. Levamisole is available as a subcutaneous injection, oral, or pour-on formulation, but evidence to date indicates great variations in absorption and anthelmintic efficiency following the pour-on route. Resistance to levamisole is becoming a significant problem on account of its overuse due to the variety of inexpensive preparations available. Severe hypersensitive-type reactions may occasionally occur following the treatment of severe cases of parasitic bronchitis with reputable products at the recommended dosage rate.

The sequential use of ivermectin at 3, 8, and 13 weeks after turnout provides strong protection against development of lungworm disease. The timing of the ivermectin treatments is based on the prepatent period of approximately 3 weeks and the findings of studies that have shown that ivermectin administered by subcutaneous injection has a prolonged action against some parasites of approximately 2 weeks. Hence, the first treatment is given after 3 weeks grazing, and further treatments are given at 5-week intervals until a maximum of 13 weeks after turnout have elapsed.

Pulsed-release boluses of oxfendazole are indicated for control of *Dictyocaulus* when given at turnout or shortly thereafter. Pulses at 3-week intervals are usually successful, and the new front-loaded oxfendazole bolus (with an extra oxfendazole tablet) provides immediate and useful control.

Control of lungworm infection in replacement heifers is not easy. One important reason is that older animals usually have a few adult lungworms that shed eggs on the pasture. This possibility is a good reason for not mixing groups of animals. Also, replacement heifers should be routinely treated with an effective anthelmintic drug.

One of the most effective drugs available for use against lungworm is levamisole. Routine treatment times vary with conditions on a given farm, but during the first 12 months of life, replacement heifer calves probably should be treated at least 3 times with the proper dose of levamisole to control lungworm infection. Lungworms are important in some areas, but the routine use of levamisole, fenbendazole, oxfendazole, albendazole, or ivermectin to control gastrointestinal parasites also controls lungworms. The morantel bolus can prevent establishment of lungworms in the host animal for up to 60 days after dosing.

29.3 LIVER FLUKE (FASCIOLIASIS) IN CATTLE

Liver flukes, *Fasciola hepatica* and *Fascioloides magna*, are common parasites. Historically, the endemic geographic areas for both parasites were rather well established, but expanded use of irrigation has changed the prevalence of *Fasciola hepatica* in recent years. This factor, together with the movement of livestock, has resulted in the appearance of *F. hepatica* in unexpected places. *Fascioloides magna* infections in cattle still occur in rather well-defined geographic areas where the reservoir hosts (deer and elk) are abundant but generally are not considered an important problem in livestock.

The common liver fluke (*Fasciola hepatica*) causes major economic losses in cattle. Fluke infections in cattle result in reduced growth rates and reduced feed efficiencies in growing animals, increased susceptibility to *Salmonella dublin* and clostridial infections of the liver, decreased reproductive efficiency in mature cattle, and increased percentage of liver condemnations in slaughtered animals.

Although losses caused by liver flukes are commonly recognized in terms of liver condemnations at slaughter, losses of far greater economic significance result from reduced conception rates in cow-calf herds, lower weaning weights, decreased feed efficiency, decreased milk production, and reduced weight gain.

LIFE CYCLE

The life cycle of the liver fluke *Fasciola hepatica* involves an intermediate host, the snail *Lymnaea truncatula*. Adult flukes live in the bile ducts of the liver. They lay eggs, which are passed out in the feces and develop into miracidia. These infect the intermediate snail host and multiply through a series of developmental stages lasting at least 5 weeks before emerging from the snail as cercariae, which encyst on blades of grass and become infective metacercariae. Following ingestion, metacercariae excyst, burrow through the intestinal wall, and migrate through the abdominal cavity to the liver. There they develop into immature liver flukes that migrate through the liver substance for approximately 6 weeks before entering the bile ducts and maturing into adult flukes 10 to 12 weeks after the ingestion of metacercariae. The epidemiology of the disease is closely linked with factors affecting the reproduction of the intermediate snail host. *Lymnaea truncatula* is essentially a mud snail that prefers soils that are saturated with water, e.g., poorly drained pastures, flushes, low-lying fields, and water meadows. Reproduction takes place during the summer months and is most successful when rainfall during this period is above average. These conditions are also the most suitable for the development and survival of miracidia, multiplication in the snail, and dispersion of cercariae on herbage.

Fluke eggs passed by infected animals during late spring and early summer develop into miracidia that infect the intermediate snail host. Multiplication in the snail takes at least 5 weeks, Cercariae then emerge, attach themselves to blades of grass, and become metacercariae. An increase in the numbers of metacercaria on the herbage occurs during the late summer and autumn and persists throughout the winter. When ingested by the grazing animal, they migrate to the liver and cause disease during the autumn, winter, and spring.

CLASSIFICATION OF DISEASE

Fascioliasis can be classified into two basic types. Acute fascioliasis is usually seen during autumn and early winter. This form of the disease is caused by the ingestion of several thousand metacercariae by the grazing animal, thereby resulting in extensive damage to the liver as young flukes migrate through its substance. In severe infections, the animal may be found dead without showing any clinical signs. Young cattle rarely suffer from acute fascioliasis; it is more commonly seen in sheep.

Chronic fascioliasis is usually seen during late winter and spring and is the usual form of the disease seen in cattle. Clinical signs are attributable to damage caused by the adult liver fluke in the bile ducts. Characteristically, loss of weight, inappetence, and anemia occur in affected animals. The flukes that live in the bile duct ultimately cause a blockage of the duct caused by the thickening of the walls. Because the cow requires the daily production of large volumes of bile to aid in the digestion of the fatty acids that come from the rumen, impairment of liver function causes serious consequences in the efficiency of the entire ruminant digestive system.

Cattle apparently have a higher natural resistance to infection with *Fasciola hepatica*, and the clinical syndrome usually seen is that of the chronic form. Clinical signs of chronic fascioliasis in cattle are loss of body weight and pallor of the mucous membranes; submandibular edema and ascites are seen less frequently.

Acute fascioliasis is primarily seen in sheep, although in years of high fluke challenge, it may also be seen in young cattle. The major sign is sudden death. The animal dies within about 6 weeks of ingesting massive numbers of metacercariae, which are on the pasture. When more than 1000 early immature flukes are present, they produce extensive damage to the liver tissue and severe hemorrhage that result in the death of the animal.

In the subacute form of the disease, the animals become infected over a longer period or are infected with fewer metacercariae than in acute fascioliasis. Deaths occur 10 to 20 weeks after the initial infection, and clinically a severe anemia, with pale mucous membranes, develops. Postmortem examination of dead animals and clinical examination with fecal egg counts and blood tests to confirm anemia in the surviving animals establish a diagnosis.

The most frequently encountered form of the disease in both sheep and cattle is chronic fascioliasis. The presence of 100 to 200 mature parasites in the bile duct is sufficient to cause a chronic anemia and a progressive loss in body condition in the affected livestock. Sometimes the classic sign of submandibular edema, known as bottle jaw, is visible, but in any case, diagnosis can be confirmed by finding fluke eggs in the feces and performing blood tests to establish the presence of anemia.

Treatment of fluke-infected sheep and cattle can lead to better fertility rates, with an increase in multiple births in sheep and fewer inseminations and reductions in calving intervals in cattle.

Most but not all of the flukicides available for use in cattle are not effective against the parenchymal stages, but rather against the mature form in the bile ducts. The drugs available are mainly salicylanilides and substituted phenols, benzimidazoles, or modified sulfonamides.

FLUKICIDES

Of the range of benzimidazoles, albendazole is active against mature flukes at twice the dosage rate recommended for roundworm therapy. Triclabendazole is a useful addition to the range currently available because it displays high efficacy against mature and immature flukes and yet displays a high margin of safety. Netobimin is also effective against mature flukes at a high dosage similar to that of albendazole (it is a prodrug of albendazole) (Table 29–4).

Albendazole is effective (75 to 95%) against adult flukes but not against immature migrating forms. Clorsulon is highly effective (>99%) against adult flukes and 95% effective against late immature (8-week-old) flukes, Clorsulon is only effective against *F. hepatica* and would ordinarily be given with a broad-spectrum anthelmintic, e.g., with ivermectin in a form such as Ivomec-F. Clorsulon is not significantly effective against *Fascioloides magna* or *Paramphistomum* in cattle at 7 mg/kg.

In addition to albendazole, netobimin and triclabendazole are other useful drugs. Treclabendazole is effective against all fluke stages, including migrating forms less than 2 weeks old.

Albendazole is one of the major benzimidazoles used in cattle in the United States. At elevated doses, albendazole is effective against mature flukes but these high dosages must be avoided during early pregnancy because albendazole is teratogenic

TABLE 29–4
FLUKICIDAL DRUGS FOR CATTLE

Chemical	Drug	Route	90% efficacy at recommended rate		
			10-wk Adult flukes	6 to 10-wk flukes	<6-wk flukes
Salicylanilides and	Nitroxynil	Subcutaneous	+ +	+ +	+
substituted	Rafoxanide	Subcutaneous or Oral	+ +	+ +	+
phenols	Oxyclozanide	Oral	+ +	+	−
	Niclofolan	Oral	+ +	−	−
Benzimidazoles	Albendazole	Oral	+ +	−	−
	Netobimin		+ +	−	−
	Triclabendazole	Oral	+ +	+ +	+ +
Miscellaneous	Clorsulon	Oral	+ +	+ +	−

Note: Increasing the normal therapeutic dosage rate can increase the susceptibility of the younger parasitic stages, for a number of drugs.
+ + = Highly effective; + = moderately effective at normal dosage rates; − = relatively ineffective.

(especially in sheep). The active metabolite released in the body is albendazole sulfoxide. Albendazole has a long withdrawal time, and is effective only against adult flukes. Treatment with albendazole has merit, however, and it is recommended each per year (7.5 mg/kg) for herds infected with *F. hepatica*. Administration should occur prior to placing the cattle on pastures in the spring of the year. Treatment for *Fascioloides magna* in cattle is seldom recommended because of the difficulty in diagnosing the infection. When indicated, albendazole can be used on an emergency basis.

Clorsulon (Curatrem) (4-amino-6-trichloroethenyl-1,3-benzenedisulfonamide), a relatively recent compound, is a sulfonamide derivative that inhibits certain glycolytic pathways of trematodes. Clorsulon inhibits the glycolytic enzyme phosphoglyceromutase in *Fasciola hepatica* by competition with 3-phosphoglycerate and 2,3-diphosphoglycerate.

Clorsulon controls immature and adult liver flukes by inhibiting these two enzymes that are essential for production of energy by the fluke. Without its energy supply, the fluke soon dies. The immature and adult stages controlled by clorsulon are the most destructive stages in the fluke life cycle. At about 8 weeks, the flukes move into the bile ducts and triple in size. Their intake of blood leads to anemia as iron stores are exhausted. Spines on the fluke cause tissue destruction and bile duct irritation. Between 10 and 14 weeks of age, the adults begin to lay eggs. Control of the egg-laying adults prevents new infestation of the pasture.

Unlike previous drug treatments, clorsulon has a wide margin of safety and exhibits no undesirable side effects at the recommended dose levels. In trials, no toxic reactions have been observed even at a level 25 times that of the label dose. Beef cows may be treated at any stage of pregnancy, and studies have not shown any adverse effects on breeding bulls. In addition to effective fluke removal from the host, clorsulon displayed a "stunting" effect on flukes that remained posttreatment.

The recommended clorsulon treatment schedule in the United States is to treat all cattle (cows, calves, and bulls) at the end of the pasture season (November–December). Treating cattle on pasture earlier than this time (September–October) is of little value, because a high proportion of infective larvae (metacercariae) are ingested during the late grazing season. A repeat treatment in late January–February eliminates any remaining flukes. Thus, the main source of year-to-year transmission (egg contamination in pasture) is greatly reduced.

Nitroxynil is one of a few injectable flukicides available in many countries and

TABLE 29–5
ANTHELMINTICS FOR PARASITIC GASTROENTERITIS IN SHEEP

Chemical Group	Drug	Gut Worms*		
		A	DL	AL
Benzimidazoles	Luxabendazole	+	+	+
	Thiabendazole	+	+	+
	Oxibendazole	+	+	+ −
	Parbendazole	+	+	+ −
	Mebendazole	+	+	+ −
	Fenbendazole	+	+	+
	Oxfendazole	+	+	+
	Albendazole	+	+	+
Probenzimidazoles	Febantel	+	+	+
	Thiophanate	+	+	+
	Netobimin	+	+	+
Imidothiazoles	Levamisole	+	+	+
	Morantel	+	+	+ −
Avermectins	Ivermectin	+	+	+

*A = Adult; DL = Developing Larva; AL = Arrested Larva.

possesses activity not only against adult flukes, but also against the parenchymal stages, i.e., flukes of more than 4 weeks of age. Rafoxanide may be given by the oral or subcutaneous route and is highly effective also against adult flukes and the later parenchymal stages. Both of these compounds have withholding times. Nitroxynil also displays a stunting effect against early immature larvae and hence reduces pasture contamination by suppressing egg output. The usual dosage for nitroxynil is 10 mg/kg. by subcutaneous injection.

Oxyclozanide (a salicylanilide) possesses activity against adult flukes only, but at elevated dosage levels, some activity against the later parenchymal stages may be observed. Transient scours may accompany its usage. It has a short withdrawal period in animals for slaughter and is one of the few flukicides that may be used, in some countries in lactating cattle on account of its short withholding times.

Brotianide, and closantel, also belong to this chemical family. Brotianide is frequently combined with thiophanate, Closantel is effective against mature and immature fluke, displaying a stunting effect against fluke less than 4 weeks old. Like nitroxynil and rafoxanide, it is highly protein bound and has a long half life. It is available

for sheep. Niclofolan, like oxyclozanide, is highly effective against adult flukes at a dose of 3 mg/kg. Niclofolan is available as an injectable solution, as a drench, or in the bolus form. Toxicity can occur at two times the recommended dosage rate.

In out-wintered stock, two doses of anthelmintic may be necessary: the first in December to remove adult and immature fluke burdens acquired from the autumnal flush of pasture metacercariae and the second in late April or early May to prevent pasture contamination and snail infection.

When cattle must be treated in late autumn and winter, a time when infections consist of both adult and immature flukes, rafoxanide and nitroxynil are useful because they possess activity against 4 to 12-week-old flukes. Triclabendazole is a potent flukicide that can be safely used also at early stages of the fluke infestation period.

29.4 PARASITIC GASTROENTERITIS IN SHEEP

The common gastrointestinal nematodes of sheep include *Haemonchus contortus*, *Ostertagia*, and *Trichostrongylus axei* in the abomasum; *Trichostrongylus*, *Nematodirus*, *Cooperia*, *Strongyloides papillosus*, and *Buno-*

stomum in the small intestine; and *Chabertia,
Trichuris,* and *Oesophagostomum* in the large
intestine. The tapeworm *Moniezia expansa*
can cause unthriftiness, if the infection is
very heavy.

Since the introduction of broad-spectrum
benzimidazoles, sheep or goats specifically
rarely are treated with a narrow-spectrum
anthelmintic for a particular species of parasite because a multiplicity of parasites may
be present in the alimentary tract. The exception probably is *Nematodirus battus* infestation in lambs, which commonly necessitates a specific therapy.

The range of anthelmintics available for
sheep is broadly similar to the range for cattle. Several anthelmintics that are relatively
ineffective against hypobiotic larvae in cattle display relatively higher activity in
sheep because of the shallower mucosa and
higher gut-penetrating ability in sheep than
in cattle.

Also, the kinetics of benzimidazoles differ between species of ruminant. Thiabendazole reaches higher plasma levels in
sheep than in cattle. This characteristic
may reflect a reduced capacity for biotransformation of thiabendazole in sheep. The
consequent reduction in the amount of
pharmacologically inactive metabolite (5-
hydroxythiabendazole) formed may explain why thiabendazole has higher activity
against *Dictyocaulus* and inhibits *Ostertagia*
in sheep.

At the manufacturer's recommended
dosage rates, the benzimidazoles, levamisole, and ivermectin are all highly effective
against the adult and developing larval
stages of the gastrointestinal nematodes
that parasitize sheep (Table 29–5) Few characteristics can help to differentiate among
them when selecting an anthelmintic for the
treatment of parasitic gastroenteritis in
lambs during the summer months. In general, the benzimidazoles, probenzimidazoles (thiophanate, febantel, and netobimin), levamisole, and ivermectin also
possess high activity against the adult and
immature larvae of *Nematodirus battus,* although the activity of some of the earlier
benzimidazoles against developing larvae
can be variable. Luxabendazole is a new
bendimidazole effective against nematodes
of the gastrointestinal tract, lungworm, and
fluke in sheep. It is not available in all countries.

Ivermectin drench has been introduced
for use in sheep. At a dose of 200 μg/kg,
ivermectin drench provides effective control against *Haemonchus contortus, Ostertagia
circumcincta, Trichostrongylus, Cooperia, Nematodirus, Strongylus, Oesophagostomum,
Chabertia* adult and immature lungworms
(*Dictyocaulus filaria*), and all larval stages of
the nasal bot (*Oestrus ovis*). The high efficacy and residual activity of ivermectin are
significant advantages. Also, it possesses a
unique action against many important ectoparasites.

The arrested fourth-stage larvae of the
abomasal nematodes of sheep are susceptible to a wider range of anthelmintics than
are those of cattle. In addition to fenbendazole, oxfendazole, luxabendazole, albendazole, and ivermectin, levamisole, (together with febantel, thiophanate, and
thiabendazole at increased dosage rates) is
effective against arrested fourth-stage larvae and therefore can be used in the treatment and control of winter scours in sheep.
The use of anthelmintics, which lack activity against arrested larvae, may require repeated treatment because anthelmintics,
only remove adult worms and developing
larvae. Arrested larvae remain to resume
development and damage the stomach lining.

As with cattle, the activities of some benzimidazoles may be subject to variation because of the operation of the esophageal
groove reflex. Because the worm eggs
passed by the ewes after lambing represent
an important source of pasture contamination for the lambs later in the year, consideration should be given to treating the ewes
at lambing time to reduce their egg output.
Where ewes and lambs are to be turned out
onto clean pasture after lambing, the ewes
should be treated with an anthelmintic active against arrested fourth-stage larvae immediately before being given access to the
pasture.

29.5 FASCIOLIASIS IN SHEEP

Live fluke disease in sheep may occur in the
acute, subacute or chronic form. The acute
form is caused by the migration of young
flukes in the parenchyma for as soon as 6
weeks after ingestion. Subacute fascioliasis

is attributable to parenchymal and biliary activity by the flukes, and the chronic condition is the result of the anemia produced by adult flukes in the bile ducts. The best control in sheep requires a drug that not only removes adult flukes, but also kills a large proportion of immature larvae so that the contamination can be kept low. Rafoxanide nitroxynil diamphenethide and closantel are useful drugs in this respect, Triclabendazole chloro-5-(2,-phenoxy-2-methyl thio benzimidazole) is particularly effective against all parasitic fluke stages, including the 1-week-old fluke. Diamphenethide has excellent activity also, against the immature stages but must be used at double dose rates to kill the adult fluke. The anthelmintics currently available for ovine fascioliasis include brotianide, albendazole, diamphenethide, nitroxynil, closantel, oxyclozanide, rafoxanide, and triclabendazole. Netobimin, oxyclozanide, niclofolan, rafoxanide, nitroxynil, brotianide, triclabendazole, and albendazole (the latter at an increase dosage rate) are all highly effective against adult flukes and therefore are suitable for the treatment of chronic fascioliasis in late winter and spring. Some of these drugs are effective against the young stages also.

Diamphenethide is effective against young flukes (1 to 6 weeks of age) and hence is indicated in acute fascioliasis. The high efficacy of this compound results from the deacetylated metabolite formed locally in the liver of the sheep. This metabolite is responsible for the activity against the liver parenchymal stages. This safe preparation is well tolerated by sheep and has a short withdrawal period.

Triclabendazole is a novel benzimidazole with high efficacy when given orally and displays high activity against early stages of liver fluke, including the very young stages in the liver parenchyma. It is useful for acute fluke disease also.

In subacute fascioliasis, diamphenethide, nitroxynil, closantel triclabendazole, rafoxanide, or brotianide may be recommended. Oxyclozanide, niclofolan, and albendazole can be considered for chronic fluke disease only. Several products are marketed for the combined treatment of gastrointestinal nematodes and liver fluke infections in sheep. With the exception of albendazole, which must be used at increased dosage rates for this combined purpose, all the products contain a mixture of chemicals, one active against gastrointestinal nematodes and the other active against liver fluke. Combinations available include levamisole/oxyclozanide, oxibendazole/oxyclozanide, thiabendazole/rafoxanide, and thiophanate/brotianide.

29.6 BOVINE COCCIDIOSIS

Coccidiosis is a major bovine disease that affects primarily young cattle. The clinical signs, severity, and losses resulting from coccidiosis are variable and may be related, in part, to stress factors, such as changes in weather, weaning, and crowding. The magnitude of the problem is often unrecognized, however, because many of the infections are subclinical and largely ignored by producers and veterinarians. Occurrence of clinical disease can be dramatic and cause obvious economic losses in feedlots, young dairy calves, and overwintering beef cattle. Isolated cases occur in pasture. The subclinical form of the disease is also of economic importance, and evidence suggests prophylactic treatment may be worthwhile.

The epidemiology of the clinical disease suggests beef cattle are not severely exposed until they are removed from pastures late in the year and grouped in intensive feedlots in overwintering quarters. Dairy units, on the other hand, experience problems all year with younger calves. Maximum exposure occurs early in life, and older animals apparently become sufficiently resistant to avoid showing clinical signs.

The severity of coccidiosis in beef and dairy cattle has been well known among parasitologists for some time. Yet, within only the last few years has coccidiosis been recognized as a major health problem in the feedlot. In addition to the economic losses associated with weight loss, treatment cost, and death of the acutely affected animal, significant more subtle costs are associated with the often unrecognized subclinical form of the disease: showing immunosuppression and susceptibility to other infections.

Of the 14 species of bovine coccidia, only 2, *Eimeria bovis* and *Eimeria zurni*, are frequently of clinical significance. The host specificity of all coccidial species is notable. Of the food animals, only sheep and goats have some species of coccidia that cross-infect. Although a disease primarily of animals from 3 weeks to 1 year of age, older animals apparently are becoming increasingly affected. In most cases, the older animals are symptomless carriers of the disease that provide a constant source of infection for the younger animals with which they come in contact.

The complex life cycle of coccidia is comprised of both an asexual and sexual phase within the host, plus a required incubation period outside the host. Although much of the 21- to 28-day life cycle of coccidia is not entirely understood, researchers already know in general how it works. The ingested coccidia-oocyst ruptures in the rumen, releasing eight sporozoites, which move to penetrate the cell walls of the small intestine. The sporozoites continue to divide into many schizonts, which themselves divide into massive numbers. At this point (i.e., about 18 days into the cycle), no clinical sign can be seen. By the time diagnosis can be established, the critical stage has passed and treatment of coccidiosis may not be effective. Treatment may be necessary, however, to ward off secondary diseases that might otherwise be invited by the weakened condition of the animal. Feed efficiency is severely altered, and death sometimes occurs.

Eimeria bovis and *Eimeria zurni* are generally accepted as the two most pathogenic strains of the species known to infect cattle. All species may contribute to both subclinical and clinical problems. Coccidiosis in cattle is usually deceptive. Clinical signs are often not demonstrated until 3 to 8 weeks following initial infection. In severe clinical cases, marked diarrhea occurs, with feces containing stringy masses of mucus and clotted blood. This sign is often accompanied by a loss of appetite, dehydration, general weakness, and loss of vigor. The disorder produced by coccidia in cattle is either the direct or the indirect result of the tremendous multiplication of coccidia in the epithelium lining of the lower small intestine, cecum, colon, or rectum. Gross lesions include loss of surface epithelium, mucosal thickening, diffuse hemorrhage,

catarrhal enteritis, and destruction of intestinal glands. In this weakened state, the animal is subject to all types of secondary disease, such as pneumonia, bacterial enteritis, and viral infections. Coccidiosis causes large economic losses from death, labor and treatment cost, and morbidity, along with loss of feed conversion and diminished weight gain in calves and cattle following classic outbreaks. Low-level or subclinical infections are more prevalent and costly than with previously thought. The classic clinical signs are bloody diarrhea and severe weight loss, but coccidiosis often can be inapparent, with only nonspecific clinical signs of a loose, foul-smelling stool. Coccidiosis can strike a feedlot, resulting in high morbidities. Few mortalities may result. The major effects of the disease, the intestinal lesions, are severe enough to require several weeks for the animal to recover normal body weight and feed consumption. Immunosuppression and predisposition to other diseases is a major feature of bovine coccidiosis.

CONTROL

Coccidia thrive in the environment, and coccidiosis is a disease that results from poor sanitation. Therefore, the enforcement of rigid sanitation programs is the best control. Calves should not be confined in close quarters in groups but rather in individual pens. Unfortunately, even when housed in individual pens, some calves occasionally show symptoms of coccidiosis. Attempts to control coccidiosis in cattle have been based on good hygiene, treatment of clinical cases as they appear, and use of preventive drugs.

Although good hygienic practices provide some benefits, they may be insufficient to control coccidia. The oocyst wall provides sporozoites excellent protection against harsh chemical disinfectants. (Coccidia even have been observed sporulating in fixed, stained slides cultured in 2 to 5% dichromate or 1% chromate solution.) Oocysts are ubiquitous and rarely destroyed in nature. Therefore, total control of coccidiosis by treating the external environment, especially in feedlots, is not feasible. Sanitation and minimization of stress are

TABLE 29–6
COCCIDIOSTATS FOR CATTLE

Drug	Dose	Administration
Amprolium		In feed, in water
	5 mg/kg	21 days (prevention)
	10 mg/kg	5 days (treatment)
Decoquinate	0.5 mg/kg body weight	In feed for 28 days (prevention)
Sulfaquinoxaline	8–15 mg/kg	Daily in water for (treatment) 3–5 days
Lasalocid	1 mg/kg body weight	30–45 days (prevention) in feed
Monensin	10–33 ppm (feed) or 1 mg/kg body weight	In feed for 20–30 days (prevention)
Sulfadimethoxine	55 mg/kg	Intravenously (treatment)
Sulfamethoxypyridazine	22 mg/kg	Intramuscular/Subcutaneous (treatment)

obvious objectives vital to the minimizing of losses caused by this disease. Under feedlot conditions, these objectives cannot always be achieved. Most feedlot operations are, therefore, high-risk operations in regard to coccidiosis. In light of the hidden and apparent costs associated with this disease, routine use of a prophylactic anticoccidial preparation is advisable, especially in calf feeding operations. Removal of bedding and use of slatted floors assist in removing the reservoir of infection in the environment. Slatted units usually show a relatively lower incidence than bedded units.

PREVENTION

The most effective control method is prevention via continuous medication in the feed or drinking water. Ionophores (monensin, salinomycin, lasalocid), amprolium, decoquinate, and sulfonamides have all been used to control coccidiosis (Table 29–6). When in-feed medication is used, one must always evaluate the medicating agent with regard to:

1. Its palatability in the ration
2. Its safety margin (to allow for mixing errors)
3. Its efficacy
4. Its cost effectiveness

Ionophores, such as lasalocid and monensin, have value as preventive anticoccidial drugs in cattle and sheep. Lasalocid and monensin, used as feed additives, are the only ionophores currently approved for the control of coccidiosis in beef cattle. They are not generally of significant value for the treatment of clinical outbreaks. Surveys of large feedlots have indicated significant reductions in feedlot deaths resulting from coccidiosis coinciding with the advent of the routine use of monensin as a feed additive.

The ionophores are more likely to have value in controlling *E. bovis* than *E. zurni*. Monensin is commonly used in feedlot rations to improve feed efficiency. The initial dose in the ration is low and is gradually increased until a dose of 200 to 300 mg/head/day is reached. Monensin also inhibits coccidiosis; however, a somewhat higher level of intake may be necessary for this effect. One can assume that 200 mg/head/day are fed for increased feed efficiency, and that an additional 50 mg are fed for the purpose of control. Field experience has shown that monensin tends to lower the incidence of coccidiosis; however, severe clinical outbreaks have been reported in cattle receiving monensin and lasalocid at the recommended level of 200 to 300 mg/head/day, as approved for improvement of feed efficiency in the United States.

Lasalocid is a relatively effective iono-phore coccidiostat that must be administered orally at a rate of 1 mg/kg body weight. Significant increases in average daily weight gain have been reported from feedlots that routinely use lasalocid. Amprolium has been reported in some cases to mitigate a severe outbreak of diarrhea associated with a severe *E. zurni* infection.

Amprolium, and decoquinate apparently are cost-effective medicants under most conditions and are widely used drugs approved for prevention of coccidiosis in cattle. Amprolium, is a coccidiostat feed additive used daily as a supplement to calf rations for 21 days. It is also available in water. It is well tolerated but must be withdrawn before slaughter. Several times the recommended dose of 5 mg/kg have been used without adverse effects.

Decoquinate (4-hydroxyquinoline) was the second drug to be cleared by the U.S. Food and Drug Administration (FDA) as a coccidiostat in cattle. Decoquinate is highly effective against the most pathogenic species of bovine coccidia. It attacks the parasites early in their asexual cycle, thereby preventing clinical disease, inhibiting oocyst production, and in turn preventing spread of infection. In ruminating calves with induced *E. bovis* and/or *E. zurni* infection, decoquinate fed at 0.5 mg/kg body weight daily prevents clinical signs of disease with complete suppression of oocyst production. Decoquinate is an active coccidiostat when fed daily at 0.5 mg/kg body weight during periods of oocyst exposure or when experience indicates coccidiosis is likely to be a hazard. For prevention, feeding should be continued for at least 28 days.

Indications are that the decoquinate is carried into the cell on the surface of the sporozoite, where it kills the microorganism by interfering with the DNA synthesis at the thymidine synthetase step. Other coccidiostats work later in the cycle and permit much greater damage to the intestinal tract.

All cattle in a pen should be put on medication for at least 28 days to prevent the cycling of coccidia in the pen. Because stress somehow triggers coccidiosis cycles, many feedlot operators start their programs when the cattle are brought in. Weather and ration changes, crowding, and other external forces introduce stress. If conditions are such that a severe outbreak is highly likely, a decoquinate program should be immediately instituted and continued until the danger period has passed. A follow-up 28-day feeding period, interrupted by a 14-day nonmedicated period, is good added insurance against future outbreaks. Numerous program variations can be worked out for specific situations and conditions. For dairy calves, the recommended program lasts from the first dry feed until the animal weighs 400 lbs.

TREATMENT

Oral sulfonamides have long been used as coccidiostatic drugs, for therapy. Sulfadimethoxine injection (Albon) followed by oral sulfadimethoxine boluses can give good results. Long slaughter withdrawal times must be observed with this sulfonamide. Other long acting sulfonamides such as sulfamethoxypyridazine are used by injection to treat clinical outbreaks.

Upon recognition of clinical symptoms (especially bloody scours), prompt treatment must be instituted with drugs and replacement fluids. Although sulfonamides and/or amprolium can be used in these cases, ancillary therapy must include kaolin/pectin absorbents and aggressive fluid therapy in severe cases. Clinically affected animals should be treated with sulfa drugs and then, with penmates, receive decoquinate at 0.5 mg/kg body weight in the feed to prevent further cycling. Additional cases may occur for about 10 days until the coccidian reproductive cycle is interrupted. The medication should be fed for 28 to 56 days, or longer if deemed necessary from past experience. All incoming cattle should be given decoquinate for at least 28 days. Medication of cattle in adjoining pens, or even of the total feedlot, for 28 days should be considered. An adequate dietary level of vitamin A must also be provided. Many feedlot veterinarians use a 28-day decoquinate feeding program for all incoming cattle to guard against costly disease that can devastate a feedlot. The ionophores monensin and lasalocid when fed at the approved levels are equivalent to decoquinate in ability to reduce oocyst numbers and prevent clinical outbreaks.

29.7 CRYPTOSPORIDIOSIS

Cryptosporidiosis was first diagnosed in calves in 1971, but was not clearly accepted as a primary intestinal pathogen until the mid 1980s. Although an important pathogen in many species, it is more commonly reported in calves than in any other domestic species. *Cryptosporidium parvum* apparently is the main species affecting the entire intestinal tract of calves. *C. muris* has been identified in the abomasal glands of calves. Taxonomically, *Cryptosporidium* is assigned to the subclass Coccidia; hence, it is related to the more familiar protozoan parasites *Eimeria, Isospora, Sarcocystis,* and *Toxoplasma.*

Cryptosporidium in neonatal calves can cause severe diarrhea that may last from 1 to 2 weeks. Calves between 5 and 20 days of age are most commonly affected. Calves become infected by ingesting material that has been contaminated with feces containing sporulated oocysts. Young animals are more prone to infection and clinical illness than are adults. Adults develop immunity to infection by *Cryptosporidium* but apparently do not transfer it to offspring. Cryptosporidia have been found with rotavirus, coronavirus, and *Escherichia coli* in the intestines of calves with acute neonatal diarrhea. Whether cryptosporidia cause or only contribute to enteric disease because of the presence of other enteropathogens is not known. Cryptosporidia have been found in diarrheic calves as young as 2 days of age, but are more common in calves at about 5 to 12 days of age. It appears that cryptosporidia may be a primary cause of diarrhea in newborn farm animals or may be part of a mixed multiple infection that causes acute neonatal diarrhea. Persistent clinical signs and shedding of *Cryptosporidium* oocysts have been observed in immunodeficient humans and horses. Both intrinsic and acquired immunodeficiency syndromes have been associated with increased susceptibility to cryptosporidiosis as has immunosuppressive chemotherapy.

LIFE CYCLE

The *Cryptosporidium* life cycle begins with the ingestion of a sporulated oocyst by a susceptible host. In the gastrointestinal tract, where this parasite is usually confined in mammals, the organisms do not invade the cytoplasm of the host epithelial cell. Instead, they attach to and develop within the microvilli (brush border) at the cell surface. The sporozoites liberated from oocysts complete the asexual and sexual cycle in the microvillous border on the surface of epithelial cells of the small intestine. The parasites are most numerous in the lower small intestine and have been associated with villous atrophy and crypt epithelial hyperplasia.

Because the organisms reside within the brush border of the intestinal absorptive cells, the primary mechanism for diarrhea appears to be malabsorption. A secretory mechanism of diarrhea is also possible as indicated by the large volume of stool and the persistence of diarrhea even after the animal has stopped eating and drinking. These mechanisms of infection allow for rapid spread of the organism along the intestinal tract and consequent impairment of digestion and absorption. Damage to the intestinal lining, diarrhea, and poor nutrition result for the calf. The diarrhea is commonly yellow to yellowish-brown and of creamy texture. The decrease in absorption of fluids, electrolytes, and nutrients is debilitating to the calf and compromises its immune system. This debilitation is especially lethal to the calf when combined with other stressors, such as wet and cold. The calf's metabolic rate is stimulated to maintain normal body temperature. Reserves are depleted because of insufficient caloric intake. Damage to the intestinal lining and a depressed immune system also result in susceptibility to superinfection by other viral or bacterial pathogens that might be present in the calf. Concurrent infections may increase the severity of disease and result in higher mortality. Adequate intake of quality colostrum (at least 10% of body weight in the first 24 hours) helps to prevent infections with other agents.

CLINICAL PRESENTATION

The clinical presentation of cryptosporidiosis in calves is typical of an enterocolitis. Calves have diarrhea characterized by an increased number of defecations of a yellow, creamy stool. The calves show signs of tenesmus, weight loss, anorexia, depression, weakness, and dehydration. Diarrhea usually persists as long as oocysts are detected in clinical cases. Dehydration is occasionally noted. Unlike other infectious causes of calf diarrhea, high mortality within herds is not usually a feature of cryptosporidiosis, although morbidity can be high. Fever is seldom recorded in association with the disease. Subclinical infections with *Cryptosporidium* occur and may be a major factor in predisposing calves to other viral and bacterial intestinal infections. Diagnosis of cryptosporidiosis is either by examination of fecal smears for oocysts with Giemsa stain or by a fecal flotation method. The organisms can also be detected by examination of scrapings of ileal mucosa. Demonstration of numerous oocysts in the feces of animals with clinical signs of enteritis is the most reliable means of diagnosis. *Cryptosporidium* oocysts are small (4.0 to 4.5 μm), but with experience, the examiner can readily recognize them in methanol-fixed smears. Cryptosporidiosis can be spread from infected animals, including calves, to humans. The disease is serious in humans, especially if the immune system is depressed. The infective sporulated oocyst that passes with the feces is extremely stable and resistant to many common disinfectants. Formal saline (10%) and ammonia (5%) are effective in destroying the infectivity of cryptosporidia.

THERAPY

At present, no available treatment is effective against cryptosporidia. Spiramycin, and quinine combined with clindamycin, have given some relief in humans. Affected calves should be warmed and supplemented with intravenous fluids containing electrolytes and nutrients. They should be immediately removed from the vicinity of other calves to prevent fecal contamination and infection of other calves. Supportive therapy is the best means of minimizing mortality resulting from cryptosporidiosis. Parenteral fluid therapy should be used to combat dehydration, restore electrolyte balance, and provide a source of energy in severe cases. Supply of energy is of critical

importance because many calves may succumb to the effects of hypoglycemia.

Dextrose and parenteral fluid therapy is clearly indicated. The acidotic state of the dehydrated animal must be addressed, and fluids preferably should contain precursors of bicarbonate (i.e., citrate and lactate). Because the villous brush border and its complement of disaccharidase enzymes have been lost, disaccharides, such as lactose must not be given to affected calves because doing so could establish a fermentative diarrhea.

Ensurance of adequate intake of early colostrum is essential. Several available colostrum supplements claim to possess high amounts of antibodies specific to the causative agents of calf scours. Such products are derived from colostrum of cows hyperimmunized with specific antigens and are given to calves in the first 24 hours of life. Other colostral substitutes are concentrates of immunoglobulins from large numbers of naturally exposed cows.

Coating the mucosa of the alimentary tract with absorbents, demulcents, and protectants can be beneficial. The nonsteroidal anti-inflammatory drugs are of some therapeutic value. No known antimicrobials effectively treat cryptosporidiosis, and although more than 40 antimicrobials have been tried, none is effective. Drugs used have included decoquinate amprolium, sulfadimidine, sulfadiazine-trimethoprim, dimetridazole, metronidazole, ipronidazole, quinacrine, monensin, and lasalocid. Of these, lasalocid has given some positive results, but only at a dose which is toxic in calves. Spiramycin is the only antibiotic that appears to show promise. In reports on treatment of human patients with persistent cryptosporidiosis associated with the acquired immunodeficiency syndrome, two drugs, furazolidone and spiramycin, appeared to afford some protection in alleviating diarrhea and in reducing oocyst shedding after prolonged treatment.

In summary, specific treatment of and control measures for cryptosporidiosis have not been established. Because effective drugs are not available and the life history is poorly understood, recommendations are difficult. Treatment of clinical signs accompanied by good sanitation to prevent consumption of many oocysts by susceptible calves is of some value. Actual prevention of cryptosporidiosis, however, requires the development of an effective chemotherapeutic agent or perhaps a vaccine. Many veterinarians who have encountered the condition agree that it can contribute to disease susceptibility quite significantly, that no specific treatment is commercially available, and that, once established in a herd, the problem continues indefinitely.

SELECTED REFERENCES

Armour, J., and Bogan, J.: Anthelimintics for ruminants. Br. Vet. J., *138*:371, 1982.

Armour, J., and Urquhurt, G.: Helminth diseases of cattle. In Practice, March, 1983.

Armour, J., Bairden, K., and Preston, J.M.: Anthelmintic efficacy of ivermectin against naturally occurring acquired bovine gastrointestinal nematodes. Vet. Rec., *107*:226, 1980.

Aurich, J.E., Dobrinski, I., and Grunert, E.: Intestinal cryptosporidiosis in calves on a dairy farm. Vet. Rec., *127*:380, 1990.

Berry, G.W., Ernst, J.V., and Crawley, R.R.: Anthelmintic efficacy of ivermectin against gastrointestinal nematodes in calves. Am. J. Vet. Res., *44*:1363, 1983.

Briscoe, M.G., and Coles, G.C.: The speed of action of anthelmintics. Vet. Rec., *106*:58, 1980.

Coles, G.C.: Anthelmintic resistance in sheep. Vet. Clin. North Am. (Food Anim. Pract.), 2:423, 1986.

Courtney, C.H., Shearer, J.K., and Whitten, R.D.: Safety and efficacy of albendazole against cattle flukes. Mod. Vet. Pract., Nov., 1984.

Craig, T.M., and Huey, R.L.: (1984) Efficacy of triclabendazole against *Fasciola hepatica* and *Fascioloides magna* in naturally infected calves. Am. J. Vet. Res., 45:1644, 1984.

Current, W.L.: Cryptosporidiosis. J. Am. Vet. Med. Assoc., *187*:1334, 1985.

Dobbins, E.: Comparison of the effect of some *Fascioloides* against immature liver fluke in calves. Vet. Rec., *111*:177, 1982.

Elliott, D.C.: The effect of fenbendazole in removing inhibited early fourth stage *Ostertagia ostertagi* larvae from yearling cattle. N.Z. Vet. J., 25:145, 1977.

Ernst, J.V., and Benz, G.W.: Intestinal coccidiosis in cattle. Vet. Clin. North Am. (Food Anim. Pract.), 2:283, 1986.

Fawcett, A.R.: A study of a restricted program of strategic dosing against *Fasciola hepatica* with triclabendazole. Vet. Rec., *127*:492, 1990.

Fetterer, R.H.: The effect of albendazole and triclabendazole on colchicine binding in liver fluke. J. Vet. Pharmacol. Ther., *9*:49, 1986.

Foreyt, W.J.: The role of liver fluke in infertility of beef cattle. Bovine Proc., No. 14, April, 1982.

Foreyt, W., Rice, D., and Wescott, R.: Evaluation of lasalocid as a coccidiostat in calves. Titration efficacy and comparison with monensin and decoquinate. Am. J. Vet. Res., 9:2031, 1986.

Fox, J.E.: Results of recent field trials using decoquinate coccidiostat. Agric. Pract., *4(10)*:19, 1983.

Fox, J.E.: Bovine coccidiosis—a review including field safety studies with decoquinate for prevention. Mod. Vet. Pract., Aug., 1978.

Gibbs, M., and Herd, R.: Nematodiasis in cattle. Vet. Clin. North Am. (Food Anim. Pract.), 2:211, 1986.

Heinrichs, A.J., and Bush, G.J.: The effect of feeding decoquinate or lasalocid on coccidia levels, feed intake, and growth of neonatal dairy calves. J. Dairy Sci., *72*:414, 1989.

Heinrichs, A.J., Swartz, L.A., Drake, T.R., and Travis, P.A.: Influence of decoquinate fed to neonatal dairy calves on early and conventional weaning systems. J. Dairy Sci., 73:1851, 1990.

Herd, R.H.: Strategies for nematode control in cattle. Mod. Vet. Pract., Oct., 1985. 66:741, 1985.

Herd, R.P., Streitel, R.H., McClure, K.E., and Parker, C.F.: Control of hypobiotic and benzimidazole resistant nematodes in sheep. J. Am. Vet. Med. Assoc., *184*:726, 1984.

Hoblet, K.H., Charles, T.P., and Howard, R.R.: Evaluation of lasalocid and decoquinate against coccidiosis resulting from natural exposure in weaned dairy calves. Am. J. Vet. Res., *50(7)*:1060, 1989.

Holste, J.E., Wallace, D.H., and Hudson, D.B.: Reproductive performance of beef cows treated with ivermectin before calving. Mod. Vet. Pract., *67*:462, 1986.

Hoover, R.C., Lincoln, J.D., and Hall, R.F.: Seasonal transmission of *Fasciola hepatica* in cattle in North Western United States. J. Am. Vet. Assoc., *184*:695, 1984.

Jacobs, D.E., and Fox, M.T.: Control of bovine parasitic gastroenteritis and parasitic bronchitis in a rotational grazing system using the morantel sustained release bolus. Vet. Rec., *110*:399, 1982.

Jones, R.M.: Therapeutic and prophylactic efficacy of morantel when administered directly into the rumen of cattle on a continuing basis. Vet. Parasitol., *12*:223, 1983.

Lopez, J.W.: Rotavirus and *Cryptosporidium* shedding in dairy calf feces and its relationship to colostrum immune transfer. J. Dairy Sci., *71*:1288, 1988.

Malone, J.: Efficacy of clorsulon for treatment of mature, naturally acquired and 8 week old, experimentally induced *Fasciola hepatica* infections in cattle. Am. J. Vet. Res., *5*:851, 1984.

Malone, J.B.: Efficacy of albendazole for treatment of naturally acquired *Fasciola hepatica* in calves. Am. J. Vet. Res., *43*:879, 1982.

Malone, J.B., and Craig, T.M.: Cattle liver flukes. Risk assessment and control. Compend. Contin. Educ. Pract. Vet., *12(5)*:747, 1990.

Marriner, S.: Anthelmintic drugs. Vet. Rec., *118*:181, 1986.

McKellar, Q.A.: Strategic use of anthelmintics for parasitic nematodes in cattle and sheep. Vet. Rec., *123*:483, 1988.

McKellar, Q.A., and Kinabo, L.D.B.: The pharmacology of flukicidal drugs. Br. Vet. J., *147*:306, 1991.

Meleney, W.R., Wright, F.C., and Guillot, F.S.: Residual protection against cattle scabies afforded by ivermectin. Am. J. Vet. Res., *43*:1767, 1982.

Middleberg, A., and McKenna, P.B.: Oxfendazole resistance in *Nematodirus spatiger*. N.Z. Vet. J., *31*:65, 1983.

Miller, J.I., Baker, M.N., and Rarver, T.: Anthelmintic treatment of pastured dairy cattle in California. Am. J. Vet. Res., *47*:2036, 1986.

Miner, M.L., and Jensen, J.B.: Decoquinate in the control of experimentally induced coccidiosis of calves. Am. J. Vet. Res., *37*:1043, 1976.

Mohammed-Ali, N.A.K., Bogan, J.A., Marriner, S.E., and Richards, R.J.: Pharmacokinetics of triclabendazole alone or in combination with fenbendazole in sheep. J. Vet. Pharmacol. Ther., *9*:442, 1986.

Moon, H.W., Woode, G.N., and Ahrens, F.A.: Attempted Chemoprophylaxis of cryptosporidiosis in calves. Vet. Rec., *110*:181, 1982.

Moore, D.A.: Minimizing morbidity and mortality from cryptosporidiosis. Vet. Med., Aug., 1989.

Myers, G., and Taylor, R.: Ostertagiasis in cattle. J. Vet. Diagn. Invest., *1*:195, 1989.

Nouri, M., and Toroghi, R.: Asymptomatic cryptosporidiosis in cattle and humans in Iran. Vet. Rec., *128*:358, 1991.

Prichard, R.K.: Anthelmintics for cattle. Vet. Clin. North Am. (Food Anim. Pract.), *2*:489, 1986.

Reinemeyer, C.R.: Prevention of parasitic gastroenteritis in dairy replacement heifers. Compend. Contin. Educ. Pract. Vet., *12(5)*:761, 1990.

Roth, J.A., Jarvinen, J.A., Frank, D.E., and Fox, J.E.: Alteration of neutrophil function, associated with coccidiosis in cattle. Influence of decoquinate and dexamethasone. Am. J. Vet. Res., *50*:1250, 1989.

Snyder, D.E., Floyd, J.G., and Di Pietro, J.A.: Use of anthelmintic and anticoccidial compounds in cattle. Compend. Contin. Educ. Pract. Vet., *13*:1847, 1991.

Taylor, M.: Liver fluke treatment. In Practice, Sept., 1987.

Wallace, D.H., Kilgore, R.L., and Benz, G.W.: Clorsulon: a new fasciolicide for cattle. Mod. Vet. Pract., Nov., 1985.

Watkins, L.E.: The prophylactic effects of monensin fed to cattle inoculated with *Coccidia* oocyst. Agric. Pract., *7(6)*:18, 1986.

Williams, J.: Efficacy of fenbendazole against inhibited larvae of *Ostertagia ostergagi* in yearling cattle. Am. J. Vet. Res., *45*:1989, 1984.

Wohlgemuth, K., Melancon, J.J., Hughes, H., and Biondini, M.: Treatment of North Dakota beef cows and calves with ivermectin: some economic considerations. Bov. Pract., *24*:61, 1989.

Yazwinski, T.A., Featherstone, M.S., Presson, B.L., et al.: Efficacy of injectable clorsulon in the treatment of immature bovine *Fasciola hepatica* infections. Agric. Pract., *63*:6, 1985.

30

THERAPY OF BOVINE RESPIRATORY DISEASE

30.1 Economic Losses
30.2 Causative Agents
30.3 Respiratory Defense Mechanisms
30.4 General Therapy Principles
30.5 Antimicrobials for Bovine Respiratory Disease
30.6 Penicillins
30.7 Sulfonamides
30.8 Tetracyclines
30.9 Macrolides
30.10 Cephalosporins—Ceftiofur
30.11 Quinolones—Enrofloxacin
30.12 Tilmicosin
30.13 Inflammation and Anti-inflammatory Drugs
30.14 Immunomodulators
30.15 Mucolytic Therapy
30.16 Bronchodilators
30.17 Fluid/Acid Base Balance and Oxygen Therapy
30.18 Pasteurellosis—Shipping Fever
30.19 Acute Bovine Pulmonary Edema and Emphysema

30.1 ECONOMIC LOSSES

Since the early 1900s, bovine respiratory disease has been referred to as "stockyard pneumonia," "transfer fever," hemorrhagic septicemia, or "shipping fever." More recently the term "bovine respiratory disease complex" or simply "bovine respiratory disease" has been used to reflect the complexity of this disease, which involves stress as well as viral and bacterial infections. Pneumonic pasteurellosis is another term used to describe the disease because *Pasteurella haemolytica* is usually involved. The economic losses attributable to shipping fever have been reported frequently and are substantial in terms of both mortality and morbidity.

Bovine respiratory disease is still the most costly disease of feedlot cattle in North America. A major component in the pathogenesis of bovine respiratory disease is immunosuppression caused by stress and/or viral infection. The lungs of these immunocompromised animals are susceptible to infection by strains of bacteria that possess virulence factors that further impair host defense mechanisms.

Respiratory disease has become an important source of economic loss through mortality and morbidity in the beef industry. This problem is frequently encountered in young calves brought together to specialized farms and beef lots. Enzootic calf pneumonia causes extensive loss in terms of reduced weight gain, but the acute onset of pneumonia also is responsible for death or severe irreversible lung damage. Calves are usually depressed, anorexic, and tachypneic, and coughing can be a dominant clinical feature. If the disease is to be avoided, prevention must begin as soon as the calf is born by ensuring the prompt early intake of colostrum rich in maternal antibodies. Enzootic pneumonia occurs in housed calves usually from 1 month of age with either an acute or an insidious onset. Affected animals may display a range of respiratory symptoms, the extent of which usually depends on the severity of the infectious process.

30.2 CAUSATIVE AGENTS

Bovine respiratory infections are commonly discussed together as the respiratory disease complex. This complex includes shipping fever and epizootics in feeder cattle and in cattle herds. The cause is complex and includes a combination of viral, chlamydial, or bacterial infections and stress. The incriminated viral agents are parainfluenza 3 virus and infectious bovine rhinotracheitis virus; however, *Pasteurella multocida* and *P. haemolytica* are so common that they should be given primary consideration with respect to therapy.

Enzootic calf pneumonia is caused by many of the infective agents just listed. Chlamydiae are reportedly a more common primary cause in calves, indicating a potential preference for use of tetracyclines in early therapy. *Pasteurella* organisms are the most common bacteria isolated.

Stress plays a major initial role. Housing, transport, mixing, management, ventilation, and nutrition interact with various microbiologic agents to trigger off the condition, which is highly infectious. Numerous viral, bacterial, and mycoplasmal agents are implicated in the disease process. Whether an individual calf succumbs to these organisms depends to a large extent on the interaction between the immunologic status of the animal and external stress factors (Tables 30–1 and 30–2).

The cause of bovine respiratory disease apparently is influenced also by environmental factors, such as weather and ventilation. It is also exacerbated by the "stress" of overcrowding and transportation. The pathologic processes are associated essentially with microorganisms, of which parainfluenza 3 virus, respiratory syncytial virus, *Mycoplasma bovis*, *M. dispar*, and *Pasteurella haemolytica* are the most important. Synergism occurs between *Mycoplasma bovis* and *Pasteurella haemolytica*, and the inoculation of these two organisms induces pneumonia experimentally in both gnotobiotic and conventionally reared calves.

The disease complex is poorly defined in terms of cause, pathogenesis, and effective treatment. Viruses, mycoplasma, and bacteria are included in this complex disease. These organisms can be demonstrated in the upper and lower respiratory tracts of affected animals and can cause a range of pulmonary lesions.

TABLE 30-1
SUMMARY OF CALF PNEUMONIA

THE DISEASE—ENZOOTIC PNEUMONIA

Viruses: P13, BVD, IBR, RSV, + Stress

Interference with Defense Mechanisms→ mucociliary clearance suppressed
                                    ↘ suppression of alveolar macrophages

Secondary Bacterial Invasion

Pasteurella → Toxins produced → Colonization—more bacteria

Corynebacterium
Streptococcus/Staphylococcus Hemophilus
Escherichia coli
Mycoplasma
Chlamydia

Clinical Signs

VIRUSES

Predominant causative agents have been viruses, including infectious bovine rhinotracheitis virus, bovine syncytial virus, and parainfluenza 3 virus. Infectious bovine rhinotracheitis virus and bovine syncytial virus produce respiratory disease that can be distinguished from bovine respiratory disease, and parainfluenza 3 virus produces a mild pneumonia considered clinically insignificant. Preinfection of cattle with respiratory disease viruses, especially infectious bovine rhinotracheitis virus, followed a few days later with a *P. haemolytica* challenge, has been utilized effectively for the induction of pneumonia. These viruses, certain mycoplasma, and possibly other agents are thought to facilitate the establishment of *P. haemolytica* in the lung by impairing the functions of alveolar macrophages and other host defenses.

Viruses frequently recovered from outbreaks of pneumonia include P13 bovine respiratory syncytial virus, infectious bovine rhinotracheitis, and bovine viral diarrhea/mucosal disease. In the United States, many calf units display high levels of antibodies to these viruses. Although other viruses may also be implicated (reovirus, rhinovirus, enterovirus, adenovirus, BAV 1/2), the

P13 and respiratory syncytial viruses apparently are the most important precipitating agents in terms of causing necrosis of bronchiolar epithelial cells and destruction of cilia.

A combined primary P13 and bovine respiratory syncytial virus viral infection often occurs, with resultant physical impairment of lung defense mechanisms and secondary bacterial colonization causing a fever. Secondary bacterial infection with *P. multocida* after bovine respiratory syncytial virus infection is common. Replication of parainfluenza 3 virus causes loss of the protective action of alveolar macrophages and epithelial cells. Similar histopathologic changes have been reported for bovine respiratory syncytial virus infection. Functional integrity of virus-damaged cells is restored by 21 days for Para Influenza 13 (PI 13) and by day 30 for bovine respiratory syncytial virus. In mixed viral infections, involvement of Para Influenza 13 virus does not significantly change the clinical picture.

Regardless of the specific causative virus(es), the initial virus-induced respiratory tract damage is then subsequently extended by invasion by mycoplasmae, chlamydiae, and secondary bacteria (especially *Pasteurella*).

BACTERIAL AGENTS

Pasteurella haemolytica has emerged as the key pathogenic infectious agent in bovine pneumonia. *P. haemolytica* is a gram-negative, bipolar-staining, encapsulated, weakly hemolytic, rod-shaped bacterium. *Pasteurella* were first described and cultured more than a century ago, but the names *P. haemolytica* and *P. multocida* were not proposed until 50 years later. Numerous *P. haemolytica* serotypes are based on soluble or extractible surface antigens. The two distinct subtypes, A and T, are based on fermentation of arabinose and xylose. *P. haemolytica* serotype 1, biotype A (A1) is the predominant bacterium found in bovine pneumonia.

Although recognized as being involved in pneumonia in cattle, *P. haemolytica* gained attention only when experimental inductions resulted in severe chronic clinical pneumonia in calves. The consistent isolation of *P. haemolytica* from pneumonic lung tissue in cattle with bovine respiratory disease and the increased understanding of the pathogenesis of *P. haemolytica* in pneumonia, have resulted in acceptance of this agent as the primary bacterial cause of bovine respiratory disease.

P. multocida and *P. haemolytica* are consistently recovered from animals with pneumonia and can be considered major bacterial pathogens in the syndrome. *Hemophilus somnus, corynebacterium pyogenes (A. pyogenes), streptococci, staphylococci, Escherichia coli*, and *Salmonella* may be involved also.

Pasteurella haemolytica is widespread in the cattle population, and fulminating acute fibrinous bronchopneumonia caused by this organism is one of the most important bacterial pneumonias seen in feeder calves. (Feedlot cattle encounter numerous stresses, including infectious agents [*Pasteurella*, mycoplasmas, viruses], weaning, crowding, feed and water deprivation, and environmental factors during transportation.)

P. haemolytica releases a soluble cytotoxin in the lungs that lyses alveolar macrophages and other white blood cells, thus defeating one of the primary defense mechanisms of the lungs (Table 30–2). The colonization and replication of the organisms in the lungs are then facilitated, thereby giving rise to clinical signs of pneumonia. A synergistic effect has been demonstrated between *P. haemolytica* and *Mycoplasma bovis*. This is of major pathogenic significance, and is also of great relevance in choice of therapeutic agents.

Pasteurella produces a neuraminidase that is mucolytic, thus allowing more easy spread of the bacterium and less efficient trapping. It also possesses an antiphagocytic capsule. The capsule forms are most common in the early multiplying culture phase, which apparently are more invasive and more immunogenic than are the nonencapsulated cultures. These characteristics, plus the fact that A1 is the main serotype of importance in pneumonic lesions, suggest that this capsule is a virulence factor.

Pasteurella haemolytica contains an endotoxin, which is released when the bacterium dies. This Endotoxin has a wide range of biological effects, including complement activation, coagulation and chemotaxis, which result in edema, and thrombosis. The role of this endotoxin is associated with the neutrophil response of the host. Toxemia can be a major factor in bovine respiratory disease. In bovine respiratory disease the presence of a protein toxin of *P. haemolytica* that kills alveolar macrophages, monocytes, neutrophils, and lymphocytes is of major significance. This leukotoxin is apparently specific for ruminants. Because *P. haemolytica* is pathogenic primarily for ruminants, this factor seems of major importance in the pathogenesis of the disease. The toxin is a soluble glycoprotein that is produced by log-phase cultures.

Another pathogen *Hemophilus* is deceptively important in the cause of bovine respiratory disease. *H. somnus* is the etiologic agent of thromboembolic meningoencephalitis, a usually fatal disease in which this bacterium is found in the central nervous system and other tissues. Hemophilus meningitis is, of course, of major significance in human medicine, especially in young children, where it is a very serious condition. *H. somnus* pneumonia may either follow thromboembolic meningoencephalitis or appear in cattle that have not had the disease. It may be found in cases of acute fibrinohemorrhagic pneumonia and fibrinous pleuritis resembling pneumonia associated with *Pasteurella haemolytica*.

The incidence and importance of *Hemophilus somnus* as a cause of pneumonia were

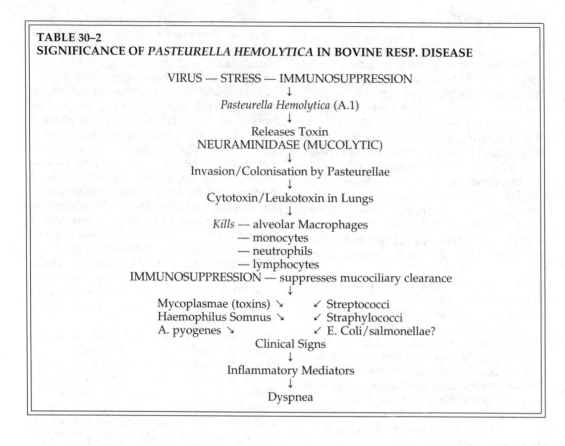

TABLE 30–2
SIGNIFICANCE OF *PASTEURELLA HEMOLYTICA* IN BOVINE RESP. DISEASE

VIRUS — STRESS — IMMUNOSUPPRESSION
↓
Pasteurella Hemolytica (A.1)
↓
Releases Toxin
NEURAMINIDASE (MUCOLYTIC)
↓
Invasion/Colonisation by Pasteurellae
↓
Cytotoxin/Leukotoxin in Lungs
↓
Kills — alveolar Macrophages
— monocytes
— neutrophils
— lymphocytes
IMMUNOSUPPRESSION — suppresses mucociliary clearance
↓
Mycoplasmae (toxins) ↘   ↙ Streptococci
Haemophilus Somnus ↘   ↙ Straphylococci
A. pyogenes ↘   ↙ E. Coli/salmonellae?
Clinical Signs
↓
Inflammatory Mediators
↓
Dyspnea

formerly thought to be considerably less than those of *Pasteurella haemolytica*. However, *Hemophilus somnus* is a particularly virulent organism that recently has assumed much greater significance as a pathogen in bovine respiratory disease.

Other pathogens frequently implicated are the mycoplasmas. Originally these spirochetes were viewed primarily as definite secondary invaders. At present, depending on the immune status of the host animal, mycoplasmas can be regarded as occasional primary pathogens. They are also believed to be toxin producers.

Mycoplasmas are the cause of insidious onset of pneumonia in housed calves. Although this insidious onset is characteristic of *Mycoplasma dispar* and *Ureaplasma*, the clinical disease seen when calves are affected with *Mycoplasma bovis* is often more acute.

Secondary bacterial invasion increases the severity of the primary lung damage caused by the viruses and mycoplasmas.

M. dispar and *M. pneumoniae* locate on the respiratory epithelium of tracheal organ cultures to exert their pathogenic effect. *M. bovis* can penetrate between the cells of the respiratory epithelium into the lamina propria below. Because *M. bovis* is a possible toxin producer, can cause acute mastitis in cattle, and has invasive potential into the blood stream, it is one of the most pathogenic mycoplasmas for cattle. It can cause focal areas of coagulative necrosis and infiltration by mononuclear cells.

M. dispar, *M. bovis*, and *Ureaplasma* are frequently recovered from the upper and lower respiratory tracts of calves in both early and late stages of pneumonia outbreaks. Mycoplasmas themselves can produce pneumonia experimentally when inoculated into the lower respiratory tract. These spirochetes are usually associated with a type of cuffing pneumonia characterized by a peribronchial sheath of lymphoid cells. In humans and in animals, mycoplasmae become invasive and pathogenic, when immunoincompetence and stress-related disorders are present.

30.3 RESPIRATORY DEFENSE MECHANISMS

Normal respiratory defense mechanisms include the cough reflex, mucociliary clearance mechanisms, and the presence of naturally occurring antibacterial proteins, such as lysozyme, lactoferrin, and interferon. Specific local defense mechanisms are mediated via local immunoglobulin A (IgA) antibodies, alveolar macrophages, and lymphocytes residing on the respiratory epithelium and alveoli. An initial viral insult devitalizes respiratory tract tissue, thus causing foci of necrosis or disruption of the defense mechanisms of local phagocytic cells. The way for a severe secondary bacterial invasion is thus paved.

Pulmonary alveolar macrophages constitute one of the prime defense mechanisms of the lung and are involved in the phagocytosis and killing of inhaled infectious organisms. Typically, enzootic pneumonia occurs in calves deficient in immunologic components to the causative agents. A severe aerogenous challenge may be able to overcome the immune system of the young calf. Increased susceptibility of young calves to respiratory infections can be associated with a lack of maternally derived passive immunity on the respiratory mucous membrane. These colostral proteins can gain access to the respiratory tract of the neonates where they contribute to the overall local defense mechanisms. Thus, adequate intake of early quality colostrum is important to protect not only against enteritis, but also against respiratory disease.

Calves with low serum immunoglobulin levels in the first few weeks of life are usually prone to the development of pneumonia, the severity of which relates to the virulence and types of infectious agents, environmental and stressful influences, and immunologic status.

Many secretory factors are present in both the upper and lower airways, including IgA (the main antibody type in the upper airways), IgG (the main type in the lungs), interferon, lysozymes, lactoferrin, alpha$_1$-antitrypsin, haptoglobin, transferrin, complement compounds, and various monokines and lymphokines. Many of these secretory factors have the potential to harm the host, as well as to protect against pathogens.

The stresses and management procedures obviously provide ample opportunities for depression of host defenses, for viral infection, and for enhancement of the challenge (and possibly even the virulence) or invading *Pasteurella*.

The Endotoxin of Pasteurella may play an important role in the pathogenesis of the disease by recruiting neutrophils that are then killed by the release of leukotoxin of *P. haemolytica*. The dying neutrophils release large amounts of inflammatory mediators, and proteolytic enzymes, thus resulting in tissue destruction.

The host defense mechanisms in pasteurellosis also contribute to the severe pulmonary damage. For instance complement components, coagulation cascades, bradykinin and kallikrein generation, arachidonic acid metabolism (with prostaglandin, thromboxane, and leukotriene production), the phagocyte respiratory activity (with production of free oxygen radicals), platelet activating factor release, and the release of numerous leukocyte proteolytic enzymes and inflammatory mediators, result in considerable and extensive tissue damage. Some of the major sequelae of these systems include thrombosis, disseminated intravascular coagulation, accumulation of leukocytes, increased vascular permeability inflammation and edema, vasodilation, bronchoconstriction, and pain.

Infectious stresses inactivate ciliary activity in the airways, suppress cellular resistance mechanisms, and lower resistance. Early separation from the dam, variable colostral intake, and confinement in small spaces increase susceptibility. In pneumonic pasteurellosis in dairy and veal units, morbidity and mortality increase when the animals are 2 to 5 weeks of age and again when calves are moved and placed in group pens.

Alterations in cellular and protein components of secretions that are evident with respiratory disease include an increase in local cell numbers, an increase in the percentage of neutrophils present, and an influx of protein into the lungs. Absence of proteins in the respiratory tract of calves that subsequently develop respiratory disease may indicate lack of absorption of colostral proteins from the gut and/or failure to transfer these proteins into the respiratory spaces. IgG1 and IgG2 represent the major isotypes available in the sera or lung secretions that may act directly on microorganisms (especially mycoplasma) or promote their killing by macrophages and neutrophils. Good housing conditions and adequate ventilation are important in controlling the incidence or severity of enzootic pneumonia. Low relative humidity leading to death of airborne organisms is of crucial importance because a relative humidity of less than 80% kills many aerosolized bacteria.

The local cellular defense mechanisms include the pharyngeal lymphoid tissues and bronchial-associated lymphoid tissue in the upper airways, and the various alveolar leukocytes. The alveolar macrophage is probably the most important defensive cell and comprises over 85% of the leukocytes in the normal alveolus. The alveolar macrophage has two major functions—phagocytosis of trapped particles and elaboration of numerous mediators of inflammation. Lymphocytes comprise about 12% of alveolar leukocytes and become important in the formation of helper and suppressor T cells, cytotoxic cells, and antibody-producing B cells. Neutrophils comprise about 2% of the alveolar leukocytes, and eosinophils comprise less than 1%.

ROLE OF PULMONARY MACROPHAGES IN DEFENSE

Pulmonary macrophages are mobile, phagocytic, and bactericidal cells maintain a clean and sterile environment in the respiratory components of the lung. Three types of pulmonary macrophages are alveolar macrophages within the lumen of the alveoli; airway macrophages within the large and small conducting airways; and interstitial macrophages within the connective tissues of the lung.

Macrophages and neutrophils are potent defense mechanisms against bacterial invasion of tissues, but contain numerous agents that when released can produce tissue damage in bovine respiratory disease. Activation of neutrophils, as well as activation of other macrophages, initiate the secretion of oxygen radicals and lysosomal enzymes and result in the release of arachidonic acid and the production of prostaglandins, thromboxanes, leukotrienes, and other mediators that initiate damage to lung tissues. These agents damage capillary endothelia, thereby resulting in leakage of plasma proteins and water into the interstitial spaces and hence the development of lung edema. Plasma proteins in the interstitial spaces lead to extravascular coagulation. Endothelial injury caused by infectious agents, toxins or by products of reactive cells can lead to intravascular coagulation. (via thromboxane–prostacyclin interaction). The activation of platelets in the coagulation process also plays an important role in the chemotaxis of neutrophils. After the release of platelet activating factor, a phospholipid produced by neutrophils, platelets initiate coagulation of blood thrombosis and disseminated intravascular coagulation.

This causes tissue annoxia, pain, and serves as a focus for chemotaxis. The presence of extracellular superoxide radicals activate a chemotactic factor that enables migration of neutrophils into an area of inflammation. The therapeutic use of superoxide dismutase and other agents that scavenge oxygen in extracellular fluid, thus preventing the activation of superoxide dependent chemoattractants apparently represents the basis for the anti-inflammatory activity of these agents. Dimethyl sulfoxide is one such agent that acting as a scavenger of free radicals, exhibits useful clinical anti-inflammatory activity.

30.4 GENERAL THERAPY PRINCIPLES

Therapy of bovine respiratory disease demands not only specific antimicrobial treatment directed toward the elimination of causative organisms, but also treatment aimed at alleviating symptoms and enhancing respiratory exchange.

In addition to appropriate antibiotic therapy, ancillary therapies may be of benefit in the management of the pathophysiology of bovine pneumonia, especially in the valuable individual. Good nursing care (shelter, temperature, and humidity regulation, ventilation, dust control, sanitation, and nutrition) is important in all situations. Fluid therapy and the use of nonsteroidal anti-inflammatory drugs (NSAID's) are practical measures that are likely to be of considerable benefit. Other measures may include expectorants, aerosol therapy, bronchodilators, decongestants, immune modulators (such as levamisole, ascorbic acid, or vitamin E), dimethyl sulfoxide (DMSO), heparin, and oxygen therapy. Hypertonic fluid solutions are also useful.

Antimicrobial drug therapy is directed mainly at the causative organisms. Because no effective antiviral drugs are available, such therapy is essentially the judicious selection and use of antibacterials. Two important criteria in selecting an antibacterial are the sensitivity of the organism(s) and the ability of the drug to reach the site of infection in effective concentration.

When antibiotics alone are used, the concentration achieved in the respiratory secretions diminishes rapidly as the capillary permeability decreases with improvement of the condition. Thus, after an initial apparent improvement, relapses are common because the antibiotic concentration in the respiratory system declines and may drop below the minimum inhibitory concentration (MIC). Normally most antibiotics cannot penetrate into lung tissue and bronchial secretions without grave difficulty. These kinetic difficulties are offset, however, by the process of inflammation and the increased capillary permeability that accompany the early stages of respiratory disease. As the inflammation subsides, the antibiotic once again diffuses only with difficulty into the respiratory tract secretions. Accordingly, the entrapped organisms in the respiratory mucus can flourish and replicate, thereby allowing a progressive deterioration of the condition or a relapse.

Thus, one of the great inherent problems in antimicrobial therapy of respiratory disease is attainment and maintenance of meaningful concentrations of antibiotics in the respiratory tract and its secretions. An-

other problem that arises when antibiotics alone are used is that these drugs do not alter the viscosity of the bronchial secretions; sometimes, in fact, the viscosity increases. This enhanced tackiness of the secretions renders expectoration difficult and inhibits clearance of the respiratory tree.

CRITERIA FOR SELECTION OF ANTIMICROBIALS

Important criteria for selecting antimicrobial agents include antimicrobial spectrum, pharmacokinetic properties, and bactericidal or bacteriostatic properties. Effective antimicrobial treatment depends particularly on the ability of the antimicrobial drug to attain therapeutic levels at the site of infection. Unless MICs of the drug are achieved at the infection site, bacterial growth can continue despite in vitro susceptibility of these pathogens to the antimicrobial drug. Many studies of bronchopulmonary infections in humans have shown that antimicrobial concentrations in respiratory secretions are therapeutically more important than are serum antimicrobial levels. As a rule, pharmacokinetic information is scarce on the penetration of many antimicrobial drugs into respiratory secretions. Although serum levels can be quite high, corresponding levels in the respiratory secretions may often be quite low. This difference may explain why some cases of chronic bronchopulmonary disease infection are never fully eradicated and also why relapses occur. Adequate MICs to some pathogens may never be attained in respiratory secretions with many commonly used antimicrobials. Choice of antibiotics for bovine respiratory disease has been based on the blood concentration of agents that were achieved. Additional criteria, including concentration in the lungs, should also be considered, however. High respiratory concentrations are attained and intracellular penetration is augmented with lipophilic drugs. These characteristics are important for respiratory infections, some of which are intracellular. The MIC of a drug for a particular organism is a measure of the serum concentration, which may have little relationship to the optimal concentration achieved or desired at the site of infection. This tissue concentration may be quite poor, and so response may be poor if the drug fails to reach the infected site in useful antibacterial concentrations. Such failure often occurs in bronchial secretions. The necessity to obtain concentrations equal to or greater than the MIC is important for antibacterial effect. When these levels are not attained, not only does therapeutic failure occur, but bacterial resistance also may be due to constant exposure to subeffective antibacterial concentrations. The increasing reported incidence of oxytetracycline resistance by *Pasteurella* is interesting to note in this context. This resistance presumably is caused not only by the widespread and possibly indiscriminate use of oxytetracycline in bovine respiratory disease over the last few years, but also to failure of oxytetracycline to obtain levels in excess of the M.I.C. in respiratory tissues, when used alone.

Local Concentration

The difference between antibiotics in terms of whether they kill bacteria (i.e., are bactericidal) or prevent bacterial growth (i.e., are bacteriostatic) is dictated by the dependence of both activities on the concentration of the drug relative to the sensitivity of the organism. Antibacterials must reach the infected site in high concentration to obtain clinical effectiveness. Frequently in veterinary medicine only low concentrations are found at the site of infection, thus allowing only a bacteriostatic effect to be obtained. Such low concentrations might also lead to bacterial resistance. Resistance or susceptibility is not an "all-or-none" phenomenon, but rather depends on local drug concentration. For instance, an organism susceptible to penicillin at 0.1 μg/ml is considered sensitive because such a level can be easily achieved physiologically. An organism susceptible to 10 μg/ml or more is considered resistant because such a concentration is difficult to achieve and maintain in the tissues. The bactericidal potency of oxytetracycline increases slowly as the concentration increases. The amount of drug required to kill a certain bacterial strain may vary depending on the number of organisms in the inoculum. With bacteriostatic antibiotics, the preponderance of evidence indicates

that tissue concentrations at or above the MIC should be obtained. High doses of antibiotics give a more prompt clinical cure than do low doses. With sulfonamides, although classed as bacteriostatic, a bactericidal action may be evident at high local concentrations. This is especially true of potentiated sulfonamides.

Pharmacokinetic Properties and Respiratory Therapy

Most of the currently accepted therapy protocols in antimicrobial treatment are derived from experimental work in healthy animals and sensitivity tests for bacteria using in vitro assays. The necessary dosage and dosing intervals required to maintain specific blood levels for a drug are determined from pharmacokinetic data usually in healthy animals. Although blood concentrations have been used as rough indicators of tissue levels, such factors as protein binding and lipid solubility can affect these tissues or organ concentrations. In addition, pharmacokinetic distributional properties can be altered by the disease state. The pH of fluid in areas of inflammation is often highly acidic. The activity of some antimicrobial agents is substantially reduced or abolished in this environment. Antimicrobial drugs that are less adversely affected by acid and pH include oxytetracycline, which is most active at pH 5.5, and sulfonamides.

The inherent pharmacokinetic properties of drugs have an important bearing on the host-microorganism-drug interaction and the eventual outcome of therapy. Therapeutic considerations include the degree of protein binding, degree of ionization and lipid solubility, relative passage across cell membranes, and the local pH during inflammation and infection. If the same conditions exist at the site of infection as in the plasma, concentrations should be the same across blood-alveolar membranes. The same conditions rarely exist at the inaccessible site of infection, however. The different pH at the site of infection can significantly influence the ratio of ionized to nonionized drug locally.

Factors governing distribution involve a multicompartmental system including all body compartments in contact indirect or direct with the blood. The extent of protein binding of the drugs in the blood and in the tissues, pH differences in the compartments, the lipid solubility, and the dissociation constant of the drug (pKa) strongly influence the efficacy of therapy. When the volume of distribution exceeds or even approximates total body water, antimicrobials can enter cells. Such large diffusion, which includes the respiratory tract, applies to oxytetracycline and sulfonamides. For this reason, the volume of distribution of a drug is crucial to its ability to obtain adequate concentration at the site of action. Obviously any other pharmacologic agent that can increase its local concentration (e.g., a mucolytic, such as bromhexine) appreciably changes the local susceptibility patterns in a most beneficial way. This change is reflected by enhanced clinical resolution of the disease.

The concentrations of drugs that are achieved in the plasma/serum of cattle using various dosages and routes of administration have been determined for numerous antimicrobials. Much less is known about the concentrations of antimicrobial drugs that can be achieved in other biological fluids and secretions, especially in the diseased state. Pharmacokinetic parameters support the possibility of an increased volume of distribution in the diseased state. This possibility holds true for broad-spectrum antimicrobial drugs in respiratory diseases of cattle. Mechanisms involved may include alteration of blood vessel permeability that allows passage of more protein-bound drug into the tissue space or changes in pH acting to trap ionized drug. Oxytetracycline concentrations may be higher in diseased tissue than in normal tissue.

30.5 ANTIMICROBIALS FOR BOVINE RESPIRATORY DISEASE

GENERAL THERAPY

The therapeutic and prophylactic agents currently available cannot deal adequately with the condition in a comprehensive fashion because the specific roles of the many various microorganisms have not been satisfactorily determined.

Because of the absence of effective antiviral agents, antibiotics are widely used in the treatment of febrile pneumonic calves to counter primary or secondary bacterial infections.

Additional supportive therapy may also be warranted to symptomatically improve gaseous exchange, e.g., anti-inflammatory agents, bronchodilators, mucolytics, fluids, expectorants, and perhaps respiratory stimulants (Tables 30–3 and 30–4).

In severe cases, irreversible changes in the calf's lung may render attempted treatment uneconomic.

After initiation of antibacterial therapy, the animal must be clinically assessed each day to monitor the response to treatment. Antibiotic treatments of acute respiratory disease must be continued for at least 3 days beyond apparent clinical recovery. Parenteral treatment is preferable initially, especially intravenous administration, to ensure maximal bioavailability and rapid arrival of high drug concentration in the diseased respiratory tissue.

As already stated, the bovine respiratory disease syndrome is a complex interaction between viruses, chlamydia, mycoplasmas, bacteria, and stress. *P. multocida* and *P. haemolytica* are so commonly isolated that they should be given priority in treatment. Secondary bacteria (e.g., *hemophilus*) and mycoplasmal infections, however, can be quite difficult to treat because the initial viral attack causes immunosuppression and a profound neutropenia. This reduced immune response and phagocytic activity can impair the efficacy of antibiotics, especially bacteriostatic types, and may further result in reinfection if therapy is discontinued.

Although viral tissue destruction can be dramatic, the regenerative capacity of the epithelium is such that a full recovery can be made if a secondary infection is absent or promptly treated.

ANTIMICROBIAL DRUGS

Because a suitable antiviral drug is not commercially available, therapy must be directed against primary or secondary pathogens. Additional therapy may also be warranted symptomatically to alleviate respiratory distress.

TABLE 30–3
RESPIRATORY DISEASE—GENERAL THERAPY

1) *Treat Infections (Bacterial) Cause*:
   —Oxytetracycline intravenously (broad spectrum, viruses, chlamydia, mycoplasma) or tilmicosin, subcutaneously, enrofloxalin, ceftiofur, danofloxacin flortenicol

   also

   —Potentiated sulfonamide, ampicillin (+ sublactam), amoxycillin (telavulanate), penicillin/streptomycin, tylosin/erythromycin, (mycoplasma, gram +, *Pasteurella*)
2) *Treat Symptoms*:
   Anti-inflammatories—flunixin (reduce fever, congestion oedema), aspirin Corticosteroids (rarely and carefully) Antihistamine—Tripelennamine

   Bronchodilator:

   Xanthines: Etamiphylline
   Beta$_2$ agonisis: Clenbuterol

   Mucolytic:

   Bromhexine
3) *Miscellaneous*: fluids, DMSO. expectorants, respiratory stimulants

TABLE 30–4
RESPIRATORY DISEASE—DOSAGE FOR ANTIMICROBIAL CHEMOTHERAPY IN CATTLE

DRUG	DOSAGE RATE	INTERVAL (HOURS)
Enrofloxacin	2.5 mg/kg	24
Danofloxacin	1.25 mg/kg (intramuscular)	24
Ceftiofur	1.0 mg/kg	24
Tilmicosin	10.0 mg/kg	72
Spiramycin	100,000 I.U./kg	48
Florfenicol	20 mg/kg (intramuscular)	48
Sodium penicillin G	10,000 U/kg	8
Procaine penicillin (Aqueous)	10–15,000 U/kg	24
Ampicillin sodium (Aqueous)	6 mg/kg	8–12
Ampicillin trihydrate (Susp.)	10 mg/kg	16–24
Amoxicillin (Susp.)	15 mg/kg	48
Dihydrostreptomycin sulphate	10 mg/kg	8–12
Oxytetracycline hydrochloride (propylene glycol)	7–10 mg/kg	24
Oxytetracycline (in 2-pyrollidone) L.A. (or PUP)		48–72
Erythromycin	6–10 mg/kg	12
Tylosin	6–10 mg/kg	18
Sulfametlazine sodium	100–150 mg/kg	24
Sulfadimethoxine sodium	55–100 mg/kg	24–36
Sulfadoxine/trimethoprim	30 mg/kg	24

Criteria for selection of a suitable antimicrobial drug must include:

1. The likely organism
2. The likely sensitivity pattern
3. The attainment and maintenance of an effective concentration in excess of the MIC at the focus of infection

The veterinarian must be familiar with the dosage rates, treatment intervals, cost, and, in food-producing animals, the specific tissue withholding times, and legal status (use in food animals/residue).

The function of drug therapy is to alleviate the symptoms of the disease and to prevent the disease from developing to such a point that mucolytics and bronchodilators are required.

For judicious selection of an antimicrobial agent, the results of culturing and sensitivity testing are important. The drug concentration attained in the lung is affected by the route of administration. If the MIC for a particular pathogen is high, high-dosage intravenous administration at short intervals may be preferable to intramuscular delivery because of the higher bioavailability and lung/bronchial secretion levels attained. Local inflammation can enhance penetration of certain antimicrobials, whereas the presence of purulent material can adversely affect the efficacy of sulfonamides, erythromycin, and penicillins. Abscessation and poor blood flow through consolidated, atelectatic lungs also render penetration difficult. Antibacterials have been used extensively for the treatment of cattle with bovine respiratory disease. Sulfonamides, penicillins, tetracyclines, fluoroquinolones, trimethoprim/sulfa, aminocyclitols, cephalosporins, and macrolides are, or have been, used either by oral or parenteral administration with beneficial results. Antibacterial therapy has utilized varied approaches. Treatment administered to animals beginning at the time first clinical signs of bovine respiratory disease are observed has been widely used. This type of treatment has often involved three or more consecutive daily treatments. In some feedlots, all cattle upon receipt have been treated prophylactically with an antibacterial during arrival. Use of this procedure is declining. Sometimes, antibiotics, especially chlortetracycline, have been fed at high levels for the first 3 to 4 weeks after arrival in an effort to decrease losses resulting from bovine respiratory disease.

Resistance of *Pasteurella* to antibiotics has been a problem since at least the early 1970s. Multiple R-plasmid resistance in *P. haemolytica* led to the use of mixtures of antibiotics for treatment. Nevertheless, by the mid 1980s, chloramphenicol, an antibiotic to which most isolates of *P. haemolytica* are susceptible, was used as the drug of choice by veterinarians for treatment of bovine respiratory disease. Shortly thereafter, the FDA banned the use of chloramphenicol in all meat animals in the United States. Treatment only with alternate antibiotics was necessary again. Since that time, other antibiotics, including fluoroquinolones, new macrolides, and new cephalosporins, have been introduced for the treatment of bovine respiratory disease. Concentrations of such antibiotics as ampicillin and cephalosporins tend to decrease when inflammation subsides, whereas concentrations of gentamicin, amoxicillin, and tetracyclines persist in respiratory secretions. Intracellular infection can be a particularly difficult focus to reach with many antibiotics.

Although chloramphenicol is prohibited for use in food-producing animals, a new structural analog, florfenicol, is a useful alternative that possesses a broad spectrum of antibacterial activity coupled with useful pharmacokinetic properties. Because florfenicol does not possess the *p*-nitro group, as does chloramphenicol, it is not associated with idiosyncratic aplastic anemia. Hence, florfenicol may play a future role in the therapy of respiratory disease in food animals. Florfenicol has been shown to be very effective in bovine respiratory disease, and is currently going through the regulatory clearance pipeline in many countries. Its general release is anticipated soon. Doses used have ranged from 11 to 22 mg/kg in calves. A patented formulation of florfenicol (300 mg/ml) given intramuscularly at a dosage of 20 mg/kg, repeated at 48 hour intervals, compares very favorably with oxytetracycline in cattle.

30.6 PENICILLINS

Although penicillins do not penetrate tissues well and are usually restricted to extracellular fluids, high-dosage penicillin is often relatively successful because of its high potency and because of a simple law of mass action whereby high local concentrations can assist tissue penetration. Aminoglycosides do not penetrate bronchial secretions well, and although gentamicin is broad spectrum in action, it has poor cellular penetration. This shortcoming can be offset somewhat by intravenous delivery. Spectinomycin penetrates lung tissue relatively well, and macrolides attain useful concentrations throughout the respiratory tract. Erythromycin can penetrate neutrophils and attains high tissue and pleural fluid levels. Following normal dosage of parenteral erythromycin, lung levels approximate three times serum levels.

Although *Pasteurella* have been isolated frequently from the lungs of fatal cases, doubts have been expressed as to their role as primary pathogens. Additionally, in the treatment of the condition, the antimicrobial sensitivity of *P. haemolytica* isolates differs markedly in the upper and lower respiratory tracts. The lower respiratory tracts usually tend to be more easily treated with certain antimicrobial agents.

Benzylpenicillin is effective against many *Pasteurella* isolates and gram-positive organisms. Rapid initial high levels can be attained by intravenous delivery of the soluble sodium or potassium salt. The spectrum of activity can be broadened by combining penicillin with streptomycin, gentamicin, or kanamycin.

The semisynthetic penicillins, ampicillin and amoxicillin, also have potent bactericidal action and, like benzylpenicillin, the virtue of negligible toxicity. They possess a broader spectrum of activity and penetrate tissues well. Amoxicillin displays a rapid bactericidal activity and attains high blood levels 30 minutes after intramuscular injection or 2 hours following oral administration. A depot long-acting suspension of amoxicillin now available for intramuscular use provides blood levels in excess of 24 hours.

AMINOPENICILLINS

Unlike penicillin G, aminopenicillins (ampicillin, amoxicillin, and hetacillin) can be absorbed orally and can penetrate the outer layer of gram-negative bacteria more readily, thereby increasing their activity against many gram-negative pathogens. Their activity against susceptible gram-positive bacteria is essentially equal to that of penicillin G.

Amoxicillin and ampicillin have equal activity, but amoxicillin is absorbed better orally and has more rapid action. Hetacillin is inactive as it exists in a preparation, but is more stable in gastric acid than are amoxicillin and ampicillin and therefore is absorbed best. After it enters the blood stream, hetacillin is metabolized to ampicillin and becomes active. Amoxicillin and ampicillin are two of the most widely used penicillins because of their wide range of activity. Amoxicillin and ampicillin are classified as broad-spectrum antibiotics because they are effective against various gram-positive and gram-negative organisms. They are also effective against most anaerobic organisms, except for *Bacteroides fragilis*, which produces beta-lactamases. Because the aminopenicillins are sensitive to beta-lactamases, the combination of aminopenicillins with clavulanic acid (amoxicillin) or sublactam (ampicillin) markedly reduces their MICs for numerous microbial organisms.

Ampicillin, the first of the broad-spectrum penicillins, is active against gram-positive and gram-negative bacteria. It is not active against beta-lactamase-producing staphylococci nor against *Pseudomonas*, *Klebsiella*, and indole-positive *Proteus*. Ampicillin is stable to gastric acid.

Ampicillin was first marketed in 1961 and has remained one of the most widely used semisynthetic penicillins. The forms of injectable ampicillin available are the trihydrate and sodium salts. Sodium ampicillin can be given intramuscularly or intravenously to achieve rapid plasma concentrations.

Amoxicillin has an antibacterial spectrum identical to that of ampicillin. It shows four significant advantages, however.

1. It can easily be made into a palatable oral tablet.
2. Amoxicillin gives blood levels 50 to 100% higher than those given by ampicillin after oral administration.
3. Amoxicillin has a different and much faster bactericidal action.

4. Evidence in humans shows that amoxicillin penetrates some tissues better than does ampicillin, e.g., sputum in chronic bronchitis.

Amoxicillin is formed by modifying ampicillin. Amoxicillin differs chemically from ampicillin by the addition of a hydroxyl group to the aminobenzyl side chain. Amoxicillin reportedly has increased activity against certain gram-negative bacteria and also has the advantage of high bioavailability when given orally to preruminant calves, pigs, and small animals.

Amoxicillin is available combined with clavulanic acid and is now formulated as a long-acting intramuscular suspension for respiratory use. Potentiated penicillins, such as sublactam-ampicillin, are more effective than penicillin-streptomycin combinations in the treatment of penicillin- or ampicillin-resistant strains of *Pasteurella* in feedlot calves. Such a combination given intramuscularly (3.3 mg/kg sublactam, 6.6 mg/kg ampicillin) for 3 successive days often gives a prompt clinical response. Sublactam, like clavulanic acid, is a beta-lactamase inhibitor that renders the combined penicillin effective against beta-lactamase-producing bacteria, especially staphylococci.

30.7 SULFONAMIDES

Sulfonamide combinations have a broad spectrum of activity and are commonly used either intravenously or orally for treatment of respiratory infections. They concentrate in the lung, sometimes at three to four times the plasma concentration, and distribute well into tissues and pleural fluid.

Sulfadiazine, a member of the long-established sulfonamide group, is a bacteriostatic drug that acts via competitive inhibition for uptake of para-aminobenzoic acid (PABA) by bacteria. It is well absorbed orally, attains good concentration in lung tissue, and is active against a wide range of gram-positive and gram-negative bacteria.

Potentiated sulfonamides are useful combinations for the treatment of pneumonic pasteurellosis because they possess good tissue-penetrating properties into the respiratory tract and secretions. Given intrave-

nously or once daily intramuscularly, therapy can be supported by oral administration. Trimethoprim is degraded in the rumen; thus, oral administration is restricted to young calves. The potentiated sulfonamides, utilizing a double blockade of folic acid biosynthesis, are less likely to display major resistance patterns than are the parent sulfonamides when used alone.

Sustained-release boluses of sulfadimethoxine (Albon) and sulfamethazine are available for pneumonic pasteurellosis. Given orally, these dose forms provide a steady payout of active sulfonamide for 3 to 4 days. Sulfadimethoxine (Albon Bolus) at an oral dose of 137.5 mg/kg provides effective plasma levels for 4 days. Stringent withdrawal times apply to these types of products, however, and the manufacturers' instructions in this regard should be carefully followed. Baquiloprim is a dihydrofolate reductase inhibitor that is not degraded in the rumen and, hence, is used in an orally active potentiated sulfonamide bolus in some countries. It possesses a long t 1/2 and acts for 2 days when combined with sulfadimidine.

Ormetoprim (combined with sulfadimethoxine), acting as an inhibitor of dihydrofolate reductase, is a sulfonamide potentiator under investigation for respiratory therapy.

30.8 TETRACYCLINES

Oxytetracycline, a broad-spectrum antibiotic of the tetracycline family, is active against most bacterial pathogens causing infectious disease of the respiratory system, including *Pasteurella* and, to a lesser extent, mycoplasma. For many years, oxytetracycline has been a front-line antibiotic in veterinary medicine for the treatment of respiratory disease in most species.

Because of the variety of microorganisms that may be involved, the selection of a broad-spectrum drug is logical, and tetracycline therapy is advocated. Tetracyclines readily penetrate most tissues, and their antibacterial spectrum includes chlamydia, which may often be implicated. When calves are first seen in the prepneumonic stage, oxytetracycline may be administered to the group in water or feed, and treatment for 5 to 10 days normally controls progression of the disease. Absorption of tetracyclines from the gut is hindered by calcium because chemical complexes are formed; thus, they should not be given orally with milk.

Tetracyclines have been traditionally popular for respiratory disease treatment because of their broad spectrum of antibacterial activity and their good distribution in lung tissues and respiratory secretions. They are useful in mixed infections, for which their secondary activity against mycoplasmas, chlamydiae, and rickettsiae is an added bonus. Many of the *Pasteurella haemolytica* A1 isolates are susceptible in vitro to oxytetracycline. Oxytetracycline is available for intravenous, intramuscular, or oral use, and the administration of concentrated 20% long-acting formulations provides useful cover for 4 days when given intramuscularly. When calves are inappetant, parenteral administration is necessary. With so many proprietary brands now available, the bioavailability from the intramuscular site can vary significantly. Hence, intravenous administration is preferable at the commencement of therapy. Although concentrations of oxytetracycline can be higher in diseased tissues than in normal tissues, the rate of excretion and overall body clearance can be retarded in these diseased animals also.

Increasing incidences of *Pasteurella* resistance to oxytetracycline have been reported. Such resistance is not surprising because of the extensive use of this antibiotic for respiratory conditions for which it has traditionally been regarded as a drug of first choice.

Tetracyclines are active also against *Escherichia coli*, *Enterobacter*, *Brucella*, *Francisella tularensis*, and *Pasteurella multocida*, although many strains of these bacteria have acquired resistance to the tetracyclines. *Proteus mirabilis* and *Pseudomonas aeruginosa* are resistant, but many strains of *Hemophilus* have remained susceptible. Tetracyclines are also effective against some mycobacterias, as well as many *Mycoplasma*, *Chlamydia*, and *Rickettsia*. Tetracycline resistance in bacteria is caused by a decreased uptake of tetracycline into the bacterial cell and an acquired ability of the bacteria to "excrete"

the drug out of the cell. Most of the resistance to tetracyclines, transferred by R-plasmids, increases in response to subinhibitory concentrations of tetracyclines. In vitro activity of members of this group is almost identical, but differences seen in their stability, absorption, and binding characteristics cause significant differences in their activity in vivo. In addition, variation in physical properties govern suitability of various tetracyclines for parenteral use.

A great deal of sophisticated formulation technology goes into creating stable oxytetracycline solutions for injections. Propylene glycol has been used as a base, but causes tissue irritation with pain and inflammation when given subcutaneously or intramuscularly. By the intravenous route it can cause temporary recumbency unless given slowly. Lactamide base is an improvement on propylene glycol.

Polyvinylpyrrolidone is a more recent base that has allowed the administration of more concentrated solutions (100 mg oxytetracycline/ml) with less pain and tissue damage and additionally prolongs effective blood levels following a single administration. Thus, 10 mg/kg intramuscularly using oxytetracycline 10% in polyvinylpyrrolidone maintains plasma levels above 0.5 μg/ml for 40 hours, thus making 2-day intervals between administration feasible.

The product containing polyvinylpyrrolidone as a vehicle causes much less tissue damage, and thus healing takes place more rapidly. Oxytetracycline forms a complex with polyvinylpyrrolidone and this complex is less irritant. The complex is rapidly carried away from the site of injection surrounded by P.V.P. and then released gradually, thus minimizing local irritation.

All tetracycline antibiotics, when administered intramuscularly, may cause severe tissue damage characterized by necrosis and polymorphonuclear infiltration. Oxytetracycline administered in a propylene glycol water solvent produced the least tissue damage. The clinical signs of pain and irritation after an intramuscular injection are well known.

Lesions may remain in the muscle tissue for a considerable period and, thus, injected animals should not be slaughtered for human consumption for considerable periods.

In an attempt to minimize this undesirable side effect, oxytetracycline formulated by some manufacturers incorporated polyvinylpyrrolidone as a vehicle.

A recent advance on this concept is a patented injectable formulation of Terramycin using 2-polyvinylpyrrolidone with an oxytetracycline concentration of 200 mg/ml. This formulation has allowed even smaller dose volumes without increasing tissue irritation and pain. More significant, however, is its action in prolonging blood levels. A single injection of 20 mg/kg intramuscularly maintains a therapeutic blood level over a 3- to 4-day period, which should cover the length of therapy required in most acute infections.

A depot formulation of oxytetracycline is now available. The product contains 200 mg oxytetracycline/ml, and the solvent system is based on 2-pyrrolidone. After intramuscular injection of 20 mg/kg body weight, therapeutic serum concentrations are maintained for 3 to 5 days. The mode of action depends on a controlled precipitation of the drug at the injection site.

Despite the unprecedented high concentration of 200 mg/ml, the drug is well tolerated at the site of injection and the residue profile indicates that all tissues are clear of residue 28 days after injection. The maximum lesion at the injection site consists of a small amount of fibrous tissue, which does not necessitate trimming even when animals are slaughtered immediately at the end of the withdrawal period.

The product Liquamycin LA-200 employs a unique patented solvent system based on 2-pyrrolidone, the lactam of gamma-amino-butyric acid. It occurs in low concentration in several common foodstuffs, such as tomatoes and catsup. It has the advantage of being rapidly metabolized in the animal and poses no safety or residue problems.

Broad-spectrum antimicrobial drugs that are formulated to maintain extended tissue levels have the advantage of lowering labor costs and increasing the interval between successive treatments. Long-acting oxytetracycline and sustained-release sulfamethazine boluses have long been used in the therapy of pneumonia because of this characteristic.

All tetracyclines, except doxycycline and minocycline, have similar pharmacodynamic and pharmacokinetic properties. Doxycycline and minocycline have the advantage of greater tissue penetration because of increased lipid solubility and an expanded antimicrobial spectrum.

Pharmacokinetics of doxycycline differ greatly from those of older tetracyclines. Major differences include a five- to tenfold increase in lipid solubility and more extensive protein binding. These properties enhance tissue penetration and prolong the biological half-life.

Minocycline and doxycycline are more lipid soluble than are older tetracyclines, so they more easily cross cell membranes. Thus, they are better able to penetrate tissues (e.g., the central nervous system and lungs) and to accumulate in secretions (e.g., bronchial secretions, tears, saliva, and bile) and are more effective against intracellular organisms. The lipid-soluble drugs are cleared primarily by hepatic metabolism and biliary elimination.

The antimicrobial spectrum of doxycycline is similar to that of other tetracyclines. Doxycycline has broad-spectrum activity against gram-positive and gram-negative aerobic and anaerobic bacteria. In general, doxycycline is more active against most staphylococci, streptococci, and anaerobic bacteria. Doxycycline has good activity against *Mycoplasma*, *Ureaplasma*, *Chlamydia*, and the Rickettsiaceae.

Veal calves with mycoplasmal infection have responded well to doxycycline in feed. The broad-spectrum, good oral bioavailability (lipophility), and absorption not modified by feed characteristics suggest a useful role for doxycycline in food animals. Pharmacokinetic studies, however, suggest retarded excretion rates and the formation of persistent drug residues.

Sulfonamides and penicillins, although useful and effective in many cases of pasteurellosis, possess no activity against mycoplasmas, which are becoming increasingly significant pathogens. When no clinical response is obtained to penicillins, sulfonamides, or tetracyclines (the latter possessing only weak antimycoplasmal activity), the antimicrobial regimen should be changed to more potent antimycoplasmal drugs.

30.9 MACROLIDES

Macrolides are basic drugs of high lipid solubility that attain high concentrations in the respiratory tract. Tylosin is perhaps a first line choice for mycoplasmal pneumonias, and this compound can often provide spectacular results where earlier therapies have failed. Tylosin possesses potent activity against gram-positive organisms also, although its activity against *Pasteurella*, which is normally poor, is enhanced considerably when used in combination with oxytetracycline. A combination of tylosin-oxytetracycline can provide rapid clinical improvement in pneumonic calves by covering mycoplasma, *Pasteurella*, chlamydia, and many gram-positive and gram-negative organisms.

The macrolides are a large group of structurally related antibiotics that include desmycosin, erythromycin, spiramycin, tylosin, and tilmicosin. Many of these products have been used in veterinary practice for more than 20 years and are still clinically useful.

ANTIBACTERIAL SPECTRUM

The macrolide antibiotics have a relatively broad spectrum that covers gram-positive bacteria, some gram-negative organisms, such as *Pasteurella* and *Hemophilus*, as well as *Mycoplasma*, *Rickettsia*, and *Chlamydia*. The relative efficacy against individual organisms varies with the different macrolides. Tylosin tends to display a high potency against *Mycoplasma* and gram-positive bacteria, but only moderate activity against *Pasteurella*. Spiramycin is widely used in Europe for gram-positive mycoplasmal and *Pasteurella* infections of pigs, poultry, and calves.

Erythromycin has a high efficacy against gram-positive organisms, especially penicillin-resistant *Staphylococcus* and *Streptococcus*. (*Pasteurella* and *Chlamydia* tend to be sensitive; *Mycoplasma* are moderately less sensitive.)

The most recent compound, tilmicosin, retains the high degree of efficacy against mycoplasma seen with the parent compound (tylosin) and shows a markedly improved activity against *Pasteurella*.

The clinically most important feature of macrolides is the accumulation of the antibiotic in lung and milk. Serum levels of tylosin tend to be low and are a poor indication of total tissue concentrations. Respiratory tract infections may be effectively treated with dosages that actually produce serum concentrations lower than the MIC for the offending organisms because the lung:serum ratios are in the order of 3:1 and 5:1. With erythromycin, spiramycin, and tylosin, peak serum concentrations occur 1 to 3 hours after intramuscular injection, 1 to 2 hours after intramuscular injection, and 1 to 2 hours after oral use. After intramuscular administration, peak serum concentrations are maintained for several hours and then decline slowly.

TYLOSIN

Tylosin, a fermentation product of *Streptomyces fradiae* and actinomyces, was isolated from a soil sample obtained in Thailand. The antibacterial spectrum is essentially against gram-positive bacteria. In addition, tylosin is widely recognized for its activity against *Mycoplasma*. Its toxicity is low, thus giving a high therapeutic index. Blood levels in cattle lasting beyond 24 hours from intramuscular administration at various dosages have been reported.

A feature of tylosin that is not shared by other macrolide antibiotics is the formation of desmycosin, a microbiologically active degradation product, produced by mild acid hydrolysis. Desmycosin exhibits physical, chemical, and antimicrobial properties that are similar to those of tylosin. Tylosin inhibits the growth of spirochetes and protozoa and is effective against mycoplasma. When fed to animals, the antibiotic stimulates growth. Like spiramycin, tylosin is a permitted feed additive at low inclusion rates.

This macrolide antibiotic was developed exclusively for veterinary use. Most of its therapeutic usage is directed against mycoplasmal diseases, particularly in poultry. It is also used as a growth promoter for poultry and pigs.

Tylosin is well absorbed orally. The tartrate salt is used for water medication and the phosphate for feed. It is a safe antibiotic at recommended dosage rates, but intramuscular injection may cause some tissue irritation.

ERYTHROMYCIN/SPIRAMYCIN

Erythromycin has been a popular antibiotic in human medicine for several years. It is usually the drug of choice for the treatment of gram-positive infections in persons allergic to beta lactam antibiotics. Veterinarians have found erythromycin useful for respiratory and mastitic infections as well, although some gastrointestinal problems following administration of erythromycin have been reported. Erythromycin quickly provides high levels in the respiratory tract following parenteral administration. Thus, erythromycin is especially useful for respiratory infections in cattle in which the respiratory secretion:serum ratio is uniquely high.

Two salts of erythromycin are available for intravenous administration, namely, the glucoheptonate and the lactobionate. Erythromycin is highly effective against *Pasteurella*, *Corynebacterium*, streptococci, staphylococci, and mycoplasma. It is rapidly absorbed after intramuscular injection; peak serum levels are obtained usually within 3 hours. Concentration of erythromycin in the lung tissue is 1.5 to 2.5 times that in the serum. The reported incidence of *Pasteurella* resistance has been lower for erythromycin than for oxytetracycline or penicillin.

Spiramycin is an active macrolide that gives high and sustained tissue levels. It is active in vivo, especially for respiratory and mastitic infections, and is a major therapeutic product.

Spiramycin at a dosage rate of 100,000 I.U./kg at 48-hour intervals, or as a single prophylactic injection, is a useful alternative agent. Its high activity against mycoplasma and *Pasteurella* can be explained by its excellent diffusion and concentration in the lung tissue and bronchial secretions.

Tiamulin is another antispirochetal agent effective against mycoplasma and *Ureaplasma*. (It is currently predominantly used against *Treponema hyodysenteriae* in swine dysentery.)

Lincomycin (50 mg/ml) and spectinomycin (100 mg/ml) administered by intramuscular injection (15 mg/kg for 3 to 5 days) is a combination that gives good results in many cases of enzootic pneumonia.

The combination of lincomycin with spectinomycin has attained popularity for use in respiratory tract diseases of cattle. This combination is apparently of greatest value against mycoplasma, and perhaps *Pasteurella* secondarily. The combination of lincomycin and spectinomycin may be at least additive or even synergistic because both agents apparently act on the same ribosomal step, but at different sites. In this respect, spectinomycin also may be useful in some situations in combination with a macrolide (for *Pasteurella*). The ratio of the preparation most commonly used, 1 part lincomycin to 2 parts spectinomycin (1:2), may not represent the most effective ratio against all organisms. The dosage that is used against mycoplasma may be too low when used against other organisms affected by only one of the drugs.

New additions to the long-established range of antimicrobial drugs useful in calf pneumonia include ceftiofur, enrofloxacin, danofloxacin, and tilmicosin.

30.10 CEPHALOSPORINS—CEFTIOFUR (NAXCEL [U.S.], EXCENEL [EC])

Cephalosporins possess antibacterial action similar to that of the other beta-lactam antibiotics—the inhibition of cell wall synthesis. The popularity and usefulness of cephalosporins result from their resistance to many of the beta-lactamase enzymes, their wide spectrum of activity compared to that of penicillin G, and their wide safety margin. Since the synthesis of the first cephalosporins from the fungus *Cephalosporium*, this class has expanded.

Although this group of compounds has been classified in several ways using various criteria, the term "generation" was originally devised as a means of separating the cephalosporins based solely on their in vitro antibacterial potency and spectrum of activity. The introduction of each cephalosporin generation has brought about a loss of gram-positive activity, an increase in gram-negative activity and spectrum, and an increase in resistance to beta-lactamase enzymes.

A new addition to the long-established range of antimicrobial drugs useful in calf pneumonia is ceftiofur. Ceftiofur has excellent activity against *P. multocida*, *P. haemolytica*, and *Hemophilus somnus*. At a dose rate of 1.0 mg/kg intramuscularly once daily for as many as 5 days, ceftiofur can quickly return animals to normal appetite and demeanor with rapid normalization of respiration rates. The clinical success of this compound may reflect not only the increased incidence of resistance of *Pasteurella* to traditional antibiotics, such as ampicillin and oxytetracycline, but also the emerging significance of *Hemophilus somnus* as a major pathogen in calf units.

Ceftiofur is a semisynthetic cephalosporin developed for the treatment of bovine respiratory disease (shipping fever, pneumonia) associated with *Pasteurella haemolytica*, *P. multocida*, and *Hemophilus somnus* in beef and nonlactating dairy cattle. The product has a wide spectrum of activity against gram-negative and gram-positive bacteria and is effective at low levels. Over 90% of 263 isolates of *Pasteurella haemolytica* and *P. multocida* from field trials were sensitive to 0.06 μg/ml or less of ceftiofur. This permits a dose rate of 1 mg ceftiofur/kg body weight.

Trials in the United States have demonstrated its effectiveness in treating shipping fever. In vitro ceftiofur shows significant activity against a broad spectrum of bacteria, including *Hemophilus influenzae* and methicillin-resistant *Staphylococcus aureus*. Furthermore, ceftiofur shows in vitro resistance to many beta-lactamases.

In clinical trials, rectal temperature after ceftiofur injections in cattle declined regularly and returned rapidly to normal. Appetite and attitude also rapidly returned to normal after ceftiofur injections, although respiratory rate remained elevated for a few days, even when the temperature was below 39.5° and when the animals were no longer coughing.

Pasteurella represented the main pathogen in veal calves and in older animals. *Haemophilus somnus* is a respiratory pathogen taking on increasing significance. Clinical signs of *H. somnus* infection are very similar to those of *Pasteurella*. Ceftiofur is exceptionally effective against *Pasteurella* and *Haemophilus* and, when given in accordance with the manufacturer's instructions, effective and rapid clinical resolution can be seen.

30.11 FLUOROQUINOLONES— ENROFLOXACIN

Field results from this new class of antimicrobials show it to be exceptionally useful in treating both gram-positive and gram-negative infections, especially respiratory infections caused by virulent or resistant gram-positive and gram-negative bacteria. Of the various classes of quinolones, the fluorinated products, norfloxacin, ciprofloxacin, and enrofloxacin, have received the most attention in veterinary medicine. They have proved extremely useful in bovine respiratory disease. The quinolones are related to nalidixic acid, but have fewer toxic effects. Adding a fluorine group to quinolones had improved their tissue distribution, as well as their spectrum of activity. In fact, their pharmacokinetic distributional properties render them unique as a group.

Enrofloxacin (Baytril), a chemotherapeutic agent from a group of new quinolone carboxylic acid derivatives, is indicated for respiratory disease therapy in cattle primarily because of the following properties:

1. Its broad antibacterial activity spectrum against gram-negative and gram-positive bacteria, as well as mycoplasmas
2. Its bactericidal and mycoplasmacidal activity at low concentrations, which in most cases are only twice as high as the MICs
3. Its efficacy even against organisms that are resistant or multi-resistant against beta lactam antibiotics, aminoglycosides, tetracyclines, folic acid antagonists, and other antibacterial substances
4. Its absorption after parenteral and oral application with high bioavailability in body fluids and organs (high intracellular levels)
5. Its good tolerance in all species
6. Its unique mechanisms of action (gyrase inhibition)
7. Its large volume of distribution

The in vitro activity of enrofloxacin is particularly pronounced in gram-negative bacteria (e.g., *Escherichia coli, Salmonella, Pasteurella, Hemophilus*) and mycoplasma, but also extends to gram-positive organisms (e.g., *Staphylococcus, C. pyogenes (A. pyogenes) Streptococci, Erysipelothrix*). The substance is rapidly absorbed even after oral administration. High concentrations of active ingredient are quickly achieved in body fluids and organs. Administration of the product via the drinking water presents little problem because it is highly soluble.

The spectrum of activity of the quinolones depends on the individual drug, but includes most gram-positive but especially gram-negative organisms, particularly *Escherichia coli, Salmonella, Klebsiella, Pasteurella, Enterobacter, Proteus, Pseudomonas, Citrobacter*, and *Serratia*. The spectrum of norfloxacin (a human product) is not as great as that of enrofloxacin. Ciprofloxacin has been used in human medicine for organisms resistant to norfloxacin. Most organisms sensitive to ciprofloxacin are also sensitive to enrofloxacin.

Quinolones also effectively treat *Chlamydia* and *Mycoplasma* infections, but are ineffective against most anaerobes.

Quinolones penetrate intracellularly into phagocytic cells, and enrofloxacin reaches a concentration in neutrophils seven times higher than the extracellular concentration, thereby allowing the effective intracellular killing of bacteria.

Being a quinolone carboxylic acid derivative, the antibacterial mode of action of enrofloxacin is fundamentally different from that of other antibiotics/chemotherapeutic drugs, such as beta lactam, aminoglycoside, tetracycline, and macrolide antibiotics, or even sulfonamides and trimethropim. Consequently, pathogens that are resistant to the aforementioned commonly used antibacterial substances are sensitive to enrofloxacin. Compared to other quinolone acid derivatives used in veterinary medicine (flumequine), enrofloxacin is distinguished by considerably lower MIC values (factor 20 to 50) and its efficacy against *Pseudomonas*, streptococci, and mycoplasmas.

Pharmacokinetic properties of enrofloxacin include rapid oral and parenteral absorption, high serum and tissue concentrations above the MIC for most gram-positive and gram-negative organisms, and high intracellular penetration with activity against mycoplasma. One of the outstanding factors of quinolone carboxylic acid derivatives is a unique mechanism of antibacterial action. This special mechanism of action (bacterial gyrase inhibition) rules out cross-resistance with well-established antibacterial agents commonly used in respiratory disease, e.g., beta lactams, tetracyclines, aminocyclitols, macrolides, and folic acid antagonists (sulfonamides). *Pasteurella*, coliforms, salmonellae, and mycoplasmas are sensitive to enrofloxacin. Given at a dose of 2.5 to 5.0 mg/kg once daily for at least 3 days of parenteral (subcutaneous) or oral administration, enrofloxacin can prompt a rapid return to clinical normality in respiratory disease.

The excellent tissue penetration is also evidenced by substantially higher microbiologic activities in the organs than in the serum. Because infections tend to occur primarily in organs and tissues, this fact is a major advantage in the therapeutic use of the product.

Enrofloxacin is absorbed readily and quickly both after oral and after parenteral administration. Maximum concentrations, as a rule, are reached within 0.5 to 2 hours.

When the quinolones are given orally, they usually are absorbed rapidly and almost completely, although food in the digestive tract may delay absorption. Food in the gastrointestinal tract does not significantly alter peak plasma concentrations, but it does delay the time of peak concentration. Delayed absorption does not seem to be clinically significant; thus, administration of quinolones between feedings is probably not necessary. In fact, giving the drug with food may prevent gastrointestinal upset.

The enrofloxacin serum levels after oral administration in calves are equivalent in amount to those after parenteral administration at the same dosage, thereby suggesting a good absorption of the active ingredient in the intestine. Because they can penetrate all body tissues, the quinolones are indicated for infection in any tissue caused by any gram-negative and selected gram-positive bacteria, including mycoplasma. These drugs, however, should be reserved for serious infections or for those that have failed to respond to other antibiotic therapy. Quinolones are especially useful for treating serious antibiotic-resistant bacterial infections of the respiratory tract.

Potential uses for enrofloxacin, on the basis of the microbiologic studies and the results of the clinical tests available thus far, are systemic and local infections with primary or secondary involvement of the following gram-negative and gram-positive bacteria and mycoplasmas: *Escherichia coli, Salmonella, Klebsiella, Proteus, Yersinia, Hemophilus, Pasteurella, Actinobacillus, Pseudomonas, Brucella, Moraxella, Campylobacter, Staphylococcus, Streptococcus* (except enterococci), *Erysipelothrix, Bacteroides,* and *Mycoplasma.*

One of its current major applications outside of salmonellosis in cattle is for the treatment of respiratory disease. Its high solubility, rapidity of absorption regardless of route, high lung to serum concentration (2:1), potential to enter intracellularly, unique mechanisms of action and hence lack of cross-resistance, and finally broad spectrum (*Mycoplasma, Pasteurella, Escherichia coli, Hemophilus, Pseudomonas,* and *Chlamydia*) have rendered it a useful product for therapy of bovine respiratory disease.

In simultaneous experimental infection of calves with *Pasteurella haemolytica* and *Mycoplasma bovis,* the substance proved to be highly effective when administered 3 to 5 times by the oral or parenteral route at dose rates from 2.5 mg/kg body weight.

Danofloxacin is a novel third-generation fluoroquinolone with potent in vitro activity against a broad spectrum of gram-negative and gram-positive bacteria and mycoplasma, including the principal bacterial and mycoplasmal pathogens involved in bovine respiratory disease. A dosage of 1.25 mg/kg (intramuscularly) of danofloxacin is the current accepted maximum dose for pasteurellosis in cattle. Studies of the pharmacokinetic properties of danofloxacin in cattle have shown that, after intramuscular or subcutaneous injection, the mean peak levels of the drug in lung tissue exceed those in the plasma by a factor of 4. This combination of spectrum, potency, and pharmacokinetic properties indicates that danofloxacin should be a useful treatment

for infectious respiratory disease in cattle. Many other pharmaceutical companies are researching and introducing new fluoroquinolone molecules into veterinary medicine for respiratory disease (e.g., ciprofloxacin, norfloxacin).

30.12 TILMICOSIN

Several macrolide derivatives are under development at present. Tilmicosin is one such chemically modified macrolide antibiotic that at doses ranging from 10 to 30 mg/kg displays high activity against 90% of *Pasteurella haemolytica* and *P. multocida* isolates in addition to common bovine *Mycoplasma* isolates.

This new macrolide antibiotic has been prepared by chemical modifications of desmycosin. In vitro against selected animal bacterial pathogens, tilmicosin inhibits growth of *Pasteurella multocida, P. haemolytica, Mycoplasma hyopneumonia, Actinobacillus pleuropneumonia, Streptococcus suis, Corynebacterium pyogenes (A. Pyogenes),* and certain other bacteria.

A formulation has been developed that produces therapeutic levels in the lungs for 3 or 4 days, and a single injection is expected to be sufficient to treat a clinical case.

The pharmacokinetics of the antibiotic as formulated into propylene glycol at a high concentration of 300 mg tilmicosin/ml has allowed prolonged effectiveness from a single subcutaneous injection. Extensive safety studies in laboratory animals and cattle have shown that tilmicosin (Micotil) injection is safe to cattle and does not result in unsafe residues when used as directed on the label.

Remember that tylosin, although an effective macrolide for bovine respiratory diseases, is primarily effective against mycoplasma. Tilmicosin, the new semisynthetic derivative, retains this potent antimicroplasmal activity, but in addition, the efficacy against *Pasteurella* is strengthened. Molecular modification has also resulted in achievement of higher lung concentrations and persistence of antimicrobial activity such that 1 subcutaneous injection provides antibiotic cover for 3 to 4 days.

The antibacterial activity of tilmicosin has led to its development for the treatment of bovine respiratory disease in cattle associated with *P. haemolytica, P. multocida,* and other sensitive organisms. Micotil was initially evaluated for the treatment of bovine respiratory disease in newly weaned, recently shipped feedlot beef calves in Canadian and U.S. studies with favorable results. The tilmicosin formulation used is an aqueous solution containing 300 mg tilmicosin/ml in 25% propylene glycol. The treatment consists of 10 mg tilmicosin/kg as a single injection administered subcutaneously in the neck. The use of a single injection, rather than several daily injections, is based on data that show that one injection of tilmicosin results in long-lived serum and tissue levels.

A single subcutaneous injection of Micotil at 10 mg/kg body weight in cattle results in peak tilmicosin levels within 1 hour and detectable levels (0.07 μg/ml) in serum beyond 3 days. Lung concentrations of tilmicosin in excess of the MIC of 3.12 μg/ml for *P. haemolytica* were observed, however, in 95% of animals for at least 3 days following the single injection.

For calves with enzootic pneumonia, the results of experiments indicate that tilmicosin as a single injection at levels of 10 mg/kg is an effective treatment for the pneumonia that occurs the first 4 weeks of age in calves reared on milk replacer.

The only adverse effect of tilmicosin that may be noted in cattle is transient swelling at the injection site. Hence, not more than 25 ml of this concentrated solution should be injected at any site. Because of its tardy kinetic excretory pattern, this drug is contraindicated for use in lactating animals. A withholding time of at least 28 days is recommended for meat. Unlike other macrolides, tilmicosin is not safe for use in pigs or monkeys. Fatalities in pigs may occur at doses as low as 20 mg/kg and in monkeys at 30 mg/kg. The drug is not intended for human use. The lethal dose for the primate is equivalent to a 6-ml injection in a 60-kg human.

Thus, accidental self-injection with tilmicosin is especially dangerous, and the drug must never be used carelessly by the human operator.

Favorable results with tilmicosin result from early treatment of clinical cases and the prolonged therapeutic levels of the drug in lung tissue. At necropsy, levels of tilmicosin in various experiments have been considerably higher than mean concentration in plasma.

FLORFENICOL

Mention has already been made of the successful preliminary use of florfenicol (FF) at 20 mg/kg intramuscularly for bovine pasteurellosis in cattle. Devoid of the para-nitrogroup, it does not cause irreversible aplastic anemia. Another alternative, thiamphenicol, is also under development.

30.13 INFLAMMATION AND ANTI-INFLAMMATORY DRUGS

Although antibiotics are the primary agents of therapy for bovine pneumonia, many factors other than simple bacterial growth contribute to the pathogenesis of bacterial colonization, proliferation, and tissue damage. The body's responses to the factors that predispose to colonization, and its subsequent responses to the bacterium and its products, play a major role in the degree of pulmonary damage and the eventual outcome. Pharmacologic modification of these responses can alter the severity and outcome of the disease process.

Residual scarring, atelectasis, bronchiectasis abscessation, necrosis and chronic bronchopneumonia are common sequelae. Fatalities are caused by hypoxemia and toxemia.

Calves with mycoplasmal pneumonia secrete a thicker, more acidic mucus, which is harder to remove and results in airway plugging. Airway irritation results in coughing.

The inflammatory process in the bovine lung is a complex response characterized by vasodilation, accumulation of edematous fluid and inflammatory exudate, increased permeability of capillaries, and infiltration with inflammatory cells. Several chemical mediators precipitate these reactions; arachidonic acid is especially important. Following cell injury and the release of arachidonic acid, two enzyme systems, cyclooxygenase (which is blocked by NSAIDs) and lipoxygenase (which is not blocked by normal doses of NSAIDs except ketoprofen), catalyze the conversion of the fatty acid substrate to prostaglandins and leukotrienes, respectively. Prostaglandins evoke effusion of fluid and exudate at the site of inflammation: leukotrienes mobilize leukocytes to the inflammatory focus.

In the bovine lung, however, histamine is not as important as the eicosanoids, such as prostaglandin and leukotriene. When the bovine lung undergoes infection, prostaglandins E, and F, thromboxane, and prostacyclin provokes massive congestion and outpouring of fluid that are potentially lethal to the animal. On the other hand, leukotriene mobilizes the leukocytes, which are an essential antibacterial defense.

Inhibition of prostaglandin synthesis has a secondary effect in that it may stimulate leukotriene production (possible by diversion of substrate). This is true of cyclooxygenase inhibitors such as flunixin.

Corticosteroids exert a more general and nonspecific effect in which both leukotrienes and prostaglandin synthesis are inhibited. Accordingly, although corticosteroids alleviate the pain and swelling of the lesion, they prevent the mobilization of leukocytes and macrophages to combat infection. Although they remove edematory fluid that may be compressing the bronchioles, steroids suppress local defense mechanisms. Thus, corticosteroids may be contraindicated in bovine respiratory disease because they deprive the animal of one of its most important antibacterial defenses. Corticosteroids have other additional adverse actions, including immunosuppression, and this is an immunosuppressive disorder.

In many cases of bovine respiratory disease, particularly those involving individual animals that are most seriously at risk within an affected group, additional, adjunctive therapy is often indicated quite apart from the need for prompt and widespread administration of more specific drugs, such as antimicrobials.

NSAIDs are potent inhibitors of the biological effects of endotoxin, but without the immunosuppressive properties. In addition, they are also potent analgesics and antipyretics. Flunixin meglumine is the drug of choice for endotoxemia in the horse. Kinetic studies in the cow indicate that a loading dose of 2.2 mg/kg followed by maintenance doses of 1.1 mg/kg every 8 hours should provide levels similar to those required for analgesia and prostaglandin inhibition. Aspirin is inexpensive and useful in cattle; the recommended dose is 100 mg/kg orally twice daily. The maintenance dose can be 30 mg/kg. Aspirin is also useful at low doses of 20 mg/kg for disseminated intravascular coagulation. Phenylbutazone can be given intravenously or parenterally at 6 mg/kg for loading, followed by 3 mg/kg daily for maintenance. These agents inhibit the enzyme cyclo-oxygenase, thereby decreasing prostaglandin and leukotriene production.

Following infection and inflammation, prostaglandin release provokes massive congestion and outpouring of fluid. Inhibition of cyclo-oxygenase and therefore local prostaglandin synthesis by NSAIDs is beneficial in drastically reducing the effusion of inflammatory exudate without affecting leukotriene activity. Flunixin meglumine can confer distinct and sometimes dramatic benefits in calves affected with respiratory infection and attendant inflammation. The analgesic and antipyretic effects of NSAIDs confer significant benefit to the affected animal also.

Flunixin also possesses some antiendotoxic activity, a property that may confer additional benefits in the treatment of pasteurellosis and mycoplasmosis (both toxin producers). For use in bovine acute respiratory conditions, flunixin meglumine is administered at a dose of 2.2 mg/kg intravenously and is repeated as necessary at 24-hour intervals for as many as 5 consecutive days. At this dosage rate, flunixin is effective in relieving coughing and dyspnea and in reducing areas of consolidation in the lungs. Ketoprofen is a newer and possibly more versatile NSAID.

In contrast to corticosteroids, the NSAIDs, such as flunixin, ketoprofen aspirin, phenylbutazone display no evidence of the rebound phenomenon or relapse of the condition.

Used with oxytetracycline, flunixin provides a useful first-line defense therapeutic strategy. In many cases of P13 virus and *P. haemolytica* infection, flunixin apparently does not reduce the capacity to produce certain types of circulatory antibody to these pathogens.

In contrast, the use of corticosteroids in acute pneumonias often exacerbates the condition of individual calves and increases the morbidity and mortality rates. The use of corticosteroid drugs is commonly associated with clinical deterioration and higher mortality than in cattle treated with antibiotics alone. Furthermore, in other situations, such as in acute bovine pulmonary emphysema, for which the administration of anti-inflammatory compounds per se would seem to be the current treatment of choice, the use of corticosteroids is often followed by abortion.

Corticosteroids, by acting higher up on the arachidonicacid pathway than do NSAIDs, block the synthesis of more putative inflammatory mediators, i.e., leukotrienes and prostaglandins. Thus, steroids can minimize the pain and swelling of inflammatory reactions, but they also prevent mobilization of leukocytes and macrophages (IE pulmonary macrophages) to combat infection by virtue of their leukotriene blockade. This blockade deprives the animal of its primary antibacterial defenses and can lead to worsening of the infectious process. In addition, the immunosuppressant effect is definitely an unwanted side effect.

Steroids are only occasionally indicated in severe cases when excessive inflammatory exudate blocks or compresses alveoli or shrinks airway patency. Massive exudate resulting from pulmonary inflammation blocks alveoli or shrinks airway patency, thereby nullifying the effects of bronchodilators. Steroids, however, should be regarded only as potential lifesaving drugs in extreme cases, and not as part of routine therapy. Sometimes the central nervous system effects of steroids are beneficial in the anorectic animal.

The hazards of steroid therapy include a tendency to a slower recovery rate and to relapses. As a rule, they are contraindicated because their immunosuppressant effects compound the problem; recovery from this primary viral condition largely depends on cell-mediated immunity.

Several steroids can abolish bronchospasm induced by prostaglandin release in the respiratory tract. Prednisolone sodium succinate is one such steroid, although its protective effect on the bronchi is not as potent as that of beta$_2$-agonists, such as clenbuterol. Corticosteroids may potentiate beta$_2$-receptor activity within the bronchiolar system.

If steroids are used, the short-acting, soluble, rapidly excreted steroids are preferable to the long-acting depot types, which have too many unwanted side effects. Intravenous dexamethasone or betamethasone, 20 mg, can be used in emergency situations. The injudicious use of corticosteroids may also contribute to the development of chronic pneumonia because the powerful analgesic and antipyretic properties of these drugs could improve the general demeanor of the animal even though the concurrent antimicrobial therapy has not had an effect on the causal bacteria. Corticosteroids and NSAIDs must only be administered when the fever falls as a result of antimicrobial therapy.

Flunixin meglumine is a prostaglandin inhibitor with anti-inflammatory, analgesic, and antipyretic activities. Use of this therapeutic agent may result in a reduction in bronchiolar mucosal swelling that leads to a reduction of small airway obstruction. Many NSAIDs exist, but all possess some disadvantages. Three drugs have been studied for use in cattle.

1. Salicylates, such as aspirin, help to reduce fever and inflammation, but have low potency and a relatively short half-life. High doses must be used.
2. Phenylbutazone, in contrast, has a long half-life (for cattle, 36 to 72 hours, depending on dose), but its action may be cumulative and toxic, thereby leading to a leukocytopenia.
3. Flunixin meglumine has a half-life in calves of 8 to 10 hours and is probably the most useful of all the NSAIDs. On the basis of several different approaches to evaluating the effects of therapy on pulmonary disorders (i.e., lung weights, consolidation scores, histopathology), ample evidence shows that clinical benefits are a direct result of the known ability of flunixin meglumine to limit the inflammatory response. The same compound, however, also has antiendotoxic activity, a property that may confer additional benefits, particularly in the pasteurellosis case.

Pharmacologic agents are available to combat the endotoxin of *P. haemolytica* or, more specifically, the body's reaction to it. Corticosteroids have been recommended in the past in severe cases and have been commonly used in practice. Their utility in helping to reverse endotoxic shock is generally accepted. Limited dosage may not affect immunity, and the beneficial effects in decreasing inflammation, edema, and bronchospasm and in improving attitude and appetite may hasten recovery. The use of dexamethasone, however, can be associated with a poorer response to initial therapy, a higher relapse rate, greater losses from death. Remember that steroids are immunosuppressant, and animals affected with bovine respiratory disease have a compromised immune system. Although effective anti-inflammatory therapy is needed in bovine pneumonias, the use of corticosteroids is of dubious worth save in exceptional circumstances and is frankly dangerous in others.

Overall, several anti-inflammatory agents can be considered for bovine respiratory disease, including betamethasone (20 mg), acetylsalicylic acid (100 mg/kg orally twice daily), sodium meclofenamate (20 mg/kg), or phenylbutazone/isopyrin (15 ml of solution containing 240 mg phenylbutazone and 130 mg isopyrin intramuscularly or intravenously).

Flunixin meglumine, 1.1–2.2 mg/kg, has beneficial effects in many cases (including 2 Methyl Indole intoxication) by virtue of its antiprostaglandin and anti-inflammatory activity.

Its antiendotoxic activity is significant, especially when *Pasteurella* or mycoplasmas are present.

DMSO is another compound with useful diverse anti-inflammatory properties. Its main beneficial effect is its ability to scavenge oxygen free radicals and therefore is attractive as a possible means of preventing neutrophil-mediated tissue damage in pasteurellosis. DMSO also has some analgesic effects. It reduces platelet aggregation and coagulation and improves tissue perfusion. DMSO has been used for pneumonia in the horses and cattle. Although the dosage is not well established. Doses of 1 gm/kg given as a 10% solution in 5% dextrose have

been used for cerebral edema. (DMSO possesses some antibacterial activity which may be of minor significance).

30.14 IMMUNOMODULATORS

Immunomodulators are compounds that enhance the function of the immune system. The three basic types of immunomodulators are synthetic, microbial and physiologic. *Synthetic* immunomodulators include, isoprinosine, levamisole adenine arabinoside, purine and pyrimidine sub units. *Microbial* agents include cyclosporin A, muramyl dipeptide. Inactivated poxvirus, C. parvum (propionibacterium lactum) *Physiological* types include, thymic factors, opioid peptides, interferons interleukins lactoferrin. The exogenous immunomodulators include bacteria or bacterial-derived products (e.g., bacille Calmette Guérin (BCG), endotoxin, *Propionibacterium acnes*) and synthetic chemicals (e.g., levamisole and lipoidal amines). One mechanism of action of the exogenous immunomodulators is to induce the release of endogenous immunomodulators. The endogenous immunomodulators include proteins that are produced and secreted by cells (cytokines). Some examples of their proteins include interferons, interleukins, tumor necrosis factor, and colony-stimulating factors. Genetic engineering techniques offer the potential to produce these compounds inexpensively.

Effective immunomodulating compounds that would overcome the immunosuppression associated with bovine respiratory disease should significantly reduce the economic loss associated with the disease. The bacterial agents that cause the severe economic losses associated with bovine respiratory disease (*Pasteurella haemolytica*, *P. multocida*, and *Hemophilus somnus*) also actively interfere with selected aspects of neutrophil function.

Glucocorticoids and several respiratory viruses, (infectious bovine rhinotracheitis, BVD, P13) each induce negative defects in molecular defensive function. Interferon is a critically important endogenous immunomodulator.

An experimental compound avridine induces interferon production and possibly also the synthesis of other protective response modifiers. Neutrophil function and lymphocytic secretion of lymphokines has been shown to be augmented by avridine. The induction of synthesis of gamma interferon underpins the biological activity of many immunomodulators, and the administration of recombinant bovine gamma interferon should have in vivo biological activity similar to that of avridine and other exogenous immunomodulators.

30.15 MUCOLYTIC THERAPY

Mucus is normally secreted in the respiratory tract in small amounts and acts to trap and transport microorganisms, irritants, dust, and cell debris from the lungs. A functional mucociliary system is essential for normal respiratory action.

The secretions consist primarily of mucopolysaccharide fibers, but in the presence of infection, these break down and are replaced by acidic mucopolysaccharides and DNA, which, as a result of cell destruction, is present in purulent secretions. DNA increases the viscosity of the secretion and also inhibits lysis of the tenacious secretions by proteases.

Under ordinary circumstances, mucoussecreting cells are not in small bronchioles, but during chronic inflammation, goblet cell metaplasia occurs and glycoprotein secretion can occur at the terminal bronchioles. Respiratory glycoproteins resemble a bottlebrush in their structure. They have a straight peptide backbone, with bristlelike oligosaccharide side chains radiating from the peptide. The oligosaccharides are attached to the peptide through o-glycosidic linkages between N-acetyl-galactosamine of the saccharides and threonine and serine of the peptide. The physical size of the molecule is determined by the saccharide side chains.

The viscosity and elasticity of tracheobronchial mucus are primarily the result of polymerization and aggregation of glycoproteins. Polymerization takes place through the formation of disulfide bonds involving cysteine, an amino acid found abundantly in respiratory glycoproteins. Aggregation of mucous glycoproteins by ions and sugar-sugar interactions forms a gel matrix. The ability to polymerize and aggregate depends on glycoprotein concentration (which increases in dehydration), increased salt concentration, and decreased pH.

Mucolytics, such as Bromhexine, N-acetylcysteine, and s-carboxymethylcysteine effectively depolymerize mucus and also act on DNA, the component of pus that is responsible for its viscosity. These substances act through free sulfhydryl groups that effectively open the disunited bonds of mucous glycoproteins.

The excessive production of viscous purulent secretion in infection can often overcome the system of expectoration, thus obstructing the airways and impairing gaseous exchange. Mucolytics render the sputum less viscous and more easily cleared. Bronchial secretions of less viscosity are produced, thereby assisting expectoration. Ciliary activity is augmented, and the respiratory mucous membrane increases in permeability.

BROMHEXINE

Bromhexine is a useful mucolytic agent that improves gaseous exchange in the animal suffering from impaired respiratory function by reducing airway congestion and the accumulation of tenacious mucus. Because bromhexine alters the permeability of the respiratory mucous membranes and the local capillary supply, bromhexine increases the local concentration of oxytetracycline, sulfonamides, erythromycin, spiramycin, and rifampin in respiratory secretion.

Bromhexine is an established mucolytic compound that exhibits high selectivity for the respiratory tract. It has been used in human medicine since the 1960s, and its main activities have been thoroughly documented in humans and animals. These activities consist of a stimulating effect on the bronchial secretion and a modification of the amount and quality of the secretions. Viscosity of bronchial mucus is lessened and expectoration is assisted and rendered more productive; hence, gaseous exchange is facilitated. When given simultaneously with an antibiotic/antimicrobial compound, bromhexine facilitates penetration of the antibiotic into the bronchial tree. This role is of paramount clinical importance because many antimicrobial compounds have difficulty attaining useful concentrations in excess of the MIC in the respiratory system. Even when serum concentrations are high, lung concentrations for many antibiotics can be low. Thus, clinical failure, long-term therapy, relapses, or repeat treatments are common.

Bromhexine is a synthetic derivative of the active ingredient vasicin found in plants. Early workers believed that the plant extract was a bronchodilator because of its potent respiratory action. Molecular modification of the natural compound, however, has resulted in the synthesis of a potent mucolytic and secretory drug.

In laboratory studies and multiple assessments of animals, and also in trials in humans and target animals, several useful properties have been clearly attributed to bromhexine:

1. Increase in volume of respiratory secretion
2. Reduction in secretion viscosity
3. Breakdown of the acidic mucopolysaccharide matrix of sputum
4. Enhancement of the mucociliary function and the transport of secretions
5. Stimulation of the pulmonary surfactant system
6. Increase in the relative concentrations of antibiotics/antimicrobials in bronchial secretion and lung tissue

Interestingly, the concentration of immunoglobulins, especially of the IgA and IgG fractions, is increased in bronchial secretions following bromhexine administration.

Bronchial secretions in patients with respiratory disease contain fiber systems of mucoproteins and mucopolysaccharides. Bromhexine alters the structure of the mucin net of sputum by a process of rarefaction and fragmentation. This process leads to a reduction in the viscosity of sputum. The effect is brought about by an inhibition of the cross-linking of acidic mucopolysaccharides. A direct action on the secretory cells of the respiratory epithelium enhances the volume of secretions then produced. Bromhexine also improves mucociliary function.

An important prerequisite for pathogenicity of bacteria in the respiratory tract is their deposition and residency on the surface epithelium. The coating of the respiratory epithelium with surfactant is an important factor in the local defense against infection of the airways. Bromhexine displays an inhibitory action on the process of pathogen adhesion. In addition, bromhexine stimulates the endogenous formation of surfactant and its release from the bronchiolar and alveolar region.

The local defense mechanisms against infectious organisms are strengthened by this stimulation of surfactant formation. An antiadhesive effect has also been described for bromhexine. This property inhibits pathogen adhesion to the respiratory mucous membrane.

Bromhexine increases the metabolism of mucous-producing cells as indicated by an increase in the alkaline phosphatase activity. This increased metabolism is accompanied by increases in acid phosphatase, alkaline phosphatase, nonspecific esterase, galactosidase, glucosamidase, and glucuronidase activities in goblet cells and in tracheal submucosal glands of bromhexine-treated animals.

Some antimicrobial action has been attributed to bromhexine also. Copious evidence shows that the use of bromhexine is accompanied by relatively higher concentrations of antibiotics/antimicrobials in the secretions of the respiratory tract. This increase expedites the efficacy of the antibiotic against the offending microorganisms.

The mucolytic action relieves respiratory distress, increases airway patency, relieves coughing, and facilitates greater clearance of respiratory debris and entrapped microorganisms.

A mucolytic such as bromhexine improves and augments the flow and transport of bronchial secretions. Following administration of bromhexine the fibrous matrix of acidic mucopolysaccharide in sputum becomes fragmented and its viscosity decreases. (Antibiotics alone possess no activity in sputum flow).

In addition, the mucolytic agent allows a better and more regular penetration of antibiotics/antimicrobials into the bronchial mucus. This characteristic is of critical significance. Local concentrations of antibiotic are higher than would be achieved without the mucolytic agent.

These high and sustained antibiotic concentrations in bronchial mucus and lung tissue quicken the onset of clinical recovery because of the rapid onset of antibiotic action and the maintenance of concentrations in mucus in excess of the MIC. The mucolytic effects are responsible for the more effective elimination of less viscid mucus and entrapped organisms by the processes of expectoration. Favorable results are obtained with a mucolytic-antimicrobial combination in even the most acute clinical syndromes for these reasons.

30.16 BRONCHODILATORS

A significant contribution to the dyspnea of bovine respiratory disease is produced by bronchiolar constriction, and in many cases, with increased mucous secretion and decreased mucociliary clearance, by occlusion of respiratory airways.

The respiratory tract is covered with cilia from the nasal passageways to the smallest conducting bronchioles. The action of the cilia is necessary for moving this mucus to the pharynx from which it may be coughed out or swallowed. Ciliary activity, in addition to the viscosity and elasticity of the mucus, determines the relative mucociliary clearance.

Stimulation of ciliary activation by adrenergic beta$_2$-agonists involves the activation of adenylate cyclase in the intracellular production of adenosine 3':5'-cyclic phosphate (cAMP). Drugs, such as prostaglandins and methylxanthines, increase cAMP in ciliated respiratory epithelial cells.

Beta$_2$-adrenergic agonists carry out their action through the direct generation of cytoplasmic cAMP via membrane-bound receptors, and adenylate cyclase. The usefulness of aminophylline and theophylline as bronchodilators results from their ability to inhibit phosphodiesterase, the enzyme that inactivates cAMP. These agents therefore produce a beta-adrenergic effect through secondary indirect means. Beta blockers, therefore, do not neutralize xanthines.

Selective adrenergic beta$_2$-agonists include isoproterenol, albuterol (also called salbutamol), terbutaline, and clenbuterol. Clenbuterol is a potent bronchodilator that can be used to provide prompt relief when bronchospasm and constricted airways impair gaseous exchange. Clenbuterol is a selective beta$_2$-agonist that causes increased patency of the bronchiolar tree via activation of adrenergic receptors. Experimentally it can reduce acetylcholine-induced dyspnea in calves. Clenbuterol possesses a relatively short half-life and must be given repeatedly. At high dosage levels, it can affect the beta$_1$-receptors of the heart and blood vessels. On account of it's abuse as a repartitioning agent in food animals, clenbuterol is now prohibited as a bronchodilator in cattle in many countries, on account of its residue hazards.

30.17 FLUID/ACID BASE BALANCE AND OXYGEN THERAPY

Fluid therapy for respiratory disease is extremely important but often overlooked. Rehydration improves clearance mechanisms, and volume expansion remains the foremost therapy for the toxemia and endotoxic shock associated with pasteurellosis. Therapy with lactated fluids should be vigorous, but animals should be monitored carefully for signs of overhydration and pulmonary edema in the case of hypoalbuminemia and pulmonary inflammation. Fluids also have ancillary mucolytic properties. The use of hypertonic fluids display expectorant effects.

The development of intravascular and extravascular coagulation, pulmonary edema, and obstruction of airways through accumulation of mucus produces serious deficiencies in the respiratory function of the lung. Low-dose aspirin (30 mg/kg) can be beneficially used to prevent disseminated intravascular coagulation. Heparin (40 i.u.) is commonly used for this in other species. Hypoxemia and hypercapnia result from this defect. Hypercapnia produces a respiratory acidosis and serves as a stimulus for increased respiratory rate and effort. Hypoxia results in an increased dependence of tissues on anaerobic metabolism and in the production of increasing amounts of lactic acid, thereby resulting in a metabolic acidosis.

When animals with respiratory disease are dehydrated, rehydration fluids must be administered. Respiratory acidosis is the underlying disorder. The degree of dehydration is estimated as mild (8% body weight loss), moderate (10% body weight loss), or severe (12% body weight loss). Alkalinizing fluids should preferably be given, i.e., those containing lactate or bicarbonate. To determine the quantity of fluid that is needed to restore body fluid volumes to normal, the dehydrated body weight must be known (or at least be accurately estimated).

When severe interstitial edema persists, the animal may benefit from a diuretic, such as furosemide. Care must be taken to prevent dehydration. Severe gaseous diffusion impairment can be at least partially overcome by oxygen therapy. Oxygen should be humidified and should best be used in concentration of 60–50% or less. The addition of 5% CO_2 stimulates deeper respiration and the production of thinner mucus. Although oxygen may be difficult to administer to a cow, the use of anti-inflammatory drugs as previously described may also help to reduce the interstitial inflammation and hence improve respiratory compliance and gas exchange.

PULMONARY EDEMA

Some element of pulmonary edema is involved in nearly all cases of bovine respiratory disease. This edema can compromise bronchiolar function. Decreased airway resistance, and thus more effective ventilation of functional alveoli, can be achieved through the use of bronchodilators (H_1-receptor blocking antihistaminics, beta-adrenergic drugs, glucocorticoids, and aminophylline). The use of diuretics, such as furosemide, to enhance edema fluid loss is sometimes effective.

Oxygen may be administered to treat bovine respiratory disease in particularly valuable individuals or in newborn animals when economically feasible. Oxygen is administered at a concentration of about 40–50%. This concentration is not high enough to damage respiratory tract cells, but does elevate alveolar oxygen concentrations to provide increased oxygen diffusion when the diffusion barrier is thickened by interstitial edema.

30.18 PASTEURELLOSIS—SHIPPING FEVER

Shipping fever is an acute respiratory infection of feedlot cattle that causes severe losses to the beef industry. It is caused by a complex interaction of stress, compromised host defenses, viruses, bacteria, and mycoplasma. *Pasteurella*, alone or with viruses, and/or mycoplasma are the most common microorganisms isolated in cases of shipping fever and apparently play a major role in the onset of clinical signs and lung damage. *P. haemolytica* serotype 1 is the organism most commonly implicated, and the stress of transportation is believed to cause a breakdown of host defense mechanisms resulting in rapid proliferation of *P. haemolytica*. Many viral agents (infectious bovine rhinotracheitis, P13 virus, BRSV, BVD, rhinovirus, enterovirus, bovine herpes type 4) and secondary invaders (salmonellae, streptococci, *Escherichia coli*, staphylococci, *Listeria*, *Neisseria*, *Corynebacterium pyogenes*, chlamydia, *Mycoplasma bovis*) are frequently involved, but *Hemophilus somnus* seems to be of particular significance.

Pasteurella are usually sensitive to penicillin, ampicillin, oxytetracycline, and sulfonamides at the usual recommended dosages. These antimicrobial agents usually give satisfactory clinical response if used early in the clinical course and if continued long enough. *Pasteurella* organisms are often more sensitive to some antibiotics than to others and also may develop relative or absolute resistance to some antibiotics. Therefore, lack of clinical response to any one of these antimicrobial agents dictates a change to one of the others or an increase in dosage levels. Culture and antibiotic sensitivity determination are also indicated in nonresponsive cases. Erythromycin and tylosin at large dosages also may be effective in some cases.

Oxytetracycline, sulfamethathine, sulfadimethoxine, or penicillin/streptomycin have proved to be useful antibacterials for shipping fever. Intravenous gentamicin and flunixin meglumine followed by intramuscular gentamicin and/or ampicillin is a useful regimen in younger animals. Long-acting oxytetracycline with oral administration of sustained-release sulfonamide boluses (Albon, Calfspan) is a traditional and effective treatment program for many cases of shipping fever.

ANTIMICROBIAL PROPHYLAXIS

Prophylactic use of antimicrobial drugs when calves are brought into lots is a contentious subject. Although prophylactic use of oxytetracycline, sulfonamides, tylosin tartrate, erythromycin, ceftiofur, and enrofloxacin can reduce the incidence and prevalence of respiratory infection when given at the time of maximum stress, such indiscriminate use could lead to resistance problems, as well as possibly contribute to buildup of drug residue burdens. Unless the veterinarian firmly believes that prophylactic therapy is rationally indicated, the practice should be discouraged.

30.19 ACUTE BOVINE PULMONARY EDEMA AND EMPHYSEMA

Acute bovine pulmonary edema and emphysema (fog fever) occurs naturally in many parts of the world. It causes morbidity and mortality in grazing cattle, usually after an abrupt pasture change. The syndrome arises from ruminal fermentation of tryptophane lush forage to 3-methylindole by a lactobacillus species of bacteria. The 3-methylindole produced is absorbed from the rumen, enters the systemic circulation, and causes acute lung damage to nonciliated bronchial epithelial cells and to alveolar cells. The extent of lung injury depends on metabolism of 3-methylindole by mixed-function oxidazes in the lung to a reactive intermediate that covalently binds to lung cell macromolecules. Covalent binding and toxicity are reduced by glutathione and cysteine, thus suggesting that conjugation of the reactive intermediate decreases toxicity. Pretreatment with endotoxin can protect against 3-methylindole toxicity by decreasing activation by the mixed-function oxidase system. Etiologic agents of acute atypical interstitial pneumonia of immature cattle include toxic dietary factors, hypersensitivities to fungal agents, autoimmune reactions in lungs already damaged by infectious pneumopathies, or hypersensitivity to microorganisms already settled in the lung. BRSV infection can predispose the lungs of calves to the actions of endogenous pneumotoxins. Viral antigens, such as infectious bovine rhinotracheitis, BVD, and P13 virus, and also *Mycoplasma bovis* have been implicated in the development of the syndrome. The overall lung insult ends with altered pulmonary capillary permeability, pulmonary edema, and hypoxemia. Lesions are of diffuse alveolar damage to the lobes of the lung accompanied by interstitial edema and emphysema. Treatment of this condition, when necessary, is aimed at reducing the infiltration of fluids into the alveoli and interstitial tissues of the lung. This approach can involve the use of anti-inflammatory agents, antihistamines, diuretics, and supportive therapy.

SELECTED REFERENCES

Ames, T.R., and Patterson, E.B.: Oxytetracycline concentrations in plasma and lung of healthy and pneumonic calves using two tetracycline preparations. Am. J. Vet. Res., 46:2471, 1985.

Ames, T.R., Casagranda, C.L., and Werdin, R.E.: (1987) Effect of sulfadimethoxine or metoprim in the treatment of calves with induced *Pasteurella* pneumonia. Am. J. Vet. Res., 48:17, 1987.

Ames, T.R., Larson, V.L., and Stowe, C.M.: Oxytetracycline levels in healthy and diseased calves. Bovine Proc., 15:136, 1983.

Anderson, D.B., and Young, W.B.: The treatment of pneumonia in housed calves, a field study using finacycline. In Proc. 14th World Congress Diseases of Cattle, Dublin, 1986.

Bach, P., and Leary, W.P.: The effects of bromhexine on oxytetracycline penetrance into sputum. S. Afr. Med. J., 46:1512, 1972.

Beech, J.: Therapeutic strategies involving antimicrobial treatment of the lower respiratory tract in large animals. J. Am. Vet. Med. Assoc., 185:10, 1984.

Bentley, O.E., and Cummins, J.M.: Efficacy of sulbactam a B-lactamase inhibitor combined with ampicillin in the therapy of ampicillin resistant pneumonia pasteurellosis in feedlot calves. Can. Vet. J., 28:591, 1987.

Breazile, J.E.: (1989) Ancillary (nonantimicrobial) therapy in the treatment of bovine respiratory disease. Bovine Proc., 21:148, 1989.

Breider, M.A., Walker, R.D., and Hopkins, F.M.: Pulmonary lesions induced by *Pasteurella haemolytica* in neutrophil sufficient and neutrophil deficient calves. Can. J. Vet. Res., 52:205, 1988.

Burrows, G.E., and Ewing, P.: In vitro assessment of the efficacy of erythromycin in combination with oxytetracycline or spectinomycin against *Pasteurella haemolytica*. J. Vet. Diagn. Invest., *1*:299, 1989.

Burrows, G.E., Barto, P.B., and Martin, B.: Antibiotic disposition in experimental pneumonic pasteurellosis: gentamicin and tylosin. Can. J. Vet. Res., *50*:193, 1986.

Clarke, C.R., Short, C.R., Corstvet, R.E., et al.: Interaction between *Pasteurella haemolytica* sulfadiazine/trimethoprim and bovine diarrhoea virus. Am. J. Vet. Res., *50*:1557, 1984.

Davies, C.P., and Webster, A.J.F.: The effects of a beta$_2$ agonist (clenbuterol) and antibacterial drugs (trimethoprim with sulfadiazine; oxytetracycline) on calf mucociliary clearance. J. Vet. Pharmacol. Ther., *12(2)*:217, 1989.

Farrington, D.O., Jackson, J.A., Bentley, O.E., et al.: Efficacy of sulbactam ampicillin in an induced *P. haemolytica* model in calves. Am. J. Vet. Res., *48*:1684, 1987.

Giles, C.J., Grimshaw, W.J., Shanks, D.J., and Smith, D.G.: Efficacy of danofloxacin in the therapy of acute bacterial pneumonia in housed beef cattle. Vet. Rec., *128*:296, 1991.

Gourlay, R.N., Thomas, L.H., and Wyld, S.G.: Effect of a new macrolide antibiotic tilmicosin on pneumonia experimentally induced in calves by *Mycoplasma bovis* and *Pasteurella haemolytica*. Res. Vet. Sci., *47*:84, 1989.

Henry, C.W.: Shipping fever pneumonia: a new look at an old enemy. Vet. Med., Sept. 1984.

Hjerpe, C.A.: Systemic antimicrobial therapy in beef cattle: Pharmacologic and therapeutic considerations. Bovine Proc., *15*:92, 1983.

Hjerpe, C.A.: The role of mycoplasma in bovine respiratory disease. Vet. Med. Sci. Animal Clin., Feb. 1980.

Jenkins, W.L.: Clinical pharmacology of antibacterials used in bacterial bronchopneumonia in cattle Mod. Vet. Pract., *66(5)*:327, 1985.

Kern, O.V., and Wilhelm, F.: Influence of bromhexine on blood levels of antibiotics in pigs. Abstr. 4th Assoc. Cong. Vet. Pharmacol. Toxicol., Budapest, 1988.

Larson, J.L.: Antibacterial therapy for pulmonary infections. J. Am. Vet. Med. Assoc., *176*:1091, 1980.

Lekeux, P., and Art, T.: Effect of ofloxicins therapy on shipping fever pneumonia in feedlot cattle. Vet. Rec., *123*:205, 1988.

Mechor, G.D., Jim, G.K., and Janzen, E.D.: Comparison of penicillin, oxytetracycline and trimethoprin-sulfadoxine in the treatment of acute undifferentiated bovine respiratory disease. Can. Vet. J., *29*:439, 1988.

Morter, R.L.: Antibiotic resistance of *Pasteurella hemolytica* in cattle. Mod. Vet. Pract., *64(2)*:165, 1983.

Ose, E.E., and Tonkinson, L.V.: Single dose treatment of neonatal calf pneumonia with the new macrobile tilmicosin. Vet. Rec., *123*:367, 1988.

Roth, J.A.: Immunomodulation in bovine respiratory disease. Bovine Proc., *22*:150, 1990.

Selman, I.E., Allan, E.M., and Dalgleish, R.C.: The effects of flunixin meglumine and oxytetracycline therapy alone and in combination in calves with experimentally induced pneumonia pasteurellosis. *In* Proc. 14th World Congress Diseases of Cattle. Dublin, 1982.

Selman, I.E., Allan, E.M., and Givvs, H.A.: The effect of antiprostaglandin therapy in experimental P13 pneumonia in weaned conventional calves. Proc. 13th Congress Diseases Cattle, *1*:87, 1984.

Shoo, M.K.: The treatment and prevention of bovine pneumonia pasteurellosis using antimicrobial drugs. Vet. Res. Commun., *14(5)*:341, 1990.

Steffan, J., Amedeo, J., Pergent, P., and Chaillau, J.F.: Treatment of respiratory disease in veal calves with a new cephalosporin ceftiofur. Proc. 1st Congress Diseases of Cattle, 1988.

Section C

SMALL ANIMAL

CARDIAC DISEASE

31.1 Congestive Heart Failure
31.2 Traditional Therapy
31.3 Cardiac Glycosides
31.4 Diuretics
31.5 Methylxanthines
31.6 Miscellaneous Measures
31.7 Alternative Therapeutic Approaches
31.8 Vasodilators
31.9 Therapy of Cardiac Arrhythmias
31.10 Receptor-Selective Antiarrhythmic Drugs
31.11 Classification of Antiarrhythmic Drugs

31.1 CONGESTIVE HEART FAILURE

A significant cause of heart failure in dogs is congestive heart disease attributable to valvular disorders (Table 31–1). The most frequently diagnosed form of valvular insufficiency results from chronic fibrosis of the mitral valve. Other less frequent forms of valvular insufficiency include cardiomyopathies and ventricular dilatation that causes distention of the valvular ring in certain congenital cardiac defects. Valvular degeneration and incompetence lead to chronic valvular regurgitation. Most of the resultant clinical signs are attributable to this regurgitant flow of blood. Cardiac failure may be left or right sided and may be revealed as acute or chronic syndromes. Several clinical signs may be described depending on the side of the heart primarily affected (Table 31–2). Chronic mitral valvular fibrosis is a disease of mature or aged dogs, and although signs of left heart failure occur initially, at a later stage these signs may be associated with signs of right heart failure.

Left-sided cardiac failure is caused by:

1. Mitral incompetence
2. Congenital aortic stenosis
3. Mitral dysplasia
4. Myocardial failure
5. Obstruction to aortic outflow

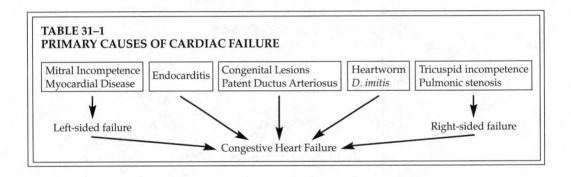

TABLE 31–1
PRIMARY CAUSES OF CARDIAC FAILURE

| Mitral Incompetence / Myocardial Disease | Endocarditis | Congenital Lesions / Patent Ductus Arteriosus | Heartworm / *D. imitis* | Tricuspid incompetence / Pulmonic stenosis |

Left-sided failure   Congestive Heart Failure   Right-sided failure

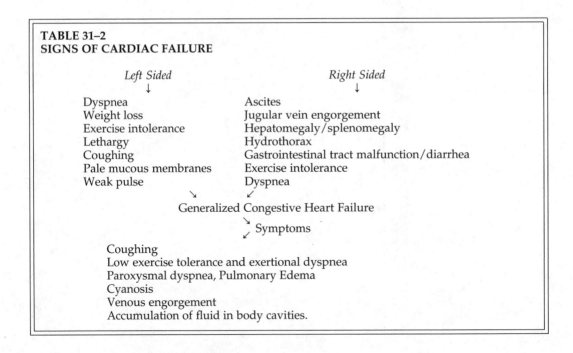

TABLE 31–2
SIGNS OF CARDIAC FAILURE

Left Sided	*Right Sided*
Dyspnea	Ascites
Weight loss	Jugular vein engorgement
Exercise intolerance	Hepatomegaly/splenomegaly
Lethargy	Hydrothorax
Coughing	Gastrointestinal tract malfunction/diarrhea
Pale mucous membranes	Exercise intolerance
Weak pulse	Dyspnea

Generalized Congestive Heart Failure

Symptoms

Coughing
Low exercise tolerance and exertional dyspnea
Paroxysmal dyspnea, Pulmonary Edema
Cyanosis
Venous engorgement
Accumulation of fluid in body cavities.

Causes of right-sided failure are:

1. Myocardial failure
2. Neoplasia
3. Heartworm infection (*Dirofilaria immitis*)
4. Cor pulmonale
5. Tricuspid incompetence

Clinical syndromes arising from cardiac failure are principally recognizable as congestive heart failure.

In general, the clinical pattern of congestive heart disease can be divided into four distinct phases.

1. Phase of compensation, when the only apparent sign is a systolic murmur.
2. Phase of early decompensation confined to the left side of the heart. Apart from the systolic murmur, a cough is present, and some respiratory embarrassment occurs after exercise or excitement.
3. Phase of left heart failure with strain on the right ventricle. Congestion of the lungs occurs after exercise and when the animal lies down or sleeps.
4. Phase of generalized congestive heart failure. Overt failure of the right and left side of the heart develops. Pulmonary edema is particularly distressing to the animal. Signs of right heart failure, ascites, pleural effusion, and enlargement of the liver become apparent. Exercise tolerance is poor. The dog becomes distressed with minimal amounts of exercise and is eventually distressed while resting. An attack of pulmonary edema frequently proves fatal.

Cardiac failure is a gradual process accompanied by activation by many of the compensatory mechanisms of the body. Few disorders are reversible, and thus, long-term medical therapy is indicated. When heart failure occurs, compensatory mechanisms include:

1. An increase in heart rate (tachycardia), during which the rapidly beating heart expels a diminished volume of blood (stroke volume) because of the shortened ventricular filling time
2. Increased myocardial contractibility leading ultimately to hypertrophy
3. Peripheral vasoconstriction to maintain circulatory blood pressure

4. Activation of the renin-angiotensin mechanism, which causes retention of water and sodium, thereby elevating the circulatory volume

The clinical signs of failure may be attributable either to the functional failure of the heart (ascites, dyspnea, coughing, cyanosis) or to the overprotective compensatory reflexes (tachycardia, cardiac enlargement).

Left-sided failure can be a consequence of mitral incompetence, myocardial disease, or congenital disorders. Mitral incompetence is associated with pulmonary congestion, chronic coughing, and exercise intolerance.

Prominent signs of right-sided failure include enlargement of the abdomen (due to hepatomegaly and splenomegaly) and dyspnea caused by hydrothorax. Right atrioventricular tricuspid incompetence, general myocardial disease, or pericardial effusions can be predisposing factors. Chronic bronchitis (cor pulmonale) may arise secondarily in response to right-sided failure.

Once progressive diminution of cardiac output becomes established, homeostatic compensatory mechanisms are activated in an attempt to maintain the integrity of the circulation and blood pressure. Thus, tachycardia, peripheral vasoconstriction, increased myocardial contractibility, and activation of the renin-angiotensin mechanism follow. Such compensatory attempts are not beneficial.

Tachycardia leads to reduced diastole and reduced ventricular filling. Vasoconstriction causes increased peripheral resistance. This increased "afterload" raises the backflow aortic pressure, thus worsening the degree of regurgitation across the incompetent valves. Increased oxygen demands are placed on the failing heart, which is already subjected to insufficient coronary blood supply. Because of the increased afterload, the valvular regurgitation, and the vasoconstriction, tissue perfusion decreases, thereby reducing renal function. Fluid accumulation in the tissues further exacerbates the peripheral resistance. In cases of left heart failure, mitral regurgitation increases the backflow of blood into the left atrium. Elevated left atrial pressure and pulmonary venous pressure result. Respiratory signs accompanying this failure therefore include alveolar and interstitial edema, which can progress to alveolar thickening and fibrosis. Severe respiratory embarrassment arises as a consequence of reduced gaseous exchange, obstruction of the bronchioles, and reduction in overall tidal volume. Clinically, respiratory embarrassment appears as an intolerance to exercise, dyspnea, coughing (especially at night), and some degree of cyanosis. Sometimes a frothy discharge accompanies the respiratory distress.

When predominant right-sided cardiac failure is present, elevation of the right atrial pressure occurs. Interference with the venous return to the heart raises the central venous pressure ("preload"), with an ensuing chronic venous congestion and peripheral edema. This cardiac malfunction is accompanied by abdominal distention (ascites, hepatomegaly), weight loss, diarrhea, pleural effusion, and dyspnea.

Although signs indicative of failure of one side of the heart may predominate initially, both sides commonly are affected to a greater or lesser degree.

Because simultaneous failure of both left and right sides is common, various features are evident, e.g., dyspnea, coughing, abdominal enlargement, lethargy, and exercise intolerance. The disorder commonly progresses from failure of one side to the other side and may be congenital, valvular, or myocardial in origin.

When left-sided failure predominates, chronic mitral regurgitation occurs. This process of regurgitation means that, at each systolic contraction, a proportion of the stroke volume is forced back into the left atrium. The left atrium then becomes enlarged because of the increased intra-atrial pressure. The accumulating pressure of blood in the pulmonary veins and capillaries causes elevation of the hydrostatic pressure of the pulmonary circulation. When the hydrostatic pressure exceeds the osmotic pressure in the capillary beds, fluid is no longer retained within the blood vessels, and thus, pulmonary edema follows.

Because of the circulatory inefficiency during congestive heart failure, the body attempts to maintain an effective circulatory system through a series of hemodynamic and neuroendocrine alterations. At normal blood pressure levels, arterial resistance to

the left ventricular ejection is not an important hindrance to cardiac output. In cases of congestive heart failure, however, vasoconstriction of the peripheral circulatory system occurs as a response to maintain circulatory efficiency. This protective mechanism is geared toward maintaining a threshold blood pressure and blood flow to important target organs and tissues (heart, brain, kidneys). Paradoxically, such an increase in blood pressure is counterproductive to a failing heart, which must pump against a greater peripheral resistance. Because of the valvular incompetence, the greater impedance to forward flow from the left ventricle creates an even greater regurgitant flow across the mitral valve into the left atrium. Thus, with each incremental increase in blood pressure, a larger proportion of the stroke volume leaks back into the already dilated atrium. As cardiac output falls still more, the vasopressor responses increase peripheral vasoconstriction. In severe heart failure, the increased release and increased concentration of catecholamines, antidiuretic hormone (ADH), and angiotensin II increasingly impede left ventricular emptying and reduce cardiac output. Increases in impedance to left ventricular forward flow result in diversion of greater amounts of the total stroke volume into the left atrium. Each decrease in cardiac output is matched by a corresponding increase in peripheral vasoconstriction. Cardiac output drops precipitously as a vicious cycle ensues. Increased workload (tachycardia, increased contractility) is placed on an already malfunctioning heart suffering from reduced coronary perfusion and hypoxia. Gross lethargy, fatigue, and exercise incompetence follow. This is the classic clinical picture.

31.2 TRADITIONAL THERAPY

Therapy for congestive heart failure has usually encompassed several key approaches (Tables 31–3, 31–4, and 31–5). The intensity of the therapeutic measures to be instituted depends on the extent and stage of development of heart failure. When exercise intolerance, dyspnea, and tachycardia develop, digitalization and diuresis are indicated. Coughing resulting from left-

TABLE 31–3
AIMS OF THERAPY

Improve Cardiac Output
↳

Increase strength of heart beat	*Reduce cardiac workload*	
	↙	↘
	Reduce volume	*Reduce pressure*
—Digoxin/Ouabain	—*Diuretics*	—*Vasolidators*
—Aminophylline	—Furosemide	—Hydralazine
—Dobutamine	—Amiloride	—Prazosin
—Milrinone	—Triamterine	—ACE inhibitors
	—Thiazides	—Nitroglycerin
	—Low-salt diet	—Isorbide dinitrate

Improve Respiration
Bronchodilation
Beta-agonists
Aminophylline/Theophylline/Etamiphylline
Cough Suppression
Codeine/Butorphanol
Rest
(± Sedation)
Sodium Restriction—Possibly
Reduction of Obesity

TABLE 31–4
GENERAL DRUG THERAPY

Reduce Volume Overload	Increase Myocardial Efficiency
	↓
• *Diuretics*	• Cardiac glycosides
Furosemide	Methylxanthines
Thiazides	
Amiloride	
Spironolactone	
Triamterene	
± Potassium supplementation	*Beta-blockers*—Propranolol (Nonselective)
↓	—Atenolol ⎫
	↓ ⎬ Selective
• *Vasodilators*	—Metoprolol ⎭
Nitroglycerin	*Cardiac stimulants (Beta agonists)*
Prazosin	Isoproterenol (Nonselective)
Hydralazine	Dobutamine (Selective)
Captopril/Enalapril	Milrinone (Phosphodiesterase inhibitor)
• *Sedatives/Antitussives*	
Diazepam	
Phenothiazine derivatives	
Butorphanol	

TABLE 31–5
TYPES OF THERAPY FOR CONGESTIVE HEART FAILURE

Traditional Therapy

Diuretics → Mobilize edema (± potassium supplementation)
Cardiac glycosides → Slow/strengthen heart beat
Xanthine derivatives → Bronchodilators (diuresis, cardiac stimulation-weak)
Corticosteroids → Relieve secondary bronchiolar inflammation

Current Therapeutic Approaches

Objective:
  Relieve volume overload, reduce peripheral resistance, and myocardial tension.

```
                                      ↗    Prazosin
1. Arteriolar vasodilators—Relieve afterload  →   hydralazine
                                      ↘   ACE inhibitors
```
                  ↓
      Increased cardiac output
                  ↓
      Increased tissue perfusion
                  ↓
      Reduce A-V incompetence and atrial overload
                  ↓
      Improve tissue perfusion
                  ↓
      Reduce mitral regurgitation

2. Venodilators—Reduce volume overload (preload) and tissue edema (prazosin/nitroglycerin)/
     Isorbide dinitrate/ACE inhibitors

3. Beta-adrenergic blockade ± Cardiac glycosides
(e.g. *propanolol*, $\beta_1\beta_2$ blocker; *Metoprolol*, β_1 —controls atrial fibrillation, tachycardia,
blocker; Atenolol, β_1 blocker).   cardiomyopathy
                                      —improved oxygen perfusion
                                      —minimizes tachydysrhythmias
                                        (e.g., propranolol)

4. Diuretics—Furosemide/Thiazides/Amiloride/Triamterine spironolactone (aldosterone antagonist) (spares potassium)

---

sided cardiac failure often responds quite well to diuresis, but severe coughing may require treatment with xanthine derivatives or cough suppressants. Cage rest, exercise restriction, a halt to stair climbing, and a salt-free diet are other key features of therapy for congestive heart failure. Exercise reduction and cage rest should be encouraged to reduce demands on the heart and encourage renal perfusion.

The major therapeutic indications for cardiac glycosides include advanced congestive heart failure, especially when associated with atrial premature beats, atrial tachycardia, fibrillation, or flutter. Any therapeutic program for congestive heart failure must also include diuretics. Current therapy is concerned with reducing the circulatory load on the heart; e.g., diuresis (to reduce volume overload), hypotensive treatment, and adrenergic blocking agents to reduce afterload, and thus lower peripheral resistance.

DIGITALIS GLYCOSIDES

Glycosides are widely and traditionally used to improve the output of a failing heart. The increased myocardial contractibility and prolongation of diastole facilitate improved ventricular filling and allows more rest for the heart.

Slowing and strengthening of the heart are beneficial, particularly when the heart rate is inefficiently high and irregular. Congestive heart failure and atrial fibrillation are major indicators for glycoside treatment. They are contraindicated in cases of heart block, multiple ventricular extrasystoles, hypertrophic myopathies, and paroxysmal tachycardia. Disadvantages include an increased demand for oxygen by an already weakened, hypoxic, and inefficient myocardium; prolongation of impulse conductance, and a consequent tendency toward dysrhythmias. Dysrhythmias can develop because of the prolonged conduction of impulses and increased irritability of the ventricular myocardium. Although the digitalis glycosides are widely used, they possess considerable potential for toxicity and can be easily misused.

Continual electrocardiogram (ECG) monitoring throughout digitalis therapy is necessary to monitor patient response and also to identify evidence of toxicity. Electrocardiographic signs of toxicity include extrasystoles (atrial or ventricular) and first- or second-degree heart block. Gastrointestinal signs, such as vomiting, diarrhea, nausea, and anorexia, and general neurologic signs of weakness, lethargy, depression, and listlessness may also be evident.

When toxic effects are observed, digitalis must be withdrawn, and in the event of dysrhythmias, the use of specific antidysrhythmic drugs, e.g., a beta-blocker, propranolol, should be considered.

Digitalis toxicity is enhanced by hypokalemia; thus, the diuretic chosen must ensure conservation of serum potassium.

Concurrent use of hepatic microsomal enzyme inducers (phenylbutazone, primidone, and phenytoin) increases the rate of metabolism and excretion of glycosides, especially digitoxin. Conversely, hepatic enzyme inhibitors (chloramphenicol, quinidine, and tetracycline) decrease the rate of metabolism and excretion and may lead to accumulation.

31.3 CARDIAC GLYCOSIDES

Cardiac glycosides increase myocardial contractility, prolong diastole, and improve ventricular filling. Indications for their use are congestive heart failure and atrial fibrillation. Little evidence shows that they effectively prevent progressive deterioration following mitral insufficiency.

Myocardial function can often be quite good in the valvular incompetence syndrome, which is a common cause of congestive heart failure. For this reason, digitalis glycosides should not always be automatically used.

A narrow safety margin exists for these compounds; the effective dosage rate is close to the toxic level. Cardiac glycosides can readily cause toxicity in cats.

Any decision to employ these potent substances must be based on clinical, radiographic, and electrocardiographic evaluation of the cardiac patient. Because of their inherent narrow safety margin, knowledge of their pharmacokinetics, mode of administration, dosages, and indications for usage is critical.

Digitalis glycosides possess positive inotropic effects, i.e., increased myocardial contractility and negative chronotropic effects (decreased heart rate). Thus, their overall clinical effects are many and varied, including retardation of the sinus rate, depression of AV conduction, and prolongation of the AV refractory period. The overall effect on the heart is a slowing and strengthening of myocardial contractility. Because the heart rate is slowed, the organ is allowed more rest, and by facilitating more diastolic filling periods, cardiac output and tissue perfusion are increased. Renal blood flow improves, edema fluids are mobilized, and the myocardium shrinks in size and in wall tension. By reducing tachycardia, the heart is allowed more rest, longer diastole, and longer filling time; myocardial contractibility consequently increases. This desired increase in cardiac output and efficiency has a secondary effect of improving coronary perfusion and myocardial oxygenation. The augmented force of cardiac contraction, however, necessitates further increases in oxygen and energy consumption in a heart that is already under severe stress. Glycosides can cause problems in animals; thus, dosage must be carefully titrated to the individual needs of each animal. Toxicity and intolerance to digitalis are common in animals, and when digitalis is used with certain diuretics, the ensuing loss of potassium may heighten the risk of glycoside toxicity. Nonetheless, glycosides still have a role as inotropic agents in cases of excessive ventricular tachycardia, atrial fibrillation, and congestive cardiac myopathies. Ectopic activity in the atria and ventricles occasionally accompanies digitalis therapy. The improved cardiac oxygenation and myocardial perfusion, however, can offset this risk and eliminate pre-existing arrhythmic foci.

DIGOXIN AND DIGITOXIN

Digitalis glycosides display a narrow margin of safety, and strict attention to dosage is necessary to avoid toxicity (Table 31–6).

Slow oral digitalization should be performed in most cases. Digoxin requires 5 to 6 days to attain the steady-state plasma level. On the other hand, digitoxin possesses a shorter half-life, and thus, effective digitalization can be attained in approximately 2 days.

Signs of effective digitalization include diminution in cardiac rate, mobilization of edema fluids, reduction of ascites and pulmonary congestion, and a stronger femoral pulse. Usually, chronic nonproductive coughing and exercise intolerance are alleviated.

Although both digoxin and digitoxin are well absorbed from the gastrointestinal tract, systemic bioavailability is better with many of the elixir formulations than with the tablet formulation.

Because of its pharmacokinetics and dosage convenience, digoxin is the preferred form of digitalis for managing congestive heart failure. Digoxin possesses much stronger negative chronotropic characteristics resulting from parasympathetic stimulation than does digitoxin. Thus, digoxin has a much greater effect on decreasing heart rate than does digitoxin. Control of heart rate is critical to the successful management of congestive heart failure.

TABLE 31–6
DIGITALIZATION PROGRAM

Drug		Program
Digoxin		Rapid Digitalization
	Dog Oral:	0.1–0.2 mg/kg, in 4 divided doses over 48 hours—digitalization dose. Reduce to 0.02 mg/kg, twice daily—maintenance dose.
	Parenteral:	0.02–0.04 mg/kg intravenously total dose. 25% given initially, then 25% every 1–6 hours to effect.
	Cat	No rapid oral digitalization. Parenteral—same as for dog.
		Slow Digitalization
	Dog	0.01–0.02 mg/kg, orally, divided twice daily.
	Cat	0.01 mg/kg, orally, divided twice daily—digitalization 0.005–0.01 mg/kg, divided twice daily (Drug must be withdrawn for at least 24 hours if signs of toxicity occur.)
Ouabain	*Parenteral*:	0.04 mg/kg, intravenously (total dose) 25% intravenously initially, then 25% every 30 minutes until desired effect or toxicity is reached.

When administered to dogs, over 10 years of age, the dosage of digoxin should be reduced. Digoxin is primarily distributed in the lean body tissue, not fat; hence, a reduction in body weight (to exclude adipose depots) should be calculated. In addition, the reduced glomerular function in older animals tends to reduce renal digoxin excretion. The concurrent use of potent diuretics also facilitates a lowering of the digoxin dosage.

Digoxin can be used alone only when animals with symptomatic atrial arrhythmias do not show evidence of congestion (pulmonary edema, pleural effusion, or ascites). If signs of congestion are evident, diuretics are clearly indicated. The early use of selected vasodilators angiotensin inhibitors, or hydralazine combined with nitrates is also indicated.

Digoxin has serum binding levels lower than those of digitoxin; therefore, digoxin displays therapeutic effects at lower serum concentrations than those of digitoxin. The half-life of digoxin is 8 to 12 hours; consequently, any toxic side effects take a long time to disappear. As already stated, cats are more sensitive to digoxin than are dogs; lower dosages are therefore recommended in cats. Digitoxin should only be administered to dogs. Also, the half-life of digitoxin is long in cats (>100 hours) and thus is not recommended in this species.

Digitoxin is extensively bound to plasma protein (80 to 90%), whereas digoxin displays plasma albumin binding of 10 to 25%. Thus, a relatively higher fraction of free unbound digoxin is available for tissue distribution. With its higher protein binding, digitoxin has a greater tendency to accumulate in the body of the animal. This characteristic is especially important when liver or kidney function is impaired. Kidney function determines the maintenance dose, and body weight governs the loading dose. If renal function is impaired, the excretion of digoxin may be reduced and the maintenance dose must be lowered.

Toxic effects are most likely with rapid digitalization or the administration of a loading dose, rather than with maintenance schedules. Toxic signs may be cardiac or noncardiac. Any disorder of rhythm that occurs in a dog receiving digoxin therapy should be regarded as a sign of toxicity until proved otherwise. One of the commonest types is the premature beat. Ventricular tachycardia may also occur, and a series of premature ventricular beats is frequently fatal. The noncardiac signs of digoxin toxicity include anorexia, vomiting, diarrhea, and colic. Sometimes fatigue, confusion, and seizures accompany the toxic state.

In the event of glycoside-induced toxicity (bradycardia, dysrhythmia, depression, anorexia, or gastrointestinal tract dysfunction), administration should be withheld for at least 24 hours. Glycoside medication should cease altogether if symptoms persist. Diuretics should also be withdrawn, especially because many of these compounds lower serum potassium levels and thus increase cardiac sensitivity to the cardiac glycosides.

In the event of serious disorders of rhythm, the administration of intravenous lidocaine may alleviate cardiac symptoms. For supraventricular dysrhythmias, such as atrial premature beats and atrial tachycardia, a beta-blocker, such as propranolol, or metoprolol/atenolol may be useful.

Digoxin is of potential value in most dogs with congestive heart failure from valvular, hypertensive, and congenital heart disease, from cardiomyopathies, and from cor pulmonale heart disease secondary to lung lesions. The drug improves impaired contractility, increases cardiac output, promotes diuresis, reduces the size of the heart, and reduces filling pressure of the failing right or left ventricle or both. Thus, vascular congestion and central venous pressure are reduced.

Digoxin is the most commonly used and most reliable glycoside. It may be given intravenously in critical emergency situations or, more usually, by the oral route, which for practical purposes is sufficiently rapid for most clinical cases. Digoxin administered by the slow oral form of digitalization is the most predictable of the cardiac glycosides and is the most uniformly absorbed orally. It is available in tablet or elixir form, and peak plasma levels occur 30 to 60 minutes after absorption. Distribution to body tissues is complete in 8 to 12 hours. Digoxin is only about 25% bound to plasma proteins and hence has a higher "free" concentration than digitoxin (90% bound).

In summary, digoxin causes:

1. Increased contractility of the myocardium (inotropic effect)
2. Stronger systole, longer diastole
3. Slowing of the heart rate
4. Decreased venous pressure
5. Improved coronary flow
6. Diuresis where edema exists

The dosage rate of digoxin depends on many factors, such as the type of heart disease, type of arrhythmia, uptake from the gastrointestinal tract, lean body weight, severity of condition, and contraindications that may be present. Dosage rate also depends on the degree of renal damage in the dog, the electrolyte disturbance, and the bioavailability of different brands. Digoxin is normally administered on a trial-and-error basis with constant assessment by clinical signs or ECG evaluation. Maximum therapeutic effects are obtained only when the point of toxicity is reached. When using cardiac glycoside therapy, the drug must be administered until the cardiac signs are alleviated or until mild signs of intoxication appear, e.g., dysrhythmias, depression, anorexia, vomiting, and diarrhea. Digitalization can be carried out rapidly by parenteral administration over a period of 24 to 48 hours for peracute conditions or slowly over 6 to 10 days by oral administration for less acute cases. Slow digitalization is satisfactory in most cases, especially when combined with cage rest and diuresis.

Rapid Oral Digitalization with Digoxin

A total initial loading dose of 0.1 to 0.20 mg/kg is computed on a body weight basis and is then given every 8 hours over a period of 48 hours until signs of effective digitalization are seen (slow heart rate, increased intervals on ECG). The drug is then withdrawn for 24 hours, and daily administration is subsequently resumed at approximately 1/8 to 1/10 of the digitalization dose.

Slow Oral Digitalization

An initial dose of 0.02 mg/kg daily digoxin is given in divided doses over a period of 1 week. This level is then gradually increased until the desired clinical response is seen. Again, administration should be withheld for about 24 hours if signs of toxicity (bradycardia, arrhythmias, depression, anorexia, or vomiting) develop. Because the precise dosage cannot be precisely computed for an individual patient, constant monitoring and observation for signs of toxicity are necessary. (Digitoxin should not be given to cats)

OUABAIN

Ouabain is a potent cardiac glycoside that has a rapid onset of action and a short half-life. Thus, its effects disappear quickly. It is very poorly absorbed from the gut and therefore is not given orally. Because ouabain is the least protein bound of the glycosides, its duration of action is short and excretion is rapid. Ouabain is indicated for treatment of emergency states by intravenous injection. (0.04 mg/kg)

OTHER DRUGS FOR POSITIVE INOTROPISM (TABLE 31-7)

Dobutamine selectively increases contractility without altering heart rate. Because of its short half-life, most of the dobutamine is metabolized or eliminated within 10 to 12 minutes. It must be given as a continuous intravenous infusion (5 to 30 μg/kg/minute). Side effects from overdosage and overstimulation of the beta$_1$-receptors include tachycardia, arrhythmias, tremors, and restlessness.

The closely related compound dopamine is the natural precursor of norepinephrine, which stimulates dopaminergic receptors (beta$_1$ and beta$_2$) and in addition causes renal vasodilation.

Amrinone and milrinone are members of a new class of inotropic drugs called bipyridine derivatives. Inhibition of the enzyme phosphodiesterase and elevation of intracellular adenosine 3':5'-cyclic phosphate (AMP) in the myocardial cells underpins their pharmacodynamic activity. In human cardiology, amrinone is quite toxic, but milrinone appears to be safer.

Milrinone has inotropic activity greater than that of digoxin and also possesses a wider safety margin. Milrinone also produces peripheral vasodilation, which fur-

TABLE 31–7
DRUGS FOR POSITIVE INOTROPISM

DRUG	ACTION	DOSE
Digoxin	Inhibits sodium, potassium, ATPase	0.008–0.02 mg/kg, orally, twice daily
Digitoxin	Inhibits sodium, potassium, ATPase	0.06 mg/kg, orally, twice daily
Dobutamine	Beta$_1$-agonist selective	5–30 μg/kg, per minute intravenously (drip)
Dopamine	Beta-agonist (High doses activate alpha-receptors)	2–10 μg/kg, intravenously
Milrinone	Phosphodiesterase inhibitor	0.5–1.0 mg/kg, orally, t.i.d.

ther facilitates adequate cardiac output. Given orally at a dose of 0.5 to 1 mg/kg, three times a day, the onset of action is about 20–40 minutes.

31.4 DIURETICS

Induction of diuresis is of critical importance in left- or right-sided failure or in generalized congestive heart failure. Diuretics reduce sodium and water retention, reduce volume overload, and reduce tissue edema. Such drugs are useful in combination with glycosides and dietary restrictions, such as salt reduction.

Furosemide, thiazides, and the aldosterone antagonist spironolactone are effective fluid-mobilizing agents. Loss of potassium and ensuing hypokalemia can be a problem with furosemide or thiazides. Hypokalemia resulting from furosemide usage can promote cardiac arrhythmias and increase the susceptibility of the patient to digitalis intoxication.

Commonly used diuretics, such as furosemide and thiazides, are most effective in mobilizing edema fluids, especially those associated with pulmonary congestion. A rapid effect is seen particularly after intravenous administration.

Diuretics have long been standard treatment for cardiac failure, edematous states, and hypertension. Loop diuretics, such as furosemide, are first-line therapy in cardiac failure of all types. The most notable side effect of both loop and thiazide diuretics is hypokalemia. Thus, dosage must always be kept carefully monitored and on the con-

servative side. Efforts to reduce the risk of hypokalemia have concentrated on the simultaneous administration of potassium supplements. Although the incidence of hypokalemia is reduced, the dosage of potassium chloride, however, is not adequate to replace losses in most instances. The usual dose of chlorothiazide is 20 to 40 mg/kg orally twice daily.

Diuretics reduce plasma volume and extracellular fluid volume once therapy is instituted. Diuretics alleviate outward pressure by reducing vascular resistance and also reduce the workload by reducing plasma and extracellular fluid volume. Furosemide (Lasix) is the most common diuretic agent used. It acts to inhibit the active reabsorption of sodium and, hence, the passive absorption of water in the tissues. Some potassium loss may occur, but furosemide is better in this regard than are most other diuretics. Oral administration is sometimes accompanied by vomiting and anorexia. Furosemide should be given intermittently according to need, not continuously. Prolonged continuous therapy induces hypokalemia, which increases the possibility of digitalis toxicity. Oral supplementation in the form of potassium chloride tablets daily may be required.

By reducing the blood volume by renal excretion of water and by dilation of veins, a diuretic such as furosemide contributes to reduction of preload and is valuable in the treatment of cardiac and noncardiac pulmonary edema.

Furosemide is useful in patients with ascites caused by right-sided congestive heart failure or with pulmonary edema caused by left-sided congestive heart failure. For cases of pulmonary edema, furosemide may be given intravenously or intramuscularly every 8 hours at a dose of 1 to 4 mg/lb. Diuretic effects last for about 2 hours after intravenous administration.

Once the initial crisis has passed, the oral route (1 to 2 mg/lb three times a day) is adequate in animals with chronic congestive heart failure.

Once congestive fluids have been mobilized, the level of diuretic should be reduced to the minimum necessary to relieve signs of cardiac failure. Once-daily or alternate-day therapy should be considered.

Following initial priming doses, maintenance doses of diuretics should be established in accordance with the individual needs of the patient. Prolonged and extensive diuretic therapy can result in refractoriness, and potassium depletion can be a serious complication, especially when cardiac glycosides are used simultaneously. Potassium-sparing agents, such as spironolactone, amiloride, or triamterene are effective in preventing potassium loss. Alternatively, oral supplementation with potassium chloride (Slow-K tablets) may be employed. This approach is not widely practiced, because of the arrival of new potassium sparing diuretics. Care should be exercised whenever potassium supplementation is given because excessive potassium may cause bradycardia, heart block, or intestinal hemorrhage. Some potassium retention is a risk with continuous spironolactone therapy. This diuretic is given at a dose rate of 2–4 mg/kg orally s.i.d.

When retained fluids are refractory to the more usual diuretics, a potassium-sparing diuretic, such as amiloride, combined with a thiazide can be considered. When furosemide is combined with amiloride, hypokalemia rarely occurs.

31.5 METHYLXANTHINES

Methylxanthines (e.g., aminophylline, etamiphylline) effect bronchodilation by a unique mechanism. These substances inhibit the enzyme phosphodiesterase. This particular enzyme is responsible for catalyzing the intracellular metabolism of cAMP, which is the intracellular second messenger for beta-receptor activation. By inhibiting the breakdown of cAMP, methylxanthines elicit bronchodilation. When combined with specific beta$_2$-agonists, they augment the bronchodilatory effects.

Xanthine derivatives, such as aminophylline, etamiphylline, and diprophylline, possess cardiac, respiratory, and diuretic properties, all of which may be of some benefit to the cardiac patient. Although their diuretic and cardiac effects are relatively weak, their major benefit is their capacity to induce bronchodilation, which alleviates dyspnea and coughing in left-sided failure. In practice, xanthine derivatives have limited cardiac potency and have restricted application. It follows from the mechanism of action, that beta blockers do not abolish the effects of the xanthines, because of their different mechanisms of action.

31.6 MISCELLANEOUS MEASURES

Corticosteroids may help to alleviate severe coughing in left-sided failure in which secondary bronchiolar inflammation may be occurring. Corticosteroids must be used judiciously, however, because they provide only symptomatic relief of respiratory signs in severely stressed patients. Additionally, this class of drugs possesses some, albeit minimal, mineralocorticoid effects; thus, sodium and water retention can be a complication of therapy. This side effect is unwanted in an edematous patient already suffering from progressively impaired renal failure.

The basic problems in congestive heart failure are increased circulating volume and a lack of forward projection of the blood. The basic therapy may be directed toward direct inotropic stimulation and/or emphasis on work reduction. High-dose diuretics consistently reduce circulating fluid volume, thereby reducing volume load on the heart (Table 31–9). They also reduce peripheral vascular resistance and, therefore, reduce the outflow pressure against which the heart must work.

Rest is an often forgotten necessity to successful therapy. Exercise creates additional cardiac stress, and therefore increased workload and need for oxygen, and so reduces cardiac reserve. With rest and a reduction of strenuous exercise and excitement, reduced cardiac demand allows bradycardia, better cardiac nutrition, and repair. Chlorpromazine and other phenothiazine tranquilizers may be quite useful because they sedate the dog and reduce the workload on the heart. In addition, they reduce blood pressure (hypotensive effect), which may be advantageous in reducing the outward pressure against which the heart must pump blood, because of their peripheral alpha$_1$ blocking effect. Although the vasodilation induced by acepromazine can be useful, hypotensive collapse can occur if a parenteral dose of 0.05 mg/kg is exceeded. Diazepam (Valium) has also been employed as a sedating agent in extreme cases, 0.2 to 1.0 mg/kg, intravenously, or 2.5–5 mg orally.

COUGH SUPPRESSION

Antitussive agents and bronchodilators are indicated to relieve distressing nonproductive chronic coughs in dyspneic dogs (Table 31–8). Codeine is the primary cough suppressant used in such cases.

Opioids, such as buprenorphine or butorphanol, can be useful when coughing is severe.

Butorphanol tartrate, orally, 0.5 mg/kg, is an effective opioid suppressant for nonproductive coughs. Mild sedation also occurs. It is contraindicated in cats.

Bronchodilators, such as aminophylline (5–10 mg/kg, intramuscularly, three times a day), may have some use if pulmonary edema is a life-threatening problem. (Afterload reduction with hydralazine should also be considered.)

Obesity should be prevented or eliminated as far as possible. Paracentesis should be considered if pressure on the diaphragm is causing dyspnea.

Broad-spectrum antibiotics may occasionally be indicated when the pulmonary edema and congestion have provided an ideal medium for bacterial growth with resultant respiratory infection.

DIETARY CONSIDERATION

It has long been believed that the intake of sodium in the diet of animals with cardiac problems must be drastically reduced, because dogs with heart failure tend to retain sodium (and consequently water), which expands blood volume and ultimately the overall workload on the heart. This is now an area of some controversy, because animals with congestive heart failure are in all probability on diuretics (natriuretics) which are causing sodium excretion anyhow. Despite this, dietary sodium excess is probably best avoided.

Sodium intake should not be exacerbated by the ingestion of added salt in the diet. Salt is present in many commercially prepared dog and cat foods, whether tinned, dried, biscuits, or meal to improve palatability. Also, salt is present in many foodstuffs intended for human consumption, such as meat (especially ham, bacon, sausages) and bread. Because fluid and sodium are retained in excessive amounts in animals with congestive heart failure because of defective renal clearance consequent to inefficient cardiac output, further salt intake must be restricted. Thus, proprietary dog/cat foods are best avoided altogether, and the meat should be directly prepared by the owner. Avoidance of canned foods especially preparation of meat without the addition of salt, and dietary supplementation of low-salt carbohydrates, such as potatoes, rice, or pasta, are therefore necessary. Several commercially prepared salt-free pet foods are now available. Such dietary control contributes to a mitigation of circulatory overload problems and may assist the animal with compensated cardiac disease.

Weight loss can be a problem in some cases of severe congestive heart failure, and thus, anabolic steroids, such as stanozolol, can be useful.

Owners of animals with congestive heart failure should be instructed to feed their pets high-fiber, low-fat, moderate-sodium diets with adequate protein of high biological value. Prescription diets for cardiac patients should be followed.

FELINE CARDIOMYOPATHIES

Therapy of cardiac failure in cats is relatively more difficult than in dogs. Dyspnea is one of the commonest clinical signs with

TABLE 31–8
MISCELLANEOUS TREATMENTS

BRONCHODILATORS

Aminophylline	5–10 mg i.m., t.i.d. or 5 mg/kg, orally, three times a day
Theophylline	2–5 mg/kg, orally, three times a day
Etamiphylline	100–300 mg, orally, three times a day
Isoproterenol	5–30 mg, orally per day (+ cardiac stim.)

COUGH SEDATIVES

Codeine/guaiacol/phosphoric acid syrup	3 ml three times a day
Codeine/aspirin tablets (codis)	2.5 mg twice daily
Diphenhydramine Hcl + codeine syrup	2.5–5 mg four times a day
Butorphanol tartrate	0.5 mg/kg two/three times a day

MISCELLANEOUS

Potassium 600-mg tablets	$\frac{1}{2}$–3 tablets/day, dog
Aspirin	25 mg/kg orally every 3rd day
Acepromazine	0.025–0.05 mg/kg/i.v.
Diazepam	0.2–1.0 mg/kg/i.v.
	2.5–5 mg orally

an accompanying pulmonary edema and hydrothorax. Aortic and iliac thromboses are frequent sequelae. The major effects of cardiac failure in cats are best treated with diuretics, which can result in marked clinical improvement. Digitalization is difficult to accomplish in this species because cats are particularly susceptible to the toxic effects of cardiac glycosides.

Cardiomyopathy in cats is often associated with thrombus formation (especially aortic thromboembolism).

The aortic trifurcation is the most common site of embolic occlusion and results in pain, paresis, a weak or absent femoral pulse, hypothermic distal limbs, and pale footpads.

Medical treatment aimed at rapid clot lysis includes systemic administration of thrombolytic enzymes (e.g., streptokinase and urokinase), heparin, or warfarin to inhibit further clot formation and of vasodilators, such as the calcium channel blocker verapamil.

Aspirin at 25 mg/kg orally every third day on a long-term basis is suggested for preventing future episodes of thromboembolism.

Serum salicylate levels needed for analgesia and antipyresis vary from 20 to 50 mg/liter, whereas anti-inflammatory effects require serum salicylate levels greater than 50 mg/liter. Inhibition of platelet aggregation requires only 1/2 to 1/5 of the levels needed for analgesia-antipyresis.

The half-life of aspirin in cats is 35 to 40 hours because of a species deficiency in conjugating drugs with glucuronic acid. Thus, a safe dosing protocol for aspirin in cats involves an increase in the interval between treatments, and a low dosage rate to avoid cumulative toxicity.

When left ventricular pressure is elevated, beta-blockers can be useful. Because of the risk of thrombosis accompanying feline cardiac disease, aspirin 25 mg/day every third day can help to minimize platelet aggregation. Heparin can also be considered, but dose titration is difficult to manage in routine practice.

The long-term prognosis for feline cardiomyopathy is not good relative to that for the canine species; collapse and sudden death frequently occur.

Cats with clinically apparent dilated cardiomyopathy sometimes may be suffering from dietary taurine deficiency. Supplementation with oral taurine may assist resolution of the condition.

In cats, dietary control is an important adjunct to medicinal therapy. Supplementation of feline diets with 200 mg taurine twice daily has been recommended, because taurine is of particular importance in cats. The supply of taurine during pregnancy and lactation must be adequate to ensure viable offspring. Taurine occurs almost solely in animal raw material. It also is required for normal vision and cardiovascular function. Because cardiomyopathy in cats can be induced by taurine deficiency, most manufacturers now routinely add taurine to proprietary cat food.

31.7 ALTERNATIVE THERAPEUTIC APPROACHES

Human cardiology has profoundly influenced current approaches for therapy of heart disease in animals. Newer approaches that facilitate reduction of the load against which the heart must pump are now being considered. These approaches include the use of adrenergic blocks to decrease heart rate and improve blood flow and of vasodilators to reduce the load on the failing heart.

Attitudes have moved toward the reduction of overload and excessive cardiovascular reflex responses, rather than the attempt to urge a failing, overloaded, hypoxic myocardium to work still harder. Cage rest and calm can reduce the activation of the renin-angiotensin mechanism.

The use of vasodilators is now in favor, and arterial vasodilators may be employed to reduce afterload or venodilators to reduce volume overload (preload) and tissue edema. Drugs that decrease preload or afterload or that increase contractility are indicated in the therapy of congestive heart failure. Such drug therapy includes various vasodilators, diuretics, and positive inotropic agents. (Tables 31–9 and 10).

Preload can be defined as the amount of myocardial fiber stretch just prior to the onset of contraction. As preload increases, stroke volume increases.

Preload is the left ventricular filling pressure, which is elevated in heart failure. In the valvular incompetent failing heart, output does not increase proportionately to the preload, and thus, filling pressure increases. Pulmonary capillary hydrostatic pressure also rises, thereby resulting in pulmonary edema.

Afterload is the resistance to left ventricular ejection and depends on several factors, including arterial vasomotor tone and left ventricular volume.

Afterload reduction in heart failure refers to reduction of the peripheral resistance, and hence arterial blood pressure, by dilating the blood vessels. The work of the heart and its oxygen demands can be reduced by decreasing this afterload.

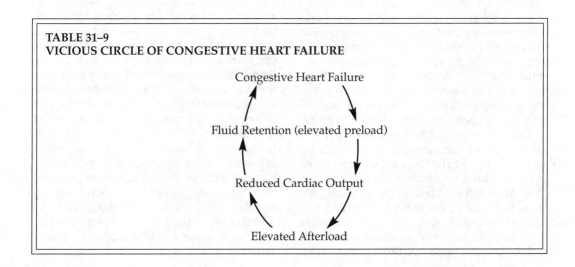

TABLE 31–9
VICIOUS CIRCLE OF CONGESTIVE HEART FAILURE

Congestive Heart Failure

Fluid Retention (elevated preload)

Reduced Cardiac Output

Elevated Afterload

TABLE 31–10
DRUG THERAPY OF PRELOAD AND AFTERLOAD

PRELOAD

Prazosin	Alpha-1 blocker (dilates arteries and veins)	0.02–0.05 mg/kg, (or 0.5–2.0 mg total dose) orally, twice daily
Captopril	ACE inhibitor (dilates arteries and veins)	0.5–2 mg/kg, orally, three times a day
Nitroglycerin	Venodilator	0.25–1 inch patch
Furosemide	Loop diuretic	1–4 mg/kg T.I.D. orally
Spironolactone		2–4 mg/kg, orally once daily
Triamterene		2–4 mg/kg, orally once daily
Chlorothiazide		20–40 mg/kg orally B.I.D.

AFTERLOAD

Prazosin	Alpha-blocker	0.02–0.05 mg/kg, orally, twice daily
Captopril	ACE inhibitor	0.5–2 mg/kg, orally, three times a day
Hydralazine	Arteriolar dilator	0.5–2.0 mg/kg orally

Vasodilators reduce afterload primarily and thus facilitate increased cardiac output against a lowered pressure gradient. Because impedance to cardiac output is reduced, generalized tissue perfusion and oxygenation are improved.

31.8 VASODILATORS

Vasodilator therapy today plays a crucial role in the management of acute and chronic heart failure in humans. These drugs are extensively used in human cardiology. Vasodilating agents can be particularly effective in alleviating dyspnea and fatigue also in small animals suffering from congestive heart failure and chronic mitral regurgitation. By reducing peripheral vascular resistance, both the preload and the afterload can be reduced, thereby alleviating the impedance to cardiac output and return. The stroke volume is allowed to pump against a reduced afterload, and forward flow from the left ventricle is therefore increased. The redistribution of the stroke volume allows relatively little regurgitated flow across the mitral valve into the left atrium. Pressure on the left ventricle and atrium decreases, and this relative cardiac shrinkage reduces the diameter of the AV valves, which are allowed to function more effectively. This outcome contributes to a diminishing of the regurgitant backflow to the atrium.

As cardiac output improves, increased perfusion and oxygenation of tissues occur also. Renal blood flow is enhanced with an attendant diuretic mobilization of sequestered fluids, a concomitant reduction in pulmonary edema, and marked alleviation of the associated clinical signs. The lessening of clinically signs is particularly noticeable in the lungs, where a marked diminution of coughing and dyspnea occurs when left atrial pressure is lowered. The frequency and severity of intractable coughing are also reduced when the swollen left atrium no longer impinges on the left bronchus.

Vasodilators are chiefly indicated when the fundamental regurgitant problem can be traced to progressive dilation of the mitral valve annulus. Vasodilators minimize AV incompetence and reduce intracardiac pressure, and myocardial tension. Although effective in augmenting a more efficient cardiac output, vasodilating agents are not without attendant risks and side effects. Reflex tachycardia, severe hypotension, and collapse are hazards accompanying their usage if individual dosage is not adequately titrated and the patient response is not carefully and continually monitored.

TABLE 31–11
LOAD REDUCERS VASODILATORS/DIURETIC THERAPY

Vasodilator Drug	Dose
Prazosin	0.02–0.05 mg/kg, twice daily, orally (or 0.5–2 mg, total dose)
Captopril	0.5–2.0 mg/kg, three times a day, orally
Hydralazine	0.5–2.0 mg/kg, twice daily, orally
Nitroglycerin	0.25–1 inch (ear) (wear gloves when applying)

Diuretic Drug	Dose
Furosemide	1–4 mg/kg three times orally
Spironolactone	2–4 mg/kg orally once daily
Chlorothiazide	20–40 mg/kg orally B.I.D.
Triamterene	2–4 mg/kg orally once daily

Vasodilators are usually indicated for use in patients with congestive heart failure unresponsive to diuretic therapy alone or in combination with digoxin (Table 31–11). Vasodilator therapy can directly modify preload and afterload and indirectly modify contractility, heart rate distensibility, and synergy of contraction (Table 31–12).

Venodilators reduce preload and can be useful in reducing pulmonary edema, pleural effusion. This type of vasodilator therapy is specifically indicated in cases of pulmonary edema. Rapid mobilization of the fluid overload by reducing circulating volume (diuretic therapy) and reduction of capillary hydrostatic pressure (venodilator therapy) is indicated. Such therapy reduces pulmonary edema and enhances oxygenation.

Preload reduction with diuretic (furosemide), a venodilator (captopril, prazosin, nitroglycerin) or both can result in dramatic

TABLE 31–12
CLASSIFICATION OF VASODILATORS

Drug	Site of Action
Prazosin	Arterial/venous
Hydralazine	Arterial
Captopril	Arterial/venous
Enalapril	Arterial/venous
Nitroglycerin	Venous
Isorbide dinitrate	Venous

clinical improvement. Overusage, however, may result in dehydration, collapse of preload pressure, and significant reduction in cardiac output. This obviously worsens the pre-existing condition.

Nitroglycerin should be deleted from the program when prazosin or captopril is used because both of these drugs possess venodilating properties in addition to their arteriolar vasodilating properties. An additive effect, with deleterious results, would be possible. Nitroglycerin is also as useful venodilator and is applied topically as an ointment to the internal surface of the pinna or as a patch applied to a shaved area before a dog is put in an oxygen cage with 40% oxygen. Venodilators, like nitrates, decrease the filling or preload pressure to allow the distended ventricle to shrink, thereby increasing flow in the coronary microcirculation and hence improving myocardial function and cardiac output.

Nitroglycerin is a potent venodilator that is applied topically to the skin. Its major effect is to reduce preload, i.e., left atrial/ventricular filling pressure. Its effects on arteriolar tension (afterload) are minimal. By reducing venous pressure, nitroglycerin alleviates pulmonary venous hydrostatic congestion and, therefore, is indicated in patients suffering from severe pulmonary edema (dyspnea, coughing, and cyanosis).

Nitroglycerin ointment has sustained action over several days. Applied to the skin of the inner ear (0.25 to 1 inch), it is well absorbed transcutaneously. For this reason, the user of the drug must wear gloves to prevent all skin contact during the application phase. (Sustained-release topical dosage forms [laminates and polymers] are available in human medicine.) These "sandwich" type patches are widely used for convenient application to the skin.

Isorbide dinitrate is another venodilator that is similar to nitroglycerin and useful for reduction of preload and accompanying tissue edema. Nitroglycerin patches are usually used on a 12 hours on 12 hours off basis.

Arterial vasodilator therapy should be considered when elevation in afterload is evident, such as with congestive heart failure secondary to dilated cardiomyopathy. Arterial vasodilator therapy can significantly assist traditional therapy (digitalis, diuretics, low-sodium diet, rest) by reducing arterial resistance and thereby facilitating an increase in stroke volume.

Arterial dilators are also clinically effective in cases of chronic severe mitral valve insufficiency, ventricular septal defects, and patent ductus arteriosus.

Compensatory vasoconstrictive responses are mediated via adrenergic agonistic stimulation or alternatively by angiotensin release.

Arteriolar dilators, such as hydralazine, can be of benefit if arteriolar constriction is disproportionately excessive in response to reduced cardiac output. Hydralazine, an arteriolar dilator, is an alpha$_1$-blocking agent. Because no two cases of heart failure are identical and because the extent and depth of hemodynamic responses in an affected patient vary, the dosage of hydralazine must be carefully computed for each patient. A normal dose is 1 to 3 mg/kg orally given twice daily. Capillary refill time and systemic arterial blood pressure are two useful working baselines from which to measure responses to therapy.

Side effects arising from the use of an alpha$_1$-blocker, such as hydralazine, include reflex tachycardia, hypotension, and tachyphylaxis. Nausea and vomiting occasionally accompany hydralazine therapy. Thus, dosage must be carefully monitored and adjusted in all patients.

Because hydralazine reduces afterload, some chance always exists of activating the renin-angiotensin mechanism, thereby re-

sulting in salt and water conservation. Thiazide diuretics (chlorothiazide), loop diuretics (furosemide), or aldosterone blockers (spironolactone) may be necessary to counter this fluid retention.

In the event of severe reflex tachycardia, digoxin can be used to reduce the heart rate. Although propranolol (a beta-blocker) might also be useful in such cases, its action is fundamentally different from that of digoxin and it may reduce total cardiac output.

Mixed arteriolar and venous dilators include the alpha-blocker prazosin and the angiotensin-converting enzymes captopril and enalapril. These drugs can be used in chronic cases of heart failure that are nonresponsive to diuretic therapy alone.

Prazosin is a postsynaptic alpha$_1$-adrenergic blocker and can be effective in chronic heart failure. The considerable refractoriness to prazosin that occurs over time limiting its long-term use.

Prazosin is a useful vasodilator for use in animals that have developed tolerance to hydralazine or in animals in which a high incidence of side effects to hydralazine are observed. An alpha-blocking agent also, prazosin is given at a relatively lower dose rate 0.02–0.05 mg/kg two or three times a day orally. Again, fluid retention and edema may complicate therapy, and in such instances, diuretics are indicated.

ACE INHIBITORS

ACE inhibitors decrease peripheral vascular resistance by inhibiting the enzyme that converts angiotensin I to the powerful vascular constrictor angiotensin II. ACE inhibitors prolong exercise tolerance, decrease left ventricle filling pressure, and increase stroke volume.

The renin-angiotensin system is stimulated by some antihypertensive drugs, notably diuretics and vasodilators, and is inhibited by others, in particular, beta-blockers and angiotensin-converting enzyme inhibitors (ACE inhibitors).

Angiotensin release can be blocked by ACE inhibitors, e.g., captopril, enalapril and lisinopril. Although these drugs act as arteriolar and venous dilators, they may also be synergistic with diuretics in inhibiting aldosterone production.

In congestive heart failure, ACE inhibitors reduce sodium and water retention by decreasing plasma aldosterone concentration and preload and afterload through venodilation and arteriolar dilation.

Captopril, launched in the late 1970s, was the first ACE inhibitor. Acting as an arteriolar dilator and venodilator, captopril is a potent, highly specific, competitive inhibitor of ACE. Plasma and renal concentrations of angiotensin II decrease, and aldosterone secretion decreases. Captopril is the most common ACE inhibitor used in humans and dogs. The usual dose is 0.5 to 2.0 mg/kg twice a day.

Enalapril is a related ACE inhibitor. (Because enalapril must be bioactivated in the liver, it can be regarded as a pro-drug.)

These ACE inhibitors are useful in the treatment of hypertension, congestive heart failure refractory to digoxin/diuretics, renal disease, and shock.

Captopril is used mainly as a vasodilator and often in combination with diuretics to reduce plasma volume. Renal failure and elevated blood urea are complications of captopril therapy.

31.9 THERAPY OF CARDIAC ARRHYTHMIAS

The sinus node is the dominant cardiac pacemaker and regulates normal cardiac rhythm. In the event of failure of normal sinus rhythm, cardiac tissue, with its own inherent rhythmicity, imparts its own rhythm to the myocardium. This takeover is especially evident if the ventricles are not activated frequently enough from the sinus node. When myocardial disease occurs, ectopic foci arise. These foci directly generate atrial or ventricular premature beats, tachycardias, or tachydysrhythmias. Ventricular fibrillation is the commonest cause of cardiac arrest.

Dysrhythmias are common because of the intrinsic rhythm of cardiac tissue and the multiplicity of internal or external factors that can provoke such dysrhythmias.

Internal factors may include myocarditis, ischemia, cardiomyopathies, neoplasia, and fibrosis.

External factors may include autonomic/endocrine disorders (adrenal, thyroid, parathyroid), metabolic disorders (hypoxia, hypothermia, acid/base/electrolyte disturbances, shock, gastrointestinal disturbances, pancreatitis, pyometra), and drug therapy (cardiac glycosides).

The ensuing dysrhythmias can be many and varied, e.g., disturbance of sinus rhythm, AV block, atrial tachycardias, and ventricular tachycardias.

Depending on the type and extent of dysrhythmia in the malfunctioning heart, various sequelae may arise:

1. Atrial fibrillation—reduction in ventricular filling
2. Ectopic beats—insufficient cardiac activity and reduced stroke volume
3. Irregular ventricular rhythm—reduction in cardiac output
4. Bradydysrhythmias—sinus arrest/ventricular bradycardia, weakness, ataxia
5. Ventricular tachycardia—fall in cardiac output

Cardiac dysrhythmias, regardless of their specific cause, result in a variable spectrum of effects, such as reduction in stroke volume, fall in cardiac output, reduced ventricular filling, diminution of tissue oxygenation and perfusion, variation in blood pressure, weakness, ataxia, collapse, and perhaps death.

If atrial fibrillation is present, a beta-blocker, such as atenolol or propranolol, may be necessary. When ventricular arrhythmias are not complicating the pattern of supraventricular tachycardia, digitalis is the drug of choice.

GENERAL PRINCIPLES OF DYSRHYTHMIA THERAPY

1. Judicious use of rationally indicated specific antiarrhythmic drugs (Table 31–13).
2. Ancillary measures that may be indicated as the individual case demands:
   a. Fluid therapy and plasma expanders in cases of toxemia or hyperkalemia
   b. Antimicrobial therapy in the presence of myocardial endocarditis
   c. Diuretics in cases of volume overload
   d. Analgesic agents
   e. Withdrawal of potentially dysrhythmic drugs (glycosides)

TABLE 31–13
SPECIFIC DRUGS FOR CARDIAC DYSRHYTHMIAS

Bradydysrhythmias (bradycardias/missed beats)

Atropine	0.2 to 2.0 mg/kg s.c. or orally
Isoproterenol	8–30 mg, three times a day, orally

Tachydysrhythmias (ectopic beats/tachycardia/fibrillation)

Lidocaine (intravenously)	1–4 mg/kg, then 25–75 mg/kg/min infusion
Tocainide	30 mg/kg, three times a day, orally
Quinidine Sulfate	5–20 mg/kg, three times a day, orally
Disopyramide	50–300 mg, three or four times a day, orally
Atenolol	Four times a day 0.5 mg/kg, orally
Metoprolol	5–40 mg, three times a day
Propranolol	0.2–1.0 mg/kg, three times a day, orally; 20–60 µg/kg, intravenously
Aprindine	0.1 mg/kg/minute for 5 minutes, intravenously; 1–2 mg/kg, three times a day, orally
Verapamil	50–150 µg/kg, intravenously for 5 minutes, repeated; 2–10 µg/kg for 30 minutes, intravenously; 0.1–0.5 mg/kg, orally three times a day
Procainamide	5–20 mg/kg, four times a day, orally; 6–8 mg/kg, intravenously over 5 minutes, then infusion of 10–40 µg/kg/minute

Cardiac Stimulants

Adrenaline	0.1 ml/10 kg (1/1000 solution), intravenously, subcutaneously
Dobutamine	5–30 µg/kg/minute, intravenously
Isoproterenol	8–30 mg/kg, three times a day, orally
Milrinone	0.5–1.0 mg/kg, three times a day, orally

f. Possible surgical intervention when pyometra or thyroid neoplasia is an underlying factor

31.10 RECEPTOR-SELECTIVE ANTIARRHYTHMIC DRUGS

Many standard antiarrhythmic drugs have been widely used by physicians and to a lesser extent, by veterinarians for many years. A new generation of cardiac drugs is proving useful, however. These alternatives are being increasingly applied to animals. Many of these drugs are taken from human medicine and, although potentially useful in veterinary medicine, are still at the clinical experimental stage and many have not yet been cleared by the veterinary regulatory agencies. Dosage thus remains on a trial-and-error basis.

This new class of antiarrhythmic drugs displays considerable variation in their pharmacodynamic and pharmacokinetic properties. Because of advances in the knowledge of autonomic pharmacology and receptor specificity, and ligand binding sites many such designer drugs are increasing in popularity.

These relatively new drugs for cardiac activity are more receptor selective and tissue specific than are older types and, accordingly, possess increased potential for directed therapeutic action accompanied by relatively fewer side effects in nontargeted organs. These cardio selective agents are widely used in human medicine.

Adrenergic receptors can be differentiated into at least four major subtypes—alpha$_1$, alpha$_2$, beta$_1$, beta$_2$. Modern second-generation adrenergic drugs are more selective in their therapeutic effects because of their greater selectivity and affinity for different receptor subtypes in target organs. Beta$_1$-selective agonists increase myocardial contractile force (inotropism) and cardiac output. Beta$_2$-selective agonists mediate bronchodilation, vasodilation, and, to a

TABLE 31–14
ANTIARRHYTHMIC THERAPY

Tissue Distribution of Beta-adrenergic Receptors

Tissue/organ	Receptor	Effect of Stimulation
Heart	Beta$_1$	Contractility ↗ Conduction velocity ↗ Dysrhythmias ↗
Vascular smooth muscle	Beta$_2$	Vasodilation
Bronchi	Beta$_2$	Bronchodilation
Intestine	Beta$_2$	Relaxation
Uterus	Beta$_2$	Relaxation

Beta-Agonist Drugs

Drug	Receptor	Agonistic effect
Isoproterenol	Beta$_1$ Beta$_2$	Cardiac/Bronchial
Dobutamine	Beta$_1$	Cardiac stimulant
Metaproterenol	Beta$_2$	Bronchial dilator
Terbutaline	Beta$_2$	Bronchial dilator
Clenbuterol	Beta$_2$	Bronchial dilator
Salbutamol	Beta$_2$	Bronchial dilator
Dopamine	Beta$_1$ Beta$_2$	Vasodilator, cardiac stimulant

Beta-Blockers

Drug	Beta$_1$	Beta$_2$	Blocking effect
Propranolol	+	+	Nonselective, heart/bronchi
Metoprolol	+	−	Selective, heart (Beta$_1$)
Atenolol	+	−	Selective, heart (Beta$_1$)
Nadolol	+	+	Nonselective, heart/bronchi
Timolol	+	+	Nonselective, heart/bronchi
Pindolol	+	+	Nonselective, heart/bronchi
Sotalol	+	+	Nonselective, heart/bronchi
Oxyprenolol	+	+	Nonselective, heart/bronchi

lesser extent, vasolidation and hypotension. At excessive doses, however, receptor selectivity cannot be considered absolute. Nonselective beta$_1$, beta$_2$-agonists combine both types of receptor effects. Alpha$_1$-selective blocking agents evoke peripheral vasodilation with less reflex tachycardia than do the nonselective alpha$_1$, alpha$_2$-blockers because the alpha$_1$-blockers spare the prejunctional alpha$_2$-receptors involved in the autoinhibition of norepinephrine release from the sympathetic neurons. Second-generation adrenergic drugs are more selective in their therapeutic actions because of their greater affinity and selectivity for specific receptor subtypes in target organs.

BETA-AGONISTS (TABLE 31–14)

Isoproterenol is a potent beta-agonist with positive inotropic effects on cardiac muscle. Because it affects beta$_1$- and beta$_2$-receptors indiscriminantly, however, its use is accompanied by tachycardia and beta$_2$-vasodilation. Use of isoproterenol, therefore, can be accompanied by hypotension and decreased coronary perfusion.

Dobutamine is a synthetic catecholamine with high selectivity and affinity for beta$_1$-cardiac receptors only. It increases myocardial contractability (inotropic effects) without accompanying beta$_2$ activation signs of vasodilation as unwanted side effects. Dobutamine, at a dose rate of 5 to 30 $\mu g/kg$, provides for reliable and selective cardiac inotropism. Like all receptor selective drugs, this selectivity is not absolute and can be lost at very high doses.

On the other hand, bronchodilatory activity is frequently desired for cardiac patients with compromised respiratory functioning. Beta$_2$-agonists are indicated in such instances. For nonselective beta$_1$, beta$_2$-agonists, such as isoproterenol, bronchodilation is accompanied by potent beta$_1$ activity, such as cardiac excitation and tachydysrhythmias. Relaxation of the uterus and intestine also occurs.

Clenbuterol, salbutamol, terbutaline, and metaproterenol are useful selective beta$_2$-bronchodilators. Salbutamol, a frequently used beta$_2$-agonist, improves airway conductance and gaseous exchange by causing bronchodilation following a single intravenous injection. Other transient beta$_2$ effects, such as vasodilation and hypotension, can accompany its use, however, and lead to a brief reflex tachycardia.

Dopamine is a beta$_1$-agonist that increases both myocardial activity and contractile strength. Dopamine activity also subserves vasodilatory activity in the coronary, visceral, renal, and cerebral vascular beds. Vasodilation mediated by dopamine can sometimes be useful in cardiac disease by augmenting cardiac activity and improving blood flow to organs in which circulatory shock is present. A dose of 8 to 10 $\mu g/kg/minute$ is useful in dogs for selective vasodilation, but higher dosages can precipitate vasoconstrictor effects.

Beta-blocking agents control cardiac dysrhythmias generated by hyperactivity of the sympathetic nervous system. Nonspecific beta$_1$, beta$_2$ blockers, such as propranolol, effectively suppress cardiac activity. Because blockage of beta$_2$-receptors also occurs, cardiac suppressant activity is accompanied by bronchoconstriction and changes in systemic blood pressure. Cardioselective beta$_1$-blockers decrease inotropic and chronotropic activity, reduce cardiac workload, and lower the myocardial demands for oxygen. Such a selective beta$_1$-blocker (e.g., atenolol or metoprolol) is useful for controlling cardiac dysrhythmias without attendant beta$_2$-mediated effects (bronchoconstriction and blood pressure effects).

ALPHA-BLOCKERS (TABLE 31–15)

Alpha-blocking drugs exert profound effects not only on vascular smooth muscle but also initially on cardiac reflex mechanisms. Nonselective alpha$_1$, alpha$_2$ blockers inhibit not only alpha$_1$-receptors of blood vessels but also alpha$_2$-receptors of the noradrenergic nerve endings. Prejunctional alpha$_2$-receptors control feedback inhibition of norepinephrine and epinephrine release mechanisms. Blockage of these receptors reduces the level of suppression of the nonadrenergic neuron and adrenal chromaffin tissue cells. This activation of reflex mechanisms can increase the outflow of catecholamines, thus increasing the activity of the beta$_1$-cardiac receptors with resultant cardiac excitation.

Prazosin is a selective alpha$_1$-adrenergic receptor blocker. Because the extrasynaptic alpha$_2$-receptors of vascular smooth muscle remain functional, vasoconstrictor receptors remain operational and assist in maintaining some degree of vasomotor tone. With such a selective alpha$_1$-blocker, reflex cardiac excitation is a rarely seen. Prazosin is a useful peripheral vasodilator for reducing cardiac workload without initiating reflex tachycardia.

Drugs that block alpha$_1$-receptors are used to reduce vasoconstriction in the treatment of peripheral vasospasm, hypertension, and visceral ischemia during circulatory shock. Nonselective alpha$_1$, alpha$_2$-blockers, such as phenoxybenzamine and phentolamine, can result in reflex cardiac excitation because of the generalized hypotensive response to inhibition of alpha-receptor mediated vasoconstrictor tone.

31.11 CLASSIFICATION OF ANTIARRHYTHMIC DRUGS

Traditionally, depending on the pharmacodynamic mechanism of action, four major categories of antiarrhythmic drugs have been defined.

Class Ia   Drugs that lengthen the action potential duration and the QT interval of the ECG.

Class Ib   The local anesthetic type.

Class II   Beta-adrenergic blocking drugs.

TABLE 31–15
ANTIARRHYTHMIC THERAPY (ALPHA)

Tissue Distribution of Alpha-adrenergic Receptors

Tissue/Organ	Receptor	Effects of Stimulation
Central nervous system	$Alpha_1$, $Alpha_2$	Neurotransmission/sedation
Kidney	$Alpha_1$	Inhibits renin release
Noradrenergic nerves	$Alpha_2$	Inhibits norepinephrine release
Vascular smooth muscle	$Alpha_1$, $Alpha_2$	Vasoconstriction
Liver	$Alpha_1$	Glycogenolysis
Uterus	$Alpha_1$	Smooth muscle contraction

Alpha-Agonists

Phenylephrine	$Alpha_1$	
Clonidine	$Alpha_2$	
Epinephrine	$Alpha_1$ $Alpha_2$ + ($Beta_1$ $Beta_2$)	
Norepinephrine	$Alpha_1$ $Alpha_2$ + ($Beta_1$)	
Xylazine	$Alpha_2$	
Detomidine	$Alpha_2$	

Alpha-Blockers

Prazosin	$Alpha_1$	Peripheral vasolidation
Phenoxybenzamine	$Alpha_1$ $Alpha_2$	Peripheral vasodilation, cardiac stimulation
Phentolamine	$Alpha_1$ $Alpha_2$	Peripheral vasodilation and cardiac stimulation

Class III   Agents that prolong the action potential duration without altering the rate.
Class IV   Calcium inflow inhibitors.
These are divided into subclasses:

CLASS Ia ANTIARRHYTHMIC DRUGS

These membrane stabilizers lower tissue excitability and can prolong the effective refractory period. Examples are quinidine, procainamide, and disopyramide.

Quinidine

Quinidine suppresses ectopic pacemakers and slows the overall velocity of conduction by interfering with rapid sodium conductance into the myocardial cell and reducing the speed of cardiac impulse conduction.

Quinidine is useful in dogs and cats for suppression of premature ventricular beats, ventricular tachycardia, and ventricular fibrillation. Although it suppresses tachydysrhythmias in general, atrial fibrillation is rarely reduced by this drug in small animals unless the fibrillation is of recent origin.

A potential side effect of quinidine is an atropine-like vagolytic effect. If this side action supersedes its direct effect on conduction velocity, a net increase in AV impulses could reach the ventricles. This outcome is most likely after rapid intravenous injection. Vagal tone to the AV node may be enhanced by an initial administration of a digitalis glycoside to nullify the vagolytic effect. Occasionally, quinidine may potentiate digitalis toxicity by interfering with binding and renal clearance of digoxin; thus, this possibility must always be borne in mind whenever quinidine and digitalis are used together.

Oral administration of quinidine is the commonest and safest route. Maximal effect occurs in 1 to 2 hours. Duration of action varies from 5 to 8 hours, depending on the condition of the animal and the formulation of quinidine used. Normally, 5 to 20 mg/kg orally every 6 hours in the dog is the recommended dose rate. Dosage must be carefully adjusted and adjudged against the individual needs of the animal to avoid toxicity.

Quinidine toxicity can take many forms. Vomiting, diarrhea, depression, and convulsions are sometimes observed. Quinidine toxicity may also reduce myocardial contractility and cause hypotension. The hypotensive effect is attributable to vasodilation because of its alpha-adrenergic blocking effect and a mild inotropic depression. Sometimes dysrhythmias, heart block, ventricular tachycardia, or even ventricular fibrillation can result with prolongation of the QRS, QT, and PR intervals. The drug should be immediately withdrawn if toxicity is suspected. Quinidine is not effective against digitalis-induced arrhythmias.

Procainamide

Procainamide is similar in action to quinidine in that it decreases conduction velocity, prolongs the refractory period, and suppresses ectopic activity. Its therapeutic applications are similar to those of quinidine, and it is used as an antiarrhythmic drug for ectopic activity of supraventricular or ventricular origin. By increasing the refractory period, procainamide possesses useful clinical efficacy for control of ventricular arrhythmias (ventricular tachycardia or premature beats.)

Rapid bolus-form intravenous delivery can elicit hemodynamic depression, although procainamide is relatively less toxic than quinidine.

As a local anesthetic derivative, procainamide possesses a short half-life (t 1/2 = 2 to 3 hours after oral administration). Although a short half-life can give greater control and minimize the occurrence of toxic effects from persistent activity, a disadvantage is that numerous daily doses must be given to maintain effect.

Toxic effects of procainamide are characterized by vasodilation, hypotension, depression of myocardial contraction, and prolongation of the PR, QRS, and ST inter-

vals. Cardiac arrhythmias, AV block, and ventricular tachycardia may occur in severe cases of toxicity. Doses of procainamide are 5 to 20 mg/kg four times a day orally. Some sustained-release oral forms can be given less frequently. Intravenously, a loading dose of 6 to 8 mg/kg is usually followed by maintenance therapy to effect.

Disopyramide

Disopyramide is more similar to procainamide than to quinidine insofar as its main efficacy is against tachyarrhythmias of ventricular origins.

Disopyramide possesses a rather short half-life in dogs (<2 hours) and also displays atropine-like side effects. When atrial flutter or fibrillation is present, disopyramide can increase heart rate. In animals with pre-existing myocardial disease, a negative inotropic effect on the heart is quite noticeable.

Disopyramide to date has only limited application as an antiarrhythmic drug in small animals because of its short half-life and accompanying side effects. The dosage in humans varies from 50–300 mg orally 3 or 4 times a day.

CLASS Ib ANTIARRHYTHMIC DRUGS

Lidocaine

Lidocaine is a long-established antiarrhythmic agent used in both human and veterinary medicine. Its major use is as an emergency treatment in life-threatening ventricular tachydysrhythmias. Lidocaine is normally given intravenously at a loading dose of 1 to 4 mg/kg intravenously, followed by infusion of 25 to 75 μg/kg/minute. It is relatively reliable following intravenous infusion and has fewer associated side effects than does either quinidine or procainamide. Signs of systemic toxicity include central nervous system stimulation (especially in cats), seizures, and muscular fasciculations.

Following oral administration, lidocaine undergoes rapid first-pass metabolism in the liver; relatively little drug subsequently reaches the systemic circulation intact. Thus, lidocaine possesses a short half-life by the oral route (t $\frac{1}{2}$ < 1 hour). Because of its brief effectiveness, oral maintenance therapy on an outpatient basis is not feasible. Lidocaine is ineffective against most supraventricular arrhythmias.

Tocainide

Structurally related to lidocaine, tocainide possesses distinct advantages because of its contrasting pharmacokinetic properties. It is not as rapidly metabolized following oral use, has higher oral activity, and has a longer duration of action.

Animals responsive to intravenous lidocaine are usually also highly responsive to oral tocainide. Because of its higher oral bioavailability when compared to that of lidocaine (its different structure spares the first-pass effect), therapeutic concentrations are maintained for approximately 12 hours after oral administration. Side effects of tocainide are fewer than, but similar to, those of lidocaine. Its primary indication is in the treatment of ventricular arrhythmias. The normal oral dose for tocainide is 30 to 40 mg/kg twice daily.

Mexiletine

This compound is similar to tocainide in that it undergoes little first-pass metabolism after oral administration and is extensively absorbed from the gut. Like lidocaine and tocainide, mexiletine is indicated for ventricular arrhythmias. Its major potential advantage lies in its oral use for maintenance outpatient therapy of lidocaine-responsive cardiac arrhythmias. In humans, maintenance doses of 250–250 mg 3 to 4 times a day, orally, are indicated.

Encainide, Flecainide, Lorcainide

This class of antiarrhythmic drugs shares the same sodium conductance blocking effects as those of quinidine, although they do not tend to prolong the refractory period. Effective against ventricular tachycardia and premature beats of atrial or ventricular origin, they are less effective in controlling atrial fibrillation or flutter. Their major application is in arrhythmias not responsive to standard traditional drug therapy.

Aprindine

This compound can be used in dogs to control ventricular arrhythmias resistant to standard antiarrhythmic therapy. It has, however, a narrow safety margin in humans, in whom leukopenia, agranulocytosis, hypotension, depression of myocardial function, and prolongation of PR, QRS, and QT intervals have been noted. Because of this narrow therapeutic-toxic ratio, aprindine is regarded as a drug of last choice in veterinary therapy. Although similar to lidocaine in many ways, aprindine possesses a relatively broader range of cardiac activity. It is effective against premature ventricular beats, ventricular tachycardia, and supraventricular premature beats. A related compound, indecainide, possesses more potency and fewer side effects than does aprindine.

CLASS II ANTIARRHYTHMIC DRUGS

This class of antiarrhythmic agents is comprised of the beta-adrenergic blocking agents. They inhibit the sympathoadrenal excitation of the beta$_1$-cardiac receptors.

Propranolol

Propranolol, a non-selective beta$_1$, beta$_2$-adrenergic blocker, has been used in dogs and cats to slow the ventricular response to atrial fibrillation and flutter by virtue of its depressant effects on the AV node conduction velocity. Atrial ectopic beats, supraventricular tachycardia, and ventricular ectopy or tachycardia are also responsive to propranolol. Sinus tachycardia and increased cardiac contractility in cats suffering from thyrotoxicosis can be treated with propranolol. Because of its blocking effects on the beta$_2$-receptors also, side effects of propranolol include hypotension, bronchoconstriction, and reduced cardiac output. When used concomitantly with digitalis, varying degrees of heart block may ensue.

Propranolol is usually given by slow intravenous injection 20 to 60 µg/kg several times per day to effect. The conventional oral dose for dogs and cats is 0.2 to 1.0 mg/kg. Extensive and rapid hepatic biotransformation (first-pass effect) by this route, however, renders the effective half-life short (1 to 2 hours). Thus, multiple oral administration is necessary for maintenance therapy.

Metoprolol

Metoprolol is a selective beta$_1$-blocker and, hence, is devoid of most of the beta$_2$-receptor-mediated side effects seen with propranolol. For this reason, metoprolol has many advantages over propranolol (the beta$_1$, beta$_2$ nonselective blocking action of propranolol precipitates undesirable side effects).

To date, metoprolol has been used almost exclusively in human medicine with little or no information available on its use in small animals. Human doses are from 50 to 300 mg/day given orally. Dosage in animals is 5 to 40 mg orally, three times a day.

Nadolol

Nadolol, which is related to propranolol, possesses distinct pharmacokinetic advantages in that it has a longer half-life following oral use and, therefore, necessitates fewer daily administrations than does propranolol. Other non-selective beta blockers include pindolol, timolol, sotalol, and oxyprenol. Atenolol is another beta blocker. The normal human dose is 50 to 100 mg/day, taken orally. In animals, 0.5 mg/kg given orally, four times daily, has been suggested as a useful dose.

CLASS III ANTIARRHYTHMIC DRUGS

These drugs induce prolongation of the action potential duration and refractory period. They have no effect on normal sodium conductance; do not affect the beta-adrenergic receptors, and do not directly alter the heart rate.

Bretylium

This drug blocks release of norepinephrine from adrenergic neurons. It prolongs the refractory period in ventricular muscle and Purkinje's fibers, but has little effect on the atria. Bretylium is, therefore, useful for ventricular, but not supraventricular, arrhythmias. Although used in humans, bretylium has little clinical use in dogs. Bretylium can cause cardiovascular excitation initially from the release of norepinephrine from adrenergic nerves before blockage. Bretylium is also contraindicated with halogenated hydrocarbons. The recommended human dosage rate is 5 to 10 mg/kg intramuscularly.

Amiodarone

Another drug used in humans, amiodarone has received little use in domestic animals. It selectively prolongs the action potential and refractory period, thus leading to prolongation of AV conduction time and increase in atrial and ventricular refractory periods. The recommended minimum effective dose in humans is 200 mg/day, orally.

CLASS IV ANTIARRHYTHMIC DRUGS

This group is comprised of drugs that are calcium channel blockers, which are of great significance and clinical importance in human medicine. Calcium-channel-blocking drugs reduce the influx of calcium through cell membrane channels in excitable tissues, thereby inhibiting the slow inward current during the cardiac action potential. The antiarrhythmic potential is mainly directed toward the sinoatrial and AV tracts, where they slow intensive excitability and decrease impulse conduction velocity. Calcium entry blockers cause vasodilation and improvement in tissue perfusion. Reduction in myocardial contractility, vasodilation in coronary and peripheral arterial beds, reduced resistance to left ventricular ejection, and slower AV impulse conduction result from use of calcium channel blockers.

Verapamil, nifedipine, nicardipine, and diltiazem are calcium channel blockers used for antianginal therapy in humans.

Verapamil

Verapamil, a papaverine derivative, is a Class IV antiarrhythmic drug used to control supraventricular tachyarrhythmias and to promote coronary vasodilation. It has been approved for antiarrhythmic use. Verapamil reduces the ventricular rate in the presence of atrial fibrillation or flutter. It also re-establishes sinus rhythm in patients with supraventricular tachycardia. In human medicine, verapamil is now the drug of choice for management of supraventricular tachyarrhythmias. Bioavailability is low after oral use because of extensive and rapid first-pass hepatic biotransformation. In dogs, intravenous doses for verapamil range from 50 to 150 μg/kg given slowly over a period of 5 to 10 minutes, followed by intravenous infusion of 2 to 10 μg/kg over a period of 30 minutes. Side effects associated with its use include hypotension, bradycardia, heart block, and a deterioration of congestive heart failure. The human dosage is 40 to 120 mg/day, t.i.d., or 5 mg intravenously over 5 minutes.

Verapamil has been successfully used in the dog for the treatment of atrial tachycardia. Recommended oral doses of verapamil in animals range from 0.1–0.5 mg/kg orally three times a day. This slow calcium channel blocker inhibits inward movement of calcium across the cell membrane and slows sinus rate in atrial tachycardia.

Nifedipine

Nifedipine, although similar to verapamil, can elicit profound hypotension because of its potent peripheral vasodilating action. This hypotension then leads to reflex sympathetic activation of the heart. Human doses are from 5 to 20 mg, orally, three times a day.

Diltiazem

Diltiazem possesses antiarrhythmic activity in supraventricular tachycardias.

SUMMARY

Although many useful compounds from human medicine are now receiving considerable attention with respect to their potential veterinary applications, the major drugs for veterinary antiarrhythmic therapy remain the well-established compounds, such as quinidine, procainamide, lidocaine, and propranolol. Because of their pharmacokinetic advantages, such drugs as tocainide provide the veterinary clinician with alternative and useful choices. Tocainide may become quite useful for orally active lidocaine-like activity in managing ventricular arrhythmias refractory to conventional therapy with quinidine or procainamide. Aprindine may be effective for resistant ventricular tachycardias, but such side effects as blood dyscrasias and hepatic damage must always be considered. Metroprolol and atenolol, selective beta$_1$-antagonists, possess numerous advantages over the nonselective beta$_1$,beta$_2$-blockers propranolol timolol, nadolol and pindolol, insofar as undesirable beta$_2$-mediated side effects do not occur, e.g., bronchoconstriction.

Verapamil is useful for suppressing paroxysmal atrial tachycardia and for controlling ventricular tachycardia arising from atrial fibrillation and flutter. Although veterinary data are relatively sparse for many of these new compounds of human origin, they do provide the veterinary clinician with attractive alternatives. Pharmacokinetic, pharmacodynamic, and toxicologic aspects must be carefully assessed for each compound before the veterinary clinician can embark on confident therapy with some of these agents. Additionally, many of these new antiarrhythmic compounds have yet to be cleared by the regulatory authorities and have yet to receive a veterinary product license. The human dosages given here can provide a working baseline, but each case, and its severity, necessitates careful individual assessment, and dose titration. Undoubtedly these antiarrhythmic agents in time to come will find a useful niche in small animal veterinary medicine. It appears that of all of the above listed compounds, the calcium entry blockers will possibly be the most exciting developments in the veterinary domain, on account of their efficacy, broad spectrum of activity, and potential applications in very many animal conditions. One has only to look at the importance of calcium influx at the cellular level to realize the sheer breadth of applications of calcium entry blockers. To date, veropamil, nifedifine and diltiazem have experienced unparalleled success in human medicine in a relatively short time.

SELECTED REFERENCES

Adams, H.R.: New perspectives in cardiology. Pharmacodynamic classification of antiarrhythmic drugs. J. Am. Vet. Med. Assoc., 189:525, 1986.

Adams, H.R.: New perspectives in cardiopulmonary therapeutics: Receptor-selective adrenergic agents. J. Am. Vet. Med. Assoc., 185(9):966, 1984.

Adams, H.R., and Parker, J.L.: Pharmacologic management of circulatory shock: cardiovascular drugs and corticosteroids. J. Am. Vet. Med. Assoc., 175:86, 1979.

Albert, J.A., and Adams, H.R.: New perspectives in cardiovascular medicine. The calcium channel blocking drugs. J. Am. Vet. Med. Assoc., 110(5):573, 1987.

Allen, T.A., Wilke, W.L., and Fettman, M.J.: Captopril and enalapril: angiotensin-converting enzyme inhibitors. J. Am. Vet. Med. Assoc., 190(1):94, 1987.

Braunwald, E.: Vasodilator therapy—A physiologic approach to the treatment of heart failure. N. Engl. J. Med., 297:331, 1977.

Button, C., Gross, D.R., and Johnston, J.T.: Pharmacokinetics, bioavailability and dosage regimes of digoxin in dogs. Am. J. Vet. Res., 41:1230, 1980.

Chamberlain, D.A.: Digitalis—where are we now? Br. Heart J., 54:227, 1985.

Cooperative North Scandinavian Enalapril Survival Study: Effects of enalapril on mortality in severe congestive heart failure. N. Engl. J. Med., 316(23):1429, 1987.

Cruickshank, J.M.: The clinical importance of cardioselectivity and lipophilicity in beta blockers. Am. Heart J., 100:160, 1980.

Darke, P.G.: Congestive cardiac failure in small animals. In Pract., May, 1989.

Darke, P.G.: Myocardial disease in small animals. Br. Vet. J., 141:342, 1985.

Darke, P.G.: Therapy for cardiac failure in small animals. Vet. Rec., 115:329, 1984.

DiFruscin, R.: The use of digitalis glycosides in the dog and cat. Can. Vet. J., 25:135, 1984.

Dollery, C.: Drug treatment of heart failure. Br. Heart J., 54:234, 1985.

Foodman, M.S., and MacIntire, D.: Reversal of atrial tachycardia with intravenous administration of verapamil in the dog. J. Am. Vet. Med. Assoc., 6:800, 1989.

Fox, P.R.: Canine and Feline Cardiology. New York, Churchill Livingstone, 1988.

Goad, D.L.: Calcium entry blockers: a review. J. Vet. Pharmacol. Ther., 5:233, 1982.

Graham, R.M.: The physiology and pharmacology of alpha and beta blockage. Cardiovasc. Med., Spec. Suppl., April, 1981.

Graham, R.M., and Pettinger, W.A.: Prazosin. N. Engl. J. Med., 300:232, 1979.

Hamlin, R.L., and Kittleson, M.D.: Clinical experience with hydralazine for treatment of otherwise intractable cough in dogs with apparent left sided heart failure. J. Am. Vet. Med. Assoc., 180:1327, 1982.

Jacobs, G.J.: Adding cardiovascular drugs to the CHF treatment plan. Vet. Med., 84(5):499, 1989.

Keene, B.: Vasodilator therapy in clinical veterinary practice—a brief review. Acad. Vet. Cardiol. News, 6:1, 1984.

Kittleson, M.D., et al.: Oral hydralazine therapy for chronic mitral regurgitation in the dog. J. Am. Vet. Med. Assoc., 182:1205, 1983.

Kittleson, M.D., Johnson, L.E., and Oliver, N.B.: Acute hemodynamic effects of hydralazine in dogs with chronic mitral regurgitation. J. Am. Vet. Med. Assoc., 187:258, 1985.

Kuehn, N.F.: Using vasodilator agents to treat heart failure due to chronic mitral regurgitation. Vet. Med., Aug., 1986.

Levine, T.B.: Role of vasodilators in the treatment of congestive heart failure. Am. J. Cardiol., 55:32(a), 1985.

McCall, L., Kaufmann, G., and Weirich, W.E.: Oral cardiac glycoside therapy in the dog. Compend. Contin. Educ. Pract. Vet., 5:753, 1983.

Miller, M.S.: Digitalis: current concepts and clinical usage in small animals. Canine Pract., May–June, 1985.

Miller, M.S., O'Grady, M.R., and Smith, F.W.: Current concepts in vasodilator therapy for advanced or refractory congestive heart failure. Can. Vet. J., 29:354, 1988.

Muir, W.W.: Pharmacodynamics of antiarrhythmic and diuretic drugs in dogs and cats. Proc. 8th Annual Kal Kan Symp., 1985.

Novotny, M.J., and Adams, H.R.: New perspectives in cardiology: Recent advances in antiarrhythmic drug therapy: JAVMA, 189(5):533, 1986.

Pion, P.D.: Treatment of myocardial failure associated with taurine deficiency in cats. Science, 237:764, 1987.

Robie, N.W.: Controversial evidence regarding the functional importance of pre-synaptic and receptors. Fed. Proc., 43:1371, 1984.

Singskoi, S.M., Peterson, A.E., and Ross, J.J.: Pharmacokinetics of captopril in dogs and monkeys. J. Pharm. Sci., 70:1108, 1981.

Somberg, J.C.: Antiarrhythmic drug therapy: recent advances and current status. Cardiology, 72:329, 1985.

Taylor, S.H., Silke, B., and Lees, P.S.: Intravenous beta blockage in coronary heart disease. Is cardioselectivity or intrinsic sympathomimetic activity hemodynamically useful? N. Engl. J. Med., 306:634, 1982.

32

PARASITIC DERMATOSES AND OTITIS EXTERNA

32.1 Demodectic Mange (Demodicosis)
32.2 Sarcoptic Mange
32.3 Cheyletiella Infestation
32.4 Dermatophytosis (Ringworm)
32.5 Otitis Externa

32.1 DEMODECTIC MANGE (DEMODICOSIS)

The parasitic mite *Demodex canis* is a normal inhabitant of canine skin and is found in small numbers on many clinically healthy dogs. The cutaneous disease demodicosis is an external manifestation of an internal disorder. In dogs, demodicosis can be a sign of severe T cell immunoincompetence, which probably is genetically determined in young animals. Endogenous or exogenous factors (severe malnutrition, stress, debilitating disease) that predispose to immunosuppression are involved in older animals.

The blood of dogs with severe generalized demodicosis contains a humoral substance that suppresses normal T-lymphocyte response and also acts as an inhibitor of neutrophil chemotaxis.

The life cycle of *Demodex canis* (20 to 35 days) is spent entirely in the skin. The parasites reside within the hair follicles and occasionally the sebaceous glands or apocrine sweat glands of the skin. Transmission of the parasite is by direct contact, and although puppies do not harbor *Demodex* mites at whelping, they can receive their infection while nursing an infested bitch during the first few days of life. Susceptible young dogs may also contract infection from close contact with the heavily infested dog.

Most outbreaks of demodicosis occur in the first 18 months of life and are seen mainly in short-haired breeds. Appearance of the disease reflects the sudden pathogenicity of a nonpathogenic organism that is attributable either to heredity or to predisposing immunodeficiency factors.

Demodex mange mites inhabit the follicle, where they multiply and produce distention of the follicle. Disruption of the root sheath follows and hairs are shed. Multiplication of the mite in large numbers results in elaboration of a humoral substance that causes generalized T cell suppression.

Unlike sarcoptic mange, demodectic mange is not characterized by pruritus. Many clinical signs may occur, varying from small areas of alopecia to extensive areas of alopecia and hemorrhagic lesions.

Two major types of demodicosis are:

1. The localized, squamous or scaly form

2. The generalized form often accompanied by deep pyoderma

The localized form is a mild condition that usually consists of nonpruritic areas of alopecia on the face and nose. Generalized demodicosis is a far more serious condition and is the result of mite proliferation, coupled with a specific T cell defect that prevents the host from mounting an immunologic attack on the parasite. Large regions of alopecia, edema, erythema, and seborrhea are common. In generalized demodectic mange, up to approximately 50% of all animals display marked pruritus and diffuse alopecia, especially on the ventral half of the body.

Although most cases occur in dogs younger than 2 years of age, isolated cases can occur in the geriatric animal. The skin in this condition becomes markedly thickened with numerous pustules, papules, and nodules. Secondary pyoderma with invasion by coagulase-positive staphylococci, *Proteus*, or *Pseudomonas* occurs in a high proportion of generalized demodicosis cases. The presence of pseudomonal pyoderma indicates a poor prognosis because deaths have been directly attributed to pseudomonal septicemia and abscess formation in multiple organs. This type of pyoderma can be very difficult to treat properly, because only a few antibiotics are effective.

TREATMENT

Localized Demodicosis

Before using any miticide, the affected animal should be prepared by clipping the hair and washing the skin with a keratolytic and antiseborrheic shampoo.

Although most dogs with localized demodicosis self cure and recover in 4 to 8 weeks, few localized cases progressively worsen and become generalized. (Localized demodicosis is rarely pruritic, but the generalized form of the condition is severely pruritic when associated with secondary pyoderma. Skin scrapings must be taken from all cases of superficial or deep pyoderma.)

Several miticides have been used to treat localized demodicosis e.g., 1% rotenone, selenium preparations, benzoyl peroxide, or benzyl benzoate. These preparations are applied topically to the affected areas, and treatment is continued until negative skin scrapings are obtained and hair regrowth is evident. Following cleansing of the lesions, the miticides are applied to the affected areas once daily and rubbed in well. Rotenone is applied once daily, and can cause some alopecia before the condition improves.

Local lesions can be treated with 25% emulsion of benzyl benzoate worked well into the affected lesions. (Benzyl benzoate must not be used in cats.) Benzyl peroxide is widely used in human medicine and is now a popular choice for skin infestations in small animals.

Oral cythioate therapy and topical benzene hexachloride also have been used with varying success to treat localized demodectic mange.

Generalized Demodicosis

Treatment of generalized demodicosis traditionally has been unsatisfactory, frustrating, and disappointing. The deep-seated location of mites, immunodeficiency, and secondary pyoderma render successful therapy difficult.

A program of treatment must be directed against not only the ectoparasitic infestation, but also the accompanying deep-seated bacterial infection of the skin. Lack of attention to the pyoderma can result in death of the animal from septicemia or multiple abscess formation.

Severe malnutrition, debilitating conditions, dietary deficiencies, and endo and ectoparasitic infestation can result in immunodeficiency. All these aspects must be evaluated and corrected to maximize patient responsiveness. Stanozolol, an anabolic steroid, may be useful as ancillary therapy in treating the emaciation associated with the condition.

Deep pyoderma develops in more than 50% of cases of generalized demodicosis and is likely to occur secondary to the immunodeficiency state induced by the mites.

Treatments have included 4% ronnel in propylene glycol, selenium-sulfide, benzoyl peroxide, cythioate, and arsenicals. None of these treatments is completely satisfactory,

and numerous side effects are seen, particularly with organophosphates. Although many products have been tried and evaluated for treatment of generalized demodicosis, only a few have been clinically effective and reliable. Ronnel in propylene glycol and amitraz have been among the most effective miticides for treating generalized demodectic mange. Ronnel is no longer available in many countries.

When available, it is the organophosphate of choice in a 4% solution made by adding 180 ml of ectoral emulsifiable concentrate (33% ronnel) to 1000 ml of propylene glycol, which acts as a solvent, vehicle, and disinfectant. This mixture is stable for approximately 1 month. Ronnel is irritating, malodorous, and potentially toxic, and the solution must be well shaken before use.

After clipping the patient, the solution is rubbed into not more than one third of the body surface area daily on a rotational basis. Care must be exercised when using this preparation. The handler should wear plastic or rubber gloves to avoid skin contact, and an ophthalmic ointment should be used to protect the animal's eyes when dressing the anterior part of the body.

The average duration of treatment by this method is 12 to 15 weeks, and weekly skin scrapings should be taken after 5 weeks of therapy to assess the response. Saline may be better than potassium hydroxide for examining the skin scraping because the potassium hydroxide kills the mites and hence makes clinical evaluation different. Although ronnel is consistently effective for treatment of chronic generalized demodicosis, attending hazards are present. Side effects include mild to moderate erythema, scaling of the skin, and mild to moderate weight loss. Other effects of organophosphate treatment, e.g., anorexia, vomiting, diarrhea, and trembling, can be observed from time to time in small breeds of dogs. A particularly serious toxic effect of ronnel is hepatotoxicity, which, although rare, must not be overlooked.

In 1982, Amitraz (Mitaban Liquid Concentrate) received approval from the U.S. Food and Drug Administration (FDA) for treatment of generalized canine demodicosis. Amitraz is now the treatment of choice for *Demodex* infestation. It is also safe and easy to administer. Amitraz results in excellent clinical improvement in most cases, but apparently does not result in an equally high percentage of permanent cures in animals with generalized demodicosis. This inability to effect a permanent cure must always be considered when discussing a prognosis because a life-long dipping program may be necessary to control the disease in severe cases. (Amitraz is not approved for use in cats.) Although classed as a monoamine oxidase inhibitor Amitraz is a formamidine compound introduced as an ixodicide for use on livestock and fruit plants. Used as a stock solution of 250–500 ppm, whole-body application of amitraz is carried out every 7 to 14 days.

Prior to treatment, the coats of animals with long, medium, or matted hair should be clipped. The area surrounding affected lesions and the interdigital spaces also should be clipped. Dogs with seborrhea or exudative pyoderma must first be cleansed with an antiseborrheic shampoo and then towel dried. A degreasing agent such as benzoyl peroxide may be useful.

The solution of amitraz is made by mixing 1 bottle of the miticide (10.6 ml) in 2 gallons of warm water (0.025%). Skin contact with amitraz must be avoided by the handler; thus, plastic or rubber gloves should be worn. The solution must be used immediately because the drug undergoes degradation and loss of potency within a few hours when mixed with water.

Amitraz solution should be poured on and sponged into the animal's skin (whole-body application). Standing the animal in a bathtub facilitates better treatment of the interdigital spaces and prevents drainage. Particular attention should be paid to the face and chin when saturating the patient with amitraz. The entire animal should be thoroughly and completely wetted with amitraz. The treatment solution is not rinsed off the animal, but is allowed to air dry. The solution is discarded after each patient.

Side effects include sedation, bradycardia, vomiting, and polyuria. Hyperglycemia may also be induced. Hence, diabetic dogs are not good subjects for amitraz therapy. Side effects of amitraz treatment in dogs, such as lethargy, transient vomiting, or diarrhea, are minimal and occur mainly within 24 to 48 hours of the first treatment.

Owners should be advised of this possible post-treatment depression in the first day or two. Amitraz may alter the animal's ability to maintain homeostasis, and hence, treated patients should be kept free of stress for 24 hours posttreatment.

Inhalation of the fumes of amitraz can cause dizziness in some people. If owners are on anti-hypertensive therapy (often mono amino oxidase inhibitors they are more susceptible to amitraz toxicity).

Treatment is performed at 14-day intervals until 2 consecutive negative skin scrapings are obtained. The 14-day interval is critical to interrupt the 20- to 35-day life cycle of the mite. Up to 12–14 treatments may be necessary in severe cases.

Between whole-body amitraz treatment, small problemmatic areas (demodectic pododermatitis) can be spot treated using 0.6 ml amitraz in 30 ml water, mineral oil, or propylene glycol.

When the 2 consecutive negative skin scrapings are obtained, amitraz treatment can be stopped. The dog is then rescraped in 1 month. If live mites are found at this stage, an additional treatment period is commenced. Usually, a treatment series consists of a minimum of 3 and a maximum of 6 individual whole-body applications.

Animals with generalized demodicosis that involves the feet, including interdigital pyoderma and edema, tend to respond more slowly to amitraz therapy than do those without pedal lesions.

If large areas of skin are ulcerated and denuded benzoyl peroxide shampoo soaps are indicated on the affected areas to encourage healing.

Rotenone can be slightly more effective than amitraz in bringing about a long-term cure. A regimen used frequently is an initial clipping followed by bathing in 1% selenium sulfide or 2.5% benzoyl peroxide. One third of the body then is treated daily with 0.75% rotenone diluted 1:3. Feet must be treated every day.

Toxic effects are rare with rotenone, although drug contact on the eyes of the animal should be avoided. Sometimes depression, anorexia, and vomiting follow rotenone treatment.

The end point of therapy with any araricide is the finding of a negative skin scraping on 3 successive occasions.

When secondary infection and pyoderma are established, aggressive antibiotic therapy must be instituted because death attributable to septicemia can readily occur. Antibiotics should be given for 6 to 8 weeks when deep pyoderma is present. Bactericidal drugs are preferable because of the immunoincompetence of the animal. See also Chapter 33.

Stanozolol at 0.25 mg/kg orally may be useful to counteract the emaciation associated with severe mite infection.

Because T cell suppression accompanies generalized demodicosis, the use of immunostimulants (e.g., levamisole, thiabendazole) has been advocated. To date, such pharmacologic agents have not proved beneficial. Biological agents have been used with some success as immunostimulants.

The bacterium *Propionibacterium acnes* can act in vivo as a nonspecific stimulator of immunologic responsiveness and as a potent stimulator of the recticuloendothelial system. Some preparations of the bacterium modulate antibody formation. The net results of these activities include enhanced resistance to bacterial and viral infections. Injections of *P. acnes* increase the number of active T-lymphocytes and cause an interferon-induced enhancement of their natural killing function.

The combination of conventional therapy with an immunomodulator can result in the alleviation of symptoms resulting from chronic dermatitis and may enhance the treatment regimen for the immunocompromised veterinary patient. Immunostimulation with levamisole is not particularly effective. Some animals may benefit from the immunomodulatory effects of vitamin E supplementation (200 mg given 4 to 5 times a day). A wide range of immunodilators, biological and nonbiological, (isoprinosine, avridine) can be considered on experimental and theoretical grounds.

Corticosteroid usage is contraindicated in generalized demodicosis. Anti-inflammatory steroids must never be used in this generalized condition. Many cases of localized demodicosis can easily be converted into fulminating generalized demodicosis with the use of corticosteroids. Thus, the temptation to use these glucocorticoids must always be resisted.

Extralabel usage of ivermectin must be discouraged; apparently, ivermectin has little or no long-lasting effect anyway.

Feline demodicosis is an inflammatory parasitic skin disease only rarely reported. The causative mite, *Demodex cati*, is smaller than *D. canis*. Feline demodicosis has been reported in association with concurrent FeLV infection and diabetes mellitus.

In cats, demodicosis usually causes localized nonpruritic alopecia with a facial predilection for the eyelids, periocular skin, and bridge of nose. Generalized feline demodicosis is rare; most of the occurrences are in the localized form.

Localized feline demodicosis requires treatment with 2.5% lime sulfur dips (every 10 days), local application of rotenone, selenium preparations, or carbaryl shampoos, or dilute organophosphates. (Fenchlorphos or phosmet can be toxic in cats.)

Whole-body application of 0.025% amitraz, a favored treatment in dogs, can cause problems when used in cats. Use of even 0.0125% amitraz solution causes reduced food intake and passage of semifluid malodorous feces for 24 hours. Hence, amitraz is not approved in cats.

Weekly washes with selenium-sulfide preparations, continuing treatment for 2 weeks beyond apparent clinical cure, and negative scrapings (up to 10 weeks) are highly effective for this condition in cats.

32.2 SARCOPTIC MANGE (SCABIES)

Sarcoptic mange is an intensely pruritic scaling dermatitis caused by infestation with *Sarcoptes scabiei* var canis. Although all ages of dogs may be affected, the disease is more commonly seen in young animals. The disease is non-seasonal, highly contagious and pruritic.

The life cycle is approximately 21 days, and the mite can survive for only a few days off the host, 2 to 3 days at most.

In sarcoptic mange, pruritus is a primary symptom; the mite prefers areas of the body that are sparsely covered with hair. Hyperkeratosis, thinning of hair, erythema, and papules are typically seen. Lesions usually begin around the borders of the pinnae, elbows, and hocks. With progression of the disease, the legs and trunk become involved.

Self-inflicted damage, with exudation of serum and blood, and secondary infection are common. The disease is transmissible to humans; approximately 50% of cases are transmitted to the owners. The condition is also highly contagious to other dogs.

Scabies lesions usually first appear on the muzzle, around the eyes, and on the ears, elbows, and chest, lesions later spread to the back and abdomen. Failure to treat infestation adequately allows the condition to become generalized first to the elbows, hocks, and ventral parts and eventually to the entire body.

TREATMENT

Overall therapy necessitates treatment of dogs in contact and spraying of kennels with an insecticide, such as iodofenphos/dichlorvos. With effective treatment, complete resolution of the condition can be expected in most cases.

Treatment consists of clipping the entire animal, cleansing the patient with a keratolytic and antiseborrheic shampoo, and applying a miticide. Multiple treatments are necessary to achieve consistent results with organophosphates and other preparations.

After 3 weeks of treatment, the dog should be reexamined. If no improvement is apparent, a change to another insecticide may be needed for an additional 3 shampoos at weekly intervals.

In dogs, several acaricides have been successfully used as therapy for sarcoptic mange, e.g., lindane (gamma benzene hexachloride), rotenone, ronnel, phosmet, malathion, sulfurated lime, and amitraz. Several acaricides in combination have also proved successful, e.g., carbaryl-lindane, malathion-lindane, and benzyl benzoate-rotenone-lindane. Lindane is potentially toxic, especially in puppies and cats.

Acaricidal preparations that are effective against *Sarcoptes* include 4% sulfurated lime solution, phosmet, malathion, and lindane. These dips must be applied to the dog's body every 5 to 7 days for at least 5 weeks.

Many of the chlorinated hydrocarbons (such as lindane) are particularly toxic to cats. Accordingly, other agents must be used in this species, e.g., rotenone, sulfurated lime washes, or topical sulfur soaps or solutions.

Severely affected areas should be clipped, and crusts should be removed by soaking in warm water. General parasiticidal treatment should be commenced with topical application of a suitable parasiticide, such as lindane. Lindane is effective and, when combined with a surfactant agent that aids penetration of the drug through the scale and crust, is one of the treatments of choice.

Topical organophosphates, such as phoxim, can be given at intervals of 7 days. Other organochlorines, such as bromocylen, can be repeated twice at 5-day intervals. Bromocylen has now been withdrawn in several countries. Benzyl benzoate emulsion can be applied topically to lesions at 3- to 6-day intervals depending on the response of the patient. Several topical sulfur preparations are also suitable, e.g., monosulfiram. This has been a traditional treatment for many years.

Amitraz, which is available to veterinarians for treatment of demodicosis, is also highly effective against scabies. For scabies treatment, the optimal concentration is 250 ppm every 2 weeks for 2 or 3 applications. Because some mites can survive beneath the heavy crusts, severely affected dogs may require 2 or more treatments with amitraz. Some dogs harboring *Cheyletiella* or *Otodectes* mites are cleared of these infestations after treatment with amitraz for scabies.

The most frequently observed side effect of amitraz treatment is transient sedation.

The parasiticide ivermectin has been used successfully for sarcoptic mange in dogs at a dose of 200 μg/kg orally or subcutaneously (repeated 2 weeks later). MSD AgVet, however, stresses that they do not endorse the use of this drug for any purpose other than those specifically described in the directions provided with the product. Veterinarians must check the legality of using products in a manner other than that specified in the directions provided by the manufacturer. The animal's heartworm status must be evaluated before ivermectin is used. Ivermectin is a microfilaricide and could induce occult heartworm disease.

If a decision is made to use ivermectin for treatment of sarcoptic mange in dogs, the owner should be informed of the intent, and possibly, a signed disclaimer should be obtained.

The numerous reports of toxic reactions to ivermectin in some dogs forbid its use in Rough Collies or their crosses.

Intensive therapy utilizing a potent acaricide should result in a dramatic alleviation of the pruritus and should reduce the necessity for resorting to corticosteroids. Because the condition is highly pruritic and can be worsened by extensive self-inflicted injury, corticosteroids can be considered to reduce the pruritus. These drugs, however, should be reserved for advanced and extreme cases.

Short-term treatment (7 days) with glucocorticoids is usually adequate. Treatment for a longer period can mask successful therapy. Adjunct therapy for sarcoptic mange can include prednisone or prednisolone, 0.5 mg/kg orally twice daily for the first 3 to 4 days.

32.3 CHEYLETIELLA INFESTATION

Cheyletiella infestation in dogs is seen most commonly in young animals of the short-coated breeds. It is highly contagious and is commonly a pet shop or kennel problem.

Cheyletiella may parasitize cats and dogs, rabbits and humans, and is a relatively common cause of pruritus. In dogs, especially puppies, extensive pityriasis of the dorsum is seen with mild pruritus ("walking dandruff"). Cats sometimes do not exhibit clinical signs. Owners may develop a characteristic pruritic rash in areas of contact.

Adult dogs and puppies infested with this mite are usually brought to the veterinarian with the complaint of dandruff and itching. Mild crusting and white scab are commonly seen around the head and along the dorsal midline.

Cheyletiella is an obligate parasite that lives in the keratin layer of the epidermis in pseudotunnels. Its' life cycle is usually completed in 3 to 4 weeks.

Because the disease is often asymptomatic in animals, the only evidence may be the papular response in the owners. Some dogs exhibit hyperesthesia and intense pruritus with a scurfy and slightly oily coat over the back.

TREATMENT

Cheyletiella mites are eradicated relatively easily because they are susceptible to most insecticides, including those used for flea control.

Successful treatment may be achieved with derris washes or dusts, the topical use of benzyl benzoate-lindane solution, or potassium tetrathionate shampoo with lindane. Pyrethrin, malathion, fenthion, phoxim, carbaryl, rotenone, and sulfurated lime dips are also effective.

Animals should be washed in a cleansing or antiseborrheic shampoo (e.g., benzoyl peroxide) prior to treatment. All animals in the household must be treated. Dogs with heavy coats are best dipped to ensure complete penetration of the insecticide.

Severe *Cheyletiella* infestation is occasionally resistant to treatment with parasiticides in powder or aerosol form because the tunnels excoriated by the mites in dermal debris provide protection from the drugs.

Dogs should be bathed thoroughly in lindane solution, preferably in combination with a surfactant to aid penetration.

Animals can be treated weekly for 6 to 8 weeks if using lindane, pyrethrin, malathion, or sulfurated lime dips. Amitraz (5.3 ml/gal) or ivermectin (0.2 mg/kg subcutaneously) are alternative effective treatments. In one study, ivermectin was reported to be safe and effective against *C. blakei*. Cats with cheyletiellosis given 2 subcutaneous injections, 300 μg/kg, of the Ivomec cattle product, 35 days apart, responded positively to the treatment.

Because benzene hexachloride is toxic to cats, they should be bathed in selenium-sulfide washes that combine parasiticidal and antiseborrheic activities. The coat must be rinsed thoroughly after treatment. This preparation may also be used on dogs. In both species, the baths should be repeated at least 3 times at weekly intervals. Therapy can be terminated when neither the mite nor its eggs are visible in microscopic sections.

Although the mites do not live off the host for more than a few days, the environment should be cleaned and sprayed with an insecticide. Routine treatment of the environment with iodofenphos/dichlorvos is advisable.

32.4 DERMATOPHYTOSIS (RINGWORM)

Superficial fungal infections known as ring-worm can be seen in all ages and breeds of dogs and cats. The disease tends to be more common in young animals, which possess a lower fatty acid content. (Fatty acids themselves possess some fungistatic activity.) Vitamin A deficiency, immunity, and hypersensitivity also play an important role in the development of the disease.

Dermatophytes invade only the dead keratinized layers of the skin and its adnexa—the stratum corneum, hair, and nails. Infection causes breakage of the hairs with a resultant patchy alopecia. Although pruritus is not a common feature of the condition, the skin becomes dry and scaly, sometimes with a secondary bacterial infection. Lesions may have an irregular diffuse appearance or, more frequently, a circumscribed annular appearance on the head and legs. Occasionally, larger areas of the trunk are involved.

In dogs, approximately 65% of cases of ringworm are caused by *Microsporum canis*, 25% by *M. gypseum*, and 10% by *Trichophyton mentagrophytes*. In cats, practically all cases are caused by *Microsporum canis*.

Although over half *M. canis* infections fluoresce with Wood's lamp, because of a tryptophan metabolite the other species, *Trichophyton mentagrophytes* and *Microsporum gypseum*, do not. Hence, negative findings with Wood's lamp do not rule out the possibility of ringworm infection. Ointments or powders containing oxytetracycline may also fluoresce, thus giving rise to false positives. Fungal culture is a more specific means of diagnosis.

Kittens are most commonly affected with focal lesions of alopecia, scaling, and crusting. Lesions are localized around the mouth with secondary lesions elsewhere. The condition can become generalized with alopecia.

Generalized dermatophytosis is rare in the dog unless accompanied by an immunodeficiency state (including corticosteroid therapy), and lesions can become inflamed in dogs.

Ringworm is transmissible to man, and many cases of human dermatophytosis are of animal origin. Owners of infected animals must always be advised of the zoonotic potential of the condition.

TREATMENT

When treating the condition, environmental contamination must be reduced because fungal spores can remain viable for years in the surrounding premises. Disinfection with bleach, formalin, or enilconazole is recommended.

Thorough vacuum cleaning and disposal of material in contact with the affected animal are indicated. All bedding must be burned and replaced regularly.

Before commencement of animal treatment, infected keratin should be removed by close-clipping, and the hairs should be burned. The entire body then should be treated with topical antifungal solution once or twice weekly for as long as systemic therapy is required. The most commonly used systemic agent is griseofulvin. Topical compounds include sulfurated lime, chlorhexidine, povidone-iodine, captan powder, and sodium hypochlorite.

Systemic Therapy

Therapy for generalized dermatophytosis involves treating the entire body and local lesions topically, and long-term systemic antifungal products (Table 32–1). For chronic or severe cases of dermatophytosis, oral therapy with griseofulvin is indicated. After oral administration, griseofulvin is deposited in the newly formed keratin of the hair and skin, thereby making it resistant to fungal attack. Dosage range for griseofulvin tend to be wide, with up to 150 mg/kg sometimes being used.

The absorption of griseofulvin can be increased by administering it with a fatty meal or by using formulations with polyethylene glycol or micronization.

The dose for microsize griseofulvin is 25–50 mg/kg/day; for the ultramicrosize, the dose is 10–30 mg/kg/day. The concentration of griseofulvin in the keratinized tissue depends on continual administration. Hence, it is administered over an extended period.

In the dog, a daily dose of approximately 30 mg/kg should be given preferably after a fatty meal. Fat promotes absorption of the drug, and the addition of 5 to 10 ml of corn oil to the diet may be beneficial. Therapy extends over a period of weeks and must be

TABLE 32–1
DERMATOPHYTOSIS THERAPY

Drug	Dose	Route of Administration
Griseofulvin	20–50 mg/kg	Orally, twice daily
Ketoconazole	10 mg/kg	Orally, twice daily
Miconazole	Local lesion	Topically, twice daily
Clotrimazole	Local lesion	Topically, twice daily
Thiabendazole	Local lesion	Topically, twice daily
Chlorhexidine	0.5–0.2% solution	Once or twice weekly (whole body)
Sulfurated Lime	0.5% solution	Once or twice weekly (whole body)
Captan	1:300 solution	Once or twice weekly (whole body)

continued for at least 2 weeks after the clinical cure or negative fungal culturing. In extreme cases, a course of treatment of as many as 12 weeks may be needed, although usually a course of 3 to 4 weeks is sufficient.

The animal should be carefully re-examined and reclipped at the end of 1 month. Treatment continues until the animal is clinically free of symptoms and cultures are negative.

The efficacy of griseofulvin is increased when used in conjunction with topical therapy. Treatment is continued until at least 1 follow-up fungal culture is negative (i.e., usually 3 to 4 weeks of treatment).

Efficacy of griseofulvin may be impaired by concurrent administration of such substances as phenylbutazone and certain sedatives that induce activity of metabolizing enzymes. Other drugs should be used with caution in animals receiving griseofulvin, especially drugs metabolized by the liver. Animals with impaired liver function should not be given griseofulvin because its metabolism will be reduced and toxic levels could be reached.

Adverse reactions to griseofulvin include leukopenia, bone marrow suppression, lethargy, vomiting, and diarrhea. Vomiting, nausea, and diarrhea can be best avoided by giving griseofulvin with food and dividing the treatment into 2 or 3 daily doses. The combined use of ketoconazole and griseofulvin can cause hepatotoxicity. Griseofulvin is teratogenic and must not be used in pregnant animals. The maximum dose for use in cats is 60 mg/kg because of the possibility of bone marrow toxicity at higher dosage rates. Resistance to griseofulvin can occur.

Ketoconazole is an orally administered antifungal drug that is well absorbed from the bowel. The recommended dose is 10 to 20 mg/kg once daily. Ketoconazole is often successful in cases of dermatophytosis that do not respond to griseofulvin. Ketoconazole, a synthetic imidazole is also safe and effective for systemic fungal disease, although side effects such as anorexia can be seen in cats. It is teratogenic in laboratory animals. Itraconazole is a relatively new antifungal drug that is effective in the treatment of feline dermatophytosis. Itraconazole, like ketoconazole, has fungistatic and fungicidal activity against various fungal organisms. Aspergillosis is included in its spectrum of activity. In addition to enhanced efficacy, compared with that of ketoconazole, itraconazole achieves greater therapeutic drug concentrations in many tissues. Preliminary results suggest that itraconazole may become a most effective antifungal drug for various fungal diseases. Itraconazole appears to be well tolerated in cats; adverse effects are limited to anorexia, which resolves when treatment is discontinued.

Topical Application

Ringworm can also be treated by topical application of antimycotic agents. Because dermatophytes extend into the hair follicle, crusts must be removed before employing such drugs. Topical treatments include chlorhexidine, povidone-iodine, sodium hypochlorite miconazole, enilconazole, clotrimazole, thiabendazole, the sodium salt of benzuldazic acid, sulfurated lime, and captan.

When using miconazole, lesions are cleaned and clipped, and a thin ribbon of miconazole 2% cream is applied daily to the infected site and surrounding area.

In the case of enilconazole, a 0.2% emulsion is applied to the animal 4 times at 3-day intervals.

Clotrimazole is applied topically twice daily. Chlorhexidine shampoo followed by chlorhexidine solution is particularly suited for topical application in cats (15 ml of 2% stock solution/gallon of water).

Sulfurated lime can also be used after a chlorhexidine shampoo. Vomiting after licking of the solution can be a problem in cats, however. Captan applied as a whole-body application is a commonly used antifungal preparation supplied as a 45% wettable powder (5 ml/quart applied weekly). Dilutions of 1:300 are also quoted.

When multiple lesions are present, 0.5% sulfurated lime or 1:300 captan solution can be used as a rinse once or twice weekly.

Povidone iodine at a 1:4 dilution in water and sodium hypochlorite at a 1:20 dilution in water applied daily are also effective and readily available topical agents for dermatophytosis.

Difficult cases may require treatment for 6 weeks or more, and medication should be continued until laboratory examination proves that the infecting organisms have been eradicated.

In immunocompromized animals, ringworm tends to be more generalized, more recurrent and poorly responsive to treatment. Vitamin A deficiency is believed to be a contributory factor in some species.

32.5 OTITIS EXTERNA

ETIOLOGY

Inflammation of the external ear canal, known as otitis externa, is a common problem that regularly affects small animals. Otitis media may result from neglect or from severe chronic infections.

Etiologic factors involved in otitis externa are numerous, and the inflammatory reaction of specific causative agents varies from animal to animal. The condition is characterized by a combination of signs including pruritus, pain, erythema, exudation, and malodorous discharge. Shaking of the head and intense rubbing and scratching of the ears are prominent, and frequently alopecia of the pinna, excoriation, or auricular hematoma may be a sequela of the scratching.

The normal shape of the ear predisposes dogs and cats to ear problems because moisture, foreign debris, and glandular secretions tend to be easily trapped. The presence of many sebaceous and ceruminous glands, which produce large amounts of secretions, and the presence of hair or polyps within the ear canal, especially in dogs with long pendulous ears, can lead to poor ventilation of the ear canal. The greater susceptibility of long-haired pendulous-eared breeds to otitis externa contrasts sharply with that of breeds possessing short erect ears, which are better ventilated.

The presence of concomitant skin disease is a significant causative factor. The lining of the external ear canal is an extension of the skin, and hence, any generalized skin conditions, especially pyodermas inflammations and allergies, can result in otitis externa. Dermatoses can involve the pinna, the external ear canal, or both, and the presence of the seborrhea complex, endocrinopathies, allergies, or immune-related disorders can also be reflected in the development of otitis externa. Allergic otitis can result from inhalant contact or food allergies. Sometimes allergic contact otitis develops from the repeated use of neomycin in otic preparations. Atopic dermatitis is likely to lead to the development of otitis externa.

Inflammation of the pinna and hyperplasia of the epidermis, dermis, or sebaceous or apocrine glands lead to an increased volume of secretions and decreased ventilation of the canal. Consequently, the canal itself becomes narrowed, thus creating an optimum environment for the proliferation of bacteria and yeasts.

If the epithelium of the ear canal is damaged, subsequent infection with staphylococci, streptococci, *Proteus*, *Pseudomonas*, and yeasts can develop and contribute to the overall severity of otitis externa.

Treatment of allergic otitis follows the general lines of therapy for any suspected allergic condition, i.e., elimination of the suspected offending cause and judicious use of systemic corticosteroids (prednisone and prednisolone) to control the inflammation and pruritus.

Numerous potentially pathogenic bacteria, fungi, and yeasts are components of the normal ear flora, and when the environment within the ear canal is altered to favor the propagations of these bacteria and yeasts, a severe secondary infection is usually established.

Bacterial infection is associated with the presence of a noticeable discharge, and the color of the exudate is often related to the type of bacteria present. A predominantly gram-positive infection produces a brownish exudate, whereas a yellowish discharge is observed with many gram-negative and yeast infections. Greenish discharges are observed with *Pseudomonas* infections.

Most infections tend to be mixed, and yeasts are frequently isolated with various gram-positive and gram-negative organisms. In cats, *Pasteurella multocida* can be recovered from a high percentage of infected ears.

Whether bacteria or yeasts/fungi are causative agents of the condition, their elimination is usually followed by a full recovery.

Malassezia pachydermatis (*Pityrosporum canis*) is a yeast that has been isolated from both normal and inflamed ear canals. Significant *Malassezia* growth occurs when the environment in the ear canal is altered by excessive cerumen production or a rise in pH following bacterial infection. (Occasionally, *Candida* or *Aspergillus* species are isolated as pathogens from cases of otitis externa.)

Although chronic otitis externa was originally believed to be caused by bacteria, *Malassezia* is now known to be at least a secondary cause in many cases and perhaps a primary pathogen in severe nonresponsive chronic cases in dogs.

Clinical otitis externa can be induced by instilling *Malassezia*, into the ear, and yeasts are generally found in considerably greater numbers in diseased rather than in apparently healthy ears. Occasionally, *Microsporum canis*, *M. gypseum*, or *Trichophyton mentagrophytes* can cause ringworm on the convex surface of the ear pinna.

Infestation with the ear mite *Otodectes cynotis* is the commonest cause of otitis externa in cats (approximately 50% of feline cases), but a less common cause in dogs (10 to 15% of cases). Cats often serve as a source of infestation for dogs, and the mites are highly transmissible. The life cycle of the mite is 3 weeks, during which they feed on cellular debris and initiate aural irritation and inflammation. When otodectic infestation is present, typical brown-black crusts and flakes result from accumulation of epithelial debris, cerumen, and serum. Mites inhabit the lower part of the ear canal and prefer darkness and humidity, but not wetness. After triggering an inflammatory reaction, the mites often evacuate the ear when conditions become unfavorable, thus making their diagnosis more difficult. Although young animals are more susceptible than older animals, dogs are always sensitive to the presence of only a few mites in the ear, and bacterial growth is favored by the inflammatory response caused by the presence of *Otodectes cynotis* within the ear canal. A dog shows severe irritation and head shaking in the presence of only a few mites, whereas a cat with many ear mites may show only occasional head shaking. *Demodex canis*, *Sarcoptes scabiei* var canis, *Notoedres cati*, and *Cheyletiella* may also be found in some cases of otitis externa.

TREATMENT

The causes of otitis externa are many and varied, and proper management of the condition necessitates complete physical and clinical examination of the animal, thorough cleaning of the ear, and full client cooperation. To successfully treat any case, one must address all the contributory factors. Many cases that are apparently primary bacterial or yeast otitis externa are in fact secondary to anatomic features (pendulous ears, excessive moisture, hair within the canals) or to the other generalized conditions (hypothyroidism, allergies, seborrhea).

Underlying causes must be identified and treated prior to initiation of specific ear therapy. If causes cannot be identified or corrected, symptomatic therapy and good management practices must be instituted.

Among the many possible causes of otitis externa that should be investigated are foreign bodies (weed awn seeds, dried wax); trauma (often self inflicted); parasites (mites, ticks); excessive moisture; ear tumors; hyperplasia of the epidermis, dermis, and glandular structures; hair within the ear canal; endocrinopathies; hypothyroidism; Zinc-responsive dermatosis Sertoli's cell tumors, and ovarian imbalances.

For effective therapy, numerous important guiding principles must be recognized and addressed.

1. Predisposing causes must be identified and corrected whenever possible. This step is a prerequisite for subsequent successful specific treatment. Foreign bodies, plant material, dirt, soil, and ear secretions must be carefully removed and the symptoms treated accordingly.

Application of irritant soaps or medication by the owner may also induce severe inflammation within the ear canal, and this possibility must not be overlooked.

2. Thorough cleaning of the ear to remove debris, exudate, hair, and moisture is essential to facilitate an accurate diagnosis and to facilitate effective activity of instilled drugs. The entire ear canal must be treated. Often the entire animal and all animals in contact with the affected animal must be treated with parasiticides to eliminate mites not living in the ear. Flea control products are useful.
3. Bacterial culture and sensitivity testing should be performed to permit choice of a rationally indicated suitable narrow-spectrum antibiotic. If broad-spectrum antibiotics are used needlessly, bacterial resistance and fungal overgrowth may become difficult problems during the course of therapy. Chronic infectious cases, especially those attributed to *Pseudomonas* or Proteus, require aggressive long-term therapy with specific anti-pseudomonal antibiotic agents.
4. Single appropriate therapeutic agents, rather than polypharmaceutical products, should be used. Most currently available products, however, are combination drugs containing one or more of the following: antibacterial, antiparasitic, antifungal, anti-inflammatory, cerumi-

---

TABLE 32–2
DRUGS USED IN TREATMENT OF OTITIS EXTERNA
Antibacterials
Antimycotics
Antiparasitics
Anti-inflammatories
Local anesthetics
Ceruminolytics/Cleansers

---

nolytic, or local anesthetic agents (Table 32–2). Nonetheless, selection of combination drugs should be rational for each condition. If a broad-spectrum antibiotic is used, an antifungal agent, such as nystatin, may have to be incorporated.

5. Topical otic corticosteroid products are normally indicated to treat the severe inflammation associated with otitis externa. Short-acting systemic corticosteroids may be indicated when severe inflammation, associated perhaps with a generalized dermatosis, is present. Systemic use of antimicrobials is indicated in animals displaying a febrile response.
6. Attention must always be paid to the possibility of tumors of the ear in any chronic case of otitis externa that does not respond to appropriate therapy. Sebaceous gland adenomas or adenocarcinomas, mast cell tumors, chondrosarcomas, fibrosarcomas, and papillomas all have been reported in dogs and cats.
7. Response to therapy should be monitored by regular examination of the ear and culturing and evaluation of cytologic smears.
8. Complete ear care and successful therapy are related to the quality of client education and the degree of client compliance. The importance of the client's role cannot be overstated.

Ear Cleaning/Examination

Detailed examination of the ear canal with an otoscope is necessary for diagnosis of otitis externa and evaluation of the extent of the disease process.

In severely inflamed or dirty ears, or with fractious animals, general anesthesia and syringing of the ear canal may be necessary. Such examination may reveal dark waxy material often associated with mite infestation or purulent discharges associated with infection. Purulent material should be swabbed and cultured when possible.

After thoroughly examining the animal, an otoscopic examination should be performed to assess the condition of the ear canal, the characteristics of the cerumen, the type of debris present, the condition of the tympanic membrane, and the degree of mite infestation.

Prior to commencement of therapy the ear must be thoroughly cleaned. Inadequate ear cleaning often leads to therapeutic failure. The cleaning process must be complete, but minimally irritating to the inflamed and infected ear.

Irrigation of the ear must be continued until all debris has been removed and the tympanum is visible. When using a suction bulb catheter or syringe, care must be exercised not to exert excessive pressure on the tympanum. A diseased eardrum easily ruptures, thereby leading to possible middle ear infection.

Ceruminolytic agents help to soften and emulsify secretions. After installation, the ear should be massaged to assist the distribution of the agent to help the overall cleaning process (Table 32–3).

Ceruminolytics can be instilled 3 to 4 times a day for 2 to 3 days. They are best given some minutes before the physical cleaning process. The ear can be cleaned by gentle irrigation of povidone-iodine solution or chlorhexidine diluted 1:3 with warm water. Particles of debris may have to be removed with an alligator forceps.

The ear canal must be thoroughly dried after the cleaning process. Irrigation fluid must be removed by gentle suction through a catheter. Cotton wool swabs or astringents, such as aluminum acetate or alcohol, facilitate the drying process.

Cleaning of the auditory canal must always precede antimicrobial therapy. Once the ear canal has been cleaned, the overall condition of the integument can be assessed.

Antibiotic Therapy

Topical antibiotic therapy is indicated for both primary and secondary bacterial infections. Culture and sensitivity testing are al-

| TABLE 32–3 |
| CLEANSERS/CERUMINOLYTICS/ |
| KERATOLYTICS |

Glycerin
Chlorhexidine
Povidone-iodine
Propylene glycol
Malic acid
Benzoic acid
Salicylic acid
Turpentine oil
Menthol
Sodium stearate
Sodium lauryl sulfate
Isopropanol
Squalene
Xanthan gum
Resorcinol

ways advisable to facilitate choice of the most appropriate and selective antimicrobial agent. Imprudent use of antibiotics can readily exert a selection pressure for resistant strains of the more pathogenic microorganisms. Resistance results from injudicious use of broad-spectrum antibiotics when more specific drugs with a narrow spectrum of activity might have sufficed.

In cases involving gram-positive cocci, otic preparations of neomycin, polymyxin, fucidin, gentamicin, thiostrepton, or chloramphenicol are indicated. For gram-negative rods, polymyxin, neomycin, or gentamicin should be considered. Anaerobes usually respond to penicillin G or tetracyclines (Table 32–4). (Metronidazole or clindamycin are drugs of choice for anaerobes.)

Topical corticosteroids are useful in the initial treatment process because they help to reduce inflammation, exudation, and glandular secretions. In the absence of a laboratory diagnosis, topical neomycin is a rational initial choice in conjunction with a topical corticosteroid, such as betamethasone, dexamethasone, prednisolone, or triamcinolone. By alleviating the inflammation, corticosteroids reduce the risk of self-inflicted injury and consequent exacerbation of the condition (Table 32–5).

TABLE 32–4
ANTIBACTERIALS USED TO TREAT OTITIS EXTERNA

General Choices:

Neomycin	Colistin
Chloramphenicol	Sulfacetamide
Cuprimyxin	Bacitracin
Cephalonium	Thiostrepton
Amoxicillin	Fusidate sodium
Penicillin G	Novobiocin
Streptomycin	

For Proteus/Pseudomonas:	*For Anaerobes*:
Gentamicin	Penicillin
Carbenicillin	Tetracyclines
Ticarcillin	Chloramphenicol
Amikacin	Metronidazole
Polymyxin B	Clindamycin
Tris buffered EDTA	
1–2% Acetic acid	
1% Silver sulfadiazine	

Neomycin combined with dexamethasone is a commonly used combination. Because organisms vary widely in their sensitivity, therapy should be based ideally on in vitro determination of the sensitivity of the strains involved. The same antibiotic is employed for both local and systemic therapy.

Chronic or resistant cases of otitis externa are usually caused by infections with *Proteus* and *Pseudomonas*, and such cases warrant intensive and aggressive therapy. *Proteus* and *Pseudomonas* species are resistant to most commonly used antimicrobial agents, including ampicillin, framycetin, tetracycline, chloramphenicol, and potentiated sulfonamides.

Topical preparations of polymyxin B or silver sufadiazine (1%) can be used in such instances, but usually specific potent antipseudomonal antibiotics, principally gentamicin (or carbenicillin, ticarcillin, amikacin), must be employed (see Table 32–3). Alternative options for *Pseudomonas* infections are topical 2% acetic acid or tris buffered EDTA.

Antibiotic therapy for most cases of otitis externa usually requires a minimum treatment period of 10 days. Chronic cases, especially those in which *Pseudomonas* is involved, may need a longer treatment period. Care should be exercised when using aminoglycosides because of their potential ototoxicity. Their long-term usage is contraindicated in patients with a ruptured tympanic membrane. The presence of pus can inactivate the sulfonamides and aminoglycosides, especially gentamicin. Thus, thorough ear cleaning is a necessary step prior to antibiotic medication. Concurrent use of ceruminolytics with antibiotic therapy is beneficial in many cases.

When infection is present within the ear canal, a necessary adjunct to antimicrobial

---

TABLE 32–5
ANTI-INFLAMMATORIES USED TO TREAT OTITIS EXTERNA

Betamethasone sodium phosphate
Dexamethasone sodium phosphate
Prednisolone
Hydrocortisone acetate
Triamcinolone acetonide in propylene glycol
Fluocinolone acetonide with DMSD

LOCAL ANESTHETICS

Benzocaine
Amethocaine
Promethazine
Lignocaine

therapy is the provision of improved drainage and ventilation by clipping and cleaning.

If the animal is febrile or the eardrum is inflamed, antibiotics should be administered parenterally for 5 to 7 days. Topical antibiotics and steroids should be continued for at least 7 days as deemed necessary by clinical and laboratory assessment.

Antiparasitic Therapy

When mites, especially *Otodectes*, are involved, treatment with parasiticides must continue for a minimum of 30 days because of the life cycle of the parasite.

Instillation of mineral oil or a ceruminolytic agent into the ear canal followed by gentle massage kills many of the parasitic mites and cleans the ear canal at the same time.

Once a thorough cleansing has been performed, a miticide, such as rotenone, pyrethrin, benzene hexachloride, dimethyl phthalate, or thiabendazole, can be applied. A ceruminolytic combined with a miticide can be effective. Because mites do not like moisture, oily solutions can also be quite effective by killing the parasites and mechanically flushing them out of the ear. Some proprietary otic preparations are miticidal by "drowning" and flushing out the mites.

Otodectes cynotis can inhabit sites on the skin other than the ear canal and may cause an immediate hypersensitivity reaction. A diagnosis is usually easy to make because the mites are easy to see on ear swabs and can occasionally be seen during otoscopic examination.

Traditional therapy has consisted mainly of commercial otic medications, such as thiabendazole (Tresaderm), carbaryl (Mitox Liquid), rotenone in oil (Canex Solution), or a combination of amitraz (Mitaban Liquid Concentrate) and mineral oil (Table 32–6).

Ivermectin has been used with no apparent side effects to treat ear mite infestation in cats. It is extremely effective in eliminating almost all mites. Reported doses range from 200 to 400 µg/kg of Ivomec (ivermectin) 1% Injection for Cattle; injections are given subcutaneously and repeated in 2 weeks. This is an extra label use and is not recommended by the manufacturer. Treatment of mites, however, must not be re-

---

TABLE 32–6
ANTIPARASITICS USED TO TREAT MITES

Xenodine polyhydroxydine
Rotenone
Thiabendazole
Pyrethrins
Piperonyl butoxide
Carbaryl
Lindane (gamma benzene hexachloride)
Monosulfiram
Benzyl benzoate
Amitraz
Ivermectin

---

stricted solely to the parasites within the ear canal; the entire body of the animal must be treated also. Infested animals, and animals living on the same premises, must be treated weekly to kill mites living outside the ear canal. Such treatment prevents a reservoir of infection from developing. Because ear mites are not species specific, clients must be instructed to treat all animals and to continue topical miticide therapy for at least 30 days.

Topical flea control products in the form of a powder dip or foam can be used to treat the entire body and to prevent reinfection from mites living outside the ears.

Antibiotics and steroid ointments may be necessary after such treatment to attend to the accompanying inflammatory and infectious changes. A protective astringent or ointment should be applied if the epithelium is acutely inflamed, hyperemic, and raw.

Antimycotic Therapy

Aspergillus, Penicillium, and *Rhizopus* molds are found in both diseased and healthy ears, as are yeasts, such as *Pityrosporum* and *Monilia.*

Significant growth of yeasts and fungi is likely when the internal microclimate of the ear canal is altered, thereby favoring their proliferation. Many bacterial infections favor yeast growth by increasing the pH of the ear canal. The fungi/yeasts must be killed and the underlying cause eliminated

TABLE 32–7
ANTIMYCOTICS USED TO TREAT
OTITIS EXTERNA

Imidazoles:
 Miconazole
 Thiabendazole
 Clotrimazole
Cuprimyxin
Nystatin
Amphotericin B
Povidone iodine
Acetic acid
Chlorhexidine
Natamycin
Thimerosal
Tannic acid

TABLE 32–8
IRRIGATING/CLEANING/DRYING
SOLUTIONS

Active Ingredient
Chlorthymol
Malic benzoic salicylic acids in alcohol
Polyhydroxydine solution
Isopropanol
Alcohol boric acid
Propylene glycol
Chlorhexidine 2%
Cetrimide 0.5%
Acetic acid 2% in aluminum acetate
5% Acetic acid 2% colloidal sulfur
5% hydrocortisol acetate 40% alcohol
Menthol
Povidone iodine 1%
Sodium stearate/sodium lauryl sulfate
Also
Warm Water
Isotonic saline
Hypertonic 3% saline

TABLE 32–9
CERUMINOLYTICS

Active Ingredient
Squalene
Glycerin
Docusate sodium solution
Dioctyl sodium sulfosuccinate,
ureaperoxide, lidocaine
Carbamide peroxide
Dioctyl sodium sulfosuccinate
Dioctyl calcium sulfosuccinate
Triethanolamine polypeptide oleate

to successfully treat the otitis. Although *Malassezia pachydermatis* (*Pityrosporum canis*) is undoubtedly the most significant of these organisms, sometimes *Candida* and *Aspergillus* can be isolated as pathogens also.

Topical application of products containing miconazole, nystatin, thiabendazole, or clotrimazole are indicated for superficial fungal and yeast problems. *Malassezia* infections can be treated also with cuprimyxin, acetic acid and tannic acid. In many fungal infections, a lowering of the local pH may be sufficient to effect a marked clinical improvement (hence, the use of lactic acid or sometimes cultures of lactobacillus organisms).

With fungal infections (otomycosis), treatment requires elimination of moisture and humidity from the ear canal. Ventilation of the canal must be ensured, and the interior must be cleansed of all scaly deposits by using alcoholic phenylmercuric nitrate solution (1:1500). Fungicidal ointments or thymol should be applied (Tables 32–7, 32–8, 32–9). In chronic cases of otitis externa, aural resection may be necessary to ensure adequate constant ventilation and drainage.

SUGGESTED REFERENCES

For Suggested References, see Chapter 33, "Pyoderma & Flea Infestation."

PYODERMAS AND FLEA INFESTATION

33.1 Canine Pyoderma
33.2 Types of Pyoderma
33.3 Treatment of Pyoderma
33.4 Antimicrobial Therapy
33.5 Therapy of Specific Pyodermas
      Flea Infestation
33.6 Classes of Insecticides
33.7 Insecticidal Formulations
33.8 Principles of Therapy: The Environment
33.9 Principles of Therapy: The Animal
33.10 Miscellaneous Skin Therapy

33.1 CANINE PYODERMA

Pyoderma is a bacterial infection of the skin in dogs. Although common, pyoderma is frequently misdiagnosed or improperly treated. Quite often, a presumptive diagnosis of another disease, such as flea allergy, food allergy, atopy, or seborrhea, obscures the identification of a secondary pyoderma. Factors predisposing to the development of pyoderma tend to be local rather than systemic. Underlying causes can include pendulous skin folds, atopy, pressure points, hypothyroidism, demodicosis, various hypersensitivities to dietary constituents, ectoparasites or contact allergens, or hyperadrenocorticism. Poor grooming practices, immunoincompetence, and injudicious use of corticosteroids may be other contributory factors. Pyoderma results when trauma and tissue damage from differing sources permit subcornual penetration of pathogenic bacteria and their subsequent colonization in sufficient numbers.

Staphylococci are the major causative organisms of skin pyodermas. Although coagulase-positive *Staphylococcus aureus* was originally believed to be the primary pathogen, the coagulase-positive *S. intermedius* is now regarded as perhaps the major causative agent.

In deep pyodermas with mixed bacterial infections, secondary invaders, such as *Escherichia coli*, *Proteus*, and *Pseudomonas*, are also involved. Anaerobic organisms, such as clostridia and *Bacteroides fragilis*, may be found in abscesses, deep fistulous tracts, and devitalized tissues.

Pyoderma may be classified by location, depth of infection, whether the bacteria are primary or secondary, and types of invading organisms. Pyodermas are generally categorized as surface, superficial, or deep. The deeper the level of infection, the more difficult the condition is to treat and the more aggressive the chosen therapy must be.

Immunodeficiencies often lead to skin infections and eruptions. The cutaneous infections most likely to follow, from an immunodeficiency are deep bacterial pyodermas. In dogs, pyoderma is most frequently caused by *Staphylococcus intermedius*; in cats, the most common pathogens are *S. intermedius* and *S. aureus*. Pyodermas in immunocompromised dogs also involve gram-negative bacteria (e.g., *Proteus*, *Pseudomonas*, *Escherichia coli*).

33.2 TYPES OF PYODERMA

SURFACE PYODERMAS

This type of pyoderma involves infection of the outermost layer of the skin with generally minimal bacterial involvement, e.g., acute moist dermatitis. The common underlying causes include flea allergy dermatitis (Table 33–1).

Only the superficial skin layers are involved in surface pyodermas. Bacterial infection in such cases extends through the epidermis to the dermis and hair follicle. It is an inflammatory reaction involving primarily the epidermis, where colonization but not severe invasion occurs. Lesions are usually secondary to irritation or trauma.

TABLE 33–1
POSSIBLE UNDERLYING CAUSES OF PYODERMAS

SURFACE PYODERMAS	SUPERFICIAL PYODERMAS	DEEP PYODERMAS
Flea allergy	Flea allergy	Demodicosis
Otitis externa	Food allergy	Dermatophytes
Superficial wounds	Seborrhea	Hypothyroidism
Anal sac impaction	Malnutrition	Immunosuppression
Bad grooming	Hypothyroidism	Corticosteroids
Anatomic defects	Unhygienic surroundings	

Acute moist dermatitis, skinfold pyoderma, juvenile pyoderma and interdigital pyoderma are examples of this surface infection.

Acute moist dermatitis can occur secondary to self-inflicted trauma from pruritus and is common in longhaired breeds. The presence of ectoparasites, otitis externa, or bacterial hypersensitivity, contributes to lesion formation.

Skin fold pyodermas occur in breeds with exaggerated skin folds, e.g., spaniels and setters. Whereas juvenile pyoderma occurs most frequently in pups younger than 4 months of age. Interdigital pyoderma consists of interdigital cysts, which can become suppurative with fistulous tracts.

SUPERFICIAL PYODERMAS

Superficial pyodermas are among the most common bacterial skin diseases. Often, intense pruritus, without marked skin changes, and the presence of some pustules or papules are evident. In such infections, bacterial involvement extends to the level of the intact hair follicle. Impetigo and folliculitis are examples of superficial pyodermas.

DEEP PYODERMAS

Deep pyodermas involve bacterial infections deeper than the hair follicles. Immunodeficiency, demodicosis, hypothyroidism, or hyperadrenocorticism may be predisposing causes.

Deep pyodermas begin as superficial pyodermas, and deep-seated infections occur as a result of the formation of fistulous tracts. Pruritus can be variable, but deep pyodermas tend to become diffuse and can spread widely. Improper use of corticosteroids can result in deep pyoderma.

33.3 TREATMENT OF PYODERMA

Any successful therapeutic strategy must be built not only on treating the bacterial pathogens involved, but also on identifying and treating predisposing factors when such exist (Table 33–2).

The underlying cause must always be identified if the condition is to respond favorably to pharmacologic therapy. Demodicosis is often overlooked, thus resulting in failure of antimicrobial treatment. Other underlying causes, such as hypothyroidism, atopy, or immune-related diseases, should always be investigated.

Hypersensitivity reactions to ectoparasites or to staphylococci, by way of repeated infections, may appear as erythematous papules, cysts, or pustules, which can rupture to produce unsightly lesions. The host response to staphylococci and staphylococcal products, such as protein A, can prematurely initiate the cascade of comple-

---

TABLE 33–2
PRINCIPLES OF PYODERMA THERAPY

- Treat underlying cause
- Use correct dosage rate of correct antibiotic
- High dose rates commensurate with safety are usually required
- Maintain therapy for adequate duration of time (weeks)
- Ensure high oral bioavailability of antibiotic
- Avoid corticosteroids unless absolutely necessary
- Choose narrow-spectrum antibiotics
- Avoid beta lactamase-susceptible antibiotics
- Coagulase-positive staphylococci are present in most cases
- Avoid use of narrow safety margin antibiotics
- Avoid antibiotics susceptible to beta-lactamase cleavage
- Immunosuppression may be present—avoid bacteriostatic drugs in such cases
- Surface pyodermas may not require antibiotics—use topical antiseptic formulations
- Examine each case for presence of possible underlying cause

ment, thereby producing inflammation and intense pruritis.

The response of the host animal to bacterial skin invasion is also determined by the presence of other inflammatory mediators, such as leukosidin, hemolysin, and epidermolytic toxin. Such hypersensitive responses to staphylococcal products can adversely affect the permeability of the skin barrier, thus promoting the inward migration and colonization of bacteria.

Susceptibility to infection is increased once the immune system has become compromised. Contributory factors may include defects within the complement system itself or deficiencies of neutrophil or lymphocyte production. Inherited complement deficiency syndrome and the granulocytopathy syndrome have been associated with the Brittany Spaniel and Irish Setter breeds, respectively.

Improper use of corticosteroids topically and parenterally can be a primary cause of the persistence of superficial pyodermas, especially those associated with flea allergy. Corticosteroids, although often used, may actually exacerbate deep pyodermas as a result of possible links with immunodeficiency.

Although corticosteroids may symptomatically reduce or arrest pruritis, they do not cure skin disease. They are contraindicated in treatment of superficial or deep pyodermas. By producing a false sense of security with a temporary alleviation of clinical symptoms, they may lead to incorrect associated treatment or premature cessation of therapy. They are also immunosuppressant, and immunoincompetence can be a key factor in many clinical subjects. Steroids reduce the inflammatory response and the production of sebum, thus favoring the spread of infection. When steroids are withdrawn, a rebound effect often is seen with a consequent worsening of the infectious process.

When therapeutically indicated, glucocorticoids should be used in the smallest dosage possible, preferably employing short-acting steroids, such as prednisolone, on an alternate-day basis to minimize unwanted side effects. Long-acting steroids, high dosage rates, and repository formulations must be avoided. The long-term use of steroids should be restricted to accurately diagnosed steroid-responsive conditions for which their use can be justified, e.g., atopy. Appropriate antibiotic therapy to treat pruritus should eliminate the underlying cause of skin infection, hence avoiding the necessity to resort to steroids, which mask symptoms and cause varied side effects.

Sometimes intense pruritus is associated with bacterial hypersensitivity, in such instances, systemic corticosteroids must be considered. If the pruritus responds dramatically to steroid therapy, the primary cause may be flea, inhalant, or food allergy with an accompanying secondary pyoderma.

Immunotherapy can be considered when relapses occur after antibiotics are withdrawn. Immunostimulants have been used with varying effects to augment immune function in severe pyoderma. Levamisole has been used in the dog at a dose of 2 mg/kg on alternate days. Levamisole has a narrow safety margin in the dog, and doses in excess of 2 mg/kg on alternate days may induce immunosuppression. Vomiting, salivation and bronchoconstriction/dyspnea are signs of levamisole toxicity.

Cimetidine, a H_2 blocker for ulceration, has been recommended for staphylococcal pyoderma in dogs at a dose of 3 to 4 mg/kg twice daily. It acts to block the H_2 receptors on lymphocytes. Although safer than levamisole, it is more expensive and requires long-term use.

Immunomodulatory bacterins have received by far the most extensive study. Staphage-lysate (SPL) is a commercially available staphylococcal bacterin product licensed for use in dogs. This lysate of *Staphylococcus aureus* does possess some immunostimulatory properties, especially in superficial pyodermas.

If an effective clinical response is not evident within 3–4 months, then the therapy must be discontinued.

Propionibacterium acnes bacterin, commercially available as Immunoregulin, is prepared from killed *P. acnes* (*Corynebacterium parvum*). This product has been available for many years as a nonspecific immunostimulant, and at a dose of 0.25 to 2 ml intravenously twice weekly, it does provide beneficial adjunct treatment for recurrent pyoderma.

Levamisole is a nonspecific immune system stimulant, which increases phagocytosis by macrophages and stimulates antibody production. Levamisole can be given at a dose of 1 mg/lb on alternate days over a period of weeks to effect. Antibiotics can be given during the first 4 weeks of immunotherapy.

Staphylococcal vaccines containing determinants of *Staphylococcus aureus* and a bacteriophage stimulate populations of T and B cell lymphocytes. The usual dose of vaccine is 1 ml subcutaneously per week for 4 weeks followed by 2 ml subcutaneously per week for a further 4 to 8 weeks. If an effective response is not evident within 10 to 12 weeks, the therapy must be discontinued.

The most common reasons for therapeutic failure in cases of canine pyodermas involve a misdiagnosis, incorrect choice of antibiotic, incorrect dosage of antibiotic, inadequate duration of therapy, or injudicious use of corticosteroids.

Dosage errors with antibiotics are common; all dogs must be weighed prior to dosage computation. Therapy must be long enough to effect a full bacteriologic cure, not just an apparent clinical remission. For superficial pyodermas, antimicrobial therapy must be maintained for at least 3 weeks. In the case of deep pyodermas, duration of therapy is also long term, intensive, and aggressive. Antibiotics must be administered for at least 2 weeks after abatement of clinical symptoms.

As a general rule, narrow-spectrum antibiotics are preferable because of the long-term nature of therapy. The chosen agent must be available in a suitable oral formulation that displays high oral bioavailability with minimal side effects because treatment in most cases is on an outpatient basis. This renders the aminoglycosides of little use because they are not absorbed from the bowel. Because some animals may be immunodeficient, bactericidal antibiotics are preferable. Improper antibiotic administration is a common error. Deep infections require higher and longer dosage regimes. Therapy must be long enough to ensure complete bacteriologic cure rather than just transient regression. Because most superficial and deep pyodermas are secondary in origin, the central objective of therapy is to find the underlying cause and to treat it successfully.

Deep pyodermas can be difficult to recognize, and the depth of infection necessitates prolonged therapy. These pyodermas run deeper than the level of the hair follicle and include furunculosis, cellulitis, nasal pyodermas, and anal furunculosis. Infections in deep-seated dermatoses, skin wounds, and abscesses require systemic and oral antimicrobial therapy combined with debridement, drainage, and palliative measures as necessary. In cases of deep pyoderma, skin scrapings must always be taken to check for demodicosis. Insufficient dosages of antibiotics for insufficient periods of time may also result in failure, thus allowing progression from superficial to deep pyodermas.

33.4 ANTIMICROBIAL THERAPY

Antimicrobial therapy is the essential component of any treatment program for superficial and deep pyoderma.

Canine pyoderma is the most common staphylococcal infection. Because staphylococci are commonly beta-lactamase producers, the antibiotic sensitivity pattern of *Staphylococcus intermedius* is crucial to successful therapy. More than 50% of staphylococcal isolates usually are resistant to beta lactam antibiotics. The incorporation of clavulanic acid, however, ensures activity against beta-lactamase-producing strains.

Successful therapy of skin pyoderma requires high dosage of antibiotic over a relatively long period of time. The severity of the condition and depth of skin involved largely determine the type of treatment needed. Duration of therapy usually extends for a minimum of 10 days, and often for 3 to 4 weeks, to completely eliminate the infection.

Topical therapy with such antiseborrheic agents as benzoyl peroxide, povidone iodine, or chlorhexidine should usually accompany antimicrobial therapy (Table 33–3).

The presence of pus in the affected lesions and the relatively poor perfusion and distribution of many antibiotics into the skin

---

TABLE 33–3
USEFUL ANTIMICROBIAL DRUGS FOR CANINE PYODERMA

ANTIBIOTIC	ORAL DOSE RATE
Amoxicillin-Clavulanate	14 mg/kg, twice daily
Amikacin	5 mg/kg, three times a day
Cefadroxil	10–20 mg/kg, twice daily
Cephalexin	22 mg/kg, twice daily
Chloramphenicol	50 mg/kg, three times a day
Erythromycin	10–15 mg/kg, three times a day
Gentamicin	2 mg/kg, three times a day
Lincomycin	20 mg/kg, twice daily
Nafcillin	20 mg/kg, three times a day
Ormetoprim/Sulfadimethoxine	27 mg/kg, once a day
Oxacillin	10–20 mg/kg, three times a day
Trimethoprim-Sulfadiazine	30 mg/kg, twice daily
Enrofloxacin	2.5 mg/kg, twice daily
Clindamycin	5.5–11 mg/kg, twice daily

---

are critical factors to be taken into account. Some antimicrobial compounds are less active in the presence of pus. Anaerobic organisms require specific treatment.

Mild superficial pyodermas must be treated for a minimum of 10 days, whereas deeper infections, such as folliculitis, require 3 to 4 weeks of intensive antimicrobial therapy.

In deep chronic pyodermas, especially those involving bacterial hypersensitivity, maintenance of therapy for weeks beyond the date of apparent clinical cure is usually essential.

Therapy may be empirical or, preferably, based on the results of bacterial culture and sensitivity tests. The most likely effective antimicrobial drugs include oxacillin, clavulanate potentiated amoxicillin, trimethoprim-sulfonamide combinations, lincomycin, erythromycin, enrofloxacin, chloramphenicol, cephalexin, and cefadroxil. Potentiated sulfonamides, erythromycin, and chloramphenicol are useful in empirical therapy. Penicillins, ampicillins, amoxicillins, and tetracyclines are usually poor choices because beta-lactamase production increases the risk of bacterial resistance.

Many strains of *Staphylococcus* are sensitive to chloramphenicol, clindamycin, erythromycin, fluoroguindones, lincomycin, and potentiated sulfa drugs. Amoxicillin clavulanate oxacillin, lincomycin, clindamycin, and cephalexin are excellent choices both for initial and for long-term therapy. Bactericidal antibiotics are a better choice than bacteriostatics because of the compromised immune system and the possible use of steroids.

Although narrow-spectrum drugs are preferable, medium- or broad-spectrum antibiotics may be necessary to treat mixed infections. Pending the results of sensitivity tests, initial antimicrobial therapy must be directed at the most likely pathogens—staphylococci and streptococci.

First-line antibiotics include lincomycin, clindamycin, erythromycin, potentiated sulfonamides, and amoxicillin-clavulanate. In severe deep pyodermas, cephalexin can be highly effective. Clindamycin penetrates better than lincomycin. Colitis is not seen with this drug in the dog, although it is in man.

When staphylococcal infection is suspected and an initial empirical regimen must be instituted prior to culture and sensitivity testing, beta-lactamase-resistant penicillins, such as cloxacillin, oxacillin, dicloxacillin, nafcillin, or potentiated penicillins provide excellent therapeutic benefit.

Gastric acid degradation is minimal, and absorption from the alimentary tract is good.

Semisynthetic penicillins, such as ampicillin or amoxicillin, may be useful when gram-negative involvement is substantial. These compounds, however, are also inactivated by beta-lactamase. If sensitivity culturing patterns indicate their potential usefulness, ampicillin or amoxicillin can be used. Because they are stable to gastric acid, oral medication can be instituted.

Resistance to beta lactam antibiotics occurs via decreased drug penetration into the bacteria, intracellular enzymatic drug inactivation, and development of alternative enzymatic pathways.

Clavulanate potentiated amoxicillin protects amoxicillin from degradation by staphylococcal beta-lactamase and, hence, is the most preferable semisynthetic penicillin with broad-spectrum activity. The most effective beta lactam antimicrobials are those of the beta lactam class that are resistant to inactivation by beta-lactamase. These can be subdivided into 3 groups: (1) amoxicillin combined with beta-lactamase inhibitor clavulanic acid, (2) first-generation cephalosporins (cephalexin, cephalothin), and (3) beta-lactamase-resistant penicillins (cloxacillin, dicloxacillin).

Many of the cephalosporins are highly effective against *S. intermedius*, *Proteus*, and *Pseudomonas*. Cephalexin is particularly useful for deep pyoderma, and many apparently refractory cases respond to it. Because of the cross-allergenicity that exists between cephalosporins and penicillins, extreme caution must be exercised when using cephalosporins in animals with suspected hypersensitivity to penicillin molecules. Some of the modern third-generation cephalosporins, such as moxalactam, are best reserved for specific cases necessitating systemic therapy.

Cephalexin is indicated for deep pyodermas because of the severity of the condition, the sensitivity of *Staphylococcus aureus* to the antibiotic, and the safety of the drug at high dose rates for lengthy periods (500 mg twice daily orally). An initial 3-week period of therapy for deep pyoderma must be maintained before re-evaluating or changing the antibiotic.

Macrolide antibiotics (e.g., erythromycin) possess a directed spectrum against gram-positive bacteria, including the staphylococcal group. Erythromycin is a reliable antibiotic against coagulase-positive staphylococci; a high proportion of isolates are usually sensitive to erythromycin. It may be given systemically or, more commonly, orally over a long-term period. Vomiting has occasionally been associated with the oral dosage form. Erythromycin and trimethoprim-sulfadiazine possess good ability to penetrate cells.

Of the lincosamides, lincomycin alone scores highly as a drug of choice for many chronic nonresponsive bacterial skin conditions. It is often a successful agent in clinical conditions for which many other antibiotics have failed. Highly effective against staphylococci and streptococci, lincomycin is potent against skin pathogens responsible for chronic dermatitis. Although suppurative lesions caused by pyogenic bacteria are resistant to many of the beta lactam antibiotics, lincomycin is effective in many such cases and penetrates tissues effectively.

Erythromycin and lincomycin are suitable choices for first-line therapy, although resistance to them can develop. Clindamycin has been approved for veterinary use for therapy of not only staphylococcal infection but also anaerobes.

Both clindamycin and lincomycin are well distributed throughout most body tissues, including skin, bones, and teeth, and thus are suitable for treating infected wounds, abscesses, and skin infections.

The fluoroquinolones, which include enrofloxacin and ciprofloxacin, are potentially useful drugs for staphylococcal pyoderma because of their excellent absorption from the gut, large volume of distribution, unique mechanism of action, and broad spectrum of antimicrobial action. Quinolones work especially well in deep pyodermas (and most infections of the epidermis). However, enrofloxacin possesses side effects. It causes arthropathies in puppies and must not be used in pups under 8 months of age, hence, other drugs might be preferred as a first choice.

Aminoglycoside antibiotics are not commonly indicated for pyodermas because of their narrow gram-negative spectrum of action, the likelihood of toxicity, and the possibility of the rapid induction of resistance. Gentamicin possesses high activity against staphylococci, *Proteus*, *Pseudomonas*, and *Escherichia coli*, and if employed judiciously, it may control many infections where secondary *Pseudomonas/Escherichia coli* invasion is causing a problem.

Although aminoglycosides (gentamicin, streptomycin, amikacin, and tobramycin) display good in vitro sensitivity to causative organisms; they are however impractical choices for therapy because they are not absorbed from the gut and they can be quite toxic on long-term therapy.

If staphylococci and *Proteus* are involved, broad-spectrum therapy is indicated. Trimethoprim-sulfonamides, clavulanate potentiated amoxicillin, and cephaloxin are especially useful.

Potentiated sulfonamides combinations are a popular and reasonably inexpensive choice for first-time treatment of pyoderma. Potentiated sulfonamides, e.g., trimethoprim-sulfadiazine in oral or parenteral form, provide high skin concentrations, and because of their broad spectrum of activity against staphylococci and gram-negative rods, they have been extensively and successfully used in canine pyodermas. Trimethoprim-sulfonamides combinations should not be employed for longer than 4 weeks because of the risk of development of keratoconjuctivitis sicca.

Potentiated sulfonamides are well absorbed from the gut and well distributed to the tissues. In cats, megaloblastic anemia may occur when high dosages of the drug are given over the long term. Treatment with folic acid (2.5 mg/kg/day) counteracts this effect.

In summary, lincomycin, erythromycin, and oxacillin are the preferred narrow-spectrum antibiotic agents. In the event of mixed infections, potentiated sulfonamides, clavulanate-amoxicillin, or chloramphenicol should be considered. Cephalexin is effective if laboratory investigation has indicated its selection. Cephalexin, oxacillin, clindamycin, and fucidin penetrate well into fresh abrasions. Dapsone, a useful compound for superficial pyodermas, reaches higher concentrations in diseased rather than normal skin.

Gentamicin, amikacin, carbenicillin, or ticarcillin should be reserved for pseudomonal infections. Anaerobic complications are best treated with metronidazole clindamycin, or as with penicillin or tetracycline, the cheaper alternatives.

Although for many clinical presentations some improvement can be noted in as few as 7 to 14 days, antimicrobial therapy normally must be maintained for at least 3 weeks and, in extreme chronic cases, possibly for 10 weeks.

Tetracyclines are not a good routine choice for pyoderma because of staphylococcal resistance to them. Doxycycline is a better choice.

33.5 THERAPY OF SPECIFIC PYODERMAS

Surface pyodermas, such as acute moist dermatitis, often respond to the elimination of the underlying factors (e.g., flea allergy). Skin scrapings should be taken to examine for the possible presence of demodicosis or occult neoplasia. Deep furunculosis may be present in some breeds. Uncomplicated surface pyodermas require palliative therapy, including clipping, cleansing, and topical application of a corticosteroid cream in conjunction with systemic corticosteroid therapy for several days.

Antibacterial shampoos commonly contain benzoyl peroxide, organic iodine compounds, chlorhexidine, or triclosan as active ingredients. Benzoyl peroxide has a relatively long residual activity on the skin (48 hours approximately). Chlorhexidine possesses residual activity for about 24 hours.

Although iodine compounds are widely used topically, they can be quite irritant, and their activity is reduced in the presence of organic matter. When the pyoderma is on the surface and quite mild, shampooing with 3% benzoyl peroxide (twice weekly) may be adequate.

Benzoyl peroxide shampoos are useful for many surface pyodermas, including skin fold pyoderma. In cases of acute moist dermatitis, systemic antibiotics, a bucket or Elizabethan collar, and corticosteroid may be necessary. Ectoparasites, otitis externa, or bacterial hypersensitivity may induce a pruritic reaction, and if the pruritis is intense, systemic corticosteroids may be needed for 2 to 5 days. Food allergies, inhalant pollen antigens, or hypothyroidism should not be overlooked as predisposing causes if the condition recurs frequently.

Impetigo, a superficial pyoderma, rarely necessitates systemic antibiotics. Topical application with a soap incorporating hexachlorophene or chlorhexidine is often successful.

Juvenile pyoderma often responds to systemic antibiotic therapy and prednisolone therapy (0.25 to 0.5 mg/lb/day). Cleansing of lesions with warm water and hexachlorophene can be beneficial. The dosage of prednisolone should be gradually decreased and ultimately phased out over a 2 to 3 week period.

Skin fold pyoderma associated with moisture, inflammation, and offensive odor should be treated with topical drying agents. Topical clindamycin sulfate solution (s.i.d.) can be beneficial with or without corticosteroid application.

Nasal pyoderma is best treated with systemic antibiotics, such as oxacillin or cephalexin. Cleansing of the lesions with warm water and chlorhexidine or povidone iodine solutions is indicated also. As with many skin infections, self-inflicted trauma may occur. The use of an Elizabethan collar or bucket may be necessary.

Occasionally, if cases are refractory to antimicrobial treatment, dermatophytes, such as *Trichophyton mentagrophytes*, should be checked out as predisposing factors.

Staphylococci are often isolated from interdigital pyodermas and narrow-spectrum beta-lactamase-resistant antibiotics should be administered systemically if the case is identified as a primary pyoderma. Fluoroquinolones (enrofloxacin) can also be useful here. The possibility of mite infestation should not be overlooked, nor should involvement of hypothyroidism, hypersensitivity, or immunodeficiency.

Marked pruritus, papules, and skin changes are common features of superficial pyodermas. Superficial pyodermas do not automatically dictate choice of an antibiotic agent. Such skin infections usually respond adequately to topical antiseptics, such as hexetidine or chlorhexidine shampoos, lotions, or creams. These possess a wide antibacterial range and are cheaper than antibiotics. Mild antiseptic soaps or washes containing chlorhexidine are adequate for topical treatment of impetigo.

For many superficial infections, the topical application of antibiotics rarely used systemically—neomycin, polymyxin B—is favored. Alternatively oral and parenteral antibiotic therapy for 3 or 4 weeks may be required, and topical dressing of the lesions with benzoyl peroxide shampoos is a beneficial palliative measure.

Refractory or recurrent cases should be further investigated to reveal potential underlying problems. Atopy, seborrhea, hypothyroidism, inflammatory disease, or incorrect usage of corticosteroids may be implicating factors. Impairment of host defense mechanisms can cause many conditions to recur.

Seborrhea is a chronic skin disease characterized by a defect in keratinization with increased scale formation. Changes in the nature and flow of sebum result in the reduction of the normal defense mechanism of the skin against potential disease-causing bacteria, e.g., *Staphylococcus intermedius*. Such bacteria then colonizes the skin, thereby causing pustules, inflammation, and itching. Seborrhea can result from ectoparasites, pyoderma, fungal infection, allergy, local irritants, neoplasia, or environmental factors. Therapy involves killing bacteria, thus eliminating infection, removing excessive oil or grease, and reducing inflammation, scaling, and itching.

Benzoyl peroxide is a broad-spectrum antibacterial follicle-flushing agent that possesses some antipruritic and antifungal activity. Its degreasing and keratolytic properties help to treat various pyodermas and seborrhea. This non-steroidal, topical agent removes excess sebum, removes dead skin (keratolytic), is bactericidal, can be used long-term, and is antipruritic.

Superficial burns often become contaminated with staphylococci, *Proteus*, and *Pseudomonas*. A localized infection after such trauma can often become septicemic. Application of a 1% cream of silver sulfadiazine is useful against *Pseudomonas* and yeasts and does not appear to interfere with subsequent healing. Parenteral gentamicin may be necessary to complement topical therapy.

In deep pyodermas, various underlying problems are likely, and their occurrence can be a sequela to hypothyroidism or immunoincompetence. Demodicosis is an important consideration in the cause of deep pyoderma. Recurrence of deep pyoderma is common when underlying causes have not been identified. Long-term antibiotic therapy is mandatory and should be continued for at least 7 to 14 days beyond the adjudged clinical resolution of the condition.

Clipping of lesions and topical application of benzoyl peroxide shampoo, dilute iodine-povidone, or chlorhexidine solution are necessary supportive measures.

Immunomodulators, such as staphylococcal lysates or levamisole, 2 mg/kg orally on alternate days, although worthy of consideration are of debatable benefit.

When deep pyoderma is associated with *Pseudomonas* infection, therapy is restricted to gentamicin, ticarcillin, or carbenicillin because *Pseudomonas* is resistant to most other antibiotics. Gentamicin given by injection is a potentially toxic compound, and therapy should be limited to a maximum of 7 days.

Cats are frequently brought to the clinic with bite wounds or abscesses. Organisms commonly isolated from the mouths of cats (*Pasteurella multocida*, beta hemolytic streptococci, and fusobacterium) are contaminants of many such feline skin lesions. Short-term treatment with penicillin G Procaine, penicillin G benzathine, oral ampicillin or amoxicillin is usually sufficient in conjunction with debridement and surgical drainage.

FLEA INFESTATION

Fleas are the commonest cause of canine and feline skin disease, and many clinical problems can occur in association with flea infestation, e.g., pruritus, pyoderma, seborrhea, otitis externa, hypersensitivity reactions, and certain systemic changes. Dermatitis is common in temperate climates during the warmer months and is manifested by a transient pruritic dermatitis. In general terms, dogs with fleas can be subdivided into two major groups: (1) dogs with relatively uncomplicated flea infestation and (2) dogs with flea bite hypersensitivity. Although pruritis is common to both groups, the intensity and extent can be markedly different. The original work on guinea pigs suggested that the flea allergen was present in saliva and was a simple chemical (a hapten). The release of histamine from mast cells, which generates the

skin wheal, results from the bridging of two adjacent molecules of IgE on the mast cells' surface. This cannot be accomplished physically by a simple chemical of low molecular weight. A major fraction of the flea antigen is protein and has a molecular weight in excess of 5000.

When fleas bite, their mouthparts release small quantities of saliva that contains anticoagulants (to facilitate bloodsucking) and hyaluronidase and proteolytic enzymes. Some of the salivary components are antigenic or are haptenogenic but become antigenic following coupling with dermal collagen or other skin proteins. A low molecular weight hapten and at least two other larger allergens are known to be present in flea saliva.

Hypersensitivity reactions to flea saliva invoke type I (immediate—IgE mediated), type IV (delayed—lymphocyte mediated), and, possibly, cutaneous basophil hypersensitivity reactions. A late onset IgE mediated hypersensitivity is also involved.

If the dog has not previously been sensitized to the allergens in flea saliva, the response is minimal compared to the intense pruritus exhibited by dogs with flea bite hypersensitivity. In hypersensitive dogs, sensitization results in extreme diffuse irritation and considerable self-mutilation. Hypersensitivity may appear clinically as diffuse erythema, alopecia, seborrhea, lichenification, and recurring pyodermas. The intensity of the clinical signs is related more to the degree of hypersensitivity to flea saliva than to the number of fleas present.

The presence of a secondary pyoderma is of crucial importance in terms of therapeutic strategies employed. Secondary superficial pyodermas can often be misdiagnosed as ringworm or simply treated as an allergy. Sudden development of seborrhea is quite often the first indication that ectoparasites are involved.

One of the most common mistakes made in treating dogs with flea infestation is not recognizing the existence of a secondary pyoderma and using only corticosteroids to control the flea-induced pruritus. Flea control alone cannot curb the irritation caused by an underlying pyoderma. This condition must always receive specific antimicrobial therapy.

Although some dogs with flea infestation may show a generalized pruritus, more usually the pruritus is marked along the dorsum, with localized and associated excoriation in the interscapular and lumbar regions. A marked scratch reflex is present together with alopecia and thickening of the predilection sites.

In hypersensitive animals, one flea bite may produce extensive pruritus and reactivate latent lesions. Flea allergy dermatitis becomes more severe clinically as animals age, with common onset at 3 to 6 years.

Although fleas may be found on an animal of any age, the dramatic reactions seen in allergic individuals are uncommon in animals younger than 6 months of age because repeat exposure to the salivary antigen is a prerequisite for sensitization.

Many therapeutic strategies fail because of poor veterinarian-client communication followed by poor client compliance. Also, quite often the family cat is not treated and serves as a reservoir for infestation of the dog.

Client education is of acute importance in the initiation of any effective flea control scheme. Clients must be educated and instructed to read carefully the label instructions of dispensed insecticides. Quite frequently, toxicity can result from carelessness in use, improper dosage, or incorrect storage, especially with organophosphates. The importance of removing other pets (fish, rodents, birds) and children from the premises during environmental treatment must receive particular attention.

A control program is aimed at ridding both the animal and its environment of fleas and at preventing or minimizing reinfection.

Because fleas spend most of their life cycle in the environment, a suitable pesticide must be applied to sites where eggs, larvae, and pupae are found. The number of fleas present on any one animal is directly related to the rate that ectoparasitic reinforcements are acquired from the environment and the speed at which fleas are killed. Thus, insect growth regulators (methoprene) and controlled-release (microencapsulated) insecticides are of great value.

Sleeping quarters of the animal must be primary targets for application of insecticides because flea feces, eggs, larvae, and pupae accumulate there. Bedding must be washed or removed, and the entire area must be kept clean by scrupulous vacuum cleaning, paying particular attention to cracks, crevices, floors, and carpets. If pets are permitted to rest on furniture, the furniture should be regularly dusted with an appropriate insecticide.

Flea collars or powders can be placed in the vacuum cleaner bag to ensure killing of fleas. All animals in an owner's household should be treated for fleas. Selection of an insecticide and the proper vehicle of administration vary with the owner, the degree of infestation, and the nature of the animal.

The overall success of any treatment regime depends on the inherent potency of the insecticide used, the frequency and thoroughness of its application, its efficiency and residual properties the habits of the affected animal, and the environment in which it lives.

Clients must be informed of the role of fleas in the transmission of disease and of the possibility that several flea species found on dogs or cats may be transferred to humans.

Fleas also play a vital part in spreading tapeworms from one animal to another. The tapeworm *Dipylidium caninum* is the commonest tapeworm of dogs and cats and can also infect humans. The flea acts as an intermediate host for the tapeworm, and swallowing of infected fleas leads to tapeworm infestation in domestic pets. Thus, veterinarians and their clients must be fully aware of the zoonotic implications of flea infestation.

33.6 CLASSES OF INSECTICIDES

The primary desireable features of any acaracide for flea control include:

1) High safety margin
2) High selective toxicity
3) Residual activity
4) Quick knockdown and kill
5) Pleasant and odorless
6) Safe to puppies and especially cats
7) Convenience of application
8) Safe to the handler and young children
9) Affects many stages of the flea's life cycle
10) Safe near food, and in confined spaces

Major classes of insecticides include botanicals, organophosphates, chlorinated hydrocarbons, carbamates, synthetic pyrethroids, and insect growth regulators. These agents are available in the form of collars, shampoos, dusting powders, dips, aerosols, tablets, sprays, foggers, and sustained-release microencapsulated products.

BOTANICALS

These older products of plant origin include rotenone, derris, and pyrethrum. Botanical products generally degrade quickly to provide a rapid knockdown effect with minimal residual activity. Although rapidly acting, pyrethrins are very sensitive to light; their synthetic counterparts (pyrethroids) are significantly more photostable. Botanical agents possess a high safety margin, are rapidly metabolized, and less toxic to mammals. Insects cannot detoxify these compounds, and symptoms of central nervous system convulsions and paralysis follow. The pyrethroids are slightly more residual than are natural pyrethrins. Potentiation is achieved by incorporation of the synergistic agent piperonyl butoxide. Pyrethroids such as fenvalerate, resmethrin and permethrin offer increased stability and residual action.

Of the major classes pyrethrin is one of the desirable chemicals for flea control. Pyrethrin is highly insecticidal but labile when exposed to sunlight. Safe and rapid-acting, the efficacy of pyrethrin is enhanced by microencapsulation.

Rotenone, derived from derris and *Lonchocarpus* plant species, paralyzes insects by causing cardiovascular, neural, and respiratory depression in affected arthropods.

D-Limonene, an extract of citrus fruits, possesses insecticidal properties and were first developed into parasiticidal dip for small animals in the late 1970s. It is safe, and effective against all stages of the flea's life cycle, and does not have the residual property of microencapsulated pyrethrin.

ORGANOPHOSPHATES AND CARBAMATES

Organophosphates are toxic to insects by virtue of their ability to irreversibly bind acetylcholinesterase. Binding of the enzyme permits continued cholinergic stimulation in the affected parasite, which then becomes paralyzed. Organophosphate insecticides may be classed as aliphatic (linear structure), heterocyclic, or a phenyl derivative. Residual effects vary from slight for the aliphatics to significant for the heterocyclic compounds. Organophosphates produce a relatively stable drug-enzyme complex that may take days to dissociate, thus leading to a prolonged recovery. Carbamates possess a shorter duration of activity because the enzyme-carbamate complex is more susceptible to spontaneous dissociation.

Carbamates (Carbaryl, propoxur and Bendiocarb) are anticholinesterase residual pesticides that kill insects fairly rapidly. Carbaryl is one of the commonest carbamate insecticides. Toxicity varies according to the concentration used, and resistance is a possibility. Staining of fabrics and animal fur can result at high dosage levels. Propoxur is used in some flea collars.

Organophosphate toxicity can occur in domestic pets if they are exposed to overdosage or to simultaneous multiple use of this class of compound in the form of flea collars, sprays, dips, oral cythioate, or dichlorvos anthelmintics. Cats are particularly susceptible to organophosphates, and if these agents are to be used in cats, great caution should be exercised. Greyhounds also appear to be especially sensitive to organophosphate drugs.

Because toxicoses can be associated with the use of organophosphates and carbamates, clients must always be instructed to read all labels carefully for proper dilution and application instructions. The importance of accompanying environmental control must be stressed. Children must not have access to these potent and toxic pesticides.

Treatment of organophosphate toxicity involves intravenous administration of atropine to elicit mydriasis and cessation of salivation. Further doses of atropine at 1 to 5 mg/lb subcutaneously may need to be administered to effect as the individual case dictates.

Pralidoxime (2-PAM) is the specific antidote for organophosphate poisoning. Doses of 10 mg/kg are necessary every 4 to 6 hours in dogs for reactivation of the enzyme complex. Organophosphates possess a higher acute toxicity potential for domestic pets than that of organochlorines, and residual activity is less also.

Fenthion is a commonly used organophosphate that has been registered by the Environmental Protection Agency (EPA) as a pesticide and by the Food and Drug Administration (FDA) as a drug for use in livestock. Fenthion is a systemic insecticide and is excreted through the sebaceous glands. It is applied topically in "Spot-on" form in dogs and cats every 3 to 4 weeks. Because this lipid-soluble drug has appreciable potential for acute toxicity, gloves must be used when applying this compound. Owners must be notified of possible oil stain on the pet's coat and of the noxious odor following use of the drug. With fenthion, the specified label instructions must be adhered to strictly, animals must always be checked for heartworm, and other anticholinesterase products must be avoided. No side effects are to be expected following applications of the recommended dosages. In some cats, the typical smell of the active ingredient (a weak garlic-like odor) may cause salivation, restlessness, and defense responses. Incompatibility reactions to acute overdoses correspond to the symptoms of parasympathetic irritation. Spontaneous vomiting and diarrhea may occur. Neurologic symptoms with fibrillary muscular twitching in the head and neck regions are reversible. In normal circumstances, incompatibility reactions disappear without antidote therapy.

Administration of 0.2 to 0.5 mg/kg of atropine intravenously or intramuscularly treats acute toxicologic reactions in dogs and cats. If no effect occurs after 15 to 20 minutes following intramuscular application, the treatment should be repeated. Oximes should not be used to reactivate intoxicated cholinesterases, if necessary, until potentially fatal symptoms (bronchial spasms, laryngospasms) have been overcome. Obidoxime, 5 mg/kg, intravenously or intramuscularly, and pralidoxime, 10 mg/kg, intravenously or intramuscularly, are used to counter toxic reactions.

Cythioate is an organophosphate compound used orally for systemic control of fleas. It is normally given at a dose of 30 mg/20 lbs orally, or 1 ml (1.6% solution)/10 pounds body weight. As a rule, cythioate is inferior to fenthion for controlling signs of flea allergy dermatitis.

Cythioate is rapidly absorbed from the animal's stomach and intestine. When distributed to the skin, it kills fleas via the bite. Because cythioate is given orally, it has the advantage of accurate dosage. At an oral dose of 30 mg/20 lbs twice daily, cythioate can help to treat some cases of flea allergy dermatitis. Cythioate possesses a short half-life in dogs and is rapidly biodegraded. Cythioate is particularly useful when combined with the less acutely toxic botanical insecticides. The drug should not be used in Greyhounds or in stressed, pregnant, or postsurgical animals.

Malathion is a relatively safe organophosphate. It is one of the few organophosphates that can be used on cats. A noticeable odor may persist for 48 to 72 hours following its use. Other useful organophosphates include dichlorvos and fenitrothion. Like malathion and fenthion, these may be used in cats. Chlorpyrifos is a popular spray for topical use on dogs; it also may be used in the environment. Sometimes chlorpyrifos is combined with methoprene for insecticidal action against both adults and larvae.

Diazinon is a particularly potent organophosphate that is used in powdered form in premises for environmental control of small areas. For animal use, diazinon is available as a microencapsulated product.

CHLORINATED HYDROCARBONS

These are among the longest established of the synthetic pesticides (e.g., chlorophenothane [DDT], lindane). They are characterized by moderately low acute toxicity for mammals, but display high residual activity for insects. One of the great problems with the chlorinated hydrocarbon group is their tendency toward bioaccumulation and buildup in food chains. They may also be carcinogenic. They persist in body fat and in the environment for long periods of time. This class of chemical is being phased out in many countries, and a number of products have already been withdrawn, e.g., Bromocyclen. In insects, they affect motor neurons, thereby causing convulsions before death. Toxicity in mammals usually causes neurologic signs that may include hyperexcitability, seizures, and pyrexia.

Therapy for host toxicity is nonspecific and consists of the removal of the insecticide from the coat by bathing and also the prevention of subsequent absorption from the gastrointestinal tract by the use of activated charcoal, fluid therapy, and the barbiturates to control seizures. Many of the chlorinated hydrocarbons are toxic in cats, persisting in the adipose tissues for a long time before eventually being deactivated by the liver.

INSECT GROWTH REGULATORS

Insect growth regulators are hormone-like substances that influence metamorphosis and development of insects.

Two larvicides, methoprene and fenoxycarb, are available for the environment. Both prevent larval fleas from maturing into adults, and display long residual activity, up to 3 months.

Methoprene, a synthetic juvenile hormone, has been a significant breakthrough in the area of environmental control. Methoprene is degraded by sunlight and is only for indoor use, whereas fenoxycarb is more photostable and can also be used indoors. Because of its high residual potency and stability, methoprene possesses important applications in the environmental control of many insect pests. The application of methoprene as fog at an average rate of 3.6 mg/m^2 results in near total suppression of the emergence of adult fleas for considerable periods after application. Because methoprene cannot kill adult fleas, it is usually combined with pyrethrin for total control of premises.

Methoprene acts on the fourth instar larvae and prevents development to the pupal stage.

Insect growth regulators disrupt the endocrine balance and metabolic process in the invertebrate species. Such agents, when used for flea control, interfere with the normal progression of metamorphosis of the insect by disrupting development from the larval to the pupal stage. When combined with an adulticide, methoprene is an effective way to kill both adults and larvae and offers better premises control. Methoprene persists in the environment for up to 75 days if not removed.

33.7 INSECTICIDAL FORMULATIONS

Various formulations exist for flea control in dogs—dips, sprays, powders, shampoos, spot-ons, collars, microencapsulation, and oral (systemic) medication.

Agents for use as baths are in the form of shampoos, creams or emulsifiable concentrates. They are difficult to apply in cats. The shampoo usually is applied to dogs, and after rinsing with water, the animal is damp dried with a towel allowing the coat to dry naturally. Treatment is best repeated at 10 to 14 days (depending on the product).

Powders are generally safe to use on small animals and are also easy to apply. Some of them, however, if licked from the coat especially by cats can precipitate toxicity. The commonly used powders are those containing BHC permethrin, and Derris. Pybuthrin and permethrin are synthetic pyrethrins called pyrethroids and these are characterized by high insecticidal activity and low mammalian toxicity. Derris is another safe insecticide but which acts less rapidly and is less persistent than the pyrethrum family. Pyrethrin powder is usually applied every 7 to 10 days.

"Spot on" preparations such as Fenthion are applied to the skin in the interscapular area where they are absorbed. Some of these preparations can remain active up to 3 to 4 weeks. These can be used in dogs and cats; organophates can be toxic, and can be absorbed through the skin of the handler. Client education is important here.

Many insecticidal sprays are now on the market and while simple to apply they can cause some problems in cats. Inhalation can be a problem if used in confined spaces—the eyes and mouth must be avoided. Cats generally dislike sprays. Most sprays contain either organophosphates, carbamates or pyrethroids (fenvalerate, permethrin, cypermethrin). The manufacturer's instructions should be followed carefully when using sprays. Dichlorvos/fenitrothion should be sprayed from a distance of 6 to 8 inches. The manufacturers recommend raising the animal's coat first and then applying the spray from tail to head. It should be applied in a well ventilated atmosphere. Animals less than one month old should not be treated with organophosphates and the spray vapor should be kept well away from people, other animals, foodstuffs and fish.

Oral systemic medication usually involves organophosphates such as cythioate or ronnel in tablet form. Oral treatment is usually continued over a period of weeks. Most organophosphate products are not recommended for use in pregnant or sick animals and should not be used simultaneously with other cholinesterase inhibiting products such as flea collars.

Collars:

Several manufacturers have flea collars on the market. These are usually strips of polyvinyl chloride impregnated with volatile organophosphorous agents (either dichlorvos or diazinon), Carbamates (propoxur) or pyrethroids (fenvalerate, permethrin, Cypermethrin) on the animal's hair to contact the parasites. Care is necessary to prevent children's chewing or handling the collars. Contact dermatitis is sometimes a problem in the animal and the organophosphate collars should generally be removed before bathing. Organophosphates are contraindicated in sick, stressed or convalescing animals and also should not be used concurrently with other systemic organophosphates. Release rates vary for up to 4 to 5 months.

COLLARS

The insecticide in collars, is incorporated into a slow-release matrix (usually vinyl chloride plastic) giving a sustained release over a period of months. Vapor generators release volatile pesticides that recrystallize over the entire length of the animal's body and environment, e.g., dichlorvos. Such collars provide relatively uniform distribution of the insecticide over the generators releasing the drug as a dust in the neck area only, e.g., carbaryl. Liquid-release collars release drugs of low volatility (e.g., chlorpyrifos, diazinon), which are then distributed over the animal's body by movement and grooming.

Flea collars are popular because of their convenience. They are generally inade-quate, however, for the treatment of flea infestation associated with flea allergy dermatitis. Flea collars are usually ineffective as the sole means of flea control, and can cause local dermatitis.

Organophosphate flea collars or medallions provide activity for as long as 6 months, depending on the individual producer, but great care must be exercised in their use, especially when young children are present. The collar must be removed when bathing the animal.

EMULSIFIABLE CONCENTRATES

These agents are applied as dips, sprays, or sponging solutions for use on animals or premises. Oils are used as carriers; emulsifiers facilitate mixing of the active insecticide with water. Because they are more concentrated, they can also be more toxic.

Dips and sprays are still relatively popular. Dips are usually applied after a medicated bath. Dips containing potent insecticides should not be used on debilitated animals.

SPRAYS

Sprays contain both a solvent and a propellent system. Emulsifiers may be included if the insecticide is not soluble in the carrier used. In recent years, more attention has been paid by the regulatory authorities to the environmental impact of propellants used in aerosol sprays. Special additives may be incorporated in the formulation to retard or inhibit pesticide breakdown or degradation of the emulsification system.

Penetration of pesticides from spray preparations can be quite poor in long-haired breeds, and the hissing sound may frighten some animals, especially cats.

Quick-drying alcohol-based sprays appear to have a quicker knockdown effect, although the alcohol itself can be irritating to the animal's skin if used over the long term.

Topical spray products, when dispensed to the owner, are useful adjuncts in a flea control program, especially when augmented with dipping. Many aerosols evaporate quickly, however, and do not provide adequate concentration on the skin. As a rule, cats dislike sprays, and such applications should not be used in enclosed areas to avoid inhalation.

For pressured particulate delivery, hand-held pump sprays or mists achieve higher and more lasting concentration. Many organophosphates can be safely used in dogs and cats, once manufacturers' recommendations are followed, e.g., dichlorvos and fenitrothion.

Probably the safest sprays contain pyrethroids, pyrethrins, or carbamates. Pyrethroids, such as permethrin or fenvalerate, offer longer residual effects. D-Limonene or microencapsulated pyrethrins are often used in sprays. Pyrethrins and methoprene in spray form are particularly effective.

POWDERS

Dusting powders in which the active ingredient is mixed with talc or pyrophyllite clay are of low toxicity to the host animal. Inhalation of active ingredients or undue skin contact could be a problem for the applicator in some cases, especially in confined spaces. An advantage of dusting powders is that the area dressed with the insecticide can be visualized. Low skin absorption and slow evaporation rate render dusting powders suitable for light infestation. Powders or dust preparations, however, tend to dry the animal's coat unduly and fall off quickly into the environment.

Most available flea powders contain either carbamates or pyrethrins. Some insecticidal preparations contain desiccants, such as silica and diatomaceous earth, that cause chaffing to the insects cuticle and result in a leakage of body fluids.

CONTROLLED-RELEASE FORMULATIONS

Microencapsulation is a useful means of extending the effectiveness of rapidly acting insecticides, such as pyrethrins.

Although synergized pyrethrins, synthetic pyrethroids, carbamates, and organophosphates all have their place, new controlled-release formulations, such as microencapsulated agents, extend the residual effect of the active ingredient while reducing toxicity.

The process traps the insecticide within the small nylon or polyurea capsules. The active ingredient slowly diffuses through the capsule and is absorbed by the animal. Such microencapsulation technique increases the stability of the pyrethrins by providing controlled release for as many as 5 weeks on the animal or in the environment. This allows a safe, non-residual insecticide to become residual.

Microencapsulated pyrethrins using an interfacial polymerization reaction provide a stabilized polyurea shell around core material containing pyrethrin. Such microcapsules continue to release lethal doses of pyrethrins from 1 day to 5 weeks, depending on the concentration of active ingredient. The microcapsules adhere to carpets, furniture, bedding and fur, thereby allowing extended protection and release of insecticide.

Spray and foam formulations of microencapsulated pyrethrins provide a rate-controlled release of stable drug with high efficacy, high safety, and residual activity.

Microcapsules break down over a period of time. The drug is released by a process of diffusion, thereby resulting in a sustained outpouring of the active ingredient. With this technique, nonresidual material can be rendered residual, and accordingly, the risk of oral or other toxicity from accidental exposure is minimized. Diazinon is available in microencapsulated form to reduce acute toxicity and provide sustained effect.

When microencapsulated insecticides are used in combination with a rapid-acting product, fleas in the environment can be killed quickly and the microencapsulation technique extends duration of effect.

Microencapsulated pyrethrins prolong the activity of the active ingredient but may take 24 to 48 hours to act.

33.8 PRINCIPLES OF THERAPY: THE ENVIRONMENT

General therapy in the animal hinges on the eradication of fleas, along with other appropriate measures to control secondary pyoderma, pruritus, seborrhea, or pyotraumatic dermatitis. Additional therapy for flea control involves medical therapy to control pruritus and skin changes.

Any overall flea control program must be directed primarily against the elimination of flea infestation in the house, the outdoor premises, and on animals, including other animals in contact with the affected animal. Treatment must be prophylactic. The appearance of fleas on a household pet indicates that infestation of the premises has already occurred.

Failure of general therapy is usually the result of inadequate client communication and poor environmental control. Because most of the life cycle of the flea is spent off the host, environmental control must receive priority attention.

Environmental control must be aimed at reducing the infestation in the animal's bedding. (Paper or disposable bedding is desirable, especially for cats.) Weekly treatments must be continued over at least 1 month, bearing in mind that all the early stages of the flea live off the host. Only the adult flea is parasitic.

Environmental foggers and sprays contain various insecticides, including organophosphates, carbamates, pyrethrins, and pyrethroids. The home environment must be treated by a combination of powders, foggers, aerosols, hand-held pump sprays, or hand-held spray lamps. Use of combinations of insecticides possessing different mechanisms of action is preferable so that development of parasite resistance is minimized and all stages of the life cycle are attacked. Before environmental application of the insecticide, the entire premises should be thoroughly cleaned. Rugs and carpets require vigorous vacuum cleaning or steam cleaning.

For environmental control, residual sprays or 5 to 12% carbaril dust are useful. Synthetic pyrethroids are safe for the environment and, in combination with carbamates, provide an instantaneous kill with some residual activity.

In cases of flea bite hypersensitivity, every effort should be made to prevent reinfestation by regular dusting or spraying. Insecticide-impregnated strips suspended over the animal's basket may be a useful supportive measure.

Chlorpyrifos sprays for large outdoor areas, or an organophosphate dust (e.g.,

diazinon) for smaller areas, are useful for outdoor premises.

The frequency of environmental treatment depends on the degree of flea infestation and the type of products used. When malathion is used, the environment should be sprayed every 2 weeks for 3 treatment periods, and then monthly during the flea season.

The combination of an adulticide with methoprene reduces the need for frequent spraying. A useful regime with this combination requires treatment of the environment twice at weekly intervals and then repeat treatments every 2 to 3 months as needed.

Alternatively, methoprene plus a quick-kill and residual insecticide can be applied indoors followed in 2 to 3 weeks by a residual agent, such as chlorpyrifos. Numerous products now combine pyrethrins with insect growth regulators for control of every stage of the insect's life cycle.

Another safe and effective flea control program includes treatment of the pet with D-limonene and treatment of the environment with an adulticidal/larvicidal combination of microencapsulated pyrethrins and methoprene.

33.9 PRINCIPLES OF THERAPY: THE ANIMAL

The primary aim of therapy is removal of the parasite. Once the flea has been removed, the secondary problems caused by the infestation can be attacked. In terms of overall flea control, safe residual products are preferable to knockdown types.

In problem cases, combinations of insecticides possessing different modes and speed of action may be required to provide comprehensive control against the major stages of the parasite.

The formulation and method of application govern the kill rate, residual effect, and overall clinical activity of insecticides. For instance, when rapidly acting pyrethrins are microencapsulated, they possess a greater residual action and are less likely to be toxic. Flea control can be achieved using insecticidal powders, sprays, mists, or dips. Sprays, mists, and powders are applied by brushing the animal's hair backward and then applying the product to the skin. Many flea shampoos, although potent, lose much of their residual effect when rinsed off.

Dipping or bathing is the most thorough method of flea control. Rubber gloves should be worn to avoid contact with the drug. After bathing and wetting the coat, the dip is allowed to air dry on the animal without rinsing.

Depending on the manufacturer's recommendations, aerosols can be used 2 to 3 times per day, powders and dust preparations twice weekly, and mists and dips every 5 to 7 days.

When a flea problem exists in young animals, regular bathing with a mild insecticidal shampoo to remove fleas mechanically may suffice, together with specific pesticide treatment of the environment and the dam.

For routine insecticidal treatment of infected animals, a residual dip can be used weekly; supplementary pyrethrins for rapid effect can be used daily if necessary.

Lindane (gamma benzene hexachloride) is suitable for dogs, but is contraindicated in cats because of its potential toxicity. A useful alternative for cats is pyrethrum. A combination of dichlorvos and fenitrothion is effective in both cats and dogs, usually in spray form.

Routine therapy for flea allergy dermatitis includes the use of appropriate flea sprays or collars, cythioate tablets (Proban), and judicious administration of corticosteroids.

Topical fenthion 10–20% (Spot-on) is widely used on animals suffering from flea allergy dermatitis.

Fenthion, a potent organophosphate when applied dermally, acts as a systemic flea control agent. Following dermal application on the dorsal neck, it is rapidly absorbed and disrupts the life cycle of the flea when the adults feed on the insecticide-containing fluids of the host prior to reproduction. Fenthion is convenient to use, potent, and provides flea control for up to 1 month. Disadvantages are its relative toxicity to the user and precise dosage. Accurate dosage is critical, and human skin contact must be avoided.

Because topical absorption takes from 6 to 8 hours, skin contact with the dog must be avoided for at least that period. Fenthion must not be used on cats under a year old, on sick, stressed, convalescent cats, or within 7 days of expected parturition.

Unlike other insecticides, the fenthion parasiticide does not take effect immediately. After a few hours, when the active ingredient has been almost completely absorbed, the systemic effect can be observed as affected fleas fall off the animal. A significant reduction in the level of flea infestation can be observed after only 4 hours; complete eradication of all the fleas on a dog may require 2 days.

Fenthion induces lethal inhibition of cholinesterase activity in the flea. Because of its spatial configuration, the active ingredient molecule binds ideally to the insect cholinesterase. Because of the molecule shape and weaker membrane penetration, fenthion has less inhibitory effect on mammalian cholinesterase. For this reason, enzyme inhibition is considerably less pronounced in warm-blooded organisms. This selective action results in a combination of highly effective parasite destruction and low mammalian toxicity. The cholinesterase inhibitions occurring at higher concentration levels are fully reversible.

When flea allergy is present, oral corticosteroids may be used to augment the acaricide. Oral prednisone 5 mg/kg prednisolone (0.5 mg/kg) daily for 4 days followed by half of this dose for another 7 days can be considered. For outpatient care, depending on client compliance in refractory cases, the prescribing of corticosteroids, cythioate tablets, sprays, or collars may be indicated.

Bromocyclen in talc form on the animal's back or bedding is a reliable agent for flea allergy hypersensitivity together with prednisolone on a reducing dosage. This organochlorine is no longer available in some countries.

When cats are affected with flea bite dermatitis, education of the client regarding pet and environmental control, and also regarding the sensitivity of cats to insecticides, is important. Because pruritus is a common problem with flea infestation, short-acting oral corticosteroids can be used on an alternate-day basis.

A significantly high number of pruritic animals receiving corticosteroids may develop urinary tract infection. Another consideration is that corticosteroids must be withdrawn for a certain number of days before intradermal tests can be performed. Alternate-day oral corticosteroid therapy must cease at least 4 weeks before intradermal testing. Nonsteroidal anti-inflammatory drugs may have some advantages insofar as they do not have serious side effects and can be used safely for relatively long periods of time. Also, diabetes mellitus may rule out the use of corticosteroids.

Antihistamines, such as chlorpheniramine maleate (2 to 4 mg/kg three times a day) or hydroxyzine (2 mg/kg three times a day) are useful agents for initial therapy of chronic nonspecific pruritus. Sedation is common with antihistamine usage and may be a beneficial factor in alleviating self-inflicted injury. If such empirical therapy elicits no advancement, essential fatty acid products containing eicosapentanoic acid can be used.

The tranquilizers diazepam (1 to 2 mg twice daily) or acepromazine (0.1 mg/kg) can help to relieve anxiety, calm the animal, and reduce self-inflicted injury.

Antihistamines are therapeutically not as effective as corticosteroids because of the great complexity of the immunopathogenic response involved in flea bite hypersensitivity. Antihistamines may be indicated when the client is reluctant to administer steroids or when the animal is usually sensitive to corticoid side effects.

Food allergy dermatitis represents less than 5% of all dermatoses encountered in veterinary practice. Sometimes it can be confused with flea bite hypersensitivity. After instigation of a flea control program and the nonseasonality and incomplete response of pruritus to corticosteroids, a hypoallergenic prescription diet may be needed if symptoms persist. Hypersensitivity to beef and/or cow's milk and dairy byproducts can be responsible for 80% of canine food allergies. Mutton and rice-based hypoallergenic diets are often successful in these instances.

SEBORRHEA AND ANTI SEBORRHEIC AGENTS

Seborrhea refers to excessively dry or greasy skin. Most seborrhea is secondary to an underlying skin disease. Some primary (or metabolic) seborrheas are breed specific, or may be genetically mediated.

Secondary seborrheas, on the other hand, are related to underlying causes that can be identified and treated. Ectoparasites, low environmental humidity and external inflammatory stimuli can trigger seborrhea. Hormonal and nutrient deficiencies can also play an important role (Table 33–4).

For many primary scaling disorders, the role played by abnormalities in essential fatty acid metabolism in the skin, either in the basic pathogenesis or in the develop-

---

TABLE 33–4
SEBORRHEAS

Types of Seborrheas	Cause
Primary Seborrhea	Breed susceptibility
	Dietary lipid (E.F.A.s)
	Fat deficiency
	Lipid metabolism disorders
	Pancreatic disease/malabsorption
	Zinc deficiency
	Enzyme deficiency
	Thyroid disfunction
Secondary seborrhea	Pyoderma
	Allergy/inflammation of skin
	Ectoparasites, fleas
	Mycotic infection

ment of clinical signs, is unclear. Some dogs with idiopathic seborrhea may have essential fatty acid deficiencies or increased requirements of fatty acids in the skin. Commercial fatty acid supplements (Evening Primrose Oil) contain variable amounts of omega-6 and omega-3 fatty acids, such as linoleic and eicosapentanoic acid. These may redirect fatty acid metabolism away from production of proinflammatory eicosanoids toward those with antiinflammatory action in the skin.

Although the efficacy of some of these oils (such as Evening Primrose Oil) is under considerable debate, dietary changes and supplementation must be given over a sustained period of weeks before any unequivocal determination of efficacy can be made.

If the animal is fat deficient because of an unbalanced diet, pancreatic deficiency, or gastrointestinal malabsorption, essential fatty acid supplementation may be necessary. Topically applied essential fatty acids can sometimes rectify the epidermal changes associated with fatty acid deficiency.

Clinically, seborrhea can be of two types—seborrhea oleosa and seborrhea sicca. In seborrhea oleosa, excessive sebum is produced, thereby resulting in increased epithelial cell turnover rate, greasy matted hair, odor, pruritus, and bacterial infection. The dry form, seborrhea sicca, results in insufficient sebum production, increased epithelial cell turnover rate, slough, dryness, pruritus, and bacterial infection.

Therapy of seborrhea involves the correction of predisposing causes. Although primary seborrhea cannot be cured, life-long symptomatic therapy with tar shampoos, benzoyl peroxide, or shampoos containing essential fatty acids may be necessary.

Antiseborrheic shampoos improve the appearance of the skin rapidly because of their keratolytic effects. These shampoos also contain keratoplastic components.

Common antiseborrheic agents include quaternary ammonium surfactants, chlorinated phenols, salicylic acid, sulfur, selenium sulfide, coal tar, and benzoyl peroxide.

Selenium sulfide is keratolytic, keratoplastic, and degreasing. It controls scale by depressing epidermal cell turnover rate and interferes with hydrogen-bond formation in keratin.

The keratolytic and antibacterial actions of sulfur based products are accomplished by the formation of hydrogen sulfide and pentathionic acid. Sulfur has a drying effect, is keratolytic, and keratoplastic, but it is also antifungal, antibacterial, antiparasitic, and antipruritic. Salicylic acid is keratolytic, keratoplastic, antipruritic, and bacteriostatic.

Tar is a commonly used antiseborrheic agent. It is keratoplastic, antipruritic, degreasing, and vasoconstrictive. Tar-based shampoos have good degreasing properties and usually also contain sulfur and salicylic acid. These products stain light-colored fur and leave a tar odor on the coat.

Seborrhea may also benefit from oral therapy with vitamin A and 13-cis/retinoic acid.

The term "retinoids" refers to the entire group of naturally occurring and synthetic vitamin A derivatives. Retinoids have various effects that result in their usefulness for treatment of various dermatoses. Such compounds as retinol, etretinate, and isiotretinoin all have been used with varying success rates in idiopathic seborrheic dermatitis and vitamin A responsive dermatosis. They are potentially teratogenic compounds and must not be used in breeding animals.

Administration of 13-cis-retinoic acid orally at a dose of 0.25 mg/kg twice daily has been reportedly effective in eliminating seborrheic lesions after 4 weeks of therapy. Dosage and duration of treatment are important factors governing response to this compound. Conjunctivitis and cheilitis are apparently dosage-related side effects.

When pyodermas and the seborrhea complex are present, benzoyl peroxide can be considered. The gel formation (5%) is applied once or twice daily to the localized lesion, whereas the shampoo can be used daily for pyoderma or every 4 days for seborrhea. Irritancy and erythema are seen at the 10% concentration of benzoyl peroxide. Many human preparations are at the 10% strength and should not be used in dogs.

Benzoyl peroxide possesses broad-spectrum antimicrobial activity, topical anesthetic effects, and promotes healing. As a degreasing agent, it is keratolytic, has considerable astringent and debriding properties, and flushes out the follicles. It is also a potent bleach.

Secondary seborrheic conditions usually disappear once the primary flea infestation and/or secondary pyoderma has been eliminated.

Benzoyl peroxide is useful in treating demodicosis, flea infestation and scabies. Although medicated shampoos, such as benzoyl peroxide or tar-sulfur-salicylic acid combinations, are often used, extensive long-term use of some antiseborrheic shampoos can be irritating to the skin, thereby causing flaking and excessive drying. An emollient rinse may be necessary after application.

33.10 MISCELLANEOUS SKIN THERAPY

Several zinc-responsive deficiencies have been identified in dogs, and zinc is of critical importance for optimum skin and hair coat condition in dogs and in cats. Zinc-responsive dermatosis is characterized by crusting and scaling of the mouth, ears, and perianal area. Animals do not usually have pruritus, but a history of high calcium supplements is often present. Secondary zinc deficiency often results because of high levels of dietary calcium, which competes with zinc for absorption. Hair loss and thickening of the skin accompany the deficiency. Flaking, hyperkeratosis and erythema at the elbows, hocks, and periocular area accompany this deficiency in puppies.

Puppies with zinc deficiency may require zinc supplementation until they are adults. Both zinc sulfate and zinc methionine have been used successfully to treat zinc deficiency dermatosis. Zinc sulfate tablets at a dose of 1–2 mg/kg/day over a period of 2–6 weeks is usually recommended. Sometimes emesis may accompany this dosage. Zinc should not be used in pregnancy.

ESSENTIAL FATTY ACIDS

Essential fatty acids (EFA) in the skin are found principally in the phospholipid fractions of cells. The degree of unsaturation of these acids gives cell membranes the mobility to allow changes to occur. In addition, these acids serve as substrates for production of local prostaglandin hormones, thromboxanes, and leukotrienes. A defi-ciency of EFA locally in skin results in hyperkeratosis.

The EFAs are required for the manufacture of cell membranes and prostaglandins that exert a major influence on many aspects of physiology and metabolism. In dogs, linoleic acid, found mainly in vegetable oils, is regarded as the major EFA. Cats require arachidonic acid. Deficiencies of EFAs are characterized by coarse dry brittle hair, dandruff, poor wound healing, and scaly skin in dogs.

Primary EFA deficiency is most likely to manifest itself when low-fat diets without vegetable oil supplementation are given.

Secondary EFA deficiencies are more likely to occur when fat intake is normal, but the ability to absorb it is reduced, e.g., because of pancreatic problems.

Adequate amounts of EFAs are found in almost all diets. Abnormalities of EFA metabolism, however, may occur in epidermal disorders. In addition, many similarities exist in the clinical syndromes associated with EFA deficiency and zinc deficiency, i.e., alopecia, hyperkeratosis, and delayed wound healing.

Zinc-deficient animals may have decreased absorption of triglycerides from the gastrointestinal tract. Zinc can also mobilize fatty acids from membrane stores and enhance PGI synthesis.

Dietary manipulation of the levels of specific fatty acids can alter the amount of each available for incorporation into cell membrane phospholipids.

The delta-6-desaturase enzyme is vital for the conversion of linoleic acid and alpha-linolenic acid to their metabolites. Loss or inhibition of this enzyme may mean that, although the animal may be consuming adequate quantities of linoleic acid (in the cis form) and adequate alpha-linolenic acid in the diet, the animal cannot make use of these acids as functional EFAs. Supplementation of the diet with gamma-linolenic acid and eicosapentanoic acid bypasses the delta-6-desaturase enzyme. Evening primrose oil provides a rich source of biologically active gamma-linolenic acid and other EFAs. It has been used in treating atopy in humans.

The skin depends on the continued formation of EFAs, and cutaneous symptoms of EFA deficiency include scaly skin, sebaceous gland hypertrophy, increased sebum viscosity, increased epidermal skin tumor rate, and weak cutaneous capillaries that rupture easily. In atopic dogs, evening primrose oil, which contains gamma-linolenic acid and linoleic acid, has been reported to effect an improvement in the clinical condition.

Although antihistamines and nonsteroidal anti-inflammatory drugs have also been tried to suppress inflammation and antibody production in atopy, best results are usually attained with prednisolone 1 to 2 mg/kg S.I.D. for 7 to 10 days.

Given the importance of EFAs to the skin and the apparent association of many skin problems with abnormalities in EFA metabolism, such as decreased delta-6-desaturase activity, supplementation with gamma-linolenic acid could possibly be of clinical benefit. Insofar as prostaglandins and leukotrienes act as mediators of inflammation and pruritus in the skin, supplementation with various EFA substrates may redirect and alter the types and ratios of prostaglandins and leukotrienes produced.

SELECTED REFERENCES

Alexander, M.M., and Ihre, P.J.: *Cheyletiella* dermatitis in small animal practice: a review. Calif. Vet., 36(3): 9, 1982.

August, J.R.: Otitis externa: A disease of multifactorial etiology. Vet. Clin. North Am. (Small Anim. Prac.), 18:731, 1988.

Baker, B.B.: Bacterial dermatoses in dogs. Mod. Vet. Pract., Sept./Oct., 1987.

Baker, K.P.: Observations on allergic reactions in arthropod parasites. Ir. Vet. J., 28:65, 1974.

Baker, K.P.: Observations on demodectic mange in dogs. J. Small Anim. Pract., 9:621, 1968.

Baker, N.: Managing flea allergy dermatitis. Vet. Med., August, 1984.

Becker, A.M., Janik, T.A., and Smith, E.K.: *Propionibacterium acnes* immunotherapy in chronic recurrent canine pyoderma. An adjunct to antibiotic therapy. J. Vet. Intern. Med., 3:26, 1989.

Beeman, R.W.: Recent advances in the mode of action of insecticides. Ann. Rev. Entomol., 27:253, 1982.

Bennett, G.W., and Lund, R.D.: Evaluation of encapsulated pyrethrins (Sectrol) for German cockroach and cat flea controls. Pest Control, Sept., 1977.

Berg, J.M., Wendell, D.E., and Vogelweid, C.: Am. J. Vet. Res., 45:1307, 1984.

Bledsoc, B., Fadok, V.A., and Bledsoc, M.E.: Current therapy and new developments in indoor flea control. J. Am. Anim. Hosp. Assoc., 18:415, 1982.

Bussieras, J., and Chermette, R.: Amitraz and canine dermodicosis. J. Am. Anim. Hosp. Assoc., 22:779, 1986.

Campbell, K.L.: Fatty acid supplementation and skin disease. Vet. Clin. North Am. (Small Anim. Pract.), 20:1475, 1990.

Cannon, R.W.: Amitraz in treatment of canine democosis. Modern Vet. Practice. 899–900, 1983.

Carr, S.H.: Geriatric demodicosis. Canine Pract., 13(4):27, 1986.

Chalmers, S., and Medleau, L.: Evaluation of ketoconazole in the treatment of canine and feline dermatophytosis (abstract). Proc. Am. Acad. Vet. Dermatol., 1989.

Chapkin, R.S., Ziboh, V.A., and McCullough, J.L.: Dietary influence of evening primrose and fish oil on the skin of EFA deficient guinea pigs. J. Nutr., 117:1360, 1987.

Chengappa, M.A., Maddux, R.L., and Greer, S.C.: A microbiologic survey of clinically normal and otitic canine ear canals. Vet. Med./SAC, 1983.

Cox, H.U.: Species of *Staphylococcus* isolated from animal infections. Cornell Vet., 74(2):124, 1984.

Cunnane, S.C., Huang, Y.S., and Horrobin, D.F.: Role of zinc in binoleic acid desaturation and PG synthesis. Prog. Lipid Res., 20:157, 1981.

De Doer, D.J., Moriello, K.A., and Thomas, C.B.: Evolution of a commercial staphylococcal bacterin for management of idiopathic recurrent superficial pyoderma in dogs. Am. J. Vet. Res., 51:636, 1990.

De Saxe, M., and Lloyd, D.H.: Antibiotic resistance and other characters of *Staphylococcus aureus* isolates from dogs. Proc. Assoc. Vet. Clin. Pharm. Ther., 1982.

Duclos, D.: A retrospective study of canine adult-onset demodicosis. Proc. Am. Coll. Vet. Dermatol., San Francisco, 1990.

Environmental Protection Agency: Federal Register 44 (213) 62940–62943, 1979.

Fadok, V.: Challenge clients to gain control of fleas in the environment. Vet. Med./SAC, 79(8):1039, 1984.

Fenster, P.: Designing a long term flea control program. Vet. Med., 80(2):45, 1985.

Folz, S.D.: Demodicosis (*Demodex canis*). Compend. Contin. Educ. Pract. Vet., 5:116, 1983.

Folz, S.D., Kakuk, T.J., and Henke, C.L.: Clinical evaluation of amitraz for treatment of canine scabies. Mod. Vet. Pract., 65:595, 1984.

Gary, R.C., and Donahue, W.A.: Pharmacologic profile of methoprene, an insect growth regulator in cattle, dogs and cats. J. Am. Vet. Med. Assoc., 194:410, 1989.

Grant, D.I.: Long term use of cephalexin in a case of deep pyoderma in the dog. Canine Pract., 13(1):31, 1986.

Gunaratnam, P., Wilkonson, G.T., and Seawright, A.A.: A study of amitraz toxicity in cats. Aust. Vet. J., 60:278, 1983.

Halliwell, R.E.W.: Skin diseases of old dogs and cats. Vet. Rec., 126:389, 1990.

Halliwell, R.E.W.: Current therapy in recurring pyodermas. Proc. Voor. Jarsdagen., Amsterdam, 1986.

Halliwell, R.E.W.: Managing canine flea allergy. Solway Vet. Dermatol. Rep., *5(1):*7, 1986.

Halliwell, R.E.W., and Gorman, N.T.: Nonatopic allergic skin disease. *In Veterinary Clinical Immunology.* Philadelphia, W.B. Saunders, 1989.

Helton, K.A., Nesbitt, G.H., and Caciolo, P.: Griseofulvin toxicity in cats: Literature review and report of seven cases. J. Am. Anim. Hosp. Assoc., 22:453, 1986.

Henfey, J.I.: Canine demodicosis. In Practice, Sept. 1990.

Hink, W.F., and Fee, B.J.: Toxicity of D-Limonene, the major component of citrus peel oil to all life stages of the cat flea, *C. felis.* J. Med. Entomol., 23:400, 1986.

Hooser, S.B., Beasley, V.R., and Everitt, J.L.: Effects of an insecticidal dip containing D-limonene in the cat. J. Am. Vet. Med. Assoc., *189:*905, 1986.

Horrobin, D.F.: Essential fatty acids in clinical dermatology. J. Am. Acad. Dermatol., 20:1045, 1989.

Hoskins, J.D., Cox, H.A., Roy, A.F., and Newman, S.S.: What's new in bacteriology? Staphylococcal intermedius. Vet. Med., Oct. 1984.

Houston, D.M., Parent, J., and Matushek, K.J.: Ivermectin toxicosis in a dog. J. Am. Vet. Med. Assoc., *191:*78, 1987.

Hsu, W.W., and Schaffer, D.D.: Effects of topical application of amitraz on plasma glucose and insulin concentrations in dogs. Am. J. Vet. Res., 49:130, 1986.

Ihrke, P.J.: An overview of bacterial skin disease in the dog. Br. Vet. J., *143:*112, 1987.

Ihrke, P.J.: Therapeutic strategies involving antimicrobial treatment of the skin in small animals. J. Am. Vet. Med. Assoc., *185:*1165, 1984.

Indiveri, M.C., and Hirsh, D.C.: Clavulanic acid—potential activity of amoxicillin against *Bacteroides fragilis.* Am. J. Vet. Res., 46:2207, 1985.

Kunkle, G.A.: Contact dermatitis. Vet. Clin. North Am. (Small Anim. Pract.), 18(5):1061, 1988.

Kunkle, G.A.: New considerations for rational antibiotic therapy of cutaneous staphylococcal infection in the dog. Semin. Vet. Med. Surg. Small Anim., 2:212, 1987.

Kunkle, G.A.: Canine pyoderma. Compend. Contin. Educ. Small Anim. Pract., 1:7, 1979.

Kwochka, K.W.: Retinoids in dermatology. *In* Current Veterinary Therapy X. Edited by R.W. Kirk. Philadelphia, W.B. Saunders, 1981.

Kwochka, K.W.: Fleas and related disease. Vet. Clin. North Am., 17:1235, 1987.

Kwochka, K.W.: Mites and related disease. Vet. Clin. North Am., 17:1263, 1987.

Kwochka, K.W.: Rational shampoo therapy in veterinary dermatology. Proc. 11th Annual Kal Kan Symp., 1987.

Kwochka, K.W., Kunkle, G.A., and O'Neill, C.: The efficacy of amitraz for generalized demodicosis in dogs: A study of two concentrations and frequencies of application. Compend. Contin. Educ. Pract. Vet., *7(1):*8, 1985.

Lloyd, D.M.: The use of benzoyl peroxide preparations in the management of skin infections. Proc. Assoc. Vet. Clin. Pharm. Ther., 1982.

Lorenz, M.: Should you use systemic therapy to control flea allergy dermatitis? Vet. Med., Sept. 1984.

Lorenz, M.: Systemic therapy of flea allergy dermatitis. Vet. Med./SAC, *79(9):*1148, 1984.

Mason, K.V., Ring, J., and Duggan, J.: Fenthion for flea control on dogs under field conditions: dose response efficacy studies and effect on cholinesterase activity. J. Am. Anim. Hosp. Assoc., 20:591, 1984.

McDonald, J.M.: Principles of insecticidal treatment in small animal dermatology, or How to make a flea flee. 53rd Annual Meeting AAHA meeting proceedings, 1986.

McKeever, P.J., and Torres, S.: Otitis externa, Part I: Predisposing factors to otitis externa. Companion Animal Practice. 7, 1988.

Medleau, L.: Managing cases of chronic pruritis that have not responded to steroids. Vet. Med., March 1990.

Medleau, L.: Demodicosis in cats. J. Am. Anim. Hosp. Assoc., 24:85, 1988.

Medleau, L., and Miller, W.H.: Flea infestation and its control. Int. J. Dermatol., 22:378, 1983.

Melman, S., and Hutton, P.: Flea control on dogs and cats indoors and in the environment. Compend. Contin. Educ. Pract. Vet., 7:869, 1985.

Moriello, K.A.: Dermatology update: Applying recent advances to practice. Vet. Med., 160, 1990.

Miller, W.H.: Topical management of seborrhea in dogs. Vet. Med., Feb. 1990. pp. 122–131.

Miller, W.H.: Nutritional considerations in small animal dermatology. Vet. Clin. N. Am. *19:*497, 1989.

Moriello, K.A.: The return of the mites. Dermatol. Dialogue, Summer 1989.

Moriello, K.A.: Common ectoparasites of the dog. Part I. Fleas and ticks. Canine Pract. *14(2):*6, 1987.

Moriello, K.A.: Common ectoparasites of the dog. Part 3. Miscellaneous parasites. Canine Pract., *14:*23, 1987.

Muller, G.H.: Amitraz treatment of demodicosis. J. Am. Anim. Hosp. Assoc., *19:*435, 1983.

Nesbitt, G., and Helton, K.A.: The diagnosis and management of chronic canine dermatoses. Vet. Med., 1984.

Nesbitt, G., and Schnitz, J.A.: Flea bite allergic dermatitis: A review and survey of 330 cases. J. Am. Vet. Med. Assoc., *173:*282, 1978.

Paradis, M., et al.: Efficacy of ivermectin against *Cheyletiella blakei* infestation in cats. J. Am. Anim. Hosp. Assoc., 26:125, 1990.

Product Information: Mitaban (Amitraz). Liquid concentrate. The Upjohn Co., Kalamazoo, MI, 1982.

Randolph, R.W.: Antimicrobial therapy for pyodermas in dogs. Mod. Vet. Pract., Dec. 1985.

Reedy, L.M.: Fatty acids in healthy skin. Vet. Forum, Aug. 1989.

Reedy, L.M.: Common parasitic problems in small animal dermatology. J. Am. Vet. Med. Assoc., *188:*362, 1986.

Refai, M.: Dermatomycosis in cats and dogs as a zoonotic problem. 20th Annual Meeting Soc. Intl. Vet. Symp., Cairo, Oct. 1985.

Rosser, E.: Dermatology Proceedings of 18th Seminar for Veterinary Technicians. Western Vet. Conference, 1989.

Rubensomn, M.: Tiguvon (Spotton) (20%) Fenthion for flea control on dogs. Aust. Vet. Pract., 12(13):76, 1982.

Scheidt, V.J., Medleau, L., and Seward, R.L.: An evaluation of ivermectin in the treatment of sarcoptic mange in dogs. Am. J. Vet. Res., 45:1202, 1984.

Schick, M.P., and Schick, R.O.: Understanding and implementing safe and effective flea control. J. Am. Anim. Hosp. Assoc., 22:421, 1986.

Shmidl, J.A., Kohlenberg, M.L., and Cox, D.D.: Fenthion safety evaluations. Vet. Med., Suppl., July 1985.

Shmidl, J.A., Kohlenberg, M.L., and Johnson, G.L.: Assessing the safety of long term cythiate therapy. Vet. Med., Sept. 1984.

Schneck, G.: Use of ivermectin against ear mites in cats. Vet. Rec., 123:599, 1988.

Scott, D.W.: Canine demodicosis. Vet. Clin. North Am. (Small Anim. Pract.), 9:79, 1979.

Scott, D.W.: Clinical assessment of topical benzoyl peroxide in treatment of canine skin diseases. Vet. Med. Small Anim. Clin., 74:804, 1979.

Scott, D.W., and Buerger, R.G.: Nonsteroidal anti-inflammatory agents in the management of canine pruritus. J. Am. Anim. Hosp. Assoc., 24:425, 1988.

Scott, D.W., and Walton, D.K.: Experiences with the use of amitraz and ivermectin in the treatment of generalised demodicosis in dogs. J. Am. Anim. Hosp. Assoc., 21:535, 1985.

Shmielyl, J.S., Kollenberg, M.L., and Johnson, G.C.: Cholinesterase values in dogs treated with cythioate. Vet. Med./SAC, 78:1561, 1983.

Shirk, M.A.: The efficacy of amitraz in treatment for demodectic mange: a field study. Vet. Med./SAC, July 1983.

Stewart, L.J.: The role of pyoderma in pruritus. Vet. Clin. North Am., 18:1013, 1988.

Thomsett, L.R.: Fungal diseases of the skin of small animals. Br. Vet. J., 142:317, 1986.

Uvarov, O.: Recent advances in the treatment of skin diseases with special reference to griseofulvin. Vet. Rec., 73:528, 1961.

White, S.D.: Treatment of canine scabies. 11th Annual Kal Kan Symp., Ohio State Univ., 1987.

White, S.D., et al.: Generalized demodicosis associated with diabetes in two cats. J. Am. Vet. Med. Assoc., 191:448, 1987.

White, S.D., and Ihrke, P.J.: Dermatology. In Contemporary Issues in Small Animal Practice. Edited by G.H. Nesbitt. New York, Churchill Livingstone, 1987.

Wiccelink, M.A., Willemse, A., and Koeman, J.P.: Deep pyoderma in the German Shepherd dog. J. Am. Anim. Hosp. Assoc., 21:773, 1985.

Woody, B.J., and Fox, S.M.: Otitis externa: Seeing past the signs to discover the underlying cause. Vet. Med., 616. July 1986.

Wright, J.E.: Environmental and toxicological aspects of insect growth regulators. Environ. Health Perspect., 24:127, 1976.

Yazwinski, T.A., Pote, L., and Tilley, W.: Efficacy of ivermectin against *Sarcoptes scabies* and *Otodectes cynots* infestations in dogs. Vet. Med./SAC, 76:1749, 1981.

CHAPTER 34

THERAPY OF ENDOPARASITES IN DOG AND CATS

34.1 Introduction
34.2 Ascarid Infestation
34.3 Hookworms
34.4 Whipworms
34.5 Threadworms
34.6 Tapeworms
34.7 Giardiasis
34.8 Toxoplasmosis
34.9 Enteric Coccidal Infections
34.10 Respiratory Parasites

34.1 INTRODUCTION

Parasites of dogs and cats are widely prevalent and, hence, are of significance to the veterinarian involved in small animal practice. Many of these parasites cause serious clinical disease states, others result in suboptimal performance, and others cause esthetically objectionable features. Because of the ever increasing animal-human bond and the transmissibility of certain of these parasites to humans, and especially young children, the zoonotic potential of many of these infestations cannot be overestimated from the standpoint of human health. The treatment and control of these parasites require a specific knowledge of each worm's epidemiology (Table 34–1) and a thorough understanding and appreciation of its susceptibility to the many anthelmintics now commercially available. Common parasites of dogs and cats include the ascarids, *Toxocara canis, Toxocara cati,* and *Toxascaris leonina,* and the *Dipylidium* and *Taenia* tapeworms. Animals kept in close quarters or kennelled together are likely to harbor infestation with hookworms (*Ancylostoma caninum, Uncinaria stenocephala*), the whipworm (*Trichuris vulpis*), and the respiratory tract parasites (*Filaroides osleri* in the dog and *Aelurostrongylus abstrusus* in the cat) (Table 34–2). Aside from *Toxocara,* the major parasite of public health importance is the cestode *Echinococcus granulosus,* the cause of hydatid disease in humans. Certain *Taenia* for which the dog is the final host have sheep, cattle, or pigs as intermediate hosts. Such intermediate stages may be responsible for downgrading the carcasses at slaughter or may themselves cause clinical disease, such as coenurosis ("gid") in sheep.

Many of the effective anthelmintics currently available kill worms present in the animal at the time of administration. The success of this form of therapy in the long term depends on the immune status of the animal, its nutritional and disease status, and, most importantly, the opportunity for re-infestation. Control of parasitic disease therefore implies a spectrum of treatment far wider than simply anthelmintic therapy alone. Attention to environmental contamination, other animals in contact, and intermediate hosts is an integral aspect of any

---

TABLE 34–1
PATTERNS OF PARASITIC INFESTATION

Classification	Parasite	Predilection Site	Usual Mode of Infection
Ascarids	Toxocara canis	Small intestine	Transplacental/via colostrum and milk/embryonated eggs
	Toxocara cati	Small intestine	Embryonated eggs
	Toxascaris leonina	Small intestine	Embryonated eggs
Hookworms	Uncinaria stenocephala Ancylostoma caninum	Small intestine	Ingestion of infective larvae, prenatal transmammary percutaneous infection
Whipworms	Trichuris vulpis	Cecum/colon	Ingestion of embryonated egg
Lungworms	Filaroides osleri	Bifurcation of trachea	Transfer of larvae in respiratory secretions
	Angiostrongylus vasorum	Right ventricle/ pulmonary artery	Eating mollusc—intermediate host
Tapeworms	Echinococcus granulosus	Small intestine	Offal containing hydatid cysts
	Taenia	Small intestine	Offal or carcass with cysticercus
	Dipylidium caninum	Small intestine	Eating flea/louse with cysticercoid

TABLE 34–2
COMMON PARASITES OF DOGS AND CATS

Genus	Common name	Predilection Site	Susceptible Host
Ancylostoma	Hookworm	Duodenum	Puppies
Uncinaria	Hookworm	Duodenum	Young and adult dogs
Toxocara	Roundworm	Small intestine	Puppies (6 months)
Toxascaris	Roundworm	Small intestine	Young dogs, cats
Trichuris	Whipworm	Cecum	Young and adult dogs
Taenia	Tapeworm	Small intestine	All ages
Dipylidium	Tapeworm	Small intestine	All ages
Spirocerca	None	Esophagus	Adult dogs and cats
Ollulanus	Small stomach worm	Stomach	Adult cats
Strongyloides	Threadworm	Small intestine	Young dogs
Mesocestoides	Small tapeworm	Small intestine	Adult dogs

preventative scheme. Intercurrent disease must be vigorously treated. Client education is imperative not simply to minimize further re-infestation, but also to avoid human infestation, which, with certain parasites, can have serious public health consequences.

Available anthelmintics can be classed as broad spectrum or narrow spectrum (Tables 34–3 and 34–4). Broad-spectrum drugs, such as nitroscanate, fenbendazole, febantel, or mebendazole, can be used when multiple infestations are present. Use of narrow-spectrum agents is restricted to targeted helminths when a specific diagnosis has been made on the basis of clinical history and signs and the results of parasitologic investigation. Some drugs have narrower safety margins than others, numerous side effects and drug interactions may occur, and efficacy against various parasites varies. Veterinarians should familiarize themselves with such aspects before commencing any worm control program. For instance, because no one anthelmintic compound is effective against all tapeworms and roundworms, combination products that include effective cestocides formulated with one or more drugs with nemadocidal activity have been developed. Drontal Plus for dogs contains a combination of febantel, pyrantel, and praziquantel. Combinations of epsiprantel and pyrantel are available for tapeworms and roundworms.

At a dosage rate of 5.5 mg/kg, epsiprantel and 5 mg/kg pyrantel, this new combination is effective against *T. canis, T. leonina, U. stenocephala, D. caninum, A. caninum, T. hydatigena,* and *T. pisiformis.*

Because of their mode of action, benzimidazoles are most effective when the target worm population is exposed to the anthelmintic for several days. Repeat administration over a period of days increases the bioavailability of the total amount of drug administered, when compared to the amount available after administration of a single large dose, given once. Administration of benzimidazoles with food, especially fatty food, may increase plasma levels.

Benzimidazoles bind to tubulin (a structural protein), thereby preventing its polymerization to microtubules that provide the transport systems of the parasites that absorb cells. The result is incomplete absorption and digestion of nutrient particles and cellular autolysis through activation of lysosomal enzymes.

Mebendazole involves a 2-day course for ascarid control and a 5-day course for broader-spectrum activity. Mebendazole is not effective against *Dipylidium caninum.*

Febantel is a broad-spectrum probenzimidazole that is effective against *Ancylostoma caninum, Uncinaria stenocephala, Toxocara canis,* and *Toxascaris leonina* in dogs.

Fenbendazole can be used for lungworm treatment in dogs as follows: 50 mg/kg for

TABLE 34–3
GENERAL SPECTRUM OF ACTION OF ANTHELMINTICS

Active Ingredient(s)	Ascarids	Hookworms	Whipworms	Cestodes	Strongyloides
Bunamidine	−	−	−	+	−
Butamisole	−	+ +	+ +	−	−
Dichlorvos	+ +	+ +	+ +	−	−
Diethylcarbamazine	+ +	−	−	−	+
Disophenol	−	+ +	−	−	−
Dithiazanine	+	+	+	−	+ +
Epsiprantel	−	−	−	+ +	−
Febantel	+ +	+ +	+ +	+	−
Febantel + Praziquantel	+ +	+ +	+ +	+ +	−
Fenbendazole	+ +	+ +	+ +	+	−
Ivermectin	+ +	+ +	+ +	−	+ +
Mebendazole	+ +	+ +	+ +	+	+
Methyl benzene + Dichlorophene	+	+	±	+	−
Niclosamide	−	−	−	+	−
Oxfendazole	+ +	+ +	−	+ +	−
Piperazine	+ +	+	−	−	−
Praziquantel	−	−	−	+ +	−
Pyrantel	+ +	+ +	−	−	−
Thenium	+	+ +	−	−	−
Thenium + Piperazine	+ +	+ +	−	−	−
Thiabendazole	+	+	−	−	+ +

TABLE 34–4
BROAD-SPECTRUM ANTHELMINTICS FOR SMALL ANIMALS

	Toxocara canis	Toxocara cati	Toxascaris leonina	Uncinaria stenocephala	Ancylostoma caninum	Taenia	Echinococcus	Dipylidium caninum	Trichuris
Nitroscanate	+	+	+	+	+	+	±	+	−
Mebendazole	+	+	+	+	+	+	+	−	+
Fenbendazole	+	−	+	+	+	+	−	−	+
Oxfendazole	+	−	+	+	−	+	−	+	−
Praziquantel/ Pyrantel/ Febantel	+	+	+	+	+	+	+	+	+
Epsiprantel/ Pyrantel	+	?	+	+	+	+	−	+	±

7 days against *Filaroides osleri*. In cats, the dose of fenbendazole against *Aelurostrongylus abstrusus* is 20 mg/kg for 5 days.

Fenbendazole is effective in a reduced dose schedule, 25 mg/kg body weight from the fortieth day of pregnancy to 2 days after whelping, for somatic ascarids.

Nitroscanate provides wide anthelmintic activity after a single dose. This drug, however, is not effective against *Trichuris* or

Echinococcus. Nitroscanate acts faster and is significantly more effective than mebendazole against *Toxocara canis.* It is also more effective than mebendazole against *Dipylidium caninum* and *Ancylostoma caninum.*

Pyrantel is a broad-spectrum anthelmintic for dogs and cats that has been used for many years. Pyrantel pamoate at a dose of 14.4 mg/kg (5 mg/kg base) is effective against *A. caninum, Uncinaria stenocephala, Toxocara canis,* and *Toxascaris leonina.* Effective action against *Trichuris vulpis* is not claimed for pyrantel.

Products based on the ivermectin or milbemycin compounds soon may become available for treatment of ecto- and/or endoparasites.

Thus, chemotherapeutic agents are only one important aspect of a parasite control program in small animals. Whenever such agents are used, knowledge of their pharmacology, indications, side effects, and contraindications is essential. Desirable features of anthelmintic drugs include:

1. Good efficacy and wide spectrum of activity
2. Wide therapeutic index
3. Minimal side effects and contraindications
4. Ease of administration

Other factors that must be considered in designing an effective parasite control scheme include

1. Sanitation, cleanliness of the environment, disinfection
2. Avoidance of overcrowding
3. Removal of fleas and decontamination of premises
4. Good nutrition and husbandry
5. Control of intermediate hosts or exposure to intermediate hosts
6. Regular fecal examination
7. Regular deworming
8. Isolation of new animals until examination or deworming
9. Special attention to the pregnant bitch and the lactating bitch
10. Cleanliness in whelping premises
11. Client education for control of parasites in their pets
12. Client education regarding the public health hazards of many parasites transmissible to humans
13. Detailed knowledge of parasites, their life cycles, and routes of infestation
14. Supportive medical treatment for infested animals

The veterinarian has an important counseling role in any parasite control program. The safety of modern anthelmintics and the importance of early treatment must be emphasized. In addition, any zoonotic potential of a particular parasite must be stressed.

34.2 ASCARID INFESTATION

These large roundworms of dogs and cats are most commonly encountered in young puppies and kittens. Of the three major species, *Toxocara canis, Toxocara cati, and Toxascaris leonina,* the most important is *Toxocara canis. T. canis* can cause severe infections in puppies and a serious condition called visceral larval migrans syndrome in humans. Infective eggs of *T. canis,* when swallowed by older dogs, undergo extensive larval development and distribution in muscles, connective tissue, and kidneys. When a bitch becomes pregnant, these larvae migrate to the uterus, pass through the placenta, and migrate through the liver and lungs of the pups in utero. After whelping, *Toxocara* larvae continue their migration in the neonatal pup, ultimately settling in the intestine. Hence, pups can be born with appreciable burdens of parasites acquired prenatally. Some of the somatic larvae in the bitch migrate to the mammary gland and infect pups through the milk.

Ill-thrift, pot-bellied appearance, vomiting, and respiratory signs frequently accompany heavy infestation in young pups. Occasionally neurologic symptoms and death occur.

In the alimentary tract, the worms mature and produce eggs that contaminate the environment. After a few months, most of the adult worms are spontaneously expelled. Adult egg-laying *Toxocara* are found in only a small proportion of the adult dog population. At the time of parturition, the immune status of the bitch can decline, and hence, many ascarid eggs may be passed, thereby creating significant environmental contamination. Grooming and licking of the pups by the bitch may further increase the intake of ascarids through fecal ingestion by the dam.

Young pups exposed to contamination of their confined surroundings by ascarid eggs may swallow many of these eggs, which hatch into larvae in the bowel, penetrate the intestinal mucosa, migrate to the liver and lungs before being coughed up, are swallowed, and mature to the egg-laying adult in the small intestine.

Eggs of *T. canis* are sticky and resistant to many disinfectant agents; thus, they persist in the environment for many months as a future source of infestation. Prenatal immunosuppression in the bitch significantly increases the amount of egg-laying adults found in the bitch at the time of parturition.

Although *Toxocara* infestation is usually acquired within the uterus and causes signs of clinical disease in young animals, *Toxascaris leonina* infestation is acquired mainly by consumption of mammalian intermediate hosts and is seen in slightly older animals.

Infection with *T. leonina* in the dog is direct, and development is confined to the wall or lumen of the gastrointestinal tract. Accordingly, neither prenatal nor transmammary transmission is a factor. Infestations therefore tend to occur later in life; the highest prevalence occurs in the 6- to 12-month-old age group. In cats, the life cycle can be indirect with rodents as intermediate hosts.

Ascarid larvae can migrate through the tissues of many animals, including humans. Infections of humans by larvae of *Toxocara canis* is referred to as the visceral larval migrans syndrome. These larvae become associated with lesions in the liver, kidney, lungs, brain, and eyes, causing mechanical damage, granuloma formation, and eosinophilia. Disease in humans usually occurs when embryonated eggs are ingested and massive amounts of larvae invade the body.

Visceral larval migrans syndrome mostly affects children under the age of 3 years, whereas ocular larval migrans (larvae rest in the eye) is seen in older children and sometimes adults. Ocular larval migrans is an important cause of childhood blindness commonly associated with fondling of infected pups by young children or with bad hygiene practices in a home frequented by an infected pup.

Ascarid control is of prime importance in puppies and kittens. Difficulties in control are caused by larval migration and sequestration in tissues (*T. canis*) and lack of efficient larvicidal agents.

ANTHELMINTIC THERAPY

Toxocara canis

Piperazine adipate or citrate is an effective drug for treatment of intestinal ascarids when administered at an oral dose rate of 110 mg/kg. Elevated doses of 200 mg/kg are approximately 80% effective against immature prenatally acquired worms in the small intestine of pups 1 to 2 weeks of age. If the bowel is atonic, worms may not be expelled; thus, a mild laxative may be necessary to augment normal peristalsis. Piperazine has no effect against somatic larvae in the bitch (Table 34–5). (Toxicity has been reported in kittens.)

Daily doses of diethylcarbamazine citrate (also used for prevention of heartworm) reduce the risk of ascarid infection, especially when combined with a benzimidazole or strylpyridinium.

Injectable ivermectin at a dose level of 200 μg/kg expels more than 90 to 100% of adults and more than 95% of fourth-stage larvae of *T. canis*. A single oral dose of ivermectin at 100 to 200 μg/kg is also highly effective against adult *T. canis*. Using the oral formulation of ivermectin for prophylaxis of canine dirofilariasis, 6 μg/kg once per month, may also result in some ascaridal activity.

Milbemycin compounds, which are structural analogs of the avermectins, are almost 100% effective at doses of 100 μg/kg.

Benzimidazole parasiticides display broad-spectrum anthelmintic activity against a wide range of endoparasites in both large and small animals. Fenbendazole, flubendazole, mebendazole, albendazole, and febantel display high efficacy against adult and larval infections in pups and adult animals. Pups must be treated as early as possible; the first treatment is given at 2 weeks of age. Nursing bitches should be treated at the same time.

Dichlorvos, dithiazanine, nitroscanate, levamisole, and pyrantel pamoate are also effective drugs for ascarid infestation.

TABLE 34–5
SOME ANTINEMATODAL DRUGS AND THEIR SPECTRUM

Active Ingredient	Approximate Efficacy Against		
	Ascarids	Hookworms	Whipworms
Butamisole hydrochloride	−	+ +	+ +
Diethylcarbamazine citrate	+	−	−
Dichlorvos	+ +	+ +	+ +
Disophenol	−	+ +	−
Dithiazanine	+	+	+
Fenbendazole	+ +	+ +	+ +
Febantel	+ +	+ +	+ +
Glycobiarsol	−	−	+ +
Ivermectin	+ +	+ +	+ +
Mebendazole	+ +	+ +	+ +
Milbemycin	+ +	+ +	+ +
Methyl benzene	+	+	−
N-Butyl chloride	+ +	+	−
Nitroscanate	+ +	+ +	−
Oxfendazole	+ +	+ +	—
Phthalofyne	−	−	+ +
Piperazine	+ +	+	−
Pyrantel pamoate	+ +	+ +	−
Strylpyridinium	+ +	+ +	−
Thenium closylate	+	+ +	−
Toluene	+	+ +	−

+ +—Efficacy about 95%
+—Efficacy about 60–80%
— —Efficacy below 50%

Toxocara Cati

The benzimidazole carbamates mebendazole, fenbendazole, and flubendazole are 100% effective against *T. cati* when administered for 3 days at 11 mg/kg, 50 mg/kg, and 22 mg/kg, respectively. Febantel, a pro-drug of fenbendazole, is approved for use in cats and is 100% effective when given in paste formulation once daily for 3 days. Use piperazine carefully in kittens. Ataxia may follow overdose in this sensitive species.

Toxascaris Leonina

Most anthelmintics with established efficacy against *T. canis* and *T. cati* are useful also for *Toxascaris leonina*.

Piperazine adipate at a single dose of 240 mg/kg is quite effective against *T. leonina*, as is fenbendazole at a dose of 50 mg/kg daily for 3 consecutive days. Oral ivermec-tin, 100 to 200 μg/kg is useful for natural infections in dogs. Nitroscanate, a broad-spectrum anthelmintic, is 100% effective against adult *T. leonina* at a single dose of 50 mg/kg and 90% effective against early fourth-stage larvae when 2 doses of 50 mg/kg are administered. Many benzimidazoles and probenzimidazoles, such as febantel, are effective also.

The Pregnant Bitch

Several of the benzimidazole carbamate anthelmintics are effective against the somatic larvae of *Toxocara canis* in the bitch. Fenbendazole is the most potent and safest of these anthelmintics in killing tissue-dwelling larvae and preventing the occurrence of prenatal infection in the bitch. A dose of 50 mg/kg from day 40 of pregnancy to day 14 post parturition ensures ascarid-free pups. Continuance of fenbendazole therapy, however, must be maintained during the lactation period to obviate any further larval transmission.

Treatment with fenbendazole at a dose rate of 100 mg/kg for 3 days is more than 90% effective against prenatally acquired larvae. A second dose should be given 2 to 3 weeks later before patency develops in the remaining ascarid parasites.

ASCARID CONTROL PROGRAMS

Ascarid control programs must always place high priority on client education to prevent the appearance of visceral or ocular larval migrans. Control of *T. canis* must be one of the most important aims in the care of small animals, especially with the growing public concern for the associated implications for human health.

Control may be based on prevention of the prenatal transfer of larvae to the pups or on the treatment of the bitch and pups post partum. The veterinarian is responsible for clearly communicating to the client the zoonotic significance of the disease.

The best type of control is prevention, which can be relatively easy in dogs and cats that are confined or that have relatively little contact with other animals of the same species.

Because transmission patterns can be quite complicated, prophylaxis programs may need to be continued for 12 months or so before final eradication can be achieved. The following are some inherent difficulties that must be overcome when executing a successful ascarid eradication program.

1. Treating bitches with conventional parasiticides has no effect on somatic larvae lodged in tissues; thus, prenatal infection of puppies cannot be prevented with these drugs.
2. The presence or absence of eggs in the feces of adult bitches does not provide any indication of whether somatic larvae are present in the tissues.
3. Infection of the dam occurs readily at parturition because of prenatal immunosuppression, increased shedding of eggs into the environment from the dam, and reinfestation of the dam by grooming of the pups.
4. Infection of pups (already prenatally infected) can occur because of increased environmental contamination at parturition.
5. Treatment of pups may eliminate most adult worms but may not prevent other serious complications, such as respiratory distress, that accompany migratory larvae.
6. Prenatal and mammary infection must be anticipated and recognized as a source of egg contamination.
7. Pups must be treated within 2 weeks of birth to prevent prenatal infections from becoming patent.
8. Treatment with a suitable parasiticide should be repeated every 2 to 3 weeks until the pup is 12 weeks of age.
9. Bitches should be regularly dewormed to reduce environmental contamination and the risk of further reinfection with somatic larva.
10. Bitches should always be treated during lactation.
11. Strict hygiene must be observed in the premises because pups are fully susceptible to infestation following ingestion of infected eggs.
12. Feces and excreted worms must be removed daily.
13. All dogs must be treated regularly, and progress must be monitored on the basis of fecal egg counts. Ascarid eggs are particularly thick shelled and are resistant to many chemical and ovicidal compounds. They are not affected by formalin, lysol, acids, or bases, but are killed by exposure to ultraviolet light, desiccation, aqueous iodine, and high temperatures. Heat, sunlight, and dryness therefore minimize contamination of premises.

34.3 HOOKWORMS

The two major species that affect dogs are *Ancylostoma caninum*, and *Uncinaria stenocephala, Ancylostoma braziliense* occurs in warmer regions of the United States.

Both of these hookworm species live in the small intestine. Infection occurs from oral ingestion of infective larvae that mature in the small intestine. Pups can acquire infection through milk and colostrum, and *A. caninum* or *A. braziliense* may also enter through the skin. Skin penetration in puppies is followed by migration of the larvae through the blood to the lungs, where larvae are coughed up, swallowed back, and then grow to maturity in the small intestine. In older animals, migration of *A. caninum* larvae through the pulmonary tissue is followed by arrest and residency in muscular tissues. These larvae can become activated in pregnancy and accumulate in the mammary gland, thus colostral transfer. Although prenatal infection is less common, transplacental passage may occur by larvae breaking into the alveoli of the young pup. Infection and migration of *A. caninum* depends on the age of the dog. Pups acquire infection largely through the dam's milk, and larvae later migrate to the intestine. Excretion of the larvae in the milk can continue for 3 to 4 weeks after parturition. Larvae may still be excreted at the next lactation, even when reinfection of the bitch has been prevented.

Hookworm disease caused by *Unicaria stenocephala*, and *Ancylostoma caninum*, is encountered especially in kennelled animals (as is whipworm disease caused by *Trichuris vulpis*). Adult dogs are primarily affected by percutaneous entry of larvae that migrate through the somatic tissues and finally settle in the muscles. Percutaneous entry is evidenced by lesions on the parts of the body that contact the ground. The number of larvae and the immunocompetence of the animal largely determine the extent of the resulting dermatitis. Usually, footpads become soft and the interdigital spaces are erythematous. Skin lesions are marked by hyperkeratosis and acanthosis.

Ancylostoma is an avid bloodsucker that can cause a severe anemia. A hypochromic microcytic anemia may result because the iron used for hematopoiesis is lost faster than it can be replaced by absorption through feedstuffs. After feeding, the parasite leaves bleeding lesions that can be fatal in a young puppy. Intestinal effects may range from mild enteritis to severe anemia with circulatory collapse, hemorrhagic diarrhea, shock, loss of proteins, and death. This condition is clinically evident by iron deficiency anemia, lack of energy, pallor, a dull coat, and tarry feces.

Mature dogs harboring a few worms may exhibit little or no clinical signs, or perhaps a diarrhea and general ill-thrift may develop in chronic cases.

Uncinaria does not feed on blood, but can produce diarrhea and leakage of blood into the alimentary tract. Patent infections are acquired when infective larvae are swallowed, but skin penetration may provoke a dermatitis between the toes. Although less pathogenic than *Ancylostoma caninum*, severe infections by *Uncinaria* can adversely affect a dog's performance.

TREATMENT AND CONTROL

Supplementary treatment with blood transfusion and iron supplementation must always be considered in severely affected anemic animals. General measures to improve sanitation and reduce environmental contamination are also necessary, especially when many animals are kept in the same premises. Pregnant bitches must be kept away from the intended whelping area.

Prevention by way of vaccination has been attempted with varying results. Sonication and fluorouracil treatment of hookworm larvae have been utilized in trial vaccination schemes for pups, sometimes with encouraging results.

Many anthelmintics are currently available for hookworm treatment and control (Table 34–6). Treatments of choice are prob-

---

TABLE 34–6
SOME DRUGS FOR HOOKWORMS IN DOGS/CATS

Butamisole
Dichlorvos
Dichlorophene
Disophenol
Febantel
Febantel/Praziquantel
Fenbendazole
Ivermectin
Mebendazole
Milbemycin
N-Butyl chloride
Oxfendazole
Oxibendazole—diethylcarbamazine
Pyrantel pamoate
Strylpyridinium—diethylcarbamazine
Thenium
Nitroscanate

ably pyrantel pamoate, ivermectin, and milbemycin, although many other chemotherapeutics, such as butamisole, thenium, dichlorvos, nitroscanate, fenbendazole, mebendazole, febantel, piperazine, dithiazanine iodide, bephenium hydroxynaphthoate, and disophenol, can be considered also.

Piperazine dosage should be increased by 50% for *Uncinaria* infections.

Pyrantel pamoate is also effective against ascarids and hookworms. It is available as a chewable tablet (Nemex) and in a paste form or suspension in some countries.

Fenbendazole given continuously to pregnant bitches also reduces the incidence of hookworm infestation in the litter.

Prophylaxis with strylpyridinium and diethylcarbamazine citrate is useful for both hookworm and heartworm infection. Oxibendazole-diethylcarbamazine citrate for heartworm control also confers benefit against hookworms.

Ivermectin given orally at a dose of 0.0006 mg/kg is up to 50% effective against the adults of *U. stenocephala*, but is up to 90% effective against the adults of *Ancylostoma caninum* at the same level. Milbemycin oxime, at 0.5 mg/kg, is highly effective against *A. caninum*, but *Uncinaria stenocephala* is more resistant to it. When milbemycin oxime is given monthly as a heartworm preventative, it is also highly effective against adult *Ancylostoma caninum* in the intestines.

Sodium borate is a useful decontaminant for infected runs. Hookworm larvae are fairly susceptible to various sprays (VIP hook-spray). Sunlight is also detrimental to the survival of larvae.

Overall control must be aimed at treatment of the pregnant bitch, treatment of the bitch during lactation, administration of medication to all animals and new animals on a regular basis, monitoring of fecal egg counts, clinical observation of kennelled animals (anemia, foot lesions), maintenance of scrupulously clean whelping and suckling areas, and routine cleaning and sanitation of preferably concrete kennels and runs two or three times a week.

34.4 WHIPWORMS

The major whipworms of small animals are *Trichuris vulpis* in the dog and *T. campanula* and *T. serrata* in the cat. Whipworms exhibit a direct life cycle, and dogs and cats become infected by consuming food or water contaminated with larvated worm eggs. After hatching, the larvae burrow into the crypts of Lieberkühn, where they reside for several days before progressing from the small intestine to the large intestine, where development to the adult stage takes place. Adult whipworms occasionally penetrate to the underlying lymphoid tissues. *T. vulpis* is located in the cecum, where it lies with its long narrow neck buried in the superficial mucosa. Infections are often tolerated without apparent ill effects, but weight loss and intermittent diarrhea may be seen.

Canine whipworms feed on the blood, tissue fluids, and dissolved mucosal epithelium. Eggs passed out in the feces usually become infective after 2 to 4 weeks in a warm moist environment. Such eggs can persist in the environment as long as 1 year.

Heavy infestation may cause colitis and periods of diarrhea intervening with periods of normal feces. Weight loss, dehydration, and anemia can be observed in severe cases with blood or mucus in the feces.

TREATMENT AND CONTROL

Phthalofyne is a useful and highly selective drug targeted against whipworms. It is given intravenously at a dose rate of 250 mg/kg. Vomiting, drowsiness, and ataxia may accompany such treatment. Oral phthalofyne has fewer of these side effects, but vomiting may sometimes occur. Phthalofyne is contraindicated in dogs with nephritis, hepatitis, or cardiac insufficiency.

Glycobiarsol orally in tablet form or crushed in feed is effective at 220 mg/kg for 5 consecutive days. In aged or debilitated animals, a lower dose rate of 110 mg/kg is recommended.

Dichlorvos at 27 mg/kg in the dog and 11 mg/kg in the pup possesses broad-spectrum activity against whipworms, ascarids, and hookworms. It is contraindicated in dogs with heartworm or in animals suffering from chronic hepatitis, nephritis, or cardiac insufficiency.

Butamisole hydrochloride is an injectable anthelmintic (2.4 mg/kg) effective against hookworms and whipworms. It possesses a relatively narrow safety margin of 4:1, may cause local irritation, and should not be used concurrently with bunamidine hydrochloride or in animals with heartworm or those that are debilitated.

Broad-spectrum anthelmintics useful against whipworms include mebendazole, fenbendazole, and febantel. Mebendazole is given daily in food for 3 days at a dose of 22 mg/kg. It affects hookworms, some tapeworms, and ascarids.

Fenbendazole is available in tablet or granular form for addition to moist food. At a dose of 50 mg/kg for 3 consecutive days, fenbendazole is effective also against hookworms, ascarids, and *Taenia* tapeworms. Febantel is another benzimidazole effective against *Trichuris vulpis*. It is commonly combined with praziquantel to affect *Ancylostoma caninum*, *Uncinaria stenocephala*, *Toxocara canis*, *Toxascaris leonina*, *Dipylidium*, and *Taenia*. The dose rate for this combination is 1 g paste/3.4 kg body weight for 3 days. (10 mg/kg febantel and 1 mg/kg praziquantel for 3 days.)

Although not recommended for such use on the label, ivermectin is effective therapy for *Trichuris vulpis* infection with 100% success against this parasite at a dose of 100 μg/kg. Prior to using the drug in this unauthorized fashion, the client must sign a release form. Milbemycin is also effective. Ivermectin is contraindicated in Collies or collie-type crossbreeds.

Animals should be monitored routinely at 12-week intervals to prevent establishment of new patent whipworm infection. Because of the extended prepatent period of *T. vulpis*, dogs should be retreated 3 months after initial therapy with suitable anthelmintic agents.

Diarrhea may require symptomatic control with locally acting gut protectants, such as Kaopectate or bismuth salts; antibiotics are rarely indicated.

Owners must be advised that, following treatment, expulsion of whipworms can take a relatively long time (72 hours or so). Whipworms can also be implicated as rare causes of visceral larval migrans in children, and the significance of this possibility should always be communicated to the owner.

Daily removal of feces from kennels, use of concrete floors/runs, avoidance of overcrowding, and maintenance of dryness of the surroundings are the necessary standard control measures. Excreted eggs take about 1 month to develop and are resistant to chemical agents. The use of flame guns is an effective method of decontaminating the environment.

34.5 THREADWORMS

These small nematodes, *Strongyloides stercoralis* in the dog and *Strongyloides tumefaciens* in the cat, parasitize the mucosa of the anterior small intestine. They are usually found in warm, wet, unsanitary, crowded, small animal premises. Infection takes place by oral ingestion or skin penetration. Oral infection may lead to systemic migration with the larvae appearing in the lungs before being coughed up and swallowed back into the small intestine. Penetration by infective third-stage larvae into the skin may produce erythema and pruritus at the site of entry. Verminous pneumonia may result from larval penetration of the lungs, whereas, blood-stained mucoid diarrhea is characteristic of heavy infestations in young animals during hot humid weather.

Four major anthelmintics are effective in threadworm infestations. Thiabendazole 50 mg/kg to 75 mg/kg daily, for 3 days is a useful first choice, but emesis may accompany use. Diethylcarbamazine 100 mg/kg, dithiazanine 5 mg/kg daily for 10 days, and pyrvinium pamoate 20 mg/kg daily for 5 days are alternate effective choices. Experimental use of broad-spectrum mebendazole has also been successful. (Ivermectin and milbemycins display high activity against strongyloides.)

General control measures include avoidance of overcrowding, regular disposal of feces, routine fecal examination, routine deworming, and attention to improvements in general sanitation. Direct sunlight and desiccation are deleterious to survival of free larval stages, and application of concentrated lime or salt solutions can be beneficial for impervious surfaces. *S. stercoralis* in dogs may cause human infestation (and vice versa). Clients should be advised accordingly.

34.6 TAPEWORMS

The life cycle of the tapeworm consists of three major stages, the adult, the oncosphere, and the larva. Adult tapeworms in dogs and cats are found attached to the wall of the small intestine by holdfast organs, i.e., hooks or suckers. Adults in the small intestine produce eggs containing the oncosphere, which then becomes infective to the intermediate host by ingestion. Different types of larvae develop in the intermediate hosts and become infective for the final host by ingestion. Depending on the species of tapeworm, these intermediate stages (bladder worms) can be found in various hosts in the forms of cysticercoids, coenuri, strobilocerci, or hydatids. A wide range of cestodes can parasitize small animals, but among the most common are *Taenia, Dipylidium, Echinococcus, Mesocestoides*, and *Diphyllobothrium*. Of these, *Taenia* and *Dipylidium* are more routinely found in dogs and cats. The life cycles among these species differ primarily because of dissimilarities in their intermediate hosts. Fleas or lice on cats and dogs are intermediate hosts for *Dipylidium*, and small or large vertebrates serve as intermediate hosts for *Taenia*. Because most domesticated urban dogs ingest prepared foods and have limited access to wild prey, ectoparasites (mainly fleas) serve as the primary source for *Dipylidium caninum* infestation. *Echinococcus*, a parasite of particular public health significance, can be acquired from ingestion of meat or offal of sheep, horses, cattle, swine, deer, or rodents.

Adult cestodes in the intestine of dogs and cats do not usually cause symptoms of serious disease unless the worm burden is particularly severe. Clinical signs can vary from ill-thrift, bad coat, and listlessness to colic, emaciation, diarrhea, and seizures. By competing for uptake of nutrients, malabsorption and anemia may be observed in extreme cases.

Diagnosis of infestation is based on identification of proglottids or eggs in the feces.

Taenia are large tapeworms that can develop to lengths of 60 cm to 100 cm or more depending on species. *Taenia multiceps* is acquired from ingestion of uncooked or undercooked sheep heads, *T. hydatigena* from offal, and *T. ovis* from meat.

Sheep may be infested with the coenurus stage ("gid") by grazing pasture contaminated by dog feces. Other *Taenia* can be responsible for financial losses at slaughterhouses because of the presence of intermediate cystlike stages in the tissues of food animals.

Dipylidium is the commonest tapeworm in the dog. Eggs develop when eaten by a flea larvae or biting louse of the dog. Completion of the life cycle occurs when the intermediate host is swallowed. Many of these tapeworms may be present in the small intestine of a single dog.

Association with infected dogs may result in human infection with metacestodes of *Echinococcus granulosus, E. multilocularis, Taenia multiceps, T. serialis, T. crassiceps*, or *Dipylidium caninum*.

Echinococcus granulosus is the cestode responsible for hydatidosis in humans, horses, and meat animals. In the dog, this cestode penetrates deeply into the bases of the villi of the small intestine, and the hundreds or thousands of eggs in the affected dog all release gravid segments that are passed with the feces. Tapeworm eggs are immediately infective and, when ingested by an intermediate host (horses, humans), develop into an hydatid cyst. A fertile cyst contains thousands of protoscolices, each capable of bearing an adult tapeworm if ingested by a dog.

In addition to causing economic damage to farm livestock, deaths, reduction of wool and slaughter quality, and contamination of offal, hydatidosis is of great importance in human medicine because the cysts can develop in humans. During the latent stage, hardly any symptoms are present, whereas in the manifest stage, the growing cysts cause atrophy and displacement manifestations. Finally, in the completion stage, the clinical picture is dominated by perforations, embolisms, infections and sepsis, anaphylactic reactions, and intoxication. Surgery performed at this stage is often too late. The treatment of choice is prevention of disease and death in humans and of damage to farm livestock by the systematic treatment of dogs with a cestocide that has complete activity against all developmental stages in the intestine (Table 34–7). Praziquantel is the drug of choice for this parasite.

Successful chemotherapy of cestode infections requires complete and total elimination of the embedded scolex from its intestinal attachment sites. Older cestocidal compounds, such as arecoline hydrobro-

TABLE 34–7
ANTICESTODAL DRUGS

Active Ingredient	Administration	Efficacy Against		
		Taenia	*Dipylidium*	*Echinococcus*
Bunamidine hydrochloride	Oral	+ +	+	+
Dichlorophene	Oral	+	+	−
Drocarbil	Oral	+	+	−
Fenbendazole	Oral	+	−	−
Mebendazole	Oral	+	−	−
Nitroscanate	Oral	+ +	+ +	±
Niclosamide	Oral	+ +	+ +	
Praziquantel	Oral/injectable	+ +	+ +	+ +
Epsiprantel	Oral	+ +	+ +	±

+ +—Efficacy > 90%
+—Efficacy 60 to 80%
− —< 50%
±—highly variable

mide and arecoline acetarsol, are still used despite their lack of efficacy against the scolices and their cholinergic type of side effects. These older compounds act primarily to remove the proglottids while leaving the embedded scolex free to bud off new segments in the intestine.

Praziquantel is the most efficacious cestocide currently available against the larvae and adult stages of *Taenia, multiceps, M. corti,* and *Dipylidium caninum.* It is the drug of choice for *D. caninum* and *Echinococcus granulosus* infestation. A single 5 mg/kg oral or subcutaneous dose of praziquantel eliminates 100% of both immature and adult stages of these major parasites. It is effective in various animal species, including humans.

Bunamidine is highly effective against *Taenia, Dipylidium,* and *Mesocestoides corti* and is the drug of choice against *Spirometra* and *Diphyllobothrium* infestation. Food must be withheld for 3 hours prior to use, and the entire unbroken tablets are given on an empty stomach. Normal dose is 25 to 50 mg/kg up to a maximum dosage of 600 mg. Ventricular fibrillation, vomiting, and diarrhea are reported side effects, and the drug should not be used concurrently with butamisole. Treatment must not be repeated within 14 days. Bunamidine is contraindicated in unweaned pups or kittens, in ani-

mals with pre-existing cardiac or hepatic disease, or in male dogs within 28 days of breeding.

Niclosamide can be given after an overnight fast to dogs and cats. It is reasonably effective against *Taenia* in dogs and cats, but is somewhat less effective against *Dipylidium* and *Echinococcus.* Vomiting and diarrhea are occasional side effects. The normal dose rate is 157 mg/kg.

Mebendazole, at 22 mg/kg for 5 days, and fenbendazole, at 50 mg/kg for 3 days, are effective against *Taenia,* as well as the other common nematode parasites of dogs and cats. Mebendazole is not effective against *Dipylidium caninum,* and elevated dosages are required to treat adult *Echinococcus.*

In summary, mebendazole, fenbendazole, niclosamide, bunamidine, and praziquantel are all effective against *Taenia.* Bunamidine is the first drug of choice against *Spirometra, Diphyllobothrium,* and *Mesocestoides.* Overall, however, praziquantel is undoubtedly the primary cestocide for infestation with *Echinococcus* and *Dipylidium.*

Epsiprantel (Cestex) is a compound related to praziquantel that is presented in tablet form for dogs and cats and provides excellent activity against *Dipylidium caninum, Taenia taeniaeformis,* and *T. pisiformis.* This drug has no known contraindications, but it should not be used in kittens or puppies younger than 7 weeks of age.

A combination of epsiprantel with pyrantel provides added cover against roundworms and hookworms.

Drontal Plus (Vercom Plus) for dogs is a broad-spectrum anthelmintic containing a combination of the active ingredients praziquantel, pyrantel embonate, and febantel. The combined formulation has several advantages:

1. Comprehensive spectrum of activity including roundworms and tapeworms
2. Activity enhancement by the synergistic action of pyrantel and febantel.

Praziquantel kills mature and immature developmental stages of tapeworms in the intestine after a single treatment. Within a few seconds of coming into contact with praziquantel, the interaction of the tapeworm with phospholipids and proteins causes damage to the integument. The inflow of calcium ions results in an immediate contraction of the entire strobilia, thereby leading to a reduction of glucose intake and an accelerated depletion of energy reserves.

Pyrantel is a member of the tetrahydropyrimidine group of compounds that act similar to levamisole by inducing neuromuscular blockade. As a cholinergic agonist, pyrantel acts as an excitatory neurotransmitter at the nicotinic receptors and thus causes spastic paralysis of the parasite.

The action of febantel is primarily based on interference with the carbohydrate metabolism of the parasite. The suppression of mitochondrial reactions inhibits the fumarate reductase, and interference with glucose transport acts not only on all developmental stages of the helminths, but also on the eggs containing the larvae.

34.7 GIARDIASIS

Giardia species are flagellate protozoan parasites inhabiting the mucosal surface of the small intestine, where they replicate by binary fission. *Giardia canis* in the dog and *Giardia cati* in the cat can be responsible for chronic diarrhea, especially in immature animals. Following ingestion of the cyst stage of the parasite, encystation occurs in the duodenum. In the upper small intestine in dogs and the lower small intestine in cats trophozoites become attached to the brush border of the villous epithelium at the base of the villi. Replication is asexual, with cysts and trophozoites excreted through the feces.

Because of the predilection sites of the parasites, malabsorption and maldigestion are common sequelae of infection. Blunting of villi with inflammatory infiltration of the villous lamina propria, exfoliation of enterocytes, and impairment of active transport mechanisms follow. Pale malodorous stools, steatorrhea, and chronic diarrhea with maintenance of normal appetite typify this malabsorption state. Adult animals may be slightly affected clinically, but can serve as asymptomatic carriers.

THERAPY

Several drugs are effective for treatment of this protozoan condition (Table 34–8).

Quinacrine, 6.6 mg/kg orally twice daily for 5 days, is useful, although vomiting,

---

TABLE 34–8
DRUGS FOR GIARDIASIS

Host	Drug	Dose schedule
Dog	Metronidazole	10–25 mg/kg, orally, twice daily for 5 days
	Quinacrine	4–6.6 mg/kg, orally, twice daily for 5 days
	Tinidazole	44 mg/kg, orally, once daily for 3 days
	Furazolidone	2–4 mg/kg, orally, twice daily for 7 days
	also Paromomycin, used experimentally in man.	
	Albendazole, used experimentally in mice.	

lethargy, and dark-stained urine may accompany its use.

Nitroimidazoles (ipronidazole, metronidazole) may also be considered. Ipronidazole in water, 126 mg/liter daily for 7 days, has proved successful, but fresh water must be replaced daily. Metronidazole, 10 to 25 mg/kg orally for 5 to 7 days, although relatively expensive, is useful in both dogs and cats. Rarely seen side effects are primarily neurologic.

Furazolidone is less expensive than the nitroimidazoles and can be given more conveniently as a suspension, 4 mg/kg orally twice daily for 7 days.

Overall control also depends on dryness of surroundings, prompt removal of feces, and disinfection of surfaces with Lysol or dilute chlorine bleach.

Some evidence shows that cross-infection from animals to humans (and vice versa) may take place.

Because metronidazole and furazolidone are suspect carcinogens, they should not be administered to pregnant animals. Skin contact with these drugs should be avoided.

34.8 TOXOPLASMOSIS

Toxoplasma gondii is an obligate intracellular protozoan parasite that affects many animals, including humans. Infection in cats is of particular significance because the feline species can serve as a reservoir of human infection.

Cats can acquire infection by carnivorous activity, primarily through ingestion of feces, or by congenital infection. *T. gondii* can parasitize small animals without producing significant clinical signs, although focal areas of necrosis can occur in many tissues. Age, sex, number of parasites, host species, and strains of *T. gondii* may be responsible for differences in the severity of the infectious process. Oocysts may penetrate the intestinal epithelial cells and multiply in the intestine, thereby spreading to the local mesenteric lymph nodes and distant organs via the blood and lymph. In young animals, especially puppies and kittens, signs include fever, anorexia, dyspnea, diarrhea, and central nervous system signs. Oocyst formation is greatest in 6 to 14-week-old cats. Following shedding, these oocysts can survive in the environment for many months and are resistant to disinfectants, freezing, and drying. A major zoonotic hazard is the presence of infected cats in the household of pregnant women, because transplacental toxoplasmosis can readily occur in humans.

THERAPY

Sulfadiazine and pyrimethamine are the two synergistic drugs commonly used to treat toxoplasmosis in humans. These drugs act in sequential blockade fashion by blocking folinic acid synthesis necessary for replication of the parasite. In humans, the dose rate is 73 mg/kg sulfadiazine and 0.44 mg/kg pyrimethamine. Sulfadiazine alone (60 to 120 mg/kg) is also successful. In dogs, clindamycin phosphate, 150 mg/kg intramuscularly 4 times per day, and sulfonamides potentiated with trimethoprim or pyrimethamine may be useful. When bone marrow depression is induced by these antifolate agents, folinic acid can be employed successfully as a reversing agent. Pyrimethamine, 1 mg/kg daily, may also be considered for infected animals.

34.9 ENTERIC COCCIDIAL INFECTIONS

ISOSPORA

Among the coccidial parasites that infect dogs and cats, *Isospora* (also called *Cystisospora*) are most commonly encountered. The fecal-oral transmission life cycle involves ingestion of sporulated oocysts, which develop into sporozoites, trophozoites, schizonts, and merozoites. A sexual cycle then develops with expulsion of oocysts in the feces.

Signs attributed to *Isospora* infection include diarrhea, dehydration, abdominal pain, vomiting, anorexia, and weight loss. Coccidial oocysts often are found in association with diarrheic stools in pups and kittens. Usually the condition is associated with other infectious agents, immunosuppression, or stress. Some animals can spontaneously eliminate *Isospora* infections, but numerous chemotherapeutic agents are also effective.

Sulfonamides, such as sulfaguanidine 100 mg/kg three times a day for 5 days, sulfadimethoxine 50 mg/kg for 10 days, sulfadiazine-trimethoprim 30 to 60 mg/kg for 6 days, or sulfadimethoxine 55 mg/kg and ormethoprim 11 mg/kg for 21 days, are relatively successful.

Amprolium 300 to 400 mg/kg for 5 days or amprolium 150 mg and sulfadimethoxine 25 mg/kg for 14 days are useful alternatives. Amprolium is probably the most useful compound, especially in newborn pups. Nitrofurazone, 20 mg/kg day, is also coccidiostatic. Supportive fluid therapy is essential in dehydrated young animals. Strong ammonium hydroxide solution or heat treatment is the most effective method of destroying oocysts in the environment. Feces must be regularly removed and contamination of food and water avoided.

CRYPTOSPORIDIUM

Although most commonly a disease affecting ruminants, a few reports of *Cryptosporidium* infections in dogs and cats have appeared. Cryptosporidia are minute protozoan parasites transmitted by the oral-fecal route. Their mean incubation period is 3 to 4 days. In dogs, the parasites locate in the brush border of the small intestine, especially the ileum, whereas in cats, the organisms may be found also on the cecal epithelium. Many of these infections in dogs and cats resolve spontaneously, and hence, only supportive therapy may be required. Animals with immunosuppression are more susceptible to severe infections and the development of more apparent clinical signs. Spiramycin, 50 to 75 mg/kg, has been used with variable results against canine cryptosporidiosis, as also has clindamycin, but usually fluid therapy and supportive care oriented toward enteritis are adequate. In man, spiramycin and furazolidone have provided some relief in affected human cases of cryptosporidia. Dogs and cats can serve as reservoirs of infection for humans, and accordingly, this parasitic disease has some zoonotic potential. Oocysts in the environment may be killed with 5% ammonia solution.

34.10 RESPIRATORY PARASITES

FILAROIDES OSLERI

This tracheal parasite is usually found in thin-walled nodules at the bronchial bifurcation. The life cycle of the nematode requires no development outside the definitive host. Hence, because of this direct life cycle, an infected bitch can transfer infection to her litter during licking and grooming. The condition of verminous nodular bronchitis arises once the larvae enter the blood and are carried to their predilection sites in the bronchial bifurcation. Transmission can occur through ingestion of regurgitated stomach contents, feces, or tissues containing first-stage larvae. Lungworm infection (*F. osleri*) may be underdiagnosed as a cause of coughing in dogs and cats. Clinical signs of respiratory distress are accompanied by a characteristic persistent dry hacking cough.

Numerous anthelmintics display varying degrees of efficacy against *F. osleri*.

Levamisole 7.5 mg/kg orally for 10 days; benzimidazoles such as thiabendazole 32 mg/kg orally twice daily for 21 days; oxfendazole 50 mg/kg and albendazole 25 mg/kg have also been employed as a daily treatment for 1 week. Arsenamide 2.2 mg/kg intravenously for 2 to 3 weeks has led to resolution of nodules. Ivermectin at a single dose of 0.4 mg/kg is perhaps one of the more promising drugs.

Fenbendazole can be used for *Filaroides* infection in dogs at a dose of 50 mg/kg for 7 days.

Parasitic tracheobronchitis is mainly associated with dogs bred in kennels where *F. osleri* is endemic.

FILAROIDES HIRTHI

Filaroides hirthi, a nematode parasite related to *F. osleri*, is found in the lung parenchyma in colonies of Beagle dogs, in which it can pose serious problems.

Oral albendazole, 25 mg/kg given twice daily for 5 days, has been successful in the treatment of *F. hirthi*. Fenbendazole, 50 mg/kg for 14 days, has also been relatively successful.

AELUROSTRONGYLUS ABSTRUSUS

This nematode parasitizes the lung parenchyma of the cat, thereby causing the condition of feline verminous pneumonia. It is the commonest lungworm of the cat in the United States and Europe. Eggs deposited in lung tissue develop into first-stage larvae, which are carried up to the tracheobronchial tree and appear in the feces. Further development occurs only if first-stage larvae enter various snails or slugs. Birds or rodents may serve as vectors of encysted larvae.

Coughing, dyspnea, wasting, and pulmonary rales are associated with this infestation, although small to moderate infections may not be revealed by clinical signs.

Oral levamisole, 8 mg/kg three times daily at 2-day intervals, can be quite effective in arresting fecal larval output. Fenbendazole, 20 mg/kg orally for 5 consecutive days, has also been effective in mitigating clinical signs and controlling parasitologic development. Variable results have been obtained with fenbendazole at 50 mg/kg daily for 3 to 7 days. Successful treatment for many of these conditions, however, is quite difficult, and results can be quite erratic.

CAPILLARIA AEROPHILA

Capillaria aerophila, usually found in the nasal cavities, frontal sinuses, trachea, and larger bronchi, parasitizes dogs, cats, foxes, and numerous carnivorous species.

The life cycle is direct in dogs, which become infected by ingesting feed or water contaminated with larvated eggs.

Although capillariasis of dogs and cats can be asymptomatic, a chronic harsh cough is sometimes associated with the condition. Sneezing and nasal discharge may also be observed. Such infection in fur farm foxes is not uncommon. Although levamisole and fenbendazole can be used in treatment, best results are obtained with a single oral dose of 0.2 mg/kg of ivermectin.

LINGUATULA SERRATA

Linguatula serrata is a specialized arthropod that parasitizes the nasal passages and frontal sinuses of dogs and carnivores. A blood-sucking pentastomid, *L. serrata* usually responds to systemic organophosphorous medication or intranasal instillation of insecticides.

BLOOD-BORNE PARASITES

Important rickettsial and protozoan parasites of canine and feline erythrocytes include *Haemobartonella canis, H. felis, Babesia canis,* and *B. gibsoni.*

Haemobartonella canis causes canine haemobartonellosis, an infectious hemolytic anemia. It usually occurs as a secondary pathogen that complicates the course of some other primary infectious disease. Listlessness, pale mucous membranes, and small to moderate anemia characterize the infection.

Therapy involves blood transfusion in severe cases, identification and treatment of the primary predisposing disease, and employment of specific drugs, namely tetracyclines, to eliminate the rickettsial infection. Oral tetracycline, 22 mg/kg three times a day for 2 weeks and oral oxytetracycline, 25 mg/kg three times a day for 10 days, are the drugs of choice. Oral prednisolone (1 mg/kg) for 1 week may be useful in restricting the lysis of parasitized erythrocytes in the monocyte-macrophage system.

Similar to *H. canis, H. felis* causes feline infectious anemia characterized by hemolytic anemia, weakness, anorexia, and depression. As an opportunist pathogen secondary to primary causes (like *H. canis*), modes of transmission include blood-sucking ectoparasites, blood transfusions, congenital infections, cat bites, or milk.

Oxytetracycline is the primary drug of choice; an alternate is tetracycline. Chloramphenicol should be avoided in cats because it tends to cause hematopoietic suppression in an already anemic animal. Blood transfusions and oral prednisolone may be employed as ancillary therapy.

Babesia canis, a protozoan blood parasite, is not amenable to therapy with chemotherapeutic agents effective against *Haemobartonella.* Drugs of choice for canine babesiasis include imidocarb dipropionate, diminazene aceturate, and phenamidine isethionate (Table 34–9). Rehydration, blood trans-

TABLE 34–9
DRUGS FOR BLOOD-BORNE PARASITES

	Drug	Route	Dose
Dog			
Babesia	Imidocarb dipropionate	Intramuscularly	5 mg/kg, once daily as a single dose
	Phenamidine isethionate	Subcutaneously	10–15 mg/kg, on 2 successive days
	Diminazene	Intramuscularly	2.0–3.5 mg/kg, once per day
Haemobartonella canis	Tetracycline	Orally	22 mg/kg, 3 times a day, 8–12 days
	Oxytetracycline	Orally	25 mg/kg, 3 times a day, 8–12 days
	Chloramphenicol	Orally	25 mg/kg, 3 times a day, 8–12 days

fusion, and correction of acidosis with bicarbonate-containing solutions are indicated.

Control of ticks is essential to prevention. *B. canis* is easier to treat with the previously mentioned compounds than is *B. gibsoni*.

SELECTED REFERENCES

Abbith, B., Huey, R.L., Eugster, A.K., et al.: Treatment of giardiasis in adult greyhounds using iproni-dazole medicated water. J. Am. Vet. Med. Assoc., *188*:67, 1986.

Allen, L.J., Marshall, J.R., Nall, L.A., et al.: Compendium of chemotherapeutic agents for parasitic protozoa and helminths of dogs and cats. VM/SAC, Aug. 1976.

Anderson, D.L., and Roberson, E.L.: Activity of ivermectin against canine intestinal helminths. Am. J. Vet. Res., *43*:1681, 1983.

Arundel, J.H.: Veterinary anthelmintics. Veterinary Review No. 26. University of Sydney, Post-Graduate Foundation in Veterinary Science, Sydney, N.S.W.

Bennett, D.: The diagnosis and treatment of *Filariodes osleri* in the dog. Vet. Ann., *15*:256, 1975.

Bogan, J., and Duncan, J.L.: Anthelmintics for dogs, cats and horses. Br. Vet. J., *140*:361, 1984.

Boray, J.C., Stong, M.B., Allison, J.R., et al.: Nitroscanate: a new broad spectrum anthelmintic against cestodes and nematodes of dogs and cats. Aust. Vet. J., *55*:45, 1979.

Bowman, D.D., Lin, D.S., Johnson, R.D., et al.: Effects of milbemycin oxine on adult *A. caninum* and *U. stenocephala* in dogs with experimentally induced infections. Am. J. Vet. Res., *52*:64, 1991.

Bowman, D.S.: Hookworm parasites of dogs and cats. Comp. Cont. Educ. Pract. Vet., *14*:585, 1992.

Bowman, D.S.: Anthelmintics for dogs and cats, effective against nematodes and cestodes. Comp. Cont. Educ. Pract. Vet., *14*:597, 1992.

Burke, T.M., and Roberson, E.L.: Fenbendazole treatment of pregnant bitches to reduce prenatal and lactogenic infections of *Toxocara canis* and *Ancylostoma caninum* in pups. J. Am. Vet. Med. Assoc., *183*:987, 1983.

Corwin, R.M., et al.: Dose titration of febantel against *Ancylostoma caninum* and *Trichuris vulpis* infections in dogs. Am. J. Vet. Res., *43*:1100, 1982.

Davidson, R.S.: The treatment of giardiasis. Am. J. Gastroenterol., *79*:256, 1984.

Evinger, J.V., Kazocos, K.R., and Cantwell, H.D.: Ivermectin for the treatment of nasal capillariasis in a dog. J. Am. Vet. Med. Assoc., *186*:174, 1985.

Genchi, C., Traldi, G., and Manfredi, M.T.: Field trials of the anthelmintic efficacy of nitroscanate and mebendazole in dogs. Vet. Rec., *126*:77, 1990.

Greene, C.G., Cook, J.R., and Mahoffey, E.A.: Clindamycin for the treatment of *Toxoplasma* in a dog. J. Am. Vet. Med. Assoc., *186*:631, 1985.

Grieve, R.B.: Parasite infections. Vet. Clin. North Am. (Small Anim. Pract.), *16*:6, 1987.

Hass, D.K., Collins, J.A., and Flick, S.C.: Canine parasitism. Canine Pract., *2*:42, 1975.

Hopkins, T.J., Gyr, P., and Hedeman, P.M.: Nematocidal and cesticidal efficacy of a tablet formulation containing febantel, pyrantel, and praziquantel in dogs. Vet. Med. Rev., *59*:71, 1988.

Hopkins, T.J.: Efficacy of a tablet containing pyrantel embonate, febantel and praziquantel against *T. canis* in dogs. Vet. Rec., *128*:331, 1991.

Hurley, K.J., Bowman, D.D., and Frongillo, M.K.: Experimental infections with *Uncinaria stenocephala* in young dogs. Treatment with nitroscanate. Proc. Am. Assoc. Vet. Parasitol., *42*:199, 1990.

Jacobs, D.E.: Control of *Toxocara canis* in puppies: A comparison of screening techniques and evaluation of a dosing program. J. Vet. Pharmacol. Ther., *10*:23, 1986.

Jacobs, D.E.: Helminths of the dog—Treatment and control. In Practice, Jan. 1984.

Jacobs, D.E., Fisher, M.A., Pilkington, J.G., et al.: J. Small Anim. Pract., *31*:59, 1990.

Kelly, P.J., and Mason, P.R.: Successful treatment of *Filaroides osleri* infection with oxfendazole. Vet. Rec., *116*:445, 1985.

Kirkpatrick, C.E.: Feline giardiasis—A review. J. Small Anim. Pract., *27*:69, 1986.

McKellar, Q.A., Harrison, P., Galbraith, E.A., and Inglis, H.: Pharmacokinetics of fenbendazole in dogs. J. Vet. Ter., *13*:386, 1990.

Portnoy, D., Whileside, M.E., and Buckley, E.: Treatment of intestinal crytosporidiosis with spiramycin. Ann. Intern. Med., *101*:202, 1984.

Rew, R.S.: Mode of action of common anthelmintics. J. Vet. Pharmacol. Ther., *1*:183, 1978.

Roudebush, P.: An updated guide to the chemotherapy of small animal intestinal parasites. Canine Pract., *12*:5, 1985.

Schantz, P.M., Stehr-Green, J.K., Toxocacaral larva migrans. J. Am. Vet. Med. Assoc. *192*:28, 1988.

Sharp, M.L., and McCurdy, H.D.: The anthelmintic efficacy of combining febantel with praziquantel in dogs. J. Am. Vet. Med. Assoc., *187(3)*:254, 1985.

Sharp, M.L., Sepesi, J.P., and Collins, J.A.: A comparative cuteal assay of canine anthelmintics. Vet. Med., Feb. 1973.

Staffman, A.E., and Braithwaite, A.: A piperazine overdose in a kitten. Can. Vet. J., *17*:140, 1976.

Takiguti, H., Mashima, O., and Okuda, M.: Milbemycin, a new family of macrolide antibiotics. Fermentation, isolation and physicochemical properties. J. Antibiot., *33*:1120, 1983.

Todd, A.C.: Pyrantel pamoate against internal parasites of dogs. VM/SAC, *70*:936, 1975.

Zajac, A.M., Giardiasis, Key Facts. Comp. Cont. Educ. Pract. Vet., *14*:604, 1992.

Zimmer, J.F., and Burrington, D.B.: Comparison of four protocols for the treatment of canine giardiasis. J. Am. Anim. Hosp. Assoc., *22*:168, 1986.

35

HEARTWORM DISEASE

35.1 Introduction
35.2 Life Cycle of *Dirofilaria Immitis*
35.3 Pathology of *Dirofilaria Immitis* Infection
35.4 Diagnosis of Heartworm Disease
35.5 Therapeutic Considerations
35.6 Chemotherapy
35.7 Supportive Therapeutic Measures

35.1 INTRODUCTION

Dirofilaria immitis is an epizootic filarial parasite that causes heartworm disease in domestic dogs and occasionally in cats. In endemic areas, heartworms are a major cause of acquired heart disease. Adults of *D. immitis* occur in the right ventricle and pulmonary artery; microfilaria are present in the blood. Chronic infections cause pulmonary hypertension and can progress to right-sided congestive heart failure. The presence of adult parasites in the posterior vena cava is associated with the clinically significant posterior caval syndrome. Many complications may occur in heartworm-infected dogs. These are mainly preventable, and the disease process is curable if diagnosis and filaricide treatment are timely.

The prevalence of *D. immitis* infection varies greatly among regions. In the coastal areas of the Southeastern United States, the infection rate of adult dogs that do not receive prophylactic therapy approaches 90%. High mosquito populations are naturally associated with greater prevalence rates.

The average age of heartworm-infected dogs is 6 to 7 years, and in general terms prevalence is higher in larger breeds and in working and sporting dogs. Pets kept predominantly indoors tend to be infected less frequently.

35.2 LIFE CYCLE OF *DIROFILARIA IMMITIS*

Unsheathed embryos produced by adult female heartworms can take up to 190 days to appear in detectable numbers in the bloodstream. The life span of the microfilaria in the blood is 1 to 3 years, and a single generation of adult parasites can continue to release microfilariae over a 7-year period. These microfilariae complete their development to the infective third stage larvae only in a suitable mosquito vector.

Within the mosquito, the infective larval stage is attained in about 2 weeks. Infective third stage larvae are transmissible to dogs during feeding by infected mosquitos. These immature stages are deposited in the intramuscular fascia, fat, or subserosal tissues and molt to fourth stage larvae 3 to 5 days after infection and to the fifth stage

larvae 70 to 80 days after infection. Arrival in the right ventricle and pulmonary arteries occurs 2 to 4 months after infection. After an additional 2 to 3 months, the cardiac parasites reach full maturity. The prepatent period of *D. immitis* is 6 to 7 months, with microfilaria released into the blood approximately 6 months after infestation.

Prenatal infection can sometimes occur when a pregnant bitch is inoculated with infective third stage larvae. Bitches with patent *D. immitis* infections and an accompanying microfilaremia can give birth to pups with low numbers of circulatory first stage microfilaria.

Adult heartworms have a predilection for the pulmonary arteries, where the primary pathologic lesions occur. At times they are found in the right ventricle. Lung parenchymal tissue is also adversely affected. When large numbers of adult worms are present in the hepatic veins and caudal vena cava, hepatic syndromes also develop. Primary lesions occur in the pulmonary arteries and lung parenchyma (intravascular parasites).

Microfilariae in the bloodstream—although playing only a relatively minor pathogenic role—may contribute to the overall development of pneumonitis and glomerulonephritis. Hypersensitivity to microfilariae frequently develops, and depending on the severity, intensity, and duration of infection, a variety of clinical syndromes can be associated with heartworm infection, viz., cor pulmonale, pulmonary pneumonitis, liver failure, and nephropathy with hemoglobinuria and proteinuria. The syndrome of occult heartworm disease is another frequently encountered clinical entity. Pulmonary hypertension is one of the most important pathologic effects of heartworm disease.

35.3 PATHOLOGY OF *DIROFILARIA IMMITIS* INFECTION

Pulmonary hypertension is the most common sequel of chronic heartworm infection. Endarteritis and thromboembolism with living and dead adult parasites are the most constant changes in the pulmonary arteries, resulting in elevation of blood pressure in the pulmonary vessels and secondary right heart enlargement (cor pulmonale). Sudden elevations in pulmonary arterial pressure are associated with embolic showers induced by heartworm death resulting from either drug treatment or natural causes. Heartworms can physically block some arteries, but more commonly, intimal proliferation and embolic worm fragments trigger thrombosis. The greatest number of worms and the most severe lesions usually occur in the caudal lobal arteries. Initial contact between the parasite and the arteries results in intimal thickening and narrowing of the vessel lumen. The resultant endarteritis and villous projections create a favorable climate for the formation of thromboemboli. Such obliterative endarteritis causes impedance to pulmonary blood flow. Thrombosis and thromboembolism compromise pulmonary circulates still further.

Pulmonary artery dilation, reduction in the pulmonary collateral circulation, and focal alterations in the ventilation/perfusion ratio all develop because of the occlusive vascular changes.

Pulmonary hypertension results in compensatory right ventricular hypertrophy and ultimately right-sided congestive heart failure. Therefore, infestation with *D. immitis* is a major contributing factor to right-sided cardiac failure. With heavy infections, pulmonary hemosiderosis, increased erythrocytic fragility, and interstitial pneumonitis can occur. The success rate of a given therapeutic program in restoring pulmonary arteries to their former normal condition depends on the level and duration of parasitic infection.

The vascular lesions cause several deleterious effects in the dog:

1. Exercise intolerance lassitude.
2. Greater pressure and work load must be generated by the right ventricle to maintain a normal blood flow through the constricted arteries.
3. Right-sided ventricular dilation, hypertrophy, and failure can develop in response to pulmonary hypertension.

Liver failure can occur when large numbers of worms accumulate in the right atria, vena cava, and hepatic veins. Heavy infections causing the caval syndrome are most common in dogs less than 3 years of age. This syndrome is marked by acute-onset, a rapidly fatal course if not promptly treated and by hemolysis causing gross hemoglobinuria and hemoglobinemia. Although most of these animals also have pulmonary vascular disease, the most severe damage occurs in the liver. Central venous pressure is elevated, which is due to tricuspid incompetence caused by heartworms at the valvular orifice. Hepatic damage resulting from direct contact with the parasites is compounded by passive congestion. Caval obstructions cause enlarged hepatic venules, thickening of hepatic veins, and centrilobular necrosis. Disseminated intravascular coagulation (DIC) may occur in dogs with the hepatic failure syndrome, with increased fragility of erythrocytes. Disintegrating worm fragments can also stimulate an inflammatory reaction in the tunica intima. This adversely affects pulmonary blood flow, and resultant hypoxia.

The glomerulus is the primary site for heartworm-related renal disease. Dogs with high microfilaremic counts show a thickened undulating capillary basement membrane. The kidneys may also show evidence of hemosiderosis of the convoluted tubules with heme casts in the medulla. Some evidence supports an immune-mediated cause of membranous glomerulonephritis in heartworm-infected dogs. Immune complex deposits have also been incriminated in the establishment of glomerular lesions in dogs with occult dirofilariasis. Severe nephrosis and proteinuria result from glomerulonephritis, and minor glomerular damage can be caused by dead microfilaria following microfilaricide treatment.

Heartworm disease may be present without evidence of circulatory microfilaria (occult, or amicrofilaremic, conditions) for several reasons:

1. Heartworms are immature and not yet producing microfilaria (prepatent infection).
2. Drug-induced heartworm sterility.
3. The worms may be of one sex or sterile.
4. The immune response may eliminate the microfilaria but leave adult heartworm intact in the heart.

Many animals (up to 25%) with severe forms of clinical heartworm disease—lung damage, congestive heart failure, and the vena caval syndrome—suffer from occult dirofilariasis (no detectable levels of circulatory microfilariae in the blood). Dogs harboring adult female heartworms with microfilaria in utero, or dead microfilaria within small vessels of the lung where they are trapped within granulomatous lesions, may have microfilariae counts of zero.

In long-standing occult heartworm disease, an interstitial pattern can develop in the lung. Dogs with cardiopulmonary disease are primary candidates for diagnosis with occult heartworm disease. The prevalence of occult infection can be as high as 80% in dogs manifesting advanced signs of clinical disease. Microfilaremia may not be detectable as a result of immaturity of the parasites (prepatent infection), the presence of adult worms of only one sex, or suppression of microfilaria with microfilaricides. In some dogs with gravid female heartworms, microfilaria can disappear spontaneously after a variable period of patency. In sensitized animals, released microfilaria can become rapidly entrapped in the microcirculation, especially of the lung, with consequent granulomatous reactions.

The sequestration and destruction of large numbers of microfilaria in the pulmonary capillaries of dogs with immune-mediated occult infections can produce severe allergic pneumonitis and respiratory distress. This is manifested radiographically by intense dense pulmonary infiltration. An eosinophilic infiltration surrounds the degenerating microfilaria in the pulmonary capillaries. Pulmonary hypertension results from the capillary hyperplasia and hypertrophy and embolized microfilaria. Because of the usual high frequency of occult heart disease, some dogs with congestive heart failure may be mistakenly diagnosed with primary heart failure only. This obviously can lead to improper therapeutic management. Microfiliaria once released can often become trapped in the microcirculation, especially in the lung.

35.4 DIAGNOSIS OF HEARTWORM DISEASE

A provisional diagnosis of heartworm infection can be made based on history, clinical signs, and identification of *D. immitis* in the blood. The parasite can be isolated and identified in fresh blood by centrifugation (modified Knott's technique) or by millipore or nucleopore filters.

Serologic tests (indirect fluorescent antibody test, e.g. "Track test XI," [IFA], hemagglutination inhibition, [HI], or enzyme-linked immunosorbent assay [ELISA] tests) coupled with typical clinical signs and thoracic radiographs confirm the diagnosis. ELISA tests (Filarochek, Dirocheck, and "CITE") are accurate to varying degrees.

Because up to 20% of infected dogs do not exhibit microfilaremia, the term *occult infection* applies.

Many factors will assist in diagnosis of *D. immitis* infection, including the following:

HISTORY

Reduced exercise tolerance
Weight loss, lack of appetite
Coughing
Syncope and episodic weakness
Hemoptysis

CLINICAL EXAMINATION

Increased audibility of heart sounds on right thorax
Splitting of second heart sound
Tachypnea/dyspnea
Abnormal respiratory sounds
Right-sided congestive heart failure
Tachyarrythmias

Clinical signs vary with the severity and chronicity of the infection.

ANCILLARY AIDS

1. Thoracic radiography
2. Electrocardiography
3. Angiography

Thoracic radiographs are recommended in dogs manifesting clinical signs of heartworm infection. Most infected dogs show right ventricular enlargement.

Specific indication for heartworm infection is the enlargement of the main pulmonary artery and of the cranial lobar pulmonary arteries. Abnormalities of the caudal lobar pulmonary arteries are seen in heartworm-infected dogs. Interstitial and alveolar abnormalities are most prevalent in the right caudal and accessory lobes of heartworm-infected dogs.

Thoracic radiography in severely affected dogs usually reveals enlargement of the right ventricle, increased prominence of the main pulmonary artery, enlargement of lobar pulmonary arteries, and right ventricular hypertrophy.

DIAGNOSIS

Heartworm infection can be diagnosed when microfilaria are detected in the peripheral blood, either by microscopic examination of a wet blood smear or hematocrit capillary tube or by the Knott or filter concentration tests. Concentration tests such as the filter and Knott tests are more sensitive and specific, generally, 10 to 15% more sensitive than microscopic examination. However, when adult heartworms have already made their way to and are sexually reproducing in the right ventricle and pulmonary artery, microfilaria can be detected only by microscopic examination.

The number of circulatory microfilaria does not necessarily correlate directly with the number of adult heartworms present, but it can be affected by the seasons, the immune status of the animal, stage of infection, and previous drug therapy. Microfilaria periodicity in peripheral blood of infected dogs is variable; peak levels occur during late evening and early morning.

Diagnosis of infection can be carried out by way of direct blood smear, buffy coat examination, the Difil test, or serologic examination. Blood urea nitrogen (BUN) and serum glutamate pyruvate transaminase (SGPT) should also be checked before and sometimes after therapy to monitor the patient's response. The absence of microfiliarae does not rule out heartworm infection.

A modified Knott's test can be used to diagnose overt heartworm infection, or dyspnea. Dogs with a positive filter test can be examined radiographically to assess the thorax for lesions.

A complete blood cell count (CBC), urinalysis, and chemistry screen can be used to determine the need for pretreatment to improve the dog's condition before definitive treatment is initiated.

If the dog has clinical signs of heartworm infection and microfilaria cannot be seen, blood samples should be assayed for occult infection. Testing for occult infection is reserved for dogs with cardiopulmonary disease refractory to treatment as well as for any dog or cat with undiagnosed illness.

DIAGNOSTIC TESTS

Most diagnostic tests for canine heartworm disease have depended on the presence of circulating microfilariae in the blood stream. Microfilariae can only be detected by microscopic examination when adult *D. imitis* are reproducing in the right ventricle and pulmonary artery.

It is possible that severe heartworm disease can be present without circulating microfilariae. Occult heartworm disease may arise from:

1. Drug-induced adult parasite sterility, or
2. Immune responses may eliminate microfilariae but leave adults in the heart.

Several commercial test kits are available to assist the diagnosis. Diagnosis of infection can be carried out through direct blood smear, buffy coat examination, serologic examination, blood urea nitrogen examination, or serum glutamate pyruvate transaminase. This is done before and sometimes after therapy to monitor the animal's response.

Before prescribing preventive medicine, the dog must not be infected with microfilariae. Otherwise it may react severely and die.

Proprietary Test Kits:

The "Difil" Test contains a reusable membrane holder, lysing solution, dispenser, and plastic tray plus, microfilariae stain, lysing solution and filter membranes for 50 canine heartworm tests.

The Modified Knott's Test is performed by mixing one mL of whole blood with 9 mL of 2% formalin and centrifuging it for 5 to 8 minutes. The supernatent is discarded and the sediment is stained with methylene blue and then viewed microscopically. This is useful in routine yearly examinations, before beginning a prevention program. The Modified Knotts' Test is one of the best for examining the morphology of the microfilariae.

Indirect Fluorescent Antibody ("Track Test XI") This I.F.A. test detects circulatory host antibody to the microfilarial cuticular antigen. It is useful in detecting occult antigens. 80 to 90% of immunologic occult infections are usually positive to this test.

Enzyme-linked Immunoabsorbent Assay (ELISA). "Dirotect" and "Dirokit" have been withdrawn in some U.S. states. They tended to have low accuracy rates. Also, a complicating feature was their cross reactivity to *D. reconditum* and various other intestinal nematodes.

The diagnostic tools for occult heart disease are the CBC, thoracic radiography, and the IFA test or an ELISA.

Commercially available immunodiagnostic tests assist in diagnosis of occult heartworm disease, which occurs in approximately 10% to 20% of all infections diagnosed.

SEROLOGY

Many commercial tests are available to detect either antibodies produced in response to infection or antigens of *D. immitis*. Some ELISAs give false-positive results, which are due to false-positive results for *Dipetalonema reconditium* and other intestinal helminths. Nonetheless, a negative ELISA for antibody is usually solid evidence that a dog is not harboring adult heartworms.

Dirocheck for heartworm antigens usually has a sensitivity of >60%, a specificity of >95%, and an overall occurrence of more than 85%. The accuracy of the ELISA is roughly similar to that reported for the latex agglutination test (Dirokit Latex, Mabco Ltd.), which also detects heartworm antigens. Both tests are more useful for confirming diagnosis of heartworms in dogs with clinical disease rather than as a screening test, because false-negatives can occur. ELISAs for detection of antibodies to *D. immitis* can often be relatively inefficient. More specific tests are those that detect adult-associated *D. immitis* antigens. Cross-reactivity and the risk of false-positives are rare with these tests (Filarochek, Dirocheck). Detection of filarial antigen as distinct from antiflarial antibody has a high positive predictive value, (e.g., CITE test).

35.5 THERAPEUTIC CONSIDERATIONS

After establishing the presence of heartworm infection, treatment of the animal should be carried out. Untreated animals serve as a reservoir of infection for other animals. Any heartworm treatment regimen can be divided into five steps (Table 35–1).

1. Pretreatment evaluation
2. Stabilization
3. Adulticide treatment
4. Microfilaricide treatment
5. Prophylaxis

The type of therapy will be determined by the severity of the animal's condition and may consist of the following:

1. Chemotherapy only: the sequential application of adulticides, microfilaricides, and heartworm prophylactic drugs.
2. Supportive or symptomatic treatment: any signs of congestive heart failure must be stabilized (e.g., with cardiac glycosides/diuretic) before specific therapy is instituted.

The following must be remembered:

1. Compromised hepatic and renal functioning can adversely impair adulticide metabolism with consequent toxic reactions.
2. Asymptomatic dogs with dirofilariasis are not necessarily free of pathologic changes (occult heartworm).

TABLE 35–1
CONTROL PROGRAM

1) Therapy Protocol
   Treatment to destroy adult worms
   Complete rest is essential after treatment
   Treatment to destroy microfilariae
   Surgery to remove as many adult worms as possible
   Other treatments: antibiotics, special diets, diuretics, digitalis, aspirin
2) Prevention Protocol
   Treatment to destroy infective larvae
   Regular testing for microfilariae
   Mosquito control
3) ELISA Tests to Detect Dirofilaria Immitis Antigens e.g., "Filarochek", (or Antibodies)
4) Regular Testing Serology
5) Mosquito Control (if feasible?)

Elimination of heartworm infections in dogs can be effected by a variety of chemotherapeutic agents. Unfortunately, however, no single drug, is effective against all stages of the parasite. General control strategies therefore necessitate the use of sequential stage-specific drugs of variable efficacy and safety in a dosing program. Usually, this consists of

1. adulticide therapy followed in 3 to 4 weeks by
2. a suitable microfilaricide, after which
3. chemoprophylaxis may be commenced.

Such an approach is necessary because microfilaricides are ineffective while gravid female adults are present and because of the frequent and serious anaphylactoid reactions that occur when preventive drugs are administered to microfilaremic dogs. The sequence of adulticide and microfilaricide therapy is controversial; some believe that prior removal of microfilaria reduces the risk of adulticide therapy.

Any treatment program must address the following factors:

1. The dog is the main definitive host.

2. High populations of dogs may exist in areas where suitable vector species (mosquitoes) are present.
3. The long prepatent period for *D. immitis* complicates early treatment and diagnosis.
4. Adult *D. immitis* can survive in adult dogs for up to 5 years.
5. Circulatory microfilaria persist for very variable periods in affected dogs.
6. The immune system of infected dogs does not effectively deal with *D. immitis* infection.
7. The possibility of prenatal infection of young dogs by infectious third stage larvae and the possibility of transplacental migration of noninfective microfilaria must always be recognized.
8. The ubiquitous distribution and feeding habits of mosquitoes, nocturnal or diurnal, render control of the intermediate vector host very difficult.

Chemotherapy can be highly effective in the control of either the adult or microfilarial stages of *D. immitis*. **Preventive therapy is the most successful strategy**. The most effective means of breaking the transmission of *D. immitis* from mosquito vector to final host rests on either (1) elimination of principal vector species (very difficult) or (2) treatment of infected dogs with safe and effective drugs.

3. Therapy with an adulticide can result in severe thromboembolism in an animal with pre-existing cardiopulmonary lesions.

PATIENT ASSESSMENT

The critical criterion in the pathogenesis of the disease is the degree of parasitism. The intensity of the vascular response depends on the number of *D. immitis* parasites present.

Treatment is directed toward

- destruction of adult heartworms
- microfilarial therapy when necessary
- an ultimate preventive strategy to prevent re-infestation.

Before initiating any heartworm therapy, it is essential to thoroughly examine the patient with particular reference to cardiopulmonary, hepatic, and renal functioning:

1. Physical examination
2. Thoracic radiography
3. Complete urinalysis

Before deciding on a treatment program, the veterinarian must examine all aspects of the animal's history and physical status to ascertain its ability to withstand therapy.

Relevant history, the animal's geographic location, and prophylactic treatment can all influence the likelihood and severity of infection.

Clinical signs, such as coughing, exercise intolerance, weight loss, dyspnea, syncope, and epistaxis, are indicators of possible heartworm infection, and pre-existing compromise of cardiac function.

Pulmonary arterial disease occurs in a high percentage of cases, with resultant coughing, pulmonary crackles, or a split in the second heart sound. Systolic murmurs (and valvular incompetence) can be detected in up to 10% of affected animals.

A data base should be collected including a CBC, BUN measurement, and urinalysis in young dogs. Young animals that have been tested annually for microfilaremia and that are also asymptomatic do not require as detailed a laboratory investigation as older untested dogs.

Middle-aged to older animals that display clinical signs or that have occult infections necessitate the acquisition of a broader data base including CBC, serum, chemistry profile, urinalysis, and thoracic radiographs. The electrocardiogram (ECG) fre-quently contributes little vital information. Glomerulopathy is often associated with heartworm infection, and if proteinuria and hypoalbuminemia are present, a 24-hour quantitation of urinary protein provides an approximation of the extent of urinary damage. A sulfabromophtalein (BSP) clearance test assists in the estimation of hepatic insufficiency.

In examination of clinical pathology, neutrophilia is seen in about 20% of dogs with a mild infection. Up to 75% of dogs with severe infection have a neutrophilia, frequently with a left shift. Most dogs with heartworm disease have an eosinophilia, and over half show a basophilia. This is especially typical of occult infections. (Endoparasites also generate this hematologic response.)

Platelet counts tend to be lower in heartworm-positive dogs, and this decrease is most marked when pulmonary arterial damage is present.

Proteinuria attributable to glomerulopathy occurs in up to 30% of infected dogs and is directly related to the severity of the infection. Azotemia is also detected in a small number of infected dogs with elevated BUN levels. Increased serum liver enzyme activity occurs in a small percentage of infected dogs.

CHEMOTHERAPEUTIC PROGRAMS

Adult heartworms are eliminated before the microfilaria because the adults are the source of the microfilaria. The sequence of initial treatment is administration of an adulticide followed in 4 to 6 weeks by a microfilaricide if the animal still has circulatory microfilaria.

In an alternative approach, microfilaricides (e.g., dithiazanine) are administered first, followed in 3 weeks by an adulticide.

All heartworm-infected dogs must be carefully evaluated before a course of adulticide is initiated; very few dogs should not receive this treatment.

The first step in heartworm control is a blood examination for microfilaria. Because *D. immitis* is not the only filarid parasite of the dog, the species must be carefully identified. Assays for heartworm antigen have a high predictive value and assist in diagnosis of occult infections. Testing for occult heartworm infection is reserved for dogs with cardiopulmonary disease unresponsive to treatment.

The modified Knott's test can be used to diagnose overt infection.

Adulticides

Adulticide treatment can begin immediately after stabilization of the patient. Therapy should commence with adulticides. Microfilaricide drugs are only partially effective before adulticide administration. Adulticides given at the time of the last larval molt interrupt the heartworm life cycle by preventing maturation of the precardiac larvae.

Exercise restriction is very important with concurrent adulticide treatment, particularly in dogs with extensive pulmonary vascular disease. After adulticide therapy the animal can be highly susceptible to thromboembolism and may experience sudden dangerous increases in pulmonary blood pressure.

Two drugs have been widely used as adulticides, levamisole and thiacetarsamide. Levamisole has a narrow safety margin in dogs and is not always dependable. Thiacetarsamide is the drug of choice for adults. After adulticide treatment close confinement is necessary for 3 weeks, and exercise should be restricted for another 3 weeks. Temperature rise, pneumonia and respiratory embarrassment may occur within the first 2 weeks as adult parasites die and their fragments lodge in the terminal branches of the pulmonary artery.

Thiacetarsamide is approved as an adulticide at 2.2 mg/kg body weight. It must be given at intervals not less than 6 to 8 hours and no more than 15 hours. Toxicity includes vomiting, lethargy, and anorexia. Repetition of these symptoms is an indication to cease therapy. Hepatotoxicity and renal dysfunction are attendant hazards.

As mentioned, pulmonary thromboembolism is a major complication of adulticide treatment. In dogs with advanced heartworm disease, adulticide treatment therefore should be delayed until signs of heavy coughing, hemoptysis, and heart failure have been controlled.

Adulticide treatment should begin when the cardiopulmonary disease is controlled and when side effects of embolism are minimized. An indication of the success of adulticide therapy can be obtained from the rate of disappearance of circulatory parasite antigens. Heartworm age and sex are determinants to successful thiacetarsamide therapy—females are more resistant.

Acute adulticide toxicity is not related to the number of circulatory microfilaria, and thus the chances of toxicity do not differ for dogs that receive adulticide or microfilaricide treatment first.

Asymptomatic dogs with little radiologic evidence of pulmonary vascular disease are unlikely to experience serious cardiopulmonary complications as a result of adulticide treatment.

If toxicity to thiacetarsamide occurs, the adulticide should be discontinued and supportive treatment given. Prednisolone, 20 mg intramuscularly (IM), as a single dose or ascorbic acid, 25 mg, two to four times daily, can be useful in such states. The concurrent use of anti-inflammatory drugs in conjunction with adulticide treatment is recommended by some veterinarians to obviate the inflammatory reactions to dead parasites in the lungs.

Dogs should be checked for pneumonia at 10 days after adulticide therapy and then treated for microfilaria for 1 month.

Adulticide therapy need not kill all heartworms to succeed, if appropriate steps are taken to prevent reinfestation.

Pulmonary thromboembolism as a common sequel of adulticide treatment is most common 7 to 17 days post-treatment, but clinical signs of embolism have been reported up to 30 days post-treatment. These signs include cough, dyspnea, pulmonary crackles, fever, and tachycardia. Animals showing radiographic evidence of severe pulmonary parenchymal disease are more likely to experience clinical signs of thromboembolism. Ancillary treatment is necessary in such cases.

Microfilaricides

The major microfilaricides are dithiazanine iodide, diethylcarbamazine citrate (DEC), levamisole, ivermectin, and fenthion. All have potential side effects.

Microfilaremia is treated 6 weeks after adulticide therapy with oral dithiazanine iodide, 6–11 mg/kg, or levamisole, 11.0 mg/kg, for 6–15 days.

Occasional treatment failures occur with combined adulticide and microfilaricide therapy. Persistence of microfilaria may be due to persistence of adult heartworms, especially the young female.

When a low concentration of microfilaria persists after repeated adulticide and microfilaricide treatment, DEC can be used to prevent additional infections. Because DEC can precipitate adverse reactions in dogs positive for microfilaria, these animals should be hospitalized until medication is complete.

Animals harboring adult dirofilaria are more likely to develop side effects to levamisole.

Adverse reactions to microfilaricidal doses of ivermectin include a shocklike syndrome, attributable to the rapid killing of many microfilaria. This can be alleviated by fluid, electrolyte, and steroid therapy. (These adverse reactions occur only at the extralabel microfilaricidal dosage rate, not at the approved preventive dosage rate.)

Prevention

Prevention is the best form of heartworm treatment. Because mosquito control is not feasible, the normal approach is daily administration of DEC before and for 2 months after the mosquito season. Dogs living in zones with endemic mosquito populations require year-round treatment.

Asymptomatic dogs are usually given DEC and are checked for microfilaria by direct blood smear. Biannual treatment for adult worms with thiacetarsamide is an alternative means of control. Preventive drugs such as DEC should not be used until microfilaria are eliminated. DEC should be given for a minimum period of 30 days, daily, at 6.0 mg/kg to effectively destroy fourth stage larvae over 30 days. (Alternatively, ivermectin can be used for prophylaxis.) Adverse effects to DEC in heartworm-negative dogs are negligible, although sterility in male dogs has been suggested.

An alternative preventive approach is twice-yearly treatment with thiacetarsamide, 0.1 ml/lb intravenously (IV), bid for 2 consecutive days (i.e., 0.2 mg/kg).

Daily administration of mebendazole protects against artificial infection with *D. immitis*, beginning 2 days before infection and continuing for 28 days. The dosage range is 40 to 80 mg/kg, and treatment is effective against developing heartworm larvae with very few side effects.

General Control

When *D. immitis* infection is endemic, the most effective medical approach is daily dosage of DEC citrate (11.0 mg/kg), year-round. Therapy should commence 1 month before the mosquito season and continue for at least 2 months after the season ends. Blood examination for microfilaria should be performed every few weeks. (Alternatively, ivermectin or milbemycin oxime can be administered orally at monthly intervals.)

In *D. immitis*-positive dogs, the adult worms should be treated with sodium thiacetarsamide, 2.2 mg/kg of 1% solution IV, bid for 2 days. Monitoring of temperature is essential, and any elevation should be treated with prednisolone (20 mg, IM) and possibly antimicrobial drugs. The remaining microfilaria can be treated 4 to 6 weeks later with levamisole 11.0 mg/kg daily for 10 days until blood tests are microfilaria negative.

Daily dosage of DEC or ivermectin can begin as soon as the animal is microfilaria negative on the basis of two blood examinations using the concentration methods 1 week apart.

Clients must be advised that a previously infected dog may have migratory preadult stages that will mature in 2 to 6 months after adulticide and microfilaricide administration. A second treatment program may be required because DEC eliminates only third and fourth stage larvae.

For occult heartworm disease dogs must be stabilized, receiving at least 1 week of supportive treatment, before adulticide administration. Supportive care alone is not sufficient if adult heartworms are not eliminated. Most dogs with occult disease have signs associated with pneumonitis; the vena caval syndrome also may be present.

Treatment of occult heartworm disease extends over 30 days. If no complications occur during therapy with an adulticide, a concentration test for microfilaria should be performed 3 weeks after treatment. If no microfilaria are present, a microfilaricide is not indicated, and a preventive program may begin. Elimination of the heartworm from the host animal is complicated by the absence of a single filaricide that is effective against both the precardiac and cardiac life cycle stages.

35.6 CHEMOTHERAPY

ADULTICIDES

Sodium thiacetarsamide is approved by the FDA for young adult heartworm infection. Although it possesses a relatively narrow safety margin, this organo arsenical is an adulticide of choice. Thiacetarsamide is rapidly cleared from the body following IV administration, and, although widely distributed to the host's tissues, its concentration is greatest in the adult heartworm. Duration of exposure to effective blood levels, rather than transient fluctuating plasma levels, is a key factor governing efficacy. Hence, daily doses should be given every 8 hours, and the overnight interval should not exceed 16 hours. Heartworm age and sex are major variables affecting susceptibility. Not every adult heartworm is killed by thiacetarsamide, and so the clinical efficacy can vary among animals. It is less efficacious in eliminating immature heartworms, but as the cardiac stages mature, worms become more susceptible to the adulticide. Female worms appear to be more resistant than male adults, and, therefore, although the overall number of heartworms can be substantially reduced, some animals can be left with a residual female heartworm infection. Thiacetarsamide is highly effective at the final molt stage during the final precardiac migration. Following treatment with this adulticide, the chances of late precardiac stages reaching the circulation are quite remote.

The regimen of treatment is 2.2 mg/kg of 1% sodium thiacetarsamide solution IV bid for 2 days as the method for eliminating adult heartworms in dogs. It is then given at 6-month intervals in areas where mosquitoes exist all year, and annually where the mosquito season is limited by weather.

As an arsenical compound, sodium thiacetarsamide is potentially nephrotoxic and hepatotoxic. Perivascular deposition results in necrosis, ulceration, and a painful and edematous swelling. The drug is therefore sometimes administered through an indwelling catheter.

Vomiting, lethargy, and anorexia are side effects commonly seen after the first injection, and their persistence is an indication to suspend thiacetarsamide treatment. Other toxic effects in heartworm-infected dogs include fever, diarrhea, tubular casts in urine sediment, jaundice, bilirubinemia, and sometimes death.

Arsenicals can produce degeneration and vacuolation of the renal tubular epithelium. Before treatment is initiated, clinical evaluation, urinalysis, CBC, and serum chemistry profile should be performed, and the animal must be weighed very accurately for precise dosage computation. Therapy is discontinued in the presence of jaundice, persistent vomiting, depression, fever, and anorexia. Dogs with adverse reactions can be re-treated with the adulticide 2 to 3 weeks later.

Pulmonary thromboembolism is the most frequent and potentially serious sequel to thiacetarsamide administration and may result from destruction of adult worms. Dead or dying heartworms produce thrombosis granulomatous arteritis, perivascular edema, and hemorrhage. Caudal and accessary lobes of the lung are most commonly affected. Postadulticide thromboembolic disease can be seen 5 to 30 days after commencing treatment and is manifested clinically by coughing, dyspnea, pulmonary crackles, weakness, and tachycardia—signs of impeded blood flow.

Adverse renal or hepatic function directly increases the risk of host toxicity, which can also be related to the onset of pre-existing pulmonary valvular disease from accumulation of worm debris.

Cage rest is generally advisable during adulticide treatment. Therapy for adverse reactions is supportive with fluid and electrolyte supplementation plus oral glucocorticoid medication.

Although thiacetarsamide will kill adult worms, it is now recognized that migratory developing microfilaria in organs such as the kidney can cause considerable damage. At any stage of heartworm infection, sudden death can result from infarction of capillary beds in various organs and tissues, which is caused by accumulation of microfilaria or adult worms.

To reduce the incidence of adverse effects, it is generally preferable to remove circulatory microfilaria with a suitable microfilaricide before commencing adulticide with thiacetarsamide. For this reason alone, an argument exists for microfilarial treatment being started before adult treatment.

While the normal high adulticide dosage can be up to 2.2 mg/kg IV bid for 2 days, in endemic areas this should be repeated after 6 months. This treatment eliminates *D. immitis* parasites before a sufficient number develops to maturity.

MICROFILARICIDES

These drugs destroy first stage (L_1), third stage (L_3), fourth stage (L_4), and fifth stage (L_5) microfilaria. Detectable microfilaremia is always due to the presence of first stage microfilaria in the blood.

In general, microfilaricides should not be administered earlier than 4 to 6 weeks after adulticide therapy. If the pulmonary thromboembolism syndrome is suspected, a microfilaricide should not be used for at least 4 weeks after full recovery. Earlier administration may cause adverse reactions that clinically resemble pulmonary thromboembolism.

The dog should have no significant disease when the microfilaricide is administered. Microfilaria numbers are easy to reduce markedly with these drugs but can be difficult to eliminate completely, as determined by successive blood concentration tests.

Dithiazanine

Dithiazanine is an FDA-approved microfilaricide. It is effective against microfilaria of *D. immitis* but not the precardiac larvae or adult stages. It is also effective against *Toxocara canis, Toxascaris leonina, Ancylostoma Caninum, Uncinaria stenocephalia, Strongyloides* and *Trichluris*. Dithiazanine is a blue cyanine dye, is poorly soluble in water, and is given as a powder or tablet. Although absorption from the alimentary tract is poor, enough is absorbed to stain body tissues faintly blue. Much of the drug remains within the bowel lumen and stains the feces and vomitus a blue-purplish color. Systemic toxicity therefore should not be seen at the recommended dosage rate or treatment duration. The dosage is 6 to 11 mg/kg for 7 to 10 days and it may be given to effect. After 5 to 7 days of treatment, microfilarial counts should usually be reduced by 90%. Very few dogs become completely free of microfilaria, as determined by the Knott concentration test. In addition to failure to totally clear the microfilaria, adverse reactions such as vomiting or diarrhea may occur. Dithiazanine can be toxic to the liver and kidney.

If microfilariae appear on follow up, a dosage of 11 to 15 mg/kg is used for an additional 7 days if no signs of toxicity occur. Feeding a meal before treatment may prevent vomiting. Clients should be warned that the vomitus and feces from treated animals will stain fabrics. Vomiting may be minimized by prior administration of antiemetic drugs (metoclopramide, anticholinergics) or by dividing the dose and giving the drug after a small meal.

On completion of the course of dithiazanine, a concentration test for microfilaria should be performed. If the dog shows negative results, it may then be started on a DEC regimen. If the dog still has microfilaremia and no adverse reactions, dithiazanine can be administered for another week. However, if microfilariae persist after extended treatment with this drug, use of another microfilaricide should be considered.

Some veterinarians use dithiazanine first followed by an adulticide in 3 weeks. This should eliminate most of the circulatory microfilaria that might impede microcirculation in the liver and kidney and predispose the animal to acute adulticide toxicity. Acute adulticide toxicity, however, is not necessarily related to the numbers of circulatory microfilaria, and thus in general the risks of adulticide toxicity do not differ significantly for dogs that receive adulticide or microfilaricidal treatment first.

Because elimination of microfilaria by preadulticidal administration with dithiazanine is difficult, this drugs popularity has waned significantly with the clinical use of levamisole and especially ivermectin and milbemycin.

Levamisole

Levamisole has been used with considerable success as a microfilaricide. Levamisole (the L-isomer of tetramisole) is primarily authorized for use as a broad-spectrum parasiticide effective against a wide range of intestinal and pulmonary helminths. Additionally, it exhibits activity against microfilariae, precardiac larvae, and adults of D. immitis. In general, however, it is employed solely as a microfilaricide.

Levamisole paralyzes parasites primarily by its cholinergic activity at the ganglia and neuromuscular junction. It has a narrow working safety margin in small animals.

Levamisole kills adult heartworms and sterilizes the females, and hence adult female worms do not contain microfilariae in utero following a combination of adulticide and levamisole treatment. Levamisole's major use is as a microfilaricide after adulticide therapy. Used alone, levamisole can produce a negative microfilarial state even when sterile adult females survive. Therefore, after treatment, repeated microfilarial concentration tests are required to determine if an adult infection still exists.

Sometimes dead microfilaria can become trapped in the liver sinusoids and at other sites within the microcirculation. Microgranulomas can form around degenerating microfilaria, which are subsequently destroyed by macrophages.

Given at a dosage rate of 10 to 11 mg/kg orally for 10 days, a 90% clearance of microfilaria is usually anticipated. Levamisole is an effective L_1 microfilaricide, and if microfilaremia persists after treatment, the course can be repeated.

Although effective against adult heartworms, levamisole is not as effective as sodium thiacetarsamide. Levamisole appears to have a preferential effect against male adult D. immitis but possesses little prophy-lactic activity. Its major application is in eliminating microfilaremiae before DEC prophylaxis or adulticide treatment with thiacetarsamide.

Levamisole has a narrow safety margin in dogs, even at the normal dosage of 10–11 mg/kg. Toxic signs include reduced food intake, weight loss, diarrhea, vomiting, and particularly central nervous system (CNS) dysfunction (ataxia, paresis). Hemolytic anemia and thrombocytopenia have also been reported. Many signs are referable to cholinergic agonistic activity. Anticholinergic agents such as atropine may reduce the incidence of vomiting, but treatment must be suspended at the first signs of CNS disorders such as muscle tremors, ataxia, and incoordination. Parenteral fluids, electrolytes, and atropine can be administered as antidotes. Unfortunately, reduction of levamisole dosage to minimize toxicity also reduces its effectiveness.

Levamisole is used as a microfilaricide at a dosage of 11.0 mg/kg daily per os for 15 days. Blood should be examined 1 week after commencing treatment, and levamisole can be discontinued if the concentration test is negative. Dogs must always be closely monitored for signs of CNS disturbance, which indicate withdrawal of levamisole. After 15 days of therapy and if microfilaremia still persists, levamisole should be replaced with another microfilaricide.

As with other microfilaricides, levamisole is usually only partially effective if adult heartworms have not been eliminated.

Milbemycin oxime (Interceptor) and ivermectin (Heartgard) are the most recent introductions for microfilarial treatment. Prophylaxis should begin immediately after clearance of the microfilaremia if exposure to infected mosquitoes is possible.

Collies and Collie-mixed breeds are particularly susceptible to ivermectin toxicity, but at the monthly prophylactic dose of 6 mcg/kg, toxicity is rare. It can be given to microfilaremic animals without adverse reactions. This is a great advantage when heartworm infection is asymptomatic and when age or concurrent illness makes treatment a great risk.

Dirochek canine heartworm antigen test kit facilitates detection of the condition despite the fact that many heartworm-infected dogs do not exhibit microfilaria.

PROPHYLACTIC DRUGS

Diethylcarbamazine Citrate

DEC is one of the major, long-established, FDA-approved drugs for heartworm prophylaxis (ivermectin and milbemycin oxime are now approved as once-a-month prophylactic agents).

A piperazine derivative, oral DEC is rapidly absorbed from the gastrointestinal tract and widely distributed throughout the body. It is used exclusively against precardiac adults and is almost 100% effective in preventing heartworm infection. It is also effective against ascarids and when combined with styrlpyridinium chloride or oxibendazole helps prevent hookworm infection.

Administration of DEC should commence at the start of the mosquito season and continue for 2 months past the end of the season. In warm climates DEC should be given year-round. Given as tablets, chewable tablets, or liquid poured over the dog's food, the normal daily dose is 2.5 to 3.0 mg/lb (13 mg/kg), which is equivalent to 1.25 mg/lb of DEC base. The importance of maintaining daily administration must always be emphasized to the client. Puppies can receive DEC when they are 6 to 9 weeks old.

DEC is a safe drug and can be given at levels exceeding the filaricidal dose. Given at four times the therapeutic dose (22 mg/kg), started as late as 60 days after infection, it can be beneficial when prophylaxis has been interrupted or neglected. DEC is prescribed immediately after successful microfilaricide treatment. After administration of DEC for several weeks, a second check for microfilariae from surviving adults should be performed. Dogs with occult heartworm infection should be started on DEC as soon as diagnosed and while being treated with an adulticide.

DEC should not be used as an L_1 microfilaricide. Doses as low as 4.5 mg/kg may induce anaphylactic reaction, shock, and death in animals with detectable microfilaremia. DEC is effective against L_3 and L_4 microfilariae, and the minimum effective dose is 6.25 mg/kg.

Dogs that have microfilaremia while on DEC therapy can be maintained on DEC while being treated with microfilaricides and an adulticide.

Normally, after adulticide and microfilaricide treatment of dogs with microfilaria, the patient is started on DEC as soon as free of microfilaria, as determined by concentration tests. This test should be performed promptly after completion of the microfilaricide treatment because the continued presence of microfilaria indicates a definite need for continued treatment.

Once DEC prophylaxis begins, a concentration test is usually repeated in 2 to 3 months. Testing for microfilaria before initiation of DEC administration is imperative because dogs positive for microfilariae are highly likely to experience adverse reactions to DEC. DEC has an approved efficacy claim against the L_3 (infective stage) microfilaria and the subsequent tissue migratory stages.

The following important points must be borne in mind when commencing with DEC prophylaxis.

1. The drug must be given daily. DEC is rapidly absorbed after oral administration and completely excreted within 24 hours. There is effectively no carryover or residual activity from day to day.
2. Care must be given to ensure the recommended dosage rate is given. Proprietary preparations are available as either the citrate salt or the base. The availability of the active drug in the citrate form is approximately 50% of the base.
3. DEC must never be given to microfilaremia-positive dogs. Shocklike syndromes or disseminated intravascular coagulopathy (often fatal) can occur in these animals (even at doses as low as 4.4 mg/kg). It is essential that microfilaria be removed from the blood with dithiazanine or levamisole before DEC prophylaxis.
4. DEC can be used prophylactically at three monthly intervals by oral administration of the drug at a dose rate of 60 to 65 mg/kg.

Adverse reactions to DEC in dogs without circulatory microfilaria are rare because the drug has a high safety margin.

Adverse reactions are a definite problem when DEC is administered to microfilaremic heartworm-infected dogs. Depression, lethargy, vomiting, and diarrhea may occur together with cardiovascular signs of bradycardia. An increase in liver enzyme counts and a decline in platelet numbers are other occasional side effects. There may be some correlation between the level of the microfilaremia and the severity of the reaction. Following DEC administration the number of circulating microfilaria peaks very rapidly, and this may be due to the mobilization of pooled microfilaria. The greatest increase in microfilaria occurs in dogs exhibiting the most severe reactions and those patients that have been microfilaremic for more than 12 months. Histopathologic changes may appear in the liver, and the microfilariae tend to become quite numerous in the liver sinusoids. Adverse reactions occur within 1 or 2 hours of DEC administration and either resolve or become life-threatening within 3 to 5 hours. Death may occur in 5 to 20% of reacting dogs.

The severity of the host reaction is influenced by the degree of host sensitization and the amount of antigen released by DEC from the surface of the affected microfilaria. High IgG concentrations arise in response to both adult and microfilarial antigens, and adverse reactions usually occur only when many microfilaria and antibodies are present. As the antigen-antibody reaction proceeds between either the microfilaria or soluble circulatory antigen, IgG concentrations tend to decrease, and the disseminated intravascular coagulation syndrome is triggered.

Adverse reactions do not occur when DEC is administered to dogs with occult infections. Thus, the adult parasite apparently is not an important source of released antigens following DEC administration. Reactive dogs usually do not continue to respond adversely to DEC if microfilaria can be destroyed with a suitable microfilaricide.

Although DEC need not necessarily be discontinued in dogs that develop a very low level of microfilaremia while on treatment, nonetheless, if treatment is interrupted even for a few days, therapy cannot be safely resumed without first eliminating the microfilaria. If adverse reactions occur, fluids and corticosteroids may be employed to counteract hypovolemic shock.

DEC and oxibendazole in combination (Filaribits Plus, Norden) are highly effective against both hookworms, heartworms and whipworms.

With the introduction of monthly heartworm products, heartworm prevention has become an even more common practice. The establishment of a routine is the key to any preventive medication program.

Ivermectin

Ivermectin is a combination of macrocyclic lactones produced by fermentation of an actinomycete streptomyces avermitilis.

Several of the original injectable formulations of ivermectin contained polysorbate 80 (for micelle formation), and the extralabel use of these products in dogs frequently elicited a histamine-like reaction. Ivermectin is now available in tablet form for dog as a heartworm preventive drug (Heartguard).

Ivermectin can interrupt the life cycle of *D. immitis* at the microfilarial and third and fourth larval stages but possesses no apparent direct effect on adult worms. Ivermectin does, however, adversely affect reproduction of the parasite by inhibiting maturation and release of microfilaria. This accounts for the unusually long suppression of microfilaremia following treatment of dogs harboring adult parasites. Because it is a large macrocyclic lactone molecule, ivermectin does not cross the blood-brain barrier, and so it possesses a very high safety factor. Collies and collie crosses are, however, particularly susceptible to ivermectin-induced adverse reactions at the normal dosage employed for endo- and ectoparasitic effects.

Ivermectin is extremely sensitive against fourth stage larvae, although the sensitivity declines as the fourth stage matures, and the precardiac stage is relatively resistant. Early studies with ivermectin demonstrated its very high efficacy when given approximately 6 weeks after thiacetarsamide therapy. Doses as low as 0.05 mg/kg cleared microfilaria, while in clinical cases dosages of 0.2 mg/kg consistently eliminated microfilaria.

Ivermectin is so potent that only minuscule doses are necessary as a heartworm prophylactic. The prophylactic dose is lower than the microfilaricidal dose, but if microfilaria numbers become reduced to an occult state, diagnosis of heartworm-induced cardiopulmonary disease can be difficult. Accordingly, a regular concentration test for microfilaria should be done for dogs that will receive ivermectin for heartworm prophylaxis.

The extremely high sensitivity of fourth stage larvae provides ivermectin with its greatest potential: administration as infrequently as every 60 days. The conventional presentation of ivermectin now available for dogs (Heartguard-30 MSD) is a once-a-month heartworm disease prevention tablet.

At the recommended dosage rate (6 mcg/kg), the drug possesses a wide margin of safety in dogs including pregnant or breeding bitches or stud dogs. It is approved for use in all breeds more than 6 weeks of age.

All dogs should be tested and clear of existing heartworm infection before they are placed on prevention treatment with ivermectin.

Mild hypersensitivity, ataxia, cough, fever, listlessness, and transient diarrhea have infrequently been reported after treatment of dogs that have circulatory microfilaria. This is a reaction to death of a few microfilaria. To maintain an effective protection program, clients should be advised to include regular testing as part of the total protection course. Ivermectin generates some antigenic stimulation arising from repetitive termination of fourth stage larval development.

Because tissue migration and development into adults requires 60 days or more, monthly treatment will prevent development of adult heartworms. The disease prevention dose is 6 mcg/kg. Heartworm larvae in tissues are sensitive to ivermectin, but a dosage of 200 mcg/kg can cause a severe reaction in Collie-type breeds. This reaction is not seen at a dosage of 50 mcg/kg, and the chosen prophylactic dosage of 6 mcg/kg is effective and safe in all breeds. Nonetheless, Collies and Collie mixed breeds ought be kept under close watch.

The ivermectin tablet should be given on the same day of each month during the mosquito season. The first dose should be given within a month of the dog's initial exposure to mosquitoes and the final dose within 30 days after last exposure. Ivermectin is not effective against adult heartworms and is not recommended for use in heartworm-positive dogs. Consequently, routine testing for heartworms is important. Ivermectin does not immediately affect the number of circulatory microfilariae in dogs before administration of thiacetarsamide but may gradually depress the number with continued monthly treatment. In dogs treated with thiacetarsamide, ivermectin displays rapid activity, with most microfilariae disappearing within 24 hours. Persistence of microfilariae beyond a few days after ivermectin administration is usually associated with the presence of adult heartworms.

Filaricidal doses may be accompanied by mild vomiting or diarrhea. As with any drug at microfilaricidal dose rates, this is related to the rapid destruction of large numbers of microfilaria. Reactions to ivermectin are seen only at dosages higher than the prophylactic dose (6 mcg/kg) or in dogs when stages other than microfilaria are present.

Ivermectin possesses the significant advantages of efficacy and once-a-month dosing—a better option to DEC when clients find daily dosing too inconvenient. Once-a-month prophylactic dosing also is associated with less risk of compliance failure.

As mentioned, ivermectin is not recommended for use in heartworm-positive dogs. It is not recommended for use in dogs less than 6 weeks of age. It is not effective against adult microfilariae. A mild hypersensitivity reaction occasionally occurs in dogs, which is presumably due to dead or dying microfilariae.

Although Collies are sensitive to ivermectin at doses of 200 μg/kg or greater, clients are advised to observe Collies closely for at least 8 hours after dosing at the much smaller heartworm dosage.

Milbemycins

Milbemycins, a family of macrolide antibiotics similar to the avermectins, are now commercially available for heartworm prophylaxis. Milbemycin oxime (Interceptor) is a once-a-month tablet that prevents heart-

TABLE 35–2
DRUGS FOR HEARTWORM DISEASE

	Drug	Dosage
Adults	Thiacetarsamide (0.1% solution)	0.2–2.2 mg/kg bid IV, 2 days. Can be toxic.
Microfilariae	Dithiazanine	6–11 mg/kg po for 7 to 10 days
	Levamisole	11 mg/kg po for 15 days. Can be toxic.
	Ivermectin	50 μg/kg
	Fenthion	15.0 mg/kg topically/3 treatments
Precardiac Larvae	Diethylcarbamazine	1.25 mg/kg po 60 days
	Ivermectin	6.0 μg/kg po monthly
	Milbemycin oxime	0.5 mg/kg po monthly

worm disease and controls hookworms in dogs.

A rising dose-response reaction was noted with milbemycin oxime in one of 14 Collies (characterized by ataxia pyrexia recumbency) treated at 12.5 mg/kg (25 times the monthly heartworm prophylactic rate).

These tablets are used not only to prevent heartworm disease caused by *D. immitis* but also hookworm disease caused by *Ancylostorum caninum*. Milbemycin oxime tablets are given orally, once a month, at a dose of 0.23 mg/lb body weight (0.5 mg/kg) (Table 35–2).

35.7 SUPPORTIVE THERAPEUTIC MEASURES

Supportive therapeutic measures are critically important before and after filaricide treatment to ensure satisfactory clinical response, particularly in advanced clinical cases.

Exercise restriction and cage rest are essential, especially during adulticide treatment and in dogs with extensive pulmonary vascular disease. Exercise must be discouraged for 3 to 4 weeks after treatment, when the worms are disintegrating. Following adulticide treatment the patient is susceptible to thromboembolism and can experience sudden severe elevations of pulmonary blood pressure.

Aspirin and prednisolone may be useful to prevent thromboembolism and to reduce the severity of lesions caused by the parasites.

Adulticide therapy should not be started before treatment of right-sided congestive heart failure. Digoxin can be quite useful, as can diuretics, although the latter could further weaken the patient by contribution to hypovolemia.

ASPIRIN

Aspirin therapy commenced 1 week before and continued 4 to 6 weeks after adulticide therapy reduces pulmonary arterial disease and thromboembolic complications and improves the patient's chances of survival.

Aspirin can assist in partial regression of pulmonary arterial lesions in concurrently infected dogs. When aspirin is administered (5–10 mg/kg) during the first 4 weeks following adulticide, severity of lesions and the patency of pulmonary arteries usually improve. This is related to the importance of blood platelet formation in the pathogenesis of heartworm-induced pulmonary vascular disease (Table 35–3).

Aspirin possesses analgesic antipyretic and anti-inflammatory effects, mediated via cyclooxygenase inhibition. Platelet blockade, aspirin's most important effect in treating heartworm disease, is produced by a very low dosage. This antithromboxane ef-

TABLE 35–3
RESPIRATORY SUPPORTIVE DRUGS

Drug	Dosage
1) Aspirin	5–10 mg/kg po daily
2) Prednisone or prednisolone	0.5–2.0 mg/kg po daily
3) Aminophylline	10.0 mg/kg po tid (IV)
4) Captopril	0.5–2.0 mg/kg po
5) Butorphanol	0.5 mg/kg po
6) Terbutaline	0.1 mg/kg tid

[Cimetidine H_2 blocker may be necessary after prolonged aspirin therapy to minimize the incidence of gastric ulceration cimetidine dose: 20 mg/kg three times daily orally.]
Other ancillary respiratory supportive therapies

7) Antibiotics: ampicillin, tetracyclines, potentiated sulfonamides
8) Oxygen and Cage Rest

fect is also accompanied by depression of platelet adhesion to damaged vascular surfaces. These effects reduce the intimal proliferation that occurs when heartworms die.

Dogs with either congestive heart failure or severe arterial disease produced by heartworm infection can be given aspirin at a dosage rate of 5 to 7 mg/kg daily, although dosage as low as 3 mg/kg every 6 days has been shown to impede platelet aggregation. Aspirin should be given at least 2 weeks before adulticide administration. Dogs are prone to developing gastrointestinal hemorrhage with nonsteroidal anti-inflammatory drug (NSAID) therapy, and aspirin appears to be the safest in the dog. (Histamine receptor 2 blockers, e.g., cimetidine and ranitidine may be occasionally indicated.)

Buffered aspirin tablets tend to produce fewer gastrointestinal side effects. Aspirin must not be given to dogs with pre-existing liver disease, and if gastrointestinal hemorrhage is suspected, the drug must be discontinued. The animals should be observed closely for gastrointestinal bleeding, and concurrent use of cimetidine or oral protectants is advisable.

Aspirin can be valuable in reducing pulmonary arterial and parenchymal disease without any apparent effect on the heartworm kill rate or the inflammatory clearance of worm fragments. Aspirin 5 mg/kg

daily is beneficial in dogs with pulmonary arterial and parenchymal disease together with enforced cage rest. Gastric ulceration may accompany its long-term usage.

Dogs without severe clinical and radiologic pulmonary changes do not require aspirin.

CORTICOSTEROIDS

Corticosteroids are not indicated when the clinical signs are mild. They are indicated when the clinical and radiographic signs are severe; prednisolone, 0.5–2.0 mg/kg/day, can be given.

Corticosteroids, although often prescribed, are not routinely indicated for patients without clinical signs. They may be indicated in pulmonary disease on the basis of clinical and radiologic evidence.

Glucocorticoids such as prednisolone are effective in controlling respiratory distress that is due to allergic pneumonitis and thromboembolism.

Prednisolone should be employed primarily in response to not in anticipation of, clinical signs, because prednisolone can retard the degradation of worm fragments, thereby increasing the risk of thrombosis by inhibiting granulocyte phagocytic and fibrinolytic activity. The pulmonary blood flow impedance can be increased by routine use of glucocorticoids.

Prednisolone is commonly given at a dosage of 1.1 to 2.2 mg/kg/day. Treatment should be of short duration; withdrawal is indicated by resolution of the clinical and radiologic signs of lung damage.

When functional alveolar disease is present, prednisone or prednisolone, 0.5 to 2.0 mg/kg daily for 1 week, can alleviate the signs of pulmonary heartworm disease.

Corticosteroids are indicated primarily for treatment of pulmonary parenchymal disease secondary to pulmonary arterial disease and for the treatment of pneumonitis.

If signs occur, prednisolone should be administered at a dose of 1 to 2 mg/kg until clinical and radiographic signs have been resolved. Corticosteroids should be used only if signs of thromboembolism occur. They will decrease the efficacy of thiacetarsamide, and more seriously, may exacerbate the degree of arterial disease and promote thromboembolism, periarterial fibrosis, and decreased pulmonary blood flow.

Prednisolone 1.1 mg/kg bid is indicated on the basis of radiographic evidence of marked interstitial and alveolar lung infiltrations in cases of severe reactions.

Coughing, crackles, dyspnea, and fever may be evident before, but more commonly following, adulticide therapy.

Corticosteroids are not recommended prophylactically or for minor clinical signs such as occasional coughing or mild temperature elevation.

Corticosteroids inhibit the inflammatory clearance of heartworm fragments and the overall resolution of heartworm disease. These steroids therefore must be prescribed only when significant clinical signs appear and for as brief a period as possible (3 to 5 days). Steroid therapy should be phased out after clinical and radiologic evidence of the resolution of parenchymal lung disease are noted.

Allergic pneumonitis associated with occult heart disease is another indication for corticosteroids. This syndrome occurs in 15 to 20% of dogs harboring occult infection but is not associated with severe arterial disease.

Following prednisolone therapy, 1.1 mg/kg bid, and resolution of the pulmonary infiltrations, thiacetarsamide can be administered within a few days.

TABLE 35–4 CARDIOVASCULAR SUPPORTIVE DRUGS	
Drug	Dosage
Digoxin	0.11 mg/kg bid
Aspirin	5 mg/kg po daily
Hydralazine	1 mg/kg po bid
Furosemide	2–4 mg/kg IV or po tid

CARDIAC SUPPORT

Dogs with cardiovascular disease, as determined by circulatory microfilarial counts, but without clinical symptoms should be treated with an adulticide (thiacetarsamide). Exercise must be restricted, and the patient must be confined for at least 3 weeks after commencing therapy. Death of heartworms can produce acute pulmonary hypertension with the right ventricle subjected to an increase in work load.

Dogs displaying clinical signs with exercise generally do not require specific treatment for congestive heart failure.

Response to treatment generally improves if these dogs are given aspirin 5 mg/kg for 2 weeks before adulticide therapy. Elimination of the heartworm alone does not automatically reduce pulmonary hypertension.

Dogs with clinical signs of congestive heart failure at rest require specific therapy for cardiac disease (Table 35–4):

1. Aspirin
2. Low sodium diet
3. Furosemide
4. Digitalis or possibly hydralazine

Adulticide treatment is indicated but not until the dog is stabilized and responding to supportive treatment. An adulticide is necessary to eliminate the parasite, which is the primary stimulant for the development of the vascular lesions.

Furosemide is given at a dosage of 2 to 4 mg/kg IV or orally. This diuretic reduces plasma volume and venous pressure. By alleviating venous pressure and mobilizing fluids, the failing heart increases its contractility and rate. Cage rest, a low-salt diet, and aspirin also assist in eliminating excess fluid.

Digoxin should be restricted to those cases that do not respond to the preceding regimen before adulticide therapy. Digoxin slows the heart by slowing the sinus rate and atrioventricular A-V impulse conduction time. This is effected by inhibition of the sacrolemma $NA^+ K^+$ adenosine triphosphatase pump, which alters the amount of CA^{++} available for excitation-contraction coupling of myocardial cells. In heartworm patients, no digoxin loading dose is necessary in most cases. A dosage rate of 0.11 mg/kg divided into two treatments each day is usually adequate, provided the cardiac changes are monitored by ECG. Heart block, escape beats, and severe bradycardia are evidence that the dosage rate is too high.

In advanced cases of *D. immitis* infection, severe pulmonary hypertension may ultimately lead to right-sided congestive heart failure. Lowering of pulmonary blood pressure is beneficial, particularly following postadulticide thromboembolism.

Alpha-blocking drugs such as hydralazine have been employed to lower blood pressure in such cases but with mixed results. Use of hydralazine is accompanied by a general lowering of systemic blood pressure and a compensatory increase in cardiac output to correct the induced hypotension. The overall response can be increased pulmonary blood flow as a direct response to the increased systemic venous return arising from the peripheral arteriolar dilation. The pulmonary blood vessels cannot accommodate this rising flow, and thus an increase in the right ventricular work load occurs. This is obviously counterproductive.

Drugs acting as venodilators (such as captopril or nitrates) can be relied on to be more beneficial to the animal than arteriolar dilators. Venodilators increase the systemic venous capacitance, lower the right heart filling pressure, and thus to some extent, alleviate the major problem of right-sided congestive heart failure. Hydralazine therapy can be quite dangerous and should be avoided unless systemic blood pressure can be monitored regularly. (For further detail see Chapter 31, on cardiac disease.)

Bronchodilators may be indicated in the patient affected by severe respiratory distress. Asthma-type chronic cases can be treated with oral bronchodilators several times per day. Beta-agonists act on the $beta_2$-bronchial muscle receptors and increase the intracellular concentration of cyclic adenosine monophosphate (cAMP). Xanthine derivatives, on the other hand, also elevate intracellular cAMP by inhibiting the enzyme phosphodiesterase responsible for cAMP breakdown.

Aminophylline 10 mg/kg bid or tid (IV or IM) is a useful bronchodilator in conjunction with cage rest, sedation, and possible oxygen therapy in extreme cases.

Antimicrobial drugs are rarely indicated routinely, but respiratory infections can occur in long-standing cases. If a positive culture is obtained, it is generally indicative of a preponderant gram-negative infection, and ampicillin, tetracycline doxycycline, chloramphenicol, or potentiated sulfonamide may be indicated. Gentamicin is best reserved for resistant non responsive cases.

SELECTED REFERENCES

Barragry, T.B.: A review of the pharmacology and clinical uses of ivermectin. Can. Vet. J., *28*(8):512, 1987.

Bennett, D.G.: Clinical pharmacology of ivermectin. J. Am. Vet. Med. Assoc., *189*:100, 1986.

Blair, L.S., Williams, E., and Ewancin, D.V.: Efficacy of ivermectin against third stage Dirofilaria immitis larvae in ferrets and dogs. Res. Vet. Sci., *33*:386, 1982.

Collins, G.H., and Pope, S.E.: An evaluation of an ELISA test for the detection of antigens of Dirofilaria immitis. Aust. Vet. J., *64*:318, 1987.

Calvert, C.: Confirming a diagnosis of heartworm infection in dogs. Vet. Med., March:232, 1987.

Calvert, C.A.: The best tests for evaluating the heartworm-infected dog. Vet. Med., March:238, 1987.

Calvert, C.A.: Indications for corticosteroids and aspirin administration in canine heartworm disease. Canine Pract., *14*(2):19, 1987.

Calvert, C.A.: Treating for heartworm disease and its complications: preventing infections wherever possible. Vet. Med., March:264, 1987.

Calvert, C.A.: Coping with canine heartworm disease. Vet. Med., Suppl., August:39, 1986.

Calvert, C.A., and Thrall, D.E.: Treatment of canine heartworm disease co-existing with right-sided failure. J. Am. Vet. Med. Assoc., *180*:1201, 1982.

Carlisle, C.H. et al.: The toxic effects of thiacertarsamide sodium in normal dogs and in dogs infected with D. immitis. Aust. Vet. J., 50:204, 1986.

Hamilton, R.G., Wagner, E., and April, M.: Firofilaria immitis: Diethylcarbamazine-induced anaphylactoid-induced reactions in infected dogs. Exp. Parasitol., 61:405, 1986.

Holmes, R.A., McCall, J.W., and Prasse, K.W.: Thiacetarsamide in dogs with Dirofilaria immitis. Influence of decreased liver function in drug efficacy. Am. J. Vet. Res., 47:1341, 1986.

Hsu, W.H.: Toxicity and drug interaction of levamisole. J. Am. Vet. Med. Assoc., 176:1166, 1989.

Jackson, R.F.: Levamisole in Dirofilariasis in dogs. J. Am. Vet. Med. Assoc., 176:1170, 1980.

Jackson, R.F., Seymour, W.G., and Beckett, R.S.: Lower dose of ivermectin as a microfilaricide, 00.05 mg/kg. In Proceedings of Heartworm Symposium 1986. Edited by G.F. Otto. Washington, D.C., American Heartworm Society, 1986.

Knight, D.H.: Heartworm infection. Vet. Clin. North Am. Small Anim. Pract., 17L(6):1463, 1987.

McColl, J.W. et al.: Of experimentally-induced heartworm and hookworm infection in dogs. Mod. Vet. P., 68:417, 1987.

Montgomery, R.D., and Pigeon, G.L.: Levamisole toxicosis in a dog. J. Am. Vet. Med. Assoc., 189:684, 1986.

Pulliam, J.D. et al.: Investigating ivermectin toxicity in Collies. Vet. Med., 6:33, 1985.

Rawlings, C.A. et al.: Effect of acetyl salicylic acid on pulmonary arteriosclerosis induced by one year and low level vacular injury. Arteriosclerosis, 5:355, 1985.

Rawlings, C.A. et al.: An aspirin prednisolone combination to modify post-adulticide lung disease in heartworm-infested dogs. Am. J. Vet. Res., 45:2371, 1984.

Rawlings, C.A. et al.: Aspirin and prednisolone modification of post-adulticide pulmonary arterial disease in heartworm infected dogs. Am. J. Vet. Res., 44:821, 1983.

Schaub, R.G., and Keith, J.C.: Effects of aspirin on vascular damage and myointimal proliferation in canine pulmonary arteries. Fed. Proc. Abstr., No. 3206, 1981.

Sheen, D., Sweeney, K., and Jones, C.K.: Heartworm testing: comparing the results of ELISA with filter techniques and necropsy findings. Vet. Med., January:49, 1985.

Whiteley, H.W.: Your diagnostic protocol. Dirofilaria immitis infection in dogs. Vet. Med., April:328, 1988.

APPENDIX

STEPS TO DIAGNOSIS OF HEARTWORM INFECTION

---

1) Detect microfilariae filter test and Knotts' test.
2) Serodiagnostic tests
   Immunodiagnostic tests diagnose occult heartworm
   (a) ELISA tests to detect antibodies against D. immitis
       —false-positives to cross reactivity can occur.
       Negative ELISA gives good evidence of absence of heartworm.
   (b) ELISA tests to detect D. immitis antigens
       —more specific and more sensitive
       —cross reactivity does not occur.
3) Clinical signs in affected animal.
4) Evidence:—X rays
            —ECG
            —angiocardiography
            —blood chemistry
            —urinalysis.

CHAPTER

36

CANCER CHEMOTHERAPY

36.1 Introduction
36.2 Chemotherapy
36.3 Side Effects of Chemotherapy
36.4 Classes of Anticancer Drugs
36.5 Alkylating Drugs
36.6 Antimetabolites
36.7 Plant Alkaloids
36.8 Steroids
36.9 Miscellaneous
36.10 Immunotherapy
36.11 Therapy Protocols
36.12 Oncogenes and Cancer

36.1 INTRODUCTION

All cellular neoplastic events change nuclear DNA, enabling its transmission from a cell to its daughter cells. Carcinogenesis is a complex, multistaged process. The tumor or initiation stage is followed by a promoting event, which allows the potentially neoplastic cells to develop. Promoting agents can include such diverse factors as hormones, the immune status, nutrition, viral infections or tissue injury, chronic irritation of the tumor, or faulty DNA repair systems. An adequate immunologic function in which transformed cells are normally kept in check by the immune response can result in proliferation of a tumor unchecked if immunosuppression exists. Radiation—through its ability to cause local tissue damage as well as immune suppression—may both initiate and promote neoplastic transformation.

The incidence of neoplasia tends to increase as dogs age. The longer life span of dogs kept under good conditions therefore means that more are now at risk of neoplastic disease. This is because the cells of older dogs have undergone more cell cycles and have been exposed to genotoxic and epigenetic carcinogens for a longer time than have the cells of younger dogs.

Among the most common tumors of young dogs (particularly those 1 or 2 years old) are histiocytomas and skin papillomas, which are seldom seen in older animals. Lymphoma and osteosarcoma are frequently seen in elderly dogs but also occur in young dogs.

Genetic influences appear to be important in the development of bone tumors in Saint Bernards and Rottweilers.

Many laboratories now specialize in histologic diagnosis, and knowledge for prognosis has greatly increased. Many owners are now prepared to pay for specialist services, especially if remission or worthwhile prolongation of a quality life can be ensured. Different types of therapy can be used to counteract neoplasia.

Surgery, a common cancer treatment in veterinary medicine, should normally be used to treat local neoplastic lesional disease. Cryotherapy and radiation therapy occasionally may be used to treat selected local tumors. The most widely-used systemic therapy includes chemotherapy, hormonal therapy, or immunotherapy, all of which are appropriate when treating disseminated cancers.

The first choice in the treatment of malignant tumors is surgery. Other treatment regimens are applicable in various circumstances. The other major therapeutic approaches involve radiotherapy, either by irradiation, implantation of radioactive materials, hyperthermia, immunotherapy, or chemotherapy.

In practice, radiotherapy may not be popular because of the expensive equipment and radiation risks. The application and efficacy of hyperthermia are not clear.

Results with immunotherapeutic approaches offer considerable promise. Bacillus, Calmette-Guérin (BCG) vaccine administered intravenously to dogs after surgery for osteosarcoma and malignant mammary tumors has resulted in some success in a very limited number of cases.

Surgery remains the first-choice treatment against most cases of cancer in the dog; electrocautery and cryosurgery have proved very useful. Radiotherapy, although very useful, requires expensive and specialized equipment. Chemotherapy is being used more often and with more confidence. Immunotherapy—or the use of modifiers and manipulators of the immune system—is a major growth area that will undoubtedly increase in significance. The hyperthermic approach is an interesting area, and the combination of radiotherapy with hyperthermia shows good promise.

Adjuvant chemotherapy is the use of cytotoxic drugs immediately following surgery, when all detectable tissue has been removed but the risk of micrometastasis is high.

The use of immunostimulants such as BCG or levamisole at the end of a treatment program may have possible benefits, but their effects have not been adequately assessed.

Immunotherapy (biologic response modification) has been used to treat lymphoma in dogs.

All forms of cancer therapy are toxic to some degree, and it is the veterinarian's professional responsibility to ascertain and clinically assess if the patient can survive therapy. A complete blood cell count (CBC) and blood chemistries are necessary before a treatment regimen is started.

Surgery is perhaps the first therapy to be considered for many solid accessible tumors, or simply to debulk the tumor and provide biopsy specimens. The theory behind cryosurgery is that rapid freezing ($-20°C$) and slow thawing destroy viable tumor cells remaining after curettage. Cryosurgery is a popular method of therapy for some neoplasia. Cryosurgery can be used to treat tumors not easily treated with conventional surgical techniques.

Hyperthermia is an alternate method of killing residual tumor cells after curettage or in conjunction with radiotherapy. The potential advantages of hyperthermia are as follow:

1. Heat suppresses the ability to repair radiation damage.
2. Tumor cells may be more heat sensitive than normal cells.
3. Hypoxic cells are more heat sensitive than aerobic cells.

Radiotherapy is also commonly used as an adjunct to surgery, cryosurgery, or hyperthermia, but it is expensive. In human medicine, radiotherapy plays a major role in cancer treatment. It is now also being used more often to treat tumors in dogs.

Radiation is usually administered by using either ortho-voltage x-rays or cobalt or cesium to deliver gamma-radiation. The principal rays used in radiotherapy are x-rays and gamma-rays. Beta-rays and electrons are also used; beta-rays are used for very superficial tumors. Radiation kills both normal and cancer cells; side effects of radiation therapy are very common. A narrow safety margin exists with radiotherapy—normal cells are easily damaged and dosage sufficient to kill neoplastic tissue will probably damage normal tissue. High dosages given over a brief interval are more likely to permanently damage normal surrounding tissue. The success of radiotherapy depends on the interrelationship between tumor type, its site, the total amount of radiation given, and the rate at which it is given.

There may be some advantages to combining radiotherapy with other treatment regimens in dogs with neoplasia. Localized hyperthermia can prove beneficial in veterinary oncology when combined with radiotherapy. In cases of lymphosarcoma that have become resistant to chemotherapy, radiotherapy applied to the lymph nodes nearly always reduces the size of the node.

Radiotherapy can be effective for local or regional cancers but not always for metastases. Tumor cells are disrupted following exposures of the cell contents to suitable doses of radiation. Effectiveness of radiation is affected by several factors: oxygen levels within the cancer cells, the type of cancer cells, and the accessibility of the cancer sites. For some malignant tumors (e.g., squamous cell carcinoma of the gum tissue), radical surgery or radiotherapy can be recommended with confidence.

Another technique of radiotherapy is the intravenous (IV) injection of radioisotopes. This radiates therapy from inside the entrapped lesion. Immunotherapy, or immunopotentiation, is an attempt to enhance the body's own immune response. It can be used alone or as an adjunct to other therapy. BCG, mixed bacterial vaccine (MBV), or levamisole has been used as an adjuvant therapy intralesionally. Efficacy is equivocal, and side effects include fever, chills, nausea, and vomiting. Administered parenterally or intralesionally, this entails fairly long-term treatment. The possibility of using immunotherapy with chemotherapy is attractive, because the immunosuppression resulting from chemotherapy is reversible on discontinuation of therapy.

In the management of animals with neoplastic disease, surgery remains the treatment of choice for most solid tumors. However, when a localized tumor is inoperable or surgical excision has been incomplete, radiation therapy may be used.

The rationale of radiotherapy depends on the fact that ionizing radiation destroys replicating tissue to a greater extent than normal tissue.

Many neoplasms are systemic and are metastatic at the time of diagnosis. Systemic diseases include the leukemias, many lymphosarcomas, and myelomas, and these are best treated by chemotherapy. Osteosarcomas, hemangiomas, and oral melanomas—having a very high incidence of undetected metastases at diagnosis—are best managed by a variety of means, including surgery, chemotherapy, radiotherapy, or immunotherapy.

Before embarking on a program of cancer chemotherapy, an understanding of the cell division cycle is essential. The cell cycle has five conventional stages or phases, as follows:

1. At the beginning of the cycle, mitosis, the chromosomes attach to the mitotic spindle and separate into two daughter cells. This "M" phase lasts 30 to 90 minutes.
2. The Gap 1 (G1) phase can last for variable periods, and is the period of RNA synthesis.
3. The synthesis phase (S) lasts up to 6 hours and is the period of DNA synthesis.
4. Gap 2 (G2) is the second period of RNA and protein synthesis.
5. The gap 0 (G0) phase is a resting state; cells are inactive.

Hence the somatic cells undergoing rapid replication are most susceptible to the effects of antineoplastic drugs. Thus, chemotherapy is most likely to succeed against rapidly growing tumors. Antineoplastic drugs are most effective during the early stages of rapid growth, when pyrimidines and nucleic acid are being utilized for cell replication. Conversely, cells in the resting phase are generally refractory to chemotherapy. Tumor size is also significant. Small tumors usually have a larger number of cells in the multiplying state and hence display a rapid turnover time. Once the tumors enlarge, the number of dividing cells is smaller, volume doubling time is prolonged, and spontaneous cell death occurs. The normally expected increased growth of tumors following surgery sometimes can be used to advantage, because in this stage neoplasms are most sensitive to chemotherapeutic interruption of their growth acting against the substrates of cellular replication.

Advances in the use and availability of chemotherapeutic antineoplastic agents have resulted in their routine use in treating disseminated or inoperable cancer, prolonging survival and improving the quality of life of many patients. The aim of antineoplastic chemotherapy is to control a problem. Few neoplastic states can be considered fully curable. Aside from the low selective toxicity of most antineoplastic drugs, a fundamental difference exists between the therapeutic regimens employed in veterinary or human medical oncology: The financial limitations on nursing care and facilities in veterinary medicine often preclude adequate duration of therapy.

Protocols for the use of chemotherapeutic agents in neoplastic diseases of animals are difficult to obtain. Information on drug dosages and treatment intervals may derive in some cases from clinical trials, or more especially from human therapy.

Recommendations for drug protocols should be regarded primarily as guidelines—flexible regimens that may require adjustment according to the individual clinical case.

As mentioned, cures should not be expected with chemotherapy; it is a palliative approach that at best provides remission. Sometimes, as in lymphoid tumors, complete remissions occur, and the quality of the animal's life is improved significantly.

The dosages of antineoplastic agents are best based on body surface area (dose per square meter) rather than weight (pounds or kilograms). This method prevents underdosing very small dogs and cats as well as overdosing giant breed dogs. Slight dosage adjustments may be needed because of individual animal variations in drug tolerance. Thus all drugs are given in mg/M². (Table 36–1)

The major aim of cancer chemotherapy is to obtain maximum efficacy with minimum toxicity. When the toxicity of anticancer agents is compared in several species, large differences in the maximum tolerated doses are observed—that is, if doses are computed on a milligram per kilogram body weight basis—but the doses are approximately the same if based on a surface area basis, in milligrams per square meter. In practice, small dogs dosed on a square meter system receive more drugs when assessed on a body weight system than large dogs.

Before initiating chemotherapy, one must address several key questions.

1. The general health of the animal, especially its kidney function.
2. The likely rate of remission.
3. The quality of life conferred on the animal by the therapy (side effects vs. neoplastic process).

TABLE 36–1
CONVERSION TABLE OF WEIGHT (kg) TO BODY SURFACE AREA (m²) FOR DOGS

kg	m²	kg	m²
1.0	0.10	22.0	0.78
2.0	0.15	24.0	0.83
3.0	0.20	26.0	0.88
4.0	0.25	28.0	0.92
5.0	0.29	30.0	0.96
6.0	0.33	32.0	1.01
7.0	0.36	34.0	1.05
8.0	0.40	36.0	1.09
9.0	0.43	38.0	1.13
10.0	0.46	40.0	1.17
12.0	0.52	42.0	1.21
14.0	0.58	44.0	1.25
16.0	0.63	46.0	1.28
18.0	0.69	48.0	1.32
20.0	0.74	50.0	1.36

4. Whether the tumor has been adequately removed and if the risk of metastasis is high.
5. The reliability of the owner with respect to drug therapy compliance.

Clients should be informed by the veterinarian about the following points regarding embarkation on a cancer therapy protocol.

1. Cancer occurs more frequently in dogs than in humans.
2. Because some forms of cancer can be controlled, early diagnosis is advantageous.
3. Clinical signs of cancer in animals are extremely diverse.
4. Because dogs now have a longer lifespan, cancer incidence has shown a relative increase.

The treatment of human patients with chemotherapy usually differs in degree from the treatment in dogs, even though the same drugs may be used.

36.2 CHEMOTHERAPY

More than 20 to 30 anticancer drugs are commercially available, and they all work at specific stages of neoplastic division or interfere with specific cellular reactions to slow or stop tumor cell proliferation. Chemotherapy is extensively used and succeeds in many cases, but the veterinarian and clients should understand that the objective of chemotherapy is to control, not to cure, the condition.

Every antineoplastic drug is a potent, toxic agent. Bone marrow suppression, is a crucial indicator of toxicity, and occurs frequently. Granulocytopenia and thrombocytopenia may make the patient unable to respond to normal bacterial flora or minor infections. Sepsis or hemorrhage can therefore cause death. Therefore, when the white blood cell (WBC) count drops below 4,000/μl or the platelet count below 100,000/μl, a change in drug dosage or interval may be necessitated.

Perivascular administration of many chemotherapeutic drugs will cause tissue necrosis. If doxorubicin hydrochloride (HCl) is given perivascularly, the site should immediately be infiltrated with 5 ml of 8.4% sodium bicarbonate and 4 mg of dexamethasone.

As mentioned, drug dosages are expressed on a milligram per square meter of body surface area, because this correlates best with physiologic parameters such as blood volume and urea clearance.

Conversion tables are available for converting milligram per kilogram dosages into milligram per square meter of body surface area.

Most, if not all, chemotherapeutic anticancer drugs are toxic to all dividing cells, and there can be a fine line between therapeutic and toxic doses. It is therefore imperative that all animals undergoing chemotherapy be closely monitored for toxic side effects, because, additionally, most patients with neoplasia are older animals. Monitoring should consist of physical examinations, CBC, serum chemistry, and renal function tests every 7 to 10 days.

The general physical condition of an animal is important, especially kidney function in old dogs and cats and the presence of any existing anemia in leukemia patients.

Remission times vary from 6 to 12 months, and while this may be disappointing to the owner, it should be viewed in the context of its proportion of the animal's life span.

Oncologic complications can be induced or aggravated by the side effects of cancer chemotherapy. The specificity of cancer chemotherapy against neoplastic cells is not high, and nearly all chemotherapeutic agents, even when properly administered, can cause substantial host toxicity. The benefits of a therapeutic regimen therefore must be weighed against the anticipated toxic side effects.

Some drugs possess very short half-lives, and their toxicity is dose related (e.g., myelosuppression with cyclophosphamide). With other drugs the toxicity is related to the total cumulative dose of the drug and is less predictable (e.g., cardiomyopathy with doxorubicin HCl).

Side effects may be accentuated by medical problems such as hepatic, renal, cardiac, or bone marrow dysfunction. Vincristine, vinblastine, and doxorubicin are excreted by the biliary system and are therefore more toxic in the patient with hepatic disease.

If myelosuppressive drugs such as cyclophosphamide and doxorubicin HCl are used in animals with poor marrow reserve, they can cause increased myelotoxicity. Similarly, in patients with underlying infection, myelotoxic drugs increase the infections morbidity.

Frequent clinical examination and a minimal data base that includes determination of packed cell volume, plasma protein concentration, WBC count, platelet count, creatinine or BUN concentration, and a urinalysis allow early detection and reversal of serious chemotherapy-induced complications.

Hematologic abnormalities are most commonly observed in cancer patients with lymphoid, myeloid, and erythroid leukemias and in chemotherapy-induced myelosuppression.

The primary side effects follow:

1. Decreased circulatory blood cells, either leukopenia, anemia, thrombocytopenia, and pancytopenia
2. Hyperviscosity caused by erythrocytosis or leukocytosis
3. Disseminated intravascular coagulation

The cell specificity of the drugs is dependent primarily on the high rate of cellular turnover of the neoplastic cells. Useful indices of toxicity are the effects on bone marrow, the gastrointestinal tract, skin, and the reproductive tract, all of which have high cellular turnover rates.

Leukopenia is the single most important factor predisposing cancer patients to infection. Infection risk is very high when the granulocyte count drops below 3000–4000 μl. Broad-spectrum IV bactericidal antibiotics are indicated. Severe anemia, on the other hand, may be an indication for blood transfusion. Cross-matching is recommended, particularly because of the likelihood of several transfusions in some cancer patients. Cimetidine, 5 mg/kg, orally or slowly IV tid is useful to reduce hemorrhage from gastroduodenal ulcers.

Disseminated intravascular coagulation (DIC) is associated with thrombophlebitis, microinfarcts, and arterial thromboemboli of the brain and lung. Heparin (250–400 IU/kg subcutaneously tid) with close monitoring of clotting time may be indicated.

Combination chemotherapy, either simultaneously or sequentially, results in prolonged remissions and survival. The advantage of using combination chemotherapy instead of single-drug therapy is that a combination of drugs with different mechanisms of action and toxicities kills more cells more effectively, produces a marked decrease in the emergence of chemoresistant cells, and may minimize the incidence of toxic side effects.

It is essential that any veterinarian about to embark on cytotoxic chemotherapy be fully conversant with the pharmacodynamics, pharmacokinetics, dosage, schedules, and toxicities of these very potent and toxic chemicals. Dosage rates computed on body surface area (M^2) are usually evaluated on a trial and error basis.

Cancer-drug-related toxicities can be subdivided according to the criteria of (1) predictability of adverse reactions (2) frequency, and time delay at which toxicity occurs following administration. Some drugs have extremely short half-lives, and hence their toxicities are dose-related (e.g., myelosuppression with cyclophosphamide). With other drugs, the toxicity is related to the total cumulative dose of the drug (longer half life) and is less predictable e.g., cardiomyopathy with doxorubicin HCl (Adriamycin, Adria). Sometimes immediate side effects occur within the first 24 hours after administration; these can include anorexia, vomiting, phlebitis, skin rash, drug fever, and anaphylaxis. Such early toxic side effects can begin within days to weeks and include leukopenia, thrombocytopenia, anemia, renal failure, and diarrhea. Delayed effects occur within weeks to months after administration; an example is cardiomyopathy induced by doxorubicin HCl. If myelosuppressive drugs, such as cyclophosphamide and doxorubicin HCl, are used in animals with poor marrow reserve, they can cause increased myelotoxicity. Cumulation, incorrect dosage, health status of the animal, all contribute to this form of delayed host toxicity.

Most cytotoxic drugs act by interfering nonspecifically with DNA synthesis or mitosis. The cell selectivity of most of these drugs depends on a high growth rate of malignant cells. Such drugs, however, do not distinguish between the high replication rate of other tissues such as hematopoietic system and the villus epithelium of the alimentary tract. These organs and tissues are therefore most prone to the toxic effects of cytotoxic drugs. Patients can be monitored for the extent of bone marrow suppression by regular blood counts.

A course of treatment with a drug or combination of drugs will kill a certain percentage of tumor cells. It will not kill all such cells in the body, because the cytotoxic effect of the drug relies on active cell growth. Some proportion of the neoplastic cells will be in the resting phase.

If the kill rate is sufficiently higher than the growth rate, after several treatment courses, a small population of resistant cells will persist. Occasionally, the patient's immune system may be able to destroy these residual cells.

There are two primary approaches to therapy, depending on the disturbance and type of neoplastic growth:

1. When surgery is not an option, as in myeloproliferative malignancies (lymphosarcoma and leukemias), chemotherapy is usually relied on alone.
2. When a tumor cannot adequately be removed because of its site or invasiveness, chemotherapy is used, possibly in conjunction with some surgery.

36.3 SIDE EFFECTS OF CHEMOTHERAPY

Most antineoplastic drugs rely on the fact that tumor cells are fast growing and rapidly dividing. Normal tissues are spared from toxic effects only because they are slower in mitosis and development. Normal cells, such as bone marrow progenitor cells and intestinal epithelium, are very rapidly dividing; they divide faster than many tumors. They are thus highly susceptible to damage by chemotherapy. Most chemotherapeutic drugs therefore have a low therapeutic index (i.e., narrow therapeutic/toxic ratio). Also, rapidly dividing cells such as marrow cells and intestinal cells are most susceptible to cytotoxic effects. (Table 36–2)

As long as the bone marrow suppression effects are predominant, the patients can be monitored for that side effect by regular WBC counts, and overt side effects can be avoided. Many drugs have their own characteristic side effects, which may develop during treatment, particularly after prolonged use.

All antineoplastic drugs are inherently toxic agents. Their safety margin is very low, and their selective toxicity margin is very narrow. Because they are designed to

---

TABLE 36–2
COMMON SIDE EFFECTS OF CYTOTOXIC DRUGS

1) Myelosuppresion: This is usually dose related. Neutropenia is highly significant as it can lead to rapid bacterial infection that can be fatal.
2) Gastrointestinal effects: Vomiting, Diarrhea
3) Alopecia/Thinning of hair.
4) Perivascular Irritancy: Many irritant drugs may cause severe tissue necrosis, which in extreme cases could require skin grafting.
5) Infertility: Reproductive germ cell proliferation is seriously impaired by cytotoxic agents given in adulthood.
6) Pulmonary Effects: e.g. Bleomycin
7) Kidney Effects: Especially with excretion of irritant chemicals through the bladder leading to cystitis.
8) Cardiotoxicity: e.g. Adriamycin
9) Skin: Patchiness/Bloating of skin
10) Mucosal Inflammation: Oral candidiasis may follow from neutropenia.

---

arrest host cell replication, they also tend to affect those host tissues displaying a rapid rate of cellular turnover.

Induced myelosuppression is the dose-limiting toxicity of most cytotoxic drugs and is an accepted consequence of combination regimens given to treat leukemia and lymphoma in humans. It is dose-related and is more common in elderly patients and in those who have received previous radiotherapy or chemotherapy.

Bone marrow depression leading to lymphopenia, granulopenia, and thrombocytopenia can often occur. If the WBC count is less than 4000 µL or lymphocytes are less than 100,000 µL of normal values, drugs should be withdrawn or severely reduced. This can lead to a dramatic increase in infection. Blood transfusion may be necessary when anemia is severe. Granulocytopenia and thrombocytopenia may make the patient unable to respond to minor infections. Normal clotting may not be possible.

Old patients should be evaluated for kidney function before therapy; nephrotoxicity can occur, especially following alkylating agents in all animals, particularly cats.

HAZARDS TO THE HANDLER

The safety of the person administering cytotoxic drugs must be addressed. The risk of hypersensitization, carcinogenicity, and toxicity to personnel handling these drugs

has prompted specific guidelines for use, decontamination, and disposal. These agents should be treated like the hazardous chemicals they are. It is a scientific paradox that these anti-cancer agents, whether alkylating, radiation or whatever, are among the most potent carcinogens for the handler.

The handler should avoid contact with these drugs because many, such as the alkylating agents are carcinogenic. Drugs should be avoided in pregnant or breeding animals. Some drugs are particularly irritant, and great care should be exercised during IV injection; vincristine is a notable example. Hemorrhagic cystitis may occur in patients receiving cyclophosphamide. Gloves should be worn by the user and all exposure to unprotected skin avoided. Some cytotoxic drugs, including doxorubicin and vincristine, are chemically irritant and can cause severe tissue necrosis. This can be persistently painful, progress widely, and require skin grafting.

Fertility is largely unaffected by chemotherapy given in childhood but will be impaired by most intensive, cytotoxic regimens given in adulthood.

Because rapidly multiplying cells are more susceptible to the effects of antineoplastic agents, it is not surprising that cells of the bone marrow, lymphoid system, gastrointestinal tract, epidermis, and reproductive tracts are equally susceptible. Bone marrow suppression is manifested by hemorrhage and sepsis. Neutropenia and thrombocytopenia precede anemia and occur very rapidly because of the very short life span of these blood elements. Should the neutrophils fall below 4000 μL, or the platelets below 50,000 μL, the therapy should be stopped.

Bone marrow toxicity, as reflected by thrombocytopenia or granulocytopenia, is very common, and such adverse effects may render the patient unable to respond to minor infections. Blood clotting may be severely affected. Hence, a range of sequelae from septicemia to hemorrhage can occur with a possible fatal outcome. Baseline hematology values therefore must be obtained and maintained. If platelets drop below 50,000/μl or WBC below 4,000/μl, the dosage may need to be reassessed or the treatment interval re-evaluated.

If bone marrow failure is related to the side effects of chemotherapeutic agents, cancer therapy must be instantly ceased or changed, depending on the degree and intensity of toxicity to the bone marrow.

Hematologic abnormalities are most commonly observed in cancer patients with lymphoid, myeloid, and erythroid leukemias and with myelosuppression caused by chemotherapy.

Leukopenia, (neutropenia and lymphopenia,) is a result of (1) bone marrow invasion by the tumor (2) myelotoxicity associated with chemotherapeutic drugs, and (3) decreased survival of circulating blood cells. Leukopenia is probably the single most important factor predisposing cancer patients to infection. The frequency of infections is inversely related to the number of circulating granulocytes; that is, the incidence of infection dramatically increases when the granulocyte count drops below threshold levels.

DISSEMINATED INTRAVASCULAR COAGULATION (D.I.C.)

DIC occurs as a consequence of the cancerous process itself but may also be a complication of drugs used in cancer chemotherapy. Alimentary tract disorders associated with antitumor drugs include anorexia, vomiting, and diarrhea. These signs may appear soon after beginning therapy.

Cisplatin, ifosfamide, IV cyclophosphamide, doxorubicin, mustine, and dacarbamazine are most likely to produce marked vomiting.

Whereas alopecia is a frequent sequel of chemotherapy in humans, it is less common in domestic animals, although occasionally the poodle may display it. Reversible alopecia is an inevitable consequence of treatment with doxorubicin in humans. It is common also following cyclophosphamide, vincristine, mustine, and etoposide and can occur with many other cytoxic drugs.

Immunosuppression following chemotherapy is due to decreased leukocyte numbers and impaired humoral and cell-mediated immunity. It is usually reversible following cessation of therapy.

As mentioned, dosages of antineoplastic drugs are conventionally based not on body weight but rather on body surface area (dose per square meter), which prevents under- and overdosing.

Many antineoplastic drugs are available, but the toxicity of most is very high and the expense of others precludes their use in routine veterinary therapy.

Drug combinations are used to increase therapeutic potency and to reduce toxicity. In most cases, because these drugs act on different phases of the cell cycle, toxicity is not additive. The tumoricidal effect therefore is maximized, while not appreciably increasing the toxic hazard. Drug combinations also may delay the emergence of resistance. When drug combinations are used, however, no advantage is obtained by mixing drugs of similar mechanisms of action.

Before using drugs in combination, it should be established that each drug is specific for the particular malignant cell line. Combination therapy, however, is not always indicated nor indeed more effective than individual drug therapy. Single-agent therapy occasionally results in limited remission and increased survival times. When the tumor fails to respond, switching to another class of drug with a different mechanism of action may be necessary. Sequential drug therapy is easy to administer and inexpensive, but survival times are short and prolonged remissions rare.

Because the selective toxicity margin of antineoplastic drugs is not wide, killing of

TABLE 36–3
ANTINEOPLASTIC DRUG CLASSIFICATION

Alkylating agents	Cyclophosphamide
	Chlorambucil.
	Melphalan
	Busulphan
	Thiotepa.
Antimetabolites	Methotrexate
	5-Fluorouracil; 6-Thioguanine
	Cytosine Arabinoside
	6-Mercaptopurine
Plant Alkaloids	Vincristine
	Vinblastine
Hormones	Estrogens; Antiestrogens: Tamoxifen
	Androgens
	Corticosteroids
Enzymes	L-asparaginase
Miscellaneous	Mitotane (DDT Congener)
	Hydroxyurea; Dacarbamazine

Other Approaches:
• Immunotherapy
• Cryosurgery
• Hyperthermia
• Radiation therapy
• Injection of Isotopes

tumor cells often results in the death of some normal cells. Toxicity is a predictable sequel of antineoplastic chemotherapy. However, judicious drug and dose selection as well as protocol planning can significantly reduce the risk of life-threatening toxicity.

Occasionally, it is necessary to change from the original cytotoxic agent to one that is less toxic and perhaps slower acting, e.g., switching from cyclophosphamide to chlorambucil. Cyclophosphamide quite often produces hemorrhagic cystitis. Withdrawal of the drug is then necessary. Perivascular deposition or leakage of many drugs can cause severe local tissue necrosis (doxorubicin [adriamycin] is one such agent). Doxorubicin can interact with many drugs including heparin. To avoid precipitates of doxorubicin HCl, it is always advisable to flush catheters with normal saline before and after giving IV doxorubicin. Other problems that occasionally may arise include severe decline in platelet levels. Blood transfusion or broad-spectrum antimicrobial therapy may then be indicated.

Paradoxically, antineoplastic drugs are carcinogenic. Contact with these agents therefore should be avoided. Equally, they may cause hypersensitivity or direct toxicity. Strict guidelines should be followed with regard to their use and disposal. Skin contact must be avoided, and latex gloves should be worn. The veterinarian must inform clients of the inherent dangers of these highly toxic substances.

Monitoring during therapy is vital. Weekly total WBC counts, platelet counts, and routine blood biochemistry (blood urea nitrogen [BUN], serum glutamate pyruvate transaminase [SGPT]) are essential. When serious side effects occur, the dosage should be reduced, the drug withdrawn, or alternatively, symptoms treated. Blood transfusions, fluids, antidiarrheals, or IV antibiotic therapy may be warranted. However, caution must be exercised when using antibiotics with agents such as methotrexate, because occupation of binding sites in the plasma will increase the effective free unbound level of methotrexate with serious side effects.

36.4 CLASSES OF ANTICANCER DRUGS

Complete familiarity with the pharmacologic mechanism of action of these drugs is essential, because quite often combinations are necessary to deliver a more potent effect by virtue of their complementary pharmacodynamics.

Antineoplastic drugs are classified according to their mechanisms of action into alkylating agents, antimetabolites, plant alkaloids, antibiotics, enzymes, hormones, and miscellaneous agents. (Table 36–3)

36.5 ALKYLATING DRUGS

Alkylating drugs are derived from mustard gases, which in addition to their vesicant action on the skin, produce atrophy of lymphoid tissue and bone marrow. Different alkylating agents have differing specificities for selected neoplasms, primarily because of differences in reactivity that alter the pharmacokinetic profile.

These cytotoxic drugs act by adding alkyl group radicals to DNA. This is similar to the effect of radiation. All alkylating agents suppress the bone marrow and can cause gastroenteritis. Alkylating agents replace the hydrogen atom with an alkyl group in the DNA molecule, particularly in the guanine locus. By inserting this alkyl radical for a hydrogen ion, the alkylating drugs prevent the cross-linkage of DNA, which then interferes with DNA replication and transcription. These are therefore classed as cytotoxic drugs.

Alkylating agents include chlorambucil, cyclophosphamide, busulfan, and melphalan. They are inherently cytotoxic agents that act by transferring their alkyl groups to various cellular constituents. Although alkylation of DNA is the main effect, they also react chemically with sulfhydryl, amino, hydroxyl, carboxyl, and phosphate groups of all cellular nucleophils. The major site of reactivity is alkylation within DNA at the guanine locus, although other bases are also alkylated to lesser degrees. These interactions may occur on a single strand or both strands of DNA because most alkylating drugs possess two reactive groupings. Miscoding through abnormal base pairing with thy-

mine or depurination by excision of guanine are the usual consequences of drug-DNA interaction, with DNA strand breakage quite common. Refractoriness to alkylating agents involves increased DNA repair capacity by the affected cell.

These highly reactive drugs exert their effects on DNA by causing breaks or inappropriate cross-linking of DNA strands. This leaves DNA unable to replicate or transcribe. Because the end result is cellular death, these agents are said to be cytotoxic. This is also one of the modes of action of ionizing radiation; therefore, these agents are also radiomimetic.

The major toxic side effect of alkylating agents is dose-related suppression of myelopoiesis in the bone marrow. This prevents DNA replication, and cell death follows.

Cyclophosphamide is a commonly used antineoplastic drug that is inert until transformed by the liver. Administration oral or IV, and as an alkylating agent cyclophosphamide is highly toxic to replicating tissue through its DNA reactivity. Accordingly, it is used to treat carcinomas, malignant lymphoma, lymphocytic leukemia, and multiple myeloma.

Cyclophosphamide can be used singly or in combination with other drugs to treat lymphoid tumors, mast cell tumors, and transmissible venereal tumors in dogs. Because the drug must be activated by hepatic microsomal enzymes, its use must be reconsidered in animals with liver insufficiency. Cyclophosphamide exerts its cytoxic effects at many phases in the cell cycle, and its most important side effects are myelosuppression and hemorrhagic cystitis.

Monitoring of the platelets and leukocytes is necessary drug therapy to minimize the side effects of neutropenia or thrombocytopenia. If the platelet count drops below 100,000 μl or the WBCs below 4,000 μl, the dosage should be decreased by 25% and dosage intervals increased. Over 90% of cyclophosphamide is excreted unchanged via the kidneys, and irritation of the bladder mucosa and resultant hemorrhagic cystitis are not uncommon. Use of diuretics to ensure frequent urination is necessary if this condition arises.

Several other side effects accompany the use of alkylating agents including nausea, vomiting, and alopecia. Cyclophosphamide is more immunosuppressive than most other alkylating agents. It is inappropriate for use in animals with liver disease.

Hemorrhagic cystitis often occurs after several months' therapy (or at high dosage rates), and in such cases the drug should be withdrawn. As well as being a useful drug in lymphosarcoma, it can also produce temporary regression in few cases of tubular adenocarcinoma of the mammary gland.

For cyclophosphamide (the more widely used alkylating agent), the dosage schedules are 50 mg/m² orally on alternative days or 300 mg/m² IV every 3 weeks.

Chlorambucil, another nitrogen mustard derivative and alkylating agent, is a slow-acting oral agent similar in activity to cyclophosphamide, which may be substituted for it when a tolerance problem arises. Given orally, chlorambucil is free of the hemorrhagic cystitis problem of cyclophosphamide. However, other unwanted effects such as hepatotoxicity, gastrointestinal dysfunction, and myelogenous suppression may follow its use.

Chlorambucil has an oral dosage rate of 0.2 mg/kg daily for 4 to 6 weeks. It is one of the least toxic of the alkylating agents and can be used with reasonable safety without monitoring WBC counts. It can be used alternatively at a dosage of 2 mg/m².

Chlorambucil is useful for chronic lymphatic leukemia and lymphosarcoma and often is combined with prednisolone and vincristine. Myelosuppression is a major and significant side effect of chlorambucil.

MELPHALAN

Melphalan is a drug of significance in human medicine for the treatment of melanomas, myelomas, and testicular seminomas. Its use is not widely documented in the veterinary literature, but side effects of leukopenia, thrombocytopenia, anemia, and gastrointestinal upset accompany its use.

TRIETHYLENE THIOPHOSPHAMIDE (THIOTEPA)

Thiotepa is used in humans in cases of bladder cancer; it can produce complete remission in up to one third of such cases. Its ma-

jor use generally has been local infusion for transitional cell carcinoma of the bladder following surgical excision. Thiotepa in a 100- to 300-ml solution is instilled locally by catheter, not exceeding a dose of 30 mg/m². It is then drained out of the bladder via catheter. Doses can be repeated depending on the incidence and severity of hematologic side effects.

36.6 ANTIMETABOLITES

Antimetabolite drugs are structural analogues of substances required for normal cell function and replication. They act by competing with normal metabolites and thereby cause dysfunction of key biochemical pathways in the cell. Antimetabolites interfere with synthesis of nucleic acids by inhibiting enzyme function or by substituting abnormal molecules for normal nucleotides and cause misreading of the genetic code. Antimetabolites are cell phase-specific drugs because they exert their cytotoxic effects at one stage of the cell cycle—the S phase.

Methotrexate blocks dihydrofolate reductase, a key enzyme necessary for the formation of folinic acid, which is needed for DNA synthesis. It has been commonly used to treat canine osteosarcoma. Side effects include myelosuppression, vomiting, and diarrhea. Other antimetabolites include 5-fluorouracil, 6-thioguanine, and cytosine arabinoside.

METHOTREXATE

Methotrexate has a particularly narrow safety margin in animals. The structure of methotrexate resembles folic acid, and the drug produces competitive inhibition of the conversion of folic acid to folinic (tetrahydrofolic acid) acid by the enzyme dihydrofolate reductase. Myelosuppression, hepatic necrosis, and severe desquamation of the intestinal epithelium accompany its use, and therefore it is best given for short periods only. Severe enteritis accompanies its use.

Methotrexate inhibits the enzyme dihydrofolate reductase by competing for its folate binding sites. By inhibiting this enzyme, tetrahydrofolic (folinic) acid production is suppressed and hence purine and pyrimidine synthesis is suppressed also. The net result is inhibition of nucleic acid synthesis and thus an antimitotic effect. A high concentration and prolonged exposure of methotrexate are necessary for satisfactory clinical response to facilitate entry of unbound methotrexate into the cell and to compete successfully for the reductase enzyme.

The major toxic effect of methotrexate is marked irritation of the mucosal lining of the alimentary tract. This is manifested as severe villous damage, infiltration of the villous lamina propria, and a frank hemorrhagic enteritis. Intravenous administration carries less risk of adverse effects than the oral route.

The cytotoxicity of methotrexate can be reversed by supplying folinic acid or leukovorin (citrovorum factor), the terminal metabolite of the reductase pathway, which is inhibited by methotrexate.

A common side effect of the methotrexate therapy in dogs is severe hemorrhagic enteritis. Some drugs interact with methotrexate to alter its cellular uptake or secretion (aspirin, vincristine, sulfonamides, corticosteroids). Malignant lymphoma responds best to methotrexate.

Methotrexate can be give orally, IV, or intramuscularly (IM). High doses of methotrexate can be given with citrovorum factor over a few hours to protect normal cells.

The main side effect of methotrexate is severe gastroenteritis. Longterm treatment may cause liver damage. Methotrexate can be useful for carcinomas and lymphosarcoma.

CYTARABINE

Another drug useful for malignant lymphoma is cytarabine. This is a nucleotide analogue of cytidine and acts as a DNA polymerase inhibitor. Because of its very short half-life, it must be given frequently (IV) or by prolonged infusion. As with methotrexate, side effects are manifested primarily at sites of rapid cellular proliferation, namely, the bone marrow and gastrointestinal tract.

Cytosine arabinoside is a pyrimidine derivative and is given IV at a dosage of 100 mg/m^2 daily for 4 days in conjunction with other drugs to treat lymphoreticular tumors.

This compound inhibits DNA polymerase by competitive inhibition of deoxycytidine triphosphate. Although often used in combination therapy, the drug is of most value in cases of lymphosarcoma.

5-FLUOROURACIL

The cytotoxic effect of 5-fluorouracil is blockade of thymidylate synthetase. The major toxic effects are diarrhea, leukopenia, and alopecia. (Table 36–4)

36.7 PLANT ALKALOIDS

Plant alkaloids interfere with formation of the mitotic spindle and prevent cell division. Vinca alkaloids, vincristine and vinblastine, are phase-specific, acting at the M phase, and have minimal effect on the bone marrow. Vinca alkaloids are used to manage specific neoplastic and immune-mediated diseases of humans and animals. The cytotoxic effects of vinca alkaloids are caused by their ability to bind to tubulin and to inhibit mitosis.

Vincristine has been widely used to treat canine lymphoid tumors, mast cell tumors, and transmissible venereal tumors. Localized necrosis follows extravascular injection of vinca alkaloids, so due care must be taken to ensure complete IV delivery.

Vincristine sulfate is possibly the most commonly used anticancer drug in veterinary practice. It is highly irritant to tissues if deposited perivascularly; hence, careful IV injection is indicated. An antimitotic agent, vincristine interferes with spindle activity during metaphase. It is excreted in the feces, is highly protein bound in plasma, and fails to cross the blood-brain barrier.

To date, vincristine has been successfully employed to induce remission of canine and feline malignant lymphomas and also to treat transmissible venereal tumors. Monitoring of blood is necessary during therapy. Sometimes, neurodermatitis and muscular weakness accompany its use.

TABLE 36–4
SOME ADVERSE EFFECTS OF SPECIFIC ANTINEOPLASTIC DRUGS

DRUG	SIDE EFFECTS
Adriamycin	Anorexia, Mouth Lesions, Leukopenia, Myelosuppression, Highly Toxic, Irritant, Perivascular Sloughing, Hemorrhagic Diarrhea, Discolors Urine (orange), Cardiotoxicity, Alopecia. Take care if combined with Radiotherapy or other Agents.
L-Asparaginase	Leukopenia, Pancreatitis
Bleomycin	Pulmonary fibrosis (Dose Dependent), Mouth Lesions, Skin Patching
Cisplatin	Vomiting, Diarrhea, Kidney/Bladder Dysfunction
Corticosteroids	Gastroenteritis, Water Retention, Cushing's
Chlorambucil	Myelosuppression, Hepatotoxicity, Alimentary Tract Disturbance
Cyclophosphamide	Hemorrhagic Cystitis, Irritant Excretion, Neutropenia, Thrombocytopenia, Myelosuppression, Infertility, Nausea, Vomiting, Alopecia/Thinning of hair
Cytarabine	Bone Marrow Suppression, Alimentary Tract Disturbance
Daunobubicin	Dose-dependent Cardiotoxicity
5-Fluorouracil	Mouth Lesions, Diarrhea, Alopecia, Leukopenia
Ifosfamide	Vomiting/Kidney Dysfunction
Melphalan	Gastrointestinal Dysfunction, Leukopenia Thrombocytopenia
Mitotane	C.N.S. Depression
Mustine	Vomiting, Alopecia, Infertility
Methotrexate	G.I.T. Irritation, Vomiting, Hemolytic Disorders, Hepatic Necrosis, Mouth Lesions, Kidney Dysfunction, Myelosuppression.
Vincristine	Thrombocytosis, Increases Fragility of Megakaryocytes, Muscular Weakness, Alopecia. Highly irritating perivascularly
Vinblastine	Greater hematopoietic toxicity; local necrosis after perivascular leakage

Vincristine is an antimitotic agent that prevents mitosis by abolishing spindle formation. It must be given slowly and very carefully IV at a dose rate of 0.5 mg/m^2. Any perivascular leakage can cause serious local problems. Its main use is in the treatment of lymphosarcoma. Side effects are rarely seen at this dose rate and are bone marrow suppression and constipation.

Antibiotics such as doxorubicin, bleomycin, and actinomycin prevent the synthesis of DNA and RNA by the formation of stable complexes with DNA. Such antibiotic antineoplastic drugs are more expensive than many other antineoplastic agents.

ADRIAMYCIN (DOXORUBICIN)

Doxorubicin is an anthracycline antitumor antibiotic isolated from *Streptomyces peucetius var caesius*. The drug acts at all phases of the cell cycle. Cytotoxicity is induced by inserting double-stranded DNA, which blocks DNA, RNA, and protein syntheses. Adriamycin inhibits DNA-dependent RNA synthesis. It can be quite cardiotoxic in dogs, more so than in humans, and therefore a total cumulative dose of 300 mg/m^2 should not be exceeded. Blood counts should be regularly carried out to monitor the effect on the bone marrow. The usual dosage of adriamycin is 30 mg/M^2.

Doxorubicin is used in lymphosarcomas and also in canine osteosarcoma. It is expensive, and side effects such as myelosuppression, anorexia, and cardiomyopathies accompany its use. Hair loss is common after doxorubicin administration and can also occur after cyclophosphamide administration. Although alopecia is a common side effect of antineoplastic drugs in man, in animals the side effect is usually restricted to a generalized thinning of the hair coat.

Doxorubicin, an anthracycline antibiotic, displays greater toxicity than conventional alkylating agents. A dose-dependent generalized myocardial degeneration is the most serious adverse effect. Careful cardiac monitoring by electrocardiogram (ECG), auscultation, and radiography is always advisable during doxorubicin treatment.

Hepatic and cardiac disease can be made worse by doxorubicin. The drug should given IV by catheter; it is an irritant to tissues. Slow IV delivery tends to minimize histamine-induced reactions such as hives or pruritus. Hemorrhagic enteritis is sometimes noticed shortly after treatment. Temporary reddish discoloration of urine accompanies therapy, and owners should be forewarned. Doxorubicin is additive to previous radiation or chemotherapy, and concurrent therapy with other anticancer drugs will further narrow its safety margin. Although it is a new and relatively expensive drug, its clinical application offers considerable promise, because it possesses a broad and versatile range of activity against thyroid carcinomas, malignant lymphomas, soft-tissue sarcomas, and transmissible venereal tumors.

Doxorubicin HCl is more toxic than most alkylating agents. Even though mild bone marrow suppression, alopecia, and allergic reactions may occur, the most serious problem is cardiotoxocity. Despite these problems, doxorubicin HCl has one of the widest spectrums of activity of the antineoplastic agents. Doxorubicin is commonly administered IV to dogs but a cumulative dosage of 300 mg/m² of body surface area must not be exceeded. A lower dosage regimen of 30 mg/M² of body surface area given every three weeks intravenously has been used in the treatment of lymphoma.

36.8 STEROIDS

Prednisone orally or prednisolone by injection may have some cytotoxic effect, especially in lymphoreticular neoplasms. Prednisone is often routinely used in drug combinations. Prednisone is generally given in a 28-day cycle: 7 days at 20 mg/m², then 14 days on half the dose, and 7 days on a quarter of the starting dose.

Commonly used corticosteroids include dexa- and betamethasone, prednisone, prednisolone, and triamcinolone. These are all antimitotic and lympholytic on lymphoid tissue. Side effects include polydypsia, polyuria, and increased appetite, while prolonged use can lead to a Cushing-type (iatrogenic) syndrome. Steroids are usually given orally in cases of lymphosarcoma and mastocytoma, but IV injection of large doses (150 to 200 mg) of hydrocortisone may be necessary in cases of severe lymphosarcoma.

Estrogens are excellent for most cases of perianal adenoma and rare prostatic carcinoma. Almost all cases of mammary neoplasia can be prevented by ovariohysterectomy early in the dog's life. Anti-estrogens such as tamoxifen are used in human medicine for breast cancer.

36.9 MISCELLANEOUS

For cases of lymphosarcoma and mast cell tumors, enzymes such as L-asparaginase have been used to deplete the body stores of asparagine. Malignant neoplastic cells lack the enzyme asparagine synthetase, necessary to make the essential amino acid asparagine, while normal cells have the enzyme to synthesize additional asparagine. Anaphylaxis can occur following L-asparaginase injection, but this is rare with IM administration.

Mitotane has been used to manage adrenal carcinoma that is due to pituitary neoplasms. It can cause necrosis of the zona reticularis and zona fasciculata of the adrenal cortex but does not damage the primary tumor in the pituitary. Mitotane is chemically related to DDT.

Cisplatin, a platinum complex, is useful in human patients for metastatic ovarian cancer and testicular cancer but has yet to be thoroughly evaluated in veterinary medicine. It has been useful in canine squamous cell carcinomas and thyroid carcinomas, but cost and nephrotoxicity limit its usefulness. Although it possesses severe pulmonary toxicity in cats, it has been widely used for the treatment of osteosarcoma in dogs. Cisplatin has recently gained extensive popularity among veterinary oncologists.

Dacarbazine can be used to treat melanoma and with adriamycin in osteosarcoma. It is given IV at a dosage of 200–300 mg/m² for 5 consecutive days every 3 weeks. Patients should be premedicated with atropine to prevent vomiting and may experience slight pain on injection.

Hydroxyurea exerts its effect on the S phase of the cell cycle, inhibiting DNA synthesis. Its major side effects are targeted toward the bone marrow, and its limited usefulness is in cases of lymphosarcoma and mastocytoma. Other drugs in human medicine include ifosfamide, mustine, dacarbazine, mitozantrone, carboplatin, bleomycin, epirubicin, and daunorubicin.

36.10 IMMUNOTHERAPY

Immunomodulators include BCG, *Corynebacterium parvum*, levamisole, and muramyl dipeptide. Although early results with BCG looked promising, more recent results in canine mammary tumors have been disappointing. BCG cell wall preparations given 3 to 5 weeks before mastectomy may improve tumor-free survival times when compared with surgery alone. *C. parvum* has been of some effect in dogs with advanced melanoma.

Interferon and interferon inducers have been used for cancer therapy in humans; but toxicity has sometimes been severe, and results have been variable.

Other agents acting on the immune system are currently being assessed: lymphokines, chalones, macrophage stimulation factor, tumor necrosis factor, T-cell growth factor, and interleukin 2.

Autologous tumor vaccines, murine derived, anti-canine lymphoma. Monoclonal antibody has also been evaluated.

Immunotherapy has been investigated for sarcoids in horses. Sarcoid is perhaps the most common skin tumor of horses. Because of its similarity to several other skin conditions, it is relatively refractory to different treatments. Equine sarcoid thus represents a major therapeutic challenge to veterinary practitioners.

Intralesional injection of immunotherapeutic agents, most specifically a cell wall preparation of BCG, have resulted in high remission rates in equine sarcoids with minimal side effects.

The cell wall preparation consists of a BCG cell wall skeleton plus trehalose dimycolate, a mycolic ester. When combined these 2 components work synergistically to produce an extensive granulomatous reaction, and tumor regression. Such a preparation does not induce suppressor activity and thus facilitate tumor growth, as does whole BCG. In equine sarcoid therapy with such a preparation, lymphodenopathy, malaise, and anorexia can occur but are transient. Localized BCG has been successful against tumors with increased antigenicity and may inhibit viral carcinogenesis. The mechanism by which intralesional injection of BCG cell wall skeleton and trehalose dimycolate cause regression of equine sarcoid is not known. However, this form of localized immunotherapy possibly involves the induction of nonspecific cellular cytoxicity, specific tumor immunity, and some type of antiviral immunity, both locally and within the regional lymph nodes.

The application of 13-cis retinoic acid, which has been proposed to influence the immune response may have a role in enhancement of antitumor activity.

36.11 THERAPY PROTOCOLS

Doses of antineoplastic drugs are varied. They possess a narrow safety margin and each neoplastic condition will require individual dosage of single or combined drugs. Table 36–5 gives an approximate guideline for some drug dosages. The commonest tumors to respond to therapy are lymphosarcomas, leukemias, and mastocytomas. Transmissible venereal tumors may also respond quite well. Malignant tumors such as oral melanomas or osteosarcomas show little or no response to treatment. (Table 36–5)

Systemic anticancer therapy is the treatment of choice for canine lymphomas. Variable success has been achieved with several drugs used either singly or in combination, such as corticosteroids, prednisone, cyclophosphamide, chlorambucil, vincristine, L-asparaginase, cytosine, arabinoside, doxorubicin, methotrexate, vinblastine, and 6-mercaptopurine.

As a general rule, drugs should be given intermittently, 4 weeks on, four weeks off. This allows the bone marrow to recover and resting tumor cells to recommence active growth and thus become susceptible to the cytotoxic drugs.

TABLE 36–5
GENERAL DOSAGE RATES FOR ANTINEOPLASTIC DRUGS

Adriamycin	30 mg/m²
Chlorambucil	2–5 mg/m²
Cyclophosphamide	50 mg/m²
Busulfan	4 mg/m²
Cisplatin	30 mg/m²
Cytosine Arabinoside	100–200 mg/m²
Dacarbazine	200–300 mg/m²
5-Fluorouracil	100–200 mg/m²
Melphalan	1.5–7.0 mg/m²
Methotrexate	5.0 mg/m²
Prednisone	20 mg/m²
Thiotepa	30 mg/m²
Vincristine	0.5 mg/m²

For specific applications, Dosage Rates, Routes of Administration and Type of Regimen, Refer to Text.

Tumors treated by chemotherapy include lymphosarcoma, leukemia, mastocytomas, and reticular cell sarcomas. Among the drugs most commonly used are cyclophosphamide, chlorambucil, vincristine, and cytosine arabinoside.

Lymphoma (also known as malignant lymphoma and lymphosarcoma [LSA]) is commonly diagnosed in dogs. It is important to remember that, although multicentric lymphoma in dogs is fatal if untreated, most dogs will respond well to treatment. One of the most valuable drugs for treatment of lymphomas is vincristine, which is frequently combined with cyclophosphamide and prednisolone in the treatment of multicentric lymphosarcoma.

Chemotherapy is the primary treatment of the management of lymphoma. The dog's age, weight, and gender have been considered as possible prognostic factors. The blood picture should always been monitored during therapy.

In general, combination chemotherapy is the most widely used approach and is considered the most efficacious. Doxorubicin and corticosteroids have been used as single agents.

Complete cures are rarely if ever obtained, and the median survival approximates 6 to 7 months in many cases. Even when the lesions become resistant to antineoplastic drugs, they can still respond to radiotherapy, and combinations of radio-therapy and chemotherapy can be quite efficacious. Low doses of radiation often result in rapid tumor remission and can be used successfully when a neoplasm, e.g., a central nervous system lymphoma, is causing mechanical damage by compression.

Lymphomas represent over 80% of all hematologic malignancies in dogs. Some evidence shows that canine lymphoma cells contain high activity of reverse transcriptase, which is an enzyme found in oncogenic retroviruses, and hence the postulation that lymphomas may have a viral-based cause.

Lymphoma is a fatal disease in the dog if untreated but, fortunately, is also responsive to therapeutic intervention. Although treatment is rewarding, it should not be undertaken without a clear understanding of two important factors: (1) the toxicity of chemotherapeutic agents, which ultimately limits the amount of chemotherapy, and (2) potential risk of exposure to those handling the drugs.

Local therapy (e.g., surgery, radiotherapy, or hyperthermia) for a solitary lymphoma should be followed by adjuvant systemic chemotherapy. Systemic anticancer chemotherapy is the treatment of choice for canine lymphomas. Drugs commonly used include corticosteroids, cyclophosphamide, chlorambucil, vincristine, L-asparaginase, cytosine arabinoside, methotrexate, vinblastine, and 6-mercaptopurine.

TABLE 36–6
DRUGS COMMONLY USED FOR LYMPHATIC TUMORS

Corticosteroids (Prednisone 10–20 mg/m².)
Vincristine 0.5 mg/m²
Chlorambucil 2–5 mg/m²
Adriamycin 30 mg/m²
Methotrexate 5.0 mg/m²
Cytosine Arabinoside 100 mg/m²
Cyclophosphamide 50–100 mg/m²

1. Combination therapy of the above is often used successfully.
2. Prednisolone, vincristine and cyclophosphamide are commonly used together for lymphomas.
3. Adriamycin and Corticosteroids have both been used as single agents for lymphomas.

"Lymphoma" or "lymphosarcoma" refers to a lymphoid neoplasm that primarily affects solid organs. "Lymphoid leukemia" refers to a malignancy in which the cells originate primarily in the bone marrow. Lymphomas generally should be considered as systemic neoplasms and thus treated with systemic antineoplastic therapy. For a solitary lymphosarcoma, local therapy (surgery, radiotherapy, or hyperthermia) should be attempted, followed by adjuvant systemic chemotherapy.

Cutaneous lymphoma usually does not respond well to antineoplastic therapy. Individual lesions should be surgically excised and chemotherapy given for probable disseminated disease. Dogs developing cutaneous malignant lymphoma secondary to a generalized lymph node neoplasia respond better to chemotherapy than those initially presenting with only cutaneous lesions. Doxorubicin HCl, 30 mg/m², IV, every 3 to 4 weeks, or various combinations

of cyclophosphamide, vincristine sulfate, prednisone, cytarabine, and methotrexate have been most effective from reports to date.

THERAPY OF SPECIFIC NEOPLASMS

Lymphosarcoma

Lymphosarcoma is the most frequently encountered neoplasm in the dog. In the majority of patients, the disease progression is rapid if left untreated, with death occurring in 3 to 4 months.

Many protocols have been used for the treatment of lymphosarcoma. Combination chemotherapy results in complete remission in up to 80% of cases. Survival times range from 6 to 8 months. Usually, there is a fairly intensive induction schedule with frequent, high doses followed by less intense maintenance therapy.

A useful protocol is oral cyclophosphamide 50 mg/M² for 3 consecutive days/ week. This therapy can be continued throughout the dog's life. If hemorrhagic cystitis develops at this dosage, chlorambucil can be substituted. Vincristine is given at a dosage of 0.5 mg/M² once weekly for the first 3 weeks then every 3 weeks. Prednisone is given orally at a dosage of 10 mg/ M² daily for the first week. (Tables 36–6 and 36–7)

Lymphosarcoma treatment protocols are well established, and 75% of animals show significant remission. The usual therapy is

---

TABLE 36–7
LYMPHOSARCOMA

(1) Cyclophosphamide 50 mg/m²
     +
(2) Vincristine 0.5 mg/m²
     OR
(3) Prednisone 10 mg/m²
     +
(4) Chlorambucil 2–5 mg/m²

vincristine, cytosine arabinoside, cyclophosphamide, and prednisone. Generally, the combination of cyclophosphamide and prednisone is the most cost-effective treatment for lymphosarcoma, with chlorambucil and prednisolone as second choice.

In the event of severe hemorrhagic cystitis developing as a side effect of cyclophosphamide, repeat flushing of the bladder with 1% formalin and tranquilization with acetylpromazine often assist the situation.

It is vitally important that hematology must be monitored during therapy and dosage adjusted downward if necessary. Vincristine can be withdrawn if good signs of incipient remission are observed. Cyclophosphamide, 50 mg/m^2, three times per week, can be combined with methotrexate, 2.5 mg/m^2, orally, twice on 1 day at weekly intervals. Cytarabine, 100 mg, IV, daily for 2 to 4 days, can also induce remission in cases of lymphosarcoma.

Dogs that develop cutaneous malignant lymphoma secondary to generalized lymph node disease may respond to doxorubicin HCl 30 mg/m^2 IV every 21 days or to various combinations of cyclophosphamide, vincristine sulfate, prednisolone, cytarabine, or methotrexate.

Skin tumors of dogs are diagnosed more frequently than any other canine tumor and account for 25 to 30% of all neoplasms. Approximately 20% of skin tumors are malignant.

Mast Cell Tumors

Mast cell tumors of dogs are usually malignant or benign. They frequently present clinically as circumscribed, raised, or hairless nodules. For inoperable mast cell tumors, prednisone, vinblastine, doxorubicin HCl, and cyclophosphamide, either singly or in combination, have been used, with prednisone generally being the most effective (Table 36–8). Following a prednisone dosage of 20 mg/m^2, orally, once daily until maximum regression is seen, the dosage can be reduced to 5 mg on alternative days to maintain tumor regression. Cimetidine, 10 mg/kg, orally, is recommended when intestinal bleeding develops.

The use of glucocorticoids may result in short-term remission if administered intralesionally (triamcinolone) or systemi-

---

**TABLE 36–8
MAST CELL TUMORS**

Glucocorticoids (Intralesionally.)
or a combination of
Prednisone/Vinblastine/
Cyclophosphamide/Adriamycin
or
Prednisone 20 mg/m^2. (Singly Systemically)

---

cally (prednisone). Combination therapy using prednisone, vinblastine, and cyclophosphamide is efficacious and is considered to be better than the use of glucocorticoids alone. Chemotherapy is indicated for mast cell tumors when multiple dermal tumors exist.

Transmissible Venereal Tumors

Initially, surgery, radiotherapy, immunotherapy, and chemotherapy are effective against transmissible venereal tumors. Surgery is a good primary therapy, but recurrence is quite common. Chemotherapy is an effective treatment, and using a combination of vincristine, cyclophosphamide, and methotrexate, a good response can be anticipated.

Vincristine IV, is as effective as a combination therapy and has the advantage of being considerably cheaper. Vincristine, 0.5 mg/m^2, IV, each week is the drug of choice and usually is very effective. Repeat weekly for 3 to 6 weeks. Monitor CBC and platelet count on each day vincristine sulfate injection is given (Table 36–9). Maintain WBC count greater than 4,000/mcl and platelet count greater than 100,000/mcl. Adriamycin (30 mg/M^2) is a useful alternative.

36.12 ONCOGENES AND CANCER

The original evidence for specific genes having a role in carcinogenesis came from RNA tumor viruses. These viruses contain only three genes, two coding for structural protein and the third for an enzyme that produces a DNA copy of the virus, which

---

TABLE 36–9
TRANSMISSIBLE VENEREAL TUMORS

- Surgery
- Immunotherapy
- Radiotherapy
- Chemotherapy
  ↓
- Vincristine/Cyclophosphamide/Methotrexate. (Combination)

  or

- Vincristine alone. (0.5 mg/m²)

  or

- Adriamycin (30 mg/m²)

---

allows the virus to incorporate into the host DNA.

The addition or substitution of another gene to the virus enables the virus to induce tumor growth in vivo and in vitro. These transforming genes were termed "viral oncogenes," and it has since been shown that such sequences were also detectable in normal human cellular genes and have therefore also been termed "cellular oncogenes." Laboratory work in several areas has now uncovered over 30 distinct cellular oncogenes, some of which are associated with specific tumor types. Another class of genes involved in carcinogenesis is called "tumor-suppressing" genes; these appear to check cellular growth. The question of which factors induce the active expression of these genes to give rise to tumor growth (or tumor inhibition) has not yet been answered.

VIRAL ONCOGENES

Viral oncogenes have also been implicated in the cause of a small number of cancers, good examples of which are Burkitt's lymphoma (Epstein-Barr virus) and cervical carcinoma (certain papilloma viruses). They become established in the target cells, and these cells continue to carry the viral genes, which appear to have an important role in maintenance of the malignant phenotype of the cell clones.

Oncogenes cannot be used to adequately explain genetic susceptibilities to cancer that exist at the moment of conception, because these various cellular oncogene alleles arise somatically. They may act by altering the immune surveillance system or affect the rate at which exogenous carcinogens are metabolized to products that actively damage the cellular genome. Alternatively, such genes may alter normal cellular growth and differentiation.

SELECTED REFERENCES

Ackerman, L.: Cutaneous T cell-like lymphoma in the dog. Compend. Contin. Ed. Pract. Vet., *6*:37, 1984.

Barton, C.L.: The diagnosis and management of canine lymphosarcoma. Proceedings. Am. Anim. Hosp. Assoc., *50*:345, 1983.

Brick, J.O., Roenigk, W.S., and Wilson, G.P.: Chemotherapy of malignant lymphomas in dogs and cats. J. Am. Vet. Med. Assoc., *153*:47, 1968.

Calvert, C.A., and Leifer, C.: Doxorubicin for treatment of canine lymphosarcoma after development of resistance to combination chemotherapy. J. Am. Vet. Med. Assoc., *179*:1011, 1981.

Carter, R.F. et al.: Chemotherapy of canine lymphoma with histopathological correlation: doxorubicin alone compared to COP as first treatment regimen. J. Am. Anim. Hosp. Assoc., *23*:495, 1987.

Conroy, J.D.: Canine skin tumours. J. Am. Anim. Hosp. Assoc., *19*:91, 1983.

Cotter, S.M., and Goldstein, M.A.: Comparison of two protocols for maintenance of remission of dogs with lymphoma. J. Am. Anim. Hosp. Assoc., *23*:495, 1987.

Couto, C.G.: Cutaneous lymphomas. Proceedings. Kal. Kan. Symp., *11*:71, 1987.

Couto, C.G.: Toxicity of anticancer chemotherapy. Proceedings. Kal. Kan. Symp., *10*:37, 1987.

Couto, C.G.: Canine lymphomas: something old, something new. Compend. Cont. Ed. Pract. Vet., *7*:291, 1985.

Crow, S.E.: Lymphosarcoma (malignant lymphoma) in the dog: diagnosis and treatment. Compend. Contin. Ed. Pract. Vet., 4:283, 1982.

Crow, S.E., Madewell, B.R., Weller, R.E., and Henness, A.M.: Cyclophosphamide-induced cystitis in the dog and cat. J. Am. Vet. Med. Assoc., 171:259, 1977.

DeVita, V.T., Jr. Young, R.C., and Canelos, G.P.: Combination versus single agent chemotherapy: a review of the basis for selection of drug treatment of cancer. Cancer, 38:98, 1978.

Fisher, R.I. et al.: Adjuvant immunotherapy or chemotherapy for malignant melanoma. Surg. Clin. North Am., 6:1267, 1981.

Friend, S.J., Dryja, T.P., and Weinberg, R.A.: Oncogenes and tumour-suppressing genes. N. Engl. J. Med., 318:618, 1988.

Golden, D.L., and Langston, V.C.: Uses of vincristine and vinblastine in dogs and cats. J. Am. Vet. Med. Assoc., 193(9):114, 1988.

Henness, A.M., Theilern, G.H., Park, R.D. and Buhles, W.C.: Combination therapy for canine osteosarcoma. J. Am. Vet. Med. Assoc., 170:1076, 1977.

Hess, P.W., MacEwen, E.G., and McClelland, A.J.: Chemotherapy of canine and feline tumors. J. Am. Anim. Hosp. Assoc., 12:350, 1976.

Knudson, A.G., Jr.: Mutation and cancer: statistical study of retina blastoma. Proc. Natl. Acad. Sci. USA, 68:820, 1971.

Legendre, A.M., Spaulding, K., and Krahwinkel, D.J.: Canine nasal and paranasal sinus tumours. J. Am. Anim. Hosp. Assoc., 19:115, 1983.

Leifer, C.E., and Matus, R.E.: Canine lymphoma: clinical considerations. Semin. Vet. Med. Surg (Small Anim.), 1:43, 1986.

MacEwen, E.G.: Cancer chemotherapy. In Current Veterinary Therapy VII. Edited by R.W. Kirk. Philadelphia, W.B. Saunders, 1980.

MacEwen, E.G. et al.: Evaluation of the effects of levamisole and surgery on canine mammary cancer. J. Biol. Resp. Mod., 4:418, 1985.

MacEwen, E.G. et al.: Levamisole was adjuvant to chemotherapy for canine lymphosarcoma. J. Biol. Response Mod., 4:427, 1985.

MacEwen, E.G. et al.: Evaluation of the effect of levamisole on feline mammary cancer. J. Biol. Resp. Mod., 5:541, 1984.

Macey, D.W.: Canine and feline mast cell tumours. Biologic behaviour, diagnosis and therapy. Semin. Vet. Med. Surg. Small Anim. Med., 1(1):72, 1986.

McKeever, P.J. et al.: Canine cutaneous lymphomas. J. Am. Vet. Med. Assoc., 180:531, 1982.

Ogilvie, G.K. et al.: Weekly administration of low dose doxorubicin for treatment of malignant lymphoma in dogs. J. Am. Vet. Med. Assoc., 198:1762, 1991.

Ogilvie, G.K. et al.: Acute and short-term toxicity associated with the administration of doxorubicin to 185 dogs with malignant tumours. J. Am. Vet. Med. Assoc., 195:1584, 1989.

Onions, D.E.: A prospective study of familial canine lymphosarcoma. J. Natl. Cancer Inst., 72:909, 1984.

Owen, L.N.: Cancer chemotherapy. Vet. Rec., 118:364, 1986.

Owen, L.W.: Identifying and treating cancer in geriatric dogs. Vet. Med., January: 55, 1991.

Page, R.L.: Acute tumour lysis syndrome. Advances in the treatment of cancer. Semin. Vet. Med. Surg. Small Anim. Med., 1(1):58, 1986.

Page, R.: Cisplatin, a new antineoplastic drug in veterinary medicine. J. Am. Vet. Med. Assoc., 186:288, 1985.

Ponder, B.A.J.: Familial cancer: opportunities for clinical practice and research. Eur. J. Surg. Oncol., 13:463, 1987.

Postorino, N.C. et al.: Single agent therapy with adriamycin for canine lymphosarcoma. J. Am. Anim. Hosp. Assoc., 25:221, 1989.

Priester, W.A.: The occurrence of tumours in domestic animals. J. Natl. Cancer Inst., 54:166, 1980.

Priester, W.A., and Mantel, N.: Occurrence of tumours in domestic animals. Data from 12 United States and Canadian Colleges of Veterinary Medicine. J. Natl. Cancer Inst., 47:1333, 1971.

Priester, W.A., and McKay, F.W.: The occurrence of tumours in domestic animals. Natl. Cancer Inst. Monogr., 54:1, 1980.

Richardson, R.C.: Lymphosarcoma. 1984 Sci. Proc. 51st Annu. Meeting. Am. Anim. Hosp. Assoc., 29–33:297, 1984.

Richardson, R.C., Rebar, A.H., and Elliot, G.S.: (1984) Common skin tumours of the dog: a clinical approach to diagnosis and treatment. Comp. Contin. Ed. Pract. Vet., 6:1080, 1984.

Rogers, K.S.: L-asparaginase for treatment of lymphoid neoplasia in dogs. J. Am. Vet. Med. Assoc., 194:1626, 1989.

Rosenthal, R.C.: Epidemiology of canine lymphosarcoma. Compend. Contin. Ed. Pract. Vet., 10:855, 1982.

Rosenthal, R.C.: Clinical applications of vinca alkaloids. J. Am. Vet. Med. Assoc., 182:1084, 1981.

Rosenthal, R.C., and MacEwen, G.E.: Treatment of lymphoma in dogs. J. Am. Vet. Med. Assoc., 195(5):774, 1990.

Rosenthal, R.C., and Miclalski, D.: Storage of expensive cancer drugs. J. Am. Vet. Med. Assoc., 198(1):144, 1991.

Strafuss, A.C.: Skin tumours. Vet. Clin. North Am. Small Anim. Pract. 15:473, 1985.

Susaneck, S.J.: Doxorubicin therapy in the dog. J. Am. Vet. Med. Assoc., 181:70, 1983.

Swanson, L.V.: Potential hazards associated with low-dose exposure to antineoplastic agents. Part I. Evidence for concern. Compend. Contin. Educ. Pract. Vet., 10:293, 1988.

Swanson, L.V.: Potential hazards associated with low dose exposure to antineoplastic agents. Part II. Recommendations for minimising exposure. Compend. Contin. Ed. Pract. Vet., 10:616, 1988.

Tams, T.R., and Macy, D.M.: Canine mast cell tumours. Comp. Contin. Ed. Pract. Vet., 3:869, 1981.

Thompson, J.M., Gorman, N.T., and Bleehen, N.M.: Hyperthermia and radiation in the management of canine tumours. J. Small Anim. Pract., *28*:457, 1987.

Thrall, E.D.: Radiation therapy in the dog: principles, indication and complications. Comp. Contin. Ed. Pract. Vet., 4:642, 1982.

Weller, R.E., Theilen, G.H., and Madewell, B.R.: Chemotherapeutic responses in dogs with lymphosarcoma and hypercalcemia. J. Am. Vet. Med. Assoc., *181*:891, 1982.

Yarbo, J.W., and Bernstein, R.S. (eds.): Oncologic Emergencies. New York, Grune & Stratton, 1981.

37

ANTIMICROBIAL CHEMOTHERAPY IN SMALL ANIMALS

37.1 Introduction
37.2 Respiratory System
37.3 Alimentary Tract
37.4 Urinary System
37.5 Bone
37.6 Central Nervous System
37.7 The Eye
37.8 Uterine/Vaginal Infections
37.9 Circulatory System
37.10 Anaerobic Infections
37.11 Skin

37.1 INTRODUCTION

In small animals practice clinicians base their choice of treatment on their clinical experience and on the likely order of frequency of causal organisms. Sensitivity testing may also be employed but has shortcomings; organisms may prove either more or less sensitive in vivo than might be expected from in vitro sensitivity testing. Despite its limitations, however, sensitivity testing remains the only guideline on which practitioners may rely when resorting to laboratory assistance.

The diagnosis and treatment of small animal infections should proceed according to the following guidelines:

1. Obtain cultures and perform bacterial antibiotic sensitivity tests.
2. Identify and treat sources of infection.
3. Identify and treat concomitant problems.
4. Treat with bactericidal antibiotics.
5. Ensure high serum antibiotic therapy by using proper recommended doses.
6. Repeat cultures after course of antibiotic therapy to ensure bacteriologic cure.

Although the primary concern is the infecting microbe, concomitant predisposing disorders should never be overlooked. Potential infection sites should always be debrided or drained. Prudent antimicrobial therapy, especially in critically ill patients, should always be initiated before culture results are available. Empirical therapy has inherent shortcomings—nevertheless, critically ill patients with infections should always be treated immediately, with subsequent antibiotic adjustments being made on the basis of culture results.

When no culture or sensitivity test results are available, the veterinarian must make a decision as to which antibacterial agent to use in a particular case until the infectious agent can be isolated. This requires knowledge of the likely pathogen, its likely antimicrobial sensitivity pattern, and a knowledge of the pharmacodynamic and pharmacokinetic properties of antimicrobial drugs. It is usually appropriate to commence antibiotic therapy with bactericidal antibiotics, which are chosen on the basis of the results of bacterial isolation and sensitivity testing. Bactericidal antibiotics are narrow spectrum, and are not heavily dependent on a functioning immune system.

Small animals with bacteremia alone should be treated for a minimum of 2 to 3 weeks. When a bacteriostatic antibiotic is included in the treatment regimen, it should be based on culture results indicating a mixed infection.

A rational choice of antibiotics can be made based on historical data, predisposing causes or other factors, the time course of infection, the likely patterns of sensitivity associated bacteria in the particular animal, and their antimicrobial sensitivity patterns. Although widespread antibiotic resistance is a common problem, trends do exist in various practices. Most strains of *Staphylococcus aureus* are sensitive in vitro to cephalosporins, aminoglycosides, clavulanate-potentiated amoxycillin, potentiated sulfonamides, lincomycin, enrofloxacin, erythromycin, and chloramphenicol; however, most are resistant to penicillin, ampicillin, and tetracyclines. Most isolates of *Escherichia coli* are sensitive to gentamicin enrofloxacin and cephalothin but resistant to ampicillin and chloramphenicol.

Beta-hemolytic streptococci usually are sensitive to penicillin, ampicillin, cephalosporins, and chloramphenicol but usually are resistant to erythromycin, aminoglycosides, and trimethroprim. The only cost effective, systemically given antibiotic currently used commonly against *Pseudomonas* spp. is gentamicin, although resistance to this drug is increasing. Polymyxin B is a cheaper but not so effective drug against pseudomonas. Ticarcillin, carbenicillin and silver sulfadiazine are more potent and more expensive alternatives.

Once an appropriate antibiotic has been rationally selected, it is necessary to attain serum levels exceeding the minimum inhibitory concentration (MIC) in the vicinity of the micro-organism (focus of infection) for a duration adequate to totally eliminate the infection. The desired effect is unlikely to be obtained unless the correct dose is administered to the patient. Antibiotic treatment commonly results in overdosage in cats and underdosage in dogs. Dosage recommendations are commonly given on the basis of milligrams per kilogram; however, these are often not easy to follow in a busy surgery, and the weighing of patients may be impractical. Errors in antibiotic dosing often occur because the clinician does not estimate the body weight correctly, and this will result in the overdosage of small patients, especially cats (with an average body weight range of 2 kg to 5 kg) and the underdosing of larger dogs. Also, only quality antibiotics should be used, strictly in accordance with the route of administration recommended by the manufacturer.

Overdosage is less serious than underdosage, which results in the selection of resistant organisms tolerating subtherapeutic levels of antibiotic with no improvement in the clinical condition. Thus, accurate weighing of animals or at least accurate weight estimation is imperative if antibiotic therapy is to succeed and the correct dosage is to be used.

The patient's condition may also influence choice of antibiotic. In debilitating or chronic disease, the activity of the host's defense mechanism may be impaired. Bacteriostatic antibiotics act in conjunction with the body's defense mechanism, and thus conditions such as septicemia, endocarditis, and chronic infections should always be treated with bactericidal agents when possible.

Regardless of how the initial antibacterial agent is selected, if the clinical response is deemed unsatisfactory after 48 hours, therapy should be reassessed and another agent employed if necessary. The most logical change is from a bacteriostatic to a bactericidal antibiotic, and if bacterial resistance is suspected, an antibiotic from a different family should be selected to avoid cross-resistance.

Combinations of antibiotics are quite popular in clinical use, and the advantages claimed for such combinations are broad-spectrum antimicrobial activity, synergistic actions, and a lower toxicity of each component drug.

The disadvantage of combinations is that antibiotics in combination may have totally different pharmacokinetic characteristics. Blood levels of procaine penicillin are maintained for 24 hours and of streptomycin are maintained for 8 to 10 hours. In cases of overwhelming infection, however, if a combination is used, a maximal dosage of each antibiotic should be used rather than a fixed dose combination; i.e., give the antibiotics

separately. Combinations should seldom be used to initiate therapy, and the practitioner should try to avoid "blunderbuss" therapy in an attempt to cover both probable and possible infections. Just as the actions of one drug against different strains of a pathogen may vary, so too may the interactions of antimicrobial drugs in combination. Regulatory authorities are currently applying very strict scientific criteria to the inclusion of combination fixed dose products.

A narrow-spectrum antibiotic with bactericidal properties should be used to initiate therapy, but if a mixed infection is thought to be present, either a combination of bactericidal antibiotics or a broad-spectrum bacteriostatic agent should be used. The penicillins, cephalosporins, and aminoglycosides are the major bactericidal drugs, whereas chloramphenicol, tetracyclines, sulfonamides, and macrolides are bacteriostatic agents. The duration of antibiotic therapy should continue until clinical signs have disappeared or a bacteriologic cure has been effected. Cessation of therapy too soon is one of the common pitfalls in practice when therapy is phased out at the first remission of symptoms. In certain diseases such as respiratory, pyoderma, or urinary tract infections (UTIs) therapy may be necessary for at least 10 to 20 days.

Although the action of the antibiotic on the causal organism is a prime factor in its selection for the therapy of a bacterial infection, its pharmacokinetic properties are of great importance also, i.e., its absorption and distribution characteristics and its persistence and excretion from the body. Although these pharmacokinetic effects are not directly within the clinician's control, the individual choice of product formulation and the route of administration are within his control and have an important influence. Minor changes in formulation may have a powerful effect on absorption rates or bioavailability; therefore, the manufacturer's recommendations regarding dosage rate, route of administration, and storage should be followed strictly. For instance, subcutaneous administration of a preparation specifically formulated for the intramuscular (IM) route may be self-defeating. Absorption from the subcutaneous site can be unreliable, and clearance from the body may proceed as rapidly as the drug is released from the injection site. Thus, therapeutic levels in the body may never be attained. Often, many antibiotics which on the basis of in vitro tests appear to be clinically indicated, are ineffective in vivo because pharmacokinetically, they cannot reach the site of infection.

To ensure that the concentration of antimicrobial agent at the site of infection remains above the desired threshold level (usually at least 3–5 times the MIC), it is necessary not only to use the correct dosage rate but also to maintain these levels for an adequate period by followup maintenance doses. In serious infections it may be advisable to administer the agent three or four times daily by the oral route, and for some of the penicillins, which are highly bactericidal, achieving high initial levels may be of more importance than the maintenance of constant levels. Absorption of drugs following oral administration is variable and depends on several intercurrent factors. Nevertheless, manufacturers take these factors into account, and the dosage interval recommendations for a specific formulation, if followed correctly, should result in the attainment of therapeutic levels. Premarket testing of drugs are specifically geared toward ensuring that dosage levels, dose intervals and bioavailability of the final formulation are optimum for clinical efficacy.

GUIDELINES FOR THERAPY

All infectious conditions warrant antibiotic intervention, although in some disease states (e.g., gastroenteritis), antimicrobial therapy may sometimes be detrimental to the animal. Before embarking on antimicrobial therapy a number of key issues must be addressed:

1. Which body system appears to be affected?—Respiratory, urinary, reproductive, etc.
2. What is the likely pathogen?—On the basis of scientific knowledge and case history.
   • Is it a mixed bacterial infection?
3. What is the pathogen's likely sensitivity to antimicrobial agents?

4. Is the process acute or chronic?
   Having answered these questions then:—
5. Select the appropriate antibiotic. Bactericidal or bacteriostatic
   • Swab, culture, isolate and determine antimicrobial sensitivity.
6. Commence therapy as early as possible.
7. Assess body weight correctly, and use the correct dosage rate.
   • Use correct route as indicated by the manufacturer
   • Ensure maintenance doses are given at correct intervals.

37.2 RESPIRATORY SYSTEM

In respiratory infections, when the bronchial tree is infected, the pharmacokinetic properties of the antibiotic (which determine its penetration across the blood-bronchus barrier) are important. Antibiotics that are unionized, lipid soluble and with a large volume of distribution enter the bronchial secretion more easily. Increased permeability resulting from local inflammation secondary to infection is known to enhance the penetration of antibiotics into bronchial secretions. Therefore, as inflammation decreases (with successful treatment), so too will the penetration of antibiotics into these secretions. The relationship between peak serum antibiotic concentration and the concentrations in bronchial (or sputum) secretions has been studied. In general, the higher the serum concentration the higher the concentration will be in the bronchial secretions. Protein binding of the antibiotic also plays a significant role here.

For respiratory infections the most important step in selecting an appropriate antimicrobial drug is to firmly establish the diagnosis of an infectious process, preferably by identifying a causative agent. In many cases, a presumptive diagnosis may be made based on clinical signs (cough, lethargy, dyspnea) and physical findings (fever, tracheal irritability, abnormal lung sounds). Additional support is often obtained from laboratory evaluation. The final diagnosis, however, should be based on the cytologic and culture results of tracheobronchial, parenchymal, or pleural secretions. The majority of canine respiratory tract infections are due to gram-negative organisms, many of which are resistant to commonly used antibiotics. Culture and sensitivity testing are recommended as the method for selecting the proper antibiotic therapy.

Lower respiratory and skin infections caused by beta-lactamase producing strains of *E. coli*, *Klebsiella*, and *Proteus* sp. can be effectively treated with potentiated penicillins such as amoxicillin/clavulanic acid or ticarcillin/clavulanic acid.

Resistant *E. coli*, *Klebsiella* sp., and indole-positive *Proteus* sp. may respond to second-generation cephalosporins, whereas *Serratia* sp. and beta-lactamase-producing *Neisseria* and *Enterobacter* sp. may respond only to amikacin, fluoroquinolones, or third-generation cephalosporins.

Combinations of amoxicillin and clavulanic acid are especially effective against infections caused by *E. coli*, *Staphylococci*, and *Klebsiella* spp. Combining ampicillin with sulbactam may help overcome infections caused by ampicillin-resistant *Pasteurella* sp. The extended spectrum antibiotic ticarcillin is usually reserved for treatment of serious gram-negative infections (i.e., *Pseudomonas* spp.); it is also available in combination with clavulanic acid.

The potentiated sulfonamides are effective against many gram-positive and gram-negative organisms. In addition, *Chlamydia* and *Actinomyces* spp. are sensitive to these agents, as are *Nocardia* spp. at high drug doses. *Pseudomonas* and *Mycoplasma* spp. tend to be resistant. Mycoplasmae infections can be deceptively common following bordetella infection in the canine respiratory tract.

Minocycline and doxycycline are more lipid soluble than older tetracyclines, so they more easily cross cell membranes. Thus, they are better able to penetrate tissues (e.g., lungs) and to accumulate in secretions (e.g., bronchial secretions) and are more effective against intracellular organisms. They represent a good alternative to traditional tetracyclines.

Tylosin is also effective against gram-positive cocci and *Chlamydia* sp., but, like erythromycin, it tends to be a second-choice antibiotic. In contrast to erythromycin, it is effective against *Mycoplasma* spp. and has been used as a first-choice antibiotic to treat upper respiratory infections in cats and dogs, when mycoplasmae are present.

The spectrum of activity of the fluoroquinolones depends on the individual drug but includes most gram-negative organisms, particularly *E. coli* and *Klebsiella*, *Pasteurella*, *Enterobacter*, *Proteus*, *Pseudomonas*, *Citrobacter*, and *Serratia* spp. The quinolones are indicated for infection in any tissue caused by gram-negative and selected gram-positive bacteria. However, these drugs should be reserved for serious infections or those that have failed to respond to other antibiotic therapy. Quinolones are especially useful for treating serious antibiotic-resistant bacterial infections of the respiratory tract. Quinolones are also effective in treating infection with *Chlamydia* and *Mycoplasma* spp. but are ineffective against most anaerobes. They are contraindicated in very young animals on account of their effects on juvenile cartilage.

Bactericidal drug concentrations with fluoroquinolones can be reached within 20 minutes of oral administration. The drugs, including enrofloxacin, are distributed very well into tissues.

While many infections of the respiratory tract in the dog are viral in origin, serious secondary bacterial infections may occur. Secondary bacterial invaders in distemper frequently respond to either benzylpenicillins or the semisynthetic penicillins such as ampicillin or amoxicillin. While ampicillin appears to have little advantage over penicillin on the basis of sensitivity patterns, however, the penetration of ampicillin into tissues is usually superior on account of its greater lipid solubility and lower plasma protein binding. Amoxicillin is even more effective and more rapidly acting in this respect. The semisynthetic derivatives, however, are usually less active than penicillin G against gram-positive organisms sensitive to penicillins. If *Bordetella bronchiseptica* is suspected as either a primary or secondary agent, tetracyclines (or doxycline) with their broad spectrum of action and good tissue diffusion are preferred.

Pasteurella organisms are highly susceptible to treatment with ampicillin (for parenteral administration) and amoxicillin (for oral use).

Infections with *Brucella*, *Pasteurella*, or *Hemophilus* spp. are often treated effectively with tetracyclines, penicillins, or chloramphenicol. More resistant isolates may respond only to the combination of sulbactam and ampicillin or the aminoglycosides.

Tetracyclines attain effective concentrations in the respiratory tract. Their antibacterial spectrum includes *Bordetella bronchiseptica*, probably the most significant bacterial pathogen of the bronchial tree of dogs and cats, and also mycoplasmae, but streptococcal resistance is not infrequent. Doxycycline is a fairly new tetracycline that has certain pharmacokinetic advantages over established drugs of that group. It has a high degree of lipid solubility, penetrates more effectively into inflamed respiratory tissue, and when it is administered orally, absorption is inhibited by food to a much lesser extent than tetracyclines.

Broad-spectrum antibacterial alternatives to tetracyclines that concentrate effectively in the respiratory tract are trimethoprim/sulfonamide, broad-spectrum penicillins, and cephalosporins. Amoxicillin attains higher concentrations in bronchial tissue than ampicillin. Chloramphenicol, gentamicin, and erythromycin are frequently also useful against infections with *Bordetella* spp. Combinations of sulfonamide and trimethoprim are useful broad-spectrum agents for respiratory infections in dogs, whereas tylosin and erythromycin are effective in gram-positive infections associated with mycoplasmae. Gram-negative respiratory infections may be treated with aminoglycosides such as streptomycin or, indeed, gentamicin, which although expensive, is useful against *Pseudomonas* infection. Combinations of beta lactam antibiotics with aminoglycosides may often be indicated for mixed infections.

37.3 ALIMENTARY TRACT

Antimicrobials have been traditionally used by veterinarians to treat acute and chronic diarrhea in dogs and cats. Little evidence exists, however, that bacterial infection is a major cause of diarrhea or that antimicrobials are in any way effective in its treatment. To date it appears that these compounds are of little proven benefit in treating acute or chronic diarrhea in dogs and cats and hence are best avoided. Most animals with enteritis appear to recover faster without antibiotics. Certain antimi-

crobials, such as neomycin, erythromycin, and ampicillin, may also induce or prolong diarrhea by decreasing nutrient absorption, disrupting motility by inducing bacterial resistance or in some cases by direct irritation of the bowel mucosa.

Antimicrobial therapy is indicated only in very definite and specific bacterial infections or with severe gastrointestinal (GI) mucosal damage. Even with mucosal damage, bacteria or their toxins may penetrate the intestinal wall and exert a deleterious systemic effect. Parenteral antimicrobial therapy is probably more appropriate than oral therapy in such animals, assuming a bacteremia or septicemia is present or the drug is secreted in a stable form into the bowel.

Antimicrobials are routinely used indiscriminately by many clinicians to treat animals with any form of acute enterocolitis, but their use is simply not warranted in patients with an intact GI mucosal barrier. Indeed, antimicrobials may be harmful in that they disturb the distribution of normal flora and may prolong the return of normal intestinal function and homeostasis. Many cases of enteritis in dogs are attributable to malabsorptive or dietary problems not susceptible to antibiotic therapy.

Parenteral antibiotics, however, may be indicated in patients with hemorrhagic diarrhea with loss of the intestinal mucosal barrier and therefore potential for bacterial invasion and septicemia. These drugs are particularly indicated if leukopenia is also present, such as in parvovirus infection or when the presence of leukocytosis and pyrexia may suggest systemic bacterial invasion. Penicillin derivatives or chloramphenicol can be useful in such instances. Antimicrobial therapy can be warranted in the treatment of bacterial overgrowth (stagnant loop syndrome) or if exocrine pancreatic insufficiency has been ruled out or if correction of the underlying condition has not resulted in clinical improvement.

Although many enteric diseases in the dog are not always attributable to infectious causes, nonetheless even when infection exists, the use of an antimicrobial agent is not necessarily indicated. The antibiotic may act iatrogenically, inducing bacterial resistance, irritating the gut mucosa, and inhibiting the normal flora, leading to superinfection with resistant bacteria or fungi. Viral agents, toxemias, or malabsorptive states, which may produce a variety of clinical symptoms referable to the gut, are not amenable to antibiotic therapy.

One of the main reasons antibiotics are not indicated for the majority of cases of diarrhea in small animals is because improper diet is the most common cause of chronic or recurrent episodes, and most acute cases are self-limiting. In such cases food should be withheld for 24 hours and fluid intake encouraged. These measures, together with conservative antispasmodic or adsorbent preparations and fluid and electrolyte therapy are sufficient in many cases. Antibiotics are indicated in cases that fail to respond or when evidence indicates systemic infection.

When longterm broad-spectrum therapy with chloramphenicol or oxytetracycline is indicated, consideration must be given to the inclusion of the nonabsorbable antifungal agents such as nystatin to prevent intestinal overgrowth with *Candida* sp. in the gut.

Doxycycline's high intestinal concentrations and high oral bioavailability are advantageous when treating primary intestinal infections, especially those caused by enterotoxigenic *E. coli*.

When infection is not confined to the gut, there is a choice of broad-spectrum drugs for oral administration that are formulated to exert an effect in the gut and are sufficiently well absorbed to combat systemic infection. For example, oxytetracycline, fluoroquinolone trimethoprim/sulfonamide, ampicillin, and amoxicillin fulfill this criterion. The broad-spectrum penicillins are particularly useful when the patient is vomiting. They can be administered parenterally and attain therapeutic concentrations in the small intestine because they are concentrated in the bile and then secreted into the gut. Similarly, for fluoroquinolones, it is axiomatic that gastric acid stability and high oral bioavailability are prerequisites for orally administered antimicrobial agents.

As general therapeutic agents to gastroenteritis in the dog, the semisynthetic penicillins such as ampicillin or amoxicillin/clavulanate should be considered first-line defense agents. These possess a rela-tively broad spectrum of activity; remain active in the gut following administration as tablets, capsules, or syrup; have high oral bioavailability; are unaffected by foodstuffs, are rapidly bactericidal in action; and are secreted into the gut following parenteral administration. Trimethoprim-sulfadiazine can also give favorable clinical results, as does chloramphenicol, streptomycin, enrofloxacin gentamicin, and tylosin.

With no evidence of systemic infection, it is reasonable to select drugs that when administered orally are poorly absorbed from the gut, thus attaining a high lumenal concentration at the site of infection. The gut-active sulfonamides (phthalylsulfathiazole, succinylsulfathiazole) gentamicin and neomycin are common examples, and commercial formulations are available that incorporate adsorbents and or antispasmodics with these antibacterial agents.

Gram-negative coliform bacilli from the gut are usually implicated in peritonitis, and frequently this condition can be successfully treated with ampicillin doxycycline or oxytetracycline. If anaerobic species such as *Bacteroides* sp. are believed to be involved, aminoglycosides (streptomycin, neomycin, gentamicin) should not be used. Anaerobes are frequently found to be sensitive to sulfonamides, tetracyclines, doxycycline, or penicillins, whereas *Clostridia* sp. are sensitive to high doses of penicillins. For mixed infections with *Bacteroides* spp. in the oral cavity, penicillin is indicated and useful, but those anaerobic infections that fail to respond to standard antibiotic treatment such as infective gingivitis or oral ulceration may be treated more successfully with clindamycin or metronidazole. Remember, a number of species of bacteroides produce beta lactamase, and so penicillins would not be good choices.

STOMATITIS/PERIODONTAL DISEASE

Mycotic stomatitis *(Candida albicans)* usually responds to topical nystatin applied three or four times daily for 2 weeks. Ulcerative stomatitis and gingivitis associated with fusobacterium are indications for treatment with metronidazole or clindamycin.

TABLE 37–1
COLITIS

TYPE OF COLITIS	Causative Organism	Treatment
Bacterial colitis	*Campylobacter jejuni* Other	Erythromycin or oral neomycin/ Kanamycin.
Protozoal colitis	*Entamoeba histolytica* *Balantidium coli* *Giardia lamblia*	Metronidazole, po, (15 mg/kg/ daily for 5–7 days)
Whipworm colitis	*Trichuris vulpis*	Appropriate anthelmintic.
Pseudomembranous enterocolitis	Clostridial exotoxin e.g. *C. difficile*	Metronidazole; cholestyramine (1/4 to 1 gram t.i.d. in water
Histoplasmosis	*Histoplasma capsulatum*	Amphotercin B/Ketoconazole
Idiopathic chronic canine colitis lymphocytic-plasmacytic colitis; relapsing ulcerative colitis	Unknown	Dietary therapy. Metronidazole. Sulfasalazine./Diet
Lymphosarcoma	Unknown/?	Appropriate chemotherapy.

Clinical signs in mild cases of vegetative stomatitis include slight salivation and formation of oral vesicles. Severe cases are usually characterized by profuse salivation, anorexia, fever, and oral ulcerations. Differential diagnoses include infection with *Candida* or *Nocardia* spp. stomatitis, ulcerative necrotic stomatitis, and stomatitis associated with periodontal disease.

Clindamycin hydrochloride is effective against the organisms associated with canine dental infections; staphylococci, streptococci, and anerobes. In addition, clindamycin penetrates bony tissues and thus is effective in treatment of alveolar bone infection, a condition frequently involved in canine dental infections.

Periodontal disease is caused mainly by plaque, which primarily is made up of bacteria. Plaque that develops above the gumline comprises mostly nonmotile, gram-positive, aerobic, coccoid microbial flora. These bacteria cause the first stage of periodontal disease, a reversible condition called "gingivitis."

When the infection invades the gingival sulcus and enters an anaerobic environment (where aerobic bacteria cannot survive), the bacterial composition changes to a more motile, gram-negative, rod-shaped, anaerobic flora. At this point, the animal has periodontitis, which is the second stage of periodontal disease. This change in bacterial composition can occur if bacterial plaque is allowed to accumulate between the teeth and the gingiva. Anaerobic infections therefore frequently fail to respond to conventional treatment. Aminoglycoside antibiotics, such as streptomycin, neomycin, or gentamicin, are not effective in an anaerobic environment, because they require an oxygen-dependent transport across the bacterial cell wall. Also, a common anaerobe, *Bacteroides fragilis*, produces a beta-lactamase that renders penicillin and other beta-lactam antibiotics ineffective. Metronidazole and clindamycin are the primary drugs for anaerobic infections. In addition, treatment with daily oral flushes of 1% hydrogen peroxide and use of an antibiotic-corticosteroid combination sometimes resolve the condition.

CANINE COLITIS

Successful management of dogs with chronic large bowel diarrhea requires an accurate diagnosis, dietary manipulation, and multiple therapeutic trials with various drugs. Other agents implicated include trichuris vulpis, entamoeba histolytica, balantidium coli, giardia, histoplasma. A variety of other causes include lymphocytic plasmacytic colitis, histiocytic colitis, and pseudomembranous colitis.

Bacterial causes of chronic large bowel diarrhea are uncommon in dogs. Fecal or

---

TABLE 37–2
ANCILLARY DRUGS USED IN CANINE COLITIS

Drug	Dose	Frequency	Route
Diphenoxylate	0.1–0.2 mg/kg	bid–tid	Oral
Clidinium bromide and chlordiazepoxide chloride	0.5 mg/kg	bid-qid	Oral
Loperamide	0.1 mg/kg	qid	Oral
Metronidazole	15–30 mg/kg	sid	Oral
Paregoric	0.05–0.06 mg/kg	bid/tid	Oral
Propantheline	0.25–.5 mg/kg	bid/tid	Oral
Sulfasalazine	12.5 mg/kg	qid	Oral
Tylosin	10–25 mg/kg	tid	Oral

---

mucosal culture may identify pathogens such as *Salmonella* sp., *Campylobacter jejuni*, *Clostridium perfringens*, and *Yersinia enterocolitica*. Protozoa and parasites may also be involved. *Campylobacter jejuni* has emerged from obscurity as a veterinary pathogen to recognition as a leading cause of enteritis in humans. A series of experiments of antibiotic sensitivity patterns of *C. jejuni* determined that high concentrations of ampicillin, penicillin, tetracycline, and metronidazole were required to inhibit growth. Because *Campylobacter* sp. are believed to produce beta-lactamase, most strains are relatively resistant to ampicillin and other related antibiotics. (Erythromycin is the drug of choice for therapy in humans.)

Symptomatic drugs used to treat canine colitis are motility modifiers, antimicrobial agents, and immunosuppressive drugs. Abnormal colonic secretory patterns are rarely specifically treated, but therapeutic agents such as sulfasalazine, opioids, anticholinergic agents, and corticosteroids that are employed to treat other aspects of colitis also enhance absorption and inhibit secretion of water and electrolytes and may help return secretory function to normal (Table 37–1).

Clinical relief from colitis may be obtained with narcotic drugs that increase colonic segmentation, such as diphenoxylate (Lomotil, 0.1 to 0.2 mg/kg, tid) or loperamide (Imodium, 0.1 mg/kg, bid, tid, or qid). Other examples include the anticholinergic drug propantheline bromide (Pro-Banthine, 0.25 to 0.5 mg/kg, tid) and the anticholinergic, antianxiety combination librax, 2.5 mg of clidinium bromide and 5 mg of chlordiazepoxide hydrochloride (Table 37–2).

There is no indication for routine use of antimicrobials in chronic disease. Antibiotic-associated pseudomembranous colitis has been induced by several drugs (lincomycin, clindamycin, tetracycline, neomycin, and erythromycin). Pseudomembranous colitis (a potentially fatal disease of the large bowel caused by antibiotic-induced colonic overgrowth of cytotoxic strains of *Clostridium difficile*) is the most severe adverse effect of clindamycin in humans. In dogs, gastrointestinal disturbances (vomiting, partial anorexia) appear to be the most common adverse effect of clindamycin treatment.

Spiramycin, a macrolide antibiotic, has had variable effectiveness in reducing the clinical signs of an oocyst shedding or intestinal cryptosporidiosis in people with acquired immune deficiency syndrome. Spiramycin is not clinically available in the United States, but clindamycin is used because of its known anticoccidial effectiveness.

Antimicrobial administration can alter normal intestinal microbial flora and delay re-establishment of normal flora following gastrointestinal disease. The only indication for antimicrobial use in treatment of colitis is in acute cases with damage to the mucosal barrier. In these cases, antibiotics are used systemically to control bacterial invasion through the gut wall and to control septicemia. Nonabsorbable antibiotics are not beneficial; to control bacterial invasion and dissemination, the antibiotic must be present systemically.

Antimicrobials have a separate, very limited role in treatment of chronic diarrhea. Compounds such as tylosin, tetracycline, neomycin, trimethoprim-sulfadiazine, or metronidazole are useful to control bacterial overgrowth or as an adjunct to treat other malabsorptive disorders. Sulfasalazine is the drug of choice for treatment of colitis.

Sulfasalazine is a combination of sulfapyridine and 5-acetylsalicylic acid (ASA), which is cleaved by colonic bacteria, resulting in the sulfa component being absorbed and ASA excreted in feces. ASA is probably the active ingredient which is due to antiprostaglandin activity. The exact mechanism, however, is unknown. The drug is indicated primarily for ulcerative and granulomatous colitis. The mechanisms of action of this drug are unknown but appear to be unrelated to its antimicrobial activity. Its effectiveness may be due to the antiprostaglandin effects of 5-aminosalicylic acid. Sulfasalazine should be administered at a dose of 12.5 mg/kg qid, for 3 to 4 weeks. If the dog improves after 2 weeks, the dose may be halved. In patients requiring longterm therapy, the minimum effective dose should be used to prevent side effects such as gastrointestinal upset, allergic dermatitis, cholestatic jaundice, and keratoconjunctivitis sicca. Concurrent use of corticosteroids may help to bring about remission in cases not responding to sulfasalazine alone. The drug has been used in cats at half the dose rate, but there is a risk of toxicity resulting from ASA; therefore, the drug should be used cautiously in cats.

If colitis cannot be resolved with the normal dosage of sulfasalazine, corticosteroids can be used concurrently or tried independently. Initial dosages of prednisone range from 1 to 2 mg/kg, sid. The dose should be gradually diminished until the dog is receiving the lowest dose every other day that still controls the clinical signs. Combination therapy with lower doses of sulfasalazine and prednisone may successfully manage diarrhea without side effects from either drug.

Tylosin is one of the most effective compounds for control of inflammatory bowel disease and bacterial overgrowth in the canine small intestine. Longterm treatment is frequently required, and the minimum dose required to control signs is determined empirically.

Metronidazole (e.g., Flagyl, Searle) is another antibacterial drug that has proved most useful in treating chronic diarrhea associated with inflammatory bowel disease or bacterial overgrowth. In addition to its antiprotozoal action, metronidazole suppresses cell-mediated immune reactions and has been used to treat granulomatous enteritis in humans. The drug also has a protective effect against experimentally induced colitis and is occasionally of use in patients that do not respond to sulfasalazine. Metronidazole is particularly effective against anaerobic bacteria and has proved useful in the treatment of anaerobic infections. In many dogs the favorable response to metronidazole may be due to elimination of undiagnosed protozoal infection. The antiprotozoal dosage is 30 mg/kg/day orally for 5 days, but treatment with lower dosages (10 mg/kg) for longer periods effectively controls bacterial overgrowth. The mechanism of action is not known but probably includes antiprotozoal action against *Giardia* sp., alteration of immune-mediated reactions in the bowel, and antibacterial action against anaerobes.

The food's fat content should be low because bacterial hydroxylation of fatty acids can promote large bowel diarrhea. Homemade diets can also be formulated from rice, low-fat cottage cheese, and chicken. Many dogs improve when fed a hypoallergenic diet.

37.4 URINARY SYSTEM

Antimicrobial treatment for UTI must accomplish two things if it is to be effective. First, the treatment must control bacterial growth in the urinary system. Second, control of microbial growth must be maintained until host defense mechanisms can prevent colonization of the urinary tract, without further administration of the drug.

With several antimicrobials, very high levels may be attained in glomerular filtrate, urine, or interstitial renal tissues, which is due to the local concentration of the drug as it is excreted through the kidney. Concentrations of many antimicrobials are many times higher in urine than in plasma which is due to normal renal concentrating mechanisms and additionally to renal tubular secretion. The fractions of drug excreted in the urine in the unchanged pharmacologically active form will also influence the antibacterial and thus the clinical effect. Drugs such as penicillins, which are excreted unchanged, attain very high levels in the kidney, and because of this high concentration, they may be present in concentrations sufficiently high to kill even insensitive bacterial species such as *E. coli*. The penicillins, streptomycin, erythromycin, gentamicin, nitrofurantoin, and the more soluble sulfonamides attain satisfactory concentrations, whereas oxytetracycline is less well concentrated (it is excreted largely via bile). Only 10% of an administered dose of chloramphenicol is excreted in an active form in the urine. Potential nephrotoxicity of an antimicrobial agent will also influence choice of drug, especially in dogs with impaired renal function. The potentiated sulfonamides are widely used for UTI, and the synergistic effect of trimethoprim allows for a low dosage of soluble sulfonamide in such preparations. Among the more commonly isolated organisms from clinical cases of UTI are *E. coli*, *Proteus* spp., *S. aureus*, *Streptococcus* spp., *Klebsiella pneumoniae*, and *Pseudomonas*, sp. (Table 37–3). In terms of frequency of occurrence, the following organisms are the more usual causes of UTI:

1. Mixed infections, with coliforms invariably involved
2. Pure coliform infections
3. *Proteus/Pseudomonas* infections
4. Beta-hemolytic streptococci

Potentiated sulfonamides, ampicillin, amoxicillin, or higher doses of penicillin G could be regarded as first-choice antibiotics in clinical cases of UTI. Second-choice antimicrobials are nitrofurantoin (in acid urine) and streptomycin or gentamicin (in alkaline urine). For refractory infections with *pseudomonas* spp. gentamicin is the antibiotic of choice.

It is always important, especially in UTIs, to attain high antibiotic concentrations, exposing the organisms to a continuous high dose of antibiotic. This may necessitate giving the antibiotic at a high dosage rate three or four times daily. High doses of potassium penicillin G or ampicillin have been used with reported high clinical cure rates. Amoxicillin—with its more rapid antibacterial effect and higher urinary concentrations than ampicillin—is now probably the semisynthetic penicillin of choice for UTIs. In practice, sensitivity tests or clinical assessments are employed in the selection of antimicrobial agents, and usually gram-negative infections tend to predominate in the urinary tract of the dog.

Surprisingly few new antibiotics have been introduced into veterinary practice since the early 1980s, fewer still are those specifically intended for treating UTI in dogs and cats. The two most recent examples are clavulanate potentiated amoxicillin and cephalexin, both of which have been developed for therapy of small animal infections, including UTI. Other antibiotics currently gaining wider acceptance for this indication include gentamicin, nitrofurantoin, nitroxoline, nalidixic acid, and the potentiated sulfonamides.

Newer members of the fluoroquinolone antibiotic family (i.e., enrofloxacin, norfloxacin) show promise in treating UTI. They are excreted primarily by the kidneys and achieve high urine concentrations. They also have a broad spectrum of antimicrobial activity (including *Pseudomonas aeruginosa*) and are bactericidal. These are especially useful in treating the causes of UTI in cats and dogs. The therapeutic strategy depends on the location and evolution of the UTI and on certain characteristics of the infected animal.

Three criteria must be taken into account when choosing urinary tract medication:

Active urinary elimination
The spectrum of activity, depending on the clinical picture, or the antibiotic sensitivity test
Urinary pH

Concentrations achieved in urine with fluoroquinolones, ampicillin, amoxicillin, tetracycline, chloramphenicol, cephalexin, trimethoprim/sulfonamides, and aminoglycosides are several-fold higher than the concentrations achieved in plasma after an equal dose. Bacteria resistant to these anti-

TABLE 37–3
SUGGESTED ANTIBIOTICS FOR CANINE BACTERIAL INFECTIONS

Site of Infection	Causal Organisms	First choice Antibiotic	Second choice Antibiotic
Respiratory Tract	Streptococci, Staphylococci, Bordetella,	Amoxycillin Benzyl Penicillin Cephalexin Doxycycline	Ampicillin Lincomycin, Tylosin, Chloramphenicol Erythromycin
	E. Coli/Klebsiella.	Streptomycin/Enrofloxacin	Gentamicin
Urinary Tract	Mixed Infection with Coliforms,	Potentiated Sulphon. Cephalexin	Nitrofurantoin
	Pure Coliform Infection,	Amoxycillin (Penicillin)	Streptomycin Gentamicin
	Proteus/ Pseudomonas,	Doxycycline	
	β-Haemolytic Streptococci.		Nalidixic Acid
Bone	Staph. Aureus, Mixed Infections	Lincomycin Sod. Fusidate Clindamycin	Ampicillin Amoxycillin Gentamicin
C.N.S.	Mixed infections	Chloramphenicol Doxycycline	Potentiated Sulphon. Oxytetracycline Ampicillin Penicillin Cephalosporin
G.I.T.	Coliforms,	Ampicillin Neomycin Doxycycline	Streptomycin
	Salmonella	Potentiated Sulphon. Chloramphenicol	
Eye	Staph. Pyogenes, Staph.-β, Haemolytic Strep. Mixed Infection with Coliforms	Neomycin) Penicillin) Topical Tetracycline, Doxycycline. Chloramphenicol (Penetration)	Framycetin
Skin	Staph. Pyogenes, Staph.-β, Haemolytic Strep, Mixed-including Gram-positive, Pure β-haemolytic Strep.	Potentiated Sulphonamides Amoxycillin/ Clavulanate Lincomycin Enrofloxacin	Tetracyclines (Doxycycline) Clindamycin Pure β-haemolytic Cephalosporin
Vagina	B-haemolytic Strep. Sulphonamide Coliforms, Mixed Infection	Potentiated Sulfonamides	Ampicillin Amoxycillin Tetracycline
Uterus	Gram-negative with Coliforms	Tetracylines Doxycycline	Nitrofurazone Potentiated Sulphonamide
Circulatory System	Streptococci Mixed Infections Leptospira	Penicillin Cephalosporin	Tetracycline Streptomycin Amikacin

TABLE 37–3
CONTINUED

Site of Infection	Causal Organisms	First choice Antibiotic	Second choice Antibiotic
Otitis Externa	S. Pyogenes	Neomycin	Framycetin
	β-haemolytic		Nystatin
	Strep.		
	Gram-negative		Cloxacillin
	Pseudomonas	Polymyxin	Erythromycin
	Yeasts/Fungi	Gentamycin	Sod. Fusidate
			Tetracycline
Deep-seated	Staph. Pyogenes	Penicillin	Pot. Sulphon.
Dermatoses	β-Haemolytic	Lincomycin/Clindamycin	
	Strep.,	Erythromycin	
	Mixed (incl.	Penicillin/OTC	
	Gram-ve)	Doxycyline	
	Bacteroides	Enrofloxacin	
Oral Cavity	Mixed infections	Penicillin	
	Bacteroides	Metronidazole/(Clindamycin).	Doxycycline

microbials in a systemic infection may be susceptible if they are exposed to the concentrations achieved in urine.

The urinary pH should preferably be measured before initiating any therapy, and the anti-infectious agent must be chosen with reference to its activity in urine at that pH (Table 37–4). Modification of urine pH

TABLE 37–4
USEFUL ANTIMICROBIAL DRUG DOSAGES FOR CANINE PYODERMA

Antibiotic	Oral Dosage Rate
Amoxicillin-Clavulanate	14 mg/kg B.I.D.
Amikacin	5 mg/kg T.I.D.
Cephadroxil	10–20 mg/kg B.I.D.
Cephalexin	30 mg/kg B.I.D.
Chloramphenicol	50 mg/kg T.I.D.
Erythromycin	10–20 mg/kg T.I.D.
Enrofloxacin	2.5–5 mg/kg B.I.D.
Gentamicin	2 mg/kg T.I.D.
Lincomycin	20 mg/kg B.I.D.
Nafcillin	20 mg/kg T.I.D.
Oxacillin	15 mg/kg T.I.D.
Clindamycin	5.0 mg/kg B.I.D.
Trimethoprim-Sulfadiazine	15 mg/kg B.I.D.
Doxycycline	10 mg/kg Daily

in treatment of UTI generally is intended to induce direct pH effects on bacterial growth in the urine or to enhance the action of antimicrobial drugs in the urine. Although an acid pH can impair bacterial growth, bacteriostatic and bactericidal urine pH values are near physiologic limits (<5) and are difficult to sustain. Some antimicrobials are more effective at an alkaline pH. For instance the urine of dogs and cats usually is slightly acidic, and only aminoglycosides, which are not preferred for initial treatment, are more active in alkaline urine.

Animals with UTI should be treated for a minimum of 14 days. Treatment for 3 to 6 weeks often has been suggested. The urine should be re-examined approximately 7 to 10 days following the first dose to evaluate the success of therapy.

THERAPY

Urine concentrations of antimicrobial agents are much more important than are serum concentrations in the successful management of UTI. Most antimicrobial agents commonly used in the treatment of UTI are present in the urine in active form at concentrations that exceed peak serum concentrations manyfold. This is the basis for the effective use of drugs such as penicillin in the treatment of UTI caused by gram-negative bacteria such as *Proteus mirabilis*, a species that is typically resistant to the concentrations of penicillin attained elsewhere in the body.

Urine concentrations of antimicrobial drugs, rather than blood concentrations, correlate best with the efficacy of agents used to treat UTI. Efficacy of a therapeutic regimen (i.e., drug, dosage, route, and frequency of administration) depends largely on its ability to provide a drug concentration in the environment of the bacteria (in vivo) that exceeds the MIC of the drug for the infecting organisms. Generally, antimicrobial drugs that are effective for treatment of UTI are excreted by the kidneys and found in much higher concentrations in the urine than in blood or tissues. The most effective antimicrobials are those that do not undergo substantial biodegradation to pharmacologically inactive metabolites in the liver.

Standardized disk diffusion methods often are used to evaluate bacterial susceptibility to antimicrobial agents. Relative to UTI, such methods have an important pitfall because results (i.e., zone-of-inhibition diameters that indicate susceptible or resistant) usually are interpreted on the basis of expected drug concentrations in blood rather than urine. Consequently, organisms may be judged to be resistant to the drugs because of the infection's location in the urinary tract.

Staphylococci are second only to *E. coli* as the most frequent bacterial isolates in canine UTIs. Also, there tends to be a relationship between urease-producing bacteria and struvite urolithiasis. Urease-producing bacteria (staphylococci, *Proteus* sp.) infecting the urinary tract often precede development of struvite urolithiasis in the dog.

Staphylococcal isolates should be sensitive to beta-lactamase-resistant beta-lactam antibiotics, such as cephalosporins, cloxacillin, dicloxacillin, and amoxicillin/clavulanic acid combinations.

Antimicrobial concentrations achieved in urine are much higher than the levels normally attained in plasma after an equal dose. Quite often, bacteria resistant to antimicrobials in a systemic infection may become susceptible if they are exposed to the concentrations achieved in urine. Many coagulase-positive staphylococci isolated from UTIs are susceptible to high urinary concentrations of ampicillin, amoxicillin/clavulanate, trimethoprim/sulfonamide, cephalexin, chloramphenicol, gentamicin, and kanamycin. Even when the staphylococci are beta-lactamase producers, the concentrations of ampicillin or amoxicillin achieved in urine may be sufficiently high to overcome enzyme inhibition and cure the infection.

Ampicillin and trimethoprim/sulfonamide are also highly effective for the treatment of UTI caused by *E. coli* and nonenteric streptococci.

For sensitive infections or for most UTIs caused by *E. coli*, *Klebsiella* spp. or *P. mirabilis*, therapy with ampicillin, amoxicillin, or a first-generation cephalosporin is appropriate.

For highly susceptible strains of *E. coli* infecting the urinary tract, chloramphenicol can be considered. Tetracyclines should usually be regarded as second choices in patients who cannot be given other antimicrobials.

In cases of more resistant strains of *E. coli* or *Klebsiella* spp. or for deep-seated infections in tissues where penicillins or cephalosporins do not concentrate, the ureido penicillins (e.g., carbenicillin, ticaricillin) or aminoglycosides should be employed.

Antimicrobial drug susceptibility of some pathogens is influenced greatly by whether antibiotic treatment (any drug for any reason) has been given recently. In dogs, the success rate for treating *E. coli* UTI with penicillins is about 75% when antibiotics have not been given in the preceding 2 months, but the success rate is less than 30% when antimicrobial drugs have been given within the preceding 2 months. This phenomenon probably is caused by transfer of resistance among organisms in R-plasmids.

Generally, aminoglycoside drugs should not be used as a first choice for treatment of UTI. Although organisms that cause UTI often are highly susceptible to aminoglycosides, drugs in this class are potentially nephrotoxic and are often inconvenient because they must be given by injection. Additionally, treatment duration tends to be limited by safety, expense, and convenience. Because other drugs are frequently effective for most infections, use of aminoglycosides in the treatment of UTI is generally unnecessary and is best reserved for instances when other drugs are ineffective.

The identity of the infecting organisms is the most important factor bearing on the selection of an appropriate drug to administer. Indeed, antimicrobial drug susceptibility testing often is unnecessary because the susceptibility of many common UTI pathogens to various drugs is known. Efficacy of some drugs against certain pathogens is highly predictable, with treatment efficacy approaching 100%. For example, consistent success in treatment of staphylococci and streptococci can be achieved using amoxicillin clavulanate. Although the drugs may not work all of the time, certain drug-pathogen combinations are effective so often that they are rational first choices (e.g., trimethoprim-sulfa combinations (TMP-S) for *E. coli* or *Enterobacter* spp., penicillins for *Proteus* spp., enrofloxacin for *Pseudomonas* spp., and cephalexin for *Klebsiella* spp.).

For recurrent gram-negative infection, trimethoprim/sulfadiazine is a good choice, for recurrent gram-positive infection, ampicillin/amoxicillin is a good choice. To ensure the effectiveness of the prophylactic therapy, urine cultures should be done every 1 to 2 months.

Selection of antimicrobial drugs for treatment of mixed infections (those caused by more than one type of pathogen) can be based on the identity of infecting organisms. Combinations of staphylococci and streptococci can be treated successfully with penicillins. When an animal is infected with staphylococci or streptococci and with *E. coli* or *Proteus* spp., TMP-S should be given. When a mixed infection includes any combination of *E. coli*, *Proteus* spp., *Enterobacter* spp., or *Klebsiella* spp., use of either TMP-S or cephalexin is rational. In mixed infections that include *Pseudomonas* spp., the other pathogens should be treated with the most effective agent against those pathogens, then the *Pseudomonas* spp. should be treated with tetracycline. Alternatively, an aminoglycoside may be effective against all pathogens in a mixed infection that includes *Pseudomonas* spp. Except for TMP-S combinations, simultaneous administration of two or more antimicrobial drugs should be avoided.

Pseudomonal UTI can be treated with the antipseudomonal penicillins, aminoglycosides, tetracyclines, cephalosporins, or the fluoroquinolones. The best aminoglycosides for *P. aeruginosa* infections are amikacin and tobramycin, followed by gentamicin. The fluoroquinolones (enrofloxacin) should be reserved for those *P. aeruginosa* infections that are refractory or resistant to other treatment modalities.

Clinically, fluoroquinolones are probably among the most useful drugs in animals for the treatment of UTIs, including those caused by bacteria resistant to beta-lactam antibiotics, aminoglycosides, and sulfonamides.

For most UTIs caused by *E. coli*, *Klebsiella* spp., or *P. mirabilis*, therapy with ampicillin, amoxicillin, or a first-generation cephalosporin (e.g., cefazolin) is appropriate. High-dose chloramphenicol is indicated when sensitive strains of *E. coli* invade the urinary tract. Chloramphenicol is extensively metabolized to nonactive metabolites, however. Tetracyclines should be regarded as second-choice drugs in patients who cannot be given the other antibiotics.

When more resistant strains of *E. coli* and *Klebsiella* spp. are involved or for more deep-seated infections in tissues that penicillins and cephalosporins do not reach, the ureido penicillins (e.g., ticarcillin, carbenicillin, or piperacillin) or the aminoglycosides should be considered.

When the episodes of UTI are caused by staphylococcus, streptococcus, or *P. mirabilis*, a penicillin should be used as the low-dose therapeutic agent. If the UTI is caused by *E. coli*, *Klebsiella* spp., or *Enterobacter* spp., trimethoprim/sulfonamide, nitrofurantoin, cephalexin, or nalidixic acid may be used as the low-dose therapeutic agent. Selection of one of these drugs should always be based on results of susceptibility testing of the latest isolate.

Dosages divided into several treatments daily have been recommended for numerous drugs including penicillin G (100,000 U/kg body weight), ampicillin (50 mg/kg), amoxicillin (33 mg/kg), cephalexin (20 mg/kg), chloramphenicol (50 mg/kg), nitrofurantoin (15 mg/kg), tetracycline (50 mg/kg), trimethoprim/sulfonamide (30 mg of the combined drugs/kg), sulfisoxazole (66 mg/kg), gentamicin (2.2 mg/kg), amikacin

TABLE 37–5
ANTIMICROBIAL DRUGS FOR URINARY TRACT INFECTION (U.T.I.)

DRUG	DOSE	ADMINISTRATION
Trimethoprim/sulfonamide	30	Orally B.I.D.
Tetracyclines		
Tetracycline	50	Orally B.I.D.
Doxycycline	10	
Chloramphenicol	50	Orally T.I.D.
Beta-lactams		
Ampicillin	50	Orally T.I.D.
Amoxicillin	30	Orally T.I.D.
Amoxicillin/clavulanic acid	12.5	Orally T.I.D.
Cefalexin	10–20	Orally T.I.D.
Amino glycosides		
Gentamicin	2–4	S.C. T.I.D
Quinolones		
Enrofloxacin	2.5	Orally B.I.D.
Macrolides		
Erythromycin	25–50	Orally T.I.D.

(15 mg/kg), and tobramycin (3 mg/kg), enrofloxacin (2.5–5.0 mg/kg for 3 to 5 days). In healthy dogs, most drugs must be given every 8 hours to maintain drug concentrations in the urine. The important exceptions are trimethoprim/sulfa combinations (given every 12 hours).

Treatment of UTI for 10 to 14 days is adequate to cure acute, uncomplicated urethrocystitis in dogs and cats. For various reasons, however, treatment should be extended beyond this interval (Table 37–5).

The optimum duration of antimicrobial therapy for canine UTI is unknown, but there is ample precedence for a 2-week course of treatment for uncomplicated UTI. A urine specimen of culture should be collected at about the seventh treatment day. If bacterial growth is not observed, a 14-day therapeutic course should be completed. A second urine specimen for culture should be obtained 4 to 7 days after completion of therapy. If growth of bacteria is observed, the therapy has failed and the reason(s) for this failure must be ascertained. Treatment failure in UTI should be analyzed thoroughly so that any error in management or omissions in diagnosis may be identified and corrected.

Most drugs for UTI treatment should be given orally; exceptions are the aminoglycosides, which should be given subcutaneously. Most drugs that are best used for initial treatment are effective when given orally, and the oral route is convenient, versatile, and well-tolerated.

Urinary antiseptics are antibacterial agents that cannot be used to treat systemic infections. These drugs are excreted so rapidly by the kidneys that substantial microbial effects occur only in the urinary tract. These drugs are also toxic when given in sufficient quantity to have systemic effects. Nitrofurantoin usually is effective against *E. coli*, staphylococci, and streptococci; it is well suited for protracted use in animals with normal renal function because substantial drug effects are produced only in the urine; and it often is satisfactory for prophylaxis against frequent reinfection in animals with impaired urinary tract defenses. Methenamine is given orally and is excreted in the urine. When the urine is acidic, methenamine decomposes, liberating formaldehyde, which has an antibacterial effect. Because the action of methenamine depends on an acidic pH in the urine, the drug is usually given in combination with a urinary acidifier (mandelic acid or hippuric acid). Methenamine is one of the few antimicrobial agents that is efficacious against fungal UTI. Methylene blue and nalidixic acid are other urinary antiseptics, but they are used seldom because of their narrow margins of safety; methylene blue causes Heinz body hemolytic anemias (particularly in cats), and nalidixic acid causes seizures.

Therapy with the most effective drug should be maintained for a minimum period of 14 days, but chronic or recurrent UTIs may necessitate at least 4 weeks of treatment. In dogs, clinical evidence indicates that about 70% of cases should respond to one course of proper antibiotic treatment, and about 30% require a further one or two courses. Trimethoprim is concentrated in the canine prostate when given in combination with sulfadiazine and may be of value in UTIs associated with chronic prostatitis. If sensitivity testing indicates that neither amoxicillin nor a potentiated sulfonamide are likely to be effective, it is well to remember that streptomycin, gentamicin, and trimethoprim are most effective when urine is alkaline, whereas nitrofurantoin and tetracycline are most effective in acid urine. With any antibiotic, if renal function is impaired, frequency of administration must be curtailed, especially when drugs with narrow safety margins or propensities toward nephrotoxicity such as some of the aminoglycosides are used.

Methenamine mandelate is most effective in acid urine. At a pH of 5.5 or lower, the compound dissociates to release the two active antibacterial agents mandelic acid and formaldehyde. Methenamine is available in combination with sodium acid phosphate to acidify the urine. Ascorbic acid is another useful acidifying agent, which possesses some antibacterial action itself. Alkalinity of urine in the dog seems to predispose to UTI, which is one reason why acidification itself may mitigate the symptoms.

Nitroxoline is another useful antibicrobial agent possessing a broad spectrum of activity against a wide range of pathogens implicated in UTI. Nalidixic acid is effective primarily against gram-negative organisms.

Treatment of cystitis requires an anti-infectious agent with a high urinary intraluminal concentration, i.e., quinolone, trimethoprim-sulfonamide, the beta-lactams, tetracycline, etc. A bacteriologic urine test is usually carried out on the third day after the beginning of treatment. For chronic cystitis, treatment should persist for 4 to 8 weeks. Periodic bacteriologic tests must be carried out, and the urine pH must be checked to ensure against infection with bacteria preferring an alkaline medium. Treatment of UTI for 10 to 14 days is adequate for cure of acute, uncomplicated urethrocystitis in dogs and cats.

In cases of pyelonephritis, beta-lactams with clavulanic acid or cephalosporins have sufficient local concentrations to treat the focus of the infection. Theoretically, prostatitis must be treated with fat-soluble, anti-infectious agents that are not closely linked to plasma, i.e., macrolides, trimethoprim, tetracyclines, doxycycline, chloramphenicol, or enrofloxacin.

In summary, the treatment of a primary UTI for (1) cystitis usually requires quinolone or potentiated sulfonamides (trimethoprim-sulfonamide), whereas treatment for (2) pyelonephritis requires a beta-lactam, and (3) prostatitis requires trimethoprim/sulfa or enrofloxacin.

Chronic bacterial prostatitis has only a fair prognosis for longterm cure. Drugs such as trimethoprim/sulfadiazine, nitrofurantoin, and cephalexin have been used successfully for this purpose. If longterm (3-month) antibiotic therapy is necessary, trimethoprim/sulfadiazine, beta lactam antibiotics and carbenicillin are considered the best choices. However, trimethoprim/sulfadiazine therapy has been associated with keratoconjunctivitis sicca and anemia that is due to folate deficiency. As a preventive measure, dogs receiving trimethoprim at full dosage (30 mg/kg, bid) for more than 6 weeks should also be given folic acid (5 mg/day). The fluoroquinolones (e.g., enrofloxacin, norfloxacin, and ciprofloxacin) may be promising alternatives for longterm therapy (see Table 37–5).

Digestive side effects (vomiting) may occur, especially with quinolones, whose administration during a meal or after an antiemetic considerably reduces these reactions. The animal's age also should be considered before prescribing the antimicrobial agents (tetracyclines or macrolides).

37.5 BONE

Bone infection is a serious condition, requiring highly specific antibiotic therapy. The penetration of antimicrobials into bone

---

TABLE 37–6
CONDITIONS OF ANAEROBIC BACTERIAL INFECTION

Foul-smelling discharges.
Deep infections from penetration of mucosal or cutaneous surfaces.
Necrotic tissue, gangrene, pseudomembrane formation.
Gas in tissues or exudates.
Deep abscesses.
Infections that do not respond to therapy with conventional antibiotics.
Septic pleuritis or peritonitis.
Complications following surgery on the gastrointestinal tract or for pyometra.

---

is generally poor, although the blood flow into bones and joints usually increases with inflammation. In the treatment of osteomyelitis, lincomycin and clindamycin should be considered. Clindamycin displays excellent bone penetration as well as being highly effective against anaerobic and aerobic bone pathogens. Lincomycin is a soluble antibiotic that penetrates extremely well into bone, but effective therapy with this antibiotic must be started early while the bone still retains its blood supply. Long-term administration of large doses of lincomycin can result in diarrhea in the dog. Sodium fusidate is a small molecule that also diffuses well into bone and can be clinically quite effective. Gram-positive, gram-negative, and mixed infections have been observed in cases of osteomyelitis in the dog, with *S. aureus* usually being the significant pathogen. The narrow, gram-positive-oriented spectrum of lincomycin, clindamycin, or sodium fusidate therefore is not usually a serious drawback. Semisynthetic penicillins (ampicillin, amoxicillin, methicillin) the cephalosporins, and gentamicin have also been reported to be relatively useful in the treatment of intractable bone infections. In the treatment of these infections, bactericidal agents are employed systematically, because high dosage rates to facilitate delivery of adequate concentrations of drug to the avascular bony structures as needed. They should preferably be given early in the infection, while the bone still retains its blood supply.

Osteomyelitis is inflammation of the bone, specifically involving the bone marrow, the cortex, and/or the periosteum. The age of an animal may influence the extent of periosteal and cortical involvement. Bacteria are not the only prerequisites for infection of the bone and, in fact, seldom cause osteomyelitis by themselves. Experimentally, infection must be accompanied by disruption of the blood supply to the bone or mechanical disruption of the bone marrow before osteomyelitis can occur. When bacteria are introduced into the bone and conditions are favorable for their growth, rapid destruction of the bone is possible, especially in young animals.

Anaerobic organisms are significant in osteomyelitis, either as pure culture or as a mixed infection with staphylococci. *Peptostreptococcus anaerobius* is the anaerobe isolated most frequently, while the most common genus encountered is *Bacteroides*.

Aerobic bacteria that are commonly encountered include *S. aureus*, *E. coli*, *Proteus* spp., and streptococcus. Multiple organisms are frequently isolated. It should be noted that this is primarily a gram-positive spectrum and that some of these organisms possess a plasmid-induced beta lactamase. Gentamicin is therefore useful for many staphylococcal infections.

In dogs, osteomyelitis and surgical wound infections that do not involve the alimentary canal are most commonly caused by staphylococci, particularly *S. aureus*.

Historically, bactericidal antibiotics have been used for acute osteomyelitis, and bacteriostatic antibiotics for chronic osteomyelitis. Current recommendations indicate that bacteriostatic antibiotics have no place in the treatment of osteomyelitis when bactericidal antibiotics are available. If the results of culture are not available or attainable, the use of clindamycin (Antirobe) has been advocated. It is an analogue of lincomycin and features a similar spectrum. Advantages of clindamycin include excellent bone penetration and good activity against *B. fragilis*. Side effects in 5 to 20% cases in humans have been overgrowth of *C. difficile* with subsequent diarrhea as a result of the exotoxin; this problem has not been reported in veterinary medicine. Clindamycin is primarily bacteriostatic, exerting its antibacterial effect by binding to the bacterial 50S ribosomal subunit and inhibiting synthesis of peptide bonds. Effective therapeutic concentrations are achieved in most body tissues, including bone and joints.

Clindamycin is rapidly and completely absorbed after oral administration in dogs and cats. Both clindamycin and lincomycin are well distributed throughout most body tissues, including skin, bones, and teeth, and so are suitable for treating infected wounds, abscesses, osteomyelitis, and dental infections caused by gram-positive or anaerobic bacteria. Clindamycin is concentrated in leukocytes, which enhances the bactericidal activity of these cells and may help concentrate the drug at infection sites. An important characteristic of clindamycin is its ability to penetrate to effective concentrations in walled off abscesses, and bone, surpassing concentrations achieved by chloramphenicol and the penicillins.

37.6 CENTRAL NERVOUS SYSTEM

Penetration of antibiotics into the central nervous system (CNS) occurs very slowly because penetration must take place via lipid cellular membranes because the capillaries are not fenestrated. Thus, lipoidal solubility, molecular size and configuration, and degree of plasma protein binding are important determinants for this passage.

A few of the commonly used antibacterials attain therapeutic concentrations in the cerebrospinal fluid (CSF) by standard doses and routes of administration when the meninges are not inflamed. These are chloramphenicol, doxycycline (after repeated doses), trimethoprim, and the sulfonamides, especially sulfadiazine, which is commonly combined with trimethoprim. Some of the newer beta-lactams and cephalosporins penetrate particularly well, e.g., cefoxitin and moxalactam, although the last is expensive.

The tetracyclines, chloramphenicol, and the sulfonamides penetrate best; penicillin entry is intermediate; and in the aminoglycoside group, penetration is almost nonexistent. The CSF contains little protein, so that most drugs in the CSF are in the free unbound form and thus can exert their antibacterial effect. Meningeal inflammation reduces the blood-brain barrier to entry of penicillin and so permits inhibitory concentrations to be reached in such states. As the inflammatory process declines, the penicillin penetration may be inadequate to finally eliminate the infection. Whereas many antimicrobials (e.g., penicillin) will cross an inflamed blood-brain barrier, use of an antibiotic that crosses the normal (noninflamed) blood-brain barrier is preferred and is more effective. It is best to maintain inhibitory antimicrobial levels in the CNS when the acute inflammatory phase has subsided. Penicillin and its semisynthetic derivative (ampicillin) suffer from this pharmacokinetic shortcoming. Because chloramphenicol, potentiated sulfonamides, some third-generation cephalosporins, and oxytetracycline penetrate the normal blood-brain barrier, increased concentrations of these agents are found in the CNS during inflammation, and even at the postinflammatory phase, adequate levels are still present to overwhelm the infection; hence, their clinical popularity. Sulfonamides, which become readily acetylated or undergo high protein binding (e.g., sulfadimidine), will not be free to cross the blood-brain barrier or to exert a therapeutic effect within in CNS. Sulfadiazine, which is incorporated into the potentiated sulfonamide preparations, penetrates well into the CSF, whereas trimethoprim has more difficulty attaining adequate levels. Hence it is prudent to use maximal doses to these potentiated preparations to attain effective levels of both components in the central nervous system. With penicillin it may be necessary to administer massive doses by the normal route to attain inhibitory concentrations with reasonable certainty. This technique can only be applied to relatively nontoxic beta-lactam antibiotics such as the penicillins and cephalosporins.

37.7 THE EYE

For the eye, systemic therapy is indicated for intraocular infection of the structures while topical therapy can be adequate for surface corneal inflammation or conjunctivitis. Penetration of antibiotics into the eye following topical application will occur only if the cornea is abraded. Antibiotics diffuse slowly into the structures of the eye because the capillaries in these organs are not fenestrated, and penetration must take place via lipid diffusion. Accordingly, chloramphenicol (a small molecule), tetracyclines, and macrolides penetrate best; the sulfonamides are unpredictable; and the entry of the penicillins is almost negligible following systemic administration. Chloramphenicol is probably the best antibiotic in terms of crossing the blood-aqueous barrier when given parenterally. The subconjunctival injections of aqueous solutions of appropriate antimicrobial agents can accompany either systemic or topical treatment. Although ointment formulations remain in the conjunctival sac for up to 1 hour and possess good stability and contact time, they do tend to hold exudates and add to the stickiness of the pus and mucus produced. Drops, on the other hand, are easier to instill into the eye, and do not cause blurring of vision, but they must be instilled more frequently and also are less stable than ointments. Antibiotic broad-spectrum agents such as neomycin, gentamicin, sodium fusidate, cloxacillin, or chloramphenicol (without corticosteroid) are first-line antibiotics for superficial eye infections when most infections are caused by either (1) *Staphylococcus pyogenes*, (2) beta-hemolytic streptococci, or (3) mixed infections including coliforms. Where the conjunctival sac does not contain a great deal of pus, the subconjunctival injection of an aqueous solution of penicillin, chloramphenicol, or neomycin might be preferred.

37.8 UTERINE/VAGINAL INFECTIONS

Vaginal infections in a bitch are usually caused by either beta-hemolytic streptococci or coliforms, but mixed infections can and do occur. Potentiated sulfonamides are reasonable first-choice antimicrobial agents, but ampicillin, amoxicillin, or a tetracycline also can be used. The choice of antimicrobial therefore will depend on the sensitivity of the isolated strains, and injudicious use of antibiotics may upset the normal floral equilibrium.

Whereas gram-positive and/or gram-negative infections commonly occur in the vagina, uterine infections in the bitch are usually caused by gram-negative organisms. Tetracyclines, oral or parenteral, are frequently used in conjunction with intrauterine infusions of nitrofurazone or potentiated sulfonamides. Anaerobes often complicate cases of pyometra, and hence specific antianaerobic antimicrobials should be chosen (e.g., clindamycin, metronidazole, penicillins, chloramphenicol).

37.9 CIRCULATORY SYSTEM

Streptococci are frequently isolated from cases of canine endocarditis, but aerobic or anaerobic organisms of mixed origin also can be involved. High doses of bactericidal antibiotics should be employed, selected on the basis of sensitivity tests. High plasma levels usually are needed, extending over a period of weeks, depending on clinical assessment.

Bacteremia defines the presence of bacteria in the blood, but it does not necessarily imply a disease state. When disease results from blood-borne bacteria and their toxic products, the term "septicemia" is used.

Bacteremia occurs commonly for a variety of reasons. Under normal conditions, bacteria are rapidly removed from the blood by phagocytosis with the assistance of immunoglobulin and complement activation. If this first line of defense is ineffective, septicemia is the usual result. The progression of bacteremia to septicemia depends on the bacterial factors, including the organism type, its virulence and the size of inoculum, and other host factors, including physical condition, degree of immunocompetence, and inter-current factors to determine the intensity and severity of the infection.

Any bacterial organism can be involved in bacteremia or septicemia. The most commonly reported aerobic bacteria are staphylococcus, streptococcus, and *Escherichia* spp., followed by *Klebsiella, Enterobacter,* and *Pseudomonas* spp.

Peracute bacteremia from endotoxemia is almost always associated with gram-negative microbes, predominantly *E. coli* and *Salmonella* spp. The progression of clinical signs occurs over a period of a few hours and, as a result of endotoxemia, leads to severe clinical and hemodynamic abnormalities. Similarly, acute bacteremia usually results from infection with gram-negative organisms but occasionally can result from *S. aureus* infections. Acute peritonitis, alimentary tract disorders, diarrhea and trauma can initiate bacteremia and endotoxemia.

Subacute bacteremia on the other hand usually is usually the result of gram-positive infections and progresses over a period of 2–3 weeks. Chronic bacteremia always is associated with a persistent focus of infection that either is difficult to eradicate or is caused by a micro-organism of relatively low pathogenicity. Low grade walled-off infections, difficult to eradicate, often contribute to chronic bacteremia.

Because disseminated bacterial infection is life-threatening, on account of local septic sequestration, antimicrobial therapy must be aggressive and instituted promptly. Errors in drug selection, dose, and route of administration contribute greatly to patient mortality. Disseminated bacteremia can result in a focus or multiple foci of infection being established in a variety of vital organs and tissues.

For bacteremia the parenteral route of antibiotic administration is preferred, because oral absorption cannot be relied on in seriously ill patients. Bactericidal agents are recommended for treatment of disseminated sepsis. Oral medication, even where high bioavailability is assured is not usually adequate. Ideally, the intravenous route should be employed.

The most widely recommended antimicrobial combination for disseminated bacterial infection is an aminoglycoside with a beta-lactam antibiotic. The aminoglycosides are bactericidal against a wide spectrum of gram-positive and gram-negative aerobic bacteria. The beta-lactams, also bactericidal, are mainly effective against gram-positive organisms, but modern or augmented beta-lactams have an extended spectrum of activity against gram-negative bacteria as well. A major reason for combining these two classes of drugs is that the combination is synergistic against many bacterial organisms. (Long acting potentiated sulfonamides given intravenously also possess high efficacy and bactericidal action.)

As a working rule, cephalothin, cephalexin, gentamicin, and chloramphenicol are most effective in vitro for gram-positive bacteria including staphylococci and gentamicin and cephalothin are most effective against gram-negative agents. A combination of an aminoglycoside with penicillin, amoxicillin/clavulanate, ampicillin, or a cephalosporin thus is the logical choice for treating life-threatening bacteremia in the absence of preliminary laboratory identification. Appropriate adjustments in therapy may be necessary subsequently, based on results of bacterial culture and antibiotic sensitivity. Modern fluoroquinolones enrofloxacin (possessing a wide volume of distribution) could also be considered on account of their broad spectrum of antibacterial action, and lowered risk of resistance.

Amikacin appears to be more effective against *Klebsiella* spp., and a change to amikacin is made when indicated by antimicrobial susceptibility test results. Cephalothin is quite resistant to the beta-lactamases of gram-positive organisms.

Antibiotic susceptibility tests results may indicate a change from cephalothin to another beta-lactam. Ticarcillin or carbenicillin is more active against *Pseudomonas* spp. than is cephalothin (it is also more expensive). If a resistant *Staphylococcus* spp. is encountered, a beta-lactamase-resistant penicillin, such as amoxicillin/clavulanate, oxacillin or nafcillin, may be indicated. Gram-negative bacteremia is more difficult to control when it accompanies neutropenia, hypogamma-globulinemia, diabetes mellitus, or renal failure, all of which generally predispose patients to this type of infection. Combination antibiotic therapy often is used for gram-negative infections, because they are associated with more acute progression and high mortality. Although some clinical evidence would support the use of carbenicillin or ticarcillin with aminoglycosides for severe infection *Pseudomonas* and *Proteus* spp. these drugs must be given separately because of known in vitro incompatibilities. Amikacin, unlike tobramycin and gentamicin, is not inactivated in vitro by penicillins. Continuous IV infusion of aminoglycosides has been recommended, although associated increased nephrotoxicity has been reported. Gentamicin is effective against beta lactamase producing staphylococci, and also, pseudomonas and proteus.

37.10 ANAEROBIC INFECTIONS

Anaerobic infections in veterinary medicine play a disproportionately significant role in animal disease. It is only in the last few years with the advent of more ''user friendly'' isolation laboratory equipment, and much greater emphasis in the scientific literature that the very important role of these organisms is being truly recognised. Anaerobes make up a large proportion of the normal bacterial flora, and mucous membranes are heavily contaminated with obligate anaerobic organisms. Infections that are due to anaerobes occur when a break in the primary defense barriers (possibly the gut) and normal flora contaminates tissue.

Obligate anaerobes such as *Bacteroides* species, *Clostridia* and *Fusobacteria* require true anaerobic conditions. They are present in the gut and can localize in devitalized forms devoid of oxygen. Facultative organisms on the other hand, such as E. coli, and certain streptococcal species, can survive either in anaerobic or certain aerobic conditions, depending on their enzymatic capability. Most of these anaerobes of both classes are present in the gastrointestinal tract.

Certain areas of the body are more susceptible to anaerobic infections than others. These are the oropharynx, gums, skin, deep wounds, respiratory tract, fistulae, abdomen, reproductive tract, feet, musculoskeletal system, and CNS. (Table 37–6)

Obligate anaerobes isolated most often from anaerobic infection in small animals include *Bacteroides*, *Fusobacterium*, *Peptostreptococcus*, *Clostridium*, and *Actinomyces* spp. Of these, *Clostridium* (especially *C. perfringens*) and *Actinomyces* spp. are the most oxygen tolerant.

Up to approximately 30% of infections (primarily oropharyngeal, pleuropulmonary, and intra-abdominal infections as well as infection from bite wounds) that occur in veterinary patients involve anaerobic organisms; the most common is B. fragilis. It is undoubtedly true that anaerobes, as a cause of disease, have been overlooked by veterinary clinicians for many years. Presumably, this is because routine laboratory isolation and culturing facilities have not been available for anaerobe isolation, and hence, negative results are received by the clinician.

One of the most distinctive characteristics of anaerobes is their putrid smell, and this can useful in diagnosis. Any infection associated with a foul smell, copious pus, and signs of necrosis probably has some anaerobic bacteria present. However, some anaerobic infections do not smell, and pus is not obvious, because the infection is deep-seated (i.e., fistulated). Another characteristic of anaerobic infection is the chronic disease that does not appear to respond to conventional antibiotic treatment or does so initially but recurs quickly (Table 37–7).

Anaerobic infection of soft tissues tends to extend along tissue planes often in accordance with extensive necrosis.

Abscesses in the pharynx, gingivitis, and adjacent tissues tend to have a mixed anaerobic infection. Many abscesses are caused by migration of foreign bodies or puncture wounds, which allow other bacteria easy access.

Anaerobic infection is common in the abdomen, especially in peritonitis following gut penetration. This is not surprising because of the bacterial load of the gut which is of the obligate or facultative type.

In anaerobic bone infection, various characteristics are associated with anaerobic osteomyelitis. These include infection developing after open fractures, bite wounds, or soft tissue trauma; putrid exudate, gas formation or dark discharges; an infection with a ''sterile'' culture; no response to an-

---

TABLE 37–7
SPECIMENS FOR ANAEROBIC BACTERIAL CULTURE

Surgical specimens from "normally" sterile sites.—Refractory to antibiotics
Contents of deep abscesses./Fistulae
Aspirates from chronic otitis media and interna.
Aspirates from deep wounds.
Gingivitis/Periodontal disease
Peritonitis
Mastitis

---

tibiotics specific for aerobes; and many different gram-stained bacteria in specimens.

Infection of the uterus in cats and dogs is usually attributed to coliform bacteria. The lack of proper (anaerobic) culturing is probably the reason that the role of anaerobes is not readily appreciated, and therapy is unsuccessful. Obligate anaerobes are the most likely cause of the foul odor of pyometra, which is due to the liberation of fatty acids as by-products of their metabolism.

Several classes of antibiotics are generally considered to be consistently effective against anaerobic bacteria, both in vitro and

in vivo. Penicillins remain the antibiotic used most widely for routine treatment of anaerobic infection (because of their relative inexpensiveness). Alternatives to penicillins are usually selected when antibiotic resistance is encountered or for increased tissue penetration. These antimicrobials include choramphenicol, clindamycin, metronidazole, and cefoxitin (Table 37–8).

Unfortunately widespread resistance to tetracycline has greatly limited its usefulness in treatment of anaerobic infection, although doxycycline and minocycline show more promise in this regard.

Penicillin G also has good activity against most species of *Actinomyces* and *Fusobacterium* and some species of *Bacteroides*. Several species of *Bacteroides*, however, especially *B. fragilis*, are uniformly resistant to penicillins. In the case of *B. fragilis*, production of beta-lactamases is produced which inactivates penicillin.

Because obligate anaerobes have a specialized metabolism, and enzyme systems, they are frequently not sensitive to the antibiotics used to treat aerobes. Many anaerobic infections therefore frequently fail to respond to conventional treatment. Aminoglycoside antibiotics, such as streptomycin, neomycin, or gentamicin, require an oxygen-dependent transport across the bacterial wall and therefore are not effective in an anaerobic environment. *B. fragilis* produces a beta-lactamase that renders penicillin and other beta-lactam antibiotics of no therapeutic use. Drugs of choice for anaerobic infections include metronidazole, lincomycin, clindamycin, penicillins, (in certain cases) doxycycline, and chloramphenicol.

The incidence of anaerobic bacteremia in dogs is significant, and the antibiotic sensi-

---

TABLE 37–8
ANTIBIOTICS EFFECTIVE AGAINST ANAEROBIC BACTERIA

Antibiotic
High efficacy
Ampicillin
Carbenicillin
Cefoxitin
Chloramphenicol
Clindamycin
Doxycycline
Metronidazole
Moderate efficacy
Erythromycin
Procaine penicillin
Tetracycline
Low efficacy
Gentamicin
Kanamycin
Streptomycin

tivity patterns of these microbes differ from those of aerobes. Anaerobic infections are likely in the presence of periodontal disease, gingivitis, deep abscesses, granulomas, peritonitis, osteomyelitis, septic arthritis, and septic pleural effusions.

The presence of anaerobic bacteria should be suspected in septicemic patients whenever there is abscessation, foul-smelling discharge, necrotic tissue, gas in tissues, fecal contamination, or evidence that the source of infection is from the liver, gastrointestinal tract, or bone. Penicillin originally was the preferred drug for anaerobic infections but resistance of these organisms (especially *B. fragilis*) to penicillin is increasing. Cephalothin is effective against many anaerobic organisms, but *B. fragilis*, certain other gram-negative anaerobic bacteria, and some *Clostridium* spp. are resistant. Because the aminoglycosides are ineffective against anaerobic organisms, the gentamicin-cephalothin combination will not cover the spectrum of organisms. Therefore, if anaerobic infection is suspected, another antibiotic is added—metronidazole, at 20 to 40 mg/kg (total daily dose). Metronidazole is bactericidal and is active against gram-negative anaerobic bacteria, including *Fusobacterium* spp. and *B. fragilis*. Most gram-positive anaerobic organisms, including *Clostridium* spp., are sensitive to metronidazole, even clostridial organisms that are resistant to clindamycin. Some gram-positive anaerobic cocci are resistant to metronidazole but are sensitive to cephalothin. Metronidazole is widely used in human medicine as "flagyl".

In summary drugs that effectively treat anaerobic infections in dogs and cats include the beta-lactam antibiotics, the penicillins, and the cephalosporins cefoxitin and cefotaxime, clindamycin, metronidazole chloramphenicol and the modified tetracyclines (doxycycline, minocycline).

Many anaerobic bacteria are highly susceptible to modern cephalosporins and cefoxitin and are moderately susceptible to most other cephalosporins, except ceftazidime, to which they are resistant. *Bacteroides fragilis*, (beta-lactamase producer) an anaerobic bacterium that is often resistant to penicillins and most cephalosporins, is sensitive to cefotetan and cefoxitin.

Bacteroides spp. currently are isolated from feline and canine infections with increasing frequency. *Bacteroides fragilis* is among the more difficult to treat anaerobes, partly because it produces beta-lactamases and because its resistance to beta-lactam antibiotics is increasing. Although *B. fragilis* is not the most common *Bacteroides* sp. isolated from feline infections, its increasing incidence, virulence, and sophisticated system of resistance indicate that beta-lactamase inhibitors may be the best drugs for anaerobic infections, e.g., clavulanate augmented amoxicillin.

Clindamycin and metronidazole are specifically effective at eliminating infections that are due to *Bacteroides* spp. Although chloramphenicol is very effective against most anaerobic organisms, this drug generally should not be given to cats, because of cumulation, toxicity and hematopoietic disturbance.

The efficacy of sulfonamide/trimethoprim combinations in treating anaerobic infections is debatable. Results have varied from high efficacy to quite disappointing results.

METRONIDAZOLE

The precise mechanisms of action of metronidazole are not fully understood, but its spectrum of activity includes *Clostridium* and *Bacteroides* spp. in addition to a variety of other obligate anaerobes.

Metronidazole is unique in that it is the only antimicrobial currently available with consistent bactericidal activity against *B. fragilis* and most other strains of *Bacteroides*. This has been one of the reasons for its unparalleled success in human medicine.

Oral administration of metronidazole can cause profuse salivation, vomiting, anorexia, and weight loss in cats. The drug is extremely bitter and may be more easily administered if a generic form that is not film coated is crushed and administered in a syrup vehicle. In man it has been extensively used for vaginitis, stomatitis, and in dripform for peritonitis. Brain abscesses and endocarditis are other human indications.

For treatment of anaerobic infections in humans, a metronidazole dose of 250–500 mg day, divided every 6 hours, is recommended. Clinically, 20 mg/kg has proven very effective for treatment of anaerobic infections in dogs, and neurologic abnormalities have not been observed. Metronidazole is the only antibiotic with consistent rapid bactericidal activity against *B. fragilis.* Clinically, the efficacy of treatment with metronidazole for most anaerobic infections is good to high and is equivalent to that of clindamycin and modern cephalosporins.

Indications for metronidazole include recurrent or persistent anaerobic infections that fail to respond to more traditional antibiotics (penicillins, clindamycin, and chloramphenicol), documented anaerobic brain abscesses, or endocarditis caused by *Bacteroides* spp. This drug is also very effective against anaerobic osteomyelitis and as prophylaxis for elective lower gastrointestinal surgery. Metronidazole, given at 10 mg/kg, tid, orally, has been effective for treatment of anaerobic infections of dogs and cats.

CLINDAMYCIN

Clindamycin is used in humans primarily for treatment of anaerobic infections, especially those caused by *B. fragilis.* Clindamycin was shown to be more effective than penicillin for treating pleuropulmonary infections in humans and is also effective in treating pelvic abscesses, in part because of its excellent tissue penetration. Clindamycin has also been effective for treating anaerobic pleuropulmonary infections of dogs. Like rifampin, clindamycin penetrates leukocytes and kills phagocytized bacteria. Clindamycin has recently been shown to be very effective for the treatment of staphylococcal osteomyelitis in humans and dogs. Because the drug can be administered orally, the owner can treat the animal at home. In veterinary medicine, clindamycin is used for anaerobic periodontal disease, gingivitis, and osteomyelitis. It displays high penetration into non-vascular tissues. Pseudomembranous colitis as occurs in humans has not yet been documented with clindamycin use in dogs.

37.11 SKIN

Skin infections in animals commonly require antibiotic treatment, and the organism involved is often *Staphylococcal Inter-*

medius. The incidence of beta-lactamase production by skin staphylococci is high, reaching 71% among strains isolated from referred cases of skin disease in dogs. Amoxicillin is very active against *Streptococcus Intermedius* but is susceptible to breakdown by beta-lactamase. The combination of a beta-lactamase inhibitor (clavulanate) with an effective extended spectrum penicillin such as amoxicillin may therefore be useful in the treatment of skin infections.

Antimicrobial therapy is the essential component of any treatment program for superficial and deep pyoderma. Successful therapy of skin pyoderma requires high doses of antibiotic over a relatively long period. The severity and depth will largely determine the type of treatment needed. The presence of pus in the affected lesions and the relatively poor perfusion and distribution of many antibiotics into the skin are critical factors to be taken into account.

Mild superficial pyodermas must be treated for a minimum of 10 days, whereas deeper infections such as folliculitis require 3 to 4 weeks of intensive antimicrobial therapy.

In deep chronic pyodermas, especially those involving bacterial hypersensitivity, it is usually essential to maintain therapy for weeks beyond the date of apparent clinical cure.

Oral therapy can be a distinct advantage in pyoderma therapy because treatment is usually longterm on an outpatient basis, so high oral bioavailability of the dispensed antibiotics is necessary.

Therapy may be empirically based but preferably is based on the results of bacterial culture and sensitivity tests. The most likely effective antimicrobial drugs include oxacillin, clavulanate potentiated amoxicillin, trimethoprim/sulfonamide combinations, lincomycin, clindamycin, erythromycin, chloramphenicol, enrofloxacin, cephalexin, and cefadroxil. Potentiated sulfonamides, erythromycin, and chloramphenicol are useful in empiric therapy. Penicillins, ampicillins, amoxicillins, and tetracyclines are generally poor choices because of the high risk of bacterial resistance.

Chloramphenicol can cause reversible nonregenerative anemia associated with hypocellular bone marrow. Cats tend to be more sensitive than dogs to these toxic effects, which may reflect the feline liver's reduced ability to metabolize the drug.

Many coagulase-positive staphylococci are producers of beta-lactamases, which catalyze cleavage of the beta-lactam ring of penicillins and related beta-lactam antibiotics. Accordingly, many of the penicillins are ineffective against these primary skin pathogens. Assuming that the animal patient is not immunodeficient, then either a bacteriostatic or bactericidal antibiotic may be chosen.

Although narrow-spectrum bactericidal drugs are preferred, in mixed infections, medium- or broad-spectrum antibiotics may have to be selected. Pending the results of sensitivity tests, initial antimicrobial therapy must be directed at the most likely pathogens, *staphylococci* and *streptococci*, especially *Staph. intermedius*.

First-line antibiotics include lincomycin, erythromycin, potentiated sulfonamides, and amoxicillin/clavulanate. In severe deep pyodermas, clindamycin cephalexin or enrofloxacin can be life-saving.

Inappropriate antibiotic therapy, incorrect dosage of antibiotics, inadequate duration of treatment, indiscriminate use of corticosteroids, and failure to identify the fundamental underlying cause are among the most common reasons for failure of pyoderma therapy.

When staphylococcal infection is suspected and an initial empiric regimen must be instituted before culture and sensitivity testing, beta-lactamase-resistant penicillins such as cloxacillin, oxacillin, dicloxacillin, or nafcillin provide excellent therapeutic benefit. Gastric acid degradation is minimal, and absorption from the alimentary tract is good.

Antibiotic drugs inactivated by beta-lactamase enzymes should generally be avoided because of the high frequency of involvement of staphylococci, which by producing beta-lactamase, cause cleavage of the penicillin nucleus.

Semisynthetic penicillins such as ampicillin or amoxicillin may be useful against substantial gram-negative involvement. These compounds, however, are also inactivated by beta-lactamase. If sensitivity culturing patterns indicate their potential usefulness, then ampicillin or amoxicillin can be used. Because they are stable to gastric acid, oral medication can be instituted.

Clavulanate potentiated amoxicillin protects amoxicillin from degradation by staphylococcal beta-lactamase and hence is the most preferable semisynthetic penicillin with broad-spectrum activity.

Many of the cephalosporins are highly effective against *Staphylococcus intermedius*, *Proteus* spp., and *Pseudomonas* spp. Cephalexin is particularly useful for pyoderma, and many apparently refractory cases respond to it. Because of the cross-allergenicity that exists between cephalosporins and penicillins, extreme caution must be exercised in the use of cephalosporins in animals suspected of being hypersensitive to penicillin molecules. Some of the modern (and expensive) third-generation cephalosporins such as moxalactam are best reserved for specific cases necessitating systemic therapy.

Cephalexin is indicated for deep pyodermas because of the severity of the condition, the sensitivity of *S. aureus* to the antibiotic, and the safety of the drug at high dosage rates for lengthy periods (500 mg, bid, orally). Enrofloxacin is particularly useful, but due to cartilage degenerative changes, it ought not be used on young animals.

An initial 3-week period of therapy in deep pyoderma must be maintained before re-evaluating or changing the antibiotic.

Macrolide lincosamide antibiotics (e.g., erythromycin, lincomycin) possess a directed spectrum against gram-positive bacteria including the staphylococcal group. Erythromycin has been found clinically to be a very reliable antibiotic against coagulase-positive staphylococci; a very high proportion of isolates (>80%) are sensitive to it. Erythromycin may be given systemically or more commonly orally over a longterm period. Vomiting has occasionally been associated with the oral dosage form. Erythromycin and trimethoprim/sulfadiazine possess good ability to penetrate cells.

Of the lincosamides, lincomycin is very effective as a drug of choice for many chronic nonresponsive bacterial skin conditions. It is often successful in clinical cases when many other antibiotics have failed. Highly effective against staphylococci and streptococci, it is potent against skin pathogens responsible for chronic dermatitis. While suppurative lesions caused by py-

TABLE 37–9
SUGGESTED ANTIMICROBIAL DOSAGES—SMALL ANIMALS

Drug	Dose (mg/kg)	Frequency (Hours)
Amikacin	5–10	8–12
Amoxicillin	12	12–24
Amoxicillin/Clavulanate	20	12
Amipicillin sodium	7	8–12
Ampicillin trihydrate	10–20	8–12
	7–11	12
Carbenicillin indanyl	20–30	8
Cefadroxil	11–22	12–24
Cefazolin	33	8–12
Cephalothin	10–20	5
Cephalexin	10–30	12
Chloramphenicol	50	12
Clindamycin	5.5	12
		24
		12
		24
Dihydrostreptomycin	10–20	12
Doxycycline	10	24
Enrofloxacin	2.5–5.0	12
Erythromycin	10–20	8
Gentamicin	1–3	8–12
Kanamycin	5.5	12
Lincomycin	11–22	12
Metronidazole	7.5	8–12
Norfloxacin	22	12
Oxytetracycline	10–25	8
Sulfadiazine/trimethoprim	30	12
		12
Sulfamethoxazol/trimethoprim	30	12
Tetracycline	10–25	8–12

ogenic bacteria are resistant to many of the beta-lactam antibiotics, lincomycin is very effective in many such cases and penetrates tissues effectively. Clindamycin is now available commercially as a veterinary product and like lincomycin is also effective against anaerobes. Lincomycin may cause mild diarrhea in dogs after 3 to 4 weeks of out-patient therapy.

Topical *P. aeruginosa* infections can be treated effectively with topical aminoglycosides or polymyxins.

Aminoglycoside antibiotics are not commonly indicated for pyodermas because of their narrow gram-negative spectrum of action, the likelihood of toxicity, and the possibility of the rapid induction of resistance. They cannot be given orally, because they are not absorbable into the gut. Gentamicin possesses high activity against staphylococci, *Proteus* spp., *Pseudomonas* spp., and *E. coli*. If employed judiciously, gentamicin may control many infections that are chronic as a result of secondary pseudomonal and/or *E. coli* invasion.

If staphylococci and *Proteus* spp. are involved, broad-spectrum therapy is indicated: trimethoprim/sulfonamide, clavulanate potentiated amoxicillin, and cephalexin are especially useful.

Potentiated sulfonamides, e.g., trimethoprim/sulfadiazine in oral or parenteral form, provide high skin concentrations; and because of their broad-spectrum of activity against staphylococci and gram-negative rods, they have been extensively and successfully used in canine pyodermas. Trimethoprim/sulfonamide combinations should not be employed for longer than 4 weeks because of the risk of development of keratoconjunctivitis sicca.

In summary, lincomycin, erythromycin, and oxacillin are the preferred narrow-spectrum antibiotic agents. In the event of mixed infections, potentiated sulfonamides, amoxicillin/clavulanate, enrofloxacin or chloramphenicol should be considered. Cephalexin is effective, assuming that laboratory investigation has indicated its selection. Cephalexin together with oxacillin, clindamycin, and fucidin penetrate well into fresh abrasions.

Gentamicin, amikacin, carbenicillin, or ticarcillin should be reserved for pseudomonal infections. Anaerobic complications are best treated with clindamycin, metronidazole or, as cheaper alternatives, with penicillin, tetracycline, or polymyxin B.

Although for many clinical presentations, some improvement can be noted as early as 7 to 14 days, antimicrobial therapy normally must be maintained for at least 3 weeks and possibly in extreme chronic cases for 10 weeks (Table 37–9).

SELECTED REFERENCES

Abromowicz, M. (ed.): Drugs for anaerobic infections. Med. Lett. Drugs Ther. 26:87, 1984.

Abromowicz, M. (ed.): Choice of cephalosporins. Med. Lett. Drugs Ther. 25:57, 1983.

Aron, D.N.: Pathogenesis, diagnosis and management of osteomyelitis in small animals. Compend. Contin. Ed. Pract. Vet., 1(11):824, 1979.

Bologna, M. et al.: Bactericidal intraprostatic concentrations of norfloxacin. Lancet, 2:280, 1983.

Boothe, D.M.: Drug therapy in cats: a therapeutic category approach. J. Am. Vet. Med. Assoc., 196:1659, 1990.

Boothe, D.M.: Drug therapy in cats: recommended dosing regimens. J. Am. Vet. Med. Assoc., 196:1845, 1990.

Boothe, D.M.: Drug therapy in cats. a systems approach. J. Am. Vet. Med. Assoc., 196:1502, 1990.

Boothe, D.M.: The practical aspects of treating bacterial infections in cats. Vet. Med., September:884, 1989.

Boscato, U., and Crotti, D.: Campylobacter jejuni: a major cause of enterocolitis in kennelled dogs. Clin. Vet., 53(5):303, 1985.

Braden, T.D., et al.: Posologic evaluation of clindamycin using a canine model of post-traumatic osteomyelitis. Am. J. Vet. Res., 48:1101, 1987.

Brittain, D.C.: Erythromycin. Med. Clin. North Am., 71:1147, 1987.

Brown, R.M.: Vegetative stomatitis in dogs. Mod. Vet. Pract., November: 856, 1985.

Bywater, R.J. et al.: Clavulanate-potentiated amoxicillin: activity in vitro and bioavailability in the dog. Vet. Rec., 12:33, 1985.

Cangston, V.C., and Davis, L.E.: Factors to consider in the selection of antimicrobial drugs for therapy. Compend. Contin. Ed. Pract. Vet., 11:355, 1989.

Collignon, P.J., Munro, R., and Morris, G.: Susceptibility of anaerobic bacteria to antimicrobial agents. Pathology, 20:48, 1988.

Collins, B.K., et al.: Sulfonamide-associated keratoconjunctivitis sicca and corneal ulceration in a dysuric dog. J. Am. Vet. Med. Assoc., 189:924, 1986.

Conha, B.E. et al.: The tetracyclines. Med. Clin. North Am., 66:293, 1982.

Dillon, A.R., Boosinger, T.R., and Blevins, W.T.: Campylobacter enteritis in dogs and cats. Comp. Contin. Ed. Pract. Vet., 9:1176, 1987.

Dow, S.W.: Management of anaerobic infections. Vet. Clin. North Am. Small Anim. Pract., 18:1167, 1988.

Dow, S.W., and Papich, M.G.: Keeping current on developments in antimicrobial therapy. Vet. Med., June:600, 1991.

Dow, S.W., and Papich, M.G.: An update on antimicrobials: new uses, modifications and developments. Vet. Med., July:707, 1991.

Dow, S.W. et al.: Bacteriologic specimens: selection, collection and transport for optimum results. Compend. Contin. Ed. Pract. Vet., 11:686, 1989.

Eliopoulos, G.M.: Induction of beta-lactamases. J. Antimicrob. Chemother., 22(Suppl. A):34, 1988.

Ford, R.B.: Enrofloxacin: a new antimicrobial strategy in small animal practice. In Proceedings: Quinolones Symposium. Lawrenceville, N.J., Veterinary Learning Systems, 1988.

Garg, R.C. et al.: Serum levels and pharmacokinetics of ticarcillin and clavulanic acid in dog following parenteral administration of Timentin. J. Vet. Pharmacol. Ther., 10:324, 1987.

Girard, A.E. et al.: Activity of beta-lactamase inhibitor sulbactam plus ampicillin against animal isolates of pasteurella, haemophilus and staphylococcus. Am. J. Vet. Res., 48:1678, 1987.

Greene, C.E., Cook, J.R., and Mahaffey E. A.: Clindamycin treatment of toxoplasma polymyositis in a dog. J. Am. Vet. Med. Assoc., 187:631, 1985.

Harpster, N.K.: The effectiveness of the cephalosporins in the treatment of bacterial pneumonias in the dog. J. Am. Anim. Hosp. Assoc., 17:766, 1981.

Hirsh, D.C., and Ruehl, W.W.: A rational approach to the selection of an antimicrobial agent. J. Am. Vet. Med. Assoc., 185:1058, 1984.

Holt, P.E.: The role of dogs and cats in the epidemiology of human campylobacter enterocolitis. J. Small Anim. Pract., 22:681, 1981.

Indiveri, I, and Hirsh, D.C.: Susceptibility of obligate anaerobes to trimethoprim-sulfamethoxazole. J. Am. Vet. Med. Assoc., *188*:46, 1986.

Indiveri, M.C., and Hirsh, D.C.: Clavulanic-acid-potentiated activity of amoxicillin against Bacteroides fragilis. Am. J. Vet. Res., *46*:2207, 1985.

Isenberg, H.D.: Antimicrobial susceptibility testing: a critical evaluation. J. Antimicrob. Chemother., *22*(Suppl. A):73, 1988.

Klausner, J.A., and Osborne, C.A.: Management of canine bacterial prostatitis. J. Am. Vet. Med. Assoc., *182*:292, 1983.

Lees, G.E., and Rogers, K.S.: Treatment of urinary tract infections of dogs and cats. J. Am. Vet. Med. Assoc., *189*:648, 1986.

Leib, M.S., Monroe, W.H., and Codner, E.C.: Management of chronic large bowel diarrhoea in dogs. Vet. Med., September:922, 1991.

Ling, G.V.: Therapeutic strategies involving antimicrobial treatment of the canine urinary tract. J. Am. Vet. Med. Assoc., *185*:1162, 1984.

Ling, G.V. et al.: Cephalexin for oral treatment of canine urinary tract infection caused by Klebsiella pneumoniae. J. Am. Vet. Med. Assoc., *182*:1346, 1987.

Ling, G.V. et al.: Tetracycline for oral treatment of canine urinary tract infection caused by Pseudomonas aeruginosa. J. Am. Vet. Med. Assoc., *179*:578, 1981.

Ling, G.V. et al.: Urine concentrations of five penicillins following oral administration to normal adult dogs. Am. J. Vet. Res., *41*:1123, 1980.

Ling, G.V., and Ruby, A.L.: Cephalexin for oral treatment of canine urinary tract infection caused by Klebsiella pneumoniae. J. Am. Vet. Med. Assoc., *182*:1346, 1983.

Maddison, J.E.: A guide to diagnosis and treatment of chronic diarrhoea in the dog. Aust. Vet. Pract., *20*(2):58, 1990.

Neer, T.M.: Clinical pharmacologic features of fluoroquinolone antimicrobial drugs. J. Am. Vet. Med. Assoc., *193*:577, 1988.

Neff-Davis, C.: Therapeutic drug monitoring in veterinary medicine. Vet. Clin. North Am. Small Anim. Pract., *18*:1287, 1988.

Norden, C.W.: Chronic staphylococcal osteomyelitis: treatment with regimens containing rifampin. Rev. Infect. Dis., *5*(Suppl. 3):495-S, 1983.

Olson, P.N. et al.: Disorders of the canine prostate gland: pathogenesis, diagnosis and medical therapy. Compend. Contin. Ed. Pract. Vet., *9*:613, 1987.

Ornstein, M.H., and Baird, I.M.: Dietary fibre and the colon. Mol. Aspects Med., *9*:41, 1987.

Papich, M.G.: Therapy of gram-positive infections. Vet. Clin. North Am. Small Anim. Pract., *18*:1141, 1988.

Parry, M.F.: The penicillins. Med. Clin. North Am. *71*:1093, 1987.

Prescott, J.F., and Baggot, J.D.: Antimicrobial susceptibility testing and antimicrobial drug dosage. J. Am. Vet. Med. Assoc., *187*(4):363, 1985.

Rogers, K.S. et al.: Effects of single dose and three day trimethoprim-sulfadiazine and amikacin treatment of induced Escherichia coli urinary tract infections in dogs. Am. J. Vet. Res., *49*:345, 1988.

Rudd, R.G.: A rational approach to the diagnosis and treatment of osteomyelitis. Compend. Contin. Ed. Vet. Pract., *8*:225, 1986.

Scully, B.E.: Metronidazole. Med. Clin. North. Am., *72*:613, 1988.

Senior, D.F.: Bacterial urinary tract infections: invasion, host defenses, and new approaches to prevention. Compend. Contin. Ed. Pract. Vet., *7*:334, 1985.

Shaw, D.H., and Rubin, S.I.: Pharmacologic activity of doxycycline. J. Am. Vet. Med. Assoc., *189*:808, 1986.

Sigel, C.W. et al.: Pharmacokinetics of trimethoprim and sulfadiazine in the dog: urine concentrations after oral administration. Am. J. Vet. Res., *42*:996, 1986.

Tally, F.P.: Factors affecting the choice of antibiotic in mixed infections. J. Antimicrob. Chemother., *22*(Suppl. A):87, 1988.

Tilmant, L.: Pharmacokinetics of ticarcillin in the dog. Am. J. Vet. Res., *46*:479, 1985.

Van Kruiningen, H.J.: Clinical efficacy of Tylosin in canine inflammatory bowel disease. JAAHA, *12*:498, 1976.

Watson, A.D.J.: Systemic antimicrobial drug therapy in cats. Practice, March:73, 1991.

Wilson, R.C. et al.: Pharmacokinetics of doxycycline in dogs. Can. J. Vet. Res., *52*:12, 1988.

MEDICAL THERAPY OF UROLITHS IN DOGS AND CATS

38.1 Introduction
38.2 General Therapy Principles
38.3 Canine Struvite Uroliths
38.4 Local Defense Mechanisms in the Urinary Tract
38.5 Urinary Tract Infection
38.6 Canine Cystine Uroliths
38.7 Canine Urate Uroliths
38.8 Canine Oxalate Uroliths
38.9 Feline Struvite Uroliths

38.1 INTRODUCTION

A urolith is a crystalline concretion forming in the urinary tract which contains organic or inorganic crystalloids and an organic matrix.

Urolith formation can arise through precipitation or crystallization of solutes where supersaturation of urine occurs. This triggers stone formation and growth. In some breeds a critical inhibitor of stone formation is the primary factor. Urolithiasis usually affects middle-aged or older dogs. Over 90% of stones in dogs are found in the bladder and urethra. Phosphates tend to occur more often in the bladder of the bitch, whereas urate and cystine calculi are usually found in the urethra of males.

Clinical signs associated with stone formation will obviously depend on stone location, number, size, and shape. The formation and persistence of several of crystals are influenced by pH. Different crystals tend to form and persist at different pH ranges.

Uroliths always represent a predisposing cause of urinary tract infection (UTI) and are always a predisposition to obstructive uropathy. Four major types of renal stones commonly are found in the dog: struvite, calcium oxalate, cystine, and uric acid.

In the dog, and especially in the bitch, when the main crystalline component is magnesium ammonium phosphate (struvite), there is usually a bacterial infection in the urinary tract, and the pH usually exceeds 7.0. Various urinary acidifiers have been used, varying from ammonium chloride, methionine, methenamine mandelate, and ascorbic acid.

In the cat the crystalline component most commonly encountered is struvite, although calcium oxalate, ammonium acid urate, and calcium hydrogen phosphate have been identified in individual cases.

The advent of effective medical protocols to dissolve and prevent uroliths in dogs and cats has resulted in renewed interest in detection and interpretation of crystalluria.

Evaluation of urine crystals may aid in the detection of disorders predisposing animals to urolith formation, the medical composition of the uroliths, and the evaluation of the effectiveness of medical protocols to treat or prevent urolithiasis.

Knowledge of the mineral composition of crystals is of diagnostic, prognostic, and therapeutic significance. Minerals that precipitate in urine often form crystals with characteristic shapes. The characteristic microscopic shape of mineral crystals and is commonly used as an index of crystal composition.

Factors involved in urine crystal formation include the following:

1. pH: Different crystals tend to form and persist in certain pH ranges, e.g., alkaline Ph for phosphate stones in dogs, acidic Ph for cystine stones.
2. Diet: This influences crystalluria (including water intake).

Crystalluria may also be influenced by diet, including water intake. Crystals sometimes may be drug related, and drug-associated crystals in dogs and cats include those resulting from sulfadiazine therapy. In humans drug-related crystalluria includes ampicillin, ciprofloxacin, primidone, and 6-mercaptopurine.

TYPES OF UROLITHS

Most canine uroliths are struvite; far fewer are calcium oxalate. The most commonly encountered uroliths in dogs follow:

Magnesium ammonium phosphate hexahydrate (struvite)
Calcium oxalate in the monohydrate and dihydrate forms
Uric acid and its salts (ammonium and sodium urate); calcium phosphate, cystine, and silica

With the advent of effective treatment protocols to dissolve magnesium ammonium phosphate uroliths and consistent use of quantitative methods of urolith analysis, the frequency of struvite uroliths has been declining, while that of calcium oxalate has been increasing.

38.2 GENERAL THERAPY PRINCIPLES

Although surgery has been an effective method for removal of uroliths, it is associated with several limitations:

TABLE 38–1
UROLITHIASIS—GENERAL THERAPY PRINCIPLES

(a) Surgery but
- Persistance of underlying cause
- Failure to remove all fragments
- May be necessary where medical therapy fails

(b) Medical Dissolution
- Identify urolith (X-ray diffraction/ optical crystallography
- Manipulate urine pH—to optimum level
- Treat urinary tract infection (3–6 weeks)
- Ensure copious water intake
- Induction of polyuria
- Use calculolytic/prescription diets

E.G.
Dietary management meets special needs, Most prescription diets aid in the dissolution of certain bladder stones.
—By reducing protein intake, ammonia ion concentration is reduced. Reduction of magnesium and phosphorus minimized excretion of these elements.

1. Persistence of underlying causes and the high rate of recurrence of uroliths despite surgery.
2. Patient factors that enhance adverse consequences of general anesthesia or surgery.
3. The inability to remove all uroliths or fragments of uroliths during surgery.

Surgery, however, remains the preferred initial option for certain animals, namely, the following:

1. Animals with urolith-induced obstruction to urine outflow that cannot be corrected by nonsurgical techniques.
2. Animals with uroliths that are refractory to current methods of medical dissolution (e.g., sodium calcium oxalate and calcium phosphate).
3. Animals with uroliths that are increasing in size and number despite medical therapy designed to inhibit their growth or cause their dissolution.
4. Animals with concurrent renal dysfunction for which the time required for medical dissolution would be too long.

Although surgery can play a very important role in the management of uroliths, medical therapy alone may suffice in some cases. Sometimes, if surgery is the only form of treatment, a persistent type of urinary tract disease may develop, and urolithiasis may recur.

The main objectives of medical management of canine uroliths are to promote urolith dissolution by correcting or controlling underlying abnormalities, to arrest further growth of existing uroliths, and/or to inhibit new urolith formation.

The medical management of the condition must deal with the relief of the obstruction and the normalization of the urine flow, medical dissolution of the calculi, and medical management oriented toward preventing recurrence.

For therapy to be effective, it must rehydrate the animal to induce undersaturation of the urine, increase the volume of urine, reduce the quantity of calculogenic crystalloids in the urine, and adjust pH. Medical therapy must be monitored by observation of urine pH, degree of crystalluria, and ra-

---

TABLE 38–2
FACTORS AFFECTING URINE CRYSTAL FORMATION

(1) *Diet*/Feeding Habits → Precursor of urolith concretions
(2) *pH* → Various uroliths form and persist depending on pH
(3) *Water Intake* → Affects supersaturation and concentration of crystalloids
(4) *Drugs* → Many possess tendencies towards crystalluria (depending on local pH and water balance)
(5) *Infection* → Urinary tract infection may increase rate of urolith formation
(6) *Inherited* Disorders → : Breed susceptibility
(7) *Congenital* Disorders

---

diographic or ultrasonographic evaluation of the uroliths.

General medical therapy for urolithiasis involves fluid and electrolyte therapy to increase normal water and electrolyte balance. If surgery has been necessary attention must be directed toward the induction of polyuria and the eradication of UTI. Polyuria is necessary to reduce the specific gravity of the urine, thus reducing the relative concentration of crystalloids.

Increasing the output of urine by dietary salt administration (0.4 to 8 g/day) has been used to reduce the urine specific gravity to suitable limits. Addition of water to the animal's food or wet food feeding may be necessary. Intensive antimicrobial therapy may be needed when UTI is present.

Induced polyuria is also useful to reduce the concentration of crystalloid substances. Adding sodium chloride tablets or salt to food is recommended as is the addition of water. Bladder distension and stasis of urine must be avoided and care taken to prevent infection of the urinary tract. Fluid and electrolyte therapy must be instituted when severe obstruction and postrenal azotemia occur.

38.3 CANINE STRUVITE UROLITHS

Phosphate stones are quite common, especially in association with bacterial UTI in females. The bladder is the common site of phosphate calculi. A significantly high incidence of staphylococcal UTI occurs in dogs with phosphate stones. The staphylococci in most cases are urease and coagulase positive, and it is now thought that the liberation of ammonia from urea by bacterial urease reduces the solubility of struvite and provides ammonium ions for stone formation. The major component of phosphate calculi is magnesium ammonium phosphate hexahydrate (struvite).

Struvite crystals and the subsequent formation of struvite stones occur when the precursor dietary substances are in high concentration in the urine and the urine pH is alkaline. Precursor substances include the minerals magnesium phosphorous and ammonium. The magnesium and phosphorous levels in the urine are directly related to the amount in the diet.

The important predisposing factors include UTIs with increased urease-producing microbes (especially staphylococci) and

---

TABLE 38–3
EXCESSIVE PRECIPITATION OF MINERAL SALTS IN URINE

- Unsatisfactory dietary intake
- Presence of suitable urinary pH for urolith formation
- Presence of urea-splitting pathogens from U.T.I.
- Inadequate water intake

excretion of a sufficient quantity of urea in urine. Medical therapy must be geared to modify both of these factors.

Underlying bacterial infection, especially with urease producers, must receive priority in therapy. This is because modification of urinary pH using acidifiers alone is ineffective against infection.

Following surgical removal of phosphate (struvite) stones, the medical therapy of urolithiasis consists of

1. elimination of infection,
2. induction of polyuria, and
3. acidification of the urine.

Eradication or control of UTI that is due to urease-producing bacteria is the most important factor in preventing recurrence of struvite uroliths. If chronic UTI persists, therapy with high dosage of antimicrobial agents eliminated in high concentrations in urine is indicated. These include betalactam antibiotics and trimethoprim/sulfonamide. Bacteria may remain viable within the struvite uroliths despite antibiotic therapy, antimicrobials must be continued until there is no radiographic evidence of uroliths.

Calculolytic diets designed to acidify urine can be effective for sterile canine urolithiasis.

Calculolytic diets low in high-quality protein and reduced concentrations of magnesium and phosphorous may be required. Additional sodium chloride may be useful to increase thirst and stimulate urine production.

Urea concentration must be reduced (the substrate for urease) and also that of phosphorous and magnesium.

Struvite and hydroxyapatite are more soluble in acid urine, and so acidification is desirable. Dosage of acidifiers must be adjusted daily in accordance with pH testing of urine.

Polyuria must be induced by the addition of salt to the diet, and low-phosphate, low-magnesium diet should be fed.

Dietary habits and breed predisposition can play a role in struvite urolithiasis. Miniature schnauzers are particularly susceptible.

Struvite crystals are often observed when urine pH is alkaline.

For struvite uroliths, if recurrent UTI persists, indefinite therapy with prophylactic doses of antimicrobials that are eliminated in high concentration in urine such as nitrofurantoin and trimethoprim sulfa is indicated.

It has been clearly established that in the dog and bitch in particular, when the main component of struvite is magnesium ammonium phosphate (struvite), there is usually a bacterial UTI, and normally in such cases, the pH exceeds 7.0. Apart from urinary acidifiers, induced diuresis can also be quite beneficial by reducing the concentration of ions and of the urine specific gravity and by stimulating frequent micturition, thus reducing the stagnant time of urine in the bladder.

Elimination of the underlying bacterial infection is crucial and can take a long time, and in common with therapy of most UTIs, antimicrobial therapy must be maintained for 3 to 4 weeks or so before the urine becomes sterile on bacteria culturing.

Urinary acidification is beneficial in canine medicine. Major benefits include the following:

1. Formation of acidic urine that is bacteriostatic and less suitable for bacterial growth.
2. Increased effectiveness of certain antimicrobial agents in the treatment of UTI, e.g., penicillin, other beta lactams, tetracycline, nitrofurantoin, chloramphenicol.
3. Assistance in the prevention and treatment of struvite urinary calculi.

Several acidifiers have commonly been used in dogs and cats including DL-methionine, ascorbic acid, ethylenediamine dihydrochloride, ammonium chloride, and acid phosphate salts.

Acidifiers (ammonium chloride) given every 10 to 12 hours can potentiate the action of penicillin, amoxicillin, and nitrofurantoin if the urine is initially alkaline as a result of bacterial action. However, central nervous system (CNS) and gastrointestinal tract (GIT) disturbances have been reported with the use of DL-methionine. Ascorbic acid must be given 4 times per day to maintain urine acidity. Ammonium salts induce gastric irritation, and the effectiveness of ammonium chloride is limited to short periods. Persistent diarrhea can be observed in some dogs during ammonium chloride therapy.

TABLE 38–4
URINARY ACIDIFIERS

- Ammonium chloride
- D-L methionine
- Ascorbic acid
- Ethylene diamine dihydrochloride
- Acid phosphate salts

The decline in the incidence of canine struvite urolithiasis has tended to coincide with the increasing use of a calculolytic diet.

38.4 LOCAL DEFENSE MECHANISMS IN THE URINARY TRACT

The mucosa of the urinary bladder has a thin layer of mucopolysaccharide on its surface composed of glycosaminoglycan. This layer plays a major role in the inhibition of bacterial adhesion and colonization. Water molecules bound by this layer form a barrier that prevents urine contaminants from contacting bladder epithelium. Abnormal functioning in this protective layer can occur with recurrent UTI.

Destruction of the protective layer allows bacterial attachment.

The production and secretion of the normal protective glycosaminoglycan layer appears to be under hormonal control by estrogen and progesterone.

Bacterial adhesion to uroepithelium is achieved by fimbriae, which bind to complementary receptor sites on epithelial cell surfaces.

This bacterial adherence is essential to subsequent tissue invasion, enzyme production (e.g., urease), and possibly urolith formation.

38.5 URINARY TRACT INFECTION

UTI must be identified from the results of laboratory tests; the ultimate confirmation is urine culture. The next step is to determine the anatomic site of the infection. Failure to appropriately manage UTI carries potentially serious consequences for the patient: pyelonephritis, cystitis, urethritis, or prostatitis. Struvite urolithiasis may result from UTI with urease-producing microbes such as staphylococci and *Proteus* spp. UTI may also cause bacteremia and septicemia, particularly when the kidney or prostate gland is affected.

MANAGING LOWER URINARY TRACT INFECTION

Antimicrobial agents used to treat lower UTI should be given at high dosages every 8 to 12 hours. This frequency will sustain high antibiotic concentrations in the urine.

For uncomplicated lower UTI in dogs, treatment should continue for at least 2 weeks. Shorter treatment periods (e.g., a single large dose administered once, or a 3-day duration of therapy) have been evaluated in female dogs but have met with variable success.

TABLE 38–5
INDICATION FOR URINARY ACIDIFICATION

- Prevention/treatment of struvite calculi
- Formation of acidic urine less susceptible to bacterial infection
- To increase effectiveness of certain antibiotics in the urinary tract e.g., beta lactam antibiotics, chloramphenicol, tetracyclines, nitrofurantoin, methenamine mandelate

---

TABLE 38–6
TREATING URINARY TRACT INFECTION

Ensure the antibiotic displays:
• Adequate spectrum of antimicrobial activity
• Elimination in the active form
• Activity at the urine pH
• Appropriate ion trapping/diffusion into appropriate tissue
• Lack of toxicity
• Oral bioavailability

Examples:

Cystitis	—Fluoroquinolones
	—Trimethoprim/sulfonamide
	—Tetracyclines
	—Betalactams
Pyelonephritis	—Betalactam antibiotics ± clavulanic acid
Prostatitis	—Enrofloxacin
	—Trimethoprim/Sulfonamide
	—Clindamycin
	—Doxycycline
	—Chloramphenicol
	—Erythromycin

Ancillary therapy (e.g., administration of urinary acidifiers, antiseptics, and analgesics) is not used routinely, because it is usually not needed if antimicrobial therapy is effective.

It is essential to identify the bacterial pathogen in order to make a rational antibiotic choice. Most strains of staphylococci or streptococci isolates can be successfully treated with ampicillin or amoxicillin/clavulanate. Nearly 80% of *E. coli*, *Proteus* spp., and *Klebsiella* spp. isolates can be usually successfully treated with trimethoprim/sulfadiazine, ampicillin, and cephalexin, respectively. Although *Pseudomonas* spp. are uniformly resistant to tetracycline, this drug nonetheless can sometimes be effective in pseudomonal infections because of the drug's relatively high urine concentration. Carbenicillin or ticarcillin are alternatives in pseudomonas treatment.

Newer members of the fluoroquinolone family, enrofloxacin and norfloxacin are excreted primarily by the kidneys and achieve high urine levels. They also have a broad spectrum of antimicrobial activity, including activity against *Pseudomonas* spp., and are bactericidal. They penetrate tissues well—including the prostate. From human comparative studies, the fluoroquinolones appear to be as good as trimethoprim/

sulfonamide and ampicillin and perhaps are more effective than nalidixic acid and nitrofurantoin.

For uncomplicated lower UTI in females, treatment should continue for 10 to 14 days. Intact male dogs with lower UTI should be treated for at least 3 weeks because of the possibility of prostatic infection. In both sexes the urine should be cultured 3 to 5 days after starting therapy and 10 to 14 days after stopping therapy.

For recurrent gram-negative infection, trimethoprim/sulfadiazine is a good choice; for gram-positive infection, cephalexin ampicillin/amoxicillin should be successful. Adjunctive therapy such as administration of urinary acidifiers, antiseptics, and analgesics is not used routinely because it is not needed if antimicrobial therapy is effective.

For prostate disease, basic antibiotics are largely un-ionized at blood pH and thus are better able to cross the blood prostate barrier and achieve therapeutic concentrations with the prostate gland. This category includes trimethoprim, erythromycin, and clindamycin. The newer fluoroquinolones—ciprofloxacin, norfloxacin, and enrofloxacin—also achieve high concentrations within the prostate gland. The fact that the prostatic fluid of most dogs with bacterial prostatitis is more acidic than plasma increases the degree of ionization of basic drugs, and this contributes to the ion-trapping phenomenon. When animals receive longterm sulfonamide-type medication (>6 weeks), the risk of keratoconjunctivitis sicca and folate-deficiency anemia should be considered. Folic acid, 6 to 10 mg/kg, might be useful during longterm therapy. Cephalexin is also a useful antibiotic for prostatitis although traditionally potentiated sulfonamides are the drug of choice.

38.6 CANINE CYSTINE UROLITHS

Canine cystine uroliths result from an inherited metabolic defect that allows excretion of abnormal quantities of cystine (a nonessential sulfur-containing amino acid) in urine. Because cystinuria is an inherited defect, cystine uroliths tend to recur.

Cystinuria in the dog is an inborn metabolic defect in which the renal tubules secrete abnormally large amounts of amino acids, cystine, lysine, ornithine, and arginine.

Cystine urolithiasis is mainly a problem in male dogs, with the dachshund being particularly susceptible. Cystine stones are most often found in the bladder and urethra. UTI is not invariably present when cystine stones are found.

Induction of polyuria, alkalinization of urine, and the administration of D-penicillamine underpin the medical management of this condition.

Polyuria induced by the addition of salt to the diet will reduce the relative concentration of cystine in the urine and reduce the risk of urolith formation. Because cystine is more soluble at alkaline pH than it is at acidic pH, alkalinization of urine to pH 7.5 is usually recommended. This can be brought about by administration of 0.8 to 1.2 g of sodium bicarbonate per 5 kg body weight. Low-sodium diets are useful in this condition, because dietary sodium may enhance cystinuria. Potassium citrate therefore may be preferred to sodium bicarbonate as a urine alkalinizer.

The amino acid methionine is a precursor of cystine, and hence a diet low in methionine should minimize formation of cystine uroliths. A low-protein diet, by reducing the quantity of urea formation, promotes formation of dilute urine.

Reduction in size of cystine uroliths can be effected by a protein-restricted diet and orally administered alkalinizers. Addition of 2-mercaptopropionylglycine (2-MPG) assists dissolution of uroliths. Orally administered 2-MPG (30 mg/kg) to dogs with cystine uroliths is recommended as beneficial in inducing stone dissolution and preventing cystine stone recurrence. (This drug is similar in activity to D-penicillamine but is less toxic.)

D-penicillamine can be given at a dose of 30 mg/kg divided into two doses per day. Side effects are common with D-penicillamine, most noticeably vomiting. The drug should be given with food or by using antiemetics. D-penicillamine (Distamine) used in humans allows the excretion of cystine as the soluble cystine-penicillamine complex, but this drug can have side effects such as vomiting, proteinuria, leukopenia, and loss of taste. If it is used, the dog must have continuous blood monitoring. A low methionine/cystine diet appears to be a logical practice to prevent the occurrence of this type of calculi. A combination of appropriate prescription diet with 2-MPG, 30-40 mg/kg/day, has proved successful in some cases.

Cystine calculi have a tendency to recur, and repeat surgery is often necessary. Male castrates show the highest incidence.

38.7 CANINE URATE UROLITHS

Uric acid and ammonium acid urate calculi are thought to form as a result of a renal tubular resorbtion defect. (The condition occurs frequently in dalmation dogs.)

Uric acid is a metabolic breakdown product of purines, and in most animals it is converted to allantoin enzymatically in the liver. In dalmatians, impaired transport of uric acid into hepatocytes occurs, and hence the rate of hepatic oxidation is decreased. This, together with reduced proximal tubular resorption and increased active tubular secretion of uric acid in the dalmation, may explain why the breed is more susceptible than most to urate stones. Blockage of the urethra in male dogs is the most common finding in urate urolithiasis.

Uric acid crystals form only in acid urine. Prevention keeps the urine above pH 6.5 by administration of 0.5 g of sodium bicarbonate in each meal. Addition of salt to the diet is the normal procedure for induction of polyuria and the reduction of the concentration of urates in the urine.

Bicarbonate therapy for urinary alkalinization is often recommended for urate stones, but equivocal results are often seen. Low-offal diets may contribute to a lowering of the offal load.

Allopurinol is an important drug in treating urate uroliths. Xanthine oxidase is the key enzyme that converts hypoxanthine to xanthine and xanthine to uric acid in the course of purine metabolism. Allopurinol competitively inhibits xanthine oxidase, which decreases the rate of conversion of hypoxanthine to xanthine and xanthine to uric acid, thus reducing the amount of uric acid formed. Usually, the drug is given at a dosage of 20 to 30 mg/kg divided into two daily doses for 3 weeks followed by 10 mg/kg. The dose must be carefully controlled because an overdose will produce xanthine, and xanthine calculi can then be found. Approximately 8 to 9 mg/day appears to be safe in most animals.

The efficacy of allopurinol depends on its conversion to oxypurinol in the liver, and its efficacy in reducing the formation of uric acid may therefore be reduced in ammonium urate urolith-forming patients with portovascular shunts. Allopurinol and oxypurinol are eliminated through the kidneys. In humans, the drug is often associated with adverse reactions in uremic patients. It must therefore be used with caution to animals with renal dysfunction. Urates are less soluble in alkaline urine, hence the use of bicarbonate alkalinizers, low protein diet, and induction of polyuria. Withdrawal of allopurinol can lead to recurrence of urate stones. Ammonium urates tend to be seen in animals with hepatic circulatory anomalies.

38.8 CANINE OXALATE UROLITHS

Canine oxalate uroliths may be caused by excess oxalate or excess calcium in the diet. These stones have sharp edges and can cause physical damage to the urinary tract. The animal must be encouraged to drink water, but a reduced calcium intake is necessary. Hence, high-calcium products such as milk, cheese, fish with bones, or even mammal bones should be avoided. Application of salt to the food may encourage fluid intake.

In contrast to struvite and urate uroliths, which readily dissolve when oversaturation of urine with calculogenic substances is abolished, calcium oxalate uroliths in dogs are less amenable to dissolution. These uroliths can occur in alkaline, neutral, or acidic pH urine, so manipulation of urinary pH is not of key importance. In general, medical protocols should be formatted in a stepwise fashion to reduce the urine concentration of calculogenic substances.

Thiazide diuretics should be avoided in hypercalcemic hypercalciuric patients because these drugs may aggravate the hypercalcemia.

In normacalcemic patients, oral potassium citrate and avoidance of excessive dietary calcium oxalate protein or ascorbic acid may be useful.

Attempts should be made to induce polyuria in hyper- and normocalcemic patients, excess dietary sodium supplements should be avoided.

When stone formation is due to oxalate, salt can be administered to induce polyuria, and any UTI must be treated with appropriate antimicrobial therapy.

Because oxalate crystal formation occurs over a wide pH range 4.5 to 8.0, manipulation of urinary pH is not warranted. A low-protein diet is usually recommended, and the presence of oxalate crystals arising from ethylene glycol poisoning should not be ignored.

Reduction in dietary calcium must be accompanied by reduction in dietary oxalate. Milk and milk products can augment intestinal absorption of calcium from dietary sources.

Ingestion of foods that contain high quantities of animal protein (meat, poultry, fish) may contribute to calcium oxalate urolithiasis by increasing urine calcium and uric acid concentrations and decreasing urine citrate concentrations. Excessive protein consumption should be avoided in dogs with active calcium oxalate urolithiasis.

A diet moderately restricted in protein calcium, oxalate, and sodium is usually recommended to help prevent recurrence of calcium oxalate uroliths in dogs with active urolithiasis.

Sodium salts should not be given to promote diuresis in patients with calcium oxalate uroliths. Vitamins C and D should be avoided, because as vitamin C is a precursor of oxalic acid and vitamin D may augment hypercalcemia. Also, urinary acidifiers should be avoided because they tend to augment hypercalcemia.

Complex factors included here are hypercalciuria, hyperoxaluria, and hyperuricosuria.

38.9 FELINE STRUVITE UROLITHS

The primary use of urinary acidifiers in feline practice has been to reduce struvite crystalluria and induce stone dissolution in cats with feline urologic syndrome (FUS). FUS is a disorder of the feline urologic tract characterized by the presence of mineral crystals ("or sand"), which can irritate the lining of the urinary tract or block the urethra.

Struvite is by far the most common urolith in the cat, and most cases will recur if no postobstruction treatment is given. It is therefore essential to take active measures to prevent crystalluria (e.g., urinary acidification, NaCl administration, low magnesium diet).

If surgery is necessary, the immediate postobstructive period, it is essential to administer fluids while the cat is still anesthetized. Normal saline or balanced electrolytes, 100 ml, should be given, followed by more balanced electrolytes given subcutaneously.

Longterm treatment involves medical management because a cat affected with acute urethral obstruction is more likely to be fed a dry cat food, be overweight, and drink less water.

Addition of 50 to 60 ml of water to the diet is useful to increase the urinary volume, lower the urine specific gravity, and reduce microcrystalluria. Longterm preventive treatment also includes urinary acidification and administration of chlorethamine, methionine, ammonium chloride, ethylene diamine dihydrochloride, ammonium sulfate, and ascorbic acid. Megestrol

acetate has been reported successful in controlling recurrent cystitis in cats.

In cats there are three major ways to alleviate clinical signs of struvite urolithiasis:

1. Surgery
2. Adding a sufficient amount of an effective urine acidifier such as ammonium chloride or DL methionine to a magnesium-restricted diet
3. Feeding a calculolytic diet

Ammonium chloride is the best urinary acidifier in cats but immature cats are more susceptible to toxicity with ammonium chloride and DL methionine. The recommended dose of ammonium chloride is 200 mg/kg daily, mixed thoroughly in the food to mask its very bitter taste. The use of acidifiers can be stopped when cats become accustomed to diets low in magnesium.

Feeding patterns affect urinary pH and thus the propensity to struvite crystal formation. The rise in incidence of struvite urolithiasis at the onset of adulthood is associated with a concurrent rise in urinary pH.

For feline urolithiasis, dietary management is effective unless UTI, especially UTI with urease-producing organisms, is present. This underlines the need for urine culture and appropriate antibiotic therapy.

While dietary control is an obvious approach to treatment, an alternative is to use an orally administered urinary acidifier. The cat can then be permitted to eat what it likes.

Magnesium can contribute to the formation of uroliths in cats, and hence low-magnesium diets are recommended for the avoidance of bladder stones. Magnesium is only a problem, however, if low urine acidity is not maintained. Preparing diets that increase urine acidity tends to be easier than removing magnesium from good ingredients.

Key components in inducing dissolution of most struvite uroliths in cats appear to be (1) reduction of urine pH to 6.0 or less; (2) reduction of urine magnesium or consumption of magnesium-restricted diets; (3) control of urinary tract infections; (4) use of calculolytic diets; and (5) ensure adequate water intake.

Although the term FUS covers a number of urologic diseases in cats, most clinical cases include urethral obstruction by plugs that incorporate struvite crystals. Crystals of struvite (magnesium ammonium phosphate hexahydrate) tend to form more rapidly in alkaline solution.

For struvite crystals to form, the urine must be supersaturated with the components of struvite, i.e., magnesium ammonium and ammonia phosphate. The urinary concentration of magnesium can be lowered by restricting magnesium in the diet. Excessive magnesium may be present in many commercial foods because they are made from components high in magnesium such as corn, soybean, or high ash meat and bone, fish, or poultry meats.

If the pH is low enough, struvite crystallization may be prevented without restricting dietary magnesium. Diets that produce an acid urine are no more expensive to manufacture than are urine-neutral or urine-alkalinizing diets.

Urinary acidifiers have been used to prevent struvite crystalluria and urethral obstruction in cats. They can also prevent struvite stone formation and induce the dissolution of experimental and struvite bladder stones. In cats the risk of developing struvite crystalluria decreases as the urine pH is progressively reduced below 6.6. Therefore, the ideal urinary acidifier must maintain urinary pH around 6.0.

Urinary acidifiers commonly recommended for use in cats include ammonium chloride; DL-methionine, combinations of ammonium chloride and DL-methionine and ethylenediamine dihydrochloride.

Use of urinary acidifiers has been based on the theory that preventing or minimizing struvite crystal formation favorably influences the clinical course of disease. Struvite crystals are more soluble in acidic than in alkaline urine.

All acidifiers can be toxic by inducing acidosis, and ammonium chloride also can be toxic by increasing the blood ammonium concentration. Ammonium chloride, however, is particularly useful because it can be administered over the longterm. Furthermore, the drug is inexpensive, easy to obtain, and has long-lasting effects. (Its biochemical properties are well understood.) Gelatin capsules containing 550 mg of pure ammonium chloride crystals given twice daily have proven effective in the control of this condition in cats.

Some problems exist with the use of urinary acidifiers, especially in cats. (Toxicity has occurred in kittens ingesting ammonium chloride methionine combinations.)

Because high doses of ammonium chloride occasionally irritate the GIT of carnivores, it is frequently combined with DL-methionine. The daily dose ranges from 80 to 200 mg/kg/day, of both ammonium chloride and DL-methionine. CNS and GIT disorders have been reported with DL-methionine.

Young or adult animals with impaired renal function may be more vulnerable to acidosis than healthy adult cats. A male cat that has undergone bouts of obstruction may have temporary or permanently impaired renal function and may be less capable of excreting acid than a normal cat.

Because ammonium is toxic to the CNS, an increase in blood ammonia concentration is another potential complication of use of ammonium chloride.

When part of the urinary tract system is colonized by micro-organisms, a UTI is present. Pathogens usually invade by ascending the tract. Whereas individual strains of bacteria can give rise to infection, two or more organisms are usually present in up to 20% of cases.

Cystitis in cats generally reoccurs frequently, and these attacks can be treated by short courses of the appropriate antibiotic. Frequent reinfections, however, generally require longterm antibiotic therapy. The antimicrobial drugs most suited to longterm therapy are nitrofurantoin 10 to 15 mg/kg, amoxicillin 10 to 30 mg/kg, trimethoprim/sulfa 30 mg/kg, and cefalalexin 15 to 30 mg/kg. Nitrofurantoin must be given with food to prevent nausea and can be safely given for months when used as a urinary antiseptic. Megestrol acetate 5 mg/day over one week is useful to reduce inflammation of the bladder.

SELECTED REFERENCES

Bernard, M.A.: Therapy of feline urethral obstruction. Can. Vet. J., 25:443, 1984.

Bovee, K.C.: Canine cystine urolithiasis. Vet. Clin. North Am., 16:211, 1986.

Finco, D.R., Barsanti, J.A., and Cromwell, W.A.: Characterization of magnesium induced urinary disease in the cat and comparison with feline urological syndrome. Am. J. Vet. Res., *46*:391, 1985.

Frenier, S.L., and Dhein, C.R.: Uncovering the cause of urinary incontinence in pets. Vet. Med., May:500, 1990.

Kramer, J.W.: Identification of Hippuric acid crystals in the urine of ethylene glycol intoxicated dogs and cats. JAVMA, *184*:584, 1984.

Lees, G.E., and Rogers, K.S.: Treatment of urinary tract infections in dogs and cats. JAVMA, *189*(6):648, 1986.

Lewis, L.D., and Morris, M.C.: Economics and rationale of dietary management of feline urological syndrome. Mod. Vet. Pract., October:723, 1985.

Ling, G.V.: Therapeutic strategies involving antimicrobial treatment of the canine urinary tract. JAVMA, *185*:1162, 1984.

Lloyd, W.E., and Sullivan, D.J.: Effects of orally administered ammonium chloride and methionine on feline urinary acidity. Vet. Med./SAC., *79*(6):773, 1984.

Malinverni, R., and Glauser, M.P.: Comparative studies of fluoroquinolones in the treatment of urinary tract infections. Rev. Infect. Dis., *10*:S153, 1988.

Moreau, P.M.: Disorders of the lower urinary tract in old dogs. Vet. Rec., *126*:415, 1990.

Osborne, C.A.: Crystalluria, observations, interpretations and misinterpretations. Vet. Clin. North Am., *16*:45, 1986.

Osborne, C.A. et al.: Strategy for non-surgical removal of canine struvite uroliths. *In* American Animal Hospital Association 49th Annual Proceedings. Edited by　　　　　1982.

Osborne, C.A., and Clinton, C.W.: Prevalence of canine uroliths. Minnesota Urolith Center. Vet. Clin. North Am., *16*:27, 1986.

Osborne, C.A., and Kruger, J.M.: Prospective clinical evaluation of feline struvite urolith dissolution. *In* Proceedings 4th Ann. ACVIM. 1986.

Osborne, C.A., Luylich, J.P., Bartges, J.W., and Felice, L.J.: Medical dissolution and prevention of canine and feline uroliths: diagnostic and therapeutic caveats. Vet. Rec., *127*:369, 1990.

Osborne, C.A. et al.: Analyzing the mineral composition of uroliths from dogs, cats, horses, sheep, goats and pigs. Vet. Med., August:750, 1989.

Rogers, K.S.: Effects of a single dose and three day trimethoprim-sulfadiazine and amikacin treatment of induced Esherichia coli urinary tract infections in dogs. Am. J. Vet. Res., *49*:345, 1988.

Rogers, Q.R., and Morris, J.G.: The effect of diet on feline struvite urolithiasis syndrome. *In* Proceedings of the Purina Faculty Symposium. St. Louis. 1987.

Senior, D.F.: Bacterial urinary tract infections: invasion, host defenses and new approaches to prevention. Compend. Contin. Educ. Pract. Vet., *7*:334, 1985.

Senior, D.F., Sunderstrom, D.A., and Wolfson, B.B.: Testing the effects of ammonium chloride and DL methionine on the urinary pH of cats. Vet. Med., January:88, 1986.

Shaw, D.H.: A systematic approach to managing lower urinary tract infections. Vet. Med., April:379, 1990.

Taton, G.F.: Evaluation of ammonium chloride as a urinary acidifier in the cat. JAVMA, *184*:433, 1984.

Taton, G.F.: Urinary acidification in the prevention and treatment of feline struvite urolithiasis. JAVMA, *184*:437, 1984.

Taton, G.F., Hamar, D.W., and Lewis, L.D.: Urinary acidification in the prevention and treatment of feline struvite urolithiasis. JAVMA, *184*:437, 1984.

Wilson, R.A.: Strains of Escherichia coli associated with urogenital disease in dogs and cats. Am. J. Vet. Res., *49*:743, 1988.

39

PRESCRIPTION DIETS

39.1 Diets for Obesity
39.2 Diets in Chronic Renal Failure
39.3 Diets for Feline Urologic Syndrome
39.4 Diets for Gastrointestinal Tract Diseases
39.5 Concentrated Diets: Convalescence

39.1 DIETS FOR OBESITY

Obesity is the most common nutritional disease of dogs, cats, and people, exceeding by far all deficiency diseases combined. Obesity is considered present when body weight is 15–20% more than optimum; health problems begin increasing at this weight.

On the basis of clinical examination, 30% of dogs and many cats are more than 15% overweight. Health and longevity are impaired because of locomotion and respiratory difficulties, heart disease, neoplastic diseases, hypertension, impaired hepatic function, reduced reproductive ability, reduced heat tolerance, decreased resistance to infectious diseases, increased dystocia, irritability, dermatosis, hormonal problems, surgical risk, diabetes mellitus, and mobility problems.

There are two stages of obesity: initial and static. During the initial stage, when obesity is developing, caloric intake exceeds expenditure of energy. During the static stage, caloric intake equals expenditure of energy, and excess body weight is maintained. Excess caloric intake is caused by or predisposed to by factors that interfere with either internal (physiologic) or external (environmental) signals that induce satiety.

Obesity in dogs is more common in females than males up to 12 years of age and is about twice as high in neutered as non-neutered dogs of either sex. Conversely, only about one half as many neutered as non-neutered dogs of both sexes are underweight.

Spayed females are twice as likely to be obese as are other dogs. The usual weight gain seen commonly is after ovariohysterectomy can be controlled by monitoring diet and exercise; however, hormonal factors may play a role in obesity. Estrogen has been found to inhibit the food intake of rats, sheep, and pigs and may likewise deter food intake and weight gain in intact bitches.

Large concentrations of follicle-stimulating hormone in spayed females may also contribute to obesity. In neutered males, lack of the anabolic effects of testosterone may foster obesity as a result of decreased amino acid deposition into muscle protein, with more energy going into fat. Adminis-

tration of corticosteroids can also contribute to obesity by boosting the animal's appetite.

Genetic predisposition to obesity may exist among some breeds and strains. Labrador retrievers; cairn, West Highland, and Scottish terriers; cocker spaniels; and collies all have a greater tendency toward obesity than other breeds.

As dogs age, the risk of obesity increases. This tendency of older dogs is probably due to reduction both in metabolic rate and physical activity.

PROBLEMS OF OBESITY

Obesity occurs with or predisposes to any one or combination of the following factors:

Joint or locomotion problems: More than 24% of overtly obese dogs have serious locomotion problems. Arthritis, herniated intervertebral disks, and ruptured anterior cruciate ligaments can all be caused by carrying excessive weight.

Respiratory difficulties, particularly with exercise: These problems are caused by the increased oxygen necessary to supply the increased body mass and additional mass against the chest wall, which increases respiratory effort, reduces respiratory efficiency, and may lead to alveolar hypoventilation.

Hypertension: Aggravated by obesity and reduced with weight loss. This can lead to

Congestive heart disease: Hypertension and the greater cardiac workload required to perfuse the increased tissue present with obesity are imposed on a heart that may already be weakened by fatty infiltration. Obesity can be involved in the initiation and progression of congestive heart disease.

Increased risk and severity of diabetes mellitus

Decreased heat tolerance

Increased dermatosis

Increased surgical risk: It is well documented that the elderly obese pet has a higher surgical risk and a poorer chance of survival.

Obesity can shorten the pet's life and predispose to or cause medical problems. The incidence of circulatory, locomotion, skin, reproductive, and neoplastic disease is significantly greater in overweight dogs than those at optimum body weight. The incidence of neoplasia, for example, is 50% higher in overweight dogs than in those at optimum body weight.

The best diet for reducing weight is a nutritionally complete and balanced high-fiber, low-fat, low-calorie diet. A common mistake is to feed less of a normal diet that is not specifically formulated for weight reduction, this is not a successful way of decreasing caloric intake in the obese animal. Success is rare if the animal is kept on its usual diet. The reduced food intake does not satisfy hunger as well as the consumption of an equal number of calories in a high-fiber diet and results in increased begging and scavenging for food. In addition, reducing some diets by the amount needed for achieving sufficient caloric restriction and a reasonable rate of weight loss may cause vitamin and mineral imbalances, or protein deficiencies.

Anti-obesity diets have been formulated to provide adequate amounts of all nutrients, except energy. Fat is replaced by digestible fiber, thus providing normal intake and a feeling of satiety. High fiber also benefits the management of diabetes mellitus by reducing hyperglycemia. Some hypocaloric diets replace fat with carbohydrate, or have a high water content. These do not usually promote the same feeling of 'fullness', as do the high fiber substitute diets.

When using an anti-obesity diet, the client must follow instructions explicitly and feed only the specific amount of the food prescribed. If table scraps, treats, or other foods are included in the animal's diet, reduction of caloric intake sufficient to obtain weight loss is virtually impossible.

Prescription diets are low-calorie, high-fiber diets, formulated to reduce caloric intake while providing all nutrients needed and a feeling of fullness. When used correctly, they force the animal to use excess fat to meet daily energy needs. A diet of this type reduces energy intake and induces satiety, thereby increasing compliance and weight loss.

Diets used for obese cardiac patients are usually sodium restricted. This reduces fluid retention and improves heart and lung function.

39.2 DIETS IN CHRONIC RENAL FAILURE

Feeding high-protein diets to patients with early-to-moderate renal failure can be associated with increased retention of some uremic toxins despite enhancement of renal function. There is evidence that the beneficial effects of reduced protein intake similar to those observed in rats may occur in dogs with diminished renal function.

Reduced-protein diets are clearly indicated for dogs with moderate-to-severe chronic renal failure (CRF) that are azotemic, hyperphosmatemic, and not anorectic. These diets are justified primarily by the need to reduce protein intake to control clinical signs of uremia.

The extent to which protein intake must be restricted to obtain maximal effects on the progression of renal disease is unknown. The goal of diet therapy in early-to-moderate renal failure is to minimize progression of renal dysfunction while maintaining adequate and balanced nutrition commensurate with the extent of the condition.

Before initiating protein restriction, one should evaluate the patient's renal function and nutritional status. Evaluation should include physical examination; subjective evaluation of nutritional status and hydration; determination of body weight, serum creatinine, urea nitrogen, albumin, calcium, and phosphate concentrations; complete blood count; and urinalysis. Once the diet has been introduced, this renal evaluation should be repeated at appropriate intervals.

Potential benefits of early protein/phosphate restriction in dogs with CRF include delaying or preventing progressive renal structural and functional deterioration and slowing or preventing renal osteodystrophy.

Many commercially available reduced protein diets are low in sodium content. This is a potentially beneficial modification designed to minimize arterial hypertension in patients with renal dysfunction.

If renal failure progresses despite reduced protein intake, consideration may be given to further reducing protein intake. However, further reductions in dietary protein intake should be undertaken only after considering the potential nutritional effects, and re-evaluating kidney function.

Prescription diets play an important role in the management of renal disease. Their aim is to minimize the "workload" of the kidney and to reduce the production of urea and other nitrogenous waste products, high levels of which are responsible for the clinical signs exhibited by affected animals. These accumulate when the degree of tissue damage within the organ is too extensive for it to function efficiently.

The pathologic *effects of uremia* and chronic renal failure may be summarized as follows:

Retention of nitrogenous end products (urea, creatinine) and spill over into the blood: Whereas urea is relatively nontoxic itself, clinical symptoms arise when other uremic toxins such as phenol and indole also accumulate.

Metabolic acidosis: Malfunctioning of the hydrogen ion exchange mechanism can lead to de-ossification (often associated with chronic interstitial nephritis) and systemic acidotic signs.

Anemia: Anemia can develop as a result of renal disease—the kidneys cannot produce sufficient erythroprotein—and also as a result of hyperproteinemia.

Protein-calorie deficiency: A low calorie intake (poor appetite) coupled with excessive protein catabolism, leads to metabolic disorders.

The protein restricted diet includes restricted amounts of phosphorus to minimize acidosis because the decreased phosphorus intake encourages renal reabsorption of bicarbonates. (In the same way, lower protein content is related to lower potassium levels, desirable in these cases to lessen the risk of hyperkalemia.) To compensate for the reduced palatability of a low-protein product and the poor appetite resulting from uremia, the food must be energy concentrated. (Many of these diets produce an alkaline urine to avoid urate and cystine stones.) Sodium content should be moderate, sufficient to alleviate the increased urinary losses, but not enough to encourage renal hypertension.

These diets have been formulated to assist in the management of various conditions in which protein must be mildly restricted, for example: (1) early renal failure and (2) geriatric patients with decreased renal function.

39.3 DIETS FOR FELINE UROLOGIC SYNDROME

Feline urologic syndrome (FUS) includes any inflammation of the urinary system accompanied by urolithiasis, which may cause obstruction of the urinary tract. Crystals of struvite (or magnesium ammonium phosphate hexahydrate) are the most commonly found calculi in the feline bladder and urethra.

The exact cause of this syndrome is still unknown. It has been suggested that certain viruses, bacteria, or mycoplasma may initiate the synthesis of an insoluble organic matrix, leading to the formation of struvite uroliths. Urinary pH also plays an important role in the disease; the condition is less likely to occur if urinary pH is acidic in the range of 6.0. Diets high in magnesium, in particular dry diets, have also been incriminated.

Diet is not the only cause of this disease, but it is nevertheless an important factor that should be thoroughly investigated in cats suffering from the condition.

Struvite uroliths and/or infection of the urinary tract, inducing cystitis and urethritis, are the major causes of dysuria and hematuria in male and female cats. Calculi or gelatinous plugs may obstruct the male's urethra, causing dysuria. To alleviate these clinical signs, the calculi, microcalculi, and crystals must be eliminated. This can be accomplished in three ways:

1. Surgery
2. Adding a sufficient amount of an effective urine acidifier, such as ammonium chloride or methionine, to a magnesium-restricted diet
3. Feeding a calculolytic diet, such as Prescription Diet, i.e., low in magnesium.

Feline uroliths of variable size, location, and composition are an important cause of hematuria, dysuria, and urethral obstruction. Urease-producing staphylococci can be significant in the formation of many uroliths.

Dietary management is the most effective and least expensive means of managing and preventing FUS. Feeding a calculolytic diet dissolves calculi and alleviates clinical signs of FUS in most cases. Feeding a magnesium-restricted diet that maintains a low urine pH is usually necessary to prevent recurrences.

Feline struvite uroliths can be dissolved by medical therapy. This involves reduction of urine pH to 6.0 or less (urinary acidifiers) and reduction of urine magnesium through magnesium-restricted diets.

DIETETIC ASPECTS

As stated previously, the element most commonly associated with FUS is magnesium. Diets with a high magnesium content stimulate the production of struvite in the urine. This tendency disappears when the magnesium content falls in a food with a relatively high energy (carbohydrate) concentration.

The influence of calcium and phosphorus is not yet clearly established. A higher calcium content might limit urinary excretion of phosphorus and could also be a factor in elevating the pH of the urine above 6.0.

However, it is still advisable to encourage the animal to drink to stimulate polyuria and reduce the risk of crystalluria, which can result from excessive urinary concentration. Salt is commonly included in these diets to increase urine volume.

Concentrated urine is most likely to occur when the cats' diet is changed suddenly, in particular from a moist to a dry diet. Frequently, the animal fails to increase its water intake to compensate, and so it is important to make every effort to encourage the cat to drink. In animals predisposed to FUS, diet clearly can be an important factor in both the cause of the disease and, by careful attention to diet composition, in the control of FUS.

Commercial prescription diets for feline pH control are complete foods for cats. They are specially formulated to be fed as an aid to the management of FUS.

INDICATIONS AND FEEDING RECOMMENDATIONS

FUS is a condition of complex causes, and although no single agent has been proven to be responsible for this disease, various dietary factors have been established that are important to consider in the management of clinical FUS in susceptible cats, including:

1. The water balance associated with the feeding of the diet
2. The urine pH
3. The mineral (particularly magnesium) content of the diet

Currently available diets for FUS control help to promote water intake, are low in magnesium, and produce an acid urine.

Diets for struvite stones in dogs contain reduced levels of high quality protein to reduce ammonium ion concentration. Magnesium and phosphorous levels are reduced also, and the salt level is higher than normal to stimulate drinking and increased urine formation of acidic pH.

39.4 DIETS FOR GASTROINTESTINAL TRACT DISEASES

Diarrhea is defined as an alteration in the normal pattern of defecation resulting in the passage of soft, unformed stools with increased fecal volume, increased bicarbonate, increased fecal water content, and/or increased frequency of defecation.

Diarrhea can be due to disorders of the small bowel and/or the large bowel or to other systemic disorders such as hepatic disease, pancreatic insufficiency, pancreatitis, infection, allergy or colitis.

If the feces contain predominantly split fats (steatorrhea) with no starch, and normal or increased trypsin concentration, and is particularly fatty and malodorous, then malabsorption is present. The presence of malabsorption is usually indicative of an intestinal lesion, such as villous atrophy.

If there is predominantly unsplit fat in the feces, pancreatic insufficiency should be suspected and fecal protease (trypsin) determined.

Restriction or manipulation of individual dietary components is perhaps the most important factor in treating acute or chronic gastrointestinal (GI) disturbances. Non-allergenic diets are assuming greater importance also.

FEEDING OF DOGS

Gastroenteritis

Following a gastrointestinal upset, the food offered should (1) minimize irritation of the digestive tract, (2) Encourage efficient digestion and absorption in the small intestine, and (3) reduce the undigested fraction that could ferment in the large intestine.

Pancreatic Insufficiency

In animals in which pancreatic lipase is the primary deficiency, malabsorption of fatty acids occurs. This leads to the production of steatorrheic feces diarrhea, and if trypsin is deficient, to severe weight loss despite a normal appetite.

In such animals the diet should have a low fiber content to reduce transit time, be high in energy, contain only modest quantities of fat, be rich in folate, B_{12}, and non-allergenic protein.

Hepatic Insufficiency

A variety of conditions involve hepatic insufficiency, some of which are amenable to similar dietetic treatment. In the case of reduced biliary secretion leading to bile salt deficiency and incomplete lipolysis or hepatic lipidosis, attention to fat content is important. If too little fat is given, there is a risk of a secondary deficiency of fat-soluble vitamins. Excessive fat leads to malabsorption and the attendant symptoms.

Low Fat Diets

A low-fat diet is important in treating a variety of GI diseases, though fat is a valuable source of calories and an important com-

ponent of the normal diet. Because fat retards gastric emptying, low-fat diets seem to be better tolerated in a variety of gastric diseases. A low-fat diet is also important in preventing recurrence of pancreatitis in affected animals because fat stimulates release of cholecystokinin, a potent pancreatic secretagogue.

A low-fat diet, in conjunction with use of enzyme supplements, is the treatment for pancreatic exocrine insufficiency or enteric disease. Low fat diets are indicated for animals with intestinal malabsorption.

Low-fat diets are indicated in diseases associated with disorders of fat digestion or absorption.

Complete prescription diets are formulated as an aid in the management of acute and chronic diarrhea in adult dogs and puppies. The fat level in the diet is restricted. Important features of these diets to help manage this condition include the following:

1. Restricted fat content
2. High digestibility
3. Selected carbohydrate source
4. Low-fiber content
5. Balanced nutrients
6. Induction of satiety

Nonallergenic Diets

Although there is increasing evidence for dietary allergy or sensitivity as a major cause of chronic diarrhea in dogs or cats, clinical experience and anecdotal reports suggest that it may occasionally be incriminated. For these reasons, especially when allergy is suspected ruling out other causes, an attempt should be made to feed a non-allergenic diet. Admittedly, this can be difficult, but it can be accomplished by feeding a protein to which the animal has never or only occasionally been previously exposed, such as lamb, mutton, egg, or cottage cheese. Allergies to dairy products may also occur. Commercial nonallergenic diets are available and may be worth trying when dogs and cats cannot tolerate normal commercial diets. The history in these animals usually involves varying combinations of vomiting, flatulence, borborygmi, and diarrhea, coupled with skin conditions or weight loss.

Diets for Colitis

These diets generally are fiber rich, fat reduced, highly digestible diets. They are usually hypoallergenic utilising, mutton or rice. The high fiber tends to increase water absorption from the colon, with less water being lost in the feces. Intestinal transit time is thus normalised.

Diets for Diarrhea

A highly digestible low fiber diet is indicated. Not more than 15% fat should be included and easily digestible bland carbohydrate such as rice can be included. Lactose and sucrose should be avoided. Small amounts of such a bland diet should be fed regularly.

39.5 CONCENTRATED DIETS: CONVALESCENCE

Concentrated diets are designed for dogs recovering from surgery or ill health, when the appetite may be poor; or at any other time when there is a particular need for a highly digestible, concentrated source of nutrients, e.g., pregnancy and lactation. These diets are suitable for use in veterinary hospitals when a highly palatable diet is frequently needed.

When animals are ill and anorexic, the problem is how to supply their increased nutritional needs. A sick animal eats little or not at all. Tiredness, pain, traumatic or postoperative shock can cause anorexia. If the patient's resistance is to be strengthened, this problem must be addressed by the use of suitable feed supplements. Palatability is, therefore, essential in all these nonspecific pathologic conditions.

CONCENTRATED RATIONS

If an animal's appetite is poor, bulky food is not suitable. Not only will the animal be unable to eat all of it, but it is more difficult to digest than a concentrated diet.

Convalescence often follows a period when the animal has been eating very little, if any, food, either because of surgery or from a disinclination to eat. The return to a normal diet must, therefore, be a gradual process if the risk of a digestive upset is to be avoided. Convalescent concentrated diets are beneficial for the following:

Stress situations: hospitalization, kenneling
Extra energy needs: intense and/or prolonged exertion, lactation, losing weight
Need for a low-bulk ration: pre- or postoperative periods, anorexia, digestive upsets, malabsorption

The ration not only must be concentrated in volume but it also must have a high energy content. Bulky substances likely to fill up the digestive tract, such as fats and animal proteins, must be avoided. Digestibility will be enhanced if the daily ration is fed in several small palatable meals.

SELECTED REFERENCES

Angerson, J.W.: Physiological and metabolic effects of dietary fiber. Fed. Proc. 44:2902, 1985.

Batt, R.M.: New approaches to malabsorption in dogs. Compend. Contin. Ed. Pract. Vet., 8:783, 1986.

Burrow, C.F.: Treatment of gastrointestinal disease in small animals. Mod. Vet. Pract., February:93, 1988.

Culpin, P.A.: Treatment of canine colitis. Vet. Rec., 119:311, 1986.

Eastwood, M.A.: Fiber in the gastrointestinal tract. Am. J. Clin. Nutr., 31:S30, 1978.

Foch, M.H.: The irritable bowel syndrome. The possible link between dietary fiber deficiency and disturbed intestinal motility. Am. J. Gastroent 83:963, 1988.

Hand, M.S.: Effects of low fat/high fiber in the dietary management of obesity. Sixth Ann. Vet. Int. Med. Forum. ACVIM Proc., 702, 1988.

Houpt, K.A., and Hintz, H.F.: Obesity in dogs. Canine Pract., 5:54, 1978.

Kronfeld, D.S.: Management of obesity in the dog. Vet. Med. S.A.C., 69:46, 1974.

LeBlanc, J., and Diamond, P.: The effect of meal frequency on post prandial thermagenesis in a dog. Fed. Proc., 44:1104, 1985.

Leib, M.S., Hay, W.H., and Roth, L.: Phasmacytic-lymphocytic colitis in the dog. In Current Veterinary Therapy. Edited by R.W. Kirk, Philadelphia, W.B. Saunders, 1989.

Lewig, L.D.: Obesity in the dog. J. Am. Anim. Hosp. Assoc., 14:402,1978.

Lewis, L.W. et al.: Small Animal Clinical Nutrition III. Topeka, KS, Mark Morris Associates, 1987.

Maddison, J.E.: A guide to diagnosis and treatment of chronic diarrhoea in the dog. Aust. Vet. Pract., *10*:58, 1990.

Nelson, R.W.: Dietary therapy for diabetes mellitus. Compend. Contin. Ed. Pract. Vet., December:1387, vol. 10, No. 12, 1988.

Nelson, R.W. et al.: Nutritional management of idiopathic chronic colitis in the dog. J. Vet. Intern. Med., 2:133, 1988.

Polzin, D.J., and Osborne, C.A.: Influence of modified protein diets on morbidity mortality and renal function in dogs with induced chronic renal failure. Am. J. Vet. Res., *45*:506, 1984.

Polzin, D.J., Osborne, C.A., and Leininger, J.R.: The influence of diet on the progression of canine renal failure. Compend. Contin. Ed. Pract. Vet., *6*(12):1123, 1984.

Sheffey, B.E., and Williams, A.J.: Nutrition and the ageing animal. Vet. Clin. North Am. Am. Anim. Pract., *11*:669, 1981.

Strombeck, D.R., and Guilford, W.G.: Nutritional management of gastrointestinal diseases. *In* Small Animal Gastroenterology. Davis, CA, Stonegate Publishing, 1990.

Ward, A.: The fat dog problem: how to solve it. Vet. Med. S.A.C. *79*(6):781, 1984.

40

THERAPY OF EPILEPTIC SEIZURES

40.1 Introduction
40.2 Therapy Principles
40.3 Side Effects of Anticonvulsants
40.4 Barbiturates
40.5 Primidone
40.6 Phenytoin (Diphenylhydantoin)
40.7 Benzodiazepines

40.1 INTRODUCTION

Generalized tonic clonic seizures represent the most common form of canine epilepsy. In broad terms classified as epilepsy can be primary or secondary in nature. The primary form is called "true idiopathic functional epilepsy," or "inherited epilepsy." The secondary form is referred to as "acquired epilepsy."

The precise etiology of primary (or idiopathic epilepsy) is unknown. Spread from the epileptiform focus is facilitated by a diminution in concentration and in activity of inhibitory neurotransmitters. This can be genetically mediated in some breeds.

Secondary (or acquired) epilepsy can result from trauma, infection, inflammation, or neoplasia.

Epilepsy can be inherited or acquired and manifested by recurrent seizures without the presence of an underlying disease. When recurrent seizures become continuous seizures, a "status epilepticus" is said to exist.

Epilepsy is a common disease in the dog, and although owners usually demand treatment, it is not always satisfactory. This is because variation in clinical and pharmacokinetic data for some anticonvulsants in the dog or cat and hence the difficulty in embarking on correct dosage regimens. Seizures generally arise from fluctuations in neuronal excitability. The level of neuronal excitability is controlled by a balance between excitatory and inhibitory neurotransmitter activity. If the balance is redirected towards excitation (depolarization), seizure may occur. Seizures alter the brain in a way that promotes additional excitatory activity.

Generalized seizures, such as grand mal or petit mal, involve symmetric epileptiform activity. In contrast, when the malfunctioning cells of the cerebrum constitute a small focus of misfiring neurons, a partial seizure may result in a localized body area, innervated by the affected cells.

Electrical discharge from neurons is modulated by a "checks and balances" system between excitatory and inhibitory neurotransmitters. Malfunctioning of this system, allowing for increased excitability of neurons, potentiates epileptic activity.

The underlying functional changes triggering seizures may include (1) increased activity and availability of excitatory neurotransmitters (e.g., acetylcholine); (2) decreased availability of inhibitory neurotransmitters, e.g., gamma-aminobutyric acid (GABA); (3) a change in the ratio and number of excitatory and inhibitory neurotransmitter receptor sites; and (4) a malfunction of cellular metabolism (e.g., failure of the active extrusion of sodium (sodium pump)). Primary epilepsy may result when biochemical defects in cortical or subcortical neurons episodically trigger spontaneous discharge. (This condition can be hereditary in some breeds.) A genetic factor in some breeds may be responsible for the predisposition. Breeds that possess this genetic trait include beagles, dachshunds, German shepherds, keeshonds, cocker spaniels, collies, golden retrievers, and Labradors. Primary epilepsy is often characterized by petit mal seizures associated with loss of consciousness and transient collapse. Common forms of these attacks are generalized tonic clonic seizures. Primary epileptiform seizures involve a loss of consciousness tremors, tonic clonic convulsions of the head and limbs, salivation, urination, and defecation. The extent and nature of the epilepsy depends on the extent and functioning of the affected cortical / subcortical areas. Secondary epilepsy, on the other hand, is an acquired brain disorder caused by previously acquired traumatic, metabolic, toxic, infectious or inflammatory processes. Although the neuronal damage can be minimal, it may cause no neurologic defects other than clinical seizures. When the seizure originates within the limbic system, behavioral changes occur. Clinical signs can include drowsiness, aggression, apparent blindness, barking, tail chasing, inappetence, voracious appetite, and chewing or licking movements.

40.2 THERAPY PRINCIPLES

Antiepileptic drugs are usually employed when seizures occur more frequent than once a month: if they are multiple, and clustered or if they last longer than 5 to 10 minutes. The object of using anticonvulsant drugs is to decrease the frequency or severity of seizures. Anticonvulsant therapy should aim to control seizures while avoid-

TABLE 40–1
ANTIEPILEPTIC DRUGS

Drug	Action
Phenobarbital	—Raises seizure threshold; —Central depressant. Prevents initiation of seizure
Primidone	—Mainly metabolized to phenobarbital (+ 2 other metabolites) —All 3 metabolites possess anticonvulsant activity —Largely similar to phenobarbital
Phenytoin (diphenylhydantoin)	—Membrane stabilizer —Limits spread of seizure from focus —Suppresses Na^+K^+ A.T.P.ASE pump
Diazepam Clonazepam Valproic Acid	—Potentiate inhibitory transmitter (G.A.B.A.) —Enhancement of presynaptic inhibition; reduces initiation of seizure

ing systemic or neurologic toxicity. Control, however, does not imply total elimination of the seizures, and the client must be made fully aware of this. Adverse reactions to drugs are most likely to occur when drug combinations are used. Choice of anticonvulsant drug depends on factors such as efficacy, safety, cost, ease of administration, and likely owner compliance. Rapidity of drug effectiveness and likely drug interactions are other considerations. At present the anticonvulsants most widely used in dogs are phenobarbital, primidone, phenytoin, (diphenylhydantoin), and diazepam (Table 40–1).

Client education is of critical importance before embarking on treatment (Table 40–2). If the client cannot tolerate the seizures but can medicate the dog consistently, treatment is indicated.

Points need to be clearly spelled out to the owner:

1. The nature of the epilepsy is important—careful note of the intensity of the seizures and their frequency will facilitate accurately-tailored medication.
2. Drugs do not cure epilepsy. At best, they control it, but treatment may last months to years.
3. The best that may be attainable is diminution in frequency and severity of seizures—not their total abolition.
4. Medication may have to be juggled, and medication several times a day may be necessary.
5. Abrupt cessation of therapy may lead to status epilepticus.
6. Kinetic data varies for individual drugs, and blood levels may occasionally need

TABLE 40–2
SOME CAUSES OF SEIZURES

Toxicants → Ethylene Glycol, lead, strychnine, herbicides, insecticides
Neoplasias → Primaries or metastases
Metabolic disturbances → Hypoglycemia, hypoxia, hypocalcemia, hepatic encephalopathy
Infection/inflammation → Canine distemper virus, rabies, toxoplasma gondii, meningitis, meningoencephalitis, residual brain damage
Trauma → Cranial damage
Idiopathic
Hereditary

to be taken to assess whether the correct drug dosage is being administered.

7. Tolerance to anticonvulsants is common, and many possess undesirable side effects.

It is always desirable to begin anticonvulsant therapy early in the course of epilepsy, because each seizure makes additional seizures more likely. The objectives of therapy must be made clear from the start, and the owner must be fully informed that whereas complete elimination of seizures is desirable, it is not always possible. Objectives of therapy include reduced severity of seizures and decreased duration and frequency. Very often, adjustments in dose and frequency of administration must be made as needed. Dosage regimens are usually drawn up on the basis of satisfactory serum drug concentrations. The drug half-life determines the frequency of administration; assessment of drug serum levels is the only accurate guide to dosage.

On balance, the prognosis for treatment of acquired epilepsy is better than for idiopathic epilepsy. For optimum results the most effective drug and dosage must be determined by the clinician and adjusted to suit the individual dog's particular disease. The animal's seizure dates and times must always be recorded. Many dosage adjustments will usually be necessary before the most satisfactory dose is reached on the basis of clinical response.

The available range of anticonvulsant drugs varies widely with respect to factors such as oral bioavailability, half-lives, time to reach the steady state, efficacy and of course, side effects.

Antiepileptic drugs act by a variety of biochemical and pharmacologic mechanisms to inhibit or suppress the spread of excitation and thus to mitigate the epileptic seizures. They exhibit different mechanisms of action. Some, like the hydantoins, possess a membrane-stabilizing effect; barbiturates increase the convulsive threshold of the neurons; others such as the benzodiazepines and valproic acid, increase the activity of the inhibitory neurotransmitters.

Compounds that raise the seizure threshold include barbiturates, succinimides and oxazolidinediones. These tend to prevent seizures starting. Hydantoins act by limiting the diffusion and spread of the seizures.

There are several aspects of client education that the veterinarian should always address when embarking on therapy. Inheritance plays an important role in canine idiopathic epilepsy, so it is unwise to breed from an animal with idiopathic epilepsy. Seizures are not believed to be necessarily painful to the animal, insofar as most dogs are unconscious during the seizure and they seem to experience only a few minor aches after. Seizures occurring very frequently, e.g., more than once per hour present a serious, life-threatening medical emergency. Dogs with multiple seizures, more often than one per month, can be significantly compromised in health such that they should be given daily preventive antiepileptic medication, usually for the rest of their lives. Owner compliance is necessary if longterm treatment is to be satisfactory because changing of dosage or omission of administration on the part of the owner can give rise to severe relapses.

Dosage rate, frequency of dosage, and bioavailability are critical factors for successful therapy. Furthermore, major pharmacokinetic differences exist between humans and animals with these drugs. Unsuccessful seizure therapy can result from inadequate client education, subeffective drug concentrations, progressive disease, or refractory epilepsy. Subtherapeutic serum levels often result from poor owner compliance, incorrect dosage or increased hepatic enzyme induction. Vomiting, diarrhea, or hepatic disease can adversely affect the oral bioavailability of the administered dose. Tolerance to antiepileptic drugs may also develop.

Treatment of epilepsy takes two forms: the removal, if possible, of any underlying or predisposing cause and the control of seizure frequency with antiepileptic medication. Infrequent and isolated seizures will usually not warrant medication. As mentioned, however, frequent seizures can be life-threatening to the animal as well as upsetting to the owner. As a general rule, dogs with seizures occurring more frequently than once per month should receive daily antiepileptic medication to reduce the threat of death from multiple seizures. Anticonvulsant drugs at best will only reduce the frequency of seizures and do not completely eliminate them, this should always be explained to the owner. Strict adherence to the chosen dosage regimen is critical. Owner compliance is essential because the longterm treatment is carried out on an outpatient basis.

Therapeutic drug monitoring by way of measurement of serum drug levels is a valuable aid toward designing and monitoring a successful program. Although it may sometimes be necessary to use and combine two antiepileptic drugs simultaneously, the potential for detrimental drug interaction must always be considered.

40.3 SIDE EFFECTS OF ANTICONVULSANTS

Phenobarbital, primidone, and phenytoin all can induce hepatic microsomal enzyme activity. Drugs dependent on liver metabolism for clearance are more rapidly metabolized when given concurrently with the previously mentioned anticonvulsant agents. Also, anticonvulsants (including the benzodiazepines) can increase the rate of their own metabolism. To compensate for the resultant decreased serum levels, the dosage of anticonvulsant is often increased, which may induce toxicity.

Phenytoin and phenobarbital are often given simultaneously because in some cases their complementary mechanisms of antiepileptic activity are indicated. Phenobarbital can increase the metabolism of phenytoin, but paradoxically also can decrease it's inactivation because of competition with hepatic microsomal enzymes. A variety of unrelated drugs such as chloramphenicol and cimetidine, which inhibit microsomal enzymes, can decrease the rate of metabolism of some anticonvulsants. Cumulation could therefore occur leading to the potential for toxic side effects. Many dogs receiving long term anticonvulsant therapy can develop abnormalities in serum biochemistry and hepatic function tests. (Many anticonvulsants cause elevations in hepatic enzymes.) Phenytoin and valproic acid are so rapidly eliminated in dogs that therapeutic plasma concentrations cannot be maintained even with very high doses. The elimination of phenytoin is further hastened by hepatic microsomal enzyme induction in the dog.

On the basis of pharmacokinetic studies in dogs, only phenobarbital and primidone are suited for the initial treatment of canine epilepsy. Both of these drugs can significantly reduce the rate and severity of seizures. Doses generally range from 2.5–5.0 mg/kg of phenobarbital or 30 to 55 mg/kg of primidone per day, but further dosage increases may be necessary to obtain a favorable clinical result. Sedative side effects are observed at the commencement of treatment and when dosages are increased. In most animals a high degree of tolerance develops within a few weeks. Primidone can give rise to liver damage during longterm treatment. This is reflected by increases in levels of alanine transferase. In dogs, primidone is metabolized partly to phenobarbital, which accumulates in the plasma on account of its long half-life, and most of the antiepileptic activity of primidine is due to phenobarbital. Hepatic injury is quite common with some drugs, and primidone is probably the most commonly implicated drug in this regard in dogs. (Phenytoin is most commonly implicated as hepatotoxic in humans) In dogs the incidence of phenytoin-induced hepatotoxicity is more frequent when phenytoin is administered in combination with primidone or phenobarbital.

Many of the commonly used anticonvulsants are microsomal enzyme inducers. Hepatotoxicity may result from the production of toxic intermediates or metabolites of anticonvulsants, which are formed at a rate faster than normal because of enzyme induction, particularly by phenobarbital. Direct hepatic toxicity ranging from hepatitis to cirrhosis may result. Anticonvulsant-induced hepatotoxicity can be reduced in several ways, including (1) Evaluation of hepatic function before commencing therapy; (2) using the least hepatotoxic drug that will successfully control the seizures; (3) preferably employing single-drug therapy; and (4) regular of the therapy protocol.

Human patients receiving anticonvulsant therapy may develop megaloblastic anemia that is due to folic acid deficiency. Folate deficiency may be due to interference with the intestinal absorption of folate by the anticonvulsant drugs. Most folates in the diet are in the form of folate polyglutamates, which are deconjugated by intestinal en-

---

TABLE 40–3
SIDE EFFECTS OF ANTIEPILEPTIC DRUGS

1. Most may produce behavioral changes, polydipsia, polyphagia, polyuria, tolerance.
2. Sedation with phenobarbital, primidone, diazepam, clonazepam.
3. Drug interaction (protein binding) with phenytoin, diazepam, valproate.
4. Phenytoin is extremely alkaline and so may irritate the gastric mucosa. Drug interaction a significant problem in man.
5. Hepatotoxicity with primidone and phenytoin.
6. Liver microsomal enzyme induction. Phenobarbital, phenytoin, primidone.

(Treatment with any antiepileptic drug is long and unsatisfactory).

---

zymes during absorption. Phenytoin inhibits folate deconjugase enzymes in the intestinal mucosa, thereby leading to folate malabsorption (Table 40–3).

40.4 BARBITURATES

PHENOBARBITAL

Phenobarbital is a major drug in the treatment of canine epilepsy. Its widespread usage is attributable to the fact that it is relatively safe, is quite predictable, and possesses relatively few side effects. Phenobarbital raises the threshold for seizure discharge and inhibits the initiation, diffusion, and spread, of discharge from the neuronal focus. The recommended starting dosage for dogs is 2.5 mg/kg – 5.0 mg/kg orally over 12 hours. Some dogs require much higher dosages every 12 hours (15–30 mg/kg) to maintain adequate serum concentrations.

The increases in dosage are limited by the side effects of drowsiness. The side effects with phenobarbital are dose dependent and often disappear once the dosage is lowered. Common side effects are ataxia, sedation, polyuria, polydipsia, and polyphagias. Tolerance to the side effects develops rapidly. Dogs that are initially depressed return to normal as the hepatic metabolism increases (phenobarbital is a potent inducer of hepatic microsomal enzymes). Barbiturate dependence occurs, and abrupt withdrawal of phenobarbital therefore should be avoided. (Phenobarbital is subject to Regulatory Control under the Federal Controlled Sub-

stances Act but this should not dissuade against its usage as an initial anticonvulsant.) Seizures can recur if withdrawal is too abrupt. Dosage tapering is recommended if the drug is to be discontinued. Tolerance often develops to phenobarbital, resulting in loss of effectiveness.

Blood levels of phenobarbital are clinically effective 12 to 24 hours after oral administration. When compared to primidone, phenobarbital is less toxic to the liver, the necessary doses are lower on a milligram per kilogram basis, and the drug is somewhat less expensive than primidone. Its pharmacokinetic properties also favor its usage. Phenobarbital is the most commonly used antiepileptic drug in veterinary medicine. It is effective, inexpensive, and has very few side effects. It is also recommended for use in cats, 1.1 to 2.2 mg/kg twice daily.

The antiepileptic effects of phenobarbital are the result from a number of mechanisms. The motor cortex threshold for electrical stimulation is increased. Decreased monosynaptic and polysynaptic transmission then results in reduced neuronal excitability. By raising the threshold for initiation and reducing the duration of afterdischarge, it prevents initiation, and to some extent, propagation. Phenobarbital possesses a specific anticonvulsant effect not shown by most other barbiturates, except mephobarbital and metharbital. It acts as a central depressant, with no analgesic effects, acting on the nerve cell body. Phenobarbital is metabolized by the liver to parahydroxyphenobarbital, which is an inactive metabolite excreted by the kidneys.

Some phenobarbital is also excreted unchanged. Phenobarbital alters the metabolism of several concurrently administered drugs such as digitoxin, phenylbutazone, corticosteroids, doxycycline, griseofulvin, and tricyclic antidepressants. Phenobarbital is a known potent hepatic microsomal enzyme inducer, and increased levels of serum alkaline phosphatase and serum pyruvic pyruvate transaminase are often found in dogs receiving this anticonvulsant.

As a barbiturate, phenobarbital induces considerable drowsiness or sleepiness. Sedation sets the upper limit on dosage. Pharmacodynamic tolerance occurs, involving adaptation of the central nervous system, but of more significance is the induction of hepatic microsomal enzymes, which are then responsible for rapid metabolism of the drug and development of tolerance. Onset of action is relatively fast, and the drug is of low toxicity. Side effects occasionally seen are polyphagia, polydipsia, and polyuria. If phenobarbital is not withdrawn gradually, increased seizures may be observed over the first few days. Phenobarbital is one of the few drugs suitable for the treatment of canine epilepsy on account of its pharmacokinetic properties. The drug is fairly rapidly and completely absorbed after oral doses, and maximum concentrations in plasma are reached 4 to 8 hours after administration. During longterm therapy, the half-lives decline, but therapeutic plasma concentrations can be maintained by adequate adjustment of dose. On account of its long half-life in dogs, it may take up to 2 weeks to reach the steady state.

Because hepatotoxicity is very rare with phenobarbital and because it is relatively inexpensive, phenobarbital is usually regarded as the first-choice drug for the treatment of generalized epilepsy in the dog. Phenobarbital may be of some value in the treatment of epilepsy in cats, although its half-life seems to be somewhat shorter than in dogs.

OTHER BARBITURATES

Mephobarbital is demethylated by hepatic microsomal enzymes to phenobarbital. Hence, the pharmacologic properties are much the same as those of phenobarbital.

Metharbital is demethylated by hepatic microsomal enzymes to barbital, which is thought to be responsible for the therapeutic effects. The general pharmacologic effects are similar to those of phenobarbital.

Mephobarbital is similarly demethylated in the liver, in this case to phenobarbital, with a similar resultant profile of anticonvulsant activity, as phenobarbital.

40.5 PRIMIDONE

Primidone is one of the most widely used anticonvulsants in veterinary medicine. The relatively high dosage, 55 mg/kg/day, is divided by three and given orally, tid. Primidone has a short half-life. Quite often, adjustments are necessary to maximize the effectiveness while minimizing side effects. An analog of phenobarbital, much of primidone is metabolized to phenobarbital in the liver. Thus, a higher dose rate is required with primidone, and phenobarbital and primidone are not used concurrently.

Primidone is a potent antiepileptic agent but does possess several undesirable side effects. Common side effects include transient drowsiness, ataxia, persistent polydipsia, polyuria, and polyphagia. Sedation is not an unexpected effect on account of bioactivation to phenobarbital. Hepatotoxicity is a definite risk with primidone. Primidone is not reliable in cats.

Primidone is very similar structurally to phenobarbital and possesses very similar properties to the barbiturate. Primidone is metabolized in the liver and excreted in the urine as unchanged primidone, phenylethylmalonamide, and phenobarbital, all of which possess anticonvulsant activity. Much of the antiepileptic activity of primidone is due to the phenobarbital metabolites. Although primidone's half-life is quite short, nonetheless, some cases of epilepsy are more responsive to primidone than to phenobarbital, perhaps because of the additive effects of the three dissimilar metabolites. Under steady state conditions, phenobarbital may be responsible for up to 85% of the total anticonvulsant effect of primidone medication in dogs.

Primidone possesses potential for hepatic enzyme induction, and this possibility must always be considered. Other possible side effects can include tachycardia, hyperventilation, and anorexia. Folic acid deficiency resulting in megaloblastic anemia has been associated with primidone usage in humans and also in dogs. The underlying mechanism is inhibition of conjugase activity in the intestine. This is the enzyme responsible for conversion of polyglutamates to monoglutamates before intestinal absorption. Longterm primidone usage has been associated with hepatic cirrhosis. Primidone-related hepatic toxicity is a real risk, and sometimes dogs can become restless while receiving therapy.

Assessment of correct primidone dosage can be made by assaying a blood sample for phenobarbital some hours after primidone dosage. The level of phenobarbital should be approximately 25 to 50 mcg/ml of serum to ensure optimum antiepileptic effect. Phenobarbital is assayed because most primidone is metabolized to phenobarbital in the liver. Primidone when indicated, must be taken daily for the duration of the dog's life to reduce seizure frequency. Anticonvulsant therapy with primidone can be started at daily dosages of 15 to 30 mg/kg. Although some sedative effects may be seen during the first couple of weeks, tolerance subsequently develops to these effects. Accumulation of phenobarbital to steady state levels usually takes about 14 days. Sometimes it may be necessary to elevate the primidone dosage to 60 mg/kg before a noticeable improvement in the clinical condition is seen.

Side effects can be seen with primidone therapy, especially at these high dosages. Liver function changes (increases in alkaline phosphatase, glutamate dehydrogenase, alanine transferase) or other signs such as polyphagia and polydipsia are characteristic of the induced toxicity. At very high dosages, hepatic oxidation of primidone to phenobarbital may be impaired on account of damage to liver tissue. Because phenobarbital is primarily responsible for the anticonvulsant activity of primidone, it is necessary only to monitor plasma phenobarbital concentrations to evaluate therapy.

Phenobarbital is less hepatotoxic than primidone, is less expensive and would generally be preferred. Primidone is used when seizures are non responsive to phenobarbital.

40.6 PHENYTOIN (DIPHENYLHYDANTOIN)

Phenytoin is a popular anticonvulsant in treating humans and is also frequently employed in controlling canine seizures. Drug-associated hepatotoxicity can be an attendant hazard with phenytoin. Phenytoin is usually used in dogs that are refractory to primidone or phenobarbital. It should not be used in cats, however, on account of its long half-life (41 hours), which increases the risk of toxicity in this species.

Phenytoin is a unique anticonvulsant because it does not induce depression of the central nervous system (CNS), while at the same time it prevents spread of seizures. Phenytoin acts by stabilizing neuronal cell membranes to the actions of sodium potassium and calcium ions, thus protecting nerves from the effects of repetitive activity.

It inhibits diffusion of abnormal electrical activity but does not prevent spontaneous discharges initiating from the seizure focus itself.

Phenytoin suppresses the sodium potassium adenosine triphosphatase pump, thereby changing the excitatory threshold of the neurons, which decreases the frequency of epileptic seizures. Once a seizure has begun, drugs such as the hydantoins (phenytoin), limit and suppress the spread. The drug is poorly and variably absorbed from the gut, possess a short half-life (2–6 hours in dogs), and is rapidly metabolized by the liver into inactive metabolites. The plasma levels necessary for seizure control can thus be very difficult to achieve following oral dosing, and attempts to attain higher therapeutic plasma levels can often result in phenytoin toxicity because the enzyme system responsible for phenytoin metabolism is saturable. With a consequently diminished metabolism rate, cumulation to toxic levels occurs. Because the half-life of phenytoin in dogs varies from 2 to 6 hours, the drug must be given three times daily. On account of its toxicity hazards and also its pharmacokinetic features, phenytoin should not be regarded as a primary drug to control canine epilepsy.

The pharmaceutical formulation is of critical importance in determining the oral bioavailability, and the choice between tablets, capsules, or microcrystalline suspensions can be a major determinant of the blood levels obtained. The microcrystalline oral suspension apparently is absorbed better and yields plasma levels similar to those with intravenous (IV) phenytoin. After oral administration the drug is rapidly but incompletely absorbed. A dosage of 33 mg/kg three times per day is necessary to obtain useful blood serum concentrations. There can be a lag phase before its effects are seen. Phenytoin therefore is of only limited use for the treatment of canine epilepsy.

Many drugs interact with phenytoin. Its blood levels are increased by phenylbutazone, halothane, diazepam, chlorpromazine, estrogens, and chloramphenicol. Phenytoin can enhance the metabolism of dexamethasone, increase blood levels of digitoxin, and decrease those of phenobarbital in humans. Chloramphenicol can increase the serum half-life of phenytoin, resulting in an accumulation of toxic phenytoin serum concentrations.

Phenytoin's irregular oral absorption can make accurate dosage and clinical responses difficult to predict. The main advantage of this nonbarbiturate antiepileptic drug is the absence of any undesirable sedative effects. Polydipsia and polyuria are side effects in dogs. Absorption of phenytoin from the gut in dogs is relatively poor, and difficulty can be experienced in endeavoring to maintain effective plasma levels; several days are required to achieve therapeutic plasma levels. Effective plasma levels in the dog have not been firmly established but are probably similar to the 10 to 30 μcg reported in humans.

Phenytoin seems to be a little more effective in small dogs and can be readily combined with other medications. A starting dose of 10–15 mg/kg is the minimal requirement, but doses up to 33 mg/kg, tid, may be necessary for satisfactory seizure control. The maximum daily dose is 100 mg/kg/day in divided doses. Overall, however, phenytoin is not very useful for the treatment of canine epilepsy on account of its rapid rate of elimination, which makes the maintenance of constant drug concentrations almost impossible. In addition, the bioavailability of various phenytoin formulations is variable, hence oral absorption cannot be relied on. Phenytoin can induce hepatic enzyme activity in the hepatic mi-

crosomes, thus hastening its own inactivation. The drug is strongly alkaline, so divided doses should be used to reduce local irritation. Phenytoin can be given IV for status epilepticus at a dosage of 2 mg/kg to 5 mg/kg, but its duration of action is short.

A side effect of phenytoin administration is folic acid deficiency. On account of the close structural relationship of phenytoin to folic acid, it is thought that phenytoin and folic acid may act as competitive antagonists.

In human patients, gingival hyperplasia is a frequently occurring side effect of phenytoin therapy. The incidence in veterinary medicine is considerably less.

In summary, for many reasons, phenytoin cannot be regarded as a primary drug for control of epilepsy in the dog. It could be used in cases refractory to phenobarbital or primidone.

40.7 BENZODIAZEPINES

DIAZEPAM

Diazepam enhances presynaptic inhibition. Diazepam is a hypnotic with muscle relaxant and anticonvulsive properties and is principally used in human medicine to treat neuroses and anxiety. The efficacy of oral diazepam as an anticonvulsant in dogs or cats is limited on account of its rapid first-pass metabolism. Oral absorption of diazepam is good.

Like many other benzodiazepines, diazepam has a strong anticonvulsant effect, but its practical use is limited by the likely development of tolerance. Because tolerance develops to their anticonvulsant effects within a few days, benzodiazepines such as diazepam and clonazepam are not generally suitable for routine treatment of canine epilepsy. Diazepam, however, remains the drug of choice for status epilepticus.

After oral administration in the dog, diazepam is rapidly metabolized. The bioavailability of the parent drug diazepam is low, while the total bioavailability of diazepam and its active metabolites is reported as 85%. Desmethyldiazepam temazepam and oxazepam, although active metabolites, possess only about one third of the anticonvulsant activity of the parent drug diaze-

TABLE 40–4
CANINE EPILEPSY

Drug	Dosage	Route	Frequency	Side effects
Phenobarbital	2.5–5.0 mg/kg	Oral	b.i.d.	Tolerance Sedation Long half-life Liver damage
Primidone	15–55 mg/kg	Oral	t.i.d.	Liver damage, sedation Polydipsia More expensive
Phenytoin	10–33 mg/kg	Oral	t.i.d.	Rapidly eliminated; variable absorption; of questionable value in dogs
Diazepam	0.2–0.5 mg/kg	Oral	b.i.d.	Sedation/Tolerance

pam. When animals are refractory to other drugs, oral diazepam can be employed satisfactorily at a dosage of 0.2 to 0.5 mg/kg. Oral diazepam is sometimes used in conjunction with other anticonvulsant agents to provide more effective control of epilepsy in dogs and cats. Dosages of 0.5 to 2 mg/kg three times daily have been recommended for cats when phenobarbital alone is ineffective. As in humans, physical dependence can accompany diazepam use, and sedation is a common side effect.

Clonazepam is another member of the benzodiazepine group with pharmacologic properties similar to those of the prototype drug diazepam. Although it has been used for petit mal epilepsy in humans, its use in veterinary medicine appears to be limited to date.

Diazepam's main use is for treatment of status epilepticus—seizures that occur more than once per hour. Emergency treatment is indicated, and IV diazepam slowly administered is indicated in a bolus dosage of 0.5 to 1.0 mg/kg. The IV dose may be repeated or then followed with a similar dose of diazepam intramuscularly (diazepam has a short half-life in dogs). Given IV in status epilepticus, diazepam is rapidly effective. Oral diazepam is less satisfactory because of extensive and rapid metabolic degradation to less active benzodiazepines. Clonazepam is more potent than diazepam. Doses of 0.05 to 0.2 mg/kg clonazepam IV are suitable for status epilepticus in the dog, tolerance to this drug develops more slowly. Phenobarbital 2 mg/kg, IV, Pentobarbital, 4–20 mg/kg IV, Phenytoin, IV, 2 to 5 mg/kg, or lidocaine, IV, 2 mg/kg, are alternative agents for status epilepticus. Diazepam is also useful in cats in treating epilepsy, and tolerance appears to develop more slowly. Another drug that can be usefully considered is clorazepate dipotassium.

TABLE 40–5
FELINE EPILEPSY

Drug	Dosage	Route	Frequency	Side Effects
Diazepam	0.5–2 mg/kg	Oral	t.i.d.	Sedation, short acting
Phenobarbital	1.1–2.2 mg/kg	Oral	b.i.d.	Sedation

TABLE 40–6
THERAPY FOR STATUS EPILEPTICUS

Drug	Dosage	Route
Diazepam	0.5–1.0 mg/kg	IV, slowly
		Repeat dose as necessary
Clonazepam	0.05–0.2 mg/kg	IV, slowly
Phenytoin	2–5 mg/kg	IV, slowly
Lignocaine	2 mg/kg	IV, slowly
Phenobarbital	2 mg/kg	IV, slowly
Pentobarbital	4–20 mg/kg	IV, slowly

This is a benzodiazepine prodrug that is metabolized in the gastrointestinal tract to nordiazepam (a metabolite of diazepam). Oral clorazepate therapy results in higher serum levels of nordiazepam than does diazepam therapy. It shows considerable promise as a secondary anticonvulsant. It is widely used in man.

VALPROIC ACID

Sodium valproate is a useful antiepileptic drug that can be used in combination with phenobarbital. Because of its short half-life in dogs, frequent dosing is necessary with valproate to maintain adequate serum concentrations. Although it would not be regarded as a primary anticonvulsant, it may be considered for use in combination with phenobarbital when phenobarbital alone is unsuccessful. The recommended dosage in combined therapy is 60 mg/kg orally every 8 hours. Oral sodium valproate is converted to valproic acid in the stomach and is then rapidly absorbed. In dogs elimination is rapid and it is excreted in the urine almost totally unchanged. In dogs it has been used experimentally at doses of 25 to 105 mg/kg/day in cases that were refractory to barbiturates. Sodium valproate acts by increasing the concentration centrally of GABA, which is an inhibitory transmitter. Valproic acid has a longer half-life in cats than in dogs (Tables 40–4, 40–5, 40–6).

Other anticonvulsants include (1) the oxazolidinediones. This group include trimethadione and paramethadione (2) the succinimides methsuximide, phensuximide, ethosuximide (3) tricyclic compounds carbamazepine.

These have been extensively used in human medicine, but critical clinical evaluation of them in veterinary medicine is lacking.

SELECTED REFERENCES

Al Tahan, F.O., and Frey, H.H.: Absorption kinetics and bioavailability of phenobarbital after oral administration to dogs. J. Vet. Pharmacol. Ther. 8:205, 1985.

Bruni, J., and Albright, P.S.: The clinical pharmacoloyt of antiepileptic drugs. Clin. Neuropharmacol., 7:1, 1984.

Bunch, S.E. et al.: Toxic hepatopathy and intrahepatic cholestasis associated with phenytocin administration in combination with other anticonvulsant drugs in three dogs. JAVMA, 190:194, 1987.

Bunch, S.E. et al.: Effects of long term primidone and phenytoin administration on canine hepatic function and morphology. Am. J. Vet. Res., 46:105, 1985.

Bunch, S.E., Castleman, W.L., and Hornbuckle, W.E.: Hepatic cirrhosis associated with long term anticonvulsant therapy in dogs. JAVMA, 181: 357, 1982.

Farnbach, G.C.: Seizures in the dog. Part II. Control. Compend. Contin. Ed. Pract. Vet., 7(6):505, 1985.

Forrester, S.D., Boothe, D.M., and Troy, G.C.: Current concepts in the management of Canine epilepsy. Compend. Contin. Ed. Vet. Pract., 11(7):811, 1989.

Frey, H.H.: Use of anticonvulsants in small animals. Vet. Rec., 118:487, 1986.

Frey, H.H., and Loscher, W.: Pharmacokinetics of antiepileptic drugs in the dog: a review. J. Vet. Pharmacol. Ther., 8:219, 1985.

Frey, H.H., and Loscher, W.: Pharmacokinetics of carbamazepine in the dog. Arch. Int. Pharmacodyn. Ther., 243:180, 1980.

Meric, S.M.: Canine meningitis. J. Vet. Intern. Med., 2(2):35, 1988.

Nafe, L.A., Parker, A., and Kay, W.J.: Sodium valproate: a preliminary clinical trial in epileptic dogs. JAVMA, 17:131, 1981.

Roye, D.B., Serrano, E.E., and Hammer, R.H.: Plasma kinetics of diphenylhydantoin in dogs. Am. J. Vet. Res., *44*:947, 1983.

Campbell, I. Primidone intoxication associated with concurrent use of chloramphenicol. JAVMA, *182*:992, 1983.

Sams, P.A., and Muir, W.W.: Effects of phenobarbital or thiopental pharmacokinetics in greyhounds. Am. J. Vet. Res., *49*:245, 1988.

Schwartz-Porsche, D., Loscher, W., and Frey, H.H.: Therapeutic efficacy of phenobarbital and primidone in canine epilepsy. A comparison. J. Vet. Pharmacol. Ther., *8*:113, 1985.

Shell, L.: Antiepileptic drugs. Comp. Cont. Ed. Vet. Pract., *6*:432, 1984.

Skerritt, G.C.: Canine epilepsy. Practice, *10*(1):27, 1988.

Wanev, T., and Nyska, A. Gingival hyperplasia in dogs. Comp. Cont. Educ. Vet. Pract. *13*:1207, 1991.

Yeary, R.A.: Serum concentrations of primidone and its metabolites, phenyl-ethyl-malanamide, and phenobarbital in the dog. Am. J. Vet. Res., *41*:1643, 1980.

41

DRUG THERAPY OF BEHAVIOR AND REPRODUCTIVE DISORDERS IN DOGS AND CATS

41.1 Drug Therapy of Behavioral Disorders
41.2 The Estrogens
41.3 The Gonadotropins
41.4 Androgenic Therapy
41.5 Antiandrogen Therapy
41.6 Progestins and Mammary Neoplasia
41.7 Control of Estrus
41.8 Termination of Pregnancy/Induction of Labor
41.9 Pseudopregnancy
41.10 Suppression of Lactation
41.11 Endometritis and Pyometra
41.12 Hormonally Responsive Skin Conditions
41.13 Urinary Incontinence

41.1 DRUG THERAPY OF BEHAVIORAL DISORDERS

Behavioral problems in dogs and cats are very common and are usually caused by many factors including genetic, hormonal, stress, and socially learned influences. Although dominance aggresssion in the dog and urine spraying in the cat are quite common, the precise triggering factors are largely unknown. One of the most frequent complaints by owners about dog behavior is fighting between males. A dog that is aggressive to other male dogs may be perfectly friendly toward people. There are three basic approaches to mitigating intermale aggression, a combination of which may be necessary to stop the fighting or reduce its frequency; progestin therapy, castration, or training procedures. In cases of aggression directed toward people (biting, scratching, etc.), a dietary sensitivity should be investigated. In cats especially, sensitivities have been recorded to canned and foil-container cooked foods, and these can be investigated by withdrawing all such food for a few weeks and replacing it with a simple dry chicken/fish prescription diet.

DOGS

Because many dogs affected by dominance aggression are males, it would be reasonable to assume that testosterone levels play a key role and that castration would reduce dominance aggression. Despite castration some dogs continue to display behavioral changes such as roaming, urine marking, and aggression. Most females displaying dominance aggression are spayed. It may be possible that spaying allows expression of masculine behavior traits in some female dogs. Hormonal imbalance, especially aggression dominance, is frequently implicated in conditions characterized by antisocial and aberrant behavior in male dogs. Aggression, roaming, destruction, and copulatory activity in both entire and castrated dogs can be controlled by administration of progestins such as megestrol acetate, medroxyprogesterone acetate, and delmadinone acetate. These drugs possess not only an antiandrogenic effect but also display a central effect on the cerebral cortex. These hormones suppress not only luteinizing hormone (LH) output but also follicle-stimulating hormone (FSH) output, and hence spermatogenesis will be suppressed during therapy. The effect of antiandrogenic drugs, especially delmadinone acetate, on behavior can be explained in terms of (1) a specific effect by reducing libido and androgen production, through which the dog is alleviated from the desire to be sexually active and socially dominant, and (2) the established tranquilizing, sleep-inducing, or narcotic activity of progestogenic steroids, which may result in an alteration of the sensitivity level of the central nervous system for aggression, nervousness, and seizures. The anticonvulsant sedative activity of many steroids is well established and some steroids raise the seizure threshold.

Synthetic progestogens can reduce or mitigate many male behavioral tendencies. Progestogens can be an invaluable aid while conditioning a dog to be nonaggressive in the presence of other males. During gestagen therapy, the dog's motivation to act aggressively is reduced, and the owner can train the dog. Gonadotropin output from the anterior pituitary of the dog causes normal testicular function. FSH acts on the seminiferous tubules to promote spermatogenesis, and interstitial cell stimulating hormone (LH) stimulates the interstitial cells of Leydig to produce testosterone and dihydrotestosterone. Gonadotropin release is inhibited by progesterone-type compounds, hence their use in behavioral disorders. The antiandrogenic effects combine with a central effect on the cerebral cortex. During progestin therapy, behavior training must accompany drug treatment.

Megestrol Acetate

A potent progestin, this drug possesses anti-androgenic, anti-estrogenic, and anti-inflammatory qualities. When first marketed, megestrol acetate was indicated for estrus control and the treatment of false pregnancy in bitches. Additional indications were predictable from the known pharmacology of the compound, whereas others such as the treatment of miliary eczema and eosinophilic granuloma in cats were not and were originally noted as chance clinical observations. More recently, the drug has been recognized as an aid in the control of behavioral problems in small animals.

Megestrol acetate is known to be a potent inhibitor of gonadotropin release in males and can therefore be expected to be useful in modifying behavior associated with excessive production or sensitivity to androgens. Megestrol acetate, however, will also modify the behavior of castrated dogs. The mode of action is believed not to be solely due to the suppression of male hormones and that the drug may have a direct effect at the level of steroid receptors within the cerebral cortex.

The initial dosage is 2 mg/kg/day for 7 days in dogs (depending on the response); dosage then can be decreased to 1 mg/kg/day for 14 days and then stopped in the event of improvement. An increase in dosage up to 4 mg/kg for a week may be necessary where no improvement is seen after the initial dose. Megestrol acetate has been shown to be a useful form of therapy, over a period of 3 to 4 weeks to counteract aggressive tendencies toward people, dominance aggression, fighting other male dogs, or urine marking in the house. Sometimes as the dosage tapers off, the intensity or frequency of aggression increases and some form of concurrent behavioral therapy is then required to ensure that dominance aggression does not recur after the drug is withdrawn. While most dogs are treated for 4 to 6 weeks, the dosage regimen usually is a trial and error approach and depends on the severity of the behavioral disturbance and response to treatment. Only the minimum dose necessary should be used, because side effects with progestogen therapy are not uncommon. In general, response to treatment is good, and usually the improvement in behavior is maintained for months after cessation of therapy. Occasionally, however, aggression is not always androgen dependent but may be socially reinforced. Additionally, the role of the cerebral cortex may be very dominant, and the central calming effect of megestrol acetate may not be sufficient at the dose used.

In difficult cases, a more persistent response may be achieved by combining high dosage megestrol acetate therapy with intensive retraining of the animal. A useful feature is that megestrol acetate does not appear to depress the response to training in a dog, and hence progestin therapy can be successfully linked to a training program. Many male dogs displaying marked urination, roaming, excitability, and/or destructiveness improve after therapy with megestrol acetate.

Side effects can include mammary hyperplasia, increased appetite, and lethargy. Megestrol acetate may be less successful for dogs younger than 1 year because the relapse rate tends to be higher in this age group than in older dogs. Oral therapy with megestrol acetate involves dosing over a period of 1 or 2 weeks with a gradual dose reduction over subsequent weeks. Hormonal therapy must always be regarded as an adjunct to behavior modification training.

An alternative method is the use of medroxyprogesterone acetate. Depot injections may need to be repeated every 1 to 6 months while oral therapy can be tailored to effect. It has been observed that the injection of 10 mg/kg of medroxyprogesterone acetate controls aggression in male dogs with response to treatment as noted by improved behavior usually within a few days of injection. This can be effective in ameliorating intermale fighting, at a dose of 10 mg/lb subcutaneously.

CATS

The most frequently used medical therapy for behavior modification in cats includes progestogens, antiandrogenic compounds, and sedatives, especially for dominance aggression or indoor spraying. Progestins are usually resorted to only after a failed period of behavior modification. A reducing dosage scale is used for no more than 3 to 4 weeks preferably combined with retraining. Progestogen therapy with megestrol acetate, delmadinone acetate, and medroxyprogesterone acetate have been successful in cats.

Behavioral disturbances include urine spraying, scratching, house soiling, nervousness, aggression to other cats as well as to people, overgrooming, and excessive fighting. Because progestogens tend to supress typically masculine behavior and because dominance aggression problems are clearly typically masculine behavior, it is logical to assume that administration of progestins may be an effective therapy.

When excessive house soiling is a problem, i.e., inappropriate urination or defecation, nervousness may be the core of the problem. If nervousness is the root problem, a sedative agent such as oral diazepam at 0.5 mg/day for a trial period may be beneficial. In the case of indoor marking (spraying or scratching) by cats, drug therapy is judged very much on a case by case basis. A tapered regimen of megestrol acetate, 2.5 mg, on alternate days for 1 to 4 weeks can be considered. In nervous cats, diazepam 0.5–1 mg/kg/day as needed can be tried.

Diazepam is as effective as megestrol acetate for alleviating some nervous problems in cats. Adverse effects other than mild sedation, a temporary increase in appetite, and weight gain are more likely with diazepam therapy at a dosage rate of 1 to 2 mg/kg (bid). Aggression toward other cats is very common, the cat being hyperactive and territorial. Behavioral changes may include physical attack and low threshold of arousal. Causes may range from hormonal dysfunction to hyperthyroidism, brain lesion, or diet sensitivity. Drug therapy includes tapered dosages of progesterone, megestrol acetate, or antiandrogenic injectables such as delmadinone acetate or medroxyprogesterone acetate. Such compounds may calm the animal (even if neutered), and the use of diazepam could also be considered. For aggressiveness therapy could include megestrol acetate at 2.5 mg on alternate days up to 10 days, reducing the dosage for the following 2 weeks and by easing off for the next 2 weeks. Other behavioral problems common to cats include overgrooming. Although grooming is usually harmless, sometimes when stressed, nervous, or ill at ease environmentally, cats will overgroom to the point of self-induced alopecia or self-mutilation. (Investigate allergies and flea infestation in such cases.) Behavior therapy can begin only when other medical disorders have been ruled out, e.g., flea sensitivity, atopy, or dietary allergy. Diazepam (0.5 mg) can be considered during retraining over a period of 1 month. The dosage may need to be raised to 1 mg/kg depending on the response.

When the mutilation is severe, the dosage of diazepam should be increased to 2 to 3 mg/day of oral diazepam.

Feline Behavior During Estrus

Feline behavior during estrus is a problem to many cat owners. Each estrus is generally accompanied by one or more of the following: vocalization, rolling, awkward body contortions, seeking of males, and other physical and behavioral changes. Puberty generally occurs in cats between 6 and 12 months of age. The cat is also seasonally polyestrous. Recurrent cycles of 14 days are common if mating does not occur. Estrus follows and generally lasts from 3 to 6 days. It may persist up to 10 days if the queen is not mated. Cats are reflex ovulators. They ovulate during estrus approximately 24 to 28 hours after natural or artificial stimulation of the vagina. Fertilization occurs 24 to 48 hours after copulation. Fertilized ova remain in the oviduct for up to 4 days with implantation occurring about 10 days later. The average gestation period in the domestic cat is 60 days. During the breeding season males are attracted and make their presence felt by crying, fighting, and urinating around the female's domain. Female characteristics during estrus include purring, crying, rolling, and crouching. Several alternatives are available to pet owners. Ovariohysterectomy is a permanent, nonreversible approach. Megestrol acetate, an orally active progestogen, is effective for the rapid remission of behavioral signs associated with estrus in cats. It postpones subsequent cycles as long as maintenance doses are given. However, cats must be isolated from males during the first 3 days of megestrol acetate dosing because the drug can aid conception if mating occurs during this time.

41.2 THE ESTROGENS

The major natural estrogens are estradiol, estrone, and estriol. The natural estrogens and their esters such as estradiol (benzoate, cypionate, valerate) are well absorbed from the gut but very rapidly metabolized in the liver (rapid first-pass effect), so dosage recommendations usually refer to parenteral dosing. Estradiol benzoate is a short chain ester and persists in the body for a few days, but the more complex cypionate ester lasts for weeks after intramuscular injection. Several estrogenic compounds—synthetic types—display high oral bioavailability. Stilbenes—diethylstilbestrol—are well absorbed from the gut and do not undergo rapid first-pass degradation in the liver, hence their former widespread popularity in small animal medicine for oral dosing.

Alkylation of the estrogen molecule at the site of metabolic cleavage is a method that has been exploited with many steroids to make the resultant molecule more resistant to hepatic degradation and hence more orally active. Ethinyl estradiol is one such drug and is widely used as an oral estrogen in human medicine; it is about 20 times more potent than stilbestrol. It is also used in small animal veterinary practice.

Estrogens interfere with progesterone dominance during the tubular phase development of the fertilized ova, altering transport time in the oviduct and creating a uterus hostile to continued pregnancy. Estrogens are bound to specific cytosolic receptors in the myometrium, which leads to increased syntheses of the contractile protein actomyosin and affects the membrane potential of the smooth muscle cell. Thus, there is an increase in tone and spontaneous motility of the uterus with enhanced sensitivity to oxytocin. Local vascularity is increased by estrogen. Administration of estrogen may cause the animal to continue to show signs of estrus or appear to return to estrus and thus be remated. This mating could be fertile. Although diethlystilbestrol was the major drug used for misalliance (and was highly effective on account of its high oral bioavailability), its use is now prohibited in most countries, and estradiol monobenzoate is used instead. This is generally held to be not quite as effective.

Estradiol benzoate injection or oral dosing with ethinyl estradiol can be used to control undesirable social behavior in male dogs that is due to excessive testosterone production. However, side effects during estrogen therapy can be a problem, and in any case progestogens possess superior reliability in treatment of this condition.

Ovariectomy in the bitch is often associated with urinary incontinence (see section 41.13). While the precise and specific cause is unknown, onset of the syndrome occurs after months or years. Urinary incontinence in the spayed bitch usually responds to estrogen therapy. A number of injections may be necessary to fully alleviate the condition. Prolonged estrogen therapy in itself may induce polydipsia and polyuria. Estradiol benzoate is recommended at daily intervals for 3 days with subsequent injections every third day. Oral preparations such as ethinyl estradiol are usually administered daily for 3-week periods; a response is observed after the first few days. The major actions of estrogens in this condition is on the urethra. Estrogens have long been used in the treatment of urinary incontinence. Diethylstilbestrol administered orally, 0.1 to 1.0 mg/kg for 3 to 5 days, has been recommended as the drug of choice. In recent years the role of alpha-adrenoceptor agonists in the management of urinary incontinence has been explored. Ephedrine, pseudoephedrine, phenylpropanolamine, and phenylephrine have been used with varying degrees of success. Phenylpropanolamine appears to be the most reliable alpha-agonist for treatment of urinary incontinence. Estrogens have been shown to increase urethral sensitivity to alpha-adrenoceptor agonists, and so the use of both compounds simultaneously appears to possess theoretical benefit.

Quite often, unwanted mating may occur with the attendant request for pregnancy termination. Diethylstilbestrol traditionally has been the method of choice for therapy of misalliance (1.0 to 2.0 mg/day). Estrogen induces the formation of edematous folds at the uterotubal junction, which retains the zygote in the oviduct for several days after ovulation. This is made use of in the treatment of misalliance in the bitch. Estradiol benzoate by injection at a dosage of 6 to 10 mg can be used to treat misalliance. The administration must be carried out within 3 to 4 days of alleged mating.

The use of prostaglandins to terminate pregnancy, although well justified in bovine patients, is not successful in the bitch. Prostaglandins generally are effective only if administered in late pregnancy, and their use is frequently associated with side effects. A further possible complication is the incomplete expulsion of fetuses. Tamoxifen is sometimes recommended at a dosage of 0.5 to 1 mg/kg orally. Tamoxifen inhibits implantation by blocking estrogen receptors and is widely used in human medicine in estrogen-dependent cancer chemotherapy. Antiprogesterones such as mifepristone have been investigated, and there are reports of successful use of mifepristone given orally after day 30 at a dosage of 10 to 40 mg/kg in the bitch.

The antiandrogen effects of estrogens are used in estrogen therapy in the male dog. In cases of excess libido, circum anal adenomas, and prostatic hypertrophy, castration is the ultimate cure. Delmadinone acetate and megestrol acetate can also be considered as alternatives to estrogens in these conditions (see Appendix tables). Hypogonadal obesity can be treated by injection of estradiol benzoate, but again, longterm therapy may give rise to undesirable estrogenic effects. Prolonged estrogen therapy may produce signs of bilaterally symmetric alopecia, epidermal hyperpigmentation, vulval enlargement, gynomastia, and squamous metaplasia of the prostate gland. This could lead to prostatic enlargement.

41.3 THE GONADOTROPINS

The two major gonadotropins are equine chorionic gonadotropin (ECG) and human chorionic gonadotropin (HCG). Equine chorionic gonadotropin is produced by the mare during pregnancy. It possesses mainly FSH activity, but a little LH action is present also. It favors growth and maturation of the follicle in the female and the induction of spermatogenesis in the male. Human chorionic gonadotropin (HCG) is extracted from the urine of pregnant women. Its effects mimic LH activity. Thus, it causes final maturation and ovulation of the follicles and the formation and luteinization of corpora lutea. In the male, HCG stimulates the intestinal (Leydig) cells to secrete testosterone. With some of these gonadotropins there is always the risk of some overstimulation of the ovary, undesirable multiple ovulations, cystic follicles, or prolonged estrus behavior. Other risks are induced antibody production and anaphylactoid reaction, following repeated injection of these foreign protein preparations. In small animals, gonadotropins are useful in a number of clinical situations, discussed next.

FEMALE ANIMALS

Subestrus: Gonadotropins can induce follicular development and secretion of estradiol, and estrus psychic and behavioral activity.

Prolonged Estrus: Gonadotropins can be used to mimic preovulatory LH surge and augment the final maturation of slow-growing especially ECG follicles.

Induction of Estrus and Ovulation: The best results are obtained when repeated dosing with equine chorionic gonadotropin is used to induce estrus and HCG is given to control the timing of ovulation. ECG itself will not only induce estrus where there is a long proestrus, but also induces ovulation on account of the LH surge resulting from follicular growth and estrogen production.

Conception Failure and Fetal Resorption: Bitches that fail to conceive are sometimes given HCG to induce ovulation or to assist corpus luteum formation and development, when it is inadequate.

MALE ANIMALS

Stimulation of Libido and Spermatogenesis: Equine chorionic gonadotropin stimulates spermatogenesis and HCG (interstitial cell stimulating hormone), and increases the production of testosterone. This can be useful in stud dogs displaying lack of libido and low sperm counts.

Genital Hypoplasia and Cryptorchidism: HCG can occasionally be successful in promoting descent of the testicle.

41.4 ANDROGENIC THERAPY

Various esters of androgens are available and the length and complexity of the chain, together with the rate of release of the steroid determines the duration of activity. Many injectable formulations are prepared in oily suspensions to further retard the rate of release.

Orally, the androgens are metabolized rapidly in the liver and, to a lesser extent, in the gastric mucosa. Methylation (e.g., methyltestosterone) reduces this first-pass effect and increases oral bioavailability.

In the case of mammary neoplasia, although the ultimate solution may be mammary surgery, some androgens such as testosterone propionate, methyl testosterone, drostanolone or mibolerone may be used in an attempt to ameliorate the neoplastic condition.

Progestins can also be used for mammary neoplasia. This is a decidedly complicated area insofar as progesterone can cause mammary neoplasia, yet paradoxically some progestins may be used to treat mammary neoplasia.

Testosterone must be reduced by the enzyme 5-alpha-reductase, to dihydrotestosterone before it interacts with the cytosolic receptor in the target tissue cells. Different types and locations of receptors have facilitated the design of anabolic steroid molecules possessing maximum affinity for musculoskeletal tissues and minimal (but some) affinity for tissues of the male reproductive tract. Drugs such as stanozolol, nandrolone and boldenone are well established anabolic steroids.

The aim in designing anabolic steroid molecules is to maximize the anabolic effects and minimize the virilizing effects. Methylated androgens such as 17-alpha-methyl substituted steroids, can result in hepatic dysfunction. Reports exist demonstrating the correlation between oral methyltestosterone and jaundice. Androgens suppress lactation by suppression of prolactin production. When methyltestosterone is combined with estrogen, it has been suggested that the androgen depresses prolactin production, and that the estrogen decreases responsiveness of the mammary gland to prolactin.

Virilizing effects of androgens include the development of secondary sexual characteristics and the promotion of libido and spermatogenesis. Anabolic effects stimulate protein synthesis, muscle deposition, and mineral metabolism, as well as appetite. Continuous high dosages of androgens over long periods will inhibit gonadotropin release and can lead ultimately to infertility. Various androgens (methyltestosterone and testosterone) are used for their anabolic effect in debilitated and aged dogs, and in specific endocrine deficiency states, namely,

(1) deficient libido, poor semen quality and
(2) feminization syndromes. Sertoli cell tumors give rise to feminization syndromes which may be suppressed by the antiestrogenic properties of various androgens such as testosterone, methyltestosterone, drostanolone, mibolerone, and testosterone propionate. (The ultimate solution to the condition is castration.)

Although androgens have been successfully employed in the treatment of hypogonadism and cryptorchidism, in the latter condition if treatment is successful, care should be taken not to breed from these animals because the condition is hereditary. Many cases of mammary neoplasia are estrogen dependent, and so the antiestrogenic effects of testosterone-type compounds may be availed of in therapy of certain mammary tumors. Androgens possess a range of adverse effects. In the female overdosing or prolonged therapy may produce virilizing effects such as clitoral hypertrophy and vaginitis. In prepubertal animals premature epiphyseal growth plate closure may occur. Mineralocorticoid effects such as sodium and water retention can be marked in longterm treatment. Androgens are thus contraindicated in hepatic and nephritic conditions. If given in early pregnancy, androgens may cause masculinization of female embryos. Sustained androgen therapy can lead to infertility via the negative feedback hypothalamic system.

41.5 ANTIANDROGEN THERAPY

Prostatic hyperplasia is usually a benign process mediated by androgens. When severe, the swollen gland may press on internal structures, resulting in difficulty in urinating or constipation. Gonadotropin output (especially FSH) is inhibited by the progestins, which are therefore antiandrogenic in effect. Progestins are useful in prostatic hypertrophy, can allay development in adenomas, but are obviously of no benefit in carcinomas or adenocarcinomas. Progestins have been used to reduce the size of the prostate in hyperplastic states. The mechanism of action of megestrol acetate in prostatic hyperplasia is believed to be by inhibition of the enzyme 5α reductase. In human studies, megestrol acetate prevents conversion of testosterone to dihydrotestosterone—the active androgen in prostatic tumors.

Injection of depot antiandrogenic compounds (delmadinone acetate, medroxyprogesterone acetate) can produce clinical improvement in a couple of days, with a long-lasting effectiveness. Oral megestrol acetate is similarly effective. The condition must be closely monitored because surgical intervention is often warranted. Similarly, circum anal adenomas which are androgen-dependent tumors, respond to progestogen therapy (delmadinone acetate, megestrol acetate, medroxyprogesterone acetate). Therapy with estradiol monobenzoate or ethinyl estradiol are useful alternatives. Such estrongenic compounds are also antiandrogenic by virtue of their suppressant activity on gonadotropin output. Repeated parenteral therapy with estradiol monobenzoate can reduce the size of the prostate gland. Orally active estrogens such as ethinyl estradiol can be equally effective. (Oral diethylstilbestrol has been used to reduce prostate size, but this drug is now banned in most countries.)

41.6 PROGESTINS AND MAMMARY NEOPLASIA

Major differences exist between many progestins and their capacity to induce mammary neoplasia. These differences are primarily in relation to (1) stimulation of growth hormone production and (2) induction of progesterone receptors.

Tremendous variation exists among the synthetic progestins, where only minor molecular modification can result in a disproportionately greater influence on pharmacologic and toxicologic properties. Hence, generalizations cannot be made accurately. On one hand, progestins help to control growth of certain mammary tumors, yet on the other hand some progesterone-like compounds can stimulate the formation of mammary tumors.

In some cases the induction of mammary tumors involves both a direct action on the gland, and the possible stimulation of growth hormone. Direct effect can involve increased concentrations of progesterone receptors in the myometrium.

Long term treatment with progesterone and certain progestins have caused production of benign and malignant tumors in the mammary gland of the bitch. Associated with long term treatment can be a diabetic-type syndrome and acromegaly which would indicate a growth hormone and possibly prolactin involvement.

Side effects of synthetic progestins include

- Lowering of natural blood progesterone levels
- Increased sodium and water retention
- Masculinization of female embryos
- Increase in low density lipoprotein
- Can be androgenic or anabolic
- Some can be carcinogenic

Uterine side effects of progestins are dose dependent, and also related to the particular drug and duration of therapy. The toxic effect may also be exacerbated by prior estrogen priming. Pyometra, diabetes, and coat changes may be due to overdosage of a depot preparation, given at the wrong time. Dosage rate and timing of progestin administration is of paramount importance if such side effects are to be avoided.

Progestins act by preventing release of androgens, by their antigonadotropic action, and also be exerting a specific anti-androgenic effect. In addition, progestins can have a central depressant effect on the higher centers of the brain, resulting in a mild tranquilizing effect.

41.7 CONTROL OF ESTRUS

Several types of drugs have been used to prevent or suppress ovulation. Although most of them have been used in bitches, many of them are not approved for use in cats in the United States. This situation does not obtain in Europe. The available drugs can be listed as follows:

Progestins: Megestrol acetate, medroxyprogesterone acetate, delmadinone

acetate, chlormadinone acetate, proligestone.

Androgens: Testosterone propionate,
methyl testosterone, mibolerone.

Megestrol acetate is used in the United
States to prevent estrus in bitches. It is not
approved for use in cats in the U.S., although it is used in both species in Europe.

Adverse effects seen with progestin
usage depend on the time of treatment,
dose used, and the type of progestin. In cats,
progestins can cause cystic endometritis, alopecia, polyuria, polydypsia, and varied
metabolic and endocrine changes. Frequent
treatment with progestins can increase the
risk of mammary tumors in queens.

Progestins are substances with progesterone-like activity and are widely used to
control reproductive behavior in small animals. Given orally or parenterally, they exert an extremely potent effect on the hypo-
thalamic/hypophyseal system in a negative
feedback fashion. Gonadotropin release
and cyclic activity is suppressed.

Side effects of progestogen therapy include aspermatogenesis, mammary gland
hyperplasia, and elevated blood glucose
levels. All these signs can be slowly reversible if the drug is withdrawn. Subcutaneous
injection may produce hair discoloration
and local alopecia.

Compounds used for estrus control may
be classified as derivatives either of progesterone or of 19-nortesterone. Both compounds regulate estrus by their antigonadotropic action, but their side effects are
related to the progestogenic activity in the
case of the progesterone derivatives and the
androgenic effect in the case of the 19-nor-
testerone derivatives. Compounds with
progestogenic activity affect the endometrium, causing cystic changes and thus increasing the incidence of endometritis and
pyometra. On the other hand, compounds
with androgenic activity may cause effects
such as enlargement of the clitoris, changes
in behavior, and temporary vaginal discharge.

Subcutaneous injections of long-acting
progestogens (medroxyprogesterone acetate, proligestone, progesterone) act as artificial corpora lutea, allowing continuous
slow release of progestogen, and these are
used during anestrus to prevent the subse-

quent estrus. Regular dosing will provide
longterm prevention. However, variability
in duration of action makes prediction of
the next estrus rather difficult. Injections of
some of these compounds can also be given
at proestral bleeding to interrupt a heat
period.

Progesterone provokes endometrial disturbances in the bitch, i.e., endometritis,
cystic glandular hyperplasia, and eventually mucometra or pyometra. The potential
for similar disturbances caused by any progesterone seems to exist if the dose chosen
is too high and treatment is commenced
during proestrus, estrus, or metestrus, before endometrial restoration is completed.
Delmadinone acetate in dogs treated either
during anestrus, approaching proestrus, or
treated during proestrus or metestrus resulted in no endometrial disturbances.

Progestogens possess numerous untoward side effects, which must be taken into
account before a choice between oral or parenteral therapy is made. Transient side effects during therapy include lethargy, increased appetite and weight gain,
mammary enlargement, lactation, pseudopregnancy, hair and coat changes, and temperament changes. Longterm progestogen
therapy is associated with significant risks
to the uterus, induction of cystic endometrial hyperplasia, pyometra, and mucometra. The duration of therapy is a major factor
in determining the toxicity risk, and this
risk is particularly associated with the injectable form. Usually, the depot preparations of progesterone or medroxyprogesterone acetate should be used only during true
anestrus. Proligestone, on the other hand,
although a potent antigonadotropic compound, is only weakly progestational and
so can be used at any stage of the cycle.

MEGESTROL ACETATE

Oral therapy with megestrol acetate produces a low incidence of side effects on the
uterus. Megestrol acetate is an oral progestational agent possessing antigonadotropic
properties and without any estrogenic, androgenic, or anabolic effects. Megestrol acetate is rapidly excreted, and this factor coupled with oral administration, means that
safe and effective dose regimens can be de-

veloped. The drug was originally introduced to suppress or delay estrus and to arrest pseudopregnancy in the bitch. It has also been used in the queen but is not currently approved for cats in the United States. Megestrol acetate is widely used for feline dermatologic problems, as well as for eosinophilic granuloma, feline neurodermatitis, military dermatitis, and feline endocrine alopecia. Megestrol acetate is a very potent progestogen with pronounced antiestrogenic and glucocorticoid activity. The glucocorticoid activity is believed to underpin the therapeutic activity of the drug in dermatologic conditions. Oral administration of a low dose of megestrol acetate during anestrus will postpone the subsequent estrus. Anestrus is ensured during the continuous oral treatment period. Estrus usually returns 3 months after medication, depending on the stage of anestrus when the tablets were administered. Correct timing of treatment is essential because late dosing is often inadequate to cause follicular atresia. Side effects of megestrol acetate are a result of the drug's progestational activity (mammary hyperplasia, pyometra), prolonged glucocorticoid-like effects, diabetes mellitus, weight gain, and atrophy of the adrenal cortex, and also depression of the CNS with perhaps some alteration in temperament. In cats increased appetite and weight gain are the most common side effects. Occasional cases of pyometra and diabetes mellitus have been associated with usage, and mammary neoplasia has also been reported.

MEDROXYPROGESTERONE ACETATE

An injection of medroxyprogesterone acetate can be used to prevent heat in bitches. It should be given every 5 to 6 months but only during anestrus. Medroxyprogesterone is a potent synthetic progestogen that is closely related to the natural corpus luteum hormone, progesterone. In suppressing ovulation in animals, it is 20 to 30 times more potent than progesterone. It acts as a pituitary antigonadotropin by supressing the secretion of the gonadotropin hormones via the feedback servo mechanisms. It also arrests or prevents the development of fol-

licles and corpora lutea within the ovary and possesses antiestrogenic properties.

With earlier potent progestogens, uterine side effects were of particular concern. These side effects, however, were attributable to the duration of administration and were also dose dependent. In the 1960s medroxyprogesterone acetate was associated with pyometra, diabetes, and coat changes. These side effects, however, arose because small bitches were being overdosed (a standard volume, regardless of the animal's size, was recommended), and the depot effect meant that cumulation of the compounds occurred with repeat injections. Also, because medication was recommended at any stage of the cycle, dosing often took place when the uterus had been primed by estrogens or when high endogenous progesterone levels were already present. The occurrence of these side effects was largely overcome by recommending dosing on a precise weight basis and only at specific stages of the cycle. Nonetheless, some pyometra-related problems could be associated with medroxyprogesterone acetate. Subcutaneous injection of this compound during anestrus 1 to 2 months before the expected heat usually inactivates the ovaries for 5 to 6 months. Treatment must take place during anestrus because during proestrus and estrus, the endometrium is estrogen primed and therefore most responsive to progestational stimulation. During metestrus when corpora lutea have not yet regressed, bitches still produce progesterone, and simultaneous administration of medroxyprogesterone acetate could result in excessively strong progestational stimulation. If therapy is repeated at intervals of 6 months, most bitches will be kept out of heat permanently. Treatment is generally recommended at intervals of 5 to 6 months. In bitches, when estrus has already begun (manifest symptoms of bleeding) it can be interrupted by oral dosing with medroxyprogesterone acetate tablets for 16 days. After completion of the course, heat will not return until the next normal period.

DELMADINONE ACETATE

Delmadinone acetate inhibits clinical and behavioral signs of estrus by suppressing FSH and LH secretion by direct and indirect action together with a direct effect of the hypothalamic centers. The drug is indicated for control of heat and ovulation and for suppression of hypersexuality, nervousness, epileptiform seizures, and hypertrophy of the prostate. Delmadinone acetate is a potent orally and systemically active progestin that exerts antiestrogenic as well as strong antiandrogenic effects. It may be used for (1) estrus prevention—an injection no earlier than 3 months after the last heat and no later than 2 months before the next anticipated heat—(2) suppression or shortening of proestrus or estrus. Recommended dosage is 1.5 to 2.0 mg/kg intramuscularly.

PROLIGESTONE

Proligestone exhibits strong antigonadotropic properties but is only weakly progestogenic and has no androgenic activity. Proligestone has therefore practically no effect on the endometrium, even if it is already sensitized by estrogen. It is therefore not contraindicated for use in proestrus but can be used at any stage of the estrus cycle. Efficacy with proligestone is dose dependent, and under normal conditions, effective blood levels are maintained after a single depot injection to prevent the occurrence of estrus for up to 5 months. In contrast to other injectable products, medication in proestrus is not contraindicated with proligestone. The signs of heat can be suppressed by giving a single injection as early as possible in proestrus. Vulval swelling, bleeding, and attractiveness to dogs will gradually stop within 5 days. Estrus can be prevented for long periods by giving repeat injections in anestrus. To obtain constant deferment of heat, a second dose should be given 3 months after the first and a third dose given 4 months after the second. Subsequent doses should be given every 5 months. Proligestone is also indicated for treatment of false pregnancy.

Proligestone is strongly antigonadotropic but only weakly progestogenic. Apart from being antiestrogenic, it has no other hormonal effect, and furthermore it has only a medium duration of action. These three characteristics make the compound intrinsically safer. Many of the restrictions applicable to first-generation compounds such as megestrol acetate and medroxyprogesterone acetate are no longer necessary. Proligestone can be given (1) at any stage of the cycle—estrogen priming or the presence of progesterone levels are of less consequence; (2) by injection; and (3) for suppression, temporary postponement, and permanent postponement of estrus. Repeat doses can be given without fear of cumulation.

Longterm administration of certain progestogens can result in mammary neoplasia of which some are benign mixed adenomata and some malignant carcinomas or adenocarcinomas. Medroxyprogesterone acetate (MPA) can stimulate development of hyperplastic nodules in the mammary glands; however, a number of trials with proligestone have revealed no such effects. This difference between the two progestogens may be due to stimulation of growth hormone by MPA.

Proligestone has an advantage in that it can be given to both species at proestrus to interrupt incipient heat.

Mibolerone (Cheque, Upjon) is a synthetic androgen available for the longterm prevention of estrus and treatment of false pregnancy. Mibolerone is androgenic, anabolic, anti-gonadotropic and inhibits pituitary gonadotropin release but possesses no progestational or estrogenic activity in the dog. It is not recommended for use in bitches before their first heat, nor is it recommended for use in breeding bitches. The usual dosage is 0.3 ml (30 mcg)/25 lb body weight/day, orally. The drops must be started at least 30 days before the next heat, or they may not stop the bitch from coming into proestrus.

41.8 TERMINATION OF PREGNANCY/INDUCTION OF LABOR

Drugs used to terminate pregnancy in bitches or queens act in a number of ways: (1) Delay transit time and prevent attachment (e.g., estrogens, anti-estrogens, tamoxifen). (2) Induction of luteolysis (prostaglandins). (3) Promote uterine emptying (mifepristone). Estradiol cypionate 20 to 40 mcg/kg given on day 2 of diestrus delays ovum transit time through the oviduct of bitches. A similar effect is noted 40 hours postcoitally in cats given 250 μg of estradiol cypionate. Side effects of estrogen include pyometra, cystic endometrial, hyperplasia, estrus, leukopenia, and anemia.

Prolactin inhibitors can successfully terminate pregnancy during its later stages. Bromocriptine 30 μg/kg has been used with varying efficiency for terminating feline and canine pregnancy. Most prolactin inhibitors are dopamine agonists and vomiting sometimes accompanies their use. This is true of bromocriptine and a new prolactin inhibitor, cabergoline.

Synthetic steroids acting as progesterone antagonists can be used to bind to and to block the body's gestagenic receptors. Such anti-progesterone drugs will abolish the effects of progesterone, and thus, they possess a number of useful clinical indications. Mifepristone is one such progesterone antagonist that can be used to terminate pregnancy in small animals. Dosages used have ranged from 2.5 mg/kg to 20 mg/kg orally. As of the moment, mifepristone is not commercially available for veterinary use in the United States.

Tamoxifen citrate is an antiestrogenic compound that has been used for early termination of pregnancy (mismatching/misalliance). At a dosage range of 0.5 to 1.0 mg/kg orally, tamoxifen has been experimentally useful for very early (post-coital) termination of pregnancy. Some adverse effects, like endometritis, can accompany its use.

Several hormonal drugs may be used to induce myometrial contractility. These include estrogens, oxytocin, ergot alkaloids, and prostaglandins. Oxytocin induces milk letdown by stimulating the myoepithelial fibers of the mammary gland. It also causes contraction of uterine smooth muscle. Dilation of the cervix and correct posture and presentation of the fetus are essential when using oxytocin, because its potent spasmogenic effect in the uterine muscle could lead to uterine rupture as a result of tumultuous contraction. Accordingly, oxytocin is contraindicated in obstructive dystocia because uterine rupture may result. It may also promote placental separation, which could jeopardize the survival of unborn fetuses. Because oxytocin has a very short half-life, repeated parenteral administration may be necessary. The major indications for oxytocin usage in small animal medicine follow:

1. Retention of the placenta
2. Postpartum hemorrhage
3. Postpartum endometritis

Estrogen is normally used before administration of oxytocin to sensitize the uterus to the effects of oxytocin. Ergot alkaloids and in particular ergometrine produce prolonged myometrial spasm, with relaxation after 1 or 2 hours when the uterus starts rhythmic contractions similar to those induced by oxytocin. It has been used to treat postpartum hemorrhage, postpartum endometritis, and uterine inertia.

PROSTAGLANDINS

Canine corpora lutea are refractory to prostaglandin therapy during early pregnancy. After this time repeated doses can be given, although side effects are common. Prostaglandin treatment induces uterine evacuation in cases of acute metritis. The use of prostaglandins for initiation of expulsive contraction in cases of pyometra, although reportedly successful in some cases, carries the attendant hazard of uterine rupture as a result of overstimulation of the myometrium. During pregnancy or pseudopregnancy in the bitch, treatment with prostaglandin (PgF2α) and its analogues cause luteolysis. Contrary to the experience in many other mammals, however, PgF2α-induced luteolysis in the bitch is only a temporary phenomenon, and the corpora lutea return to their capability to produce progesterone within 12 to 24 hours. Therefore, induction of abortion requires repeated treatments at 12-hour intervals for about 3 to 4 days to keep progesterone levels low long enough to trigger abortion.

Side effects seen with the treatment can be quite severe. Adverse effects to prostaglandins are very common in small animals. Signs observed are salivation, restlessness, vomiting, abdominal pain, pyrexia, tachycardia, and diarrhea. These effects occur rapidly after injection and last for up to 3 hours.

To produce a successful abortion with prostaglandins, the proper length of treatment of about six injections every 12 hours is necessary. Treatment must be delayed until mid- to late gestation because the early corpora lutea in the bitch are more refractory to PgF2α. PgF2α also induces strong myometrial contractions in the bitch, which play a role in inducing abortion, along with a decreased luteal function. Although a single injection of 1 mg/kg of PgF2α in the bitch is an effective abortifacient, side effects can be expected at this dosage. When a bitch has accidentally mated, the owner frequently wants an abortion performed. If more than 2 or 3 days have elapsed since misalliance, a mismating injection of estrogen 0.5 to 2.0 estradiol may be ineffective. A prostaglandin-induced abortion may be indicated. Assuming the dog is pregnant, it can be started on a dosage of PgF2α at 25 to 30 μg/kg every 12 hours parenterally for 72 hours (total of six treatments) starting no earlier than the 33rd day of gestation. Sometimes priming the animal with 0.1 mg of estradiol given intramuscularly 24 hours before starting the PgF2α treatment may increase the abortifacient effect. Abortion should be expected to occur approximately 60 hours after the first PgF2α injection. In the queen it has been reported that one or two subcutaneous injections of PgF2α 24 hours apart at a dosage of 0.2 to 1 mg/kg can induce abortion if given after the 40th day of gestation. Abortion occurs usually within 24 hours of the first injection or within 24 hours of the second injection. Within 15 minutes after injection, defecation and often panting occur. The PgF2α-induced abortions in cats may be due to luteolysis of the corpus luteum of pregnancy or are the result of PgF2α-induced myometrial contractions.

Prostaglandins alone or in combination with oxytocin, estrogen, or dexamethasone can induce parturition. This relates to the important role prostaglandins play in the normal physiology of parturition in the dog and the manner in which they terminate pregnancy in mid- to late gestation. PgF2α can be used to terminate gestation in the bitch and the queen. In bitches, given from day 33 to day 53 of gestation, at a dosage of either 20 mcg/kg every 8 hours or 30 μg/kg every 12 hours for 72 hours, prostaglandin will cause the fetus to abort within 50 to 72 hours after treatment begins.

41.9 PSEUDOPREGNANCY

Pseudopregnancy is a normal phenomenon that follows each non fertile estrus. Clinical signs include abdominal enlargement, mammary gland enlargement, lactation and nesting.

Androgens, estrogens, and progestins inhibit prolactin release and thus are effective in treating pseudopregnancy, or false pregnancy. Because androgens lack the estrogen/progesterone type of adverse effects on the uterus, they may be more suitable in this condition (e.g., oral or injectable methyltestosterone with or without ethinyl estradiol, testosterone phenylpropionate, testosterone implants, mibolerone). Estrogens have long been used to suppress postpartum lactation and to terminate pseudopregnancy. The negative feedback effect of estrogens on the hypothalamic/pituitary axis means that they reduce prolactin levels. Both oral diethylstilbestrol or parenteral estradiol monobenzoate have been used. Several estrogens from human medicine such as ethinyl estradiol have also been employed as diethylstilbestrol substitutes.

False pregnancy can respond quite erratically to a whole range of hormone treatments. Repeated parenteral treatment with estradiol benzoate may sometimes substitute for oral therapy with stilbenes. Ethinyl estradiol in combination with methyltestosterone or methyltestosterone alone can be successfully used. Megestrol acetate, delmadinone acetate, 1.0 to 2.5 mg/kg, bid, or an injection of proligestone can also be effective. On account of the potent antigonadotropic activity of proligestone, it can be used therapeutically to suppress the endogenous hormones responsible for pseudopregnancy. Being largely devoid of progesterone-type activity itself, proligestone does not induce any mammary development. The drug can be safely used in breeding bitches. The luteolytic effect of prostaglandins can be used for the treatment of pseudopregnancy and has successfully caused regression of galactorrhea, mammary enlargement, mothering behavior, nest building, and labor pains in clinically falsely pregnant bitches. The animals returned to normal about 7 to 8 days following the treatment. A more logical alternative might be the use of specific drugs that inhibit pro-lactin. Bromocriptine is one such inhibitor and has been used with equivocal results. Bromocriptine is a related synthetic ergot alkaloid that inhibits prolactin secretion. It is not specifically licensed for use in dogs. Daily oral administration of small doses (6 to 12 μg/kg) is often successful in the treatment of pseudopregnancy, but it may cause vomiting. This can be prevented by minimizing the dose, mixing the drug with food, or using antiemetics.

41.10 SUPPRESSION OF LACTATION

Veterinarians are often consulted about the undesirable lactation that accompanies pseudopregnancy in bitches. More than half of bitches develop this condition at least once during their lifetime, and recurrence is common. The condition is accompanied by changes in behavior (agitation, upset appetite, licking of mammary gland) and development of the mammary gland and the onset of lactation, which may be pronounced. It usually occurs 6 to 12 weeks after estrus. The condition is accompanied by hormonal changes similar to those of pregnancy. The prolactin concentration increases during metestrus, though not to the same extent as during true pregnancy. Many treatments have been suggested to suppress lactation, but in most cases their effectiveness has not stood up to rigorous evaluation. Most of the commonly employed steroid hormones can produce side effects that are unacceptable in view of the physiologic nature of the condition and the fact that it regresses slowly and without complication. Trials in women have shown that bromocriptine suppresses lactation after parturition. As mentioned, bromocriptine is a synthetic ergot alkaloid that inhibits the secretion of prolactin by the pituitary. The action is reversible. It is a dopaminergic agent that lowers the prolactin concentration in the blood. In the bitch administration parenterally of bromocriptine to lactating females inhibits lactation at dose rates between 6 and 12 μg/kg. Oral administration of bromocriptine is hampered by its emetic effect in dogs. Bromocriptine rapidly suppresses lactation and also brings about the rapid disappearance of the altered behavior that accompanies the condition. Thus, it is an effective means for treating the lactation of pseudopregnancy. Even though its effect is rapid, treatment for 14 days is recommended to avert any rebound effect. The problem of vomiting during therapy can be addressed in two ways. One is to give bromocriptine in increasing doses to accustom the bitch to the drug. The other solution is to combine bromocriptine with an antiemetic. The correct choice of drug is crucial because the phenol derivatives (haloperidol, droperidol) block the systemic transmission of dopamine and consequently oppose the action of bromocriptine. In the same way, metclopramide is a powerful stimulant of prolactin secretion.

Bromocriptine is not popular because of its emetic side effects. More promising is the longer acting compound cabergoline, which is active orally and parenterally and is without noticeable side effects.

Metopimazine has mainly peripheral action and can be administered with bromocriptine. Such a technique can supplement other regimens that use estrogens, androgens, or progestogens in view of the side effects of the latter. Bromocriptine also suppresses lactation in cats without provoking vomiting at dose rates up to 50 μg/kg. Other progestogens such as megestrol acetate, and proligestone inhibit the release of prolactin from the pituitary gland and are effective in treating false pregnancy in the bitch. Progesterone, medroxyprogesterone acetate, and delmadinone acetate are also effective. Normal behavior usually occurs within 3 days.

Androgens have been used to suppress lactation. Combined androgen-estrogen therapy has proved useful in human therapy because of a synergistic activity. Androgen depresses prolactin production, and estrogen decreases the responsiveness of the gland to prolactin.

Work from human medicine indicates that a combination of estrogen and androgen is superior for lactation suppression than either used individually. By combining androgenic and estrogenic ingredients it is possible to reduce the effective dosage of each if given separately. Combined estrogen-androgen therapy exerts a synergistic effect for the suppression of lactation. Their actions are attributable to suppression of the anterior pituitary gland and therefore prolactin production. Androgen alone only partially suppresses lactation, and in large doses, can interfere with normal uterine involution.

41.11 ENDOMETRITIS AND PYOMETRA

Progestogens are synthetic compounds that mimic the effects of progesterone. They have a multiplicity of physiologic actions that make them effective in controlling estrus as well as in many other clinical situations. Because the biologic activity of progestogens is related to the structure of the compound, it is not valid to transpose findings with one progestogen to all others. All of these compounds affect the endometrium to a greater or lesser degree. The normal appearance of the uterus can be changed dramatically by the administration of progesterone or progestogens. These pathologic changes can be classified in three main types: cystic endometrial hyperplasia, mucometra, and pyometra. The occurrence of these changes will depend on both the daily dose and the duration of administration. The administration of progestogen in bitches is therefore potentially hazardous, and thus it is important that the compound is selected with care and attention is paid to dosage rate and duration and method of administration. In practical terms this means that progestogens should be given only when safety of the method of administration is such that the amount of compound given and the duration of effect can be controlled.

With repeated doses of estrogen, ovariectomized bitches can develop experimental hyperplastic endometritis and, by simultaneous injection of progesterone, the condition of pyometra. Cystic endometrial hyperplasia (pyometra syndrome) in the bitch results from persistent uterine glandular stimulation by circulating progestogens. Progesterone induces endometrial gland proliferation and secretion while suppressing myometrial activity, allowing accumulation of these secretions, which then act as a medium for bacterial growth. The uterus becomes atonic, and the cervix remains functionally closed in most cases. Clinical signs vary with the severity of the disease, its duration, the presence or absence of bacterial infection, cervical drainage, and systemic involvement. Vaginal discharge, polydipsia, polyuria, vomiting, and fever are common signs of the condition.

Although ovariohysterectomy is the treatment of choice for canine pyometra, hormonal and antimicrobial therapies have been proposed for breeding bitches. Estrogen priming of the myometrium of the bitch has been used in the treatment of pyometra and delayed parturition, especially in conjunction with ecbolic drugs such as oxytocin. Estrogens increase the vascularity of the uterus, dilate the cervix, and increase myometrial motility. Many cases of vaginitis and acute postpartum metritis therefore are estrogen-responsive conditions. Prostaglandins are luteolytic, although in the cat and dog, the normal life span of the corpus luteum is unaltered by the absence of the uterus. Because the corpora lutea of bitches are not readily lysed by prostaglandin action, the uses of such compounds are related to their presumed ability to produce myometrial continuation and relaxation of the cervix. PgF2α has been used at dosages of 0.23 mg/kg/day for 1–4 consecutive days in pyometric bitches. Reactions after subcutaneous injection have included restlessness, hypersalivation, vomiting, defecation, panting, and uterine evacuation. These effects can last up to half an hour. Nonetheless, prostaglandins, although relatively toxic to the bitch, are effective in causing a disappearance of the hemorrhagic vaginal discharge, return of appetite, and loss of depression, polydipsia, and polyuria. The resolution of pyometra and endometritis can be assisted by PgF2α at a dose of 0.23 mg/kg. This is in addition to other appropriate therapeutic measures such as antimicrobial therapy. Within 24 hours of this dose, purulent discharge is expelled. Oxytocin can be given at the time of the evacuation to effect a complete discharge of the uterine contents. Prostaglandin treatment is not curative in most cases, but it can reduce pyometra to subclinical levels, at least temporarily. $PgF_2 = \alpha$ subcutaneously (0.23 to 5.0 mg/kg) for 3 days, intravenous (IV) fluids, and antimicrobial drugs for 3 to 4 weeks reportedly make up a good regimen for successful treatment of pyometra in the bitch.

Because no prostaglandins are specifically licensed for use in the bitch, there is no clear guideline as to specific dosages. The median lethal dose (LD_{50}) of $PgF_2\alpha$ in the dog is low (5.13 mg/kg), and so care must be taken to avoid overdosing. Doses range from 0.1 mg/kg to 0.23 mg/kg over a period of days. A regimen of two subcutaneous injections at 0.23 mg/kg given 24 hours apart has proven successful. Side effects include urination, diarrhea, vomiting, hyperventilation, salivation, anxiety, trembling, and increased heart rate. These side effects tend to be transient, last for about 1 hour, and are not dose related. Cases of open pyometra may respond to prostaglandins given for 5 days parenterally and combined with antibiotic therapy, although adverse effects may be severe and success rates variable.

Retained fetal membranes in the bitch can be treated in a number of pharmacological ways. Oxytocin, 1–8 IU, is successful as is ergometrine maleate (0.5–1.0 mg). Following retention of the fetal membrane, infection of the canine genital tract commonly occurs after the first week of parturition or abortion. Hemolytic staphylococci, E. coli, Haemophilus sp., and A. pyogenes are common primary pathogens. Proteus, Pseudomonas, and Klebsiella may become secondarily involved.

Intrauterine therapy may be indicated with antibacterial agents. Estrogens, oxytocin (10–20 units) and ergometrine (0.2 mg) can be useful in restoring uterine tone and evacuating exudate.

41.12 HORMONALLY RESPONSIVE SKIN CONDITIONS

Estrogens are potent epitheliotropic hormones. This activity is particularly useful for the treatment of alopecia following ovariectomy. The effect of the estrogen in such cases is to suppress sebum production and to promote keratinization. The dosage, however, must be kept low enough to avoid induction of generalized estrogenic behavioral effects. Eosinophilic granuloma complex is a chronic localized dermatosis involving the lips, oral mucosa, and integument. The cause is unknown, and there appears to be no breed, sex, or age predilection. Constant licking and grooming may be the cause of the complex.

Megestrol acetate is a potent oral progestogen that is rapidly excreted primarily via the feces and urine. At a dosage of 2.5 mg daily for the first week, 2.5 mg every second day for the second week, and 2.5 mg twice weekly for maintenance, megestrol acetate has been reportedly successful in the treatment of the condition. Occasionally, corticosteroids or antihistamines may be necessary to reduce the severity of the pruritus. Although side effects should be minimal, all animals on therapy should be closely monitored for untoward effects. (Common side effects in cats are increased appetite and weight gain.)

Miliary dermatitis is characterized by multiple small, dry, scaly, papular lesions. If left untreated these lesions increase in size and eventually coalesce. Pruritus erythema and alopecia are very common presenting signs. Ulceration can occur in severe cases as a result of trauma caused by repeated licking. Various causes have been proposed such as fleas, improper diet, hormone deficiencies, and food allergies. Progestogens have been found effective for treating miliary dermatitis, and some are in fact more effective than corticosteroids. Chronic miliary dermatitis in cats has been effectively controlled with megestrol acetate in doses up to 2.5 mg/kg.

Megestrol acetate offers several advangages over continuous corticosteroid therapy. Steroids are contraindicated in congestive heart failure, diabetes, osteoporosis, and viral infection. They have been known to mask the signs of bacterial infections and induce anorexia, polydipsia, and polyuria. The value of corticosteroids in treatment of miliary dermatitis is at best only palliative. Increased appetite and weight gain occasionally accompany its usage, but this can be minimized to some degree by interrupting the therapeutic dose or reducing the dosage to a maintenance level when remission of clinical signs is apparent. In cats proligestone is suitable for treatment of miliary eczema at a dosage of 1.5 times that used for estrus control. This dosage of 50 mg/kg can be repeated within 14 days, and at the same time concurrent treatment to remove ectoparasites should be considered. Megestrol acetate amd medroxyprogesterone acetate have both been shown to be effective in controlling the growth of estrogen-dependent mammary tumors. Paradoxically, they both possess the potential also to induce mammary neoplasia. Most of the progestogen-induced tumors are benign mixed adenomata, but some are malignant carcinomas or adenocarcinomas. The induction of mammary tumors by medroxyprogesterone acetate may be partially attributable to the stimulation of growth hormone and perhaps also a direct effect on the mammary gland. Major differences exist between progestogens in relation to their ability (1) to stimulate the production of growth hormone and (2) to influence progestogen receptor concentrations in mammary tissue.

The biologic activity of progestogens is related to the structure of the compound. The effects of different progestagens are therefore variable, and it is not valid to transpose findings with one progestogen to all others. Minor differences in molecular configuration have repeatedly produced wide variations in pharmacologic effects. Feline neurodermatitis has been treated with glucocorticoids, tranquilizers, vitamin mineral supplements as well as phenobarbitol and diazepam. Progestational drugs, like megestrol acetate, given in large doses sometimes control the skin lesions associated with these conditions. Combined androgen-estrogen injections or progestational drugs have been used for the treatment of feline endocrine alopecia.

41.13 URINARY INCONTINENCE

Urinary incontinence, the involuntary passage of urine, may occur when the pressure in the bladder is greater than the ability of the normal urethal sphincter to prevent emptying or the urethral sphincter is too weak to inhibit micturition. Incontinence is usually a disease of older animals, especially spayed bitches.

"Micturition" refers to the storage and voiding of urine, and many processes can disturb this function. Micturition disorders can affect voiding or storage of urine (or both), and the underlying cause may be neurogenic or non-neurogenic.

Non-neurogenic causes include such diverse causes as chronic cystitis, urethral inflammation, or urethral calculi. Neutered dogs of both sexes commonly display reproductive hormone responsive incontinence. (Estrogen and testosterone contribute to the maintenance of urethral muscle tone.) Prostatic disease and lower urinary tract infections are other predisposing causes.

Neurogenic causes include abnormal interference with the neurologic control of the detrusor muscle, urethral sphincters, or both. Different therapeutic objectives must be set depending on the underlying causes.

Sympathetic and parasympathetic innervation of the bladder and urethra governs micturition. Stimulation of beta receptors of the bladder causes the detrusor muscle to relax while stimulation of the alpha receptors of the urethra causes the urethra to contract. Stimulation of the parasympathetic receptors of the lower urinary tract causes contraction of the detrusor muscle.

The storage phase of micturition involves relaxation of the detrusor muscle (beta-adrenergic stimulation) and sphincter contraction (alpha-adrenergic stimulation).

Different classes of drugs can be used to treat urinary incontinence

1. Cholinergic agents, which increase bladder contractability
2. Anticholinergic agents, which decrease bladder contractability
3. Alpha-adrenergic agents, which increase sphincter tone
4. Alpha-adrenergic blocking agents, which decrease sphincter tone

In spayed females estrogens are used because they increase urethral tone by increasing the sensitivity of the urethra to alpha-adrenergic stimulation.

Ephedrine and pseudoephedrine are often particularly effective, especially in older animals. Acting as an alpha-adrenergic agonists, they stimulate alpha-receptors in the urethra resulting in increased urethral tone.

Phenylephrine or phenylpropanolamine are particularly useful alpha-agonists that act in the same manner. Phenylpropanolamine is one of the most useful drugs in this regard.

Urethral incompetence is commonly associated with abnormal smooth muscle function. Drugs that can increase the smooth muscle activity of the urethra include alpha-adrenergic agonists such as phenylpropanolamine. Drugs that decrease the smooth muscle activity of the urethra include alpha-adrenergic blocking agents such as phenoxybenzamine. Myorelaxing drugs such as dantrolene and baclofen or tranquilizers such as diazepam also can be considered.

Estradiol monobenzoate or testosterone propionate can be given to spayed bitches or castrated males, respectively, in which urinary incontinence is a problem.

Apart from other measures such as treating any urinary tract infection that may be present, the administration of a low-salt diet can be useful in some cases. A low-salt diet reduces water intake and will tend to reduce urine volume, and thus the internal bladder pressure.

SELECTED REFERENCES

Barsanti, J. A., and Downey, R.: Urinary incontinence in cats. JAVMA, 20:979, 1984.

Borshelt, P. L., and Voith, V. L.: Dominance aggression in dogs. Compend. Contin. Ed. Pract. Vet., 8:36, 1986.

Borchelt, P. L., and Voith, V. L.: Elimination behavior problems in cats. Compend. Contin. Ed. Pract. Vet. 8:197, 1986.

Bowen, R. A., Olson, P. N., Behrendt, M. D., and Wheeler, S. L.: Efficacy and toxicity of estrogens commonly used to terminate canine pregnancy. JAVMA, 186:783, 1985.

Brown, J. M.: Use of prostaglandin F2 in treatment of uterine diseases in the bitch. Mod. Vet. Pract., 66:381, 1985.

Bryan, H. S.: Parenteral use of medroxyprogesterone acetate as an antifertility agent in the bitch. Am. J. Vet. Res., 34:5, 1973.

Burke, T. J., and Reynolds, M. A.: Megestrol acetate for estrus postponement in the bitch. JAVMA, 167:285, 1975.

Concannon, P. W., and Hansel, W.: Prostaglandin F2 alpha induced luteolysis hypothermia abortions in Beagle bitches. Prostaglandins, 13:533, 1977.

Concannon, P. W., Meyers-Wallen, V. N.: Current and proposed methods for contraception and termination of pregnancy in dogs and cats. JAVMA, 198:1214–1225, 1991.

Concannon, P. W.: Endocrinology of canine estrus cycles, pregnancy and parturition. Proceed. Ann. Meeting. Soc. Theriogenol., 1–24, 1984.

Conley, A. J., and Evans, L. E.: Bromocryptine-induced abortion in the bitch. In Proceedings of the 10th International Congress on Animal Reproduction and A.I. Urbana, IL, 1984.

Eigenmann, J. E., and Eigenmann, R. Y.: Influence of medroxy progesterone acetate (Provera) on plasma growth hormone levels and on carbohydrate metabolism. II. Studies in the ovariohysterectomised estradiol-primed bitch. Acta Endocrinol. 98:603, 1981.

Evans, J. M.: Hypersexuality in dogs with particular reference to the role of progestogens. The postgraduate committee in veterinary science. University of Sydney, Practice, 37:19, 1978.

Gaunt, S. D., and Pierce, K. R.: Effects of estradiol on hematopoietic and marrow adherent cells of dogs. Am. J. Vet. Res., 47:906, 1986.

Gerber, H. A., and Sulman, F. G.: The effects of methyloestranelone on oestrus, pseudopregnancy and vagrancy. Nord. Vet. Med., 29:287, 1977.

Gosselen, P., Chalifoux, A., and Papageorges, M.: The use of megestrol acetate in some feline dermatological problems. Can. Vet. Med., 22:382, 1981.

Hart, B. L., and Hart, L. A.: Canine and feline behavioral therapy. Philadelphia, Lea and Febiger, 1985.

Henik, R. A., Olson, P. N., and Rosychuk, R. A. W.: Progestogen therapy in cats. Compend. Contin. Ed. Pract. Vet., 7:132, 1985.

Houdeshell, J. W., and Hennessey, B. S.: Megestrol acetate for control of estrus. Vet. Med. S.A.C., 6:1013, 1977.

Jochle, W., and Anderson, A. C.: The estrus cycle in the dog: review clarification and contribution. Theriogenology, 7:113, 1977.

Jochle, W., Ballabio, R., and DiSalle, E.: Inhibition of lactation in beagle bitches with the prolactin inhibitor cabergoline: dose response and aspects of long term safety. Theriogenology, IM Druck. 1987.

Jochle, W., Lamond, D. R., and Anderson, A. C.: Mestranol as an abactifacient in the bitch. Theriogenology, 4:1, 1975.

Krawiec, D. R., and Rubin, S. I.: Urinary incontinence in geriatric dogs. Compend. Contin. Ed. Pract. Vet., 7:566, 1985.

Line, S., and Voith, V. L.: Dominance aggression of dogs towards people. Behaviour profile and response to treatment. Appl. Anim. Ethol., 16:77, 1986.

Meyers-Wallen, V. N.: Prostaglandin F2 treatment of pyometra. JAVMA, 189:1557, 1986.

Neville, P.: Treatment of behaviour problems in cats. In Practic. Suppl. to Vet. Record., March 1991, p. 43.

Nakao, T., et al.: Induction of estrus in bitches with exogenous gonadotropins and pregnancy rate and blood progesterone profiles. Jpn. J. Vet. Sci., 47:17, 1985.

Olson, P. N., Husted, P. W., Allen, T. A., and Nett, T. M.: Reproductive endocrinology and physiology of the bitch and queen. Vet. Clin. North. Am. Small. Anim. Pract., 14:927, 1984.

Olson, P. N., Johnston, S. D.: New developments in small animal population control. JAVMA, 202:904–909, 1993.

Os, J. L., Von Laar, P. H., Oldenkemp, E. P., and Verschoor, J. S. C.: Oestrus control and the incidence of mammary nodules in bitches; a clinical study with two progestogens. Vet. Q., 46, 1981.

Paradis, M., Post, K., and Mapletoft, R. J.: Effects of prostaglandin F2 on corpora lutea formation and function in mated bitches. Can. Vet. J., 24:239, 1983.

Romatowski, J.: Use of megestrol acetate in cats. JAVMA, 194(5):700, 1989.

Rosin, A. E., and Barasanti, J. A.: Diagnosis of urinary incontinence in dogs. Role of the urethral pressure profile. JAVMA, 178(8):814, 1981.

Rosin, A. H., and Ross, L.: Diagnosis and pharmacological management of disorders of urinary continence in the dog. Compend. Contin. Ed. Pract. Vet., 3:601, 1981.

Rubin, S. I.: Pharmacologic management of urinary incontinence. In Proceedings ACVIM, Blacksburg, VA, 1988.

Sokolowski, J. H.: Reproductive features and patterns in the bitch. J. Am. Anim. Hosp. Assoc., 9:71, 1973.

Turner, D. C.: The ethology of the human-cat relationship. Schiveiz. Arch. Tierheilk., 133, 1991.

APPENDIX

APPENDIX 41–1
DRUGS FOR REPRODUCTIVE THERAPY

PROGESTOGENS

Proligestone
Progesterone
Megestrol acetate
Medroxyprogesterone acetate
Delmadinone acetate
Chlormadinone acetate

ANDROGENS

Methyltestosterone
Testosterone phenylpropionate
Testosterone
    Propionate
    Decanoate
Drostanolone propionate
Mibolerone

ANTIANDROGENS

Delmadinone acetate
Megestrol acetate
Medroxyprogesterone acetate
Proligestone
Estrogens

ANTIESTROGENS

Tamoxifen

ANTIPROLACTIN

Bromocriptine
Cabergoline

APPENDIX 41–2
HORMONALLY RESPONSIVE CONDITIONS

Urinary Incontinence:
    Estrogens
    Alpha-adrenoceptor agonists/antagonists
    Cholinergic agonists/antagonists

Pseudopregnancy
    Estrogens
    Androgens
    Prostaglandins
    Progestins: megestrol acetate, proligestone
    Medroxyprogesterone acetate
    Bromocriptine

Misalliance: Termination of Gestation
    Estrogens
    Megestrol acetate
    Tamoxifen
    Prostaglandins
    Mifepristone, Bromocriptine/cabergoline

Estrus Prevention/Suppression
    Progesterone
    Megestrol acetate
    Proligestone
    Medroxyprogesterone acetate, delmadinone acetate
    Mibolerone

Suppression of Lactation
    Bromocriptine/cabergoline
    Estrogens
    Megestrol acetate
    Proligestone
    Delmadinone acetate

Benign Prostatic Hyperplasia
    Delmadinone acetate
    Megestrol acetate
    Medroxyprogesterone acetate
    Estrogens

Dominance Aggression
    Delmadinone acetate
    Megestrol acetate
    Medroxyprogesterone acetate

Endometritis/pyometra
    Estrogen
    Oxytocin
    Prostaglandins
    (Antimicrobials, etc.)

Induction of Labor
    Prostaglandins
    Estrogens
    Oxytocin
    Ergot alkaloids

APPENDIX TABLE 41–3
SUPPRESSION OF OVULATION

1) *Progestins*
   Megestrol acetate, medroxyprogesterone acetate, delmadinone acetate, chlormadinone acetate, proligestone

2) *Androgens*
   Mibolerone is approved in the United States for use in dogs but not in cats

(Vaginal discharge, clitoral enlargement and masculinization of female embryos are potential side effects of mibolerone treatment.)

(Intramuscular testosterone propionate given weekly or oral administration of methyl testosterone has also been used successfully to prevent estrus in bitches)

APPENDIX 41–4
THERAPEUTIC OBJECTIVES FOR URINARY INCONTINENCE

Pharmacologic Objective ↓	Drug Effect ↓
I URETHRAL MUSCLE	
(a) Increase tone of muscle (Alpha agonists)	Contraction in urethral incompetence.
(b) Decrease tone of muscle (Alpha blockers)	Used if urethral blockage is present.
II BLADDER	
(a) Increase tone of detrusor muscle (Cholinergic agonist)	Bladder muscle constriction and urinary elimination
(b) Decrease tone of detrusor muscle (Cholinergic antagonist)	Inhibits tone of spastic bladder muscle contraction.

APPENDIX TABLE 41–5
PHARMACOLOGICAL CLASSIFICATION OF DRUGS USED FOR URINARY INCONTINENCE

- Alpha Agonists
  - — Phenylpropanolamine
  - ↘ Ephedrine
- Alpha Adrenoceptor Antagonists — Phenoxybenzamine
- Cholinergic Agonists — Bethanecol
- Cholinergic Antagonists — Propantheline
  - ↘ Flavoxate
  - ↘ Oxybutynin
  - ↘ Dicyclomine

APPENDIX TABLE 41–6
DRUGS FOR URINARY INCONTINENCE

A Effects on Bladder Drug Action	Dose	Pharmacologic effect
(a) *Reduced detrusor activity*		
• Dicyclomine	10–15 mg (orally) (t.i.d.)	Parasympatholytic
• Flavoxate	80–200 mg (orally) (t.i.d.)	Parasympatholytic
• Oxybutynin	3–6 mg	Parasympatholytic
• Propantheline	12–35 mg Orally (t.i.d.)	Parasympatholytic
(b) *Increased detrusor muscle contraction*		
• Betanechol	2–15 mg s.c. t.i.d.	Cholinergic Agonist
B Effects on Urethra		
(a) *Increased urethral tone*	Dose	Pharmacologic effect
• Phenylpropanolamine	10–40 mg t.i.d. (To effect)	Alpha$_1$ agonist
• Imiprimine	3–20 mg b.i.d.	Alpha/beta agonist
• Pseudoephedrine	20–30 mg (3–4 days)	Alpha$_1$ Agonist
• Ephedrine	3–50 mg (4 days)	Alpha$_1$ Agonist
• Diethylstilbestrol	0.2–1.0 mg (orally 5 days)	Hormone supplementation
• Testosterone propionate	2.0–2.5 mg/kg (I.M. twice weekly)	Hormone supplementation
(b) *Decreased urethral tone*		
• Phenoxybenzamine	0.25–0.75 mg/kg	Alpha 1 blocker
• Baclofen	1.0–2.0 mg/kg	Muscle relaxant
• Dantrolene	0.5–6.0 mg/kg	Muscle relaxant
• Diazepam	0.1–0.2 mg/kg	Muscle relaxant, anti anxiety

APPENDIX TABLE 41–7
SUMMARY OF EFFECTS OF ESTROGENS

- Suppression of Lactation (Androgens Also)
- Induction of Estrus—Behavioral and Histological changes
- Mismating in Bitches— 1) Edema at utero tubal junction
  2) Endometrial Motility
- Urinary Incontinence Treatment
- Edema of the Reproductive Tract and Genitalia
- Myometrial Stimulation—Enhances Sensitivity to Oxytocin
- Hypogonadal Obesity Treatment
- Epitheliotropic Activity—Skin, Endometrium, Mammary Gland
- Release of Prostaglandins at Parturition
- Metabolic Actions—Increased Insulin and Growth Hormone, Anabolic Activity, Fat
  Deposition
- Anti-androgenic Effects in Males

Suppresses $\begin{cases} \text{Excessive Libido} \\ \text{Circum Anal Gland Tumors} \\ \text{Prostatic Hyperplasia} \\ \text{Behavioral Changes} \end{cases}$

Index

Entries followed by a t refer to tabular matter.

Abamectin, 104–105
  effect on larval *Diptera*, 110
Abomasum
  disorders, 183
  nematodes in, 86
Abortion
  in dogs, 1006
  in horses, 483–484
  prostaglandin-induced, 1014
  salmonellosis and, 149
  toxoplasma and, 729
Abscesses, 258
Absorbents, 136, 143
Acepromazine
  anxiolytic activity, 873
  dosage, 137, 201t
  indications
    emesis, 137
    furazolidone poisoning, 206
    laminitis, 467, 468t
    metaldehyde poisoning, 209
    spasmodic colic, 143, 414
  JECFA evaluation, 377
  tranquilization with, 937
  warfarin and, 461t
Acetaminophen
  in bovine respiratory diseases, 128
  poisoning, 209
Acetic acid, 204
Acetylcysteine, 124
  nebulized, 489
Acetylpromazine. *See* Acepromazine
Acetylsalicyclic acid. *See* Aspirin
Acid-base balance, 168

Acidosis, 168–171
  causes of, 183
  in cattle, 183
  metabolic, 169–170, 985
  poisoning and, 202, 202t
  respiratory, 170–171
  tetracyclines and, 270
  treatment of, 183–185
Acquired immunodeficiency syndrome, 68
Actinomycosis, 304
Activated charcoal, 197–199
Actomyosin, estrogen and, 1006
Addisonian shock, 186
Adenoma, perianal, 933
ADEQUAN. *See* Polysulfated glycosaminoglycan
Aditoprim, 301
Adrenal carcinoma, 933
Adrenaline. *See* Epinephrine
Adrenergic agents, 120. *See also* Alpha adrenergic
        agonists; Beta adrenergic agonists
  receptors, classification of, 639–640, 640t
Adria. *See* Doxorubicin
Adriamycin. *See* Doxorubicin
Aelurostrongylus abstrusus infection, 895
Aflatoxins, 73, 216
Agression, dominance, 1003
Agriculture, genetic engineering in, 62
AIDS, 68
ALBACILLAN. *See* Penicillin, novobiocin combined
        with
Albendazole
  absorption, 88
  antiparasitic spectrum, 89t, 762
    in ruminants, 91t, 763t

Albendazole, *continued*
  carcinogenicity, 373
  efficacy, 765t
  electronic bolus, 85
  embryotoxicity, 99
  in cattle, 764t
  indications
    fascioliasis, 768–769, 769t
    Filaroides hirthi infection, 894
    liver fluke, 87
    lungworm infection, 894
    ostertagiasis, 92, 763
    parasitic gastroenteritis, 770t
    tapeworm infection, 762
  in ruminants, 48, 91t, 763t
  in sheep, 335, 770t
  JECFA evaluation, 378t
  liposome formulations, 44
  mechanism of action, 82t
  metabolism, 87, 94
  metabolites, 86, 97
  residues, 96, 356
  ruminal delivery of, 48
  synthesis, 86
  teratogenicity, 768–769
    in sheep, 96, 335, 336
  withdrawal period, 769
ALBON-SR. *See* Sulfadimethoxine
Albuterol, 121
Aldosterone, 138
Aldrin, 212
Alimentary tract infections
  antimicrobial agents in, 946–950
Alkaline phosphatase, 73
Alkalosis
  abomasal disorders and, 183, 185
  poisoning and, 202t
  treatment, 185
Alopecia
  antineoplastic agents and, 932
  chemotherapy and, 927
  feline endocrine, 1011, 1018
  following ovariectomy, 1017
Alpha adrenergic agonists, 1006. *See also* specific
      agents
  antisecretory activity, 144, 155
  as sedatives, 414
  estrogens and, 1006
  in antiarrhythmic therapy, 833t
  in urinary incontinence, 1018
Alpha adrenergic blocking agents, 832
  in urinary incontinence, 1018
Alpha chloralose poisoning, 207
Alpha-naphthylthiourea, 210
Aluminum salts, 162
Ames test, 329–331
AMIGLYDE V. *See* Amikacin
Amikacin, 247
  antibacterial spectrum, 246
  dosage, 247

  small animal, 967t
  gentamicin vs, 510
  indications
    calf scour, 152
    canine pyoderma, 860t
    colic, 424t
    endometritis, bacterial, 474t, 476, 477, 478t
    genital tract infections, 247
    metritis, contagious equine, 480
    respiratory infections, in foals, 505t
    Rhodococcus equi pneumonia, 488
    salmonellosis, 510
    septic arthritis, 458t
  in foals, 496t
  in horses, 247, 496t
  minimum inhibitory concentration, 245
  nephrotoxicity, 251
  ototoxicity, 247
  resistance, 245
  toxicity, 247, 251
  uterine infusion, 480
Amino acids, 45
Aminoglycoside(s). *See also* specific agents, e.g.
      gentamicin, netilmicin, etc.
  absorption, 243
  anaerobiosis and, 704
  bacterial resistance to, 242
  elimination, 243
  half-life, 243
  indications, 245–246
  intramuscular, 243
  intraperitoneal, 243
  lipid solubility, 243
  mechanism of action, 243–244
  penicillin G combined with, 498
  penicillins combined with, 480
  pharmacokinetics, 242–243
  pleural fluid level, 243
  protein binding, 243
  resistance, 244–245
  subcutaneous, 243
  toxicity, 251
  urine levels, 951
Aminopenicillins, 227–228, 792–793. *See also* specific
      agents, e.g. Ampicillin, amoxicillin, etc.
Aminopentamide, 157
  in canine emesis, 137, 141
Aminophylline
  in cardiac disease, small animals, 823, 824t
  indications
    chronic obstructive pulmonary disease, 492t
    pneumonia, 489
  in heartworm infection, 917
  mechanism of action, 121
Amiodarone, 836
Amitraz, 841–842, 844
Ammonia toxicosis, 203–204
Amoxicillin, 221
  ampicillin vs
    absorption, 228

onset of action, 792
tissue penetration, 793
antibacterial spectrum, 227, 228, 792
bacterial sensitivity to, 237t
blood levels, 792
clavulanic acid combined with, 224, 228
 in bovine respiratory disease, 793
 in canine pyoderma, 860, 860t
 in small animals, 228, 967t
 in urinary tract infections, 951
 long-acting suspension, 793
clavulanic acid vs, 223
dosage, 238t
in cattle, 238t
indications
 calf scour, 152, 154
 colibacillosis, 579
 respiratory disease, bovine, 790t, 792
 respiratory tract infections, 226
 septic arthritis, 458t
 septicemia, in foals, 498
 skin infections, 226
 urinary tract infections, 226
in foals, 496t
in horses, 238t, 496t
minimal inhibitory concentration, 224
onset of action, 951
penicillin vs, 228
residues, 367
urine levels, 951
AMP-EQUINE. *See* Ampicillin
Amphetamine, 202t
Amphotericin B, 130
in endometritis, bacterial, 478t
Ampicillin, 225
absorption, 228
allergy, 346
amoxicillin vs
 absorption, 228
 onset of action, 792–793
 tissue penetration, 793
antibacterial activity, 227, 228
bacterial sensitivity to, 237t
cloxacillin combined with, 661
dosage, 227, 238t
dosage, small animal, 967t
E. coli resistance, 233
Escherichia coli resistance to, 942
esters, 228
excretion, 228
gastric acid and, 792
H. influenza resistance, 235
in cattle, 227, 238t
indications
 calf scour, 152
 colibacillosis, 579
 colic, 424t
 endometritis, bacterial, 474t, 476, 478t
 metritis, contagious equine, 480
 pleuropneumonia, swine, 576

respiratory disease, 790t, 792
respiratory tract infections, 226
respiratory tract infections, in foals, 505t
salmonellosis, 587
septic arthritis, 458t
septicemia, in foals, 498
skin infections, 226
summer mastitis, 680
urinary tract infections, 226
uterine infections, 706
in foals, 496t
in horses, 238t, 496t
lipid solubility, 945
plasma protein binding, 385
residues, 367
resistance, 233
Staphylolcoccus aureus resistance to, 942
sulbactam combined with, 224
 in *Pasteurella* infections, 793
tissue penetration, 793, 945
urine levels, 951
AMPROL. *See* Amprolium
Amprolium, 726
as feed additive, 727, 775
ethopabate combined with, 727
indications
 coccidiosis, 774t
 ovine coccidiosis, 726, 727, 727t
in poultry, 306
laminar cortical necrosis and, 727
residues, 376
sulfonamides combined with, 306, 894
Amprolium hydrochloride, 150
Amrinone, 820
Anabolic steroids, 1008
residues, 627
Anaerobic infections, 962–965
clindamycin in, 965
cultures from, 963t
metronidazole in, 964–965
penicillins in, 963
Anaerobic mastitis, 682
Analgesics, 408–410
Anaphylactic reactions, 266
Anaphylaxis, 123
Androgenic therapy, 1007–1008
Androgen(s)
adverse effects, 1008
anabolic effects, 1008
esters, 1007
estrogens combined with, 1015
infertility and, 1008
lactation suppression, 1008, 1015
metabolism, 1008
mineralocorticoid effects, 1008
virilizing effect, 1008
Andromedotoxin, 214
Anemia, 202t
aplastic, 279–280
hemolytic, sulfonamides and, 309

Anemia, *continued*
 renal failure and, 985
 urinary antiseptics associated with, 956–957
Anesthetics, 58
 enzyme induction and, 347
Anestrus, 697
Angiotensin-converting enzyme inhibitors, 828–829
Antacids, 510–511
ANTHELCIDE. *See* Oxibendazole
Anthelmintic(s), 55. *See also* specific agents
 abomasal administration, 83, 84
 absorption, 85–86
 administration, 48–49, 83–85
 antiparasitic spectrum, 91t
 chemistry, 88, 90, 92
 classification, 881
 combination products, 881
 dosing paste syringes, 84
 drench and paste preparations, 84
 efficacy, 86
 environmental impact of, 441
 for *Strongylus* larvae, 415, 416t
 in cattle, 764t
 in feed preparations, 84
 in foals, 511
 in horses, 511
 injectable preparations, 84
 in parasitic gastroenteritis, 770t
 in ruminants, 48–49, 91t
 in thromboembolic colic, 415
 long term administration, 45
 mechanism of action, 81–83, 82t
 paste formulations, 84, 438
 pharmacokinetics, 86–87
 poisoning, 198
 prophylactic use, 438, 439–441
 resistance, 114–115, 438
 ruminal delivery systems, 48–49
 safety margins, 88
 sustained-release formulations, 47t, 84–85
 topical, 84
 withholding times, 87–88
Anthraquinones, 144
Antiandrogen therapy, 1008
Antiarrhythmic agents, 832–837
Antibiotics. *See* Antimicrobial agents
Antibiotics, ionophore. *See* Ionophore antibiotics
Antibodies, 55, 67
Anticestodal agents, 881, 891t
Anticholinergic agents. *See also* specific agents, e.g.
  Atropine
 in canine emesis, 137, 138
 in colitis, 146
 in gastrointestinal disorders, 138, 141–142, 146
 in urinary incontinence, 1018
 mechanism of action, 138
Anticoagulant(s). *See also* specific agents, e.g.
  Warfarin
 in endotoxemia, 419
 in navicular disease, 459–461

NSAIDs and, 518
 poisoning, 202t
Anticonvulsants, 201t. *See also* Antiepileptic drugs
 in foals, 502, 502t
Antidotes, 197–199, 202t, 202–203
Antiemetics, 135, 136
 central, 137–138
Antiepileptic drugs, 991, 992t
 hepatoxicity and, 994
 long term use, 996
 mechanism of action, 993
 side effects, 994, 995
Antifreeze. *See* Ethylene glycol
Antihistamines
 indications
  chronic obstructive pulmonary disease, 494
  motion sickness, 139
  placenta, retained, 484
  pruritus, 873
 in respiratory disorders, 129
 warfarin interaction with, 461t
Anti-inflammatory agents, 127–129
 for otitis externa, 852
 in doping, 562–563
 in racing horses, 562–563
Antimicrobial agents, 33, 151. *See also* specific agents
 as growth promoters, 569–570
 bacterial resistance to, 589
 boluses, 52–55
 CNS penetration, 959
 combinations, 943, 945
 diarrhea and, 946
 dosage, 942
  over vs under, 943
 duration of therapy, 943
 estrogens combined with, 704
 for otitis externa, 851–853
 guidelines for therapy, 944
 in alimentary tract infections, 946–950
 in calf scour, 152–154
 in canine bacterial infections, 952t–953t
 in canine pyoderma, 859–862
 in cats, 942
 in dogs, 942
 in foals, 496t, 504–505
 in gram-negative sepsis, 424t
 in milk, tests for, 366, 367
 in respiratory tract infections, 944–946
 in skin infections, 965–968
 intrauterine, 703–706, 1017
 in urinary tract infections, 950–951, 953–957
 limitations, 704
 liposomal-associates, 44
 manufacture of, 33
 microencapsulated intramammary, 58
 poisoning, 198
 prophylactic use, 809
 residues, 337–338, 347–351, 591–592
 sustained release, 47t, 52–55
 uterine absorption, 704

withdrawal period, 578, 589
Antimycotic agents, 853–854, 854t
Antinematodal agents, 885t
  for cattle, 765t
Antineoplastic agents. *See also* specific agents, e.g.
        Doxorubicin
  alimentary tract disorders associated with, 927
  alopecia and, 932
  antibiotic, 932
  carcinogenicity, 928
  classification of, 928t, 929
  combination therapy with, 927
  mechanism of action, 925
  protocols for administration of, 934–936
  risks to persons administering, 926–927
  safety margin, 925
  side effects of, 925–928, 926t, 932t
Antiparasitic agents, 853, 853t
Antipseudomonal penicillins, 229–230
ANTIROBE. *See* Clindamycin
Antiseborrheic shampoos, 874
Antisecretory agents, 143–144, 155–156
Antiseptics, 713
Antispasmodics, 526
Antistaphylococcal penicillins, 230
Antiulcer drugs, 135
ANTU. *See* Alpha–naphthylthiourea
Aplastic anemia, 279–280
Apnea, 200
Apomorphine, 134
Appetite stimulants, 146–147
Apramycin, 154, 381
  antibacterial spectrum, 248
  bactericidal activity, 249
  chemical structure, 249
  dosage, 249
  indications
    colibacillosis, 579, 721
    E. coli infection, 246
    salmonellosis, 246, 248, 587
  in lambs, 721
  intramuscular, 249
  mechanism of action, 248
  minimum inhibitory concentration, 248–249
  neomycin vs, 249
  oral, 721
  "postantibiotic effect," 249
  resistance to, 248–249
  streptomycin vs, 249
Aprindine, 830t, 835
Aprotinin, 192
Aqua polymers, 58
Arecoline, 217t
Arsenamide, 894
Arsenic, 212
  in racing horses, 552
  poisoning, 202t, 205
Arthritis, 247
  infectious, 588
Ascarid(s), 880, 880t

control programs, 886
  infestation, 883–886
Ascorbic acid, antibacterial activity, 957
Aspergillosis, nasal, 130
Aspergillus, 216t
Aspirin, 128, 405
  half-life, in cats, 824
  heartworm infection and, 914–915
  in diarrhea, 155
  indications
    laminitis, 425, 466, 468t
    septic arthritis, 458t
  in equine laminitis, 425
  in horses, 425, 451
  poisoning, 208–209
  prostaglandin synthesis and, 144, 151
  sulfapyridine combined with, 146
  toxicity in cats, 217t, 824
Astringents, 137, 197
Atrophic rhinitis
  in pigs, 570–573
Atropine
  diphenoxylate combined with, 141
  glycopyrrolate vs, 493, 494
  indications
    cardiac dysrhythmias, 830t
    chronic obstructive pulmonary disease, 122,
        492t, 493
    diarrhea, 145
    emesis, 137
    organophosphate poisoning, 202t, 204, 211,
        867
  in horses, 493, 505t
  mechanism of action, 138, 142, 493
  spasmolytic activity, 156, 157, 422
Attapulgite, 143, 154
Aujeszky's disease, 70, 74
  deleted subunit vaccines and, 75–76
  testing for, 73
AUREOMYCIN. *See* Chlortetracycline
AUTOWORM/REDIDOSE. *See* Oxfendazole
AVATEC. *See* Lasalocid
Avermectin(s), 104–109. *See also* Ivermectin
  antinematodal activity, 765t
  antiparasitic spectrum
    in ruminants, 91t
  chemistry, 104–105
  in sheep, 770t
  mechanism of action, 83, 104–108
  toxicity, 104–108, 109–110
Avoparcin, 570, 605
Azlocillin, 221, 229

Babesiasis, 895–896
Bacillus, Calmette-Guerin vaccine, 920
Bacillus, 67
Bacitracin, as growth promoter, 599t
Baclofen, 1019
Bacteremia
  anaerobic, 963

Bacteremia, *continued*
  etiology, 960
  gram-negative, 961
  pathogens in, 960
  preacute, from endotoxemia, 961
  predisposing factors to, 961
  progression to septicemia, 960
  subacute, 961
Bacteria, beta-lactamase producing, 237t
Bacterial overgrowth, 946
  tylosin in, 950
Bacterial resistance, 338–343
Bacterial toxins, 198
Bacteroides nodosus, 71
BACTRIM. *See* Sulfonamide, combined with
      trimethoprim
Balling guns, 51
Bambermycin, 570, 606–607
BANAMINE. *See* Flunixin meglumine
Baquiloprim, 300
  half-life, 301
  sulfamethazine combined with, 302
  sulfonamides combined with, 301, 302, 793
Barbiturate(s), 205, 993
  in metaldehyde poisoning, 209
  in rodenticide poisoning, 210
  poisoning, 202t, 217t
  warfarin interaction with, 461t
Barriers, summer mastitis control and, 680
BAYNIX. *See* Coumaphos
BAYTRIL. *See* Enrofloxacin
Becampicillin, 228
Bemegride, 201t
  in barbiturate poisoning, 202t, 211
BENADRYL (diphenhydramine), 129
Bentonite, 155
BENYLIN EXPECTORANT (diphenhydramine/
      ammonium chloride/sodium citrate/
      menthol), 129
Benzathine, 58
BENZELMIN. *See* Oxfendazole
BENZELMIN PLUS. *See* Oxfendazole, trichlorfon
      combined with
Benzene hexachloride, 841
Benzetimide, 141, 157, 422
Benzimidazoles. *See also* specific agents, e.g.
      Albendazole, oxfendazole, etc.
  abomasal administration, 84
  absorption, 86
  antinematodal activity, 765t
  antiparasitic spectrum, 89t
    in ruminants, 91t
  bioavailability, bound residues and, 97–99
  chemistry, 88–89
  cross resistance, 115, 439
  diethylcarbamazine combined with, 884
  extractable residues, 99–100
  food ingestion and, 881
  indications
    parasitic gastroenteritis, 770t

Trichostrongylus infection, 435
  in horses, 90
  in ruminants, 90
  kinetics, 92–93
  mechanism of action, 81, 82, 82t, 95
  metabolism, 86–87
  mutagenicity, 95
  pharmacokinetics, 92–94
  potency, solubility and, 93
  precursors, 86
  pregnant dogs and, 885–886
  residues, 97
    bound, bioavailability of, 97–99
    extractable, 99–100
  resistance, 435
  safety margin, 84
  solubility, potency and, 93
  suspensions, 84
  teratogenicity, 95–96
  tissue clearance, 96–97
  toxicity, 95–100
  tubulin binding, 95, 881
Benzoin, 123
Benzonatate, 126
Benzoyl peroxide
  antifungal activity, 863
  antipruritic activity, 863
  indications, 841, 875
  shampoos, 862
Benzyl benzoate, cats and, 217t, 841
Benzylpenicillin
  in equine metritis, 480
  JECFA evaluation, 377, 379t
  plasma protein binding, 385
Beta adrenergic agents, 639–640, 640t, 701. *See also*
      specific agents
  as repartitioning agents, 640
  cardiovascular effects, 642
  high dose, 643, 644–645
  in antiarrhythmic therapy, 831t, 831–832
  in doping, 563
  in pigs, 645–646
  mechanism of action, 641–642
  metabolic effects, 642
  physiological effects of, 642
  protein deposition and, 641
  receptor specificity, 640
  residues, 644
  respiratory effects, 642
  toxicity, 642–644
Beta$_2$-adrenergic agents, 120–121
Beta adrenergic blocking agents, 33, 316, 831t
Beta adrenergic receptors, 639–640
Beta agonists. *See* Beta adrenergic agents
Beta blockers. *See* Beta adrenergic blocking agents
beta-galactosidase, 73
Beta lactam antibiotics
  mechanism of action, 221–223
  recommended dosage, 238t
  residues, 375

Beta lactamase, 223–224
Betamethasone, 128
    dosages, 541t
    duration of action, 696
    in endotoxic shock, 420t, 426t
Betamethasone alcohol, 695
Beta-2-selective agents, 120, 640
Biotechnology, 62, 76–77
    pharmaceutical agents produced by, 67–70
Biotin, 468t
Biotransformation, 318, 319t, 320
Bismuth subsalicylate, 151
BISOLVOMYCIN. *See* Bromhexine, oxytetracycline
        combined with
BISOLVON. *See* Bromhexine
Bithionol sulfoxide
    anthelmintic spectrum, in ruminants, 91t, 763t
    mechanism of action, 82t
    peak levels, 112
Bleomycin, 932t
Blood-borne parasites, 895–896
Boldenone, 1008
Boluses, 47t, 48, 52–55
Bone infections, 957–959
    in dogs, 952t
Bordetella bronchiseptica, 945
Bots, 430, 431t, 432t, 434
BOVATEC. *See* Lasalocid
BOVILENE. *See* Fenprostalene
Bovine coccidiosis, 772–776
    control of, 773–774
    prevention of, 774–775
    therapy, 775
Bovine growth hormone. *See* Bovine somatotropin
Bovine herpes-virus-1, 74
Bovine mastitis
    acidosis and, 183
    anaerobic, 682
    causative agents, 657t
    cephalosporins for, 235–236
    coliform, 671–677
    combination antibiotic therapy for, 662
    control of, 666–668, 684–686
    fungal, 682
    intramammary therapy, 246, 660–662
    klebsiella, 682
    mammary gland defenses against, 668–669
    mycoplasmal, 681
    nocardial, 681
    parenteral therapy, 662–666
    pseudomonas aeruginosa, 682
    somatic cell count monitoring for, 685–686
    staphylococcal, 669–671
    summer, 677–681
    vaccination against, 682–684
Bovine metritis, 701–703
    acidosis and, 682–684
Bovine ostertagiasis, 760–765
    epidemiology, 761–762
    therapy, 762–765

Bovine pyometra, 711–712
Bovine respiratory tract infections
    causative agents, 781–785
    defense mechanisms against, 785–786
    fluid therapy in, 807–808
    Pasteurella hemolytica in, 784t
    pulmonary edema in, 808
    treatment, 304, 786–809
        aminopenicillins, 792–793
        antiinflammatory agents, 801–804
        antimicrobial agents, 789–801
        bromhexine, 805–807
        bronchodilators, 807
        cephalosporins, 797–798
        enrofloxacin, 798–800
        erythromycin, 797
        florfenicol, 801
        immunomodulators, 804–805
        macrolides, 796–797
        mucolytic agents, 805–807
        penicillins, 791–793
        principles of, 786–789
        spiramycin, 797
        sulfonamides, 793
        tetracyclines, 793–795
        tilmicosin, 800–801
        tylosin, 796–797
Bovine somatotropin, 634–635
    bioengineered, 631–632
    effect on dairy cows, 634–635
    JECFA evaluation, 377, 637
    liposomal delivery, 44, 58
    mastitis and, 635
    microencapsulated bolus, 58
    milk production and, 632
    safety of, 636–637
    side effects, 634–635, 635–636
    species specificity, 634
    sustained release, 33
Brackens, 212–213
    antidote, 202t
Brassica family, 213
Breast cancer, 920
    cyclophosphamide in, 930
Breeding control programs, 55
Bretylium, 836
Bromhexine, 124
    antitussive activity, 125
    dosage, 125
        in chronic obstructive pulmonary disease, 492t,
            494
    in bovine respiratory tract infections, 805–807
    in cattle, 125, 805–807
    in dogs, 125
    in horses, 125
    in respiratory disorders, 123
    mucolytic activity, 125
    oral formulation, 125
    oxytetracycline combined with, 125
    warfarin and, 461t

Bromobenzene, 347
Bromocriptine
  antiemetics and, 1015
  indications
    abortion, 1013
    pseudopregnancy, 1015
  side effects, 1015
Bromocyclen
  cats and, 212
  flea allergy and, 872
  in sarcoptic mange, 844
Bronchodilators, 120
  in bovine respiratory tract infections, 807
  in horses, 505t
  types of, 493–494
Brotianide, 88, 770
  thiophanate combined with, 772
Brucellosis, 44, 55
Bufotenine, 550
Bulk-forming laxatives, 144
Bunamidine, 114, 882t, 891, 891t
Buscopan, 142
Busulfan, 935t
Butamisole, 882t, 885t
  indications
    hookworm infestation, 887t
    whipworm infestation, 888
  safety margin, 888
BUTAZOLIDIN. *See* Phenylbutazone
Butorphanol
  antiemetic activity, 127
  antitussive activity, 127
  cats and, 823
  in horses, 409t, 410, 412t, 416t
  in pain, 202, 202t
  mechanism of action, 127
  pentazocine vs, 126
Butyl rubber, 35t
Butyrophenone, 137

Cabergoline, 1013, 1015
Calcium, 51
Calcium borogluconate, 205
Calcium channel blockers
  antisecretory activity, 155
  antisecretory effects, 143
  in bronchospasms, 129
  in shock, 192
  mechanism of action, 192
Calcium disodium edetate, 202t
Calcium gluconate, 201
Calf scour, 150–152, 304. *See also* Neonatal diarrhea
  adsorbents in, 154–155
  antimicrobial agents in, 152–154
  antisecretory agents in, 155–156
  coliform, 150–154
  colostrum and, 160–162
  fluid replacement in, 157–160
  gastrointestinal protectives in, 154–155
  motility-inhibiting agents in, 156–157

  probiotics in, 156
  prostaglandins and, 151t
  therapy package, 153t
CALF SPAN (sulfamethazine), 52, 53t
Calmodulin, 144
Calves, 248, 286
  coccidiosis in, 610
  diphtheria in, 304
  enrofloxacin in, 290, 291
  lung abscesses in, 487
  lungworm infestation in, 765–767
  mycoplasmal infection in, 795
  navel ill in, 304
  scour in. *See* Calf scour
  sulfachlorpyridazine in, 303t
  sulfathiazole in, 303t
  sulfonamides and, 309
Cambendazole
  mechanism of action, 82t
  pharmacokinetics, 97
  residues, 98
  synthesis, 90
  teratogenicity, 96, 336
Camylofine, 141
Cancer. *See* Carcinoma for cancer of specific organs
  Bacille, Calmette-Guerin vaccine in, 920
  chemotherapy in, 922, 923–925. *See also*
    Antineoplastic agents
    alopecia and, 927
    dosages, 922, 923, 923t
    immunosuppression following, 927
    infections and, 927
    protocols for, 922
    side effects of, 925–928
    therapeutic index, 925
    toxicity of, 922
  cryotherapy in, 920
  electrocautery in, 920
  immunotherapy in, 920
  metastases in, 1
  oncogenes and, 937–938
  radiation therapy in, 920
Canine heartworm. *See* Heartworm infection
Cannabinoids, 139
Captan, 847t
CAPTEC. *See* Albendazole
Captopril
  in cardiac disease, 829
    dosage, 826t, 827t
  in shock, 192
  site of action, 827t
CARAFATE. *See* Sucralfate
Carazolol, 377, 381
Carbadox, 379t
  feed medication, 379t, 587t
  indications
    salmonellosis, 587
    swine dysentery, 578, 582
  in pigs, 578, 582, 649
  JECFA evaluation, 377

premixes, 582
safety, 616
salmonellosis control, 587
swine dysentery control, 584t, 585
toxicity, 373
withdrawal period, 373, 578, 584
Carbamate(s)
  CNS effects, 217t
  insecticidal activity, 866–867
  poisoning, 210–211
  teratogenicity of, 335
Carbapenems, 230, 231
Carbaryl, 207, 210, 866
Carbazolol, 379t
Carbenicillin, 221, 229–230
  antibacterial activity, 229
  dosage, 238t
    small animal, 967t
  gentamicin combined with, 229
  in cattle, 238t
  indications
    cystitis, 229
    endometritis, bacterial, 474t, 477, 478t
  in foals, 496t
  in horses, 238t, 496t
  intramuscular, 229
  oral, 229
  ticarcillin vs, 221, 229, 230
Carbomycin, 251, 255
Carbon tetrachloride, 347
Carboxylic ionophores, 192
Carboxymethylcellulose, 35t, 39
Carcinogenesis, 627–629
  promoting factors, 920
Carcinogenicity, 320–328. *See also* Carcinogens
  diethylstilbestrol and, 315
Carcinogens, 320–325
  classification, 320–321, 321t
  DNA-reactive genotoxic, 321, 321t
  epigenetic, 321, 321t
  mechanism of action, 321t, 322t, 322–323
  screening for, 325–328
Carcinoma
  adrenal, 933
  breast, 920, 930
  squamous cell, 933
  thyroid, 933
Cardiac arrythmias, 829–837
Cardiac failure, in cats, 823–825
Cardiac glycosides, 817–821
Cardiogenic shock, 186
Cascara, 144
Castor oil, 144
Cathartics, 144, 199–200
Cats
  aggression in, 1005
  alopecia in, 1011
  aminoglycoside toxicity and, 250–251
  antimicrobial agents in, 942
  apomorphine contraindication, 134

  aspirin and, 208, 824
  as reservoirs of infection, 894
  behavior disorders in, 1005
  behavior modification in, 1004
  benzyl benzoate and, 841
  bromocyclen and, 212
  cardiac failure in, 823–825
  Cheyletiella infestation in, 845
  chloramphenicol and, 277, 278, 280, 895
  cisplatin toxicity in, 933
  clindamycin absorption in, 257
  codeine and, 217t
  cryptosporidiosis in, 894
  cystitis in, 246
  demodicosis in, 843
  drug toxicity in, 217t
  endocrine alopecia in, 1011
  eosinophilic granuloma in, 1011
  epilepsy in, 999t
  gastric acid secretion, 135
  griseofulvin and, 203
  haemobartonellosis in, 895–896, 896t
  hookworms in, 886–888
  indoor spaying by, 1003, 1004
  in estrus, 1005
  lindane and, 872
  miliary dermatitis in, 1011, 1017
  neomycin and, 217t
  neurodermatitis in, 1011
  ovariohysterectomy in, indication for, 1005
  overgrooming in, 1005
  parasites in, 881t
  parturition induction in, 1012–1014
  pregnant, drugs and, 217
  puberty in, 1005
  roundworms in, 883–886
  taurine deficiency in, 824–825
  therapy
    clindamycin, 258
    diazepam, 999, 999t, 1005
    digitoxin, 819
    emetic, 196
    enrofloxacin, 291
    etamphylline, 122
    gentamicin, 246
    levamisole, 895
    megestrol, 1003, 1011
    metronidazole, 964
    phenobarbital, 996, 999t
    phenytoin, 999t
    progestin, 1010
    propranolol, 835
    quinidine, 833
    sulfadimethoxine, 303t
    sulfonamide, 304
    sulfonamide-trimethoprim, 303t, 309
    valproic acid, 1000
    vincristine, 931
    xylazine, 134–135, 196
  thyrotoxicosis in, 835

Cats, *continued*
  urinary tract infections in, 951
  urine spraying in, 1003, 1004
  uterine infections in, 963
  verminous pneumonia in, 895
Cattle, 55. *See also* Bovine terms; Dairy cows
  abomasal disorders in, 183
  actinomycosis in, 304
  castration, alternatives to, 648
  coccidiosis in, 304, 772–776
  coccidiostats for, 774t
  copper poisoning in, 206
  cryptosporidiosis in, 776–778
  dexamethasone in, 128
  dystocia in, 701
  feed additives in, 602
  foot rot in, 246, 304, 306
  gastrointestinal obstruction in, 185
  intestinal obstruction in, 183, 185
  listeriosis in, 488
  liver fluke in, 767–770
  mastitis in, 235, 236, 246
  NSAIDs in, 128
  ovarian hormone control in, 691
  parturition induction in, 693–694, 694t
  pneumonia in, 306
  polyarthritis in, 304
  pyometra in, 698–699, 711–712
  respiratory tract diseases in, 258, 261
  respiratory tract infections in. *See also* Bovine
     respiratory tract infections
  scours in. *See* Calf scour
  shipping fever in, 246
  therapy
    amoxicillin, 238t
    ampicillin, 227, 238t
    antinematodal, 765t
    bromhexine, 125
    carbenicillin, 238t
    cefadroxil, 238t
    cephalothin, 238t
    cimaterol, 643, 644
    clenbuterol, 641, 701
    dexamethasone, 128
    erythromycin, 252, 797
    etamphylline, 122
    florfenicol, 801
    flukicidal, 769t
    gentamicin, 246
    ivermectin, 108
    kanamycin, 247
    monensin, 246
    niclofolan, 769t
    oxfendazole, 335
    oxibendazole, 762
    oxyclozanide, 769t, 770
    oxytetracycline, 265
    penicillin G, 238t
    prostaglandin, 697
    sulfabromomethazine, 303t

    sulfadiazine, 303t
    sulfadimethoxine, 303t
    sulfamerazine, 303t
    sulfamethazine, 303t
    sulfonamides, 304
    thiabendazole, 762
    thiophanate, 762
    ticarcillin, 238t
    tilmicosin, 252, 258
    zeranol, 630
  umbilical infections in, 246
  uterine control in, 691–692
  wound infections in, 246
Cefaclor, 233, 235
Cefadroxil, 232
  dosage, 233, 238t
    small animal, 967t
  half-life, 234
  in canine pyoderma, 860t
  in cattle, 238t
  in horses, 238t
  oral, 233
Cefamandole, 233, 235
Cefazolin
  antibacterial activity, 232
  dosage, small animal, 967t
  half-life, 235
  in foals, 496t
  peak plasma levels, 234
Cefonicid, 233, 235
Cefoperazone, 235, 236
Ceforanide, 235
Cefotaxime, 235
  in foals, 496t
  resistance beta-lactamases, 234
Cefotetan, 233
Cefoxatime, indications, 499, 502
Cefoxitin, 233, 235
Ceftazidime, 234
Ceftiofur, 236
  antibacterial spectrum, 798
  dosage, 798
  indications
    bovine respiratory tract infections, 797–798
    respiratory disease, 790t
  residues, 367
Ceftizoxime, 234, 235
Ceftriaxone, 234, 235
Cefuroxime, 233, 235
  indications
    bovine mastitis, 236
    pneumonia, ampicillin-resistant, 235
  tissue penetration, 236
Cell cycle, stages of, 922
Central nervous system
  effect of poisons on, 217t
  infections, 959–960
    in dogs, 952t
Cephacetrile, 662
  antibacterial activity, 236, 662

bovine udder absorption, 58
Cephalexin, 232
  antibacterial activity, 232
  dosage, 233
    small animal, 967t
  indications
    canine pyoderma, 860, 860t, 861
    colic, 424t
    gastrointestinal tract infections, 233
    pyoderma, deep, 966
    respiratory tract infections, 233
    skin infections, 233
    urinary tract infections, 951
    urogenital tract infections, 233
  oral, 233
  urine levels, 951
Cephalonium, 236
Cephalosporin(s), 146, 232–236
  allergy, 343, 346
  beta lactam compounds vs, 234–235
  boluses, 47t
  cerebrospinal fluid penetration, 234
  chemical structure, 231
  classification, 238t
  first-generation, 232–233, 238t
    second-generation vs, 233, 235
    third-generation vs, 233
  indications
    bovine mastitis, 235, 662
    prophylaxis, surgical, 235
    Staphylococcus intermedius infections, 235
  kinetics, 234–235
  pharmacokinetics, 235
  second-generation, 233, 238t
    first-generation vs, 233, 235
  therapy, 235–236
  third-generation, 231, 233–234, 238t
    first-generation vs, 233
  volume of distribution, 234
Cephalothin
  antibacterial spectrum, 232
  bacterial resistance and, 232, 235
  dosage, 238t
    small animal, 967t
  in cattle, 238t
  in foals, 496t
  in horses, 238t, 496t
  liposomal-associated, 44
Cephamycin, 235
Cephapirin, 232
  residues, 367
Cephradine, 232
Ceruminolytic agents, 851, 854t
CESTEX. *See* Epsiprantel
Cestocides, 881, 891t
Charcoal, activated, 197–199
Chelating agents, 203
CHEQUE. *See* Mibolerone
Cherry laurel, 213
Cheyletiella infection, 845

Chlamydia psittaci infection, 131
Chloral hydrate, 411t, 415
  enzyme induction, 347
  in flatulent colic, 423
Chlorambucil
  dosage, 930
    rate of, 935t
  onset of action, 930
  side effects, 930, 932t
Chloramphenicol, 396
  absorption, 276
  adverse effects, 278–281
  analogs, 281–282
  antibacterial spectrum, 275–276
  bioavailablity, in cats, 277
  blood-aqueous barrier permeability, 960
  blood-brain barrier permeability, 278, 959
  bovine udder absorption, 58
  cats and, 277, 278, 280, 895
  distribution, 277
  dosage, small animal, 967t
  drug interactions, 279
  elimination, 277
  Escherichia coli resistance to, 942
  formulations, 277
  half-life, 488
  illegal use, 316
  immunosupression, 279
  indications
    canine pyoderma, 860t
    endometritis, 704
    haemobartonellosis, 895, 896t
    metritis, contagious equine, 480
    otitis externa, 851
    Rhodococcus equi pneumonia, 488
    septicemia, in foals, 499
  in dogs, 278, 280
  in foals, 496t
  in horses, 488
  JECFA evaluation, 378t, 381
  lipid solubility, 275
  mechanism of action, 275
  metabolism, 278
  3-methylcholanthrene potentiation, 279
  parenteral, 277
  pentobarbital and, 279, 347
  pharmacokinetics, 276–278
  phenytoin interaction with, 998
  protein binding, 277, 385
  residues, 281, 374–375
  spectinomycin combined with, 259
  subconjunctival, 278
  teratogenicity, 279
  tolbutamide interaction with, 347
  toxicity, 280–281, 344, 965
    in cats, 217t
  urine levels, 951
  uterine absorption, 704
Chlorates, 202t
Chlordiazepoxide, 142

Chlorhexidine, 847t
  indications
    dermatophytosis, 847t
    metritis, contagious equine, 480
    ringworm, 848
  shampoo, 848
  uterine irrigation with, 476t
Chlorinated hydrocarbons, toxicity, 212, 867–868
  in cats, 217t
CHLORODYNE. *See* Chloroform, morphine
    combined with
Chloroform, 140
  morphine combined with, 140, 145
Chlorotheophylline, 137
Chlorothiazide, 826t, 827t
Chlorpheniramine, 873
Chlorpromazine, 137, 205
  antidiarrheal effects, 155
  in apomorphine overdose, 134
  in cardiac disease, 823
  plasma protein binding, 385
Chlorpyrifos, 867, 871
Chlortetracycline, 306
  as growth promoter, 569, 599t
  control dosages, 576
  JECFA evaluation, 377, 381
  protein synthesis and, 271
Cholestyramine, 143, 155
Cholinergic agents. *See also* specific agents
  in urinary incontinence, 1018
Cholinesterase inhibitors, 202t. *See also*
    Organophosphate(s)
Cholinolytics, 141
Chorionic gonadotropin, equine, 1007
Chorionic gonadotropin, human, 1007
Chronic obstructive pulmonary disease
  development of, 491
  environment and, 491
  in horses, 490–495
  treatment, 491–495
Chronic renal failure
  diets in, 984–985
  in dogs, 984–985
  protein-calorie deficiency in, 985
Cimaterol, 643–644
Cimetidine
  efficacy, 135
  indications
    gastric ulceration, 510, 511
    gastroduodenal ulcers, 924
    septic arthritis, 458t
  in foals, 457, 510, 511
  omeprazole vs, 136
  ranitidine vs, 510
  theophylline interaction, 493
Ciprofloxacin, 284
  distribution, 287
  in canine pyoderma, 861
Cisplatin, 927
  dosage rate, 935t

in dogs, 933
  pulmonary toxicity, in cats, 933
  side effects, 932t
CLAMOXYL. *See* Amoxicillin
Clavulanic acid
  amoxicillin combined with, 224
    in bovine respiratory disease, 793
    in canine pyoderma, 860, 860t
    in small animals, 228, 967t
    in urinary tract infections, 951
    long-acting suspension, 793
  amoxicillin vs, 223
  antibacterial spectrum, 224
  sulbactam vs, 224
  ticarcillin combined with, 224, 229, 498
Clenbuterol, 121, 396
  anesthesia and, 701
  dosage, 493
  duration of action, 701
  dystocia and, 701
  excretion, 644
  half-life, 807
  high dose, 644
  in cattle, 641, 701
  indications
    chronic obstructive pulmonary disease, 121, 492t,
      493
    pneumonia, 489
  in horses, 121, 493, 505t
  isoxsuprine combined with, 701
  mechanism of action, 641
  oxytocin antagonism of, 701
  residues, 645
  theophylline vs, 493
  therapeutic dose, 641
  tocolytic activity, 701
  warfarin and, 461t
Clidinium, 141, 142
  in canine colitis, 146
Clindamycin
  absorption, 959
    bovine udder, 58
    effect of food on, 257
  antibacterial spectrum, 253
  boluses, 47t
  bone penetration, 958
  C. difficile overgrowth and, 959
  distribution, 257
  dosage, small animal, 967t
  elimination, 258
  indications
    abscesses, 258
    anaerobic infections, 965
    canine dental infections, 948
    canine pyoderma, 860t
    cryptosporidiosis, 894
    nocardial mastitis, 681
    osteomyelitis, 258, 958
    osteomyelitis, staphylococcal, 965
    otitis externa, 851

periodontal diseases, 258
stomatitis, 947
Toxoplasma gondii infection, 258
wound infections, 258
leukocyte concentration, 959, 965
lincomycin vs, 255, 258, 860
mechanism of action, 959
metabolism, 257
peak serum concentration, 256
placental barrier permeability, 257
preparations, 257
tissue concentrations, 258
toxicity, 259, 260
Clonazepam, 992t, 999
diazepam vs, 999
Clones, 66
Clonidine, 144, 155
Cloprostenol, 696t, 699–700, 709
Clorazepate dipotassium, 999, 1000
Clorsulon
anthelmintic spectrum, 91t, 763t
in cattle, 764t
in fascioliasis, 768, 769, 769t
ivermectin combined with, 764t
mechanism of action, 82t
therapeutic index, 113
Closantel
flukicidal activity, 770
half-life, 112
in sheep, 112
JECFA evaluation, 377, 379t, 380t
protein binding, 770
Clotrimazole, 847t, 848
Cloxacillin, 221
absorption, gut, 225
ampicillin combined with, 661
indications
bovine mastitis, 661
summer mastitis, 680
oxacillin vs, 230
plasma protein binding, 385
residues, 367
Coal tar products, 211
Cobalt, 45
deficiency. *See* Cobalt deficiency
glass boluses, 51
oral administration, 745
sustained release, 47t
toxicity, 746
Cobalt deficiency
diagnosis, 745
in sheep, 50, 720
marginal, 744–745
symptoms, 744
treatment and prevention, 745–746
vitamin B$_{12}$ and, 743–744
Coccidiosis, 304
in calves, 610
in cattle, 772–776
in lambs, 610

in sheep, 719
Coccidiostats, 306
for cattle, 774t
Coccoidiosis
in lambs, 724–728
Codeine
antidiarrheal activity, 141, 145
constipatory activity, 145
in cardiac disease, 823
mechanism of action, 126
toxicity, in cats, 217t
Colchicine, 99
antitubulin activity, 95
Colibacillosis
apramycin in, 248
gentamicin in, 246
in pigs, 248, 578–580
in sheep, 719
NSAIDs in, 156
septicemic, 147–148
Colic, 402–426
aminoglycosides in, 423
analgesics in, 408–410
antimicrobials in, 423, 424, 424t
migration of *S. vulgaris* larvae in, 415
NSAIDs in, 411–413
sedatives/tranquilizers in, 414–415
shock in, 416–419, 417t
thromboembolic colic, 415
Coliform calf scour, 150–154. *See also* Calf scour
role of prostaglandins in, 151t
Coliform mastitis, 671–677
antibiotic therapy for, 676
antiinflammatory shock therapy in, 676–
677
causative agents, 671
clinical presentation, 672
control of, 673–674
endotoxic shock in, 674–676
mediators of inflammation in, 673–674
Colisepticemia, 152, 161. *See also* Calf scour
Colitis
ancillary therapy in, 949t
diets for, 988
in dogs, 142, 146, 948–950
in horses, 511–512
types of, 948t
Colitis-X, 270
Collies, 208
Colloidal dispersal systems, 58
Colonic impaction, 422–423
Colostrum, 160–161
COMBOT. *See* Trichlorfon
COMBOTEL PASTE. *See* Febantel, trichlorfon
combined with
Competitive enzyme immunoassay, 73
COMPUDOSE (estradiol), 56t
as growth promoter, 599t
COMPUDOSE 200. *See* Estradiol
COMPUDOSE 365. *See* Estradiol

Congestive heart failure, 812–814
  obesity and, 983
  therapy, 814–817. *See also* specific drug therapies
Contact lenses, medicated, 58
Contraceptive devices, 44
Controlled medication programs, 548–549
Controlled-release glasses, 33, 51
Controlled-release systems. *See also* Sustained-release
        systems
  advantages of, 33–34, 35t
  conventional delivery systems vs, 33, 34
  design of, 46
  diffusion as basic concept of, 34
  drug release from, 34, 36–39
  external application, 55
  implant, 46
  liposomal delivery, 43–44
  matrix of, 34. *See also* Polymer matrix
  oral, 46–47
  osmotic pumps, 44–45, 49
  reservoir type, 41–42, 42t
Control program, 433, 439–441
Convulsions, 502
Copper, 710
  absorption, 736
  availability and requirements, 735–736
  controlled release glass, 741
  deficiency. *See* Copper deficiency
  glass boluses, 51
  herbage concentration, 736
  injectable formulations, 741–742
  longterm delivery, 45
  oral administration, 739–740
  parenteral preparations, 750t
  poisoning, 202t, 206–207
  sustained delivery devices, 47t
  sustained release, 740
  toxicity, 742–743
Copper capsules, 51
Copper deficiency, 50
  diagnosis, 737–738
  in sheep, 719–720
  symptoms, 737
  treatment and prevention, 738–739
Copper oxide needles, 50, 740
Copper sulfate, 196, 731
CORAMINE. *See* Nikethamide
Coronaviruses, 149–150
Corticosteroid(s), 151. *See also* Steroids
  antibody production and, 192
  bacterial clearance and, 192
  contraindications, 131, 467
  cytotoxic effects, 933
  depot preparations, 532
  distribution, 532
  duration of action, 530
  healing and, 192
  heartworm infection and, 915–916
  hyaluronic acid supression by, 451
  in colitis, 950

indications, 539–542
  COPD, 492t, 494
  degenerative joint disease, 449–451
  endotoxic shock, 191, 191t
  navicular disease, 463
  otitis externa, 851
  parturition induction, 481, 690–693, 696t
  pruritus, 872–873
  septic arthritis, 456
  in endotoxic shock, 421
  in horses, 449–451, 530–542
  in lymphosarcoma, 933
  in respiratory distress, 822
  intra-articular, 538–539
  laminitis and, 537–538
  long-acting, 451, 532
  long-term therapy, 532
  miliary dermatitis and, 1017
  parturition induced by. *See* Corticosteroid(s),
        indications, parturition induction
  precautions, 541t
  prostaglandin inhibition by, 127
  reproduction control and, 316
  short-acting, 531
  side effects, 450, 539, 932t, 933
  warfarin interaction with, 461t
Corynebacterium pyogens, 54
Cough sedatives, 824t
Cough suppressants, 126–127, 823
Coumaphos
  haloxon combined with, 763t
  in cattle, 764t
  indications
    ostertagiasis, 762
  neuromuscular coordination and, 83
  poisoning, 210
Coumarin, 210
Cresols, 211
Cromolyn, 129
Cryotherapy, 920
Cryptorchidism, 1007, 1008
Cryptosporidiosis
  chemotherapy, 150
  in cats, 894
  in cattle, 776–778
  in dogs, 894
  spiramycin in, 894
CURATREM. *See* Clorsulon
Cyathostomes. *See* Strongylus infection, small
Cyclizine, 137
Cyclophosphamide, 924
  dosage, 930
    rate, 935t
  excretion, 929
  hemorrhagic cystitis and, 927
  in breast cancer, 930
  indications, 929
  in lymphosarcoma, 930, 936
  liver transformation, 929
  mechanism of action, 929

predisolone and, with vincristine, 935
   side effects, 929, 930, 932t
Cypermethrin, 55
Cyproheptadine, 193
Cystic endometrial hyperplasia, 1016
Cystisospora infection, 893–894
Cystitis, 247
   feline urologic syndrome and, 985
   hemorrhagic, cyclophosphamide and, 928
   in cats, 246
   in dogs, 246
   treatment, 957
Cysts, 699
Cytarabine
   dosage rate, 935t
   in lymphoma, malignant, 931
   side effects, 932t
Cythioate, 867
Cytochrome P-450, 347
Cytosine arabinoside, 931

Dacarbazine
   dosage rate, 935t
   doxorubicin in combined therapy with, 933
   emetic effects, 927
Dairy cows
   bovine somatotropin in, 634–635
   mastitis in, 301
   metritis in, 185
Danofloxacin
   in cattle, 800
   in pasteurellosis, 291
   in respiratory disease, 291, 790t
Dantrolene, 1019
DARAPRIM. *See* Pyrimethamine
Darrow's solution, 176–177
Daunorubicin, 932t
DDT, 212, 933
DDVP, 207
DECCOX. *See* Decoquinate
Decoquinate
   as feed additive, 775
   dosage, 729
   in coccidiosis, 774t
      ovine, 726, 727, 727t
   mechanism of action, 775
   monensin vs, 729
Deferoxamine, 152, 203
Degenerative joint disease, 447–455
   cycle of, 450t
   pathogenesis, 448–449
   treatment, 449–455
      corticosteroids, 449–451
      dimethyl sulfoxide, 454–455
      hyaluronic acid, 453–454
      NSAIDs, 451–452
      orgotein, 455
      polysulfated glycosaminoglycan, 452–453
Dehydration, 167, 171–173, 420t
   therapy, 173–177. *See also* Fluid replacement
      therapy

Dehydrocodeinone, 126
Delayed neurotoxicity, 204
Deletion mutants, 74
Delivery systems. *See* Drug delivery systems
Delmadinone acetate, 1008
   as alternate to estrogen therapy, 1007
   dosage, 1012
   indications
      lactation suppression, 1015
      pseudopregnancy, 1014
   in dogs, 1010
Dembrexine, 124, 492t, 494
Demeclocycline, 264
DEMEROL. *See* Meperidine
Demethylchlortetracycline, 264
Demodectic mange, 840–843
Demodicosis, 840–843
DEPO-MEDROL. *See* Dexamethasone, methyl
      prednisolone combined with
Dermatitis, 437
   miliary, 1011, 1017
DERMATON dog collar, 57t
Dermatophytosis, 846–848
Dermatoses, deep-seated
   in dogs, 953t
Derris, 868
Desmycosin, 796
Detomidine, 411t, 426t
   analgesic properties, 415
   duration of action, 414, 415
   in foals, 502, 502t
   in horses, 502, 502t, 562
DEXADRESSON. *See* Dexamethasone
Dexamethasone, 202t, 212
   absorption, 695
   dosage, 128, 541t
   duration of action, 694
   in cattle, 128
   indications
      chronic obstructive pulmonary disease, 492t, 494
      endotoxic shock, 191t, 420t, 426t
      parturition induction, 481, 695
   in horses, 128
   in otitis externa, 852
   JECFA evaluation, 381
   methyl prednisolone combined with, 128
   neomycin combined with, 852
   phenytoin interaction with, 998
Dexamethasone phenylpropionate
   dexamethasone sodium phosphate combined with,
      696
Dexamethasone sodium phosphate, 695
   dexamethasone phenylpropionate combined with,
      696
Dexamethasone trimethylacetate, 695–696
Dextran
   as a plasma expander, 177
   in fluid therapy, 187–188
   in shock, 202t, 426t
      endotoxic, 420t

Dextrose saline, 177, 212
Diabetes mellitus, 983
Diagnostic tests, 67
Diamfenetide, 87, 91t
    anthelmintic spectrum, 91t, 763t
    effectiveness against liver flukes, 110
    mechanism of action, 772
    metabolites, 111
Diaminopyrimidines, 299
Diamphenethide. *See* Diamfenetide
Diarrhea, 144–147
    acidosis and, 183
    antimicrobial agents and, 946
    aspirin in, 155
    chain reaction in, 152t
    diets for, 988
    hypersecretion and, 157
    hypomotility and, 157
    in horses, 185, 507
    neonatal
        in calves, 147–150
        in pigs, 291
    parasitic infection and, 511
Diaveridine, 306
Diazepam
    absorption, 998
    adverse effects, 1005
    anticonvulsant activity, 992t, 998
    bioavailability, 998
    clonazepam vs, 999
    CNS effects, 217t
    dosage, 999t, 1005
    in cardiac disease, 823
    in cats, 999, 999t, 1005
    in combined therapy, 999
    in convulsive states, 201
    indications
        motion sickness, 139
        overgrooming, in cats, 1005
        status epilepticus, 998
        urinary incontinence, 1019
    in flea infestation, 873
    in foals, 502, 502t
    in metaldehyde poisoning, 209
    in strychnine poisoning, 202t, 208
    megestrol acetate vs, 1005
    oxazepam vs, 147
    side effects, 999t
Diazinon, 207, 210, 867
Dichlorophene, 891t
    in hookworm infestation, 887t
    methyl benzene combined with, 882t
Dichlorphene
    toxicity, in cats, 217t
Dichlorvos, 82t, 210, 443t
    absorption, 102
    antinematodal spectrum, 885t
    antiparasitic spectrum, 882t
    boluses, 47t
    contraindications, 102–103

dosage, 432t
    environmental impact, 441
    formulations, 432t
    indications, 431t
        ascarid infection, 102
        bots, 102
        hookworm infections, 887t
        whipworm infections, 888
    in flea and tick control, 55, 57t
    neuromuscular coordination and, 83
    parasiticidal spectrum, 432t
    resin pellets, 49
    toxicity, 442t
Diclazuril, 726
Dicloxacillin, 230
Dicyclomine, 141, 142
Dieldrin, 212
Diethylcarbamazine, 82t, 84
    administration, 911
    adverse reactions, 911–912
    antinematodal spectrum, 885t
    antiparasitic spectrum, 763t, 882t
        in ruminants, 91t
    benzimidazole combined with, 884
    dosage, 911
    formulations, 911
    indications
        ascarid infestation, 884
        chronic obstructive pulmonary disease, 495
        heartworm disease, 914t
        threadworm infestation, 889
    mechanism of action, 113
    oxibendazole combined with, 887t, 888, 912
    prophylactic use, 888, 907, 911
    safety margin, 911
    strylpyridinium combined with, 884, 887t, 888
Diethylstilbestrol, 315, 316, 346, 396
    genotoxicity, 346, 628
    in misalliance, 1006
Diets
    for colitis, 988
    for feline urologic syndrome, 985–986
    for obesity, 983–984
    in chronic renal failure, 984–985
    in convalescence, 988
    low fat, 987
    nonallergenic, 987
Difil test, 902
Digitalis, toxicity, in cats, 217t
Digitalis glycosides, 817–821. *See also* Digitoxin;
        Digoxin
    poisoning, 202t
Digitalization program, 818t
Digitoxin
    digoxin vs, 818, 819
    mechanism of action, 821
    phenytoin interaction with, 998
    plasma protein binding, 385, 819
Digoxin
    digitoxin vs, 818, 819

dosage rate, 820
in congestive heart failure, 819
in heartworm disease, 917
in poisoning, 201
intoxication, 198–199
mechanism of action, 821
oral digitalization with, 820
serum binding levels, 819
steady-state plasma level, 818
tissue distribution, 819
Dihydrofolate reductase inhibitors, 299–300
Dihydrostreptomycin, 381
antibacterial spectrum, 246
dosage, small animal, 967t
indications
endometritis, 704
respiratory disease, 790t
procaine penicillin combined with, 461t
uterine absorption, 704
Dihydroxyanthroquinone, 426t
Diltiazem, 837
Dimenhydrinate, 137
Dimercaprol, 203, 212
dosage, 205
in poisoning, 202t, 203
Dimercaptopropane sulfonate, 205
Dimercaptosuccinate, 205
Dimethylsulfoxide. *See* Dimethyl sulfoxide
Dimethyl sulfoxide, 128–129, 192–193
analgesic effect, 455
indications
chronic obstructive pulmonary disease, 492t
degenerative joint disease, 454–455
endometritis, bacterial, 475–476, 476t
endotoxic shock, 420t
gastrointestinal disease, 425
laminitis, 466, 468t
in foals, 502, 502t
nebulized, 489
topical, 454, 468t
Dimetridazole, 396
ban on, 582
feed medication, 587t
in cryptosporidiosis, 150
JECFA evaluation, 378t
mutagenic activity, 375
premixes, 582
swine dysentery control, 584t
water medication, 586t
Diminazene, 378t
in canine babesiasis, 895–896, 896t
Dinoprost, 696t, 709
Diphacinone, 207
Diphemanil methylsulfate, 141
Diphenhydramine, 129, 137
Diphenoxylate, 144, 145, 146
antidiarrheal activity, 140
atropine combined with, 141
mechanism of action, 141
neomycin combined with, 141

oral dosage, 141
structure, 140
toxicity, in cats, 217t
Diphenylhydantoin. *See* Phenytoin
Diphtheria, 304
Dipyrone, 128
antispasmodic synergy, 526
dosage, 412t
duration of action, 526
flunixin vs, 526
hyoscine combined with, 422, 422t
in equine colic, 426t
in horses, 526
in pneumonia, 489
methindizate combined with, 143, 461t
warfarin and, 461t
Diquat, 205
Dirochek test, 910
Dirofilaria immitis infection. *See* Heartworm infection
Dirokit, 903
Dirotect, 903
Disodium cromoglycate, 129
Disophenol, 882t, 885t
in hookworm infection, 887t
Disopyramide, 830t, 834
Disseminated intravascular coagulation, 924, 927–928
heparin in, 425, 426t
Distal sesamoiditis. *See* Navicular disease
Disulfoton, 207
Dithiazanine, 882t, 914t
absorption, 909
antinematodal spectrum, 885t
dosage, 909
indications
threadworm infestation, 889
toxicity, 909
Diuretics, 821–822
DL-batyl alcohol, 202t
D-Limonene, 866
DMSO. *See* Dimethyl sulfoxide
DNA, 63, 64, 65
DNA ligases, 64, 65
DNA probes, 71
DNA synthesis, inhibition of, 932
Dobutamine, 821t, 830t
in cardiac disease, 820
in horses, 421
in shock, 187
DOBUTREX. *See* Dobutamine
Dogs
abortion in, 1006
alimentary tract infections in, 946–950
aminoglycoside toxicity and, 251
as reservoirs of infection, 894
babesiasis in, 895–896
bacteremia in, anaerobic, 963
bacterial infections in, antibiotic therapy for, 952t–953t
bacterial overgrowth in, 946, 950
behavioral disorders in, 1003

Dogs, *continued*
bone infections in, 952t
central nervous system infections in, 952t
Cheyletiella infection, 845
colitis in, 146, 948–950, 988
cryptosporidiosis in, 894
cystitis in, 246
demodicosis in, 840–843
dental infections in, 948
dermatoses in, deep-seated, 953t
diarrhea in, 988
dominance aggression in, 1003
emesis in, 137–138
endocarditis in, 960
endometritis in, 1016–1017
enteritis in, 946
epilepsy in, 991, 993
therapy for, 999t
eye infections in, 952t, 960
gastroenteritis in, 947, 987
gastrointestinal tract infections in, 952t
griseofulvin and, 336
haemobartonellosis in, 895–896, 896t
heartworm in. *See* Heartworm infection
hepatic insufficiency in, 987
histiocytoma in, 920
hookworms in, 886–888
lymphosarcoma in, 920, 932
therapy for, 935
misalliance in, 1012
neoplasia in, 920
obesity in, 983
oral cavity infections in, 953t
osteomyelitis in, 958
osteomyelitis in, staphylococcal, 965
osteosarcoma in, 920, 932
otitis externa in, 953t
ovariectomy in, 1016
pancreatic insufficiency in, 987
papillomas in, skin, 920
parasites in, 881t
parturition induction in, 1012–1014
peridontal disease in, 948
polymyositis in, 258
protein/phosphate restriction in, 984
pseudopregnancy in, 1011
pyoderma in, 856
antimicrobial therapy for, 953t
renal failure in, chronic, 984
respiratory tract infections in, 304, 946, 952t
retained placenta in, 1017
roundworms in, 883–886
sepsis in, 952t
skin infections in, 235, 304, 952t
skin papillomas in, 920
skin tumors in, 937
squamous cell carcinoma in, 933
stomatitis in, 948–949
testosterone in, 1008
therapy

acepromazine, 873
amoxicillin, 228
ampicillin, 228
antimicrobial agents, 942
benzimidazole, 885–886
bromhexine, 125
chloramphenicol, 278, 280
cimetidine, 924
cisplatin, 933
clidinium, 146
clindamycin, 257, 258, 259
delmadinone acetate, 1003, 1010
disopyramide, 834
doxorubicin, 932, 933
enrofloxacin, 288
epsiprantel in, 114
etamphylline, 122
gentamicin, 246
griseofulvin, 846–847, 847t
isopropamide, 137, 142
ivermectin, 107–108
kanamycin, 247
levamisole, 910
lindane, 872
medroxyprogesterone acetate, 1003
megestrol acetate, 1003
methotrexate, 931
methyltestosterone, 1008
mibolerone, 1012
monensin, 192
naloxone, 193
norfloxacin, 287
phenobarbital, 994, 995
phenylbutazone, 525
phenytoin, 997
primidone, 994
propranolol, 835
prostaglandins, 1014
quinidine, 833
sulfadiazine, 303t
sulfadimethoxine, 303t
sulfonamide, indications for, 304
sulfonamide-trimethoprim in, 303t
thyroid carcinoma in, 933
Toxoplasma gondii infection in, 258
urinary tract infections in, 304, 951, 952t
uterine infections in, 952t, 963
vaginal infections in, 952t, 960
valproic acid in, 1000
vincristine in, 931
vomiting in, treatment of, 137–138
whipworms in, 888–889
wound infections in, 958
Dominance aggression, 1003
Domperidone, 137, 139
Dopamine, 187, 421, 820
in hypotension, 421
inotropic activity, 821t
Doping
antiiflammatory agents in, 562–563

beta-agonists in, 563
categories of, 547
defined, 559
furosemide in, 563
legitimate therapy and, 552
"medications to lose," 550
"medications to win," 550
patterns and problems of, 559–562
prerace testing for, 561–562
sampling for, 552–559
sedatives in, 562
sodium bicarbonate in, 563
types of, 549–551
DOPRAM. *See* Doxapram
DORMOSEDAN. *See* Detomidine
Doxapram, 201t, 202t, 212
Doxorubicin, 923
    antineoplastic spectrum, 933
    cardiomyopathy and, 924
    cardiotoxicity, 932–933
    dacarbazine combined with, 933
    dosage
        in dogs, 933
        rate, 935t
    enteritis and, hemorrhagic, 933
    excretion, 924
    heparin interaction with, 928
    in combined therapy, 933
    in dogs, 932, 933
    in transmissible venereal tumors, 937, 938t
    mechanism of action, 932
    perivascular administration, 923
    radiation therapy and, 933
    side effects, 932t
    site of action, 932
    tissue necrosis and, 928
    toxicity, relative, 933
    vomiting and, 927
Doxycycline, 131, 264
    absorption, 272, 273
    antibacterial activity, 273–274, 795
    bioavailability, oral, 947
    distribution, 273
    dosage, small animal, 967t
    drug interaction, 274
    excretion, 273
    feed medication, 577, 795
    indications, 275
        pleuropneumonia, swine, 577
    lipid solubility, 272, 795, 945
    peak plasma levels, 267
    pharmacokinetics, 272–273
    toxicity, 274
DRAMAMINE, 139
Drocarbil, 891t
DRONTEL PLUS, Febantel, pyrantel and
        praziquantel combined with
Droperidol, 137
Drostanolone, 1008
Drug allergy, 343–346

Drug delivery systems. *See also* Controlled-release
        systems; Pulsed-release systems; Sustained-
        release systems
    anthelmintic ruminal devices, 48–49
    innovations in, 58
    single dose vs controlled-release, 33, 34
Drug doping. *See* Doping
Drug residues. *See* Residues
Drug(s)
    approval, role of FDA in, 18–24
    biotransformation, 318, 319t, 320
    development of, 6–10
    discovery and screening, 4–6
    fetal exposure, 333
    half-life, 394
    passage across cell membranes, 386–388
    pH and diffusion of, 388–390
    pharmacokinetics, 391–394
    placental transfer, 333
    plasma protein binding, 383–386
    regulatory clearance, 17–18
    safety, 317
    target animal studies, 15–17
    toxicity studies, 10–15
    transport processes, 390–391
Drug testing
    immunoassay-based, 557–559
Dry cow mastitis, 677–681
Dry cow therapy, 58, 661
DYREX T F. *See* Trichlorfon, phenothiazine and
        piperazine combined with
Dystocia, 480, 481
    isoxsuprine in, 701
    oxytocin and, 1013

E. coli, 143
EAR FORCE tags. *See* Permethrin
Ear implants, 55, 56t
Edema, pulmonary, 808, 809
EDTA. *See* Calcium disodium edetate;
        Ethylenediaminetetra-acetic acid
Eggs, 372
ELANCO. *See* Tylosin
Elastomer(s), 37
Electrocautery, 920
Electronic bolus, 48, 85
ELISA, 72
Embryotoxicity, 289
Emetics, 134–135, 196–197
    central, 197
    local, 196
Emphysema, 130, 809
Enalapril, 827t, 829
Encainide, 835
Endocarditis, 960
Endometritis, 471–480
    causative pathogens, 471–472
    drug-induced, 1016
    etiology, 471–472
    in dogs, 1016–1017

Endometritis, *continued*
  oxytocin in, 702t
  progestogens and, 1016
  progression to pyometra, 703
  treatment
    antibiotic, 476–478
    nonantibiotic, 478
    systemic, 473
    underlying principles of, 472–473
    uterine irrigation, 473–476
Endotoxic shock, 186, 188–189
  in equine colic, 419–421, 420t
  prostaglandins and, 189
Endotoxins, 198
Enrofloxacin, 282, 289–290
  absorption, 286, 290, 799
  antibacterial spectrum, 283, 799, 800
  chemistry, 283
  dosage, small animal, 967t
  feed mix, 575
  in calves, 290, 291
  in cats, 291
  indications, 290
    bovine respiratory disease, 798
    bovine respiratory tract infections, 798–800
    bronchopneumonia, 575
    canine pyoderma, 860t, 861
    colibacillosis, 579
    diarrhea, 291
    E. coli infections, 291
    enzootic pneumonia, 575
    MMA syndrome, 291
    pneumonia, 291
    respiratory disease, 790t
    respiratory tract infections, 291
    salmonellosis, 146, 291, 587, 800
    skin infections, 291
  in dogs, 288, 291
  in pigs, 290, 291, 575
  in poultry, 290
  JECFA evaluation, 381
  metabolism, 287
  mycoplasmacidal activity, 290
  oral, 286
  serum level, 286
  structure, 283
  teratogenicity, 289
  tissue distribution, 945
  tissue penetration, 799
  tylosin vs, 290
Enteritis
  equine colic and, 403
  hemorrhagic, doxorubicin and, 933
  in dogs, 946
  in foals, 507
  in horses, 403
  salmonellosis in, 403
  sulfonamides in, 304
    bolus, 52
Enterotoxigenic *E. coli*, 147

Enzyme immunoassays, 73–74
Enzyme inducers, 347
Eosinophilic granuloma, in cats, 1011
Ephedrine
  dosage, 123
  duration of action, 122
  epinephrine vs, 122
  in horses, 505t
  in urinary incontinence, 1018
  mechanism of action, 122
Epilepsy
  causes of seizures, 992t
  medical management of, 993
  primary, 991
  prognosis, 993
  secondary, 991
Epinephrine
  ephedrine vs, 122
  in anaphylaxis, 123
  in cardiac disease, 830t
  in cardiac dysrhythmias, 830t
Epitope, 72
Epsiprantel, 881
  anticestodal activity, 891, 891t
  antiparasitic spectrum, 882t
  in dogs, 114
  pyrantel combined with, 882t
Epsom salts, 144
Eptomycin
  gastrointestinal absorption, 152
EQUIGARD. *See* Dichlorvos
Equine chorionic gonadotropin, 1007
Equine colic
  colonic impaction in, 422–423
  enteritis and, 403
  flatulent, 423–425
  fluid therapy in, 419–421, 420t
  idiopathic, 403
  obstructive, 402
  pain, 405–407
  pathophysiology, 403–405
  peritonitis and, 403
  salmonellosis and, 403
  shock in, 416–419, 417t
  spasmodic, 402, 421–422
  thromboembolic, 402, 415
  treatment of
    acepromazine, 414
    alpha adrenergics, 414
    analgesics, 408–410
    butorphanol, 410
    chloral hydrate, 415
    detomidine, 415
    flunixin meglumine, 412–413
    ketoprofen, 413
    meperidine, 409–410
    methadone, 410
    naloxone, 410
    NSAIDs, 411–414
    pentazocine, 410

phenylbutazone, 413
principles of, 407–408
sedatives, 414–415
tranquilizers, 414–415
types of, 402–407
EQUIPAR. *See* Oxibendazole
EQUIZOLE. *See* Thiabendazole
EQUIZOLE A. *See* Thiabendazole, piperazine
    combined with
EQVALAN. *See* Ivermectin
Ergometrine, 1013
Ergonovine
in retained placenta, 714
Ergot, 213
Erythromycin, 154, 251
absorption, 257
against coagulase-positive staphylococci, 966
antibacterial spectrum, 255, 258, 662
as growth promoter, 599t
bacterial resistance and, 661
chemical structure, 252
cross resistance, 254
distribution, 256
dosage, small animal, 967t
elimination, 256
gentamicin combined with, 258
in cattle, 252, 797
indications, 255, 258
    bovine mastitis, 661
    bovine respiratory tract infections, 797
    canine pyoderma, 860, 860t, 861
    foot rot, 731
    metritis, contagious equine, 480
    respiratory disease, 790t, 796, 797
    respiratory infections, in foals, 505t
    Rhodococcus equi infection, 259
    Rhodococcus equi pneumonia, 488
    septic arthritis, 458t
    swine dysentery, 582
in foals, 488, 496t
in gram-positive infections, 253
intramammary, 662
lipid solubility, 706
lung level, 797
mechanism of action, 253
metabolism, 255
oleandomycin vs, 255, 258
oral, 256–257
parenteral, 256, 576
Pasteurella resistance, 797
peak serum concentration, 255
penicillin G combined with, 259
preparations, 256, 257
resistance, 253
ribosomal binding, 254
rifampin combined with, 488
rifampin synergy, 488
salts of, 797
theophylline interaction, 493
tissue penetration, 662

toxicity, 257, 259, 260
Escherichia coli, 67
antimicrobial resistance, 942
Escherichia coli, enterotoxicogenic, 69
Escherichia coli infections, 720–724
Escherichia coli mastitis, 676. *See also* Coliform mastitis
Esophageal groove reflux, 92
Essential fatty acids, 875–876
Estradiol benzoate
dosage, 1006
indications
    behavioral control, 1006
    hypogonadal obesity, 1007
    termination of pregnancy, 1006
    urinary incontinence, 1019
persistence in body, 1006
progesterone combined with, 56t, 599t, 619
testosterone and, 619
Estradiol cypionate, 1012
Estradiol monobenzoate, 1009, 1014
Estradiol(s), 315, 479t
as growth promoter, 33
implants, 54
progesterone combined with, 629
residues, 628
role of, 691
sustained release, 47t, 56t
with other steroids, 47t, 56t
Estrogen benzoate-progesterone implants, 622
Estrogen(s), 691, 707–708
actomyosin synthesis and, 1006
alpha adrenergic agonists and, 1006
alternates to, 1007
anabolic effects, 54
androgens combined with, 1015
antimicrobial agents combined with, 704
as growth promoters, 622
effects of, 1024t
flumethasone combined with, 482
indications, 1006
    hypogonadal obesity, 1007
in endometritis, bacterial, 474t
in male dogs, 1007
in perianal adenoma, 933
lactation suppression of, 1014
methyltestosterone and, 1008
myometrial binding, 1006
natural, 1005
oxytocin and, 1013
phagocytosis and, 479
postpartum, 478
side effects, 1006, 1007, 1013
urethral sensitivity and, 1006
urinary incontinence, 1018
ESTRUMATE. *See* Cloprostenol
Estrus
control of, 699, 700, 1003, 1009–1012
feline behavior during, 1005
induction of, 1007
Etamiphylline

Etamiphylline, *continued*
  bronchodilator activity, 121
  duration of action, 493
  in cardiac disease, 824t
Etamphylline
  formulations, 122
  in cats, 122
  in cattle, 122
  in dogs, 122
  in horses, 122, 493
Ethacrynic acid, 151
Ethanol, in ethylene glycol intoxication, 202t, 207–208
Ethinyl estradiol, 1006, 1009
  methyltestosterone and, 1014
Ethopabate, 306
  amprolium combined with, 727
Ethylcellulose, 35t
Ethylenediaminetetra-acetic acid, 203
Ethylene glycol, 217t
  poisoning, 198, 207–208
Ethylene vinylacetate copolymer, 35t, 37, 40
Etorphine, toxicity, in cats, 217t
EVA. *See* Ethylene vinylacetate copolymer
EXCENEL. *See* Ceftiofur
Exercise-induced pulmonary hemorrhage, 563
EXPAR insecticide ear tag. *See* Permethrin
Expectorants, 123
Extracellular fluid acidifiers, 176
Extracellular fluid alkalinizers, 176
Eye infections
  in dogs, 952t, 960
  in horses, 503

False pregnancy. *See* Pseudopregnancy
Fasciola hepatica, 87
Fascioliasis, 767–770
FASINEX. *See* Triclabendazole
Fatty acids, essential, 875–876
Febantel
  absorption, 86
  active metabolite, 86
  anthelmintic spectrum, 89t, 763t
    in dogs, 881
    in horses, 432t
    in ruminants, 91t
    in small animals, 882t
  antinematodal spectrum, 885t
  dosage, 97, 432t
  efficacy, 765t
  formulations, 432t
  indications, 431t
    ascarid infection, 885
    hookworm infection, 887t
    Ostertagia infection, 92
    parasitic gastroenteritis, 770t
  in horses, 432t
  in sheep, 770t
  JECFA evaluation, 377, 379t
  mechanism of action, 82t, 892
  metabolism, 92

paste formulation, 885
praziquantel combined with, 882t, 887t
pyrantel and praziquantel combined with, 881
residues, 96
safety margin, 442t
teratogenicity, 96, 336
trichlorfon combined with, 430, 443t
Feed additives
  in cattle, 602
  in pigs, 605
  in poultry, 605
  poisoning with, 198
Feed medication
  in poultry, 605
Feline calici virus, 130
Feline leukemia virus, 74
Feline respiratory disease, 130–131
Feline urologic syndrome
  clinical signs of, 985
  cystitis and, 985
  dietary management in, 985–986
  hematuria and, 985
  surgical management of, 985
  urethritis and, 985
  urinary pH and, 985
  urolithiasis and, 985
Feline viral rhinotracheitis, 130
Fenbendazole, 443t
  absorption, 88
  active metabolite, 86
  adverse effects, 442t
  anthelmintic spectrum, 89t
    in horses, 432t
    in ruminants, 762, 763t
  anticestodal activity, 891, 891t
  antinematodal spectrum, 885t
  antiparasitic spectrum, 882t
    in ruminants, 91t
  dosage, 92, 432t, 433, 433t, 434
  efficacy, 765t
  formulations, 432t
  for small animals, 882t
  in cattle, 764t
  indications, 431t
    Aelurostrongylus abstrusus infection, 895
    ascarid infestation, 885
    Filarioides hirthi infection, 894
    hookworm infestation, 887t
    lungworm infection, 437, 881–882, 894
    Ostertagia infestation, 92
    ostertagiasis, 763
    parasitic gastroenteritis, 770t
    Strongyloides westeri infection, 436
    verminous arteritis, 415
    whipworm infestation, 889
  in horses, 432t
  in sheep, 770t
  JECFA evaluation, 377, 379t
  mechanism of action, 82t
  metabolism, 87

metabolite, 92
milk level, 97
oxfendazole vs, 94
pharmacokinetics, 94
pregnancy and, 885–886
prophylactic use, 888
residues, 96
resistance, 438
safety margins, 95
solubility, 94
synthesis, 86
teratogenicity, 336
thiabendazole vs, 86
warfarin and, 461t
Fenoterol, 121
Fenoxycarb, 868
Fenprostalene, 696t, 697, 709
Fentanyl, 138
Fenthion
excretion, 867
in heartworm disease, 914t
mechanism of action, 82t
poisoning, 207
safety index, 210
structure-activity relationship, 103, 872
Fenvalerate, 55
Fetal membranes, retained, 712–715
Fetal toxicity, 336
Fetus, mummified, 700
Fibrosis, generalized, 130
FILARIBITS PLUS. *See* Diethylcarbamazine,
    oxibendazole combined with
Filarioides hirthi infection, 894
Filarioides osleri infection, 894
FINAPLIX. *See* Trenbolone
FLAGYL. *See* Metronidazole
Flatulent colic, 402, 423–425
chloral hydrate in, 423
neomycin in, 423
oil of turpentine in, 423
penicillin in, 423
Flavomycin. *See* Bambermycin
Flea collars, 869
Flea control, 55, 57t
Flea infestation, 864–865
Flecainide, 835
Florfenicol, 282
dosage, 801
indications
    pasteurellosis, 801
    respiratory disease, 790t
Flubendazole
in ascarid infection, 885
JECFA evaluation, 377, 380t
mechanism of action, 81
Fluid therapy, 173–177, 181t
adjuncts to, 174
choice of solution, 175–177, 184t
classification of fluids, 176t
composition of fluids, 175t, 176t

estimation of fluid requirement, 182t
fluid-responsive conditions, 183–185
glucose and glycine content, 178–180
guidelines for, 181–183
in bovine respiratory infections, 807–808
in calf scour, 157–160
in cattle, 807–808
in colibacillosis, 579
in diarrhea, 145
in equine colic, 419–421
in horses, 185
in laminitis, 468t
in septicemia, 500, 500t
in strangles, 490
intraperitoneal, 180–181
maintenance fluid solutions, 177
oral, 174, 177–178
routes of administration, 177–181
subcutaneous, 180–181
Flukicides, 84, 110–113
excretion, 87
Flumequine, 381
Flumethasone, 482
dosages, 541t
Flunixin meglumine, 128, 407
antiendotoxic activity, 802
dipyrone vs, 526
dosage, 528, 530
in colic, 411, 412t
indications
    chronic obstructive pulmonary disease, 492t
    colibacillosis, 155
    endotoxic shock, 420t, 426t
    equine colic, 412–413, 426t
    in calf scour, 150
    laminitis, 466, 466t, 468t
    navicular disease, 463t
    pain, 202t, 528
    pneumonia, 489
    septic arthritis, 458t
    shock, 202, 202t
in horses, 528–529
in racing horses, 563
oxytetracycline combined with, 802
potency, 528
protein synthesis and, 151
recommended dosage, 412t
Fluoroacetamide (1081) poisoning, 210
Fluoroacetate (1080) poisoning, 210
Fluoroquinolone(s), 146, 282
antibacterial spectrum, 945
distribution, 287
mechanism of action, 285
metabolism, 287–288
oral absorption, 286
resistance, 286
tissue distribution, 945
urine levels, 951
5-Fluorouracil
dosage rate, 935t

5-Fluorouracil, *continued*
  mechanism of action, 931
  side effects, 931, 9932t
Fluphenazine, 137
Fluprostenol, 479t
  in parturition induction, 481–482
Foals
  central nervous disorders in, 501–503
  diarrhea in, 507
  enteritis in, 507
  gastric ulceration in, 510–511
  gastrointestinal disorders in, 506–508
  navel ill in, 304
  nebulization in, 125, 489
  ocular infections in, 503
  osteomyelitis in, 503
  parasitic infection in, 511
  peritonitis in, 508
  pneumonia in, 487–489
  pneumonia in, bacterial, 503–506
  respiratory infections in, 504–505
  Rhodococcus equi infection in, 487–489
  sedatives in, 502, 502t
  septic arthritis in, 458t, 503
  septicemia in, 495–503
  strongylus infection in, 436
  sulfonamides and, 309
  therapy
    anthelmintic, 511
    anticonvulsant, 502, 502t
    antimicrobial, 504–505
    antimicrobial, dosage, 496t
    cimetidine, 510, 511
    erythromycin, 488
    xylazine, 502, 502t
  uveitis in, 503
Folic acid, 299
Follicle stimulating hormone, 690
  obesity and, 983
  spermatogenesis and, 1003
  suppression, 1003
Food allergy dermatitis, 873
Foot rot, 304
  in sheep, 730–731
  streptomycin in, 246
  sulfadimidine in, 305–306
  sulfonamide bolus in, 52
Formalin, 731
FSH. *See* Folicle-stimulating hormone
Fucidin, 851
Fungal mastitis, 682
Fungicide poisoning, 198
Furazolidone, 396
  carcinogenicity, 893
  indications
    colibacillosis, 579
    giardiasis, 892t, 893
    swine dysentery, 582
  JECFA evaluation, 377, 380t
  poisoning, 206

  residues, 373–374
Furosemide
  dosage, 826t, 827t
  in congestive heart failure, 821
  in doping, 563
  in racing horses, 548, 563
Fusarium, 216t

Garden pellets, 209
Gasterophilus infection, 431, 434
Gastric acid, 792
Gastric distention, 424–425
Gastric lavage, 197, 197t
Gastric ulceration
  in foals, 510–511
  treatment, 506t
Gastric ulceration syndrome, 451, 457
Gastroenteritis, 987
  in dogs, 947
  parasitic, 770–771
Gastrointestinal diseases
  diets for, 986–988
Gastrointestinal obstruction, upper, 185
Gastrointestinal protectives and absorbents, 154–155
Gastrointestinal tract infections
  cephalexin in, 233
  in dogs, 952t
  sulfonamides in, 145
Gelatin, 35t, 39
Gelatin colloidal solution, 177, 188
Gene cloning, 69
Gene deletion vaccines, 70
Gene expression, 66
Genetic engineering, 62–63. *See also* Biotechnology;
    Recombinant technology
Gene transfer, 62
Genital hypoplasia, 1007
Genital tract infections, 246–247
GENOCIN. *See* Gentamicin
Gentamicin, 246–247
  absorption, 152
  acidity and, 704
  amikacin vs, 510
  anaerobiosis and, 704
  antibacterial spectrum, 246
  bacterial resistance, 942
  boluses, 47t
  carbenicillin combined with, 229
  dosage, 246, 247
  dosage, small animal, 967t
  erythromycin combined with, 258
  gastrointestinal absorption, 152
  in cats, 246
  in cattle, 246
  indications
    calf scour, 152, 154
    canine pyoderma, 860t
    colibacillosis, 246, 579, 721
    colic, 424t
    cystitis, 246

diarrhea, 145
endometritis, bacterial, 474t, 476, 477, 478t
genital tract infections, 246–247
mastitis, 246
metritis, 246
metritis, contagious equine, 480
nephritis, 246
otitis externa, 851
placenta, retained, 484
pneumonia, 246
pyodermatitis, 246
respiratory infections, in foals, 505t
respiratory tract infections, 246
Rhodococcus equi pneumonia, 488
septic arthritis, 458t
septicemia, in foals, 499
swine dysentery, 246, 582
tracheobronchitis, 246
upper respiratory tract infections, 246
urinary tract infections, 951
uterine infections, 246, 705
wound infections, 246
in dogs, 246
in foals, 496t
in horses, 246–247
in lambs, 721
in pigs, 246, 247
in staphylococcal infections, 958
intramammary, 246
intrauterine, 246, 477, 480
JECFA evaluation, 381
minimum inhibitory concentration, 245
nebulized, 489
neomycin combined with, 579
nephrotoxicity, 251
oral, 721
penicillin combined with, 246
resistance, 245
ribosomal, 244
water medication, 586t
German shepherds, 146
Giardiasis, 892–893
gI-negative vaccines, 70
Gingivitis, 947
Glass boluses, 51
Glucocorticoids, 271
in endotoxic shock, 191, 191t
Glucorticoids, 127
Glucose-glycine-electrolyte solution, 159
Glycobiarsol, 885t, 888
Glycopyrrolate, 157
atropine vs, 493, 494
distribution, 493, 494
dosage, 493, 494
duration of action, 494
indications
chronic obstructive pulmonary disease, 492t, 493
diarrhea, 141
emesis, canine, 137
pneumonia, 489

in horses, 505t
onset of action, 493
safety margin, 493, 494
Glycosides, cardiac, 817–821
Goats
listeriosis in, 488
lymphadenitis, 487
Gonadotropin-releasing hormone, 702, 709–710
Gonadotropin(s), 1007
inhibition, megestrol acetate and, 1004
Grain overload, 198
acidosis and, 183, 203
Gram-negative sepsis, antimicrobial agents in, 424t
Granuloma, eosinophilic, 1011
Griseofulvin
absorption, 846
adverse effects, 847
antitubulin activity, 95
dosage, 847, 847t
efficacy, 847
formulations, 846
in cats, 336
in dermatophytoses, 846–847
in dogs, 336, 846–847
ketoconazole combined with, 847
phenylbutazone interaction with, 847
resistance, 847
teratogenicity, 99, 336, 847
tumorigenicity, 347
warfarin interaction with, 461t
Growth hormone, 55, 63. *See also* Bovine
somatotropin
Growth promoters, 47t, 71
antimicrobial, 569–570, 600–607
approved for beef, 599t
classification of, 600
hormonal, 616–631
classification of, 618–620
formulations, 617–618
principles in using, 617
ionophore antibiotics as, 607–615
JECFA evaluation, 378t
requirements for, 602
Guanosine monophosphate, 143
Gut antidotes, 197–199

Habronema infection, 437
HAEMACCEL. *See* Gelatin polypeptide colloidal
infusion
Haemobartonellosis
in cats, 895–896, 896t
in dogs, 895–896, 896t
Hair loss. *See* Alopecia
Halogenated anesthetics, 347
Haloperidol, 137
Haloxan
indications, 431t
Haloxon
anthelmintic spectrum, 91t
coumaphos combined with, 763t

Haloxon, *continued*
  mechanism of action, 82t
  neuromuscular coordination and, 83
  safety, 102
Hartmann's solution, 176, 426t
HAVA-SPAN. *See* Sulfamethazine
HEARTGARD. *See* Ivermectin
Heartworm infection
  assay for, 74
  cardiac support therapy in, 916–917
  clinical syndromes associated with, 899
  control program, 904t, 907–908
  diagnosis, 901–903
  prevalence, 899
  prevention, 907, 911–914
  pulmonary hypertension and, 899–900
  respiratory support therapy in, 914–916
  supportive therapy, 914–917
  therapy, 905–907, 908–910
    pulmonary thromboembolism and, 906
    supportive, 914–917
Heavy metal poisoning, 212
Hematuria, 985
Hemoangioma, 921
Hemorrhage, pulmonary, 563
Heparin, 211, 426t
  doxorubicin interaction with, 928
  in disseminated intravascular coagulation, 425, 426t
  in laminitis, 468t
Hepatic insufficiency, 987
Hepatitis B vaccine, 63
Herbicide poisoning, 198, 205–206
Herpesvirus, 73
Hetacillin, 228
  absorption, 792
  antibacterial activity, 227
Hexachlorophene
  anthelmintic spectrum, 91t
  antiparasitic spectrum, 763t
  mechanism of action, 82t
Hexoprenaline, 121
Histamine, 127
Histiocytoma, 920
Homatropine, 157
Hookworms, 880, 880t, 886–889
Hormonal growth promoters, 616–631
  biotechnology and, 631–639
  classification of compounds used, 618–619
  commercially available preparations, 619–620
  implants, 619–622
  responses to, 622–623
  side effects, 623
Hormonally responsive conditions, 1021t
  skin, 1017–1018
Hormones, reproductive, 47t
Horseradish peroxidase, 73
Horses, 84
  abdominal pain, 406–407
  abortion in, induction of, 483–484

chronic obstructive pulmonary disease in, 121, 490–495
colic, 402–426. *See also* Equine colic
degenerative joint disease in, 447–455
diarrhea in, 185
doping in. *See* Doping
endometritis in, 471–480
ephedrine in, 505t
exercise-induced pulmonary hemorrhage in, 563
eye infections in, 503
fluid therapy in, 185
Gasterophilus infection in, 434
Habronema infection in, 437
immunotherapy in, 934
intestinal obstruction in, 185
laminitis in, 464–468
large strongylus infection in, 430–434
lincomycin(s) and, 258
lungworm infection in, 430, 437
metritis in, contagious, 480
Onchocerca infection in, 437
osteomyelitis in, 456–457
Oxyuris equi infection in, 435
Parascaris equorum infection in, 434–435
parturition, induction of, 480–483
peritonitis in, 488
pinworms in, 430
polyarthritis in, 304
respiratory tract infections in, 304
Rhodococcus equi infection in, 259
salmonellosis in, 509–510
septic arthritis in, 456–457
shock in, 535–537
small strongylus infection in, 435
spasmodic colic in, 143, 414
strangles in, 304, 489–490
Strongyloides westeri infection in, 436
strongylus infection in, 430–434, 435, 436
tapeworm infection in, 430, 436–437
therapy
  amoxicillin, 238t
  ampicillin, 238t
  aspirin, 451
  atropine, 493, 505t
  bromhexine, 125
  butorphanol, 409t, 410, 412t, 426t
  carbenicillin, 238t
  cefadroxil, 238t
  cephalothin, 238t
  chloramphenico, 488
  clenbuterol, 493, 505t
  corticosteroid, 449–451, 530–542
  detomidine, 562
  dexamethasone, 128
  dimethyl sulfoxide, 454–455
  dipyrone, 526
  dobutamine, 421
  etamphylline, 122
  flunixin meglumine, 528–529
  gentamicin, 246

glycopyrrolate, 505t
hyaluronic acid, 453–454
isopropamide, 422
isoxsuprine, 461–462
ivermectin, 107, 108
kanamycin, 247
ketoprofen, 527–528
meclofenamic acid, 528
monensin, 206
naproxen, 527
niclosamide, 436
NSAID, 451–452, 519
orgotein, 455, 462–463
oxytetracycline, 269–270
penicillin G, 238t
phenylbutazone, 451, 522, 525
polysulfated glycosaminoglycan, 452–453
salicylate, 526–527
sulfadimethoxine, 303t
sulfonamide, 304
terbutaline, 505t
theophylline, 493, 505t
ticarcillin, 229, 238t
warfarin, 459–461
xylazine, 411t, 412t, 414, 426t
Trichostrongylus infection in, 435
young. *See* Foals
Human chorionic gonadotropin, 1007
HYALARTIN V. *See* Hyaluronic acid
Hyaluronic acid
commercial preparations, 453
corticosteroid supression of, 451
indications
degenerative joint disease, 453–454
septic arthritis, 458t
Hybridoma, 62, 66–67, 72
Hydatidosis, 890
Hydralazine, 826t, 827t, 828
Hydrocortisone
in endotoxic shock, 191t
in lymphosarcoma, 933
Hydrogels, 35t, 39, 40
as rate controlling membranes, 41
Hydrogen peroxide, 196, 476t
Hydroxyzine, 873
Hyoscine
antispasmodic activity, 142
dipyrone combined with, 422, 422t
duration of action, 138
in colic, equine, 421, 422t, 426t
in emesis, canine, 137
methscopolamine vs, 142
Hyoscyamine, 145, 157
Hypertension, obesity and, 983
Hyperthermia, 200
Hypocupremia, 50
Hypogonadal obesity, 1007
Hypogonadism, 1008
Hypomagnesemia, 50
Hypoplasia, genital, 1007

Hypovolemia, 200
Hypovolemic shock, 186

Ibuprofen, 128, 407
Idiopathic colic, 403
Idoxuridine, 131
Ifosfamide, 927, 932t
Imidazothiazoles, 100–101. *See also* Levamisole
in cattle, 765t, 770t
in sheep, 770t
mechanism of action, 82t
Imidocarb, 381
for blood-borne parasites, 895, 896t
Immunoassays, 72–73
Immunomodulators, 33
delivery systems, 55
in bovine respiratory disease, 804–805
pulse-release systems, 52
Immunostimulators, 33
Immunotherapy
as adjunct therapy, 921
in horses, 934
postoperative, 920
Impetigo, 863
Implant systems, 46, 54, 55
Indomethacin, 407
antiprostaglandin effect, 151
side effects, incidence of, 155
Infertility, 1008
Insecticide(s)
classes of, 865–868
collars, 869
controlled-release, 47t, 870
dips, 869
ear tags, 680
formulations, 868–870
poisoning, 198
powders, 870
sprays, 680, 869–870
sustained delivery devices for, 47t
teratogenicity, 335
Insulin, genetically engineered, 63, 68
INTERCEPTOR. *See* Milbemycin
Interferon(s), 65, 534
genetically engineered, 63, 68
in cancer therapy, 934
Intestinal obstruction, 183
acute, 185
Intestinal worms, 84
Intoxications
large animal, 203–207
small animal, 207–211
Intramammary formulations, 658–660
sustained release, 55
Iodide salts, 124
Iodine
deficiency. *See* Iodine deficiency
in laminitis infection, 468t
in pregnancy, 755–756
Lugol's, 476t

Iodine, *continued*
  role in thyroxin synthesis, 752
  sustained delivery devices, 47t
Iodine deficiency
  symptoms, 754, 755t
  treatment and prevention, 756–757
Ionophore antibiotics, 607–615. *See also* specific agents
  toxicity of, 613–615
Ipecac, 134
Ipronidazole
  in cryptosporidiosis, 150
  JECFA evaluation, 378t, 396
  toxicity, 375
  water medication, 586t
Iron, 47t
Isaverin, 143
Ischemic gut disease, 402
Isoetharine, 489
Isoflupredone, 541t
Isometamidium, 378t, 381
Isopropamide, 157
  in colitis, canine, 142
  in dogs, 137, 142
  in emesis, canine, 137
  in horses, 422
  mechanism of action, 138
Isoproterenol
  in cardiac disease, 824t
    dysrhythmias, 830t
  nebulized, 489
Isopyrin, 128
  phenylbutazone interaction with, 518
Isorbide dinitrate, 827t
Isospora infection, 893–894
Isoxsuprine, 461–462
  contraindications, 462
  dosage, 462, 463t
  indications
    dystocias, 701
    laminitis, 466t, 467, 468t
    navicular syndrome, 461
  in horses, 462
  warfarin vs, 462
Itraconazole, 847
Ivermectin, 104
  absorption, 109
  antinematodal spectrum, 885t
  antiparasitic spectrum, 763t, 882t
  clorsulon combined with, 764t
  contraindication, 889
  dosage, 432t, 433, 433t, 434
    in heartworm disease, 912
  drench, 771
  efficacy, 765t, 912
  environmental impact, 441
  formulations, 432t, 912
  half-life, 109
  in cattle, 764t
  indications, 431t
    ascarid infection, 884, 885

  bots, 434
  Habronema infection, 437
  heartworm disease, 914t
  hookworm infection, 887t
  lungworm infection, 437, 894
  Onchocera dermatitis, 437
  ostertagiasis, 763
  parasitic gastroenteritis, 770t
  prophylaxis, 430, 440, 910, 912
  sarcoptic mange, 844
  Strongyloides westeri infection, 436
  tapeworm infection, 436
  Trichostrongylus infection, 435
  verminous arteritis, 415
  in foals, 511
  injectable preparations, 84
  in sheep, 771, 894
  JECFA evaluation, 379t, 380t
  larvicidal activity, 433
  mechanism of action, 82t, 912
  oral drench, 105
  osmotic pump delivery, 44
  paralytic activity, 105
  parasiticidal spectrum, 432t
  poisoning, 208
  prophylactic use, 430, 440, 910, 912
  sustained delivery devices, 47t
  sustained-release, 85
  tapeworms and, 436
  teratogenicity, 109–110
  toxicity, 208, 443t, 910
IVOMEC. *See* Ivermectin
IVOMEC-F. *See* Ivermectin, combined with clorsulon
IVOMEC SR. *See* Ivermectin

JECFA. *See* Joint Expert Committee on Food
    Additives
Johne's disease, 73
Joint Expert Committee on Food Additives, 377. *See*
    under drug names for specific evaluations

Kanamycin, 154, 245
  antibacterial spectrum, 246, 661
  dosage, 247
    small animal, 967t
  in cattle, 247
  indications
    colic, 424t
    Rhodococcus equi pneumonia, 488
    septic arthritis, 458t
    wound infection, 247
  in dogs, 247
  in foals, 496t
  in horses, 247
  JECFA evaluation, 381
  nebulized, 489
  nephrotoxicity, 251
  penicillin G combined with, 247
  resistance, ribosomal, 244
  subcutaneous, 247

K88 antigens, 69, 578
Kaolin, 136, 143, 154
K99 *E. coli* antibody, 72
Keratitis, ulcerative, 131
Keratoconjunctivitis, infectious, 55
Keratoconjunctivitis sicca, 957
Ketoconazole
  indications
    Candida infections, 130
    dermatophytosis, 847, 847t
    nasal aspergillosis, 130
  miconazole vs, 130
KETOFEN. *See* Ketoprofen
Ketoprofen, 407, 412t
  absorption, 527
  dosage, 412t, 426t, 527
  duration of action, 527
  excretion, 527
  half-life, 527
  indications
    COPD, 492t
    endotoxic shock, 420t
    equine colic, 413, 527
    laminitis, 466t, 468t
    navicular disease, 463t
    septic arthritis, 458t
  in horses, 527–528
  mechanism of action, 527
  metabolism, 527
  phenylbutazone vs, 528
  plasma protein binding, 527
  safety margin, 527–528
Ketosis, 185
Klebsiella mastitis, 682
Knott test, 902, 903

Laburnum, 213
Lactated Ringer's solution, 426t
Lactation, suppression of, 1008, 1015–1016
  estrogens and, 1014
Lactic acid bacteria, 646
Lactobacillus, 156
Lactoferrin, 534
Lambs
  coccidiosis in, 610, 724–728
  Escherichia coli infections in, 720–724
  Nematodirus battus infection in, 771
  scours in, 718–720
Laminar cortical necrosis, 727
Laminitis, 464–468, 525
  corticosteroids and, 537–538
  heparin in, 468t
Large strongylus infection, 430–434
Larvicides, 868
Lasalocid, 150, 609t
  as feed additive, 775
  as growth promoter, 599t, 611–612
  indications
    coccidiosis, 774t
    ovine coccidiosis, 726, 727t

  toxicity, 614
L-Asparaginase
  anaphylaxis and, 933
  side effects, 932t
Laxatives, 144, 199–200
  bulk-forming, 144–145
Lead poisoning, 205, 211
  antidote for, 202t
  CNS effects, 217t
LECTADE/RE-SORB, 178
LECTADE RESORB PLUS, 159
Leukemia, 73
Leukotrienes, 127
  chemotaxis and, 521
  hyperthermia and, 533
  pain and, 533
Levamisole, 100–101
  absorption, 84
  adverse effects, 101–102, 443t
  antiparasitic spectrum, 763t
    in ruminants, 91t
  blood levels, 100
  bolus, 85
  dosage, 910
  efficacy, 765t
  gastrointestinal absorption, 100
  immunologic effects, 101
  in cats, 895
  in cattle, 764t
  indications
    Aelurostrongylus abstrusus infection, 895
    brucellosis, 101
    heartworm infection, 906, 914t
    lungworm infection, 894
    parasitic gastroenteritis, 770t
    pyoderma, 859
  in dogs, 910, 914t
  injectable preparations, 84
  in sheep, 770t
  JECFA evaluation, 379t, 381
  mechanism of action, 82t, 910
  organophosphate potentiation, 211
  oxyclozanide combined with, 772
  piperazine combined with, 432t, 443t
  residues, 100, 101
  safety margin, 906, 910
  slow-release boluses, 100
  toxicity, 101, 910
LEVASOLE. *See* Levamisole
Lidamine, 155
Lidocaine, 210, 830t, 834–835
Lincomycin(s), 252, 253
  antibacterial spectrum, 255
  clindamycin vs, 255, 258, 860
  comparative antibacterial activity, 575
  control dosage, 576
  dosage, small animal, 967t
  elimination, 257
  feed medication, 587t
  formulations, 583

Lincomycin(s), *continued*
  horses and, 258
  indications, 255
    canine pyoderma, 860, 860t, 861
    Mycoplasma hypopneumoniae infection, 574–575
    pneumonia, swine, 574–575
    salmonellosis, 587
    skin infections, 966
    swine dysentery, 582
  in-feed mix, 575
  intramuscular, 256
  metabolism, 255
  oral, 256
  parenteral administration, 575
  peak serum concentration, 256
  premixes, 583
  preparations, 257
  salmonellosis control, 587
  spectinomycin combined with
    in bovine respiratory infection, 258, 797
    in-feed medication, 587t
    in foot rot, 731
    in mycoplasmal infections, 258
    in swine dysentery, 248
    in swine dysentery control, 578
    in swine pleuropneumonia, 578
    water medication, 586t
  swine dysentery control, 584t, 585
  toxicity, 259, 260
  water medication, 586t
Lincosamides, 252, 253
Lindane, 844, 872
Linguatula serrata infection, 895
Lipiodol, 756–757
Liposomal delivery, 43–44
LIQUAMYCIN LA-200. *See* Oxytetracycline, depot formulation
Liquid paraffin, 145, 426t
Listeriosis, 488
Liver fluke, 84
  in cattle, 767–770
  in sheep, 771–772
Liver infections, 487
Local anesthetics, 58
LOMITIL. *See* Diphenoxylate
Loperamide
  antisecretory activity, 144, 155
  calmodulin binding, 141
  constipatory activity, 145
  dosage, 141
  in colitis, canine, 146
  mechanism of action, 141, 157
  naloxone antagonism, 141
  structure, 141
Lorcainide, 835
Low-salt diet, 1019
Lugol's iodine, 476t
Lung abscesses, 487
Lungworm infection
  in calves, 765–767

  in cats, 880, 894
  in dogs, 880, 894
  in horses, 437
  site of, 880t
LUTALYSE. *See* Dinoprost tromethamine
Luteal cysts, 699
Luteinizing hormone, 690–691
Luxabendazole, 763t, 770t, 771
Lymecycline, 264
Lymphadenitis, 487
Lymphoma. *See* Lymphosarcoma
Lymphosarcoma, 920
  corticosteroids in, 933
  cutaneous, 936, 937
  cytabarine in, 931
  in dogs, 932
  methotrexate in, 931
  therapy for, 936t, 936–937
    local, 935
  vincristine in, 932

Macrolide(s), 251–252
  antibacterial spectrum, 254–255, 796
  clinical application, 258–259
  elimination, 257
  indications, 258
  lung levels, 796
  mechanism of action, 253–254
  milk levels, 796
  pharmacokinetics, 255–258
  resistance, 254
  toxicity, 259
Maduramycin, 607
Magnesium, 144, 426t
Malabsorption, 986
Malathion, 207, 210, 867
Mammary tumors, 1008
  drug-induced, 1018
  ovariohysterectomy and, 933
  treatment for, 1009
Manganese, 47t
Mange
  demodectic, 840–843
  sarcoptic, 843–845
Mannitol, 212
MARMADUKE flea and tick collar, 57t
Mast cell tumors, 937
  therapy for, 937t
Mastitis
  acidosis and, 183
  anaerobic, 682
  assays for, 73
  bovine. *See* Bovine mastitis
  bovine somatotropin and, 635
  coliform, 671–677
  control policy, 684–686
  dry-cow, 677–681
  fungal, 682
  gentamicin in, 246
  in cattle. *See* Bovine mastitis

in dairy cows, 185
Klebsiella, 682
liposome-encapsulated drugs for, 55
mycoplasmal, 681
nocardial, 681
pseudomonal, 682
summer, 677–681
vaccination in, 682–684
Mebendazole, 443t
adverse effects, 442t
anticestodal activity, 891, 891t
antinematodal spectrum, 885t
antiparasitic spectrum, 881, 882t
as feed additive, 889
bioavailability, 98
dosage, 432t
formulations, 432t
for small animals, 882t
indications, 431t
ascarid infection, 885
hookworm infection, 887t, 888
lungworm infection, 437
parasitic gastroenteritis, 770t
tapeworm infection, 436
whipworm infection, 889
in sheep, 770t
mechanism of action, 81, 82t
parasiticidal spectrum, 432t
pharmacokinetics, 97
piperazine combined with, 439
prophylactic use, 907
residues, 98
resistance, 438
MECADOX. *See* Carbadox
Meclizine, 137
Meclofenamic acid, 407
bioavailability, 518
indications
COPD, 492t
laminitis, 466t
in horses, 528
in laminitis, 468t
in respiratory disease, 128
recommended dosage, 412t
Medroxyprogesterone acetate, 1004, 1009
mammary tumors and, 1018
potency, 1011
proligestone vs, 1012
side effects, 1011
sustained delivery devices, 47t
tumorigenicity, 1018
Megestrol acetate, 1010–1011
alternate-day therapy, 1005
as alternate to estrogen therapy, 1007
corticosteroids vs, in miliary dermatitis, 1017
diazepam vs, 1005
dosage, 1004, 1005
excretion, 1010, 1017
gonadotropin inhibition, 1004
in castrated dogs, 1004

in cats, 1003, 1011
indications
aggression, 1005
behavior disorders, 1004
elimination of estrus-induced behavior, 1005
estrus control, 1003
excessive grooming behavior, 1017
miliary dermatitis, 1017
prostatic hypertrophy, 1009
pseudopregnancy, 1003, 1014
maintenance dose, 1005
mechanism of action, 1009
medroxyprogesterone acetate as alternate to, 1004
oral, 1004, 1010
side effects, 1004, 1011
tapered regimen, 1005
tumorigenicity, 1018
MEGIMIDE. *See* Bemegride
Melanoma, 933
oral, 921
Melengestrol acetate, 630–631
as growth promoter, 599t
residues, 630
withdrawal period, 630
Meloxicam, 526
Melperone, 155
Melphalan, 930, 932t
dosage rate, 935t
Menadiol, 210
Meningitis, 234, 502
Mepenzolate, 141
Meperidine, 409t, 409–410, 412t
Mephobarbital, 996
Mercury, 212
Metabolic acidosis, 169–170
Metaldehyde poisoning, 209–210, 217t
Metamizole. *See* Dipyrone
Methacycline, 264
Methadone, 409t, 410
Methemoglobinemia, 202t
Methenamine, 956
sodium acid phosphate and, 957
Methicillin, 154
absorption, 230
Methindizate, 145
dipyrone combined with, 143, 461t
in colic, equine, 421, 422t, 426t
Methiocarb, 207
Methionine, 467, 468t
Methocarbamol, 201, 201t, 202t
Methoprene, 868
Methoprim, 300
Methorphan, 126
Methotrexate
citrovorum factor and, 931
cytotoxicity, reversal of, 931
dosage rate, 935t
gastroenteritis and, 931
high-dose therapy, 931
in dogs, 931

Methotrexate, *continued*
  in lymphosarcoma, 931
  long-term therapy, 931
  mechanism of action, 930–931
  safety margin, 930
  side effects, 930, 932t
Methoxyflurane, 271
Methscopolamine, 145, 422, 422t
  gastrointestinal motility and, 141, 156, 157
  hyoscine vs, 142
  in emesis, canine, 138
Methyl benzene, 885t
  dichlorophene combined with, 882t
3-methylcholanthrene, 279
Methylene blue, 202t
Methylprednisolone, 128, 451
  indications
    endotoxic shock, 191, 191t
    navicular disease, 463t
4-Methylpyrazole, 208
Methylsulfonylmethane, 129, 495
  in chronic obstructive pulmonary disease, 492t
Methyltestosterone, 1008
  estrogen and, 1008
  ethinyl estradiol and, 1014
  in dogs, 1008
Methylxanthines, 122, 822
Metoclopramide, 137, 138–139
  aldosterone release, 138
  antiemetic activity, 139
  gastrointestinal motility and, 138
  half-life, 139
  intravenous administration, 139
  mechanism of action, 138
  oral dosage, 139
  procainamide vs, 138
  prolactin inhibition, 138
  sedative effect, 138
Metopimazine, 1015
Metoprolol, 830t, 836
Metrifonate, 210
Metritis
  acidosis and, 183
  bovine, 701–703
  contagious equine, 480
  gentamicin in, 246
  postpartum, 1016
  progression to pyometra, 703
  puerperal, 704
  sulfonamide bolus in, 52
Metronidazole
  carcinogenicity, 375, 893
  dosage, small animal, 967t
  for clindamycin-resistant *C. difficile*, 260
  in cats, 964
  indications
    anaerobic infections, 423–424, 964–965
    colic, 424t
    colitis, canine, 146
    cryptosporidiosis, 150
    diarrhea, 950
    endometritis, bacterial, 476
    giardiasis, 892t, 893
    laminitis, 468t
    otitis externa, 851
    stomatitis, 947
  JECFA evaluation, 378t
  side effects, 964
  toxicity, 375
Mexiletine, 835
Mezlocillin, 221, 229
  ticarcillin vs, 221
Mibolerone, 1008
  dosage, 1012
Miconazole
  indications
    dermatophytosis, 847t, 848
    nocardial mastitis, 681
  ketoconazole vs, 130
MICOTIL. *See* Tilmicosin
Microencapsulation, 42–43, 58
Micronucleus test, 331–332
Micturition disorders, 1018
MIDICEL. *See* Sulfamethoxypyridazine
Mifepristone, 1013
Migratory strongylis, 431t, 433
Milbemycin(s), 884
  antinematodal spectrum, 885t
  indications
    hookworm infection, 887t, 888
    in heartworm disease, 913–914, 914t
Miliary dermatitis, 1011
  clinical signs, 1017
  treatment, 1017
Milk production, 632
Millophylline. *See* Etamiphylline
Milrinone, 820, 821t, 830t
Mineral oil, 145, 468t
Minerals, 33
Minocycline, 264
  absorption, 272, 273
  antibacterial activity, 274
  antibacterial spectrum, 795
  distribution, 267, 268, 273
  drug interaction, 274
  lipid solubility, 272, 795, 945
  peak plasma levels, 267
Misalliance, 1012, 1021t
MITABAN. *See* Amitraz
Mitotane, 932t
  chemical relationship to DDT, 933
  in adrenal carcinoma, 933
Mixed bacterial vaccine, 921
MMA syndrome, 291
Molluscacide poisoning, 198
Molybdenum, 202t
Monensin, 609t
  absorption, 610
  anabolic steroids combined with, 623
  as feed additive, 774

as growth promoter, 599t, 610–611
decoquinate vs, 729
drug interactions, 613
in cattle, 610–611
in coccidiosis control, 610, 774t
in cryptosporidiosis, 150
in dogs, 192
in horses, 206
in ovine coccidiosis, 727, 727t
in shock, 192
mechanism of action, 610
ruminal delivery, 49, 611
sustained delivery devices, 47t
toxicity, 613–614
Monobactams, 230, 231
Monoclonal antibodies, 62, 72
against K99 antigens, 162–163
preparation of, 67
specificity of, 66
Monocycline, 131
MONTEBAN. *See* Narasin
Mood-altering drugs, 139–140
Morantel, 47t, 49t
antiparasitic spectrum, 763t
in ruminants, 91t
efficacy, 765t
in cattle, 764t
in parasitic gastroenteritis, 770t
in sheep, 770t
mechanism of action, 82t
pyrantel vs, 104
sustained-release, 84–85
bolus, 48, 104
Morphine, 126
chloroform combined with, 140, 145
naloxone antagonism of, 138
Motility-inhibiting drugs, 156–157
MOTILIUM. *See* Domperidone
Motion sickness, 139
Moxalactam, 234
in salmonellosis, 510
Mullerian inhibitory factor, 68
Mummified fetus, 700
Mustard, 196
Mustine, 927, 932t
Mutagenicity, 289
tests, 329–332, 330t
Mutants, deletion, 74
Mycoplasmal mastitis, 681
Mycotoxins, 198, 214
Myeloid toxicity, 279

N-acetylcysteine, 124
Nadolol, 836
Naficillin, 230
in canine pyoderma, 860, 860t
Nalidixic acid, 154
bacterial resistance, 283
in urinary tract infections, 283, 951
in vitro activity, 282

mechanism of action, 285
Naloxone, 410
in dogs, 193
in hypovolemic shock, 193
mechanism of action, 193
Naltrexone, 193
Nandrolone, 1008
Naphazoline, 144, 155
Naphthyridines, 282
Naproxen, 128, 407
in horses, 527
phenylbutazone vs, 529
Narasin, 609t, 613
Narcotic analgesics, 140–141
Nasal aspergillosis, 130
Nasogastric reflux, 425
Natamycin, 130
Navel ill, 304
Navicular disease, 457–464
isoxsuprine in, 461
NAXCEL. *See* Ceftiofur
N-Butyl chloride
antinematodal spectrum, 885t
in hookworm infection, 887t
Nebulization, in foals, 125, 489
Nematocides, 881
Nematodes, 718–719
Nematodiasis, 85
NEMEX. *See* Pyrantel
Neobiotic-P, 142
Neomycin, 154
antibacterial spectrum, 246
antimicrobial spectrum, 661
apramycin vs, 249
dexamethasone combined with, 852
gastrointestinal absorption, 152
gentamicin combined with, 579
in combined therapy, 247, 661
indications, 247
colic, equine, 424t, 426t
diarrhea, 145
endometritis, bacterial, 476, 478t
in flatulent colic, 423t
metritis, contagious equine, 480
otitis externa, 852
Rhodococcus equi pneumonia, 488
JECFA evaluation, 381
nephrotoxicity, 251
salmonellosis control, 587
toxicity
comparative, 251
in cats, 217t
uterine infusion, 480
Neonatal diarrhea, 147–150. *See also* Calf scour;
 Neonatal scour
Neonatal scour
oral therapy and, 177–178
swine, 578
Neonatal septicemia, 495–503
Neoplasia, mammary, 1008, 1009

Nephritis, 246
Netilmicin
    antibacterial spectrum, 246
    nephrotoxicity, 249
    vs other aminoglycosides, 249
Netobimin, 89t, 90
    antiparasitic spectrum, 762
    efficacy, 765t
    indications
        fascioliasis, 768, 769t
        parasitic gastroenteritis, 770t
    mechanism of action, 82t
Neurodermatitis, 1011
    in cats, 1018
    vincristine and, 931
Neurogenic shock, 186
Neurotoxicity, delayed, 204
Niclofolan
    anthelmintic spectrum, in ruminants, 91t
    antiparasitic spectrum, 763t
    in cattle, 769t
    mechanism of action, 82t
    teratogenicity, 112
    toxicity, 770
Niclosamide
    absorption, gastrointestinal, 114
    anticestodal activity, 891, 891t
    antiparasitic spectrum, 882t
    indications, 431t
        tapeworm infection, 436
    in horses, 436
    mechanism of action, 82t
Nifedipine, 837
Nikethamide, 201t, 211, 551
Nitrate poisoning, 205
Nitrates, 202t
Nitrofuran(s)
    allergy, 343
    carcinogenicity, 373
    mutagenicity, 373
Nitrofurantoin, 956
    in urinary tract infections, 951
Nitrofurazone, 377, 380t, 396
    coccidiostatic activity, 894
    indications
        cryptosporidiosis, 894
Nitroglycerin, 826t, 827, 827t
Nitroimidazole(s), 396, 893
    carcinogenicity, 375
5-nitroimidazoles, 356
Nitroscanate, 114, 882, 882t
    anticestodal activity, 891t
    antinematodal spectrum, 885t
    indications
        ascarid infestation, 885
Nitroxoline, 57
    indications
        urinary tract infections, 951
Nitroxynil, 83, 84, 769t, 769–770
    absorption, 88

antiparasitic spectrum, 763t
    in ruminants, 91t
    liver level, 112
    mechanism of action, 82t
    metabolism, 111
Nocardial mastitis, 681
Nonsteroidal anti-inflammatory drugs
    additivity, 519
    anticoagulants and, 518
    antipyretic effect, 521
    antisecretory activity, 145
    classification, 407, 516t, 516–517
    clearance time, 561–562
    common features, 517, 517t
    cyclic AMP and, 144
    cyclooxygenase inhibition, 190, 147
    distribution, 518
    dosage, in horse, 530t
    gastric ulceration syndrome and, 451
    half-lives, 518
    in calf scour, 151
    in cattle, 128
    in colic, equine, 407
    indications, 528–529, 529t
        COPD, 492t, 494
        degenerative joint disease, 451–452
        endotoxic shock, 190
        laminitis, 466, 466t
        navicular disease, 463t
        placenta, retained, 484
        respiratory tract infections, 801–804
    in feline respiratory disease, 131
    in horses, 451–452, 519
    mechanism of action, 520–522
    parenteral administration, pain upon, 518
    pharmacokinetic, 517–520
    side effects, 522–524, 523t
        neonatal, 523
    toxicity, 522–524
    warfarin interaction with, 461t
Norfloxacin, 282, 283, 284
    adverse effects, 289
    dosage, small animal, 967t
    in dogs, 287
    metabolism, 288
Norgestomet, 55, 56t, 700
Noscapine, 126
Novobiocin, 661
NSAIDs. See Nonsteroidal anti-inflammatory drugs
NUMORPHAN. See Oxymorphone
Nystatin, 478t

Obesity
    congestive heart disease and, 983
    diabetes mellitus and, 983
    diets for, 983–984
    follicle stimulating hormone and, 983
    genetic predisposition to, 983
    heat tolerance and, 983
    hypertension and, 983

hypogonadal, 1007
  in dogs, 983
  locomotion and, 983
  respiratory disorders and, 983
  spaying and, 983
  surgical risk and, 983
Obstructive colic and ileus, 402–403
Ocular infections
  in dogs, 952t, 960
  in horses, 503
Ocular inserts, 58
Ofloxacin, 282, 283
Olaquindox, 377, 381
Oleandomycin, 251, 253
  chemical structure, 252
  cross resistance, 254
  erythromycin vs, 255, 258
Olivanic acids, 223
Omeprazole, 136
OMNIZOLE. *See* Thiabendazole
Oncogenes, 937–938
One-stage prothrombin time, 459
Opiates
  antiemetic activity, 137–138
  antisecretory activity, 155
  mechanism of action, 157
Opioids, 140
  contraindications, 140
Oral cavity infections, in dogs, 953t
Oral medication, 34, 46–47
Organogenesis, 332
Organophosphate(s)
  absorption, skin, 103
  antiparasitic spectrum
    in ruminants, 91t
  bound residues, 103
  contraindications, 102–103
  enzyme inhibition, 347
  intoxication, 210–211
  mechanism of action, 82t
  metabolism, 102
  poisoning, 202t, 204, 217t
  safety margin, 102
  sustained delivery devices, 47t
  teratogenicity, 335, 336
  topical, 83
  toxicity
    in cats, 217t, 866–867
    pralidoxime for, 866
Orgotein
  indications
    degenerative joint disease, 455
    navicular disease, 462–463, 463t
  in horses, 462–463
  warfarin and, 461t
Ormethoprim
  half-time, 301
  sulfadimethoxine combined with, 302
    in bovine respiratory disease, 793
    in canine pyoderma, 860t

  in coccidiosis, 894
Osmolarity, 168
Osmotic pumps, 44–45, 49
  ivermectin in, 85
Osteoarthritis, 525
Osteomyelitis
  causative organisms, 958
  characteristics of, 962–963
  clindamycin in, 258
  in horses, 455–457
  kanamycin in, 247
  septicemia and, 503
Osteosarcoma, 920
  Bacillus, Calmette-Guerin vaccine in, 920
  doxorubicin and dacarbazine in, 933
  in dogs, 932
Ostertagia ostertagi, 760–761
Ostertagiasis, bovine, 760–765
Otitis externa, 848–854, 953t
Ouabain, 820
Ovarian cysts, 699
Ovarian hormone control, 691
Ovariectomy, 1006, 1016
  alopecia following, 1017
Ovariohysterectomy
  for canine pyometra, 1016
  in cats, 1005
  mammary neoplasia and, 933
Overgrooming, in cats, 1005
Ovulation, 1022
Oxacillin, 860, 860t
  cloxacillin vs, 230
  indications
    septicemia, in foals, 498
    Staphylococcus aureus infection, 230
Oxalate crystals, 213
Oxazepam, 147, 998
Oxazolidinediones, 993, 1000
Oxfendazole, 443t
  absorption, 86, 88
  adverse effects, 442t
  anthelmintic efficacy, 94
  antinematodal spectrum, 885t
  antiparasitic spectrum, 882t
    in cattle, 762
    in horses, 432t
    in ruminants, 89t, 91t, 763t
  bolus, ruminal, 48
  dosage, 432t, 433t, 434
  efficacy, 765t
  fenbendazole vs, 94
  formulations, 432t
  for small animals, 882t
  in cattle, 335, 762
  indications, 431t
    hookworm infestation, 887t
    lungworm infection, 894
    ostertagiasis, 92, 763
    parasitic gastroenteritis, 770t
    tapeworm infection, 762

Oxfendazole, *continued*
  verminous arteritis, 415
 in horses, 432t
 in sheep, 335, 770t
 JECFA evaluation, 377, 379t
 mechanism of action, 82t
 milk level, 97
 parasiticidal spectrum, 432t
 pharmacokinetics, 94
 pulsed-release bolus, 85
 residues, 96
 resistance, 438
 ruminal delivery, 48
 safety margins, 95
 solubility, 94
 sustained delivery devices, 47t
 sustained-release, 49t
 teratogenicity, 96, 335, 336
 trichlorfon combined with, 443t
Oxibendazole
 antiparasitic spectrum, 763t
 diethylcarbamazine combined with, 887t, 888, 912
 dosage, 432t
 efficacy, 765t
 formulations, 432t
 in cattle, 762
 indications, 431t
   parasitic gastroenteritis, 770t
   prophylactic, 440
   Strongyloides westeri infection, 436
 in foals, 511
 in sheep, 770t
 mechanism of action, 82t
 oxyclozanide combined with, 772
 parasiticidal spectrum, 432t
 prophylactic use, 888
 safety, 336, 442t
 teratogenicity and, 336
Oxicams, 526
Oximes, 204
Oxolinic acid, 282, 285, 381
Oxphenbutazone, 128
Oxyclozanide
 anthelmintic spectrum, 91t
 antiparasitic spectrum, 763t
 flukicidal activity, 769t, 770
 in cattle, 769t, 770
 levamisole combined with, 772
 mechanism of action, 82t
 oxibendazole combined with, 772
 protein binding, 87, 88
Oxygen therapy, 495, 807–808
Oxymetazoline, 144, 155
Oxymorphone, 412t
Oxyphenbutazone
 in racing horses, 552
 phenylbutazone vs, 524
 plasma protein binding, 385
 potency, 519
Oxyphenonium bromide, 141

Oxytetracycline
 antibacterial spectrum, 265
 as growth promoter, 599t
 bacterial resistance to, 794
 bromhexine combined with, 125
 depot formulation, 7, 269
 distribution, 267, 706
 dosage, 265, 576, 578
 dosage, small animal, 967t
 feed medication, 793
 flunixin combined with, 802
 formulations, 268, 269, 794, 795
 half-life, 265
 in cattle, 265
 indications
   colibacillosis, 579
   endometritis, 704
   haemobartonellosis, 895, 896t
   in Chlamydia infection, 131
   pleuropneumonia, swine, 576, 577
   respiratory disease, 790t, 793
   salmonellosis, 587
   swine dysentery, 582
 in horses, 269–270
 intrauterine administration, 706
 JECFA evaluation, 377, 379t
 lipid solubility, 706
 long-acting, 571, 576, 794, 795
 oral, 267
 parenteral, 267
 parenteral administration, 575
 Pasteurella resistance to, 794
 peak plasma levels, 267
 penicillin vs, 704
 plasma protein binding, 267
 polyvinylpyrrolidone base, 794
 residues, 591
 terramycin combined with, 795
 toxicity, 270
 toxicity, in cats, 217t
 tumorigenicity, 377
 tylosin combined with, 796
 uterine absorption, 704, 706
 warfarin interaction with, 461t
 water medication, 793
Oxytocin
 dystocia and, 1013
 estrogen and, 1013
 half-life, 1013
 inactivation, 706
 indications, 1013
   parturition induction, 482–483
   retained placenta, 714
 in endometritis, bacterial, 474t, 479t, 702, 702t
 in mastitis, 661
 intramuscular, 702
 retained placenta and, 702, 706
 spasmogenic effect, 1013
 tetanus uteri, 707
Oxyuris equi infection, 435

Pain, 202t
PANACUR. *See* Fenbendazole
Pancreatic exocrine insufficiency, 146
Pancreatic insufficiency, 987
987P antigens, 69
Papillomas, skin, 920
Paracetamol, 217t
Paracetamol poisoning, 209
Paraffins, 39
Paraquat, 205, 217t
Parascaris equorum infection, 434–435
Parasite control program, 433, 439–441
Parasitic bronchitis, 765–767
Parasitic gastroenteritis, 770–771
Parasiticides, 33
  equine use, 431t
  poisoning, 198
  teratogenicity, 335
Parasitic infection
  diarrhea and, 511
  in foals, 511
  patterns of, 880t
Parasympatholytics, 122
PARATECT. *See* Morantel
Parathion, 210
Parbendazole
  antiparasitic spectrum, 89t
    in ruminants, 91t, 763t
  dosage, 92
  indications
    parasitic gastroenteritis, 770t
  in sheep, 335, 770t
  mechanism of action, 82t
  pharmacokinetics, 97
  teratogenicity, 335, 336
Parturition
  corticosteroid-induced, 690–693
  induction of
    disadvantages, 694t
    in cats, 1012–1014
    in cattle, 690–698
    indications for, 693–694, 694t
    in dogs, 1012–1014
    in horses, 480–483
  physiology of, 691–692
  postponement of, 700–701
  prostaglandins and, 1014
Parvovirus, 74
Pasteurella hemolytica, 784t
Pasteurellosis, 808–809
  danofloxacin in, 800
PAYLEAN. *See* Ractopamine
Pectin, 143, 154
Penicillamine
  in arsenic poisoning, 202t
  in copper poisoning, 203
  in lead poisoning, 211
Penicillin G, 225
  aminoglycosides combined with, 498
  antibacterial activity, 226

  dosage, 238t
  erythromycin combined with, 259
  half-life, 225
  in cattle, 238t
  indications
    colic, 424t
    endometritis, bacterial, 474t
    respiratory disease, 790t
    respiratory infections, in foals, 505t
    septic arthritis, 458t
    septicemia, in foals, 498
    Streptococcus equi infection, 490
  in foals, 496t
  in horses, 238t
  kanamycin combined with, 247
  repository preparations, 225
Penicillin(s)
  absorption, 476
  allergy, 343, 346
  aminoglycosides combined with, 480
  amoxicillin vs, 228
  boluses, 47t
  broad-spectrum, 236t
  classes of, 236t
  elimination, 225
  extended spectrum, 226–228
  fourth generation, 229
  gentamicin combined with, 246
  high doses, 226
  in anaerobic infections, 963
  indications
    bovine mastitis, 661
    bovine respiratory disease, 791–792
    endometritis, 704
    endometritis, bacterial, 476, 477, 478t
    foot rot, 731
    placenta, retained, 484
    pleuropneumonia, swine, 576
    uterine infection, 706
  in feed medication, 568
  in flatulent colic, 423
  manufacture of, 62
  natural, 224–226, 236t
  novobiocin combined with, 661
  oxytetracycline vs, 704
  penicillinase-resistant, 236t
  residues, 367
  sensitization, 338
  Staphylococcus aureus resistance to, 942
  streptomycin combined with, 246, 793
  structure, 222
  tissue levels, 226
  urine concentrations, 225
  uterine absorption, 704
Penicillin V, 225
Penicillium, 216t
Pentazocine
  butorphanol vs, 126
  in equine colic, 409, 409t, 410, 412t, 426t
  in poisoning, 202, 202t

Pentobarbital
chloramphenicol interaction with, 279, 347
in foals, 502, 502t
in poisoning, 201, 201t, 202t, 211–212
Pentobarbitone, 201t
Pentylene tetrazol, 201t
Perianal adenoma, 933
Periodontal disease, 258, 948
Peritonitis, 403
in foals, 508
in horses, 488
Permethrin
insecticidal activity, 868
sustained-release formulations, 55, 57t
Pesticides, 55. *See also* specific agents
Pethidine
in equine colic, 426t
in poisoning, 202, 202t
poisoning
heavy metal, 212
Pharyngitis, 183
Phenamidine isethionate, 895, 896t
Phenobarbital
absorption, 996
blood levels, 995
corticosteroids and, 996
digitoxin and, 996
dosage, 994, 999t
doxycycline and, 996
enzyme induction, 347
griseofulvin and, 996
half life, 996
in cats, 996, 999t
in foals, 502, 502t
onset of action, 996
overdose, 211–212
phenylbutazone and, 996
phenytoin interaction with, 998
primidone vs, 996
side effects, 994, 995, 999t
toxicity, 996
tricyclic antidepressants and, 996
tumorigenicity, 347
valproic acid combined with, 1000
Phenols, 217t
substituted, 82t, 110–113
Phenothiazine(s), 155, 205
antiemetic activity, 137
contraindications, 137
indications
prophylactic, 137
JECFA evaluation, 377
mechanism of action, 137
Phenoxybenzamine
in laminitis, 466t, 467, 468t
Phenoxymethyl penicillin, 225
Phenylbutazone
absorption, 524
antisecretory activity, 155
bioavailability, 518

chemical structure, 524
cyclo-oxygenase inhibition by, 521
dosage, 412t, 426t
formulations, 524
toxicity and, 523
griseofulvin interaction with, 847
half-life, 519, 524
indications, 524
colibacillosis, enteric, 156
degenerative joint disease, 451
equine colic, 412t, 413, 426t
laminitis, 446t, 466, 468t, 525
navicular disease, 463t
osteoarthritis, 525
pneumonia, 489
septic arthritis, 458t
strangles, 490
in dogs, 525
in gastrointestinal disease, 151
in horses, 451, 522, 525
in poisoning, 202
in racing horses, 548, 552
in respiratory system disorders, 128
intravenous preparations, 518
isopyrin interaction with, 518
ketoprofen vs, 528
mechanism of action, 407, 521
metabolism, 519
naproxen vs, 529
oxyphenbutazone vs, 524
plasma protein binding, 385
residues, 526
safety margin, 525
sulfonamide interaction with, 518
toxicity, 413, 522
formulation and, 523
in cats, 217t
warfarin interaction with, 461t, 518
Phenylephrine, 126, 1018
Phenylpropanolamine, 126, 1018
PHENYLZONE. *See* Phenylbutazone
Phenytoin, 992t
absorption, 998
chloramphenical interaction with, 998
dexamethasone interaction with, 998
digitoxin interaction with, 998
dosage, 999t
drug interactions, 998
elimination of, 994
enzyme induction, 347
folic acid deficiency and, 998
formulations, 997–998
half life, 997
hepatotoxicity, 997
in cats, 999t
in foals, 502t
mechanism of action, 997
phenobarbital interaction with, 998
serum concentration, 998
side effects, 994, 999t

toxicity, 997
Pholcodine, 126
Phosmet, 210
Phospholipids, 44
Phosphorus, 51, 212
Phoxim, 844
Phthalofyne, 885t
  contraindications, 888
  in whipworm infestation, 888
  side effects, 888
Phthalylsulfacetamide, 145
Phthalylsulfathiazole, 297
Phytomenadione, 210
Picrotoxin, 201t
Pigs, 248, 286. *See also* Swine
  arthritis in, 588
  atrophic rhinitis in, 570–573
  beta adrenergic agents in, 645–646
  beta agonists in, 645–646
  colibacillosis in, 248, 578–580
  feed additives in, 605
  in salmonellosis, 586–588
  medication of, 567–569
  pneumonia in, 304
  polyserositis in, 588
  rhinitis in, atrophic, 570–573
  scours in, 304
  therapy
    carbadox, 649
    cimaterol, 643, 644
    enrofloxacin, 290, 291, 575
    gentamicin, 246, 247
    ractopamine, 645–646
    sulfonamide, 304
Pig vaccines, 74–76
Pinworms, 430, 431t, 432t, 435
Pipenzolate, 141
Piperacillin, 221, 229
  ticarcillin vs, 221
Piperazine, 91t
  antinematodal spectrum, 885t
  antiparasitic spectrum, 882t
  ataxia and, 885
  dosage, 432t
  formulations, 432t
  in ascarid infection, 884, 885
  in kittens, 885
  levamisole combined with, 432t
  mebendazole combined with, 439
  mechanism of action, 82t, 113
  parasiticidal spectrum, 432t
  safety margin, 443t
  thenium combined with, 882t
  toxicity, 884
Piperonyl butoxide, 347
Piroxicam, 128, 526
Pival, 207
Pivampicillin, 228
Placenta, retention, 484
Placental transfer, 333

PLANIPART. *See* Clenbuterol
Plant poisons, 198, 212–214
Plasma expanders, 177
Pleuropneumonia, in swine, 576–578
Pneumonia, 306
  bacterial
    in foals, 503–506
  enrofloxacin in, 291
  gentamicin in, 246
  in foals, 487–489
  in pigs, 304
  in swine, 573–576, 576–578
  kanamycin in, 247
  sulfonamide bolus in, 52
Podophyllotoxin, 99
Podotrochlitis. *See* Navicular disease
Poisoning
  acidosis in, 202, 202t
  advanced management, 196t
  alkalosis in, 202t
  alpha chloralose, 207, 217t
  anticoagulant, 202t
  antidotes, 197–199, 202t
    guidelines for, 198–199
  antifreeze, 202t
  apnea in, 200
  arsenic, 202t, 205
  aspirin, 208–209, 217t
  barbiturate, 202t, 211–212, 217t
  bracken, 202t
  carbamate, 217t
  chlorate, 202t
  chlorinated hydrocarbon, 217t
  CNS effects, 217t
  copper, 202t, 206–207
  delayed neurotoxicity, 204
  digitalis, 202t
  early management, 196t
  ethylene glycol, 207–208, 217t
  fluoroacetate, 217t
  herbicide, 205–206
  hyperthermia in, 200
  hypovolemia in, 200
  ivermectin, 208
  large animal, 203–207
  lead, 202t, 205, 217t
  metaldehyde, 217t
  nitrate, 202t, 205
  organophosphate, 202t, 204, 217t
  phenol, 217t
  respiratory distress in, 200
  rotenone, 217t
  sedative, 217t
  shock in, 202, 202t
  small animal, 207–211
  strychnine, 202t, 208, 217t
  supportive therapy, 200–203
  treatment, 195, 200–203
  urea, 203–204
  weed killer, 217t

Polioencephalomalacia, 727
Polyacrylamide, 37
Polyactic acid, 35t, 39
Polyamide, 35t
Polyarthritis, 304
Polyclonal antibodies, 72
Polyester, 35t
Polyether, 35t
Polyether antibiotics, 607
   toxicity, 613–615
Polyethylene, 35t
Polymer matrix
   design of, 35
   desirable properties, 35, 36t
   drug release from, 36–39, 46
      factors affecting, 37–39, 38t
      filler materials and, 39
      kinetics of, 38
   hydrophilic, drug release from, 37
   laminated type, 37
   manufacture of, 35
   monolithic, 37, 41, 41t
Polymer(s). *See also* Polymer matrix
   biodegradable, 35, 39, 39t, 46
   creation of, 35t
   natural, 35
   nonbiodegradable, 39–40, 40t
   porosity of,, 37
   structure of, 35
   synthetic, 35
   types of, 35, 35t
Polymixin B, 154, 478t
   in metritis, contagious equine, 480
   in otitis externa, 851
   uterine infusion, 480
Polyorthoesters, 39
Polypropylene, 35t
Polyserositis, 588
Polysulfated glycosaminoglycan
   indications
      degenerative joint disease, 452–453
      septic arthritis, 458t
Polyvinylacetate, 35t
Polyvinylalcohol, 37
Polyvinylchloride, 35t
Polyvinyl chloride tags, 55
Polyvinylpyrrolidone, 37, 268, 269, 794
Pony, 518
Porcine somatotropin, 377, 638–639
Postpartum therapy
   in cattle, 701–711
Potassium chloride, 468t
Potassium penicillin G, 424t
Potomac horse fever, 509
Poultry, 257, 286, 306, 309
   cimaterol in, 643, 644
   enrofloxacin in, 290
   feed additives in, 605
Poultry meat, 372
Povidone iodine, 476t, 848

Pralidoxime, 202t, 866
Praziquantel, 881
   anticestodal activity, 891t
   antiparasitic effects, 113
   antiparasitic spectrum, 882t
   febantel combined with, 882t, 887t
   in cestode parasites, 113
   mechanism of action, 892
   pyrantel and febantel combined with, 882t
Prazosin, 826t, 827t, 828
Precipitants, 197
Prednisolone
   cyclophosphamide and, with vincristine, 935
   cyclotoxic effect, 933
   dosages, 541t
   indications
      chronic obstructive pulmonary disease, 492t
      endotoxic shock, 191, 191t
      haemobartonellosis, 895
      retained placenta, 714
   sulfasalazine combined with, 950
Prednisone
   cytotoxic effect, 933
   dosage rate, 935t
PRESCRIPTION DIET, 146
Primidone
   dosage, 994, 996, 999t
   folic acid deficiency and, 997
   hepatic enzyme induction and, 996
   high dose, 997
   in foals, 502, 502t
   metabolism, 992t, 996
   phenobarbital vs, 996
   side effects, 994, 996, 999t
   toxicity, in cats, 217t
PRIMOR. *See* Sulfadimethoxine, ormethoprim
      combined with
Probenzimidazoles, 85
   antiparasitic spectrum, 89t
      in ruminants, 91t
   in ruminants, 765t, 770t
   mechanism of action, 82t
Probiotics, 156, 646–648
Procainamide, 138, 210, 830t
   bolus administration, 834
   dosage, 834
   half-life, 834
   oral administration, 834
   sustained release, 834
   toxic effects, 834
Procaine penicillin, 225, 424t
   dihydrostreptomycin combined with, 461t
   indications
      endometritis, bacterial, 477
      laminitis, 467, 468t
      respiratory disease, 790t
Procaine salts, 58
Prochlorperazine, 137, 142
PROFTRIL. *See* Albendazole
Progestagen, tumorigenicity, 1018

Progesterone, 33, 47t
  endometrial proliferation and, 1016
  estradiol benzoate combined with, 56t, 599t, 619, 629
  indications
    parturition induction, 481
  in female dogs, 1010
  long term therapy, 1009
Progesterone releasing intravaginal device, 700
Progestins. *See also* specific agents
  acromegaly and, 1009
  antiandrogenic effects, 1003
  carcinogenicity, 1009
  CNS effects, 1003
  diabetic-type syndrome and, 1009
  follicle-stimulating hormone suppression, 1003
  in cats, 1010
  indications
    mammary neoplasia, 1008
    prostatic hypertrophy, 1008
  luteinizing hormone suppression, 1003
  mechanism of action, 1009, 1010
  side effects, 1009, 1010
Progestogens
  endometritis and, 1016
  indications
    miliary dermatitis, 1017
Prolactin, 138
Proligestone, 1010, 1012, 1014
  advantages of, 1012
  duration of action, 1012
  efficacy, 1012
  in lactation suppression, 1015
  medroxyprogesterone acetate vs, 1012
Promazine, 137, 377
Pronidazole, premixes, 582
Propantheline, 137, 141, 146
Propantheline bromide, 142
Propoxur, 207
Propranolol, 202t, 828, 830t
  antiarrhythmic activity, 835
  half-life, 836
  in cats, 835
  in dogs, 835
Proquamezine, 421, 422t
Prostaglandin(s), 127, 189
  abortion and, 1013
  absorption, 697, 698
  analogs, 697, 699
  calf scour and, 151t
  endotoxic shock, 189
  half-life, 696
  in cattle, 697
  indications
    abortion induction, 483–484
    anestrus, 697
    endometritis, 701–702
    endometritis, bacterial, 474t
    estrus control, 699
    parturition induction, 481–482, 698

    pyometra, 698–699, 1016
    subestrus, 697
  in dogs, 1014
  luteolytic activity, 696t, 697
  luteolytic effect, 1014
  parturition and, 1014
  pyometra and, 1013
  side effects, 697, 1006, 1013
  skin absorption, 697
  smooth muscle activity and, 698
  synthesis, 144
Prostatic hyperplasia, 1008
Prostatic hypertrophy, 1008
  treatment for, 1009
Prostatitis, 957
Protectives, 136, 143
Protein/phosphate restriction, 984
Proteoglycans, 448
Prothrombin time, one-stage, 459
PROTROPIN (human growth hormone), 68
Pruritus, 873
Pseudoephedrine, 125
Pseudomembranous colitis, drug-induced, 949
Pseudopregnancy, 1003, 1011, 1014
Pseudorabies, 74
Pulmonary edema, 808, 809
Pulmonary hemorrhage, 563
Pulmonary hypertension, 899–900
Pulmonary thromboembolism, 906
Pulsed-release systems, 33, 51–52
  oxfendazole in, 48
  principles of, 52t
  somatotropin-bovine growth hormone in, 58
Purgatives, 144
Pybuthrin, 868
Pyelonephritis, 247, 957
Pyoderma, 841
  antimicrobial therapy for, 859–862
  benzoyl peroxide shampoos for, 862
  canine, 856
  deep, 965
  nasal, 863
  skin fold, 863
  superficial, 965
  treatment of, 857–859
  types of, 856–857
Pyodermatitis, 246
Pyometra
  in cattle, 698–699, 711–712
  in dogs, 1016
  prostaglandin and, 1013
Pyometra syndrome, 1016
Pyrantel, 881, 883
  adverse effects, 442t
  antinematodal spectrum, 885t
  antiparasitic spectrum, 882t, 883
  dosage, 432t
  epsiprantel combined with, 882t
  formulations, 432t, 888
  indications, 431t

Pyrantel, *continued*
  hookworm infection, 887t
    tapeworm infection, 430, 436
  mechanism of action, 82t, 892
  metabolism, 104
  morantel vs, 104
  parasiticidal spectrum, 432t
  warfarin and, 461t
Pyrethrin, 866
Pyrethroids, 47t, 55
Pyridimines, 82t
Pyrimethamine, 300, 306
  in toxoplasmosis, 893
  sulfadiazine combined with, 893
Pyrimidines, 765t
Pyrvinium, 889

Quinacrine, 150
  in giardiasis, 892, 892t
Quindoxin, 616
Quinidine, 210, 830t
  antiarrhythmic activity, 833
  dosage, 834
  duration of action, 834
  in cats, 833
  in dogs, 833
  oral, 833
  side effect, 833
  toxicity, 834
Quinolones
  antibacterial spectrum, 284
  efficacy of action, 285
  mechanism of action, 284–286, 285
  pharmacokinetics, 286–288
  therapeutic indications, 289–291
  toxicity, 288–289

Rabbits, 304
Ractopamine, 377, 645–646
Radiation, neoplasia and, 920
Radiation therapy, 920, 921
  as adjunct therapy, 921
  low dose, 935
  rationale of, 921
Rafoxanide, 82t, 83, 88, 110, 112, 381, 769t, 770
  antiparasitic spectrum, 763t
    in ruminants, 91t
  fasciolicidal effect, 87
  thiabendazole combined with, 772
Ragwort, 213–214
RALGRO, 55, 56t. *See also* Zeranol
  as growth promoter, 599t
Ranitidine, 135, 457
  cimetidine vs, 510
  in cats, 135
  omeprazole vs, 136
Recombinant DNA, 62
Recombinant technology, 63, 66
Redworms, 430. *See also* Strongylus infection
Relay bioavailability, 351

Relay toxicity, 349
Renal failure, chronic, 984–985
Repartitioning agents, 641
Reproductive therapy, drugs for, 1020t
Reproductive toxicity, 336
Reservoir matrix systems, 41–42, 42t
Residues, 277, 281, 317
  anabolic agents, 627
  anabolic steroids, 627
  antimicrobial agents, 337–338, 366, 367
  beta adrenergic agents, 644
  clenbuterol, 645
  covalently bound, 349–351
  depletion studies, 349
  estradiol, 628
  formation, 317–318, 590–591
  in food, 356
  in milk, 366, 367
  in poultry meat, 372
  melengestrol acetate, 630
  monitoring, 24–26
  of antimicrobial agents, 591–592
  radiotracer tissue studies, 348–349
  sulfonamide, 578, 592–595
  swine production and, 588–592
  tolerances, 26–29
    guidelines for establishing, 29–30
  trenbolone, 625
  zeranol, 630
Resin collars, 55
Respiratory acidosis, 170–171
Respiratory disorders, obesity and, 983
Respiratory distress, 200
Respiratory stimulants, 201t
Respiratory tract diseases, 73
  in cattle, 258, 261
Respiratory tract infections, 226, 233, 246, 247, 291
  antimicrobial agents in, 944–946
  in cattle. *See* Bovine respiratory tract infections
  in dogs, 946, 952t
  in foals, 504–505
  lower, 945
  small animal, 130, 946, 952t
  sulfonamides in, 304
Restriction endonucleases, 64, 65
Retained fetal membranes. *See* Retained placenta
Retained placenta, 484, 702, 712–715
  in dogs, 1017
  selenium deficiency and, 710, 714
  uterine prolapse and, 714
  vitamin deficiency and, 714
Reversible anemic syndrome, 279
R factor, 245
R factor transfer, 254
Rhinitis, 304
  control and prophylaxis of, 572–573
  in pigs, 570–573
Rhodococcus equi infection, 259
  pneumonia, 487–489
RIFADIN. *See* Rifampin

Rifampicin, 665
Rifampin
    antibacterial activity, comparative, 488
    bacterial resistance, 488
    enzyme induction, 488
    erythromycin combined with, 488
    erythromycin synergy, 488
    indications
        listeriosis, 487
        liver abscesses, 487
        lung abscesses, 487
        lymphadenitis, 487
        Neisseria meningitidis infection, 488
        peritonitis, 488
        Rhodococcus equi pneumonia, 487–488
        septic arthritis, 458t, 488
        umbilical infections, 487
    in foals, 496t
    side effects, 487
    solubility, 487
Ringer's lactate solution, 217t
Ringworm, 846–848
RINTAL. *See* Febantel
RIPERCOL PIPERAZINE. *See* Levamisole, piperazine
        combined with
RNA, 63
ROBAXIN. *See* Methocarbamol
Rodenticide, 210
    poisoning, 198
Rolitetracycline, 264
ROMPUN. *See* Xylazine
Rondazole
    swine dysentery control, 584t
Ronidazole, 375
    feed medication, 587t
    JECFA evaluation, 378t, 381
    premixes, 582
    water medication, 586t
Ronnel, 210
Rosamicin, 252, 256, 258
Rotaviruses, 149–150
Rotenone, 217t, 842, 866
Rottweilers, 920
Roundworms, 431t, 432t, 434–435, 883–886
Rumen, 84
Rumen acidosis, 203
Rumen delivery systems, 46
Rumenotomy, 214
Rumen overload, 198
RUMENSIN. *See* Monensin
RUMENSIN RDD (monensin), 49
Ruminal glass bullets, 741
Ruminants, 46, 47–48
    anthelmintics in, 91t, 763t
    baquiloprim and sulfamethazine in, 302
    trimethoprim in, 301

SAFEGUARD. *See* Fenbendazole
Safety of veterinary drugs, 317
Saint Bernards, 920

Salbutamol, 120
    excretion, 644
Salicylanilides, 81, 82t
    efficacy, 111
    fasciolicidal effect, 87, 111
    plasma levels, 112
    plasma protein binding, 87
    toxicity, 112
Salicylates, 156
    in horses, 526–527
Salicylazosulfapyridine, 297
Salicylic acid
    in racing horses, 552
Salinomycin, 583
    as growth promoter, 612
    dosage, 612
    mechanism of action, 612
    metabolism, 612
    potassium and, 612
    prophylactic use, 585
    propionic acid and, 612
    synthesis, 609t
    tiamulin interaction with, 613
    toxicity, 614
Salmonellosis
    abortions and, 149
    antibiotics in, oral, 153
    apramycin in, 246, 248, 587
    cephalothin in, liposomal-associated, 44
    enrofloxacin in, 291
    equine colic and, 403
    in horses, 509–510
    in pigs, 586–588
    tests for, 73
    water medication for, 568
Sarcoptic mange, 843–845
Scabies, 843–845
S-carboxymethylcysteine, 124
Scopolamine
    gastrointestinal motility and, 145
    indications, 142
    in equine colic, 422
Scours, 304
    calf. *See* Calf scour
    in lambs, 718–720
Sebacil, 210
Seborrhea, 863, 873–875
Sedatives, 414
    in doping, 562
    in foals, 502
    in racing horses, 562
Selenium, 746–752
    bolus therapy, 51, 751–752
    glass boluses, 51
    injectable preparations, 749–751
    interaction with other elements, 746
    longterm delivery, 45
    oral, 751
    oxidant-induced muscle damage and, 746
    sustained-release, 47t

Selenium, *continued*
   toxicity, 752
Selenium deficiency, 50
   diagnosis, 748–749
   retained placenta and, 710, 714
   symptoms, 747–748
   treatment and prevention, 749–752
Semduracin, 607
Senna, 144
Sepsis, 251, 952t
Septic arthritis, 456–457
   septicemia and, 503
Septicemia
   antimicrobial therapy in, 496t, 497–499, 508–509
   bacteria commonly associated with, 496
   central nervous disorders in, 501–503
   convulsions in, 502
   fluid therapy in, 500, 500t
   gram negative, 508
     therapy for, 498t
   in foals, 495–503
   meningitis in, 502
   sedatives in, 502
   septic arthritis and, 503
   sulfonamide bolus in, 52
   supportive therapy in, 500–501
Septic shock, 186
Sesamoiditis, distal. *See* Navicular disease
Sex hormones, 316
Sex steroids, 627–628
   endogenous, 627–628
   synthetic, 628–629
Shampoos
   antibacterial, 862
   antiseborrheic, 874
Sheep
   cobalt deficiency in, 720
   coccidiosis in, 304, 719
   colibacillosis in, 719
   copper deficiency in, 719–720
   copper poisoning in, 206
   enteritis in, 304
   foot abscess in, 304
   foot rot in, 730–731
   intravaginal reproductive hormones in, 55
   listeriosis in, 488
   liver fluke in, 771–772
   lymphadenitis, 487
   nematodes in, 718–719
   parasitic gastroenteritis, 770–771
   perinatal mortality, 718
   therapy
     albendazole, 335, 770t
     closantel, 112
     febantel, 770t
     fenbendazole, 770t
     ivermectin, 106–107, 108, 770t
     levamisole, 770t
     luxabendazole, 770t
     mebendazole, 770t
     morantel, 770t
     netobimin, 770t
     oxfendazole, 335, 770t
     oxibendazole, 770t
     parbendazole, 335, 770t
     sulfonamide, 304
     tetracycline, 54
     thiabendazole, 770t
     thiophanate, 770t
   toxoplasmosis in, 728–730
Shellac, 35t, 39
Shipping fever, 246, 282
   in cattle, 808–809
   sulfonamide bolus in, 52
Shock
   endotoxic, 188–189
   fluid therapy in, 185–188
   in colic, 416–419, 417t
   in horses, 535–537
   poisoning and, 202, 202t
   surgical, 186
   thermal, 186
   treatment for, 187, 190–193
   types of, 185–186
Silicone rubber, 35t, 40, 54
   implant, 55
Sinusitis, 247
Sisomicin, 249
Skin infections
   beta lactams in, 226
   cephalexin in, 233
   cephalosporins in, 235
   in dogs, 235, 952t
   in small animals, 952t, 965–968
   sulfonamides in, 304
Skin tumors, 937
Small strongylus infection, 435
Sodium ampicillin, 227
Sodium arsanilate
   feed medication, 587t
   water medication, 586t
Sodium bicarbonate
   in acidosis, 177
   in doping, 563
   in race horses, 563
Sodium borate, 888
Sodium chloride
   as dietary supplement, in laminitis, 468t
   in emetic solutions, 196
   in uterine irrigation, 476t
Sodium cromoglycate
   in prophylactic, 492
   mechanism of action, 492
Sodium sulfate, 209
Sodium thiosulfate, 202t, 212
Sodium valproate, 1000
Somatic cell count monitoring, 685–686
Somatostatin, 633
   immunization against, 648
Somatotropin, 633–634

Somatotropin-bovine growth hormone. *See* Bovine somatotropin
Sorbitol, 198
SPANBOLET II. *See* Sulfamethazine
Sparteine, 551
Spasmodic colic, 143, 402, 414
Spasmolytic agents, 142–143, 421–422
Spectinomycin, 154, 247–248
  absorption, 247
  antibacterial spectrum, 248
  chloramphenicol combined with, 259
  feed medication, 587t
  indications
    colibacillosis, 579, 721
    endometritis, bacterial, 478t
    salmonellosis, 587
    swine dysentery, 582
  in lambs, 721
  in salmonellosis control, 587
  intramuscular, 247
  JECFA evaluation, 381
  lincomycin combined with
    in bovine respiratory infection, 258, 797
    in-feed medication, 587t
    in foot rot, 731
    in mycoplasmal infections, 258
    in swine dysentery, 248
    in swine dysentery control, 578
    in swine pleuropneumonia, 578
    water medication, 586t
  metabolism, 247
  oral, 721
  parenteral administration, 575
  preparations, 257
  resistance, 248
  toxiciity, 248
  water medication, 586t
Spermatogenesis, 1003, 1007
Spiramycin
  antibacterial activity, 255
  as feed additive, 796
  dosage, 797
  indications
    bovine respiratory tract infections, 797
    cryptosporidiosis, 777, 894
    respiratory disease, 790t
    swine dysentery, 582
  in-feed medication, 587t
  JECFA evaluation, 377, 379t
  milk level, 256
  prophylatic use, 797
  tissue levels, 255
Spironolactone, 826t, 827t
SPUTOLYSIN. *See* Dembrixine
Stagnant loop syndrome, 946
Stanozolol, 823, 1008
Staphylococcal resistance, 660
Staphylococcus aureus
  antimicrobial resistance, 942
Starch, 35t, 39

Status epilepticus
  diazepam in, 998
  therapy for, 1000t
Steatorrhea, 986
STEER-OID (progesterone/estradiol benzoate), 56t
Steroids, 190–191. *See also* Corticosteroid(s)
  adverse reactions, 540t
  anabolic, 1008
  anticonvulsant sedative activity, 1003
  contraindications, 541t, 1017
  indications, 540t
  natural, 618–619
  synthetic, 625–627
  types of, 694–696
Stilbenes, 618
  gut absorption, 1006
STOCKGUARD insecticide ear tag (flucythrinate), 57t
Stomach worms, 84
Stomatitis
  clinical signs, 948
  in dogs, 948–949
  mycotic, 947
  ulcerative, 947
Strangles, 304, 489–490
Streptococcus equi infection, 489–490
Streptococcus pyogens, 54
Streptomycin, 154
  antibacterial spectrum, 246
  apramycin vs, 249
  bacterial resistance, 246
  indications, 246
    diarrhea, 145
    foot rot, 731
    shipping fever, 246
    wound infections, 246
  JECFA evaluation, 381
  liposomal-associated, 44
  penicillin combined with, 246, 793
  pharmacokinetics, 246
  postoperative, 246
  resistance, 246
    ribosomal, 244
  toxicity, in cats, 217t
STRONGID. *See* Pyrantel
Strongylus infection
  control program, 433
  in foals, 436
  large, 430–434
    clinical symptoms, 431
    treatment, 431t
  small, 431t, 432t, 435
Strychnine poisoning, 202t, 208, 217t
Strylpyridinium, 884
  antinematodal spectrum, 885t
  diethylcarbamazine
    combined with, 887t, 888
  prophylactic use, 888
Subestrus, 697
Substituted phenols, 82t, 91t
Succinimides, 993

Sucralfate, 136, 457
  indications
    gastric ulceration, 511
    septic arthritis, 458t
Sulbactam
  ampicillin combined with, 224, 793
  antibacterial spectrum, 224
  clavulanic acid vs, 224
  mechanism of action, 222–223
Sulfabromomethazine, 303t
Sulfacetamide, 297
Sulfachlorpyridazine, 154
  in calves, 303t
  in swine, 303t
  maintenance therapy, 304t
Sulfadiazine
  CNS penetration, 959
  duration of action, 302
  in cattle, 303t
  in dogs, 303t
  in gastrointestinal infections, 145
  in swine, 303t
  metabolism, 297
  pyrimethamine combined with, 893
  trimethoprim combined with
    dosage, small animal, 967t
    formulations, 302, 303t
    in canine pyoderma, 860t
    in cattle, 303t
    in cryptosporidiosis, 150
    in dogs, 303t
    in foals, 458t
    in laminitis therapy, 468t
    in small animals, 302
Sulfadimethoxine
  amprolium combined with, 894
  blood levels, 298
  boluses, 47t
  duration of action, 52, 301
  in cats, 303t
  in cattle, 303t
  indications
    coccidiosis, 774t
    pneumonic pasteurellosis, 793
    respiratory disease, 790t, 793
  in dogs, 303t
  in gastrointestinal infections, 145
  in horses, 303t
  maintenance therapy, 304t
  ormethoprim combined with, 302
    in bovine respiratory disease, 793
    in canine pyoderma, 860t
    in coccidiosis, 894
  residues, 310
  sustained-release, 53t, 793
Sulfadimidine
  duration of action, 299
  efficacy, 305–306
  in cryptosporidiosis, 150
  in salmonellosis, 587

JECFA evaluation, 377, 378t, 379t, 381
  protein binding, 299
  safety, 299
  salmonellosis control, 587
  tylosin combined with, 571, 587
Sulfadoxine, trimethoprim combined with, 302, 790t
Sulfaguanidine, 145
Sulfamerazine
  bacteriostatic activity, 305
  in cattle, 303t
  in swine, 303t
  maintenance therapy, 304t
Sulfamethazine
  baquiloprim combined with, 302
  boluses, 52
    duration of action, 53t
  bolus preparations, 304t
  control dosage, 578
  in cattle, 303t
  indications
    ovine coccidiosis, 727t
    pneumonic pasteurellosis, 793
    respiratory disease, 790t
  in gastrointestinal infections, 145
  in swine, 303t
  maintenance therapy, 304t
  metabolism, 297
  plasma protein binding, 385
  residues, 310, 376, 590, 593
  tylosin combined with, 571, 578
Sulfamethiazine
  in endometritis, 704
  uterine absorption, 704
Sulfamethoxazole
  metabolism, 297
  trimethoprim combined with, 303t
    dosage, small animal, 967t
Sulfamethoxypyridazine
  absorption, 299
  duration of action, 299
  in coccidiosis, 727t, 728, 774t
  protein binding, 299
Sulfamezathine, 47t
Sulfamonomethoxine, 305
"Sulfa-on-site" testing, 310, 594–595
Sulfapyridine
  aspirin combined with, 146
  in gastrointestinal infections, 145
  maintenance therapy, 304t
Sulfaquinoxaline
  adverse effects, 309
  in coccidiosis, 774t
  residues, 310
Sulfasalazine
  in colitis, 146, 950
  prednisolone combined with, 950
  toxicity, in cats, 217t
Sulfathiazole
  in calves, 303t
  in gastrointestinal infections, 145

in swine, 303t
JECFA evaluation, 378t
maintenance therapy, 304t
metabolism, 297
Sulfisoxazole, 297
Sulfonamide(s). *See also* specific agents
    absorption, 145, 305
    adverse effects, 308–310
        following rapid IV administration, 308
    allergy, 343, 346
    bacterial resistance, 307–308
    baquiloprim combined with, 301, 302, 793
    boluses, 47t
    coccidiostats and, 306
    comparative bacterial activity, 305
    crystalluria and, 308
    drug interactions, 309
    goitrogenic effects, 309
    hemolytic anemias and, 309
    hypersensitivity reactions and, 309
    in calves, 309
    indications
        actinomycosis, 304
        bovine respiratory tract infections, 793
        coccidiosis, 304
        colic, 424t
        diphtheria, 304
        endometritis, bacterial, 474t, 476, 478t
        enteritis, 304
        foot rot, 304
        gastrointestinal tract infections, 145
        metritis, contagious equine, 480
        navel ill, 304
        pneumonia, 304
        polyarthritis, 304
        respiratory tract infections, 304
        rhinitis, 304
        salmonellosis, 587
        scours, 304
        skin infections, 304
        strangles, 304
        urinary tract infections, 304
    in foals, 309
    in gastrointestinal tract infections, 145
    in veterinary medicine, 303t
    kernicterus and, 309
    long-acting, 305
    long-term therapy, 309
    pharmacokinetics, 297–299
    phenylbutazone interaction with, 518
    potentiated, 302–303, 306–308
    protein binding, 298
    recommended dosages, 304t
    residues, 310–312, 376, 578, 592–595
    side effects, 308–310
    solubility, 297
    sustained-release vs conventional, 52
    therapy, 303–306
    toxicity, 308–310
        renal, 308

trimethoprim combined with, 300, 301, 306–307
    in foals, 496t
    in septicemia, 496t, 499
tumorigenicity, 310
warfarin interaction with, 461t
Sulfurated lime, 847t
Summer mastitis, 677–681
    antibiotic therapy, 680–681
    causative agents, 677
    control, 679–680
    disease transmission, 678–679
    pathogenesis, 678
    prevention, 678–679
    susceptibility, 678
    treatment, 679
Surgical shock, 186
Sustained-release systems. *See also* Controlled-release
        systems
    anthelmintics in, 47t
    antimicrobial agents in, 47t, 52–55
    boluses,, 47t, 48
    copper capsules in, 51
    design of, 46, 46t
    growth promoters in, 47t
    hormonal formulations in, 55, 56
    intramammary, 55
    plasma half-life and, 34
    reproductive hormones in, 55
    rumen devices in, 46
    sulfonamides in, 47t, 52, 53t
    topical preparations in, 58t
    trace elements in, 47t
SUSTAIN III. *See* Sulfamethazine
SUSTAIN III CALF BOLUS. *See* Sulfamethazine
Swine
    Aujeszky's disease in, 73
    colibacillosis in, 578–580
    dysentery. *See* Swine dysentery
    herpes infection in. *See* Aujeszky's disease
    pleuropneumonia in, 576–578
    pneumonia in, 573–576
    therapy
        ivermectin, 107, 108
        sulfachlorpyridazine, 303t
        sulfadiazine, 303t
        sulfamerazine, 303t
        sulfamethazine, 303t
        sulfathiazole, 303t
Swine dysentery, 580–586
    causative agents, 580
    control, 578
    feed medication for, 581, 587t
    treatment, 581–582
    water medication for, 581, 596t
Sympathomimetics, 122–123
SYNANTHIC MULTIDOSE 130 (oxfendazole), 49t
Synergistin. *See* Ampicillin, sulbactam combined with
SYNOVEX-C. *See* Progesterone, estradiol benzoate
        combined with
SYNOVEX-H. *See* Testosterone, estradiol benzoate
        combined with

SYNOVEX-S. *See* Progesterone, estradiol benzoate combined with
SYNULOX. *See* Clavulanic acid, amoxicillin combined with

TAGAMET. *See* Cimetidine
Talampicillin, 228
TALWIN V. *See* Pentazocine
Tamoxifen
    adverse effects, 1013
    dosage, 1006–1007, 1013
    mechanism of action, 1007
Tapeworms, 889–892
    albendazole against, 762
    eggs, infestation via, 890
    in dogs, 890
    in horses, 436–437
    in small animals, 880, 880t, 881t
    ivermectin and, 436
    oxfendazole against, 762
    parasiticides for, 431t, 890–892, 891t
    pyrantel against, 430, 436
    species of, 436
Taurine deficiency, 824–825
Teat sealants, 680
TELMIN. *See* Mebendazole
Temazepam, 998
Teratogenicity, 332–337
    albendazole, 335, 336
    cambendazole, 336
    carbamate, 335
    enrofloxacin, 289
    febantel, 336
    griseofulvin, 336
    mebendazole, 336
    organophosphate, 335
    oxfendazole, 335, 336
    parbendazole, 336
    testing for, 336
Teratogen(s), 334–336
    animal, 335–336
    defined, 332
    human, 334–335
Terbutaline, 121
    in horses, 505t
    in pneumonia, 489
TERRAMYCIN. *See* Oxytetracycline
Terramycin. *See* Oxytetracycline
Testosterone, 33, 54, 315
    estradiol benzoate combined with, 56t, 619
    in dogs, 1008
    sustained-release devices, 47t
    trenbolone vs, 619
Testosterone propionate, 1008
Tetracycline(s), 154
    absorption, 266
    acidosis and, 270
    allergy, 346
    anaphylactic reactions to, 266
    antibacterial spectrum, 264, 265, 794

biliary transport, 268
bolus, 47t, 54
distribution, 266, 267
dosage, small animal, 967t
drug interactions, 271–272
elimination, 266, 268
formulations, 264–265, 268–269
glucocorticoids and, 271
indications
    bovine respiratory tract infections, 793–795
    endometritis, bacterial, 474t, 476
    haemobartonellosis, 895, 896t
    metritis, contagious equine, 480
    placenta, retained, 484
injection site discomfort associated with, 268
in sheep, 54
interactions, 271
intramuscular, 268
JECFA evaluation, 377, 381
liver function and, 376
mechanism of action, 265–266
methoxyflurane combined with, 271
milk levels, 266
oral, 267
parenteral, 267
peak plasma levels, 266, 267
pharmacokinetics, 266–268
protein synthesis and, 271
residues, 376–377, 591
resistance, 265, 266
respiratory tract concentrations, 946
Staphylococcus aureus resistance to, 942
toxicity, 269–271
    colitis, 270
    hepatosis, 271
urine levels, 951
Tetrahydrocannabinal, 139
Tetrahydropyridimines, 104
Tetramisole, 82t
Thalidomide, 334
Thallium, 212
Thenium
    antinematodal spectrum, 885t
    antiparasitic spectrum, 882t
    in hookworm infection, 887t
    piperazine combined with, 882t
Theobromine, 552
Theophylline
    cimetidine interaction, 493
    clenbuterol vs, 493
    dosage, 493
    drug interactions, 493
    erythromycin interaction, 493
    in cardiac disease, 824t
    in chronic obstructive pulmonary disease, 492t, 493
    in horses, 493, 505t
    protein binding, 493
Thermal shock, 186
Thiabendazole
    absorption, 88

antiparasitic spectrum, 89t, 763t, 882t
   in ruminants, 91t
dosage, 92
   in horses, 432t, 433, 433t, 434
efficacy, 765t
fenbendazole vs, 86
formulations, 432t
in cattle, 762, 764t
indications, 431t
   dermatophytosis, 847t
   lungworm infection, 437, 894
   nasal aspergillosis, 130
   parasitic gastroenteritis, 770t
   Strongyloides westeri infection, 436
   threadworm infestation, 889
   verminous arteritis, 415
in foals, 511
in horses, 431t–432t, 433–434
in sheep, 770t
JECFA evaluation, 380t
mechanism of action, 82t
metabolism, 86
parasiticidal spectrum, 432t
piperazine combined with, 443t
plasma level, 93, 771
rafoxanide combined with, 772
residues, 96
resistance, 84, 438
safety margin, 442t
solubility, 90
warfarin and, 461t
Thiacetarsamide, 914t
   dosage, 906, 908
   in heartworm infection, 906
   prophylactic use, 907
   safety margin, 908
   side effects, 908, 909
   toxicity, 906
Thiamine, 202t, 205
Thiamphenicol, 281–282
Thiopentone, 211–212
Thiophanate
   antiparasitic spectrum, 89t, 763t
      in ruminants, 91t
   brotianide combined with, 772
   efficacy, 765t
   in cattle, 762
   ind parasitic gastroenteritis, 770t
   in sheep, 770t
   mechanism of action, 82t
   metabolism, 86
Thiostrepton, 851
Thiotepa, 930
   dosage rate, 935t
Threadworms, 431t, 432t
   in small animals, 889–891
Thromboembolic colic, 415
Thromboxane, 127
Thymidine kinase gene, 74
Thyroid carcinoma, 933

Thyrotoxicosis, 835
Tiamulin
   absorption, gastrointestinal, 577
   against *Treponema hyodysenteriae*, 797
   control dosage, 576, 578
   feed medication, 587t
   formulations, 583
   indications
      pleuropneumonia, swine, 577
      pneumonia, swine, 574
      swine dysentery, 582
   narasin interaction with, 613
   parenteral administration, 575
   premixes, 583
   salinomycin and, 583, 613
   swine dysentery control, 583, 584t, 585t
   water medication, 577, 586t
Ticarcillin, 229
   antibacterial spectrum, 221
   carbenicillin vs, 221, 230
   clavulanic acid combined with, 224
   dosage, 238t
   elimination, 230
   gentamicin synergy, 230
   in cattle, 238t
   indications
      colic, 424t
      endometritis, bacterial, 474t, 477, 478t
      metritis, contagious equine, 480
      osteomyelitis, 457
      septic arthritis, 457, 458t
   in foals, 496t
   in horses, 229, 238t
   mezlocillin vs, 221
   piperacillin vs, 221
   tobramycin synergy, 230
   uterine infusion, 480
TICILLIN. *See* Ticarcillin
Ticks, control of, 55, 896
Tilmicosin
   adverse effect, 801
   antibacterial activity, 260
   antibacterial spectrum, 800
   formulation, 261
   in cattle, 252, 258
   indications
      bovine respiratory disease, 801
      bovine respiratory tract infections, 800–801
      respiratory disease, 790t, 796
   lung levels, 261, 801
   pharmacokinetics, 260
   subcutaneous, 260
   toxicity, 261
TIMENTIN. *See* Clavulanic acid, ticarcillin combined with
Tincture of iodine, 468t
Tinidazole, 892t
TIRADE fly tags. *See* Fenvalerate
Tissue plasminogen activator, 68

Tobramycin
  antibacterial spectrum, 246
  dosage, 249
  nephrotoxicity, 251
  ticarcillin synergy, 230
Tocainide, 830t, 835t
Tocolytic drugs, 700–701
Tolbutamide, 347
  chloramphenicol interaction with, 347
Toluene, 885t
TOMANIL. *See* Isopyrin
Tonicity, 168
Topical preparations, 58
TORBUGESIC. *See* Butorphanol
Totrazuril, 727t
Toxascaris leonina, 885
Toxic mastitis, 183
Toxic metritis, 183
Toxicologic shock, 186
Toxocara canis, 884
  pregnancy and, 885
Toxocara cati, 885
Toxoplasma abortion, 729
Toxoplasma gondii, in dogs, 258
Toxoplasmosis, 728–730, 893
  vaccine, 729
Trace elements. *See also* specific minerals
  boluses, glass, 51
  delivery systems, 33, 47t
  long-term administration of, 40
  supplementation, 50–51
  sustained-release, 45
Tracheitis, 247
Tracheobronchitis, 130, 246
Track test XI, 903
Transmissible venereal tumors, 937
  therapy for, 938t
Traumatic shock, 186
Trenbolone, 625–626
  acceptable daily intake, 629
  anabolic activity, 625
  as growth promoter, 599t
  delivery systems, 33
  DNA binding, 626
  ear implants, 55, 56t
  implants, ear, 625
  in beef cattle, 315
  JECFA evaluation, 378t, 629
  metabolism, 625
  mutagenicity tests, 626
  protein binding, 625–626
  relay toxicity studies, 625
  residues, 356, 625, 629
  sustained-release, 55, 56t
    devices for, 47t
  testosterone vs, 619
  toxicity, 625–626
Treponema hyodysenteriae, 797
TRESADERM. *See* Thiabendazole
Triacetyloleandomycin, 259

Triamcinolone, 541t
Triamterene, 826t, 827t
TRIBRISSEN. *See* Trimethoprim, sulfadiazine
    combined with
Trichlorfon, 443t
  dosage, 430, 432t
  febantel combined with, 430, 443t
  formulations, 432t
  indications, 430, 434
  mechanism of action, 82t, 83
  parasiticidal spectrum, 432t
  phenothiazine and piperazine combined with, 443t
  toxicity, 442t
Trichostrongylus infection, 435
Triclabendazole
  antiparasitic spectrum, 89t, 763t
    in ruminants, 91t
  efficacy, 87
  flukicidal activity, 110, 112
  in cattle, 764t
  in fascioliasis, 768, 772
  metabolism, 94
  residues, 97
Tridihexethyl chloride, 141
Triethylene thiophosphamide. *See* Thiotepa
Trimethoprim, 300–301
  adverse effects, 301
  allergy, 346
  chemical structure, 301
  half-life, 301
  indications
    colic, 424t
    endometritis, bacterial, 478t
  in ruminants, 301
  long-term therapy, 301
  mutagenicity, 301
  oral, 301
  ormethoprim vs, 301
  rumen degradation of, 793
  sulfadiazine combined with
    anemia and, 957
    dosage, small animal, 967t
    in canine pyoderma, 860t
    in cryptosporidiosis, 150
    in dogs, 302, 303t
    in foals, 458t
    in laminitis, 468t
    in meningitis, coliform, 502
    in respiratory infections, in foals, 505t
    in *Rhodococcus equi* pneumonia, 488
    keratoconjunctivitis sicca and, 957
  sulfadoxine combined with, 302
    in bovine respiratory disease, 790t
  sulfamethoxazole combined with, 303t
    dosage, small animal, 967t
  sulfonamides combined with, 306–307
    in calf scour, 152
  tissue concentrations, 302
Troleandomycin, 258
Tumorigenicity, 323t, 324t

Tumor necrosis factor, 68
Tumors
  bone, 920
  in young dogs, 920
  malignant, 920. *See also* Cancer
    treatment of, 920
  mast cell, 937
  skin, in dogs, 937
  transmissible venereal, 937
Turkeys, 375
Turpentine, oil of, 423
Tylosin, 252–253
  absorption, oral, 252, 796
  antibacterial activity, 258
  antibacterial spectrum, 571
  as feed additive, 796
  blood levels, in cattle, 796
  control dosages, 576
  enrofloxacin vs, 290
  feed medication, 587t
  growth promoting effect, 570
  indications, 258
    atrophic rhinitis, 571
    bacterial overgrowth, 950
    bovine respiratory tract infections, 796–797
    Corynebacterium pyogenes infection, 571
    mycoplasmal pneumonias, 796
    Pasterella multocida infection, 571
    pneumonia, swine, 571, 573
    respiratory disease, 790t, 796
    salmonellosis, 587
    swine dysentery, 582
  in gram-positive infections, 945
  lipid solubility, 706
  lung-to-serum ratio, 256
  mechanism of action, 253
  oral, 256
  oxytetracycline combined with, 796
  parenteral, 256, 575
  peak serum concentration, 255
  resistance, 252
  salmonellosis control, 587
  sulfadimidine combined with, 571, 587
  sulfamethazine combined with, 571, 578
  swine dysentery control, 584t
  toxicity, 796
  water medication, 586t
Tympanitic colic, 402

Ulcerative keratitis, 131
Umbilical infections, 246, 487, 503
Upper respiratory tract infection, 246
Urea poisoning, 203–204
Urinary antiseptics, 956–957
Urinary incontinence, 1006, 1018–1019
  treatment, 1006, 1023t
    objective of, 1022t
Urinary tract infections
  antimicrobial agents in, 950–951, 953–957
    dosage, 956t

beta lactams in, 226
  in cats, 951
  in dogs, 951, 952t
  prostatitis and, 957
  sulfonamides in, 304
  urinary incontinence and, 1019
Urine spraying, 1003, 1004
Urogenital tract infections, 233
Urolithiasis, 985
Uterine atony, 702
Uterine control, 691–692
Uterine evacuation, 714
Uterine infections, 246, 703. *See also* Endometritis;
    Metritis
  coliform bacteria in, 963
  in cats, 963
  in dogs, 952t, 963
Uterine irrigation, in endometritis, 476t
Uterine prolapse, 714, 715t
Uveitis, 503

Vaccination, 162
Vaccines
  delivery systems for, 55
  gene deletion, 70
  genetically engineered, 62, 68–71
  gI-negative, 70
  recombinant, production of, 69
  safety of, 68
  subunit, 69–70, 71
Vaginal infections, in dogs, 952t, 960
Vaginitis, 1016
VALBAZEN. *See* Albendazole
VALIUM. *See* Diazepam
Valproic acid, 992t
  elimination of, 994
  in cats, 1000
  in dogs, 1000
  phenobarbital combined with, 1000
Vancomycin, 260
Vasoactive intestinal peptide, 127
Vasodilators, 826–828
Vegetable oils, 145
VENTIPULMIN. *See* Clenbuterol
VENTOLIN. *See* Salbutamol
Verapamil, 830t, 836–837
Verminous arteritis, 415
VERSENATE. *See* Ethylenediaminetetra-acetic acid
Vinblastine, 924, 932t
Vincristine
  antitubulin activity, 95
  cyclophosphamide and prednisolone with, 935
  dosage rate, 935t
  excretion, 924
  in cats, 931
  in dogs, 931
  in lymphosarcoma, 932
  in transmissible venereal tumors, 937, 938t
  mechanism of action, 931
  muscle weakness and, 931

Vincristine, *continued*
  neurodermatitis and, 931
  side effects, 932t
  teratogenicity, 99
  tissue necrosis and, 931
Virginiamycin, 615–616
  as growth promoter, 616
  feed medication, 587t
  gram positive activity, 615
  indications
    salmonellosis, 587
    swine dysentery, 582
  salmonellosis control, 587
  swine dysentery control, 584t
Vitamin B_{12}, 62, 743–744
Vitamin C, 62
Vitamin D, 205
Vitamin E, 710, 746
  therapy, 615
Vitamin K, 202t
Vitamin(s), 45
  deficiency, retained placenta and, 714

Warfarin, 459–461
  dosage, 459, 461, 463t
  drug interactions, 460, 461
  in navicular disease, 459–461, 463t
  intoxication, 207
    symptoms of, 210
    treatment of, 210
  isoxsuprine vs, 462
  long-term treatment, 460
  phenylbutazone interaction with, 518
  plasma protein binding, 460
  side effects, 460
  toxicity, 461
Water medication, 586t
Waxes, 35t, 39
Weed killers, 212
Whipworms, 880, 880t, 888–889
Wound infections, 958

clindamycin in, 258
kanamycin in, 247
streptomycin in, 246

Xanthines, 121–122, 493. *See also* specific agents, e.g.
    Theophylline
Xylazine
  analgesic properties, 414
  antisecretory activity, 144
  as an emetic, 134
  combined therapy, 411t
  in cats, 134–135, 196
  in colic, equine, 411t, 412t, 426t
  in foals, 502, 502t
  onset of action, 134

Yews, 213

ZANTAC. *See* Ranitidine
Zeranol, 626–627
  acceptable daily intake, 630
  as growth promoter, 623
  delivery systems, 33
  ear implants, 55, 56t
  estrogenic activity, 619
  implant, 626
  in beef cattle, 315
  in cattle, 630
  JECFA evaluation, 378t, 630
  long-term administration, 626
  metabolism, 626
  metabolites, 630
  mutagenicity tests, 626, 630
  no-effect level, 627
  residues, 630
  sustained-release, 47t
  toxicity, 626
Zinc bacitracin, 570
  as growth promoter, 599t
Zinc chelate, 468t
Zinc deficiency, 875
Zinc ointment, toxicity, in cats, 217t